EVIDENCE-BASED PRACTICE
of **CRITICAL CARE**

EVIDENCE-BASED PRACTICE
of CRITICAL CARE

second edition

Clifford S. Deutschman, MS, MD, FCCM
Vice Chair, Research, Department of Pediatrics
Professor of Pediatrics and Molecular Medicine
Hofstra North Shore-LIJ School of Medicine
New Hyde Park, New York
Investigator, Feinstein Institute for Medical Research
Manhasset, New York

Patrick J. Neligan, MA, MB, FRCAFRCSI
Department of Anaesthesia and Intensive Care
University College Galway
Galway, Ireland

ELSEVIER

ELSEVIER

1600 John F. Kennedy Blvd.
Ste 1800
Philadelphia, PA 19103-2899

EVIDENCE-BASED PRACTICE OF CRITICAL CARE,
SECOND EDITION

ISBN: 978-0-323-29995-4

Previous edition copyrighted 2010.

Library of Congress Cataloging-in-Publication Data

Deutschman, Clifford S., editor. | Neligan, Patrick J., editor.
Evidence-based practice of critical care / [edited by] Clifford S. Deutschman, Patrick J. Neligan.
Second edition. | Philadelphia, PA : Elsevier, [2016] |
  Includes bibliographical references and index.
LCCN 2015041109 | ISBN 9780323299954 (pbk. : alk. paper)
| MESH: Critical Care. | Evidence-Based Medicine. | Intensive Care Units.
LCC RC86.7 | NLM WX 218 | DDC 616.02/8—dc23 LC record
  available at http://lccn.loc.gov/2015041109

Senior Content Strategist: Suzanne Toppy
Senior Content Development Specialist: Jennifer Ehlers
Publishing Services Manager: Patricia Tannian
Senior Project Manager: Claire Kramer
Design Direction: Julia Dummitt

Printed in the United States of America

Last digit is the print number: 9 8 7 6 5 4 3 2

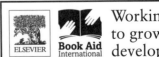

To my family:
Chris, who makes everything possible—and worthwhile
Cate, Nicki, and Beth, who are now adults, and still make us proud every day,
and Linus, who makes it entertaining.

To my former colleagues in the
Surgical Intensive Care Unit at the Hospital of the University of Pennsylvania
(including my coauthor):
For tolerating 20 years of "Teaching by Confrontation" without ever taking it personally.
To my new colleagues at
the Cohen Children's Medical Center and
the Feinstein Institute for Medical Research:
We will figure it out.

Clifford S. Deutschman, MS, MD
New York

To Diane, David, Conor, and Kate and to my parents Maurice and Dympna Neligan
for their continued support and wisdom.

Patrick J. Neligan, MA, MB, FRCAFRCSI

Contributors

Gareth L. Ackland, PhD, FRCA, FFICM
William Harvey Research Institute
Queen Mary University of London
London, United Kingdom
> Chapter 48 What Is the Role of Autonomic Dysfunction in Critical Illness?

Dijillali Annane, MD
General Intensive Care Unit
Raymond Poincaré Hospital (AP-HP)
University of Versailles SQY
Laboratory of Inflammation and Infection U1173 INSERM
Garches, France
> Chapter 71 Is There a Place for Anabolic Hormones in Critical Care?

Pierre Asfar, MD, PhD
Département de Réanimation Médicale et de Médecine Hyperbare
Centre Hospitalier Universitaire Angers
Angers, France
> Chapter 40 What MAP Objectives Should Be Targeted in Septic Shock?

John G. Augoustides, MD, FASE, FAHA
Professor
Anesthesiology and Critical Care
Perelman School of Medicine
University of Pennsylvania
Philadelphia, Pennsylvania
> Chapter 52 When Is Hypertension a True Crisis, and How Should It Be Managed in the Intensive Care Unit?
> Chapter 82 Which Anticoagulants Should Be Used in the Critically Ill Patient? How Do I Choose?

Hollman D. Aya, MD
Clinical and Research Fellow
Intensive Care Department
St. George's University Hospitals NHS Foundation Trust
London, United Kingdom
> Chapter 84 Does ICU Admission Improve Outcome?

Lorenzo Ball, MD
IRCCS AOU San Martino-IST
Department of Surgical Sciences and Integrated Diagnostics
University of Genoa
Genoa, Italy
> Chapter 8 How Does One Evaluate and Monitor Respiratory Function in the Intensive Care Unit?

Arna Banerjee, MD
Associate Professor of Anesthesiology, Surgery, and Medical Education
Department of Anesthesiology and Critical Care
Vanderbilt University Medical Center
Nashville, Tennessee
> Chapter 73 How Does One Diagnose, Treat, and Reduce Delirium in the Intensive Care Unit?

John Bates, MD
Anaesthesia and Intensive Care Medicine
University Hospital Galway
Galway, Ireland
> Chapter 24 How Do I Transport the Critically Ill Patient?

S. V. Baudouin, MD, FRCP, FICM
Department of Anaesthesia
Royal Victoria Infirmary
Newcastle upon Tyne, United Kingdom
> Chapter 36 Are Anti-inflammatory Therapies in ARDS Effective?

Michael Bauer, MD
Center for Sepsis Control and Care
Department of Anesthesiology and Critical Care Medicine
Jena University Hospital
Jena, Germany
> Chapter 68 How Does Critical Illness Alter the Liver?

Jeremy R. Beitler, MD, MPH
Division of Pulmonary and Critical Care Medicine
University of California, San Diego
San Diego, California
> Chapter 28 What Is the Clinical Definition of ARDS?

Rinaldo Bellomo, MD, FCICM
Australia and New Zealand Intensive Care Research Centre
Department of Epidemiology and Preventive Medicine
Monash University
Melbourne, Australia
> Chapter 5 Do Early Warning Scores and Rapid Response Teams Improve Outcomes?

François Beloncle, MD
Département de Réanimation Médicale et de Médecine Hyperbare
Centre Hospitalier Universitaire Angers
Angers, France
> Chapter 40 What MAP Objectives Should Be Targeted in Septic Shock?

Kimberly S. Bennett, MD, MPH
Associate Professor
Pediatric Critical Care
University of Colorado School of Medicine
Denver, Colorado
Chapter 11 Is Extracorporeal Life Support an Evidence-Based Intervention for Critically Ill Adults with ARDS?

Paulomi K. Bhalla, MD
Fellow, Division of Neurocritical Care
Neurology
Hospital of the University of Pennsylvania
Philadelphia, Pennsylvania
Chapter 63 How Should Aneurysmal Subarachnoid Hemorrhage Be Managed?

Maneesh Bhargava, MD
Assistant Professor of Pulmonary, Allergy, Critical Care, and Sleep Medicine
University of Minnesota Medical School
Minneapolis, Minnesota
Chapter 32 Do Patient Positioning in General and Prone Positioning in Particular Make a Difference in ARDS?

Alain F. Broccard, MD
St Vincent Seton Specialty Hospital
Indianapolis, Indiana
Chapter 32 Do Patient Positioning in General and Prone Positioning in Particular Make a Difference in ARDS?

Josée Bouchard, MD
Division of Nephrology
Department of Medicine
University of Montreal
Montreal, Canada
Chapter 56 How Does One Optimize Care in Patients at Risk for or Presenting with Acute Kidney Injury?

Naomi E. Cahill, RD, PhD
Department of Public Health Sciences
Queen's University
Kingston, Ontario, Canada
Chapter 67 Is It Appropriate to "Underfeed" the Critically Ill Patient?

Andrea Carsetti, MD
Anaesthesia and Intensive Care Unit
Department of Biomedical Sciences and Public Health
Università Politecnica delle Marche
Ancona, Italy
Department of Intensive Care Medicine
St George's University Hospitals NHS Foundation Trust
London, United Kingdom
Chapter 84 Does ICU Admission Improve Outcome?

Maurizio Cecconi, MD
Department of Intensive Care
St. George's Hospital
London, United Kingdom
Chapter 84 Does ICU Admission Improve Outcome?

Celina D. Cepeda, MD
Division of Pediatric Nephrology
Pediatric Department
Rady Children's Hospital
Division of Nephrology and Hypertension
Department of Medicine
University of California, San Diego
San Diego, California
Chapter 56 How Does One Optimize Care in Patients at Risk for or Presenting with Acute Kidney Injury?

Maurizio Cereda, MD
Assistant Professor of Anesthesia and Critical Care
Department of Anesthesia and Critical Care
Perelman School of Medicine at the University of Pennsylvania
Philadelphia, Pennsylvania
Chapter 10 How Does Mechanical Ventilation Damage Lungs? What Can Be Done to Prevent It?

John Chandler, MD, BDS, FDSRCS, FCARCSI
Consultant in Anaesthesia and Intensive Care
Cork University Hospital
Cork, Ireland
Chapter 24 How Do I Transport the Critically Ill Patient?

Randall M. Chesnut, MD, FCCM, FACS
Integra Endowed Professor of Neurotrauma
Department of Neurological Surgery
Department of Orthopaedic Surgery
Adjunct Professor
School of Global Health
Harborview Medical Center
University of Washington
Seattle, Washington
Chapter 61 Is It Really Necessary to Measure Intracranial Pressure in Brain-Injured Patients?

Meredith Collard, MD
Department of Anesthesiology and Critical Care
Perelman School of Medicine
University of Pennsylvania
Philadelphia, Pennsylvania
Chapter 6 What Are the Indications for Intubation in the Critically Ill Patient?

Maya Contreras, MD, PhD, FCARCSI
Department of Anesthesia
St. Michael's Hospital
Toronto, Ontario, Canada
Chapter 31 Is Permissive Hypercapnia Useful in ARDS?

David J. Cooper, MD, BM, BS
Australian and New Zealand Intensive Care–Research Centre
School of Public Health and Preventive Medicine
Monash University
Alfred Hospital Campus
The Alfred Hospital
Melbourne, Australia
Chapter 9 What Is the Optimal Approach to Weaning and Liberation from Mechanical Ventilation?

Craig M. Coopersmith, MD
Professor of Surgery
Department of Surgery
Associate Director
Emory Critical Care Center
Vice Chair of Research
Department of Surgery
Director
Surgical/Transplant Intensive Care Unit
Emory University Hospital
Atlanta, Georgia
>Chapter 46 *Is Selective Decontamination of the Digestive Tract Useful?*

David Cosgrave, MB, BCh, BAO
Anaesthesia SPR
University Hospital Galway
Galway, Ireland
>Chapter 24 *How Do I Transport the Critically Ill Patient?*

Cheston B. Cunha, MD
Assistant Professor of Medicine
Division of Infectious Disease
Medical Director, Antimicrobial Stewardship Program
Rhode Island Hospital and the Miriam Hospital
Brown University Alpert School of Medicine
Providence, Rhode Island
>Chapter 17 *What Strategies Can Be Used to Optimize Antibiotic Use in the Critically Ill?*

Gerard F. Curley, PhD, MB, MSc, FCAI, FJFICM
Departments of Anesthesia and Critical Care
Keenan Research Centre for Biomedical Science of St Michael's Hospital
St. Michael's Hospital
Department of Anesthesia and Interdepartmental Division of Critical Care
University of Toronto
Toronto, Ontario, Canada
>Chapter 39 *What Is the Role of Empirical Antibiotic Therapy in Sepsis?*

Randall J. Curtis, MD
Professor
Division of Pulmonary and Critical Care Medicine
A. Bruce Montgomery–American Lung Association Endowed Chair in Pulmonary and Critical Care Medicine
Section Head
Harborview Medical Center
Director
Cambia Palliative Care Center of Excellence
Harborview Medical Center
Seattle, Washington
>Chapter 87 *What Factors Influence a Family to Support a Decision Withdrawing Life Support?*

Allison Dalton, MD
Assistant Professor of Anesthesia and Critical Care
Department of Anesthesia and Critical Care
University of Chicago
Chicago, Illinois
>Chapter 15 *How Do I Manage Hemodynamic Decompensation in a Critically Ill Patient?*

Kathryn A. Davis, MD, MTR
Medical Director
Epilepsy Monitoring Unit
Assistant Professor of Neurology
Hospital of the University of Pennsylvania
Philadelphia, Pennsylvania
>Chapter 65 *How Should Status Epilepticus Be Managed?*

Daniel De Backer, MD, PhD
Department of Intensive Care
Erasme University Hospital
Brussels, Belgium
>Chapter 13 *What Is the Role of Invasive Hemodynamic Monitoring in Critical Care?*

Clifford S. Deutschman, MS, MD, FCCM
Vice Chair, Research, Department of Pediatrics
Professor of Pediatrics and Molecular Medicine
Hofstra North Shore–LIJ School of Medicine
New Hyde Park, New York
Investigator, Feinstein Institute for Medical Research
Manhasset, New York
>Chapter 1 *Critical Care Versus Critical Illness*
>Chapter 37 *What Is Sepsis? What Is Septic Shock? What Are MODS and Persistent Critical Illness?*
>Chapter 49 *Is Sepsis-Induced Organ Dysfunction an Adaptive Response?*
>Chapter 52 *When Is Hypertension a True Crisis, and How Should It Be Managed in the Intensive Care Unit?*

Margaret Doherty, BMedSci, MB BCh BAO, FFARCSI, EDIC
Interdepartmental Division of Critical Care Medicine
University Health Network
University of Toronto
Toronto, Ontario, Canada
>Chapter 30 *What Is the Best Mechanical Ventilation Strategy in ARDS?*

Tom Doris, MD FRCA
Department of Anaesthesia
Royal Victoria Infirmary
Newcastle upon Tyne, United Kingdom
>Chapter 36 *Are Anti-inflammatory Therapies in ARDS Effective?*

Todd Dorman, MD, FCCM
Senior Associate Dean for Education Coordination
Associate Dean Continuing Medical Education
Professor and Vice Chair for Critical Care
Department of Anesthesiology and Critical Care Medicine
Joint Appointments in Medicine, Surgery, and the School
    of Nursing
Johns Hopkins University School of Medicine
Baltimore, Maryland
> *Chapter 85 How Should Care Within an Intensive Care
> Unit or an Institution Be Organized?*

Tomas Drabek, MD, PhD
Associate Professor of Anesthesiology
Scientist
Safar Center for Resuscitation Research
University of Pittsburgh School of Medicine
Pittsburgh, Pennsylvania
> *Chapter 22 Is Hypothermia Useful in Managing Critically
> Ill Patients? Which Ones? Under What Conditions?*

Stephen Duff, MB BCh
St. Vincent's University Hospital
Dublin, Ireland
> *Chapter 9 What Is the Optimal Approach to Weaning and
> Liberation from Mechanical Ventilation?*

Eimhin Dunne, MRCS, PG Dip (Clin pharm)
Critical Care Clinical Fellow
King's College Hospital
London, United Kingdom
> *Chapter 18 Is Prophylaxis for Stress Ulceration Useful?*

Ali A. El Solh, MD, MPH
Division of Pulmonary, Critical Care, and Sleep Medicine
Department of Medicine and Department of Social and
    Preventive Medicine
State University of New York at Buffalo School of
    Medicine and Biomedical Sciences and School of Public
    Health and Health Professions
VA Western New York Healthcare System
Buffalo, New York
> *Chapter 23 What Are the Special Considerations in the
> Management of Morbidly Obese Patients in the Intensive
> Care Unit?*

E. Wesley Ely, MD, MPH
Professor of Medicine
Associate Director of Research GRECC
Center for Health Services Research
Department of Allergy, Pulmonary, and Critical Care
    Medicine
Vanderbilt University Medical Center
Nashville, Tennessee
> *Chapter 73 How Does One Diagnose, Treat, and Reduce
> Delirium in the Intensive Care Unit?*

Andrés Esteban, MD, PhD
Departamento de Cuidados Intensivos
CIBER de Enfermedades Respiratorias
Hospital Universitario de Getafe
Madrid, Spain
> *Chapter 28 What Is the Clinical Definition of ARDS?*

Laura Evans, MD
Associate Professor
Department of Medicine
New York University School of Medicine
New York, New York
> *Chapter 43 Do the Surviving Sepsis Campaign
> Guidelines Work?*

Niall D. Ferguson, MD, FRCPC, MSc
Interdepartmental Division of Critical Care Medicine
University Health Network
University of Toronto
Toronto, Ontario, Canada
> *Chapter 30 What Is the Best Mechanical Ventilation
> Strategy in ARDS?*

Jonathan Frogel, MD
Assistant Professor
Anesthesiology and Critical Care
Hospital of the University of Pennsylvania
Philadelphia, Pennsylvania
> *Chapter 53 How Does One Prevent or Treat Atrial
> Fibrillation in Postoperative Critically Ill Patients?*

Jakub Furmaga, MD
Assistant Professor of Emergency Medicine
Faculty in Medical Toxicology
University of Texas Southwestern Medical Center
Dallas, Texas
> *Chapter 79 How Do I Diagnose and Manage Patients
> Admitted to the ICU After Common Poisonings?*

Ognjen Gajic, MD
Professor of Medicine
Pulmonary and Critical Care Medicine
Mayo Clinic
Rochester, Minnesota
> *Chapter 12 What Factors Predispose Patients to Acute
> Respiratory Distress Syndrome?*

Alice Gallo De Moraes, MD
Department of Medicine–Division of Pulmonary and
    Critical Care
Mayo Clinic
Rochester, Minnesota
> *Chapter 12 What Factors Predispose Patients to Acute
> Respiratory Distress Syndrome?*

Erik Garpestad, MD
Associate Chief, Pulmonary, Critical Care, and Sleep Division
Director, Medical ICU
Associate Professor
Tufts University School of Medicine
Boston, Massachusetts
> *Chapter 7 What Is the Role of Noninvasive Ventilation in
> the Intensive Care Unit?*

Hayley B. Gershengorn, MD
Departments of Medicine and Neurology
Albert Einstein College of Medicine
Montefiore Medical Center
Bronx, New York
> *Chapter 3 Have Critical Care Outcomes Improved?*

Emily K. Gordon, MD
Assistant Professor
Anesthesiology and Critical Care
Perelman School of Medicine
University of Pennsylvania
Philadelphia, Pennsylvania
> Chapter 52 When Is Hypertension a True Crisis, and How Should It Be Managed in the Intensive Care Unit?
> Chapter 82 Which Anticoagulants Should Be Used in the Critically Ill Patient? How Do I Choose?

W. Robert Grabenkort, PA MMSc, FCCM
Director
Nurse Practitioner/Physician Assistant Residency
  Program
Emory Critical Care Center
Emory Healthcare
Atlanta, Georgia
> Chapter 86 What Is the Role of Advanced Practice Nurses and Physician Assistants in the ICU?

Guillem Gruartmoner, MD
Department of Critical Care
Corporació Sanitària Universitària Parc Taulí
Hospital de Sabadell
Universitat Autònoma de Barcelona
Barcelona, Spain
Department of Intensive Care
Erasmus Medical Center
Rotterdam, The Netherlands
> Chapter 42 How Can We Monitor the Microcirculation in Sepsis? Does It Improve Outcome?

Jacob T. Gutsche, MD
Assistant Professor
Cardiothoracic and Vascular Section
Anesthesiology and Critical Care
Perelman School of Medicine
University of Pennsylvania
Philadelphia, Pennsylvania
> Chapter 26 How Do I Diagnose and Treat Pulmonary Embolism?
> Chapter 52 When Is Hypertension a True Crisis, and How Should It Be Managed in the Intensive Care Unit?

Scott Halpern, MD, PhD
Associate Professor of Medicine, Epidemiology, and
  Medical Ethics and Health Policy
Director
Fostering Improvement in End-of-Life Decision Science
  Program
Deputy Director
Center for Health Incentives & Behavioral Economics
Department of Medical Ethics and Health Policy
Perelman School of Medicine
University of Pennsylvania
Philadelphia, Pennsylvania
> Chapter 83 How Can Critical Care Resource Utilization in the United States Be Optimized?

Ivan Hayes, MD
Consultant Intensivist
Cork University Hospital
Cork, Ireland
> Chapter 18 Is Prophylaxis for Stress Ulceration Useful?

Nicholas Heming, MD
General Intensive Care Unit
Raymond Poincaré Hospital (AP-HP)
University of Versailles SQY
Garches, France
> Chapter 71 Is There a Place for Anabolic Hormones in Critical Care?

Daren K. Heyland, MD
Department of Critical Care Medicine
Queen's University
Clinical Evaluation Research Unit
Kingston General Hospital
Kingston, Ontario, Canada
> Chapter 67 Is It Appropriate to "Underfeed" the Critically Ill Patient?

Nicholas S. Hill, MD
Investigator
Pulmonary Hypertension Clinic at Rhode Island Hospital
Providence, Rhode Island
Chief of the Pulmonary, Critical Care, and Sleep Division
  at Tufts-New England Medical Center
Professor of Medicine
Tufts University School of Medicine
Boston, Massachusetts
> Chapter 7 What Is the Role of Noninvasive Ventilation in the Intensive Care Unit?

Eliotte Hirshberg, MD, MS
Critical Care Attending Physician
Intermountain Medical Center
Associate Professor
Internal Medicine
Division of Pulmonary and Critical Care Medicine
Assistant Professor (Adjunct) Pediatrics
Division of Critical Care
University of Utah
Salt Lake City, Utah
> Chapter 11 Is Extracorporeal Life Support an Evidence-Based Intervention for Critically Ill Adults with ARDS?

R. Duncan Hite, MD
Professor and Chairman
Department of Critical Care Medicine
Respiratory Institute
Cleveland Clinic
Cleveland, Ohio
> Chapter 11 Is Extracorporeal Life Support an Evidence-Based Intervention for Critically Ill Adults with ARDS?

Steven M. Hollenberg, MD
Professor of Medicine
Cooper Medical School of Rowan University
Director, Coronary Care Unit
Cooper University Hospital
Camden, New Jersey
Chapter 54 Is Right Ventricular Failure Common in the Intensive Care Unit? How Should It Be Managed?

Richard S. Hotchkiss, MD
Professor of Anesthesiology, Medicine, Surgery, Molecular Biology and Pharmacology
Washington University School of Medicine
St. Louis, Missouri
Chapter 38 Is There Immune Suppression in the Critically Ill Patient?

Can Ince, PhD
Department of Intensive Care
Erasmus Medical Center
Rotterdam, The Netherlands
Chapter 42 How Can We Monitor the Microcirculation in Sepsis? Does It Improve Outcome?

Margaret Isaac, MD
Assistant Professor of Medicine
Attending Physician
General Internal Medicine and Palliative Care
University of Washington/Harborview Medical Center
Seattle, Washington
Chapter 87 What Factors Influence a Family to Support a Decision Withdrawing Life Support?

Shiro Ishihara, MD
Biomarkers and Heart Diseases
UMR-942
Institut National de la Santé et de la Recherche Médicale (INSERM)
Paris, France
Nippon Medical School Musashi-Kosugi Hospitals
Kanagawa, Japan
Chapter 50 How Do I Manage Acute Heart Failure?

Theodore J. Iwashyna, MD, PhD
Associate Professor, Department of Internal Medicine
Faculty Associate, Survey Research Center, Institute for Social Research
Research Scientist, Center for Clinical Management Research
Ann Arbor VA Health Services Research and Development
Co-Director, Robert Wood Johnson Foundation Clinical Scholars Program
Ann Arbor, Michigan
Chapter 4 What Problems Are Prevalent Among Survivors of Critical Illness and Which of Those Are Consequences of Critical Illness?

Gabriella Jäderling, MD, PhD
Department of Anesthesiology
Surgical Services and Intensive Care
Karolinska University Hospital
Stockholm, Sweden
Chapter 5 Do Early Warning Scores and Rapid Response Teams Improve Outcomes?

Marc G. Jeschke, MD, PhD, FACS, FCCM, FRCS(C)
Professor at the University of Toronto
Department of Surgery
Division of Plastic Surgery
Department of Immunology
Director, Ross Tilley Burn Centre
Sunnybrook Health Sciences Centre
Chair in Burn Research
Senior Scientist
Sunnybrook Research Institute
Toronto, Ontario, Canada
Chapter 76 How Should Patients with Burns Be Managed in the Intensive Care Unit?

Lewis J. Kaplan, MD
Section Chief
Surgical Critical Care
Philadelphia VA Medical Center
Associate Professor of Surgery
Division of Trauma, Surgical Critical Care, and Emergency Surgery
Perelman School of Medicine
University of Pennsylvania
Philadelphia, Pennsylvania
Chapter 75 What Is Abdominal Compartment Syndrome and How Should It Be Managed?

Scott E. Kasner, MD
Professor of Neurology University of Pennsylvania
Director
Comprehensive Stroke Center
University of Pennsylvania Health System
Philadelphia, Pennsylvania
Chapter 64 How Should Acute Ischemic Stroke Be Managed in the Intensive Care Unit?

Colm Keane, MD
Department of Anaesthesia and Intensive Care
National University of Ireland
Galway, Ireland
Chapter 41 What Vasopressor Agent Should Be Used in the Septic Patient?

Mark T. Keegan, MB, MRCPI, MSc
Professor
Division of Critical Care
Department of Anesthesiology
Mayo Clinic and Mayo Clinic College of Medicine
Rochester, Minnesota
Chapter 69 How Is Acute Liver Failure Managed?

Leo G. Kevin, MD, FCARCSI
Department of Anaesthesia
University College Hospitals
Galway, Ireland
  *Chapter 33 Is Pulmonary Hypertension Important in
  ARDS? Should We Treat It?*

**Fiona Kiernan, MB BCh BAO, B Med Sc,
FCAI, MSc**
Department of Anesthesia and Intensive Care
RCSI Smurfit
Beaumont Hospital
Dublin, Ireland,
  *Chapter 39 What Is the Role of Empirical Antibiotic
  Therapy in Sepsis?*

Ruth Kleinpell, PhD, RN, FAAN, FCCM
Director, Center for Clinical Research and Scholarship
Rush University Medical Center
Professor, Rush University College of Nursing
Chicago, Illinois
  *Chapter 86 What Is the Role of Advanced Practice Nurses
  and Physician Assistants in the ICU?*

Kurt Kleinschmidt, MD
Professor of Emergency Medicine
Division Chief and Program Director, Medical Toxicology
University of Texas Southwestern Medical School
Dallas, Texas
  *Chapter 79 How Do I Diagnose and Manage Patients
  Admitted to the ICU After Common Poisonings?*

Patrick M. Kochanek, MD, FCCM
Professor and Vice Chairman
Department of Critical Care Medicine
Professor of Anesthesiology, Pediatrics and Clinical and
  Translational Science
Director, Safar Center for Resuscitation Research
University of Pittsburgh School of Medicine
Pittsburgh, Pennsylvania
  *Chapter 22 Is Hypothermia Useful in Managing Critically
  Ill Patients? Which Ones? Under What Conditions?*

W. Andrew Kofke, MD
Professor
Director of Neuroscience in Anesthesiology and Critical
  Care Program
Co-Director Neurocritical Care
Co-Director Perioperative Medicine and Pain Clinical
  Research Unit
Department of Anesthesiology and Critical Care
Department of Neurosurgery
University of Pennsylvania
Philadelphia, Pennsylvania
  *Chapter 62 How Should Traumatic Brain Injury Be
  Managed?*

Benjamin A. Kohl, MD
Professor of Anesthesiology
Sidney Kimmel Medical College of the Thomas Jefferson
  University
Philadelphia, Pennsylvania
*Chapter 51 How Is Cardiogenic Shock Diagnosed and Managed
in the Intensive Care Unit?*

Andreas Kortgen, MD
Center for Sepsis Control and Care
Department of Anesthesiology and Critical Care Medicine
Jena University Hospital
Jena, Germany
  Chapter 68 How Does Critical Illness Alter the Liver?

John G. Laffey, MD, MA, FCAI
Department of Anesthesia
Critical Illness and Injury Research Centre
Keenan Research Centre for Biomedical Science
St. Michael's Hospital
Departments of Anesthesia, Physiology, and Inter-
  departmental Division of Critical Care Medicine
University of Toronto
Toronto, Ontario, Canada
  Chapter 31 Is Permissive Hypercapnia Useful in ARDS?

Francois Lamontagne, MD
Assistant Professor
Department of Medicine
Division of Internal Medicine
Faculty of Medicine and Health Sciences
Université de Sherbrooke
Sherbrooke, Québec, Canada
  *Chapter 34 Inhaled Vasodilators in ARDS: Do They Make
  a Difference?*

Meghan Lane-Fall, MD
Assistant Professor of Anesthesiology and Critical Care at
  the Hospital of the University of Pennsylvania
Core Faculty
Center for Healthcare Improvement and Patient Safety
Department of Medicine
Senior Fellow
Leonard Davis Institute of Health Economics
Philadelphia, Pennsylvania
  *Chapter 6 What Are the Indications for Intubation in the
  Critically Ill Patient?*

Michael Lanspa, MD, MS
Adjunct Assistant Professor
Department of Pulmonary and Critical Care Medicine
Intermountain Medical Center and University of Utah
Salt Lake City, Utah
  *Chapter 11 Is Extracorporeal Life Support an Evidence-
  Based Intervention for Critically Ill Adults with ARDS?*

David Lappin, MD
Galway University Hospitals
Galway, Ireland
  *Chapter 57 What Is the Role of Renal Replacement Therapy
  in the Intensive Care Unit?*

Michael Lava, MD
Fellow in Pulmonary and Critical Care
Emory University School of Medicine
Atlanta, Georgia
> Chapter 29 What Are the Pathologic and Pathophysiologic
> Changes That Accompany Acute Lung Injury and ARDS?

Joshua M. Levine, MD
Chief
Division of Neurocritical Care
Department of Neurology
Co-Director
Neurocritical Care Program
Associate Professor
Departments of Neurology, Neurosurgery, and
   Anesthesiology and Critical Care
Hospital of the University of Pennsylvania
Philadelphia, Pennsylvania
> Chapter 63 How Should Aneurysmal Subarachnoid
> Hemorrhage Be Managed?
> Chapter 64 How Should Acute Ischemic Stroke Be
> Managed in the Intensive Care Unit?
> Chapter 65 How Should Status Epilepticus Be Managed?

Andrew T. Levinson, MD, MPH
Assistant Professor of Medicine
Warren Alpert School of Medicine at Brown University
Providence, Rhode Island
> Chapter 2 What Lessons Have Intensivists Learned During
> the Evidence-Based Medicine Era?

Mitchell M. Levy, MD
Professor of Medicine
Chief, Division of Pulmonary, Critical Care, and Sleep
   Medicine
Warren Alpert Medical School at Brown University
Director of the Medical Intensive Care Unit
Rhode Island Hospital
Providence, Rhode Island
> Chapter 2 What Lessons Have Intensivists Learned During
> the Evidence-Based Medicine Era?

Richard J. Levy, MD
Vice Chair for Pediatric Laboratory Research
Department of Anesthesiology
Division of Pediatric Anesthesia
Columbia University College of Physicians and Surgeons
Columbia University Medical Center
New York, New York
> Chapter 49 Is Sepsis-Induced Organ Dysfunction an
> Adaptive Response?

José Angel Lorente, MD
Departamento de Cuidados Intensivos
CIBER de Enfermedades Respiratorias
Hospital Universitario de Getafe
Universidad Europea de Madrid
Madrid, Spain
> Chapter 28 What Is the Clinical Definition of ARDS?

John Lyons, MD
Department of Surgery
Emory University
Atlanta, Georgia
> Chapter 46 Is Selective Decontamination of the Digestive
> Tract Useful?

Larami MacKenzie, MD
Associate Director
Neurocritical Care
Abington Jefferson Health
Abington, Pennsylvania
> Chapter 62 How Should Traumatic Brain Injury Be
> Managed?

Anita K. Malhotra, MD
Assistant Professor of Anesthesiology
Director, Critical Care Anesthesia Fellowship
Penn State Hershey Medical Center
Hershey, Pennsylvania
> Chapter 26 How Do I Diagnose and Treat Pulmonary
> Embolism?

Joshua A. Marks, MD
Fellow
Division of Traumatology, Surgical Critical Care, and
   Emergency Surgery
Department of Surgery
Perelman School of Medicine at the University of
   Pennsylvania
Philadelphia, Pennsylvania
> Chapter 10 How Does Mechanical Ventilation Damage
> Lungs? What Can Be Done to Prevent It?

Brian Marsh, MD
Anaesthesia and Intensive Care Medicine
Mater Misericordiae University Hospital
Dublin, Ireland
> Chapter 18 Is Prophylaxis for Stress Ulceration Useful?

John C. Marshall, MD, FRCSC
Scientist
Keenan Research Center for Biomedical Science of the Li
   Ka Shing Knowledge Institute
St. Michael's Hospital
Professor
Surgery/General Surgery
University of Toronto
Toronto, Ontario, Canada
> Chapter 47 Is Persistent Critical Illness an Iatrogenic
> Disorder?

Greg S. Martin, MD, MSc
Professor and Associate Division Director for Critical Care
Division of Pulmonary, Allergy, and Critical Care
Emory University School of Medicine
Director of Research, Emory Center for Critical Care
Section Chief for Pulmonary, Allergy, and Critical Care
Grady Memorial Hospital
Atlanta, Georgia
> Chapter 29 What Are the Pathologic and Pathophysiologic
> Changes That Accompany Acute Lung Injury and ARDS?

Allie M. Massaro, MD
Resident
Department of Neurology
Hospital of the University of Pennsylvania
Philadelphia, Pennsylvania
Chapter 64 How Should Acute Ischemic Stroke Be Managed in the Intensive Care Unit?

Claire Masterson, MSc, PhD
Department of Anesthesia
Keenan Research Centre in the Li Ka Shing Knowledge Institute
Critical Illness and Injury Research Centre
Keenan Research Centre for Biomedical Science
St. Michael's Hospital
Departments of Anesthesia and Physiology
University of Toronto
Toronto, Ontario, Canada
Chapter 31 Is Permissive Hypercapnia Useful in ARDS?

Virginie Maxime, MD
General Intensive Care Unit
Raymond Poincaré Hospital (AP-HP)
University of Versailles SQY
Laboratory of Cell Death Inflammation and Infection
Garches, France
Chapter 71 Is There a Place for Anabolic Hormones in Critical Care?

Danny McAuley, MD, MRCP, DICM
Professor and Consultant in Intensive Care Medicine
Regional Intensive Care Unit
Royal Victoria Hospital
The Wellcome Wolfson Institute for Experimental Medicine
Queen's University Belfast
Belfast, Northern Ireland
Chapter 35 Do Nonventilatory Strategies for Acute Respiratory Distress Syndrome Work?

Kevin W. McConnell, MD
Department of Surgery and Emory Center for Critical Care
Atlanta, Georgia
Chapter 70 How Does Critical Illness Alter the Gut? How Does One Manage These Alterations?

Gráinne McDermott, MB BCh, FCARCSI, FJFICM
Consultant in Cardiothoracic Anaesthesia
Harefield Hospital
Middlesex, United Kingdom
Chapter 41 What Vasopressor Agent Should Be Used in the Septic Patient?

Bruce A. McKinley, PhD
Professor of Surgery
Department of Surgery
University of Florida College of Medicine
Gainesville, Florida
Chapter 25 Are Computerized Algorithms Useful in Managing the Critically Ill Patient?

Maureen O. Meade, MD
Critical Care Consultant
Hamilton Health Sciences
Professor
Department of Medicine
McMaster University
Hamilton, Ontario, Canada
Chapter 34 Inhaled Vasodilators in ARDS: Do They Make a Difference?

Alexandre Mebazaa, MD, PhD
Biomarkers and Heart Diseases
UMR-942
Institut National de la Santé et de la Recherche Médicale (INSERM)
Department of Anesthesiology and Intensive Care
Lariboisière-Saint-Louis University Hospital
Assistance Publique–Hôpitaux de Paris
Université Paris Diderot
Paris, France
Chapter 50 How Do I Manage Acute Heart Failure?

Ravindra L. Mehta, MD
Professor of Clinical Medicine
Associate Chair for Clinical Research
Department of Medicine
Director, UC San Diego CREST and Masters of Advanced Studies in Clinical Research Program
University of California San Diego Health System
San Diego, California
Chapter 56 How Does One Optimize Care in Patients at Risk for or Presenting with Acute Kidney Injury?

Jaume Mesquida, MD
Department of Critical Care
Corporació Sanitària Universitària Parc Taulí
Hospital de Sabadell
Universitat Autònoma de Barcelona
Barcelona, Spain
Chapter 42 How Can We Monitor the Microcirculation in Sepsis? Does It Improve Outcome?

B. Messer, FRCA, MRCP, DICM
Department of Anaesthesia
Royal Victoria Infirmary
Newcastle upon Tyne, United Kingdom
Chapter 36 Are Anti-inflammatory Therapies in ARDS Effective?

Imran J. Meurling, MB BCh BAO, MRCPUK
Specialist Registrar in Respiratory Medicine
Galway University Hospital
National University of Ireland
Galway, Ireland
Chapter 27 Should Exacerbations of COPD Be Managed in the Intensive Care Unit?

Rohit Mittal, MD
Department of Surgery and Emory Center for Critical Care
Atlanta, Georgia
Chapter 70 How Does Critical Illness Alter the Gut? How Does One Manage These Alterations?

Xavier Monnet, MD, PhD

Service de reanimation
Paris-Sud University Hospitals
Paris-Sud University
Orsay, France
> *Chapter 16 What Are the Best Tools to Optimize the Circulation?*

Alan H. Morris, MD

Professor of Internal Medicine
Adjunct Professor of Biomedical Informatics
University of Utah School of Medicine
Director, Urban Central Region Pulmonary Laboratories
Intermountain Healthcare
Salt Lake City, Utah
> *Chapter 11 Is Extracorporeal Life Support an Evidence-Based Intervention for Critically Ill Adults with ARDS?*

Vikramjit Mukherjee, MD

Instructor of Medicine
Assistant Director of Critical Care
NYU Langone Hospital for Joint Diseases
New York, New York
> *Chapter 43 Do the Surviving Sepsis Campaign Guidelines Work?*

Taka-Aki Nakada, MD, PhD

Chiba University Graduate School of Medicine
Department of Emergency and Critical Care Medicine
Chiba, Japan
> *Chapter 19 Should Fever Be Treated?*

Patrick J. Neligan, MA, MB, FRCAFRCSI

Department of Anaesthesia and Intensive Care
University College Galway
Galway, Ireland
> *Chapter 1 Critical Care Versus Critical Illness*
> *Chapter 41 What Vasopressor Agent Should Be Used in the Septic Patient?*
> *Chapter 58 How Should Acid-Base Disorders Be Diagnosed and Managed?*

Alistair Nichol, PhD, MB

Australian and New Zealand Intensive Care–Research Centre
School of Public Health and Preventive Medicine
Monash University
Alfred Hospital Campus
Melbourne, Australia
> *Chapter 9 What Is the Optimal Approach to Weaning and Liberation from Mechanical Ventilation?*

Sara Nikravan, MD

Clinical Assistant Professor
Director of Critical Care Ultrasound and Focused Bedside Echocardiography
Stanford University Department of Anesthesiology, Perioperative, and Pain Medicine
Division of Critical Care Medicine
Stanford, California
> *Chapter 14 Does the Use of Echocardiography Aid in the Management of the Critically Ill?*

Mark E. Nunnally, MD, FCCM

Professor
Department of Anesthesia and Critical Care
The University of Chicago
Chicago, Illinois
> *Chapter 60 How Does Critical Illness Alter Metabolism?*

Michael O'Connor, MD FCCM

Professor
Section Head of Critical Care Medicine
Department of Anesthesia and Critical Care
The University of Chicago
Chicago, Illinois
> *Chapter 15 How Do I Manage Hemodynamic Decompensation in a Critically Ill Patient?*

Stephen R. Odom, MD

Assistant Professor of Surgery
Beth Israel Deaconess Medical Center
Boston, Massachusetts
> *Chapter 59 What Is the Meaning of a High Lactate? What Are the Implications of Lactic Acidosis?*

Steven M. Opal, MD

Professor of Medicine, Infectious Disease Division
The Alpert Medical School of Brown University
Providence, Rhode Island
Chief, Infectious Disease Division
Memorial Hospital of Rhode Island
Pawtucket, Rhode Island
> *Chapter 17 What Strategies Can Be Used to Optimize Antibiotic Use in the Critically Ill?*

Anthony O'Regan, MD

Consultant Respiratory Physician
Galway University Hospital
Galway, Ireland
> *Chapter 27 Should Exacerbations of COPD Be Managed in the Intensive Care Unit?*

John O'Regan, MD

Nephrology Division
University Hospital Galway
Galway, Ireland
> *Chapter 57 What Is the Role of Renal Replacement Therapy in the Intensive Care Unit?*

Michelle O'Shaughnessy, MD

Division of Nephrology
Stanford University School of Medicine
Palo Alto, California
> *Chapter 57 What Is the Role of Renal Replacement Therapy in the Intensive Care Unit?*

Pratik P. Pandharipande, MD, MSCI

Professor of Anesthesiology and Surgery
Division of Anesthesiology Critical Care Medicine
Vanderbilt University Medical Center
Nashville, Tennessee
> *Chapter 73 How Does One Diagnose, Treat, and Reduce Delirium in the Intensive Care Unit?*

Prakash A. Patel, MD
Assistant Professor
Anesthesiology and Critical Care
Perelman School of Medicine
University of Pennsylvania
Philadelphia, Pennsylvania
Chapter 82 Which Anticoagulants Should Be Used in the Critically Ill Patient? How Do I Choose?

Andrew J. Patterson, MD, PhD
Executive Vice Chair
Larson Professor of Anesthesiology
University of Nebraska Medical Center
Omaha, Nebraska
Chapter 14 Does the Use of Echocardiography Aid in the Management of the Critically Ill?

Paolo Pelosi, MD
IRCCS AOU San Martino-IST
Department of Surgical Sciences and Integrated Diagnostics
University of Genoa
Genoa, Italy
Chapter 8 How Does One Evaluate and Monitor Respiratory Function in the Intensive Care Unit?

Anders Perner, MD, PhD
Department of Intensive Care
Copenhagen University Hospital–Rigshospitalet
Copenhagen, Denmark
Chapter 20 What Fluids Should I Give to the Critically Ill Patient? What Fluids Should I Avoid?

Ville Pettila, MD, PhD
Department of Intensive Care Medicine
Bern University Hospital (Inselspital)
University of Bern
Bern, Switzerland
Division of Intensive Care Medicine
Department of Perioperative, Intensive Care, and Pain Medicine
University of Helsinki and Helsinki University Hospital
Helsinki, Finland
Chapter 9 What Is the Optimal Approach to Weaning and Liberation from Mechanical Ventilation?

Matthew Piazza, MD
Resident
Department of Neurosurgery
University of Pennsylvania
Philadelphia, Pennsylvania
Chapter 80 How Should Acute Spinal Cord Injury Be Managed in the ICU?

Michael R. Pinsky, MD, Dr hc
Department of Critical Care Medicine
University of Pittsburgh
Pittsburgh, Pennsylvania
Chapter 16 What Are the Best Tools to Optimize the Circulation?

Lauren A. Plante, MD, MPH
Director
Maternal-Fetal Medicine
Professor
Departments of Obstetrics and Gynecology and Anesthesiology
Drexel University College of Medicine
Philadelphia, Pennsylvania
Chapter 78 How Should the Critically Ill Pregnant Patient Be Managed?

Jean-Charles Preiser, MD, PhD
Professor
Department of Intensive Care
Erasme University Hospital
Universite Libre de Bruxelles
Brussels, Belgium
Chapter 21 Should Blood Glucose Be Tightly Controlled in the Intensive Care Unit?

Peter Radermacher, MD
Institut für Anästhesiologische Pathophysiologie und Verfahrensentwicklung
Universitätsklinikum Ulm
Ulm, Germany
Chapter 40 What MAP Objectives Should Be Targeted in Septic Shock?

Patrick M. Reilly, MD, FACS
Professor of Surgery
Chief
Division of Trauma, Surgical Critical Care, and Emergency Surgery
Department of Surgery
Perelman School of Medicine at the University of Pennsylvania
Philadelphia, Pennsylvania
Chapter 74 How Should Trauma Patients Be Managed in the Intensive Care Unit?

Andrew Rhodes, MD
Professor of Intensive Care Medicine
Divisional Chair
Children's, Women's, Diagnostics, Therapies and Critical Care
St. George's University Hospitals NHS Foundation Trust
London, United Kingdom
Chapter 84 Does ICU Admission Improve Outcome?

Zaccaria Ricci, MD
Pediatric Cardiac Intensive Care Unit
Department of Pediatric Cardiac Surgery
Bambino Gesù Children's Hospital, IRCCS
Rome, Italy
Chapter 55 How Does One Rapidly and Correctly Identify Acute Kidney Injury?

Claudio Ronco, MD
Division of Nephrology and Hypertension
Department of Medicine
University of California, San Diego
San Diego, California
Chapter 55 How Does One Rapidly and Correctly Identify Acute Kidney Injury?

James A. Russell, MD, FRCP(C)
Professor of Medicine
Principal Investigator
Centre for Heart Lung Innovation
University of British Columbia
St. Paul's Hospital
Vancouver, British Columbia, Canada
   Chapter 19 Should Fever Be Treated?

Ho Geol Ryu, MD
Assistant Professor
Department of Anesthesiology and Pain Medicine
Seoul National University
Seoul, South Korea
Master of Public Health
Johns Hopkins Bloomberg School of Public Health
Baltimore, Maryland
   Chapter 85 How Should Care Within an Intensive Care Unit or an Institution Be Organized?

Noelle N. Saillant, MD
Fellow
Division of Traumatology, Surgical Critical Care, and Emergency Surgery
University of Pennsylvania School of Medicine
Philadelphia, Pennsylvania
   Chapter 72 How Do I Diagnose and Manage Acute Endocrine Emergencies in the ICU?
   Chapter 75 What Is Abdominal Compartment Syndrome and How Should It Be Managed?

R. Matthew Sailors, BE
Assistant Program Director
Department of Surgery
University of Florida College of Medicine
Gainesville, Florida
   Chapter 25 Are Computerized Algorithms Useful in Managing the Critically Ill Patient?

Danielle K. Sandsmark, MD, PhD
Assistant Professor of Neurology, Neurosurgery, and Anesthesiology/Critical Care
Division of Neurocritical Care
Hospital of the University of Pennsylvania
Philadelphia, Pennsylvania
   Chapter 62 How Should Traumatic Brain Injury Be Managed?

Babak Sarani, MD, FACS, FCCM
Associate Professor of Surgery
George Washington University
Washington, District of Columbia
   Chapter 81 When Is Transfusion Therapy Indicated in Critical Illness and When Is It Not?

Naoki Sato, MD, PhD
Cardiology and Intensive Care Medicine
Nippon Medical School Musashi-Kosugi Hospital
Kawasaki, Japan
   Chapter 50 How Do I Manage Acute Heart Failure?

James Schuster, MD
Associate Professor
Chief of Neurosurgery, Penn Presbyterian Medical Center
Director of Neuro-Trauma
Department of Neurosurgery
University of Pennsylvania
Perelman School of Medicine
Philadelphia, Pennsylvania
   Chapter 80 How Should Acute Spinal Cord Injury Be Managed in the ICU?

Mike Scully, MD
Consultant Anaesthetist/Senior Lecturer
Anaesthesia and Critical Care
National University of Ireland
Galway, Ireland
   Chapter 45 How Do I Diagnose and Manage Catheter-Related Bloodstream Infections?

Mara Serbanescu, MD
Emory University School of Medicine
Atlanta, Georgia
   Chapter 70 How Does Critical Illness Alter the Gut? How Does One Manage These Alterations?

Ronaldo Sevilla Berrios, MD
Department of Critical Care and Hospitalist Medicine
UPMC Hamot
Erie, Pennsylvania
   Chapter 12 What Factors Predispose Patients to Acute Respiratory Distress Syndrome?

Carrie A. Sims, MD, MS, FACS
Associate Professor of Surgery
University of Pennsylvania School of Medicine
Philadelphia, Pennsylvania
   Chapter 72 How Do I Diagnose and Manage Acute Endocrine Emergencies in the ICU?

Brian P. Smith, MD
Assistant Professor of Surgery
The Hospital of the University of Pennsylvania
Assistant Professor of Surgery
VA Medical Center of Philadelphia
Philadelphia, Pennsylvania
   Chapter 74 How Should Trauma Patients Be Managed in the Intensive Care Unit?

Andrew C. Steel, BSc, MBBS, MRCP, FRCA, FFICM, FRCPC, EDIC
Interdepartmental Division of Critical Care Medicine
Toronto General Hospital
University of Toronto
Toronto, Ontario, Canada
   Chapter 30 What Is the Best Mechanical Ventilation Strategy in ARDS?

Yuda Sutherasan, MD
IRCCS AOU San Martino–IST
Department of Surgical Sciences and Integrated
    Diagnostics
University of Genoa
Genoa, Italy
Division of Pulmonary and Critical Care Unit
Department of Medicine
Ramathibodi Hospital
Mahidol University
Bangkok, Thailand
    *Chapter 8 How Does One Evaluate and Monitor
    Respiratory Function in the Intensive Care Unit?*

Rob Mac Sweeney, PhD
Regional Intensive Care Unit
Royal Victoria Hospital
Belfast, Northern Ireland
    *Chapter 35 Do Nonventilatory Strategies for Acute
    Respiratory Distress Syndrome Work?*

Waka Takahashi, MD, PhD
Chiba University Graduate School of Medicine
Department of Emergency and Critical Care Medicine
Chiba, Japan
    Chapter 19 Should Fever Be Treated?

Daniel Talmor, MD
Department of Anesthesia, Critical Care, and Pain
    Medicine
Beth Israel Deaconess Medical Center
Harvard Medical School
Boston, Massachusetts
    *Chapter 59 What Is the Meaning of a High Lactate? What
    Are the Implications of Lactic Acidosis?*

B. Taylor Thompson, MD
Division of Pulmonary and Critical Care Unit
Department of Medicine
Massachusetts General Hospital
Harvard Medical School
Boston, Massachusetts
    Chapter 28 What Is the Clinical Definition of ARDS?

Aurelie Thooft, MD
Intensive Care Unit
Erasme Hospital
Brussels, Belgium
    *Chapter 21 Should Blood Glucose Be Tightly Controlled in
    the Intensive Care Unit?*

**Samuel A. Tisherman, MD, FACS, FCCM,
FCCP**
Professor of Surgery
RA Cowley Shock Trauma Center
University of Maryland
Baltimore, Maryland
    *Chapter 77 What Is the Best Approach to Fluid
    Management, Transfusion Therapy, and the Endpoints of
    Resuscitation in Trauma?*

Isaiah R. Turnbull, MD, PhD
Assistant Professor of Surgery
Washington University School of Medicine
St. Louis, Missouri
    *Chapter 38 Is There Immune Suppression in the Critically
    Ill Patient?*

Amit Uppal, MD
Assistant Professor
Division of Pulmonary, Critical Care, and Sleep Medicine
New York University School of Medicine
New York, New York
    *Chapter 43 Do the Surviving Sepsis Campaign Guidelines
    Work?*

Emily Vail, MD
Department of Anesthesiology
Columbia University
New York, New York
    Chapter 3 Have Critical Care Outcomes Improved?

Carrie Valdez, MD
Chief Resident, General Surgery
Department of Surgery
The George Washington University Hospital
Washington, District of Columbia
*Chapter 81 When Is Transfusion Therapy Indicated in Critical
Illness and When Is It Not?*

Joy Vijayan, MD
Division of Neurology
National University Hospital
Singapore
    *Chapter 66 How Should Guillain-Barré Syndrome Be
    Managed in the ICU?*

Gianluca Villa, MD
International Renal Research Institute
San Bortolo Hospital
Vicenza, Italy
Department of Health Science
Section of Anaesthesiology and Intensive Care
University of Florence
Department of Anaesthesia and Intensive Care
Azienda Ospedaliero-Universitaria Careggi
Florence, Italy
    *Chapter 55 How Does One Rapidly and Correctly Identify
    Acute Kidney Injury?*

Jean-Louis Vincent, MD, PhD
Department of Intensive Care
Erasme University Hospital
Université libre de Bruxelles
Brussels, Belgium
    *Chapter 44 Has Outcome in Sepsis Improved? What Has
    Worked? What Has Not Worked?*

Jason Wagner, MD, MSHP
Division of Pulmonary, Allergy, and Critical Care
  Medicine
Perelman School of Medicine
University of Pennsylvania
Philadelphia, Pennsylvania
  *Chapter 83 How Can Critical Care Resource Utilization in
  the United States Be Optimized?*

Criona M. Walshe, MD, FCARCSI
Department of Anaesthesia
Beaumont Hospital
Dublin, Ireland
  *Chapter 33 Is Pulmonary Hypertension Important in
  ARDS? Should We Treat It?*

Scott L. Weiss, MD
Assistant Professor of Critical Care and Pediatrics
Department of Anesthesia and Critical Care
The Children's Hospital of Philadelphia
University of Pennsylvania Perelman School of Medicine
Philadelphia, Pennsylvania
  *Chapter 49 Is Sepsis-Induced Organ Dysfunction an
  Adaptive Response?*

Stuart J. Weiss, MD, PhD
Section Chief
Cardiovascular Anesthesia
Department of Anesthesiology and Critical Care
Hospital of the University of Pennsylvania
Philadelphia, Pennsylvania
  *Chapter 53 How Does One Prevent or Treat Atrial
  Fibrillation in Postoperative Critically Ill Patients?*

Hannah Wunsch, MD, MSc
Department of Critical Care Medicine
Sunnybrook Health Sciences Center
Department of Anesthesiology
University of Toronto
Toronto, Ontario, Canada
  Chapter 3 Have Critical Care Outcomes Improved?

Debbie H. Yi, MD
Instructor of Emergency Medicine
Fellow in Neurology
University of Pennsylvania
Philadelphia, Pennsylvania
  Chapter 65 How Should Status Epilepticus Be Managed?

Felix Yu, MD
Division of Pulmonary, Critical Care and Sleep Medicine
Tufts Medical Center
Boston, Massachusetts
  *Chapter 7 What Is the Role of Noninvasive Ventilation in
  the Intensive Care Unit?*

Evin Yucel, MD
Cooper Medical School of Rowan University
Camden, New Jersey
  *Chapter 54 Is Right Ventricular Failure Common in the
  Intensive Care Unit? How Should It Be Managed?*

Nobuhiro Yuki, MD, PhD
Departments of Medicine and Physiology
Yong Loo Lin School of Medicine
National University of Singapore
Singapore
  *Chapter 66 How Should Guillain-Barré Syndrome Be
  Managed in the ICU?*

Fernando Zampieri, MD
Intensive Care Unit
Emergency Medicine Discipline
Hospital das Clínicas
University of São Paulo
São Paulo, Brazil
  *Chapter 11 Is Extracorporeal Life Support an Evidence-
  Based Intervention for Critically Ill Adults with ARDS?*

Ting Zhou, MD
Department of Neurology
Hospital of the University of Pennsylvania
Philadelphia, Pennsylvania
  *Chapter 63 How Should Aneurysmal Subarachnoid
  Hemorrhage Be Managed?*

Preface

We are delighted to present the second edition of our textbook *Evidence-Based Practice of Critical Care*. It is a bit surprising to realize that it has been 5 years since the first edition was released. It seems as if we finished our editing only a few months ago, and we were grateful to be done. The reception has also been surprising, and again, we are grateful to the many critical care practitioners who have purchased the book and complimented us on its value. What is most surprising of all is the degree to which a new edition is justified. The practice of critical care medicine has changed immeasurably in the past 5 years, and the evidence base that supports care delivery has grown with it. These changes (Chapter 2) make it imperative that the contents of this book also change.

Several basic principles that had only begun to emerge 5 years ago now appear to be more firmly established. Many generate a sense of hope and a belief that care is improving and will continue to do so.

- We may be doing better—but maybe not. Determining if outcomes from critical illness have improved is problematic (Chapter 3), and determining just what has worked and what has not (Chapter 44) may be even more difficult.
- The consistent application of proven interventions is beneficial (Chapter 43), but just what interventions should be applied (and when they should be applied) may be more difficult to determine (Chapters 10, 11, 18–22, 31, 32, 34, 36, 39, 46, 57, 61, 67, 71, 81, and 82).
- Patients survive critical illness but often at a cost (Chapter 3). Survivors may be plagued by debilitating dysfunction in their musculoskeletal and peripheral nervous systems, irreversible respiratory defects, cognitive deficits that hamper performance of the activities of daily living, and psychological abnormalities such as posttraumatic stress disorder and even delirium. Attention has now turned to understanding the problems facing survivors and to generating patient networks to support them.
- Critical illness most often develops outside of the intensive care unit (ICU), and that is where treatment needs to begin. However, success depends on identifying and intervening as early as possible, and not all attempts to make this happen have been successful (Chapter 5). For it to be successful, intervention for vascular disorders such as stroke, myocardial infarction, and cardiac arrest requires early identification of patients, and these patients should be rapidly transported to centers where the appropriate care can be provided by expert practitioners who have access to the most advanced technology (Chapters 22 and 64). New approaches to the definitions of sepsis and acute respiratory distress syndrome (ARDS) have been accompanied by identification of simple clinical criteria that improve our ability to recognize at-risk patients in the hope that we can initiate management at an earlier point in the natural history of these disorders (Chapters 28 and 37). With earlier initiation of fluids and antibiotic therapy, some at-risk patients may never require care in an ICU.
- Some of the criteria that served as key identifiers of critically ill patients are no longer germane. For example, it is now recognized that the identification of patients who have sepsis with inflammatory markers (e.g., temperature, heart rate, respiratory rate, and white blood cell count, the SIRS [systemic inflammatory response syndrome] criteria) is too nonspecific and identifies a multitude of individuals with infection or other inflammatory disorders who do not have sepsis and whose risk of having sepsis is low. One result is the derivation of new definitions for sepsis and sepsis-related diagnoses and the associated validation of better clinical criteria to better identify patients with infection who are at high risk for mortality and morbidity (Chapter 37).
- Our understanding of the pathophysiology of several key disorders, notably sepsis and ARDS, has improved. Sepsis is no longer viewed in terms of excessive inflammation; it is now recognized that there are aspects of the syndrome that reflect profound immunosuppression (Chapter 38) and others that do not involve immunology at all. Indeed, sepsis may reflect an adaptive response to a profound metabolic defect that cannot, as yet, be identified (Chapter 49). Likewise, our understanding of the effects of critical illness on specific organ systems (Chapters 10, 13, 29, 54, 55, 61, 68, 70, 72, and 81) and the way in which specific organ systems determine the development and course of critical illness (Chapters 15, 27, 50, 51, and 68) has been profoundly altered. Finally, what is "normal" in the absence of critical illness may not be "normal" when critical illness is present and vice versa (Chapters 8, 19, 21, 31, 40, 41, and 52).
- We have come to recognize that host and nonhost factors beyond the acute illness itself determine whether a patient becomes critically ill (Chapters 12, 23, and 78).
- More is not necessarily better, and in some aspects of treatment "more" may be detrimental. Although administration of fluids has been a mainstay of critical care practice since its inception, we now recognize that there are limits that, if exceeded, may make matters worse (Chapters 20, 75, 77, and 81). Overuse of mechanical ventilation is clearly detrimental (Chapters 9 and 10), and it may be best to avoid intubation altogether (Chapter 7). Intervention to maintain blood pressure or other hemodynamic measures is not always indicated (Chapter 41), and, even when appropriate, it is not at all clear when intervention needs to be instituted (Chapter 40).
- Not all of the things we monitor need to be monitored, but we also misuse monitoring tools (Chapters 8, 13, 14, 16, 58, 59, and 61).

- In aggregate, the results of many studies are equivocal, especially when the study results are negative. Examples of trials in which intervention did not significantly alter outcome but where opposite results in different subpopulations negate each other abound. For example, the results of the ALVEOLI/EXPRESS and LOVs trials indicate that use of high positive end-expiratory pressure (PEEP) did not provide a statistically significant benefit over low PEEP in the management of ARDS (Chapter 30). However, in a population of morbidly obese patients, high PEEP is likely essential (Chapter 23). Likewise, the FACTT trial suggested that liberal fluid management offered no measurable benefit over conservative fluid management, a finding that is likely correct, unless the patient has ongoing fluid losses (e.g., bleeding, ascites) that would not be adequately replaced with a conservative approach.

Thus, targeting more specific populations for intervention may be necessary.
- Making the patient an active participant in, rather than a passive recipient of, care in critical illness may be advantageous.

Finally, we would like to thank all of the authors of the chapters in this book. Reading and editing the chapters has been hugely enjoyable and thought provoking, and we finish with the realization that we are only at the beginning of our understanding of critical illness and in the development of critical care. More than anything else, that is what lies behind the excitement we feel as we present this new edition.

Clifford S. Deutschman

Patrick J. Neligan

May 2015

Contents

SECTION I
CRITICAL CARE AND CRITICAL ILLNESS

1. Critical Care Versus Critical Illness 3
   Patrick J. Neligan, Clifford S. Deutschman

2. What Lessons Have Intensivists Learned During the Evidence-Based Medicine Era? 8
   Andrew T. Levinson, Mitchell M. Levy

3. Have Critical Care Outcomes Improved? 11
   Emily Vail, Hayley B. Gershengorn, Hannah Wunsch

4. What Problems Are Prevalent Among Survivors of Critical Illness and Which of Those Are Consequences of Critical Illness? 16
   Theodore J. Iwashyna

5. Do Early Warning Scores and Rapid Response Teams Improve Outcomes? 21
   Gabriella Jäderling, Rinaldo Bellomo

SECTION II
BASIC RESPIRATORY MANAGEMENT

6. What Are the Indications for Intubation in the Critically Ill Patient? 31
   Meredith Collard, Meghan Lane-Fall

7. What Is the Role of Noninvasive Ventilation in the Intensive Care Unit? 36
   Felix Yu, Erik Garpestad, Nicholas S. Hill

8. How Does One Evaluate and Monitor Respiratory Function in the Intensive Care Unit? 43
   Yuda Sutherasan, Lorenzo Ball, Paolo Pelosi

9. What Is the Optimal Approach to Weaning and Liberation from Mechanical Ventilation? 52
   Alistair Nichol, Stephen Duff, Ville Pettila, David J. Cooper

10. How Does Mechanical Ventilation Damage Lungs? What Can Be Done to Prevent It? 61
    Joshua A. Marks, Maurizio Cereda

11. Is Extracorporeal Life Support an Evidence-Based Intervention for Critically Ill Adults with ARDS? 66
    Eliotte Hirshberg, Fernando Zampieri, Michael Lanspa, Kimberly S. Bennett, R. Duncan Hite, Alan H. Morris

12. What Factors Predispose Patients to Acute Respiratory Distress Syndrome? 75
    Ognjen Gajic, Alice Gallo, De Moraes, Ronaldo Sevilla Berrios

SECTION III
HEMODYNAMIC MANAGEMENT

13. What Is the Role of Invasive Hemodynamic Monitoring in Critical Care? 83
    Daniel De Backer

14. Does the Use of Echocardiography Aid in the Management of the Critically Ill? 88
    Sara Nikravan, Andrew J. Patterson

15. How Do I Manage Hemodynamic Decompensation in a Critically Ill Patient? 92
    Allison Dalton, Michael O'Connor

16. What Are the Best Tools to Optimize the Circulation? 99
    Xavier Monnet, Michael R. Pinsky

SECTION IV
GENERAL CRITICAL CARE MANAGEMENT

17. What Strategies Can Be Used to Optimize Antibiotic Use in the Critically Ill? 105
    Cheston B. Cunha, Steven M. Opal

18. Is Prophylaxis for Stress Ulceration
    Useful? 112
    Eimhin Dunne, Ivan Hayes, Brian Marsh

19. Should Fever Be Treated? 118
    Taka-Aki Nakada, Waka Takahashi, James A. Russell

20. What Fluids Should I Give to the
    Critically Ill Patient? What Fluids
    Should I Avoid? 124
    Anders Perner

21. Should Blood Glucose Be Tightly
    Controlled in the Intensive Care Unit? 128
    Jean-Charles Preiser, Aurelie Thooft

22. Is Hypothermia Useful in Managing
    Critically Ill Patients? Which Ones?
    Under What Conditions? 133
    Tomas Drabek, Patrick M. Kochanek

23. What Are the Special Considerations
    in the Management of Morbidly Obese
    Patients in the Intensive Care Unit? 144
    Ali A. El Solh

24. How Do I Transport the Critically
    Ill Patient? 154
    David Cosgrave, John Chandler, John Bates

25. Are Computerized Algorithms Useful in
    Managing the Critically Ill Patient? 160
    Bruce A. McKinley, R. Matthew Sailors

SECTION V

NON-ARDS AND NONINFECTIOUS RESPIRATORY DISORDERS

26. How Do I Diagnose and Treat Pulmonary
    Embolism? 169
    Jacob T. Gutsche, Anita K. Malhotra

27. Should Exacerbations of COPD Be
    Managed in the Intensive Care Unit? 175
    Anthony O'Regan, Imran J. Meurling

SECTION VI

ARDS

28. What Is the Clinical Definition
    of ARDS? 183
    *Jeremy R. Beitler, Andrés Esteban, José Angel Lorente,
    B. Taylor Thompson*

29. What Are the Pathologic and
    Pathophysiologic Changes
    That Accompany Acute Lung
    Injury and ARDS? 190
    Michael Lava, Greg S. Martin

30. What Is the Best Mechanical
    Ventilation Strategy in ARDS? 195
    *Margaret Doherty, Andrew C. Steel,
    Niall D. Ferguson*

31. Is Permissive Hypercapnia Useful
    in ARDS? 204
    *Maya Contreras, Claire Masterson,
    John G. Laffey*

32. Do Patient Positioning in General
    and Prone Positioning in Particular
    Make a Difference in ARDS? 212
    Alain F. Broccard, Maneesh Bhargava

33. Is Pulmonary Hypertension
    Important in ARDS? Should We
    Treat It? 219
    Criona M. Walshe, Leo G. Kevin

34. Inhaled Vasodilators in ARDS:
    Do They Make a Difference? 224
    Francois Lamontagne, Maureen O. Meade

35. Do Nonventilatory Strategies for
    Acute Respiratory Distress
    Syndrome Work? 229
    Rob Mac Sweeney, Danny McAuley

36. Are Anti-inflammatory Therapies
    in ARDS Effective? 239
    Tom Doris, B. Messer, S.V. Baudouin

SECTION VII

SEPSIS

37. What Is Sepsis? What Is Septic Shock?
    What Are MODS and Persistent Critical
    Illness? 249
    Clifford S. Deutschman

38. Is There Immune Suppression in
    the Critically Ill Patient? 256
    Isaiah R. Turnbull, Richard S. Hotchkiss

39. What Is the Role of Empirical Antibiotic
    Therapy in Sepsis? 262
    Fiona Kiernan, Gerard F. Curley

40. **What MAP Objectives Should Be Targeted in Septic Shock?** 278
François Beloncle, Peter Radermacher, Pierre Asfar

41. **What Vasopressor Agent Should Be Used in the Septic Patient?** 284
Colm Keane, Gráinne McDermott, Patrick J. Neligan

42. **How Can We Monitor the Microcirculation in Sepsis? Does It Improve Outcome?** 291
Guillem Gruartmoner, Jaume Mesquida, Can Ince

43. **Do the Surviving Sepsis Campaign Guidelines Work?** 297
Laura Evans, Amit Uppal, Vikramjit Mukherjee

44. **Has Outcome in Sepsis Improved? What Has Worked? What Has Not Worked?** 301
Jean-Louis Vincent

SECTION VIII
INFECTIONS

45. **How Do I Diagnose and Manage Catheter-Related Bloodstream Infections?** 307
Mike Scully

46. **Is Selective Decontamination of the Digestive Tract Useful?** 311
John Lyons, Craig M. Coopersmith

SECTION IX
PERSISTENT CRITICAL ILLNESS

47. **Is Persistent Critical Illness an Iatrogenic Disorder?** 325
John C. Marshall

48. **What Is the Role of Autonomic Dysfunction in Critical Illness?** 330
Gareth L. Ackland

49. **Is Sepsis-Induced Organ Dysfunction an Adaptive Response?** 335
Scott L. Weiss, Richard J. Levy, Clifford S. Deutschman

SECTION X
CARDIOVASCULAR CRITICAL CARE

50. **How Do I Manage Acute Heart Failure?** 343
Shiro Ishihara, Naoki Sato, Alexandre Mebazaa

51. **How Is Cardiogenic Shock Diagnosed and Managed in the Intensive Care Unit?** 347
Benjamin A. Kohl

52. **When Is Hypertension a True Crisis, and How Should It Be Managed in the Intensive Care Unit?** 353
Emily K. Gordon, Jacob T. Gutsche, John G. Augoustides, Clifford S. Deutschman

53. **How Does One Prevent or Treat Atrial Fibrillation in Postoperative Critically Ill Patients?** 361
Jonathan K. Frogel, Stuart J. Weiss

54. **Is Right Ventricular Failure Common in the Intensive Care Unit? How Should It Be Managed?** 370
Evin Yucel, Steven M. Hollenberg

SECTION XI
KIDNEY INJURY AND CRITICAL ILLNESS

55. **How Does One Rapidly and Correctly Identify Acute Kidney Injury?** 383
Gianluca Villa, Zaccaria Ricci, Claudio Ronco

56. **How Does One Optimize Care in Patients at Risk for or Presenting with Acute Kidney Injury?** 388
Celina D. Cepeda, Josée Bouchard, Ravindra L. Mehta

57. **What Is the Role of Renal Replacement Therapy in the Intensive Care Unit?** 399
Michelle O'Shaughnessy, John O'Regan, David Lappin

SECTION XII
METABOLIC ABNORMALITIES IN CRITICAL ILLNESS

58. **How Should Acid-Base Disorders Be Diagnosed and Managed?** 409
Patrick J. Neligan

59. What Is the Meaning of a High Lactate? What Are the Implications of Lactic Acidosis? 419
Stephen R. Odom, Daniel Talmor

60. How Does Critical Illness Alter Metabolism? 424
Mark E. Nunnally

SECTION XIII
NEUROLOGIC CRITICAL CARE

61. Is It Really Necessary to Measure Intracranial Pressure in Brain-Injured Patients? 431
Randall M. Chesnut

62. How Should Traumatic Brain Injury Be Managed? 441
Danielle K. Sandsmark, Larami MacKenzie, W. Andrew Kofke

63. How Should Aneurysmal Subarachnoid Hemorrhage Be Managed? 450
Paulomi K. Bhalla, Ting Zhou, Joshua M. Levine

64. How Should Acute Ischemic Stroke Be Managed in the Intensive Care Unit? 461
Allie M. Massaro, Scott E. Kasner, Joshua M. Levine

65. How Should Status Epilepticus Be Managed? 470
Debbie H. Yi, Kathryn A. Davis, Joshua M. Levine

66. How Should Guillain-Barré Syndrome Be Managed in the ICU? 475
Joy Vijayan, Nobuhiro Yuki

SECTION XIV
NUTRITION, GASTROINTESTINAL, AND HEPATIC CRITICAL CARE

67. Is It Appropriate to "Underfeed" the Critically Ill Patient? 487
Naomi E. Cahill, Daren K. Heyland

68. How Does Critical Illness Alter the Liver? 494
Michael Bauer, Andreas Kortgen

69. How Is Acute Liver Failure Managed? 497
Mark T. Keegan

70. How Does Critical Illness Alter the Gut? How Does One Manage These Alterations? 510
Rohit Mittal, Mara Serbanescu, Kevin W. McConnell

SECTION XV
ENDOCRINE CRITICAL CARE

71. Is There a Place for Anabolic Hormones in Critical Care? 517
Nicholas Heming, Virginie Maxime, Djillali Annane

72. How Do I Diagnose and Manage Acute Endocrine Emergencies in the ICU? 523
Noelle N. Saillant, Carrie A. Sims

SECTION XVI
PREVENTING SUFFERING IN THE ICU

73. How Does One Diagnose, Treat, and Reduce Delirium in the Intensive Care Unit? 535
E. Wesley Ely, Arna Banerjee, Pratik P. Pandharipande

SECTION XVII
TRAUMA, OBSTETRICS, AND ENVIRONMENTAL INJURIES

74. How Should Trauma Patients Be Managed in the Intensive Care Unit? 545
Brian P. Smith, Patrick M. Reilly

75. What Is Abdominal Compartment Syndrome and How Should It Be Managed? 551
Noelle N. Saillant, Lewis J. Kaplan

76. How Should Patients with Burns Be Managed in the Intensive Care Unit? 556
Marc G. Jeschke

77. What Is the Best Approach to Fluid Management, Transfusion Therapy, and the Endpoints of Resuscitation in Trauma? 563
Samuel A. Tisherman

78. How Should the Critically Ill Pregnant Patient Be Managed? 571
Lauren A. Plante

79. How Do I Diagnose and Manage Patients
     Admitted to the ICU After Common
     Poisonings? 577
     Jakub Furmaga, Kurt Kleinschmidt

80. How Should Acute Spinal Cord Injury
     Be Managed in the ICU? 583
     James Schuster, Matthew Piazza

SECTION XVIII

HEMATOLOGY CRITICAL CARE

81. When Is Transfusion Therapy Indicated
     in Critical Illness and When Is It Not? 595
     Carrie Valdez, Babak Sarani

82. Which Anticoagulants Should Be Used
     in the Critically Ill Patient? How Do I
     Choose? 603
     Prakash A. Patel, Emily K. Gordon, John G. Augoustides

SECTION XIX

CRITICAL CARE RESOURCE USE AND MANAGEMENT

83. How Can Critical Care Resource
     Utilization in the United States Be
     Optimized? 611
     Jason Wagner, Scott Halpern

84. Does ICU Admission Improve
     Outcome? 616
     *Andrea Carsetti, Hollmann D. Aya, Maurizio Cecconi,
     Andrew Rhodes*

85. How Should Care Within an Intensive Care
     Unit or an Institution Be Organized? 622
     Ho Geol Ryu, Todd Dorman

86. What Is the Role of Advanced Practice
     Nurses and Physician Assistants in the
     ICU? 626
     Ruth Kleinpell, W. Robert Grabenkort

SECTION XX

CRITICAL CARE ETHICS

87. What Factors Influence a Family to
     Support a Decision Withdrawing Life
     Support? 633
     Randall J. Curtis, Margaret Isaac

EVIDENCE-BASED PRACTICE
of CRITICAL CARE

CRITICAL CARE AND CRITICAL ILLNESS

1 Critical Care Versus Critical Illness

Patrick J. Neligan, Clifford S. Deutschman

Intensive care units (ICUs) were developed in the 1950s to treat patients with two distinct problems. In some cases, ICU care was required to provide an intervention to support organ dysfunction—mechanic ventilation for acute respiratory failure.[1,2] Conversely, ICUs also permitted intensive monitoring of a patient whose physiologic condition might change abruptly, that is, observation of patients undergoing a "stress response" following surgery or trauma or patients with cardiac or neurologic conditions that might suddenly change.[3,4] Over time, technologic evolution has enhanced our ability to care for both types of patients. In addition to ventilators, it is now possible to support patients with life-threatening, acute organ dysfunction with renal replacement therapy, vasoactive drugs or even ventricular assist devices, exogenous metabolic support, and more. At the same time, we can directly monitor the function of areas such as the heart, the lungs, the brain, the gastrointestinal (GI) tract, and the kidneys. Over the years, the distinction between the two forms of technology has blurred: we monitor patients who require life-sustaining therapy, and we support organs in patients who are at high risk to prevent deterioration. The difference between the two types of patients remains. There are patients who will most often have a predictable response to a major perturbation of homeostasis following high-risk (e.g., cardiac, neurologic, vascular, transplant, and upper GI) surgery, trauma, a myocardial infarction (MI) or arrhythmia, stroke, or subarachnoid hemorrhage. These patients may require intervention to allow the damage to heal, but, by and large, they require careful monitoring and observation as they traverse a course whose length, magnitude, and complications are predictable.[5,6] Conversely, patients who have sustained shock, sepsis, or direct/progressive damage to an organ system require support, and monitoring is used to determine if that support is working. In short, there are ICU patients who are at risk of becoming critically ill, and there are patients who *are* critically ill (Fig. 1-1). In this introductory chapter, we explore the differences and emphasize that the most important tasks facing modern medicine are to determine where the transition occurs and to prevent those at risk for critical illness from becoming critically ill.

THE PERIOPERATIVE/POSTINJURY STRESS RESPONSE

In contrast to critical illness, the biology underlying the stress response to surgery or trauma is well-characterized, predictable, and, absent comorbidities that may be effected, adaptive.[5,6] Cuthbertson first described the stress response over 80 years ago.[5] Since then, a number of brilliant investigators and clinicians have added to our understanding of its biology.[7-9] We now recognize that "stress" provokes inflammation and that the purpose of inflammation is restoration of a biologic "steady state," where cellular, tissue, organ system, and, ultimately, organism-wide activity fluctuates around some mean level of behavior and maintenance of interaction and cooperation on these same levels.[6] In most cases, the overwhelming imperative driving inflammation is a need to repair, replace, or compensate for damage to cells and tissues.[6] This damage may result from physical injury (trauma), from interruption of blood supply (e.g., stroke, MI), or from invasion of microorganisms that "hijack" normal cellular metabolism.

CRITICAL ILLNESS

Critical illness is characterized by acute, potentially life-threatening organ dysfunction that requires therapy. It is often precipitated by the same disturbances that provoke inflammation. The initiator may be "shock," whose origin can often, but not universally, be traced to circulatory failure or to infection that overwhelms endogenous responses. The common denominator is a profound insult to homeostasis on the cellular level that exceeds endogenous corrective responses. However, the manner in which these states result in abnormal organ function is unknown.

Critically ill patients may present to primary care, to the emergency department (ED), or on the hospital wards. They represent a small subset of patients; the vast majority of individuals with deviations from "health," for example, those with inflammation or even shock, respond to initial therapy. A few, however, become acutely critically ill. Acute critical illness is often unanticipated and may not follow a predictable stress response trajectory.

3

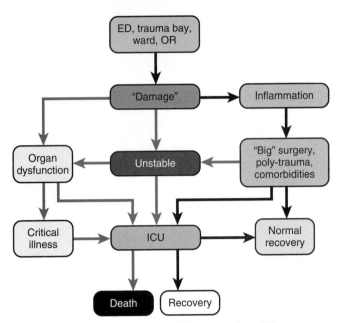

Figure 1-1 The critical care–critical illness paradigm. *ED*, emergency department; *ICU*, intensive care unit; *OR*, operating room.

With early recognition and appropriate therapy, many critically ill patients will recover. Once again, however, a subset will deteriorate further, to a state of *persistent critical illness* with multiorgan dysfunction (see Chapter 37). This state may persist for weeks and thus can appear stable, but it is also highly abnormal, with defects in most organ systems.[10,11] Once again, many patients will recover. However, it is increasingly clear that this recovery is incomplete. Many patients who have undergone a prolonged ICU course are left with persistent respiratory, cardiac, neuromuscular, and cognitive dysfunction.[12-15] Some may remain ventilator dependent; others will have a variant of posttraumatic stress disorder.[13] Recent studies suggest that, in the United States, there may be upward of 700,000 ICU survivors each year, many of whom require ongoing support, but many others whose ongoing problems escape detection.[16]

INFLAMMATION VERSUS CRITICAL ILLNESS: BIOLOGIC PERSPECTIVES

Both inflammation and critical illness are, at the core, responses to significant, and often extreme, perturbation of homeostasis, the biologic steady state. As a result, there is a tendency to assume that therapy appropriate for one will also be effective for the other. There is, indeed, some truth to this assumption. As an example, in both inflammation and critical illness, an initial imperative is the restoration of substrate delivery to and waste removal from cells. However, the profound change that differentiates inflammation from critical illness has been characterized by some as a loss of a cell's ability to use substrate, or the creation of a by-product that cannot be removed by ordinary means. Consider the cellular need for oxygen. Inadequate delivery may reflect abnormalities in the lungs, with impaired gas exchange, or in the circulation, where the cardiovascular system is

unable to transfer oxygen itself, or oxygen-containing molecules or cells, to tissues for use. Cells can often meet energy demands by means of glycolysis alone, bypassing the electron transport chain, and generating lactate and hydrogen ions. Recycling of lactate requires an intact circulation for delivery to the liver. Acidosis is corrected by buffering with the production of carbon dioxide (CO_2), which must be excreted by ventilation. Thus, a clinician's initial response would be to enhance oxygen uptake by increasing the inspired concentration, restoring the circulation with fluid, and, perhaps, increasing the oxygen-carrying capacity with red blood cells. This same fluid will restore hepatic flow and allow for the conversion of lactate to pyruvate. Improving gas removal with mechanical ventilation will facilitate CO_2 removal. This approach may be effective when directed toward inflammation secondary to tissue damage, where oxygen use is diverted to support white blood cells, the primary effectors of tissue repair, and where delivery is inadequate because damaged tissue is essentially avascular. This response is self-limiting because capillary angiogenesis takes about 4 days,[17] after which exogenous support can be weaned. However, a more profound insult, or one that is not addressed in a timely manner, may do more than limit oxygen availability or divert its use. Damage to mitochondria, which is a hallmark of sepsis, will impair the ability of a cell to use oxygen irrespective of availability.[18,19] Thus, restoration of gas exchange or cardiovascular function will not, in and of itself, be sufficient to restore homeostasis. As a result, organ dysfunction may not improve or resolve with these standard measures—a hallmark of critical illness that is often unrecognized or unappreciated. Unfortunately, the distinction between stress and critical illness is not always clinically self-evident, and this lack of distinction leads to diagnostic and therapeutic dilemmas whose resolution, for the moment, is intensely problematic.

INFLAMMATION VERSUS CRITICAL ILLNESS: THERAPEUTIC PERSPECTIVES

An unfortunate extension of our difficulties in distinguishing a stress response from critical illness is a persistent tendency to assume that what works for one group will also work for the other. Examples abound. The following is a summary of several of the most important examples, both historically and therapeutically:

- *Fluid resuscitation in sepsis:* In a landmark 2001 study by Rivers and colleagues,[20] researchers studied patients with suspected infection who were thought to have sepsis and compared fluid resuscitation using standard endpoints such as blood pressure (BP) to alternatives that focused on tissue oxygen delivery, for example, venous oxygen saturation (SvO_2) or central venous pressure (CVP). This single center study demonstrated a remarkable improvement in outcome using the latter approach. However, three recent multicenter studies applying essentially the same paradigm failed to duplicate the original findings.[21-23] A number of possible explanations have been advanced, but it is essential to note that in "inflammation," adequate resuscitation may be reflected in measures such as CVP and SvO_2. However, sepsis involves a pathologic defect in either the microcirculation or the mitochondria so that oxygen delivery or extraction cannot be corrected with fluid alone.[18,24] Unfortunately, the entry criteria in both the initial Rivers trial and the subsequent multicenter trials cannot truly distinguish inflammation and hypovolemia secondary to suspected infection for sepsis, a state of critical illness that reflects early organ dysfunction that is difficult to detect. Fluid resuscitation that is appropriate for one may be ineffective, and even excessive, for the other.

- *Ventilator management in acute lung injury/acute respiratory distress syndrome (ARDS)*: A series of studies by a network of United States–based investigators and others have examined therapeutic approaches to lung injury. The most important of these "ARDSnet" studies is the initial "ARMA" trial, demonstrating that limiting tidal volumes to 6 cc/kg body weight is associated with better outcomes than use of larger (10 to 12 cc/kg) volumes.[25] The diagnosis of ARDS was based on the standard criteria: hypoxemia, reflected in a decreased ratio of arterial oxygen tension (Pao_2) to fraction of oxygen in the inspired gas (Fio_2), the presence of bilateral "patchy" infiltrates on chest radiographs, and no evidence that the abnormalities were of cardiogenic origin. Conversely, for decades, anesthesiologists have administered tidal volumes in the 10 to 12 cc/kg range in the operating room. Many, if not most, postoperative patients have abnormal Pao_2/Fio_2 ratios and abnormal chest radiographs. This is especially true for patients undergoing cardiac surgery. Postoperatively, though, the great majority of these patients do not require more than supplemental oxygen. Even in those who are maintained with mechanic ventilation into the postoperative period, exogenous support is rarely needed for more than a short period. All surgical patients have capillary leak as part of the inflammation induced by tissue injury. This "stress response" results in mild hypoxemia and "wet" lungs. In contrast, patients with ARDS have lung dysfunction. Postoperative patients have inflammation; patients with ARDS have critical illness.

- *Determination of outcome*: The management of patients with sepsis has been an important focus of critical care practice for more than a decade.[26-28] Attempts to consolidate limited positive multicenter clinical trials in critical care have resulted in international and national clinical practice management guidelines. Perhaps the most widely disseminated involve the Surviving Sepsis Campaign (SSC) guidelines for the management of sepsis. The SSC (www.survivingsepsis.org) has been effective in increasing awareness of early sepsis and perhaps in advancing the implementation of therapy that may improve outcome.[29] Importantly, recent studies from the United States and Australasia have demonstrated that mortality from sepsis has decreased to surprisingly low levels—under 10% in one multi-institutional U.S. health system[30] and under 20% when more broadly applied over a 12-year period in Australia and New Zealand.[31] However, personal communications from intensivists in the three industrialized European countries suggest that, despite use of some or all elements of the SSC guidelines, mortality may be as high as 50%

(personal communications, Mervyn Singer, M.D.). The expressed opinion of those practicing in the United Kingdom, Germany, and Italy is that many patients diagnosed with sepsis and admitted to ICUs in the United States and Australasia would be managed in the EDs of other countries. If these patients responded to ED management, they would not be admitted to the ICU and would not be identified as "septic." To further complicate matters, Gaieski et al.[32] applied four different methods of defining "sepsis" to a single U.S. patient dataset and found a 3.5-fold variation in the incidence and a 2-fold variation in mortality. Clearly, some of the patients diagnosed with sepsis in the United States and Australasian databases were undergoing inflammation in response to infection. Again, differentiating inflammation from critical illness is profoundly important.

- *Intensive insulin therapy*: In 2001, Van den Berghe and colleagues[33] published a much sited clinical trial that randomized patients to *intensive insulin therapy* (ITT) (glucose levels maintained between 80 and 110 mg/dL), as opposed to "normal care" (glucose levels treated when above 180 mg/dL). The study was based on the knowledge that hyperglycemia is associated with a number of untoward outcomes in critically ill patients and demonstrated a statistically significant 3.4% absolute reduction in the risk of death at 28 days in the surgical ICU of a major hospital in Leuven, Belgium. The paucity of interventions that improve outcomes in critical care and the fact that insulin is inexpensive and easy to administer led to wide adoption of ITT. Although Van den Berghe et al.[33] clearly documented the need for careful monitoring of blood glucose levels and the risk of hypoglycemia, these potential complications were largely ignored. "Tight glycemic control" was even considered a key performance indicator in many ICUs[34] and became a component of the first SSC guidelines.[26] However, some elements of the study methodology suggested that the near-universal adoption of IIT might be problematic. Specifically germane to this discussion is the fact that more than 60% of the patients who entered into the study had recently undergone cardiac surgery, and virtually all were seen either postoperatively or post-traumatically. A follow-up study by the Van den Berghe group[35] applied the same protocol to patients in the medical ICU of the same institution and failed to demonstrate outcome benefits. In addition, somewhat problematic trials were stopped early because of concerns that high levels of hypoglycemia might cause harm.[36,37] Finally, the 2008 NICE SUGAR (Normoglycaemia in Intensive Care Evaluation Survival Using Glucose Algorithm Regulation) trial applied the Leuven protocol to more than 6000 patients and demonstrated that, if anything, tight glycemic control may worsen outcomes in critical care,[38] likely as a result of hypoglycemia.[39] Although the IIT episode contains many lessons, it remains a textbook demonstration of the difference between inflammation (e.g., the response to surgery, especially when cardiopulmonary bypass is involved) and critical illness, which was more likely to be represented in the population from the Leuven Medical ICU and the multicenter trials. Importantly, the mortality of untreated patients in the Leuven Surgical ICU was about 8%,[34] whereas that of the same group in the Leuven Medical ICU was 40%,[35] which clearly demonstrated that they were different.

- *Monitoring the heart*: The widely held belief that there is a need to monitor substrate delivery to tissues has led to the development of a wide variety of hemodynamic monitoring devices. Conventional monitoring of the circulation involves using heart rate (HR), mean arterial pressure (MAP), urinary output, and CVP. The optimal MAP is unknown.[40,41] CVP does not measure volume responsiveness,[42] and high CVPs have been associated with adverse outcomes.[43] More important, the meaning of a change in CVP is entirely dependent on the model of cardiovascular function used. A rise in CVP in the Frank-Starling formulation of cardiac function (which focuses on the determinants of ventricular output), where it serves as a surrogate for preload, should result in an increased stroke volume (SV).[44] However, in the Guyton model, where the focus in on ventricular filling, a similar increase in CVP will reduce the gradient for flow into the ventricle and thus will decrease SV.[45] The "normal" urinary output of more than 0.5 mL/kg/hr is actually a "minimum" hourly output and is based on theoretic calculations involving the maximal capacity to concentrate the urine and the "average" daily nitrogen load to be eliminated. There are many reasons why these numbers may not be germane either in individual patients or in the setting of either stress or critical illness. Importantly, there are no studies demonstrating that achieving this target affects the development of renal injuries.

One way in which to more accurately monitor cardiac function is to directly measure the effects of a change in volume on cardiac output (or to eliminate the effects of HR on SV).[46] For two decades, pulmonary artery catheters (PACs) were extensively used to monitor both perioperative and critically ill patients. Use has declined because a large randomized trial of PACs in ICUs failed to demonstrate a mortality benefit.[47] However, this study was performed on approximately 2000 patients undergoing high-risk surgery; the overall mortality was under 8%, likely too low to be an appropriate endpoint. Given the nature of the patient population and the low mortality, it is likely that many of the patients entered into this trial were not critically ill.

Parenthetically, the incidence of renal insufficiency in the PAC group was 7.4%, whereas it was 9.8% in the standard care group, generating a P value of .07, just above the threshold for significance. Indeed, if one more patient in the standard care group had developed renal insufficiency, or one less patient in the PAC group had not, the use of PACs might have increased.

In summary, it is imperative that critical care practitioners do not confuse inflammation and critical illness. Examples of the dangers inherent in failure to account for these differences, beyond those detailed here, abound. Both may require enhanced surveillance and intensive monitoring, but the need for intervention and, if necessary, the time course during which intervention is required are likely to be different. Inappropriately applied therapy is both expensive and potentially dangerous.

AUTHORS' RECOMMENDATIONS

- Not all patients in ICUs are critically ill; patients admitted after surgery or for monitoring may need to be managed differently than critically ill patients.
- Research data derived from the perioperative (including surgical ICUs) literature may not be applicable in critical illness.
- The perioperative realm provides a useful laboratory for new therapies or monitors; however, it is characterized by a controlled and curtailed stress response, recovery from which is predictable.
- Acute critical illness is characterized by organ dysfunction.
- Persistent critical illness likely reflects an underlying disease process that is different from either stress or acute critical illness, and interventions designed for one may be ineffective or even harmful in the other.

REFERENCES

1. Ibsen B. The anaesthetist's viewpoint on the treatment of respiratory complications in poliomyelitis during the epidemic in Copenhagen, 1952. *Proc Royal Soc Med*. 1954;47:72–74.
2. Lassen HCA. A preliminary report on the 1952 epidemic of poliomyelitis in Copenhagen with special reference to the treatment of acute respiratory insufficiency. *Lancet*. 1953;1:37–41.
3. Mosenthal WT. The special care unit. *J Maine Med Assoc*. 1957;48:396–399.
4. Grenvik A, Pinsky MR. Evolution of the intensive care unit as a clinical center and critical care medicine as a discipline. *Crit Care Clin*. 2009;25:239–250.
5. Cuthbertson DP. Observations on the disturbance of metabolism produced by injury to the limbs. *Q J Med*. 1932;1:233–246.
6. Kohl BA, Deutschman CS. The inflammatory response to surgery and trauma. *Curr Opin Crit Care*. 2006;12:325–332.
7. Moore FD, Olesen KH, MacMurray. *The body cell mass and its supporting environment: body composition in health and disease*; 1963. Philadelphia.
8. Meguid MM, Brennan MF, Aoki TT, Muller WA, Ball MR, Moore FD. Hormone-substrate interrelationships following trauma. *Arch Surg*. 1974;109:776–783.
9. McClelland RN, Shires GT, Baxter CR, Coin D, Carrico CJ. Balanced salt solution in the treatment of hemorrhagic shock. *JAMA*. 1967;199:830–834.
10. Nelson JE, Cox CE, Hope AA, Carson SS. Chronic Critical Illness. *Am J Respir Crit Care Med*. 2010;182:446–454.
11. Hotchkiss RS, Monneret G, Payen D. Sepsis-induced immunosuppression: from cellular dysfunction to immunotherapy. *Nat Rev Immunol*. 2013;13:862–874.
12. Herridge MS, Tansey CM, Matté A, et al. Functional disability 5 years after acute respiratory distress syndrome. *New Engl J Med*. 2011;364:1293–1304.
13. Bienvenu OJ, Colantuoni E, Mendez-Tellez PA, et al. Co-occurrence of and remission from general anxiety, depression, and posttraumatic stress disorder symptoms after acute lung injury: a 2-year longitudinal study. *Crit Care Med*. 2015;43:842–853.
14. Hermans G, Van Mechelen H, Clerckx B, et al. Acute outcomes and 1-year mortality of intensive care unit-acquired weakness. A cohort study and propensity-matched analysis. *Am J Respir Crit Care Med*. 2014;190:410–420.
15. Iwashyna TJ, Ely EW, Smith DM, Langa KM. Long term cognitive impairment and functional disability among survivors of severe sepsis. *JAMA*. 2010;302:1787–1794.
16. Iwashyna TJ, Cooke CR, Wunsch H, Kahn JM. Population burden of long-term survivorship after severe sepsis in older Americans. *J Am Geriatr Soc*. 2012;60:1070–1077.
17. Knighton DR, Silver IA, Hunt TK. Regulation of wound-healing angiogenesis-effect of oxygen gradients and inspired oxygen concentration. *Surgery*. 1982;90:262–270.
18. Singer M. The role of mitochondrial dysfunction in sepsis-induced multi-organ failure. *Virulence*. 2014;5:66–72.

19. Vanhorebeek I, Gunst J, Derde S, et al. Insufficient activation of autophagy allows cellular damage to accumulate in critically ill patients. *J Clin Endocrinol Metab*. 2011;96:E633–E645.
20. Rivers E, Nguyen B, Havstad S, et al. Early goal-directed therapy in the treatment of severe sepsis and septic shock. *N Engl J Med*. 2001;345:1368–1377.
21. ProCESS Investigators, Yealy DM, Kellum JA, et al. A randomized trial of protocol-based care for early septic shock. *N Engl J Med*. 2014;370:1683–1693.
22. ARISE Investigators and ANZICS Clinical Trials Group, Peake SL, Delaney A, et al. Goal-directed therapy for patients with early septic shock. *N Engl J Med*. 2014;371:1496–1506.
23. Mouncey PR, Osborn TM, Power GS, et al. Trial of early, goal-directed resuscitation for septic shock. *N Engl J Med*. 2015;372:1301–1311.
24. Edul VS, Enrico C, Laviolle B, Vazquez AR, Ince C, Dubin A. Quantitative assessment of the microcirculation in healthy volunteers and in patients with septic shock. *Crit Care Med*. 2012;40:1443–1448.
25. Brower RG, Matthay MA, Morris A, Schoenfeld D, Thompson BT, the Acute Respiratory Distress Syndrome Network. Ventilation with lower tidal volumes as compared with traditional tidal volumes for acute lung injury and the acute respiratory distress syndrome. *N Engl J Med*. 2000;342:1301–1308.
26. Dellinger RP, Carlet JM, Masur H, et al. Surviving Sepsis Campaign: guidelines for management of severe sepsis and septic shock. *Crit Care Med*. 2004;32:858–873.
27. Dellinger RP, Levy MM, Carlet JM, et al. Surviving Sepsis Campaign: international guidelines for management of severe sepsis and septic shock: 2008. *Crit Care Med*. 2008;36:296–327.
28. Dellinger RP, Levy MM, Rhodes A, et al. Surviving Sepsis Campaign: international guidelines for management of severe sepsis and septic shock: 2012. *Crit Care Med*. 2013;41.
29. Levy M, Dellinger RP, Townsend S, et al. The Surviving Sepsis Campaign: results of an international guideline-based performance improvement program targeting severe sepsis. *Intensive Care Med*. 2010;36:222–231.
30. Miller 3rd RR, Dong L, Nelson NC, et al. Multicenter implementation of a severe sepsis and septic shock treatment bundle. *Am J Respir Crit Care Med*. 2013;188:77–82.
31. Kaukonen K, Bailey M, Suzuki S, Pilcher D, Bellomo R. Mortality related to severe sepsis and septic shock among critically ill patients in Australia and New Zealand, 2000-2012. *JAMA*. 2014;311:1308–1316.
32. Gaieski DF, Edwards JM, Kallan MJ, Carr BG. Benchmarking the incidence and mortality of severe sepsis in the United States. *Crit Care Med*. 2013;41:1167–1174.
33. Van den Berghe G, Wouters P, Weekers F, et al. Intensive insulin therapy in critically ill patients. *N Engl J Med*. 2001;345:1359–1367.
34. Angus DC, Abraham E. Intensive insulin therapy in critical illness. *Am J Respir Crit Care Med*. 2005;172:1358–1359.
35. Van den Berghe G, Wilmer A, Hermans G, et al. Intensive insulin therapy in the medical ICU. *N Engl J Med*. 2006;354:449–461.
36. Preiser JC, Devos P, Ruiz-Santana S, et al. A prospective randomised multi-centre controlled trial on tight glucose control by intensive insulin therapy in adult intensive care units: the Glucontrol study. *Intensive Care Med*. 2009;35:1738–1748.
37. Brunkhorst FM, Engel C, Bloos F, et al. Intensive insulin therapy and Pentastarch resuscitation in severe sepsis. *N Engl J Med*. 2008;358:125–139.
38. NICE-SUGAR Study Investigators, Finfer S, Chittock DR, et al. Intensive versus conventional glucose control in critically ill patients (NICE SUGAR). *N Engl J Med*. 2009;360:1283–1297.
39. NICE-SUGAR Study Investigators, Finfer S, Liu B, et al. Hypoglycemia and risk of death in critically ill patients. *N Engl J Med*. 2012;367:1108–1118.
40. Walsh M, Devereaux PJ, Garg AX, et al. Relationship between intraoperative mean arterial pressure and clinical outcomes after noncardiac surgery: toward an empirical definition of hypotension. *Anesthesiology*. 2013;119:507–515.
41. Asfar P, Meziani F, Hamel JF, et al. High versus low blood-pressure target in patients with septic shock. *N Engl J Med*. 2014;370:1583–1593.
42. Marik PE, Cavallazzi R. Does the central venous pressure predict fluid responsiveness? An updated meta-analysis and a plea for some common sense. *Crit Care Med*. 2013;41:1774–1781.
43. Boyd JH, Forbes J, Nakada TA, Walley KR, Russell JA. Fluid resuscitation in septic shock: a positive fluid balance and elevated central venous pressure are associated with increased mortality. *Crit Care Med*. 2011;39:259–265.
44. Monnet X, Teboul JL. Volume responsiveness. *Curr Opin Crit Care*. 2007;13:549–553.
45. Guyton AC. Regulation of cardiac output. *N Engl J Med*. 1967;277:805–812.
46. Pinsky MR. Functional hemodynamic monitoring. *Curr Opin Crit Care*. 2014;20:288–293.
47. Sandham JD, Hull RD, Brant RF, et al. A randomized, controlled trial of the use of pulmonary-artery catheters in high-risk surgical patients. *N Engl J Med*. 2003;348:5–14.

2 What Lessons Have Intensivists Learned During the Evidence-Based Medicine Era?

Andrew T. Levinson, Mitchell M. Levy

Evidence-based medicine, in existence for just over two decades, has resulted in monumental changes in critical care medicine. In the last 20 years, practice has shifted from a reliance on expert opinion to a critical appraisal of the available literature to answer focused clinic questions.[1] Systematic examination of what works and what does not, while valuing clinic experience and patient preferences, has been a surprising and thought-provoking journey that has resulted in dramatic improvements in the care of the critically ill patient. Many of the lessons learned during the evidence-based medicine era would have never been predicted two decades ago.

In this chapter, we describe five important lessons learned in intensive care during the evidence-based medicine era:

1. We need to look beyond single randomized clinic trials (RCTs).
2. It is the small things that make a difference.
3. Accountability is critically important.
4. We often need to do less to patients rather than more.
5. It is the multidisciplinary intensive care unit (ICU) team, not the individual provider, that is the most responsible for good clinic outcomes and high-quality critical care.

LOOKING BEYOND SINGLE RANDOMIZED CONTROLLED TRIALS

By critically appraising the entire body of literature on specific interventions and clinic outcomes, we have learned many lessons about what is most important in the delivery of critical care. However, we have learned that we must wait before we immediately embrace the results of a single randomized clinic trial (RCT) with very impressive results and instead base our clinic practices on more comprehensive, cautious, and critical appraisals of all of the available literature.

The last two decades of critical care research are filled with stories of impressive findings from single-center RCTs that could not be replicated in larger multicenter RCTs. Unfortunately, in many cases, the initial positive single-center results have been embraced by early adopters, only

to have the results refuted by subsequent follow-up trials. The story of tight glycemic control in critical illness is illustrative. A single-center study of the management of hyperglycemia in a population consisting primarily of postcardiac surgical patients found that intensive glucose management with insulin infusion with a target blood glucose of 80 to 110 mg/dL dramatically reduced mortality when compared with a more lenient target blood glucose of 160 to 200 mg/dL.[2] The results of this single-center study were embraced by many intensivists and rapidly generalized to a wide variety of critically ill patents. The factors behind this rapid adoption by the field are multiple, including ease of implementation and cost. Unfortunately, a subsequent similar study of medical patients showed no significant benefit of an intensive insulin therapy protocol in the critically ill medical patient.[3] Ultimately, the most comprehensive multicenter trial of medical and surgical critically ill patients found significantly increased mortality in the group randomized to a tight glycemic control protocol, compared with targeting a blood glucose level of less than 180 mg/dL. This excess mortality was likely due to the much higher rates of severe hypoglycemia.[4]

In 2001, the era of early goal-directed therapy (EGDT) was introduced through the publication of a single-center, randomized controlled trial. EGDT was widely adopted, and multiple subsequent published trials, all prospective cohort series, confirmed its benefit.[5] More recently, two large RCTs[6,7] failed to demonstrate a survival benefit when protocolized resuscitation was compared with "usual care." It is possible that these results, at least in part, reflect the effect of the original EGDT trial; the widespread adoption of aggressive, early resuscitation; and the broad-based implementation of the Surviving Sepsis Campaign Guidelines and bundles.[8] If this continues to define usual care, then perhaps it is no longer necessary to mandate specific protocols for resuscitation because it appears that standard sepsis management has evolved to be consistent with published protocols.

The evidence for the use of hydrocortisone in the treatment of septic shock is an example of a sepsis treatment in which the initial promising study was embraced quite early,[9] only to be questioned by subsequent conflicting evidence.[10] We are still awaiting the final answer about the utility of the administration of corticosteroids as an adjunctive therapy in septic shock.

Activated protein C is an example of how little we still currently know about the pathobiology of sepsis and the difficulty in developing targeted therapies. Activated protein C as an adjunct therapy for patients with sepsis initially was thought to be quite promising,[11] but it was abandoned after subsequent randomized controlled trials failed to duplicate the original results.[12]

SMALL THINGS MAKE A BIG DIFFERENCE

The evidence-based era has taught us that small, often neglected or overlooked details of everyday bedside care can play a large role in determining whether our patients survive their ICU stay. Pneumonia that develops after the initiation of mechanic ventilation (ventilator-associated pneumonia [VAP]) is associated with high morbidity and mortality and significantly increased costs for critically ill patients. Several simple targeted interventions to address this problem have significantly reduced VAP rates. Simply keeping our intubated patients' heads elevated at least 30 degrees rather than leaving them supine (as was customary two decades ago) has resulted in major reductions in VAP.[13,14] In addition, a focus on better oral hygiene of mechanically ventilated patients via the administration of oral chlorhexidine has even further reduced the VAP rates.[15-18]

Another simple small intervention in the evidence-based era, the early mobilization of our critically ill patients, has also been found to significantly improve patient outcomes. We previously kept critically ill patients immobilized for weeks on end in the belief that this was necessary for their recovery. The result was very high rates of ICU-acquired weakness that required prolonged periods of rehabilitation in ICU survivors.[19] More recent studies have shown dramatic improvements in functional status and significantly decreased ICU length of stay (LOS) when critically ill patients are mobilized as soon and as much as possible.[20,21]

ACCOUNTABILITY IS IMPORTANT

Another important lesson learned during the evidence-based era is the importance of tracking clinic behavior through performance measures. Published reports have demonstrated a significant gap between intensivists' perceptions of their ability to adhere to current evidence-based medicine and actual practice.[22] This dichotomy has been noted in adherence to low tidal volume strategies in acute respiratory distress syndrome and other common "best ICU practices." These findings have led to the development of checklists and performance metrics to foster clinician accountability that have provided tangible improvements in clinic care. Multifaceted interventions using checklists have dramatically reduced catheter-related blood stream infections[23] as well as complications from surgical procedures.[24]

In acute situations, checklists have also been shown to improve delivery of care.[25] Continuous measurement of individual performance in the evidence-based medicine era has allowed ongoing, real-time feedback to individual clinicians and groups of providers. Application of this approach to sepsis care has resulted in significant improvement in adherence to evidence-based guidelines and in patient outcomes.[26]

DO LESS, NOT MORE

The evidence-based era has also taught us that we often should do less, not more, to and for our critically ill patients. We have learned that interrupting sedation and awakening mechanically ventilated patients each day, and thus reducing the amount of medication administered, can significantly reduce ICU LOS.[27,28] When coupled with a daily weaning trial, daily awaking of ICU patients significantly reduced mortality.[29] We have also learned that decreasing the need for mechanic ventilation by first using noninvasive strategies in specific groups of patients with acute respiratory distress can improve outcome.[30] In addition, use of smaller tidal volumes in mechanically ventilated patients has been shown to be lifesaving.[31] We have also learned that reducing the amount of blood given to patients can significantly improve outcomes.[32,33]

IT IS NOT JUST THE INTENSIVIST

Finally, we have learned that it is not the physician, but rather the entire health-care team, that is responsible for the delivery of high-quality care in the ICU. In a large observational cohort study based on the Acute Physiology and Chronic Health Evaluation IV (APACHE IV) model for predicting ICU LOS, investigators found that the key factors for predicting ICU LOS were structural and administrative. Specific APACHE IV variables of importance include reduced nurse-to-patient ratios, specific discharge policies, and the utilization of protocols. Structural and administrative factors were significantly different in high-performing ICUs with decreased LOS when adjusting for patient variables.[34,35]

In addition, the use of weaning protocols managed by respiratory therapists has resulted in significant reductions in the duration of mechanic ventilation relative to the subjective individualized assessment of an ICU clinician.[36,37] In addition, it was recently shown that staffing academic ICUs with intensivists overnight did not change clinic outcomes.[38] Finally, a recently published study found that empowering critical care nurses to intervene when they witnessed breaches in sterility was a key component in reducing catheter-related blood stream infections.[23] Taken together, these and other data strongly suggest that it is not solely the intensivist, but the entire critical care team, that is the key to high-quality care.

In summary, it seems that lessons offered by evidence-based medicine suggest that patience, keeping it simple, paying attention to detail, and working as a team are the key elements of good clinic care.

Key Points

1. Look beyond single randomized controlled trials.
2. Small things make a big difference.
3. Accountability is important.
4. Do less, not more.
5. It is not just the intensivist.

AUTHORS' RECOMMENDATION

- Single randomized controlled trials may be misleading, and the totality of evidence should be evaluated.
- Simple interventions such as head of bed elevation and early mobilization make a significant difference to outcomes.
- Measuring performance levels with checklists and audit improves outcomes. Accountability is important.
- Taking a conservative approach to interventions and therapies appears to confer patient benefit: "do less, not more."
- High-quality organized multidisciplinary intensive care improves outcomes: it is not just the intensivist.

REFERENCES

1. Smith R, and Rennie D. Evidence-based medicine–an oral history. *JAMA.* 311(4):365-367.
2. van den Berghe G, et al. Intensive insulin therapy in critically ill patients. *N Engl J Med.* 2001;345(19):1359–1367.
3. Van den Berghe G, et al. Intensive insulin therapy in the medical ICU. *N Engl J Med.* 2006;354(5):449–461.
4. NICE-SUGAR Study Investigators, et al. Intensive versus conventional glucose control in critically ill patients. *N Engl J Med.* 2009;360(13):1283–1297.
5. Rivers E, et al. Early goal-directed therapy in the treatment of severe sepsis and septic shock. *N Engl J Med.* 2001;345(19):1368–1377.
6. Angus DC, et al. Protocol-based care for early septic shock. *N Engl J Med.* 2014;371(4):386.
7. ARISE Investigators, et al. Goal-directed resuscitation for patients with early septic shock. *N Engl J Med.* 2014;371(16):1496–1506.
8. Dellinger RP, et al. Surviving Sepsis Campaign: international guidelines for management of severe sepsis and septic shock, 2012. *Intensive Care Med.* 2013;39(2):165–228.
9. Annane D, et al. Effect of treatment with low doses of hydrocortisone and fludrocortisone on mortality in patients with septic shock. *JAMA.* 2002;288(7):862–871.
10. Sprung CL, et al. Hydrocortisone therapy for patients with septic shock. *N Engl J Med.* 2008;358(2):111–124.
11. Bernard GR, et al. Efficacy and safety of recombinant human activated protein C for severe sepsis. *N Engl J Med.* 2001;344(10):699–709.
12. Ranieri VM, et al. Drotrecogin alfa (activated) in adults with septic shock. *N Engl J Med.* 2012;366(22):2055–2064.
13. Torres A, et al. Pulmonary aspiration of gastric contents in patients receiving mechanical ventilation: the effect of body position. *Ann Intern Med.* 1992;116(7):540–543.
14. Orozco-Levi M, et al. Semirecumbent position protects from pulmonary aspiration but not completely from gastroesophageal reflux in mechanically ventilated patients. *Am J Respir Crit Care Med.* 1995;152(4 Pt 1):1387–1390.
15. Shi Z, et al. Oral hygiene care for critically ill patients to prevent ventilator-associated pneumonia. *Cochrane Database Syst Rev.* 2013;8:CD008367.
16. Chan EY, et al. Oral decontamination for prevention of pneumonia in mechanically ventilated adults: systematic review and meta-analysis. *BMJ.* 2007;334(7599):889.
17. Labeau SO, et al. Prevention of ventilator-associated pneumonia with oral antiseptics: a systematic review and meta-analysis. *Lancet Infect Dis.* 2011;11(11):845–854.
18. Price R, et al. Selective digestive or oropharyngeal decontamination and topical oropharyngeal chlorhexidine for prevention of death in general intensive care: systematic review and network meta-analysis. *BMJ.* 2014;348:g2197.
19. Schweickert WD, Kress JP. Implementing early mobilization interventions in mechanically ventilated patients in the ICU. *Chest.* 2011;140(6):1612–1617.
20. Schweickert WD, et al. Early physical and occupational therapy in mechanically ventilated, critically ill patients: a randomised controlled trial. *Lancet.* 2009;373(9678):1874–1882.
21. Stiller K. Physiotherapy in intensive care: an updated systematic review. *Chest.* 2013;144(3):825–847.
22. Brunkhorst FM, et al. Practice and perception–a nationwide survey of therapy habits in sepsis. *Crit Care Med.* 2008;36(10):2719–2725.
23. Pronovost P, et al. An intervention to decrease catheter-related bloodstream infections in the ICU. *N Engl J Med.* 2006;355(26):2725–2732.
24. de Vries EN, et al. Effect of a comprehensive surgical safety system on patient outcomes. *N Engl J Med.* 2010;363(20):1928–1937.
25. Arriaga AF, et al. Simulation-based trial of surgical-crisis checklists. *N Engl J Med.* 2013;368(3):246–253.
26. Levy MM, et al. The Surviving Sepsis Campaign: results of an international guideline-based performance improvement program targeting severe sepsis. *Crit Care Med.* 2010;38(2):367–374.
27. Kress JP, et al. Daily interruption of sedative infusions in critically ill patients undergoing mechanical ventilation. *N Engl J Med.* 2000;342(20):1471–1477.
28. Hughes CG, McGrane S, Pandharipande PP. Sedation in the intensive care setting. *Clin Pharmacol.* 2012;4:53–63.
29. Girard TD, et al. Efficacy and safety of a paired sedation and ventilator weaning protocol for mechanically ventilated patients in intensive care (Awakening and Breathing Controlled trial): a randomised controlled trial. *Lancet.* 2008;371(9607):126–134.
30. Brochard L, et al. Noninvasive ventilation for acute exacerbations of chronic obstructive pulmonary disease. *N Engl J Med.* 1995;333(13):817–822.
31. Futier E, et al. A trial of intraoperative low-tidal-volume ventilation in abdominal surgery. *N Engl J Med.* 2013;369(5):428–437.
32. Villanueva C, et al. Transfusion strategies for acute upper gastrointestinal bleeding. *N Engl J Med.* 2013;368(1):11–21.
33. Jairath V, et al. Red cell transfusion for the management of upper gastrointestinal haemorrhage. *Cochrane Database Syst Rev.* 2010;9:CD006613.
34. Zimmerman JE, et al. Intensive care unit length of stay: Benchmarking based on Acute Physiology and Chronic Health Evaluation (APACHE) IV. *Crit Care Med.* 2006;34(10):2517–2529.
35. Zimmerman JE, Alzola C, Von Rueden KT. The use of benchmarking to identify top performing critical care units: a preliminary assessment of their policies and practices. *J Crit Care.* 2003;18(2):76–86.
36. Ely EW, et al. Effect on the duration of mechanical ventilation of identifying patients capable of breathing spontaneously. *N Engl J Med.* 1996;335(25):1864–1869.
37. Blackwood B, et al. Protocolized versus non-protocolized weaning for reducing the duration of mechanical ventilation in critically ill adult patients. *Cochrane Database Syst Rev.* 2014;11:CD006904.
38. Kerlin MP, Halpern SD. Nighttime physician staffing in an intensive care unit. *N Engl J Med.* 2013;369(11):1075.

3 Have Critical Care Outcomes Improved?

Emily Vail, Hayley B. Gershengorn, Hannah Wunsch

Over the past 50 years, critical care medicine has rapidly developed into a complex, resource-intensive, and multidisciplinary field. The care of patients has evolved with implementation of new monitoring devices and therapies based on the best available evidence. In addition, care has been affected by the introduction of new team members dedicated to the care of critically ill patients and specific protocols for care. In the setting of ever-changing practice, it is important to ask whether outcomes for our patients have improved.

OUTCOMES MEASURED IN CRITICALLY ILL POPULATIONS

The most consistently described outcome in both observational and interventional studies is mortality, which is variably reported as intensive care unit (ICU) mortality, in-hospital mortality, or mortality within a fixed time limit (most often between 28 and 90 days, but sometimes longer[1,2]). This chapter focuses primarily on short-term mortality, still the most commonly used measure of success.

Mortality as an outcome has the advantages of objectivity and ease of measurement, but it may not be appropriate for every study, such as in studies of palliative care when unchanged or higher mortality may be acceptable. A focus on reporting mortality can misrepresent the effect of a given intervention if the period of measurement is too short (failing to identify all related mortalities) or too long (introducing confounding from other sources of mortality). Moreover, mortality may not be the focus of an intervention or improvement initiative.

Many other endpoints have been used to assess outcome in critically ill patients (Table 3-1).[3-6] Data on these endpoints may be more difficult to obtain but may hold greater significance for patients and their caregivers. The strength of these different approaches to outcome lies in the delineation of clear administrative, policy, and economic implications and the ability to determine if these variables overlap with patient-centered outcomes (such as length of stay in the hospital).

SOURCES OF DATA

A wealth of data from various sources can be used to study critical care outcomes, including administrative data, prospectively collected clinical data, and control arms of randomized trials. Each data source has inherent strengths and weaknesses that may bias the conclusions regarding trends in mortality over time.

Administrative data are readily available from various government, public, and private sources but have important limitations. The quality of the data relies on documentation and coding by clinicians. Data acquired in this way may have low sensitivity for specific diagnoses and may be variable across individual physicians and hospitals.[7] A related concern is the potential for "upcoding," the practice of billing for more expensive diagnoses and services than provided. This (illegal) practice can create biases toward higher severity of illness.[8] Changes in coding standards or payment incentives also may alter the use of a given diagnostic code without a change in true incidence of the condition.[9,10] Finally, "extraction," the identification of certain combinations of signs, symptoms, and diagnostic terms, may be used to identify complex clinical conditions from within administrative datasets. The algorithms used in this process vary in sensitivity and specificity,[11,12] with consequences for measured incidence and outcomes.[8,12-15] Outcomes derived from administrative databases are most meaningful when their data extraction methods have been validated with multiple clinical datasets[16] and with consistent coding practices over time.

Clinical observational data can be used to study various risk factors and outcomes, but data collection is expensive and time consuming. Often, such data reflect the experience of either a single center or a few centers, and result may be poorly generalizable to other patients or institutions. Outcomes among patients randomized to receive placebo or "usual care" in controlled trials may be extrapolated to describe the natural history of a given condition. Data collected in this setting are prospective, clinically relevant, and frequently validated. However, because these patients must meet specific study inclusion criteria, they may differ significantly from the larger pool of critically ill patients with respect to severity of illness, age, comorbid disease,[17] and sites of care delivery. Moreover, such studies frequently exclude patients with poor prognoses.[18] A consistent outcome trend in all types of available data increases confidence in the conclusions drawn. When such consistency does not occur (i.e., a trend is apparent in one data type but not discernable in another), these concerns must be weighed for each study to adjudicate its quality.

Table 3-1 Selected Common Outcome Measures for Critically Ill Patients

Mortality	Processes of Care and Resource Use	Measures Related to Short- and Long-Term Quality of Life
ICU	ICU length of stay	ICU length of stay
Hospital	Hospital length of stay	Hospital length of stay
28 or 30 days	Time on a ventilator	Time on a ventilator
60 or more days	Ventilator-(or other) free days	Ventilator-(or other) free days
	Iatrogenic complications	Iatrogenic complications
	Location after acute hospital discharge	Location after acute hospital discharge
	Long-term health care utilization	Physical or functional disability
	Hospital costs	Hospital costs
	Hospital readmission	Hospital readmission
		Quality of dying and death
		Family satisfaction with ICU care

TRENDS IN MORTALITY

Critical care outcomes are generally studied with one of three approaches: examining outcomes among patients receiving ICU care for any reason, limiting evaluation to a specific subgroup of patients admitted to ICUs (e.g., septic shock requiring mechanical ventilation), or focusing on a specific critical illness that might necessitate admission to an ICU for a proportion of the patients (e.g., severe sepsis).

Trends for Patients Admitted to Intensive Care Units

Data showing trends over time for all ICU patients are sparse. Recent studies in which outcomes were examined over the past two decades have identified consistent changes in patient demographics and severity of illness. These differences must be accounted for when an attempt is made to determine whether outcomes have improved. A study by Zimmerman et al.[19] examined trends in in-hospital mortality among 482,601 patients admitted to U.S. ICUs between 1988 and 2012. Despite increases in severity of illness and patient age over the study period, the investigators found significant decreases in all-cause acute hospital mortality as well as in ICU and hospital lengths of stay. However, these observed improvements were partially attributable to higher rates of discharge to skilled nursing facilities. Mortality in such facilities is known to be high; therefore, although these data are clear in showing a decrease in acute hospital mortality for ICU patients over this period, we cannot conclusively determine whether overall short-term mortality decreased.

Likewise, in a retrospective analysis of a large ICU patient database in Australia and New Zealand between 2000 and 2012, Kaukonen and colleagues[20] observed decreased crude and adjusted in-hospital mortality and, with the exception of patients with severe sepsis or septic shock (who were more likely, over time, to be discharged home), increasing rates of discharge to rehabilitation facilities. In the United Kingdom, work by Hutchings et al.[21] demonstrated lower risk–adjusted ICU and hospital mortality for critically ill patients between 2000 and 2006 despite a constant severity of illness. This decrease in mortality was specifically attributed to changes in the system of care, including an increase in the number of ICU beds in the country and other systems interventions, such as critical care networks and rapid response teams.

Perhaps the most compelling evidence of improving short-term mortality for critically ill patients is the "drift" or "fade" of severity of illness scores over time.[22] Many of these scores (e.g., the Simplified Acute Physiology Score [SAPS][23] and the Acute Physiology and Chronic Health Evaluation [APACHE][24]) have been recalibrated multiple times over the past 20 to 30 years to maintain predictive accuracy. The model drift (in general) has been toward overprediction of mortality, leading to a progressive overestimation of predicted mortality that affects the accuracy of severity of illness adjustments between historical cohorts.[25] Although subtle shifts in case mix may account for some of these changes, this trend adds weight to the suggestion in the studies previously described that overall short-term mortality has decreased over time.

Trends for Specific Critical Illnesses

Changes in outcomes have been assessed for many ICU-specific illnesses. This chapter focuses on two common diagnoses: septic shock and acute respiratory distress syndrome (ARDS). A systematic review by Friedman and Vincent[26] published in 1998 examined trends in septic shock mortality with 131 studies published between 1958 and 1997. The authors found an overall mortality of 49.7%, decreasing mortality over time, and changes in infection site and causative organisms; however, they noted significant heterogeneity in definitions of disease and severity of illness between studies. Because the American College of Chest Physicians' and Society of Critical Care Medicine's 1991 European Consensus Conference definitions of sepsis, severe sepsis, and septic shock[27] have been widely adopted, comparison of outcomes over time has become a little easier, although patient populations in individual studies remain heterogeneous because of variable interpretation of aspects of the definition, such as "hypotension" and "unresponsive to adequate resuscitation."[28-30] An additional marker of possible decreasing mortality for patients with septic shock is that the mortality for the usual care arms of studies designed to capture this population has steadily decreased over time.[13]

As with septic shock, the assessment of ARDS mortality is confounded by changes in clinical definitions with time,[31,32] and trends for mortality associated with ARDS are even less consistent. A study by Milberg et al.[33] analyzed the etiology of ARDS and outcomes in the Harborview Medical Center ARDS registry and found decreases in crude and adjusted mortality between 1983 and 1993 despite increasing severity of illness. Since the publication of that study, our understanding of the pathophysiologic features of ARDS[34] and the role of ventilator-induced lung injury in patients susceptible to ARDS[35] has significantly grown. The resultant implications for ventilator management and adjunct interventions for ARDS may affect outcomes and outcomes assessment. Despite advances in understanding and options for care, recent evidence in temporal ARDS outcomes does not consistently demonstrate large improvements in mortality.

When randomized controlled trials are considered in isolation, short-term mortality among patients with ARDS does appear to be improving. Examining 2451 patients enrolled in ARDS Network randomized controlled trials, Erickson and colleagues[36] found decreased raw (from 35% to 26%) and adjusted 60-day mortality despite increased severity of illness; this trend was evident even with inclusion of patients who received high tidal volume ventilation (12 mL/kg), a finding that led the authors to conclude that observed decreases in mortality were due to generalized improvements in critical care delivery at participating hospitals rather than specific interventions for ARDS.

Two systematic reviews (incorporating both trial and observational evidence) on ARDS mortality provide conflicting results. One reported a 1.1% annual decrease in mortality[37] between 1994 (the year of publication of the European-American Consensus definitions[32]) and 2006, whereas the other found no significant change in mortality among 18,900 patients.[18] Moreover, an observational study of 514 patients with ARDS in Olmsted County, Minnesota, between 2001 and 2008 also failed to identify a significant change in hospital mortality over time.[38]

ARDS remains a heterogeneous syndrome involving subjective assessment and many causes. These inconsistencies may explain the conflicting conclusions in different studies. The development of electronic "sniffers"—programs that automatically process real-time clinical data from electronic medical records to alert clinicians to the potential presence of ARDS[39]—may provide more consistent identification of patients and thus a more accurate assessment of trends in mortality.

Trends for Diagnoses with Variable Admission to Intensive Care Units

The decision to admit a given patient to an ICU is multifactorial.[15,40,41] For example, many patients with severe sepsis are admitted to ICUs, but many patients with the same diagnosis are cared for in emergency departments,[42] hospital wards,[3,15,43,44] or step-down units.[45] Mortality in these alternative treatment sites may be substantial.[43,44]

Several large observational studies have described the epidemiologic features of severe sepsis in the United States over the past 30 years.[3,42] Serial analyses of the Agency for Healthcare Research and Quality's Nationwide Inpatient Sample (NIS) database,[46] which includes data from 1993 to 2010, demonstrate increases in measured incidence of severe sepsis and severity of illness, as well as decreased hospital mortality.[13,14,47-50] The largest of these studies, by Stevenson and colleagues,[13] included both NIS data collected between 1993 and 2009 and a meta-analysis of more than 14,000 patients enrolled in usual care or placebo arms of 36 multicenter randomized controlled trials worldwide. The authors observed differences in effect size between observational and trial data but consistent, significant decreases in overall mortality, regardless of data or the administrative coding method used. Likewise, in a study with clinical and administrative data sampled from a cohort of more than 1 million patients admitted to two U.S. medical centers between 2003 and 2012, Rhee et al.[12] found decreased hospital mortality among patients with severe sepsis.

A study of 92,000 adults with severe sepsis admitted to 240 ICUs in England, Wales, and Northern Ireland between 1996 and 2004 identified an increasing proportion of ICU admissions with sepsis. Mean patient age increased over time, but there was no change in severity of illness (as described by the APACHE II score) or the extent of organ dysfunction on admission. Importantly, unadjusted ICU and hospital mortality also were unchanged.[45] Data from Australia and New Zealand in which 100,000 ICU patients with severe sepsis were examined between 2000 and 2012 similarly showed an increasing rate of ICU admissions with severe sepsis. However, this study found decreasing rates of crude and adjusted mortality that paralleled overall ICU mortality trends and increased rates of discharge to home.[20]

The "Will Rogers phenomenon," in which earlier diagnosis of a given condition leads to an observed increase in measured incidence and decreased mortality,[51] may play a role in observed increases in severe sepsis incidence.[52] Growing clinician and hospital awareness of severe sepsis with an emphasis on early diagnosis and intervention[53] may decrease observed overall severe sepsis mortality because of the addition of a group of patients with less severe disease and lower expected mortality to a pool of previously identified, sicker patients. Appropriate risk adjustment may help to minimize this issue, but such a phenomenon remains a concern.

HAS MORTALITY IMPROVED?

Although difficult to tease apart, the trends across many, but not all, different groups of ICU patients suggest that overall short-term mortality for ICU patients has decreased over the past few decades. Observed improvements in general critical care outcomes likely reflect multiple contributing factors and may parallel improvements in overall medical care. For example, hospital mortality for *all* hospitalized patients in the United States decreased between 2000 and 2010.[54]

In the past 20 years, significant scientific progress has advanced our understanding and management of critical illness and its complications. Advances in technology and drug development and an emphasis on patient safety and quality improvement have resulted in the prevention of complications and improved the management of comorbid diseases. Improved care of the critically ill patient likely reflects better monitoring, treatment, and overall care. However, it is also clear that improvements may not extend to all subsets of critically ill patients. Furthermore, it will be important to enhance future evaluation with the application of consistent definitions of specific disorders and with uniform practices to identify critically ill patients, irrespective of their specific diagnosis or treatment locale.

AUTHORS' RECOMMENDATIONS

Mortality associated with critical illness is challenging to accurately compare over time and between populations. To better assess outcomes and to identify potential strategies for improvement, we recommend the following:
- Awareness of the variability in diagnostic definitions and ICU admission practices that affect reported outcomes.
- Development of more precise definitions of clinical syndromes commonly observed in critically ill patients to foster standardized comparison of outcomes among patients, hospitals, and regions.
- Use of available electronic medical record abstraction systems to provide for consistent and unbiased identification of specific types of critically ill patients.

REFERENCES

1. Winters BD, et al. Long-term mortality and quality of life in sepsis: a systematic review. *Crit Care Med.* 2010;38(5):1276–1283.
2. Wunsch H, et al. Association between age and use of intensive care among surgical medicare beneficiaries. *J Crit Care.* 2013;28(5): 597–605.
3. Angus DC, et al. Epidemiology of severe sepsis in the United States: analysis of incidence, outcome, and associated costs of care. *Crit Care Med.* 2001;29(7):1303–1310.
4. Herridge MS, et al. Functional disability 5 years after acute respiratory distress syndrome. *N Engl J Med.* 2011;364(14):1293–1304.
5. DeCato TW, et al. Hospital variation and temporal trends in palliative and end-of-life care in the ICU. *Crit Care Med.* 2013;41(6): 1405–1411.
6. Kahn JM, et al. Long-term acute care hospital utilization after critical illness. *JAMA.* 2010;303(22):2253–2259.
7. Misset B, et al. Reliability of diagnostic coding in intensive care patients. *Crit Care.* 2008;12(4):R95.
8. Whittaker SA, et al. Severe sepsis cohorts derived from claims-based strategies appear to be biased toward a more severely ill patient population. *Crit Care Med.* 2013;41(4):945–953.
9. Helms CM. A pseudo-epidemic of septicemia among medicare patients in Iowa. *Am J Public Health.* 1987;77(10):1331–1332.
10. Lindenauer PK, et al. Association of diagnostic coding with trends in hospitalizations and mortality of patients with pneumonia, 2003-2009. *JAMA.* 2012;307(13):1405–1413.
11. Iwashyna TJ, et al. Identifying patients with severe sepsis using administrative claims: patient-level validation of the angus implementation of the international consensus conference definition of severe sepsis. *Med Care.* 2014;52(6):e39–43.
12. Rhee C, et al. Comparison of trends in sepsis incidence and coding using administrative claims versus objective clinical data. *Clin Infect Dis.* 2015;60(1):88–95.
13. Stevenson EK, et al. Two decades of mortality trends among patients with severe sepsis: a comparative meta-analysis. *Crit Care Med.* 2014;42(3):625–631.
14. Gaieski DF, et al. Benchmarking the incidence and mortality of severe sepsis in the United States. *Crit Care Med.* 2013;41(5): 1167–1174.
15. Sundararajan V, et al. Epidemiology of sepsis in Victoria, Australia. *Crit Care Med.* 2005;33(1):71–80.
16. Linde-Zwirble WT, Angus DC. Severe sepsis epidemiology: sampling, selection, and society. *Crit Care.* 2004;8(4):222–226.
17. Van Spall HG, et al. Eligibility criteria of randomized controlled trials published in high-impact general medical journals: a systematic sampling review. *JAMA.* 2007;297(11):1233–1240.
18. Phua J, et al. Has mortality from acute respiratory distress syndrome decreased over time?: a systematic review. *Am J Respir Crit Care Med.* 2009;179(3):220–227.
19. Zimmerman JE, Kramer AA, Knaus WA. Changes in hospital mortality for United States intensive care unit admissions from 1988 to 2012. *Crit Care.* 2013;17(2):R81.
20. Kaukonen KM, et al. Mortality related to severe sepsis and septic shock among critically ill patients in Australia and New Zealand, 2000-2012. *JAMA.* 2014;311(13):1308–1316.
21. Hutchings A, et al. Evaluation of modernisation of adult critical care services in England: time series and cost effectiveness analysis. *BMJ.* 2009;339:b4353.
22. Kramer AA. Predictive mortality models are not like fine wine. *Crit Care.* 2005;9(6):636–637.
23. Le Gall JR, Lemeshow S, Saulnier F. A new Simplified Acute Physiology Score (SAPS II) based on a European/North American multicenter study. *JAMA.* 1993;270(24):2957–2963.
24. Knaus WA, et al. The APACHE III prognostic system. Risk prediction of hospital mortality for critically ill hospitalized adults. *Chest.* 1991;100(6):1619–1636.
25. Wunsch H, Kramer AA, The role and limitation of scoring systems. In: Webb AJ, et al. ed. *Oxford Textbook of Critical Care.* Oxford University Press.
26. Friedman G, Silva E, Vincent JL. Has the mortality of septic shock changed with time. *Crit Care Med.* 1998;26(12):2078–2086.
27. Bone RC, Sibbald WJ, Sprung CL. The ACCP-SCCM consensus conference on sepsis and organ failure. *Chest.* 1992;101(6): 1481–1483.
28. Annane D, et al. Effect of treatment with low doses of hydrocortisone and fludrocortisone on mortality in patients with septic shock. *JAMA.* 2002;288(7):862–871.
29. Briegel J, et al. Stress doses of hydrocortisone reverse hyperdynamic septic shock: a prospective, randomized, double-blind, single-center study. *Crit Care Med.* 1999;27(4):723–732.
30. Sprung CL, et al. Hydrocortisone therapy for patients with septic shock. *N Engl J Med.* 2008;358(2):111–124.
31. Ranieri VM, et al. Acute respiratory distress syndrome: the Berlin definition. *JAMA.* 2012;307(23):2526–2533.
32. Bernard GR, et al. The American-European Consensus Conference on ARDS. Definitions, mechanisms, relevant outcomes, and clinical trial coordination. *Am J Respir Crit Care Med.* 1994;149(3 Pt 1): 818–824.
33. Milberg JA, et al. Improved survival of patients with acute respiratory distress syndrome (ARDS): 1983-1993. *JAMA.* 1995;273(4):306–309.
34. Matthay MA, Zimmerman GA. Acute lung injury and the acute respiratory distress syndrome: four decades of inquiry into pathogenesis and rational management. *Am J Respir Cell Mol Biol.* 2005;33(4):319–327.
35. Slutsky AS, Ranieri VM. Ventilator-induced lung injury. *N Engl J Med.* 2013;369(22):2126–2136.
36. Erickson SE, et al. Recent trends in acute lung injury mortality: 1996-2005. *Crit Care Med.* 2009;37(5):1574–1579.
37. Zambon M, Vincent JL. Mortality rates for patients with acute lung injury/ARDS have decreased over time. *Chest.* 2008;133(5): 1120–1127.
38. Li G, et al. Eight-year trend of acute respiratory distress syndrome: a population-based study in Olmsted County, Minnesota. *Am J Respir Crit Care Med.* 2011;183(1):59–66.
39. Herasevich V, et al. Validation of an electronic surveillance system for acute lung injury. *Intensive Care Med.* 2009;35(6):1018–1023.
40. Levy MM, et al. Outcomes of the Surviving Sepsis Campaign in intensive care units in the USA and Europe: a prospective cohort study. *Lancet Infect Dis.* 2012;12(12):919–924.
41. Simchen E, et al. Survival of critically ill patients hospitalized in and out of intensive care units under paucity of intensive care unit beds. *Crit Care Med.* 2004;32(8):1654–1661.

42. Wang HE, et al. National estimates of severe sepsis in United States emergency departments. *Crit Care Med*. 2007;35(8):1928–1936.
43. Esteban A, et al. Sepsis incidence and outcome: contrasting the intensive care unit with the hospital ward. *Crit Care Med*. 2007;35(5): 1284–1289.
44. Sands KE, et al. Epidemiology of sepsis syndrome in 8 academic medical centers. *JAMA*. 1997;278(3):234–240.
45. Harrison DA, Welch CA, Eddleston JM. The epidemiology of severe sepsis in England, Wales and Northern Ireland, 1996 to 2004: secondary analysis of a high quality clinical database, the ICNARC Case Mix Programme Database. *Crit Care*. 2006;10(2):R42.
46. Healthcare Cost and Utilization Project. *Overview of the National (Nationwide) Inpatient Sample (NIS)*; September 11, 2014. Available from: http://www.hcup-us.ahrq.gov/nisoverview.jsp.
47. Dombrovskiy VY, et al. Rapid increase in hospitalization and mortality rates for severe sepsis in the United States: a trend analysis from 1993 to 2003. *Crit Care Med*. 2007;35(5):1244–1250.
48. Kumar G, et al. Nationwide trends of severe sepsis in the 21st century (2000-2007). *Chest*. 2011;140(5):1223–1231.
49. Lagu T, et al. What is the best method for estimating the burden of severe sepsis in the United States? *J Crit Care*. 2012;27(4):414 e1–9.
50. Gaieski DF, et al. The relationship between hospital volume and mortality in severe sepsis. *Am J Respir Crit Care Med*. 2014;190(6): 665–674.
51. Feinstein AR, Sosin DM, Wells CK. The Will Rogers phenomenon. Stage migration and new diagnostic techniques as a source of misleading statistics for survival in cancer. *N Engl J Med*. 1985;312(25):1604–1608.
52. Iwashyna TJ, Angus DC. Declining case fatality rates for severe sepsis: good data bring good news with ambiguous implications. *JAMA*. 2014;311(13):1295–1297.
53. Dellinger RP, et al. Surviving sepsis campaign: international guidelines for management of severe sepsis and septic shock: 2012. *Crit Care Med*. 2013;41(2):580–637.
54. Hall MJ, Levant S, DeFrances CJ. Trends in inpatient hospital deaths: National Hospital Discharge Survey, 2000-2010. *NCHS Data Brief*. 2013;118:1–8. Hyattsville, MD.

4 | What Problems Are Prevalent Among Survivors of Critical Illness and Which of Those Are Consequences of Critical Illness?

Theodore J. Iwashyna

This topic covers an area of rapidly evolving research. As such, an exhaustive approach is guaranteed to be outdated by publication. Therefore this chapter seeks to provide an approach to the problems faced by survivors of critical illness with a focus on patients surviving acute respiratory distress syndrome (ARDS) and severe sepsis.

WHAT PROBLEMS ARE PREVALENT AMONG SURVIVORS OF CRITICAL ILLNESS?

Survivors of critical illness must deal with many problems. Indeed, compared with an age-matched population, survivors of critical illness face nearly every medical complication imaginable. As is discussed in the next section, some of these problems reflect preexisting illnesses. In some cases, an exacerbation or complication of the preexisting condition led to the development of critical illness. However, regardless of when they developed, these long-term problems prevalent among critical illness survivors are real problems that survivors, their families, and their physicians need to face.

Some survivors of critical illness face a substantially elevated mortality after discharge from the hospital, a problem best documented for severe sepsis. For example, Quartin et al.[1] compared patients with severe sepsis in the 1980s to matched nonseptic patients hospitalized during the same time period. Among patients who had lived at least 180 days after their illness, patients with severe sepsis were 3.4 times more likely than controls (95% confidence interval: 2.3, 4.2) to die in the subsequent 6 months (i.e., days 181 to 365 after hospitalization). Indeed, among those who lived at least 2 full years, survivors of severe sepsis were still 2.2 times as likely as controls to die by year 5. Yende et al.[2] and Prescott et al.[3] have shown similar rates of excess postdischarge mortality among survivors of severe sepsis. In contrast, Wunsch et al.[4] looked at intensive care unit (ICU) patients with and without mechanical ventilation and compared them with the general population and with hospitalized controls; these authors suggested that there is substantial excess mortality among patients who had undergone mechanical ventilation relative to the other groups, but that excess mortality occurred largely in the first 6 months postdischarge.

The term *post–intensive care syndrome* (PICS) was coined to provide an intellectual framework for organizing the problems prevalent among those who survive this excess mortality.[5,6] A working description of PICS was developed over several years and involved extensive contributions from stakeholders—including patients, families, caregivers, administrators, and others—within critical care and throughout the broader medical and rehabilitation communities. Within PICS, it is valuable to consider three broad domains: physical health, cognitive impairment, and mental health.

Most work after critical illness has focused on the presence and persistence of neuromuscular weakness. In my opinion, enduring weakness, which can be profound and disabling, is the central patient-centered physical problem facing the population of survivors as a whole. Abnormalities of motor function, united under the useful umbrella of "ICU-acquired weakness," include myopathies and polyneuropathies.[7] The biology of this syndrome remains an active area of research, but there is little evidence that the origin (nerve or muscle) of the underlying defect affects either prognosis or specific treatment. Physical and occupational therapies are the mainstay of recovery.[8]

Other physical problems are common but less studied. Transient and enduring renal failure have been noted.[9] High rates of cardiovascular disease are reported.[10] Dyspnea and low exercise tolerance, even in the face of seemingly normal or near normal pulmonary function tests, are ubiquitous after severe ARDS.[11,12] Other survivors report subglottic stenosis and profound cosmetic changes.[10] High rates of cachexia, injurious falls, incontinence, and impaired hearing and vision have all been reported.[13]

A spectrum of cognitive impairment is also common after critical illness. Abnormalities range from dysfunction in specific tasks (defects in executive function are particularly common) to frank cognitive impairment. The prevalence seems to be high, although there is disagreement regarding how severe an abnormality must be to be "bad enough to be counted."[14-19] Patients who experience severe delirium in the ICU may be at greater risk to lose cognitive function at a later time,[20] but the duration of the cognitive dysfunction is probably months to years; therefore it is unlikely to be a simple extension of ICU- or hospital-acquired delirium.

There is also evidence that ICU survivors experience high degrees of depression, anxiety, and posttraumatic stress disorder (PTSD). Assessments of depression with the Hospital Anxiety and Depression Scale (HADS) have tended to emphasize the PTSD finding.[21-23] In contrast, more recent work by Jackson and colleagues[24] suggested that the HADS may be insufficiently sensitive to somatic symptoms of depression and that symptoms attributed to PTSD were not in fact tied to the critical illness experience. Although these issues are being addressed, it is clear that many patients have significant emotional disorders.[25,26]

In summary, survivors of critical illness face a wide array of problems. Only some of these have been adequately studied, and there are specific interventions for even fewer. These problems lead to high rates of ongoing health-care resource use and frequent rehospitalization.[3,27,28] There is growing recognition that the consequences of critical illness also place substantial strain on families of ICU survivors, who often bear the brunt of high levels of ongoing informal care.[29-37]

In the face of such high prevalence, it is understandable that critical care practitioners may develop a certain nihilism or sense of hopelessness. Obviously, this is an issue that must be addressed by each involved individual. However, it seems important to stress that the inability to save everyone does not mean that many are not fully saved. The newly appreciated prevalence of PICS represents a problem to be tackled and eventually solved, not an inevitable fate to which all ICU patients are doomed. Indeed, as Cuthbertson and colleagues noted in their longitudinal cohort of Scottish sepsis survivors, "At five years all patients stated they would be willing to be treated in an ICU again if they become critically ill… [and] 80% were either very happy or mostly happy with their current QOL [quality of life]."[38]

WHICH OF THE PROBLEMS FACED BY SURVIVORS ARE CONSEQUENCES OF CRITICAL ILLNESS?

It is sometimes rhetorically useful to frame studies of long-term consequences as extremes on a spectrum: preexisting problem or conditions caused entirely by critical illness. One unfortunate consequence of such a dichotomy is the development of a false sense of hierarchy—asking, "which is more important?" It is rather much more valuable to examine the extent to which acute changes and preexisting conditions contribute in any given patient.

Perhaps the best research on this particular problem lies in the domain of cognitive impairment after critical illness. A large group of investigators followed 5888 older Americans in the Cardiovascular Health Study, a population-based observational cohort.[19] Patients were examined every year with the Teng Modified Mini-Mental Status examination. Shah et al.[19] noted that patients who went on to have pneumonia were more likely to have lower premorbid cognitive scores and scores that had been declining more rapidly before the development of pneumonia. However, whatever their baseline trajectory, patients who contracted pneumonia had an increasingly rapid transition to dementia. Iwashyna et al.[18] found similar results with severe sepsis, and Ehlenbach et al.[39] noted this finding in a group of severely critical ill patients.

In other cases, findings have been less consistent. Wunsch et al.[25] used elegantly detailed Danish records to show that depression and other mental health disorders were diagnosed much more commonly in patients after critical illness with mechanical ventilation than in the years before the critical illness. However, Davydow et al.[26] showed that U.S. survivors of severe sepsis did not exhibit a change in the (already very high) level of depressive symptoms present before or after severe sepsis. It is possible to reconcile such findings by attributing them to the known low sensitivity of general medical practice for the detection of depression and an increased level of surveillance in the years after critical illness. The Davydow findings might also be explained by an insufficiently responsive scale for symptoms; however, the data are not yet conclusive.

In some cases—often with too few studies for there to be much conflict—it appears that the prevalent problems after critical illness are primarily the result of preexisting morbidity. Further complicating such work is the fact that older Americans are at increasing risk for both critical illness and potential complications. Thus, work in the Health and Retirement Study showed dramatic increases in rates of injurious falls and incontinence in survivors of severe sepsis relative to both the general population of older adults and even compared with the same patients when measured presepsis.[13] However, any apparent effect of sepsis disappeared when the "morbidity growth curve" of older Americans was controlled (i.e., their presepsis trajectory of increasing development of morbidity).

In summary, patients who have critical illness typically had both worse level of functioning than the general population before the development of their critical illness and were on trajectories of more rapid decline before their critical illness. However, it is common to have even worse function after critical illness. This finding is not universal; for example, no such exacerbations after critical illness were detectable for geriatric conditions such as injurious falls. It may also not be true for impaired quality of life, particularly because people may be able to adapt to their new postcritical illness deficits.

WHY DOES IT MATTER WHETHER THE PROBLEM PRECEDES CRITICAL ILLNESS OR IS A CONSEQUENCE OF CRITICAL ILLNESS?

Having established that there are substantial problems that are highly prevalent among survivors of critical illness, it is increasingly time to ask what can be done to make things better. The next section discusses specific strategies. However, there are generally three strategies that can be informed by this approach: (1) in-ICU prevention, (2) treatment and remediation, and (3) triage. In-ICU prevention strategies are only effective for problems that develop over the course of critical illness; although one can prevent it from becoming worse, one cannot prevent a problem that already exists. Therefore it is important to know which conditions present in each individual patient, as opposed to the population of survivors as a whole, did or did not preexist the development of critical illness.

"When newly acquired diagnoses are evaluated, it is essential to distinguish the degree of morbidity consequent of critical illness from complications arising from interventions to treat the disorder and support the patient. For example, ICU-acquired weakness is common in ICU survivors. However, it is difficult to determine to what extent this disability results from the critical illness itself as opposed to the treatment modalities, including prolonged bed rest; use of neuromuscular blocking agents, antibiotics, or other drugs; decreased respiratory muscle activity resulting from mechanical ventilation; and inadequate metabolic/nutritional support. Indeed, PICS is an acronym for "post–intensive care syndrome," not "postcritical illness syndrome," but health-care providers should not let this bold (but untested), implicit assertion provide false assurances as to where the problems may lie. Misattribution to management of problems that are really a consequence of critical illness itself could lead to faulty triage decisions, in which patients with a critical illness are kept out of the ICU to spare them the perceived risk of exposure to ICU-induced consequences. However, such triage would also preclude such patients from receiving ICU-possible improvements in care. However, to the extent that ICU care is of lower marginal value and prone to excess interventions, invasive monitoring, and bed rest, then such a decision would be fully appropriate. Conversely, an incorrect belief that a complication is a component of the underlying disorder may lead to overuse of therapy; for example, it appears that less sedation reduces the psychological sequelae of critical care rather than providing the preventive amnesia that some once hoped it would. There is an urgent need for objective data to inform this debate; in particular, data should not merely catalog the problems in one place but also catalog comparative effectiveness research of care in alternative settings.

GIVEN THE ABSENCE OF PROVEN SPECIFIC THERAPIES, WHAT IS A PRAGMATIC APPROACH TO IMPROVING LONG-TERM CONSEQUENCES FACED BY PATIENTS SURVIVING CRITICAL ILLNESS?

Patients surviving critical illness labor under a complex burden of problems—some newly developed as a consequence of the acute episode, some present before critical illness but exacerbated by the episode to the point of decompensation, and some preexisting in occult form that are unmasked critical illness. There are no proven therapies specifically remediating long-term problems after the ICU. There are several potentially promising approaches or interventions that could be initiated in the ICU. A pragmatic approach, which is based on the work of Margie Lachman in a different setting,[40] that the author

has found to be clinically valuable involves six steps detailed here:

1. *Prevention*: There is frustratingly little to prove that excellent in-ICU care prevents post-ICU problems. However, the physiologic rationale that minimizing the extent of critical illness is an essential step to improving the lives of patients who survive the ICU is highly compelling. It is the my practice to emphasize aggressive sepsis detection and resuscitation, low tidal volume ventilation, sedation minimization, and early mobilization of mechanically ventilated patients.

2. *Protection*: That ICU patients frequently experience discontinuities of care after transfer out of the ICU is well documented.[41] Essential home medications are never restarted. Antipsychotics intended only for short-term delirium management are continued for prolonged periods.[42,43] The receiving team is not made aware of the appearance of new radiographic findings, and follow-up does not occur.[44] There are multiple process-of-care efforts to prevent such discontinuities that would seem to be essential. Furthermore, there may be roles for early mobility, sedation minimization, patient diaries, and other yet unproven therapies that will prevent ICU patients from having new neuromuscular and emotional deficits in the first place.

3. *Treatment*: Previously unrecognized or undiagnosed problems often are uncovered in the ICU. In some cases (e.g., the patient whose diabetes first presents as diabetic ketoacidosis), there are well-established procedures not only to correct the acute problem but also to ensure appropriate follow-up, including education and communication with primary care providers. However, other conditions, in particular depression and mental health issues, are often neglected. A balanced approach to improving life after the ICU must ensure appropriate follow-up for all new problems diagnosed or likely to be exacerbated in the ICU. Good approaches to specifically ensure appropriate follow-up after the ICU are lacking, but work on transitions of care for geriatric patients may provide promising models.

4. *Remediation*: The evidence increasingly suggests that disability after critical illness is rooted in muscle weakness, cognitive impairment, and lack of social support. Many practitioners strongly recommend early and ongoing physiotherapy for all patients in the ICU, with follow-up as an outpatient when appropriate. However, the appropriate approach to physiotherapy should be one of preventing any loss of functioning while in the ICU as opposed to only treating those with demonstrable weakness. Moreover, work by Hopkins and others[45] has shown that physical therapy in the ICU may also have important cognitive and psychiatric benefits. Also, it is essential that a patient's family or other support group be intimately involved in the process of providing ICU care. Netzer[36] has defined a "family ICU syndrome." His work and others' show the incredible toll that ICUs take on families. However, if patients are critically vulnerable in the period immediately after discharge, family participation may be an essential and underused determinant of whether the patients have a trajectory of recovery or a trajectory of disability.

5. *Compensation*: Even with the best medical care and physical therapy, some patients will have new problems after the ICU. There is an ongoing struggle to find a systematic approach to evaluating their needs. The model of a Comprehensive Geriatrics Assessment may hold great promise, but it needs to be customized to the ICU.[46] In this approach, there is a structured questionnaire tied to initial interventions to assess a range of potential needs. The sort of pragmatic assistance that geriatricians routinely provide to allow weak older patients to stay in their home may be of great value to ICU patients in their recovery.

6. *Enhancement*: The next frontier of recovery of critical illness will be finding ways to empower survivors to help each other by developing innovative peer support models. This approach allows patients to become partners in discovering new approaches to facilitate recovery. Such groups have fundamentally transformed recovery from cancer, stroke, Alzheimer disease, and other disabling conditions. This powerful tool holds enormous promise for improving outcomes after the ICU.

CONCLUSION

Many, but not all, patients have a range of physical, cognitive, and emotional challenges after critical illness. There are a limited number of validated tools to identify patients at risk for PICS.[14] Likewise, critical care professionals have yet to develop specific, validated therapies to prevent or treat these multifactorial problems. However, there is reason to believe that emerging techniques in patient management and rehabilitation offer the hope of improving the lives of survivors.

AUTHOR'S RECOMMENDATIONS

- A significant proportion of patients have range of physical, cognitive, and emotional challenges after critical illness; this is known as PICS (post– intensive care syndrome).
- There is growing recognition that the consequences of critical illness also places substantial strain on families of ICU survivors, who often bear the brunt of high levels of ongoing informal care.
- Patients who have critical illness typically had both worse functionality than the general population and were on trajectories of more rapid decline before their critical illness.
- There are a limited number of validated tools to identify patients at risk for PICS. Three strategies that can be can be used to prevent PICS are (1) in-ICU prevention, (2) treatment and remediation, and (3) triage.
- Clinicians have yet to develop specific, validated therapies to prevent or treat these multifactorial problems.
- There is reason to believe that emerging techniques in patient management and rehabilitation offer the hope of improving the lives of survivors.

REFERENCES

1. Quartin AA, Schein RMH, Kett DH, Peduzzi PN. Magnitude and duration of the effect of sepsis on survival. *JAMA*. 1997;277: 1058–1063.
2. Yende S, Linde-Zwirble W, Mayr F, Weissfeld LA, Reis S, Angus DC. Risk of cardiovascular events in survivors of severe sepsis. *Am J Respir Crit Care Med*. 2014;189:1065–1074.
3. Prescott HC, Langa KM, Liu V, Escobar GJ, Iwashyna TJ. Increased 1-year healthcare use in survivors of severe sepsis. *Am J Respir Crit Care Med*. 2014;190:62–69.
4. Wunsch H, Guerra C, Barnato AE, Angus DC, Li G, Linde-Zwirble WT. Three-year outcomes for medicare beneficiaries who survive intensive care. *JAMA*. 2010;303:849–856.
5. Needham DM, Davidson J, Cohen H, et al. Improving long-term outcomes after discharge from intensive care unit: Report from a stakeholders' conference. *Crit Care Med*. 2012;40:502–509.
6. Elliott D, Davidson JE, Harvey MA, et al. Exploring the scope of post-intensive care syndrome therapy and care: engagement of non-critical care providers and survivors in a second stakeholders meeting. *Crit Care Med*. 2014;42:2518–2526.
7. Schweickert WD, Hall J. ICU-acquired weakness. *Chest*. 2007;131:1541–1549.
8. Schweickert WD, Pohlman MC, Pohlman AS, et al. *A Randomized Trial of Early Physical and Occupational Therapy in the Management of Critically Ill Patients Undergoing Mechanical Ventilation*. Toronto: American Thoracic Society; 2008.
9. Mehta RL, Pascual MT, Soroko S, et al. Program to Improve Care in Acute Renal D. Spectrum of acute renal failure in the intensive care unit: the picard experience. *Kidney Int*. 2004;66:1613–1621.
10. Griffiths RD, Jones C. Recovery from intensive care. *BMJ*. 1999;319:427–429.
11. Herridge MS, Cheung AM, Tansey CM, et al. for the Canadian Critical Care Trials Group, One-year outcomes in survivors of the acute respiratory distress syndrome. *N Engl J Med*. 2003;348: 683–693.
12. Herridge MS, Tansey CM, Matte A, et al. Functional disability 5 years after acute respiratory distress syndrome. *N Engl J Med*. 2011;364:1293–1304.
13. Iwashyna TJ, Netzer G, Langa KM, Cigolle C. Spurious inferences about long-term outcomes: the case of severe sepsis and geriatric conditions. *Am J Respir Crit Care Med*. 2012;185:835–841.
14. Woon FL, Dunn C, Hopkins RO. Predicting cognitive sequelae in survivors of critical illness with cognitive screening tests. *Am J Respir Crit Care Med*. 2012;186:333–340.
15. Hopkins RO, Weaver LK, Pope D, Orme JJF, Bigler ED, Larson-Lohr V. Neuropsychological sequelae and impaired health status in survivors of severe acute respiratory distress syndrome. *Am J Respir Crit Care Med*. 1999;160:50–56.
16. Hopkins RO, Weaver LK, Collingridge D, Parkinson RB, Chan KJ, Orme JJF. Two-year cognitive, emotional, and quality-of-life outcomes in acute respiratory distress syndrome. *Am J Respir Crit Care Med*. 2005;171:340–347.
17. Wilcox ME, Brummel NE, Archer K, Ely EW, Jackson JC, Hopkins RO. Cognitive dysfunction in ICU patients: risk factors, predictors, and rehabilitation interventions. *Crit Care Med*. 2013;41: S81–S98.
18. Iwashyna TJ, Ely EW, Smith DM, Langa KM. Long-term cognitive impairment and functional disability among survivors of severe sepsis. *JAMA*. 2010;304:1787–1794.
19. Shah F, Pike F, Alvarez K, et al. Bidirectional relationship between cognitive function and pneumonia. *Am J Respir Crit Care Med*. 2013;188:586–592.
20. Pandharipande PP, Girard TD, Jackson JC, et al. Long-term cognitive impairment after critical illness. *N Engl J Med*. 2013;369: 1306–1316.
21. Davydow DS, Gifford JM, Desai SV, Bienvenu OJ, Needham DM. Depression in general intensive care unit survivors: a systematic review. *Intensive Care Med*. 2009;35:796–809.
22. Davydow DS, Gifford JM, Desai SV, Needham DM, Bienvenu OJ. Posttraumatic stress disorder in general intensive care unit survivors: a systematic review. *Gen Hosp Psychiatry*. 2008;30:421–434.
23. Davydow DS, Desai SV, Needham DM, Bienvenu OJ. Psychiatric morbidity in survivors of the acute respiratory distress syndrome: a systematic review. *Psychosomatic Med*. 2008;70:512–519.
24. Jackson JC, Pandharipande PP, Girard TD, et al. Bringing to light the risk F, incidence of Neuropsychological dysfunction in ICUssi. Depression, post-traumatic stress disorder, and functional disability in survivors of critical illness in the brain-ICU study: a longitudinal cohort study. *Lancet Respir Med*. 2014;2:369–379.
25. Wunsch H, Christiansen CF, Johansen MB, et al. Psychiatric diagnoses and psychoactive medication use among nonsurgical critically ill patients receiving mechanical ventilation. *JAMA*. 2014;311:1133–1142.

26. Davydow DS, Hough CL, Langa KM, Iwashyna TJ. Symptoms of depression in survivors of severe sepsis: a prospective cohort study of older Americans. *Am J Geriatr Psychiatry*. 2013;21:887–897.

27. Weycker D, Akhras KS, Edelsberg J, Angus DC, Oster G. Long-term mortality and medical care charges in patients with severe sepsis. *Crit Care Med*. 2003;31:2316–2323.

28. Coopersmith CM, Wunsch H, Fink MP, et al. A comparison of critical care research funding and the financial burden of critical illness in the United States. *Crit Care Med*. 2012;40:1072–1079.

29. Cameron JI, Herridge MS, Tansey CM, McAndrews MP, Cheung AM. Well-being in informal caregivers of survivors of acute respiratory distress syndrome. *Crit Care Med*. 2006;34:81–86.

30. Chelluri L, Im KA, Belle SH, et al. Long-term mortality and quality of life after prolonged mechanical ventilation. *Crit Care Med*. 2004;32:61–69.

31. Azoulay E, Pochard F, Kentish-Barnes N, et al. Risk of posttraumatic stress symptoms in family members of intensive care unit patients. *Am J Respir Crit Care Med*. 2005;171:987–994.

32. Davidson JE, Jones C, Bienvenu OJ. Family response to critical illness: postintensive care syndrome-family. *Crit Care Med*. 2012;40:618–624.

33. Davidson JE, Daly BJ, Agan D, Brady NR, Higgins PA. Facilitated sensemaking: a feasibility study for the provision of a family support program in the intensive care unit. *Crit Care Nurs Q*. 2010;33:177–189.

34. Verceles AC, Corwin DS, Afshar M, et al. Half of the family members of critically ill patients experience excessive daytime sleepiness. *Intensive Care Med*. 2014;40:1124–1131.

35. Sullivan DR, Liu X, Corwin DS, et al. Learned helplessness among families and surrogate decision-makers of patients admitted to medical, surgical, and trauma ICUs. *Chest*. 2012;142:1440–1446.

36. Netzer G, Sullivan DR. Recognizing, naming, and measuring a family intensive care unit syndrome. *Ann Am Thorac Soc*. 2014;11:435–441.

37. Davydow DS, Hough CL, Langa KM, Iwashyna TJ. Depressive symptoms of older patients with severe sepsis. *Crit Care Med*. 2012;40:2335–2341.

38. Cuthbertson BH, Elders A, Hall S, on behalf of the Scottish Critical Care Trials Group and the Scottish Intensive Care Society Audit Group, et al. Mortality and quality of life in the five years after severe sepsis. *Crit Care*. 2013;17:R70.

39. Ehlenbach WJ, Hough CL, Crane PK, et al. Association between acute care and critical illness hospitalization and cognitive function in older adults. *JAMA*. 2010;303:763–770.

40. Lachman ME, Agrigoroaei S. Promoting functional health in midlife and old age: long-term protective effects of control beliefs, social support, and physical exercise. *Plos One*. 2010;5.

41. Bell CM, Brener SS, Gunraj N, et al. Association of ICU or hospital admission with unintentional discontinuation of medications for chronic diseases. *JAMA*. 2011;306:840–847.

42. Morandi A, Vasilevskis E, Pandharipande PP, et al. Inappropriate medication prescriptions in elderly adults surviving an intensive care unit hospitalization. *J Am Geriatr Soc*. 2013;61:1128–1134.

43. Morandi A, Vasilevskis EE, Pandharipande PP, et al. Inappropriate medications in elderly ICU survivors: where to intervene? *Arch Intern Med*. 2011;171:1032–1034.

44. Gandhi TK. Fumbled handoffs: one dropped ball after another. *Ann Intern Med*. 2005;142:352–358.

45. Hopkins RO, Suchyta MR, Farrer TJ, Needham D. Improving post-intensive care unit neuropsychiatric outcomes: understanding cognitive effects of physical activity. *Am J Respir Crit Care Med*. 2012;186:1220–1228.

46. Stuck AE, Siu AL, Wieland GD, Adams J, Rubenstein LZ. Comprehensive geriatric assessment: a meta-analysis of controlled trials. *Lancet*. 1993;342:1032–1036.

5 Do Early Warning Scores and Rapid Response Teams Improve Outcomes?

Gabriella Jäderling, Rinaldo Bellomo

The rapid expansion of medical knowledge and the advances in surgical techniques, drug treatments, and interventions make it possible to treat conditions that would have been untreatable only 50 years ago. Progress has also led to a change in demographics, with an unparalleled increase in the age of patients treated and, as a result, an increasing level of illness severity.[1]

These medical and social changes have coincided with alterations in hospital care. Such trends include healthcare budget containments, cuts in the number of beds available, shortages of trained nurses, and working time directives. These new imperatives, which are associated with fewer and less experienced staff at hand to manage a larger workload of more complex patients, do not match the rising demand for admissions. Intensive care units (ICUs) have a proportionately limited number of beds to deal with such complex patients. Furthermore, the general wards, which lack sufficient monitoring, vigilance, and staffing resources, are being asked to provide care at levels usually reserved for ICUs. As a result of these system characteristics, patients whose condition deteriorates while on the general ward may not be identified and may not receive an appropriately high level of care in a timely manner.

Rapid Response Systems (RRSs) have been adopted in different forms worldwide to address the needs of such deteriorating patients in general wards. The RRS is an organized approach to improve patient safety by bridging care across hierarchies and specialties. RRSs facilitate the delivery of intensive care knowledge outside of the walls of the ICU, benefiting ward patients regardless of their location. The purpose is to detect and treat deviating physiology in time to prevent progression to irreversible conditions such as cardiac arrest or death.

Although intuitively appealing, some have questioned the evidence on which the implementation of an RRS rests. In this chapter, we present the concept of identifying and treating patients at risk using early warning scores (EWS) and RRSs as well as the emerging body of evidence in which these systems are evaluated.

DO EARLY WARNING SCORES HELP IDENTIFY PATIENTS AT RISK?

Adverse Events

Hospitals are dangerous places. In the early 1990s, several reports highlighted the occurrence of unexpected and potentially avoidable serious adverse events in hospitals.[2-4] These reports were not confined to a specific health-care system but were emerging from different parts of the world, thus forming the picture of a global problem.[5-11] Adverse events, defined as unintended injuries or complications caused by medical management rather than by the underlying disease and leading to death, disability, or prolonged hospital stays, were identified in between 2.9% and 16.6% of hospitalizations.[2,3,5,8-11] Up to 13.6% of such events were reported to lead to death and, importantly, 37% to 70% of these complications were deemed preventable. An in-hospital cardiac arrest is an example of a serious adverse event that is likely to have dire consequences. Despite dedicated efforts to improve resuscitation routines during cardiac arrest, mortality has remained unaltered at 85% to 90% over the past 30 years.[12-16] This lack of improvement could be explained by the fact that in-hospital cardiac arrests occurring in general wards are mostly related to noncardiac processes, with the arrest representing the common final pathway of various underlying disturbances.[17] As such, it is logical to hypothesize that outcome will improve with appropriate recognition and management of the precipitating disorder. Indeed, retrospective chart reviews suggest that this approach may well make it possible to avoid cardiac arrest altogether. In many, if not most, patients, signs of deterioration such as changes in pulse, blood pressure, respiratory rate, and mental status were present many hours before an actual arrest occurred.[17] Several studies have confirmed that this slow deterioration in vital signs may be present up to 48 hours before serious adverse events such as cardiac arrest, unanticipated ICU admission, or death.[18-23] These reports imply that the development of critical illness is not so much "sudden" but rather "suddenly recognized."[24]

Early Warning Scores

The classic vital signs are temperature, pulse rate, blood pressure, and respiratory rate. Oxygen saturation, as measured by pulse oximetry, and level of consciousness may also constitute useful vital signs.[25-27] Development of a score/numerical value quantifying derangements of these easily measured physiologic markers, the so-called EWSs, thus has potential. The UK National Early Warning Score (NEWS) is shown for illustration (Fig. 5-1).

Assessment of a patient's vital signs is a routine component of in-hospital care. However, only rarely are detected abnormalities linked to specific responses. In the formulation of such a closed-loop system, it is essential to define assessment parameters that trigger a response.[28] Trigger systems can be categorized as single-parameter, multiple-parameter, aggregate weighted scoring, or combination systems.[24] The two most common are the single-parameter and the aggregate weighted scoring systems.

The first RRS was a single-parameter system.[29] The triggers were acute change in respiratory rate, pulse oximetry saturation, heart rate, systolic blood pressure, or conscious state or that the staff was simply worried about the patient because of specific conditions, physiologic abnormalities, and the subjective criterion "any time urgent help is needed or medical and nursing staff are worried." A deviation of any single parameter from its predefined cutoff level was enough to alert the team. These original RRS activating criteria are, with slight modifications, still in use in Australia, the United States, and parts of Europe. Advantages of the single-parameter system are ease of implementation and use and the provision of a binary response (call for help or not). The criteria consist of the observation of an acute change in respiratory rate, pulse oximetry saturation, heart rate, systolic blood pressure, conscious state, or that the staff are simply worried about the patient.

The subjective "worried" criterion is designed to empower the staff to activate a response whenever they are concerned about a patient. This approach relies on the intuition and experience of nurses and other providers and should not be underestimated because subtle symptoms or small changes observed by vigilant practitioners often turn out to be precursors to more objective physiologic changes.[30,31] Studies on several systems demonstrated that the worried criterion activated nearly half of RRS calls.[32-36]

In the aggregate weighted scoring systems, deviations of vital signs are assigned points. The sum of these points constitutes total scores that have been referred to as the EWS or Modified EWS.[37] Once a threshold score is reached, a response is triggered. Alternatively, a trend in the score can be followed and an increase over time can then be used to direct a graded escalation of care. However, this approach is relatively complex and time-consuming and depends on accurate calculation.[37,38] Variations of scoring systems with different triggers or additional parameters (e.g., urinary output) have been used. The Royal College of Physicians of the United Kingdom has recently proposed the application of a national standard, the NEWS,[39] to increase consistency and reproducibility.

EWS have been shown to predict the development of critical illness. Prospective prevalence studies of entire hospital populations have demonstrated that fulfilling criteria for abnormal vital signs is clearly associated with a worse outcome.[40-42] Most studies have focused on mortality, but derangements in vital signs also presage cardiac arrest and the need for ICU transfer.[43] However, the accuracy of scores can vary as a function of the chosen outcome parameter. In a comparison by Churpek et al.,[44] the areas under the curve for different EWSs ranged from 0.63 to 0.88, with prediction of mortality being the most accurate. A recent systematic review by Alam et al.[45] concluded that introduction of EWSs was associated with better clinical outcomes (improved survival and decreases of serious adverse events), although meta-analysis could not be performed because of the heterogeneity of the patient populations and lack of standardization of the scores used in the included studies.

There is no clear evidence to indicate which form of warning system is best or even what frequency of

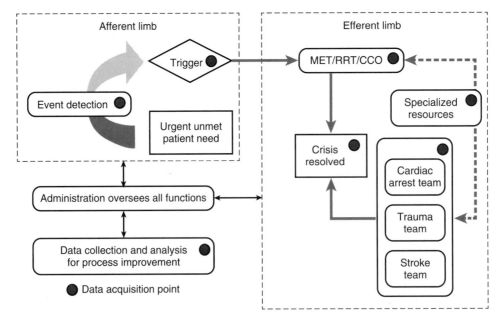

Figure 5-1. The composition of Rapid Response Systems. *CCO*, critical care outreach; *MET*, medical emergency team; *RRT*, rapid response team.

monitoring is ideal.[28] One study found a median duration of 6.5 hours for vital sign deteriorations before cardiac arrest,[46] whereas other studies found an even longer period.[18,21] Patients clearly respond better to earlier than delayed interventions.[47-50] In general, all systems provide reasonable specificity and negative predictive values but low sensitivity and positive predictive values.[51-53] Sensitivity can be improved by reducing the trigger threshold but not without compromising specificity, thus increasing workload. Including other parameters such as age,[54] comorbidities, or laboratory data[55,56] may improve predictive value.

Although many systems are in use, they differ primarily in details. Virtually all are based on the same concept: vital signs can provide clinicians with useful clues in evaluating a patient's condition or trajectory of illness. Implementing the use of any form of EWS conveys an important message: patients need to be checked. Placing the focus on monitoring and educating staff on when to react heightens awareness across the whole hospital; thus, it is likely to improve patient safety. In all probability, the value of an RRS lies not in the exact cutoffs or form of scores but rather in providing clear and objective tools to aid in assessing patients and in encouraging and empowering front-line providers to seek help when needed.

DO RAPID RESPONSE SYSTEMS IMPROVE OUTCOME?

General Principles of Rapid Response Systems

The usefulness and predictive value of EWSs must always be seen within the context of the response they can trigger. This response typically emanates from ICUs: dedicated teams that can be summoned to respond early to deteriorating patients, removing the usual boundaries of specialties and locations and centering care instead around the patients' needs.

Systems were simultaneously starting to take form in several parts of the world. An RRS is activated in Pittsburgh under the denotation "Condition C" (crisis) as opposed to "Condition A" (arrest), whereas in Australia the RRS is referred to as the "Medical Emergency Team" (MET). The first description in the literature appeared from an Australian center in 1995.[29] This report described the use of the team, its triggers, and the interventions provided. In the United Kingdom, a similar model was named the "Patient-at-Risk Team."[57] In 2005, the first international conference on METs was held in Pittsburgh, and faculty consensus findings were published. The report from this meeting defined a common nomenclature and composition and set the framework for future research.[58]

The term *Rapid Response System* refers to an entire network for responding to patients with a critical medical problem. The system comprises an afferent limb that detects the problem and triggers a response (Table 5-1). The responding team constitutes the efferent limb. This aspect may be of different designs, reflecting local culture and resources.

Teams that include physicians and nurses are traditionally called METs, whereas teams that are led by nurses are called RRSs. Critical Care Outreach teams are another model; they typically use ICU nurses as first responders and perform follow-up visits to patients discharged from the ICU. Outcome data on the superiority of one form to the other and the optimal composition of the team are lacking because there have been no studies directly comparing these different models.

Two additional components are needed to implement and maintain a successful RRS: an administrative framework and a feedback loop for quality evaluations (Fig. 5-1). These two are important because, in our opinion, only multilevel collaboration within the entire hospital organization can achieve a sustainable improvement of safety and quality in health care.

Outcome Measures

Measuring safety and monitoring success can be challenging in these complicated systems because the interventions are complex and are critically dependent on educational efforts and the context in which they are implemented.[59,60] Therefore process measures such as staff satisfaction, impact of education, or effects on end-of-life care are as important to investigate as traditional outcomes such as cardiac arrest rate, in-hospital mortality, and unanticipated ICU admission.

Table 5-1 **NEWS for United Kingdom National Health Scheme Hospitals**							
Physiologic Parameters	**3**	**2**	**1**	**0**	**1**	**2**	**3**
Respiration rate	≤8		9–11	12–20		21–24	≥25
Oxygen saturation	≤91	92–93	94–95	≥96			
Any supplemental oxygen		Yes		No			
Temperature	≤35.0		35.1–38.0	38.1–39.0	≥39.1		
Systolic blood pressure	≤90	91–100	101–110	111–219			≥220
Heart rate	≤40		41–50	51–90	91–110	111–130	≥131
Level of consciousness				A			V, P, or U

From https://www.rcplondon.ac.uk/.../national-early-warning-score-standardising-assessment-acute-illness-severity-nhs.pdf
NEWS, National Early Warning Score; *a*, alert; *P*, pain; *U*, unresponsive; *V*, voice.

RRSs have been widely adopted and endorsed by patient safety organizations, but there has been conflicting evidence regarding their value. Several "before-and-after" studies have shown a significant decrease in cardiac arrest rate, with reductions ranging from 20% to 65%.[32,61-64] Other reports have not been able to confirm an effect.[65] Evidence supporting reductions in cardiac arrests is more robust than in overall mortality[32,61,65-69] (see Table 5-2 for a summary). Most studies have been performed in single centers, but there are two reports in which hospitals are concurrently compared with and without an RRS. Bristow et al.[66] compared one hospital with an RRS to two hospitals with only conventional cardiac arrest teams and found that the RRS hospital had fewer unanticipated admissions to the ICU and high dependency unit but not a significant difference in cardiac arrest rates or mortality. Chen et al.[70] recently compared a hospital with a mature RRS to three hospitals without RRSs and found that the cardiac arrest rate was 50% lower and overall hospital mortality was 6% lower in the institution with mature RRS. In addition, introducing an RRS was associated with a 22% reduction in cardiac arrest rate and an 11% reduction in overall mortality.

Performing clinical trials of RRSs is problematic because randomization on an individual patient level (to either receive increased vigilance of deterioration with a targeted response or not) is ethically and practically unsound. However, two randomized studies have been published. Priestley et al.[69] performed a ward-based randomization of an outreach service and showed a significant reduction in hospital mortality. These studies also suggest that hospital length of stay was increased. The largest randomized trial is MERIT, a cluster randomization of 23 hospitals in Australia.[71] No outcome benefit was detected, although both trial arms improved relative to baseline. It has been argued that this study was underpowered,[72] that the teams were inadequately implemented,[73] and that there was contamination between the sites because control hospitals actually adopted RRS principles and used their cardiac arrest teams in RRS-like activities. However, an in-depth look into MERIT and its findings found that timely intervention by any team resulted in a significant reduction in cardiac arrests and unexpected hospital deaths.[48]

There have been variable reports of effects on unanticipated ICU admission. The MERIT trial did not demonstrate a difference. However, other data are equivocal. Several nonrandomized trials found a decrease,[66,74,75] two others found no effect,[76,77] and one found an increase.[61] ICU admission represents a potentially problematic endpoint because it is affected by local policies, bed numbers and occupancy, and resource availability. Such findings should be placed in context because an increase in low-acuity ICU admissions may decrease mortality rates, but it may represent a poor use of resources. Estimates of length of stay are equally difficult to interpret. Survivors may have a long length of stay, whereas the extremely ill who die shortly after admission will not. Furthermore, this measure may again be influenced by local policies in addition to medical decisions.

Two recent high-quality systematic reviews addressed RRSs.[78,79] In 2010, Chan et al.[78] identified 18 published studies, examining nearly 1.3 million admissions. Of the studies that reported team composition, 13 of 16 were led by physicians. The utilization of the team, or dose, was (in median) 15.1 of 1000 admissions (range, 2.5-40.3) in adult studies and 7.5 (range, 2.8-12.8) in pediatric studies. The analysis demonstrated a pooled risk reduction of 33.8% for adult cardiac arrest rates (relative risk [RR] 0.66, 95% confidence interval [CI] 0.54-0.80) but no significant effect on hospital mortality (RR 0.79, 95% CI 0.84-1.09). The pooled risk reduction in the five pediatric studies was 37.7% for cardiac arrest rates (RR 0.62, 95% CI 0.46–0.84) and 21.4% for hospital mortality (RR 0.79, 95% CI 0.63-0.98). The study concluded that RRSs were associated with reduced rates of in-hospital cardiac arrests but consistent evidence of improved overall hospital survival was lacking.

Winters et al.[79] conducted a systematic review in 2013 to include more recent evidence and found 26 additional studies on the effectiveness of RRSs (3 of which were conducted on children) and 17 additional studies addressing RRS implementation. The implementation processes varied widely and were driven by local needs and resources. Most studies described education as an integral part of implementation, although not all involved formal training. It has been posited that the use of an RRS may give rise to unintended consequences, some of which may be harmful. These concerns include deterioration in the resuscitative skills of ward staff, but this particular issue has been refuted in several qualitative studies. Rather, data indicate that nurse satisfaction is generally increased and that the system is highly appreciated in part because it provides a sense of security and improves patient care as well as the work environment.[80-83] Thus, this updated review supported the conclusions of Chan et al., but it also found that more recent studies reported favorable results, perhaps reflecting maturation of the systems and improvements in implementations. One study also adjusted for possible trends over time and found that reductions in cardiac arrest rates and mortality were unaffected.[36] In summary, it was concluded that the evidence supporting the use of RRSs to improve outcomes of hospitalized patients was moderately strong.

Ethical Issues

Over time, the use of RRSs has led to ethical concerns. Specifically, the deployment of an RRS often required the team to discuss and arrive at a quick conclusion regarding escalation of care. Although not an initial goal, several studies have reported the involvement of an RRS team in end-of-life care decisions.[84-88] An international multicenter study showed that one third of RRS calls were for patients in whom there were specific limitations in medical therapy. Furthermore, activation of the RRS frequently occurred after hours, and in 10% of cases the RRS was directly involved in designating patients "not for resuscitation."[86] It was also noted that the existence of a limitation in care did not exclude patients from RRS calls.[88] These findings suggest that wards need support not only in advanced care planning but also in providing comfort or appropriate treatment for patients with limitations of treatment orders. Such a patient may in fact improve as

Table 5-2 Summary of Studies Investigating the Effect of RRSs on Clinical Outcomes

Author, Year, Country	Study Design	Team Composition and Trigger System	Outcomes Studied	Results
Bristow,[66] 2000, Australia	Concurrent multicenter cohort comparison	Physician-led, single-parameter score	Cardiac arrest rate, hospital mortality, unplanned ICU admission	No effect on cardiac arrests or mortality, decreased ICU admissions
Buist,[61] 2002, Australia	Observational before-after	Physician-led, single-parameter score	Cardiac arrest rate, hospital mortality	50% reduction of cardiac arrests, no effect on hospital mortality
Bellomo,[32] 2003, Australia	Observational before-after	Physician-led, single-parameter score	Cardiac arrest rate, hospital mortality	65% reduction of cardiac arrests, 26% reduction of hospital mortality
Bellomo[68] 2004, Australia	Observational before-after	Physician-led, single-parameter score	Hospital mortality in postoperative patients after major surgery	36% reduction of hospital mortality
Kenward,[65] 2004, England	Observational before-after	Not reported, aggregate weighted score	Cardiac arrest rate, hospital mortality	No effect
Priestley,[69] 2004, England	Randomized on ward basis	Nurse-led outreach service, aggregate weighted score	Hospital mortality, hospital length of stay	48% reduction of hospital mortality
DeVita,[63] 2004, United States	Observational before-after	Physician-led, single-parameter score	Cardiac arrest rate	17% reduction of cardiac arrests
Hillman,[71] 2005, Australia	Cluster-randomized controlled trial	Physician-led, single-parameter score	Composite of cardiac arrests, unplanned ICU admission, unexpected death	No effect, both groups reduced cardiac arrests and unexpected deaths as compared with baseline
Jones,[64] 2005, Australia	Observational before-after	Physician-led, single-parameter score	Cardiac arrest rate	53% reduction of cardiac arrests
Jones,[89] 2007, Australia	Observational before-after	Physician-led, single-parameter score	Long-term mortality in postoperative patients	23% reduction in mortality at 1500 days after major surgery
Dacey,[74] 2007, United States	Observational before-after	Physician assistant-led, single-parameter score	Cardiac arrest rate, hospital mortality, unplanned ICU admission, ICU length of stay	61% reduction of cardiac arrests, no effect on hospital mortality, 16% decrease of unplanned ICU admissions
Jolley,[90] 2007, United States	Observational before-after	Nurse-led, single-parameter score	Cardiac arrest rate, hospital mortality	No effect
Offner,[91] 2007, United States	Observational before-after	Physician-led, single-parameter score	Cardiac arrest rate	50% reduction of cardiac arrests
Baxter,[92] 2008, Canada	Observational before-after	Physician-led, single-parameter score	Cardiac arrest rate, ICU admissions and readmissions, hospital mortality	38% reduction of cardiac arrests, decrease in ICU admissions and readmissions, no effect on hospital mortality
Chan,[67] 2008, United States	Observational before-after	Nurse-led, single-parameter score	Cardiac arrest rate, hospital mortality	41% reduction of non-ICU cardiac arrests, no effect on hospital mortality
Campello,[93] 2009, Portugal	Observational before-after	Physician-led, single-parameter score	Cardiac arrest rate, hospital mortality	27% reduction of cardiac arrests, no effect on hospital mortality
Konrad,[62] 2010, Sweden	Observational before-after	Physician-led, single-parameter score	Cardiac arrest rate, hospital mortality	26% reduction of cardiac arrests, 10% reduction of overall hospital mortality
Lighthall,[94] 2010, United States	Observational before-after	Physician-led, single-parameter score	Cardiac arrest rate, hospital mortality	57% reduction of cardiac arrests, trend toward lower mortality
Santamaria,[95] 2010, Australia	Observational before-after	Physician-led, single-parameter score	Cardiac arrest rate, hospital mortality, unexpected ICU admission	Significant reductions of cardiac arrests and hospital mortality, no effect on ICU admissions

Continued

Table 5-2   Summary of Studies Investigating the Effect of RRSs on Clinical Outcomes—cont'd

Author, Year, Country	Study Design	Team Composition and Trigger System	Outcomes Studied	Results
Laurens,[96] 2011, Australia	Observational before-after	Physician-led, single-parameter score	Cardiac arrest rate, hospital mortality, unexpected ICU admission	45% reduction of cardiac arrests, 24% reduction of hospital mortality, 21% reduction of unexpected ICU admissions
Beitler,[36] 2011, United States	Observational before-after	Physician-led, single-parameter score	Cardiac arrest rate, hospital mortality	51% reduction of cardiac arrests, 11% reduction in hospital-wide mortality, 35% reduction in out-of-ICU mortality
Sarani,[97] 2011, United States	Observational before-after/retrospective review	Physician-led, single-parameter score	Cardiac arrest rate, hospital mortality	40% reduction of cardiac arrests in medical patients, 32% in surgical, 25% reduction in hospital mortality for medical patients, no effect on surgical
Shah,[98] 2011, United States	Observational before-after/retrospective review	Nurse-led, single-parameter score	Cardiac arrest rate, hospital mortality, unplanned ICU admissions	No effect
Tobin,[99] 2012, Australia	Retrospective review of administrative data	Physician-led, single-parameter score	Hospital mortality	10% decrease in adjusted hospital-wide mortality 4 years after the introduction of MET
Chen,[70] 2014, Australia	Concurrent comparison of a hospital with a mature RRS and three hospitals without RRS	Not reported	Cardiac arrest rates, hospital mortality	50% lower cardiac arrest rate in RRS hospital and 6% lower mortality; after introducing an RRS, the other hospitals decreased their cardiac arrest rates 22% with an 11% drop in mortality

ICU, intensive care unit.

a result of RRS actions (e.g., by receiving antibiotics or fluids). However, the limitations for more advanced care, such as cardiopulmonary resuscitation or invasive ventilation, will not alter outcome in a favorable way and must be honored.

Therefore the manner by which RRSs decrease cardiac arrests may result from earlier detection and treatment of deteriorations; thus, they may truly prevent cardiac arrest. However, value may also arise as a result of increased discussions of the indications for treatment and of the limitations imposed at end of life, thus reducing the use of cardiopulmonary resuscitation and other resuscitative measures in terminally ill patients who have other needs.

The number of patients seen by an RRS is not proportional to an actual decrease in mortality. It may be that the RRS affects more than just the number of calls delivered. The intense educational efforts that are a part of RRS implementation increase general knowledge and awareness among the staff of failing vital signs. This change in itself may result in ancillary positive effects, providing ward staff with the tools to correctly recognize and manage early signs of deterioration,[80] thus obviating the need to call the RRS team. This potential benefit is a crucial part of the system that is difficult to quantify but nonetheless has a pivotal influence on how hospitalized patients are cared for and hence on their outcome.

AUTHORS' RECOMMENDATIONS

- All hospital patients should have an individual monitoring plan. This may be revised according to the development of a patient's clinical status during hospitalization.
- EWSs can be used to predict the development of critical illness and perform reasonably well in the identification of patients at risk. However, there is no clear evidence to indicate which form of EWS is best.
- Components of a successful RRS include adequate trigger criteria for activation (afferent limb); a response team of competent composition (efferent limb); and an administrative and quality improvement component for educating staff, collecting data, and maintaining the system.
- There is moderate strength of evidence that RRSs decrease cardiac arrest rates and hospital mortality. EWSs and RRSs promote a patient-focused safety culture and increase understanding of the importance of measuring and understanding vital signs.

REFERENCES

1. Hillman K, Parr M, Flabouris A, et al. Redefining in-hospital resuscitation: the concept of the medical emergency team. *Resuscitation.* 2001;48(2):105–110.
2. Brennan TA, Leape LL, Laird NM, et al. Incidence of adverse events and negligence in hospitalized patients. Results of the Harvard Medical Practice Study I. *N Engl J Med.* 1991;324(6):370–376.

3. Leape LL, Brennan TA, Laird N, et al. The nature of adverse events in hospitalized patients. Results of the Harvard Medical Practice Study II. *N Engl J Med*. 1991;324(6):377–384.

4. Kohn L, Corrigan J, Donaldson M. *To Err is Human: Building a Safer Health System*. Washington, DC: Institute of Medicine, National Academies Press; 1999.

5. Wilson RM, Runciman WB, Gibberd RW, et al. The quality in Australian health care study. *Med J Aust*. 1995;163(9):458–471.

6. Thomas EJ, Studdert DM, Burstin HR, et al. Incidence and types of adverse events and negligent care in Utah and Colorado. *Med Care*. 2000;38(3):261–271.

7. Vincent C, Neale G, Woloshynowych M. Adverse events in British hospitals: preliminary retrospective record review. *BMJ*. 2001;322(7285):517–519.

8. Davis P, Lay-Yee R, Briant R, et al. Adverse events in New Zealand public hospitals I: occurrence and impact. *N Z Med J*. 2002;115(1167):U271.

9. Baker GR, Norton PG, Flintoft V, et al. The Canadian Adverse Events Study: the incidence of adverse events among hospital patients in Canada. *CMAJ*. 2004;170(11):1678–1686.

10. Soop M, Fryksmark U, Koster M, et al. The incidence of adverse events in Swedish hospitals: a retrospective medical record review study. *Int J Qual Health Care*. 2009;21(4):285–291.

11. Zegers M, de Bruijne MC, Wagner C, et al. Adverse events and potentially preventable deaths in Dutch hospitals: results of a retrospective patient record review study. *Qual Saf Health Care*. 2009;18(4):297–302.

12. Peatfield RC, Sillett RW, Taylor D, et al. Survival after cardiac arrest in hospital. *Lancet*. 1977;1(8024):1223–1225.

13. Bedell SE, Delbanco TL, Cook EF, et al. Survival after cardiopulmonary resuscitation in the hospital. *N Engl J Med*. 1983;309(10):569–576.

14. Schneider 2nd AP, Nelson DJ, Brown DD. In-hospital cardiopulmonary resuscitation: a 30-year review. *J Am Board Fam Pract*. 1993;6(2):91–101.

15. Peberdy MA, Kaye W, Ornato JP, et al. Cardiopulmonary resuscitation of adults in the hospital: a report of 14720 cardiac arrests from the National Registry of Cardiopulmonary Resuscitation. *Resuscitation*. 2003;58(3):297–308.

16. Sandroni C, Nolan J, Cavallaro F, et al. In-hospital cardiac arrest: incidence, prognosis and possible measures to improve survival. *Intensive Care Med*. 2007;33(2):237–245.

17. Schein RM, Hazday N, Pena M, et al. Clinical antecedents to in-hospital cardiopulmonary arrest. *Chest*. 1990;98(6):1388–1392.

18. Hillman KM, Bristow PJ, Chey T, et al. Antecedents to hospital deaths. *Intern Med J*. 2001;31(6):343–348.

19. Franklin C, Mathew J. Developing strategies to prevent inhospital cardiac arrest - analyzing responses of physicians and nurses in the hours before the event. *Critical Care Medicine*. 1994;22(2):244–247.

20. Hillman KM, Bristow PJ, Chey T, et al. Duration of life-threatening antecedents prior to intensive care admission. *Intensive Care Med*. 2002;28(11):1629–1634.

21. Kause J, Smith G, Prytherch D, et al. A comparison of antecedents to cardiac arrests, deaths and emergency intensive care admissions in Australia and New Zealand, and the United Kingdom–the ACADEMIA study. *Resuscitation*. 2004;62(3):275–282.

22. Buist M, Bernard S, Nguyen TV, et al. Association between clinically abnormal observations and subsequent in-hospital mortality: a prospective study. *Resuscitation*. 2004;62(2):137–141.

23. Smith AF, Wood J. Can some in-hospital cardio-respiratory arrests be prevented? A prospective survey. *Resuscitation*. 1998;37(3):133–137.

24. DeVita M, Hillman K, Bellomo R. Textbook of rapid response systems – concept and implementation. In: *Book Textbook of Rapid Response Systems - Concept and Implementation*. Springer; 2011. City.

25. Mower WR, Myers G, Nicklin EL, et al. Pulse oximetry as a fifth vital sign in emergency geriatric assessment. *Acad Emerg Med*. 1998;5(9):858–865.

26. Neff TA. Routine oximetry. A fifth vital sign? *Chest*. 1988;94(2):227.

27. Flaherty JH, Rudolph J, Shay K, et al. Delirium is a serious and under-recognized problem: why assessment of mental status should be the sixth vital sign. *J Am Med Dir Assoc*. 2007;8(5):273–275.

28. DeVita MA, Smith GB, Adam SK, et al. "Identifying the hospitalised patient in crisis"–a consensus conference on the afferent limb of rapid response systems. *Resuscitation*. 2010;81(4):375–382.

29. Lee A, Bishop G, Hillman KM, et al. The Medical Emergency Team. *Anaesth Intensive Care*. 1995;23(2):183–186.

30. Cioffi J. Recognition of patients who require emergency assistance: a descriptive study. *Heart Lung*. 2000;29(4):262–268.

31. Cioffi J, Conwayt R, Everist L, et al. 'Patients of concern' to nurses in acute care settings: a descriptive study. *Aust Crit Care*. 2009;22(4):178–186.

32. Bellomo R, Goldsmith D, Uchino S, et al. A prospective before-and-after trial of a medical emergency team. *Med J Aust*. 2003;179(6):283–287.

33. Santiano N, Young L, Hillman K, et al. Analysis of medical emergency team calls comparing subjective to "objective" call criteria. *Resuscitation*. 2009;80(1):44–49.

34. Jaderling G, Calzavacca P, Bell M, et al. The deteriorating ward patient: a Swedish-Australian comparison. *Intensive Care Med*. 2011;37(6):1000–1005.

35. Hodgetts TJ, Kenward G, Vlachonikolis IG, et al. The identification of risk factors for cardiac arrest and formulation of activation criteria to alert a medical emergency team. *Resuscitation*. 2002;54(2):125–131.

36. Beitler JR, Link N, Bails DB, et al. Reduction in hospital-wide mortality after implementation of a rapidresponse team: a long-term cohort study. *Crit Care*. 2011;15(6):R269.

37. Subbe CP, Gao H, Harrison DA. Reproducibility of physiological track-and-trigger warning systems for identifying at-risk patients on the ward. *Intensive Care Med*. 2007;33(4):619–624.

38. Prytherch DR, Smith GB, Schmidt P, et al. Calculating early warning scores–a classroom comparison of pen and paper and hand-held computer methods. *Resuscitation*. 2006;70(2):173–178.

39. National Early Warning Score (NEWS): standardising the assessment of acute illness severity in the NHS. Report of a working party. In: *Book National Early Warning Score (NEWS): Standardising the assessment of acute illness severity in the NHS*. Royal College of Physicians; 2012. Report of a working party.

40. Bell MB, Konrad D, Granath F, et al. Prevalence and sensitivity of MET-criteria in a Scandinavian University Hospital. *Resuscitation*. 2006;70(1):66–73.

41. Fuhrmann L, Lippert A, Perner A, et al. Incidence, staff awareness and mortality of patients at risk on general wards. *Resuscitation*. 2008;77(3):325–330.

42. Bucknall TK, Jones D, Bellomo R, et al. Responding to medical emergencies: system characteristics under examination (RESCUE). A prospective multi-site point prevalence study. *Resuscitation*. 2012;84:179–183.

43. Churpek MM, Yuen TC, Edelson DP. Predicting clinical deterioration in the hospital: the impact of outcome selection. *Resuscitation*. 2013;84(5):564–568.

44. Churpek MM, Yuen TC, Edelson DP. Risk stratification of hospitalized patients on the wards. *Chest*. 2013;143(6):1758–1765.

45. Alam N, Hobbelink EL, van Tienhoven AJ, et al. The impact of the use of the Early Warning Score (EWS) on patient outcomes: a systematic review. *Resuscitation*. 2014;85(5):587–594.

46. Buist MD, Jarmolowski E, Burton PR, et al. Recognising clinical instability in hospital patients before cardiac arrest or unplanned admission to intensive care. A pilot study in a tertiary-care hospital. *Med J Aust*. 1999;171(1):22–25.

47. Kumar A, Roberts D, Wood KE, et al. Duration of hypotension before initiation of effective antimicrobial therapy is the critical determinant of survival in human septic shock. *Crit Care Med*. 2006;34(6):1589–1596.

48. Chen J, Bellomo R, Flabouris A, et al. The relationship between early emergency team calls and serious adverse events. *Crit Care Med*. 2009;37(1):148–153.

49. Cardoso LT, Grion CM, Matsuo T, et al. Impact of delayed admission to intensive care units on mortality of critically ill patients: a cohort study. *Crit Care*. 2011;15(1):R28.

50. Boniatti MM, Azzolini N, Viana MV, et al. Delayed medical emergency team calls and associated outcomes. *Crit Care Med*. 2014;42(1):26–30.

51. Gao H, McDonnell A, Harrison DA, et al. Systematic review and evaluation of physiological track and trigger warning systems for identifying at-risk patients on the ward. *Intensive Care Med*. 2007;33(4):667–679.

52. Smith GB, Prytherch DR, Schmidt PL, et al. Review and performance evaluation of aggregate weighted 'track and trigger' systems. *Resuscitation*. 2008;77(2):170–179.

53. Smith GB, Prytherch DR, Schmidt PE, et al. A review, and performance evaluation, of single-parameter "track and trigger" systems. *Resuscitation*. 2008;79(1):11–21.

54. Smith GB, Prytherch DR, Schmidt PE, et al. Should age be included as a component of track and trigger systems used to identify sick adult patients? *Resuscitation*. 2008;78(2):109–115.

55. Prytherch DR, Sirl JS, Schmidt P, et al. The use of routine laboratory data to predict in-hospital death in medical admissions. *Resuscitation*. 2005;66(2):203–207.

56. Loekito E, Bailey J, Bellomo R, et al. Common laboratory tests predict imminent medical emergency team calls, intensive care unit admission or death in emergency department patients. *Emerg Med Australas*. 2013;25(2):132–139.

57. Goldhill DR, Worthington L, Mulcahy A, et al. The patient-at-risk team: identifying and managing seriously ill ward patients. *Anaesthesia*. 1999;54(9):853–860.

58. Devita MA, Bellomo R, Hillman K, et al. Findings of the first consensus conference on medical emergency teams. *Crit Care Med*. 2006;34(9):2463–2478.

59. Delaney A, Angus DC, Bellomo R, et al. Bench-to-bedside review: the evaluation of complex interventions in critical care. *Crit Care*. 2008;12(2):210.

60. Hillman K, Chen J, May E. Complex intensive care unit interventions. *Crit Care Med*. 2009;37(1 Suppl):S102–S106.

61. Buist MD, Moore GE, Bernard SA, et al. Effects of a medical emergency team on reduction of incidence of and mortality from unexpected cardiac arrests in hospital: preliminary study. *BMJ*. 2002;324(7334):387–390.

62. Konrad D, Jäderling G, Bell M, et al. Reducing in-hospital cardiac arrests and hospital mortality by introducing a medical emergency team. *Intensive Care Med*. 2010;36(1):100–106.

63. DeVita MA, Braithwaite RS, Mahidhara R, et al. Use of medical emergency team responses to reduce hospital cardiopulmonary arrests. *Qual Saf Health Care*. 2004;13(4):251–254.

64. Jones D, Bellomo R, Bates S, et al. Long term effect of a medical emergency team on cardiac arrests in a teaching hospital. *Crit Care*. 2005;9(6):R808–R815.

65. Kenward G, Castle N, Hodgetts T, et al. Evaluation of a medical emergency team one year after implementation. *Resuscitation*. 2004;61(3):257–263.

66. Bristow PJ, Hillman KM, Chey T, et al. Rates of in-hospital arrests, deaths and intensive care admissions: the effect of a medical emergency team. *Med J Aust*. 2000;173(5):236–240.

67. Chan PS, Khalid A, Longmore LS, et al. Hospital-wide code rates and mortality before and after implementation of a rapid response team. *JAMA*. 2008;300(21):2506–2513.

68. Bellomo R, Goldsmith D, Uchino S, et al. Prospective controlled trial of effect of medical emergency team on postoperative morbidity and mortality rates. *Crit Care Med*. 2004;32(4):916–921.

69. Priestley G, Watson W, Rashidian A, et al. Introducing Critical Care Outreach: a ward-randomised trial of phased introduction in a general hospital. *Intensive Care Med*. 2004;30(7):1398–1404.

70. Chen J, Ou L, Hillman K, et al. The impact of implementing a rapid response system: a comparison of cardiopulmonary arrests and mortality among four teaching hospitals in Australia. *Resuscitation*. 2014;85(9):1275–1281.

71. Hillman K, Chen J, Cretikos M, et al. Introduction of the medical emergency team (MET) system: a cluster-randomised controlled trial. *Lancet*. 2005;365(9477):2091–2097.

72. Chen J, Flabouris A, Bellomo R, et al. Baseline hospital performance and the impact of medical emergency teams: modelling vs. conventional subgroup analysis. *Trials*. 2009;10:117.

73. Cretikos MA, Chen J, Hillman KM, et al. The effectiveness of implementation of the medical emergency team (MET) system and factors associated with use during the MERIT study. *Crit Care Resusc*. 2007;9(2):206–212.

74. Dacey MJ, Mirza ER, Wilcox V, et al. The effect of a rapid response team on major clinical outcome measures in a community hospital. *Crit Care Med*. 2007;35(9):2076–2082.

75. Ball C, Kirkby M, Williams S. Effect of the critical care outreach team on patient survival to discharge from hospital and readmission to critical care: non-randomised population based study. *British Medical Journal*. 2003;327(7422):1014–1016A.

76. Leary T, Ridley S. Impact of an outreach team on re-admissions to a critical care unit. *Anaesthesia*. 2003;58(4):328–332.

77. Garcea G, Thomasset S, McClelland L, et al. Impact of a critical care outreach team on critical care readmissions and mortality. *Acta Anaesthesiol Scand*. 2004;48(9):1096–1100.

78. Chan PS, Jain R, Nallmothu BK, et al. Rapid response teams: a systematic review and meta-analysis. *Arch Intern Med*. 2010;170(1): 18–26.

79. Winters BD, Weaver SJ, Pfoh ER, et al. Rapid-response systems as a patient safety strategy: a systematic review. *Ann Intern Med*. 2013;158(5 Pt 2):417–425.

80. Jones D, Baldwin I, McIntyre T, et al. Nurses' attitudes to a medical emergency team service in a teaching hospital. *Qual Saf Health Care*. 2006;15(6):427–432.

81. Galhotra S, Scholle CC, Dew MA, et al. Medical emergency teams: a strategy for improving patient care and nursing work environments. *J Adv Nurs*. 2006;55(2):180–187.

82. Salamonson Y, van Heere B, Everett B, et al. Voices from the floor: Nurses' perceptions of the medical emergency team. *Intensive Crit Care Nurs*. 2006;22(3):138–143.

83. Shapiro SE, Donaldson NE, Scott MB. Rapid response teams seen through the eyes of the nurse. *Am J Nurs*. 2010;110(6):28–34. quiz 35–26.

84. Chen J, Flabouris A, Bellomo R, et al. The Medical Emergency Team System and not-for-resuscitation orders: results from the MERIT study. *Resuscitation*. 2008;79(3):391–397.

85. Jones DA, McIntyre T, Baldwin I, et al. The medical emergency team and end-of-life care: a pilot study. *Crit Care Resusc*. 2007;9(2):151–156.

86. Jones DA, Bagshaw SM, Barrett J, et al. The role of the medical emergency team in end-of-life care: A multicenter, prospective, observational study. *Crit Care Med*. 2012;40(1):98–103.

87. Parr MJ, Hadfield JH, Flabouris A, et al. The Medical Emergency Team: 12 month analysis of reasons for activation, immediate outcome and not-for-resuscitation orders. *Resuscitation*. 2001;50(1):39–44.

88. Jaderling G, Bell M, Martling CR, et al. Limitations of medical treatment among patients attended by the rapid response team. *Acta Anaesthesiol Scand*. 2013;57(10):1268–1274.

89. Jones D, Egi M, Bellomo R, et al. Effect of the medical emergency team on long-term mortality following major surgery. *Crit Care*. 2007;11(1):R12.

90. Jolley J, Bendyk H, Holaday B, et al. Rapid response teams: do they make a difference?. *Dimens Crit Care Nurs*. 2007;26(6): 253–260. quiz 261–252.

91. Offner PJ, Heit J, Roberts R. Implementation of a rapid response team decreases cardiac arrest outside of the intensive care unit. *J Trauma*. 2007;62(5):1223–1227. discussion 1227–1228.

92. Baxter AD, Cardinal P, Hooper J, et al. Medical emergency teams at The Ottawa Hospital: the first two years. *Can J Anaesth*. 2008;55(4):223–231.

93. Campello G, Granja C, Carvalho F, et al. Immediate and long-term impact of medical emergency teams on cardiac arrest prevalence and mortality: a plea for periodic basic life-support training programs. *Crit Care Med*. 2009;37(12):3054–3061.

94. Lighthall GK, Parast LM, Rapoport L, et al. Introduction of a rapid response system at a United States veterans affairs hospital reduced cardiac arrests. *Anesth Analg*. 2010;111(3):679–686.

95. Santamaria J, Tobin A, Holmes J. Changing cardiac arrest and hospital mortality rates through a medical emergency team takes time and constant review. *Crit Care Med*. 2010;38(2):445–450.

96. Laurens N, Dwyer T. The impact of medical emergency teams on ICU admission rates, cardiopulmonary arrests and mortality in a regional hospital. *Resuscitation*. 2011;82(6):707–712.

97. Sarani B, Palilonis E, Sonnad S, et al. Clinical emergencies and outcomes in patients admitted to a surgical versus medical service. *Resuscitation*. 2011;82(4):415–418.

98. Shah SK, Cardenas Jr VJ, Kuo YF, et al. Rapid response team in an academic institution: does it make a difference? *Chest*. 2011;139(6):1361–1367.

99. Tobin AE, Santamaria JD. Medical emergency teams are associated with reduced mortality across a major metropolitan health network after two years service: a retrospective study using government administrative data. *Crit Care*. 2012;16(5):R210.

BASIC RESPIRATORY MANAGEMENT

6 What Are the Indications for Intubation in the Critically Ill Patient?

Meredith Collard, Meghan Lane-Fall

The specific indications for endotracheal intubation are difficult to define, in part because large-scale studies examining the question are lacking and in part because clinical practice is evolving. Although a seasoned practitioner is usually able to identify a patient who requires intubation, it is challenging to explain the precise parameters used to arrive at this decision. In addition, advancements in oxygen delivery systems and noninvasive forms of ventilation have changed the decision-making process in recent years. In this chapter, we describe strategies for diagnosing respiratory failure and deciding whether endotracheal intubation is needed for support. We also briefly discuss reasons to avoid endotracheal intubation.

We divide indications for intubation into two broad categories: patients with physiologic compromise currently in need of support ("actual need") and those at high risk of decompensation ("impending need"). Actual need for intubation occurs when the patient is physiologically unstable as a result of impaired gas exchange (e.g., hypoxic respiratory failure or hypercarbic ventilatory failure). Impending need is present when respiratory compromise can be reasonably anticipated (e.g., impaired consciousness, airway edema). These two general indications are based on accepted practice, with few or no data available to support specific guidelines. This poor evidence base is reflected in Marino's statement that "...the indication for intubation and mechanical ventilation is thinking of it."[1]

As with any invasive procedure, informed consent for endotracheal intubation should be obtained from the patient or proxy if possible. Advanced directives should be consulted to ensure that intubation is consistent with the patient's goals of care, and patients and families should be counseled about the expected duration of mechanical ventilation. Previous intubation records should be reviewed when possible to determine whether difficulty in securing the patient's airway is likely to occur.

ACTUAL NEED FOR INTUBATION

Signs and Symptoms

Acute hypoxic respiratory failure results from inadequate exchange of oxygen across the pulmonary alveolar-capillary membrane. This impairment leads to a decrease in arterial oxygen tension (hypoxemia) and insufficient delivery of oxygen to tissues and cells (hypoxia). In addition, because oxygen delivery is the product of arterial oxygen content and cardiac output, hypoxia can also occur secondary to decreased cardiac output, anemia, or abnormal oxygen-hemoglobin binding affinity. In the medical literature, hypoxic respiratory failure is often described as type I failure when hypoxemia is present without hypercarbia. When associated with hypercarbia, this is described as type II respiratory failure.

In contrast, acute ventilatory failure (and subsequent hypercarbia and respiratory acidosis) results from inadequate removal of gas from distal alveoli. Mild ventilatory failure can exist alone or, when impairment is more severe, may be associated with hypoxemia. Ventilatory failure can result from a primary lung process such as chronic obstructive pulmonary disease, or it can occur secondary to disorders in the cardiac, neurologic, metabolic, or other systems.

Both the symptoms and signs of hypoxia and hypercarbia are nonspecific and are noted in Table 6-1. In addition, the signs and symptoms of hypercarbia also depend on the patient's baseline $Paco_2$ (partial pressure of carbon dioxide in arterial blood) the absolute value of $Paco_2$, and the rate of change. Unlike hypoxemia, chronic hypercarbia may be well tolerated. Eliciting a history of chronic CO_2 retention and performing careful serial evaluations of arterial pH are essential because hypercarbia with a near-normal pH is a sign of chronic compensation and often does not reflect an acute disorder. Symptoms of acute hypercarbia may include respiratory fatigue and suggest that the patient soon may be unable to achieve the minute ventilation required to maintain a normal pH.

Many disease processes can lead to type I failure (Table 6-2) or type II failure (Table 6-3). These processes can be divided into pulmonary and nonpulmonary processes. Although they are presented separately, there is some overlap in these two types of respiratory failure. For the purposes of this chapter, respiratory and cardiac arrest are included as ventilatory (type II) failure.

Table 6-1 Symptoms and Signs of Hypoxia and Hypercarbia

Hypoxia	Hypercarbia
Symptoms	*Symptoms*
Confusion	Confusion
Dyspnea*	Dyspnea
Exhaustion	Exhaustion
Headache	Headache
Irritability	
Signs	*Signs*
Agitation	
Central cyanosis	Accessory respiratory muscle use
Coma	Cardiovascular collapse
Increased work of breathing	Coma
Lethargy	Flapping tremor
Seizures	Increased work of breathing
Somnolence	Lethargy
Tachypnea*	Seizures
	Shallow or small tidal volume breathing
	Somnolence
	Tachypnea

*May or may not be present depending on the cause of the hypoxia.

Table 6-2 Causes of Hypoxemic Respiratory Failure*

PULMONARY DISORDERS
Intrinsic lung disease
Lung consolidation (e.g., tumor)

Pathophysiologic state
Acute respiratory distress syndrome (ARDS)
Atelectasis
Lung consolidation (e.g., hemorrhage)
Noncardiogenic pulmonary edema
Pneumonia
Transfusion-related acute lung injury (TRALI)

NONPULMONARY DISORDERS
Cardiac disorders
Cardiogenic pulmonary edema

Vascular disorders
Pulmonary embolism

Toxins
Carbon monoxide

*These are causes of type I respiratory failure (hypoxia without hypercarbia).

Table 6-3 Causes of Hypercarbic Ventilatory Failure

PULMONARY DISORDERS
Intrinsic lung diseases
Asthma
Chronic obstructive pulmonary disease

Pathophysiologic state
Airway obstruction (functional or mechanical)
Obstructive sleep apnea

NONPULMONARY DISORDERS
Neurologic disorders
Brainstem or medullary stroke
Central sleep apnea
Critical illness myopathy or polyneuropathy
Myasthenia gravis, Guillain-Barré syndrome
Obesity-hypoventilation syndrome
Opiate or sedative overdose
Phrenic nerve dysfunction

Cardiac disorders
Cardiac arrest
Cardiogenic shock
Heart failure

Vascular disorders
Pulmonary embolism

Metabolic disorders
Hypomagnesemia
Hypophosphatemia

Diagnosis of Respiratory Failure

Hypoxemia is usually defined as a Pao_2 (partial pressure of oxygen in arterial blood) of less than 60 mm Hg (8 kPa). The gold standard test for diagnosing hypoxemia is arterial blood gas testing. However, pulse oximetry, being continuous and inexpensive, is more commonly used for detection of decreased oxygen levels. However, it is important to note that pulse oximetry measures the saturation of hemoglobin, not Pao_2 (a reflection of oxygen dissolved in the blood) or oxygen content (a reflection of both bound and unbound O_2). Thus, pulse oximetry may be unreliable in cases in which the patient may have a normal Pao_2 but a low available O_2 content, such as in severe anemia, carbon monoxide poisoning, methemoglobinemia, or peripheral vasoconstriction.

Normal Pao_2 levels are 80 to 100 mm Hg in a healthy patient breathing room air and can exceed 500 mm Hg in a patient breathing 100% oxygen. Pulse oximetry values may remain normal until Pao_2 decreases from normal values to less than 60 mm Hg. For this reason, the alveolar-arterial oxygen gradient should be evaluated in patients receiving a high Fio_2 (fraction of inspired oxygen) because a widening alveolar-arterial oxygen gradient is a sign of worsening hypoxemia. Therefore, the decision to intubate must take into consideration that low pulse oximetry values coincide with significant hypoxemia, but normal oxygen saturation does not exclude hypoxemia, especially in patients receiving a high Fio_2.

Hypercarbia, commonly defined as a $Paco_2$ of more than 45 mm Hg (6 kPa), should also be diagnosed with arterial blood gas sampling. Noninvasive diagnosis of hypercarbia is problematic. End-tidal CO_2 monitoring is used in operating rooms, but accurate reflection of $Paco_2$ requires a sealed airway and consistent tidal volumes: gas leakage, dead space ventilation, and low cardiac output may provide misleading data. Pulse oximetry should not be used to gauge the adequacy of ventilation because normal oxygen saturation can be found in the presence of significant hypoventilation, providing false confidence.

With both hypoxia and hypercarbia, it is important to follow Pao_2 and $Paco_2$ changes over time, which may provide more information than absolute values.

In addition to instruments and tests being used to detect worsening ventilatory failure, it is essential to evaluate the patient's clinical condition for signs of fatigue and impending respiratory collapse on a continuous basis. Clinical assessment, combined with medical experience, is the most important tool for identifying patients requiring early intubation. Signs of impending collapse often include worsening dyspnea, tachypnea, use of accessory breathing muscles, and rapid shallow breathing. Planned endotracheal intubation in a controlled setting is always preferable to emergent airway management.

Treatment of Acute Respiratory Failure

The initial treatment of all actual or impending cases of respiratory failure is the same: ensure a patent airway, adequate ventilation, and adequate fraction of inspired oxygen. Little research has been performed on minimal safe Pao_2 levels in critically ill patients. Pao_2 values of 50 to 60 mm Hg (6.5 to 8 kPa) or arterial oxygen saturation of 88% to 90% are often anecdotally suggested as minimum acceptable values during treatment of hypoxemia. However, for patients in shock states, with acute myocardial ischemia or after brain injury, higher arterial oxygen content levels would appear advantageous. Except in patients with right to left shunt greater than 30%, hypoxemia will improve with delivery of high Fio_2.

Not all patients with respiratory compromise require intubation and mechanical ventilation. Initial treatment of hypoxemia often starts with low-flow nasal cannula and escalates to 100% with a nonrebreather mask or high-flow O_2 therapy. Indeed, high-flow oxygen therapy shows promise in avoiding noninvasive ventilation in patients with mild to moderate respiratory failure.[2] If hypoxemia fails to reverse with supplemental oxygen and the patient is symptomatic, noninvasive assisted ventilation may be attempted.[3] If a patient is still unable to maintain minimal oxygen saturation while breathing 100% Fio_2, endotracheal intubation and mechanical ventilation will be required to improve oxygenation. During the process of intubation, high oxygen tensions should be maintained when possible. High-flow oxygen may be superior to nonrebreather face masks for maintaining oxygen saturation during the process of intubation.[4]

In cases of hypoxemia persisting despite intubation, mechanical ventilation with progressive levels of positive end expiratory pressure, and administration of high inspired oxygen tensions, additional therapeutic modalities such as continuous neuromuscular blockade, prone positioning, inhaled nitric oxide or nebulized prostacyclin, or extracorporeal membrane oxygenation should be considered.

It is crucial to diagnose the underlying cause of type I or type II failure so that adequate therapy such as antibiotic administration or surgical source control can be instituted. However, with type II failure, immediate management may also be affected by the etiology of the derangement. Cases in which ventilatory failure is not the primary disorder may require ventilatory support, but promptly administered definitive therapy can rapidly reverse respiratory compromise. For example, opioid or benzodiazepine overdose can be treated with reversal agents, and ventilatory failure secondary to cardiogenic shock can improve with inotropic agents and diuretics.

When specific medical therapies are not applicable or not successful in increasing ventilation, or when ventilatory failure is the primary problem, treatment is focused on providing a means to increase minute ventilation. Most often, this support is provided with either noninvasive positive-pressure ventilation or endotracheal intubation and mechanical ventilation. Therapy is often initiated when hypercarbia is associated with worsening hypoxemia or when the patient experiences cardiac or neurologic failure secondary to effects of elevated CO_2. The assisted ventilation provided from noninvasive positive-pressure therapy (i.e., steroids, bronchodilators, diuretics, nitrates) can provide additional time for treatment of underlying medical conditions. Using this approach to manage exacerbations of chronic obstructive pulmonary disease[5,6] and congestive heart failure[7,8] (both level of evidence A) is well supported by evidence showing improved morbidity and mortality for patients managed noninvasively.

When optimal medical management and/or noninvasive ventilation fail, or when there is a contraindication to the use of noninvasive ventilation (e.g., obtundation, recent esophageal anastomosis), endotracheal intubation and mechanical ventilation are indicated.

Impending Needs for Intubation

In the absence of frank respiratory failure, endotracheal intubation may still be appropriate if respiratory failure can be reasonably anticipated (Table 6-4). For example, patients with traumatic injury or swelling of the face, neck, or airway are at risk for airway obstruction. Patients with significant aspiration of particulate matter may be candidates for brief endotracheal intubation to facilitate bronchoscopy and lavage. In cases of metabolic acidosis, the respiratory drive to correct acidemia may lead to increased work of breathing and respiratory failure. When the underlying metabolic process, such as neuroleptic malignant syndrome or septic shock, cannot be reversed quickly, intubation and mechanical ventilation may be needed to increase pH.

Impaired consciousness with inability to protect the airway is another often-described indication for endotracheal intubation. Neurologic indications for endotracheal intubation are important because intubation for impaired consciousness and presumed airway protection may account for 20% of patients intubated in the intensive care unit (ICU).[9] The trauma and neurologic literature often cites a Glasgow Coma Scale (GCS) value of 8 or less as a

Table 6-4 Potential Indications for Endotracheal Intubation in the Absence of Respiratory Failure

AIRWAY OBSTRUCTION (ACTUAL OR IMPENDING)
Angioedema
Foreign body
Hemorrhage
Metabolic acidosis
Secretions
Trauma

LOSS OF PROTECTIVE REFLEXES (ACTUAL OR IMPENDING)
Coma
Pharmacologic sedation
Seizure

IMPENDING RESPIRATORY FAILURE (TYPE I OR TYPE II)
Asthma exacerbation
Metabolic acidosis

specific indicator for endotracheal intubation.[10] The GCS criterion for intubation is not based on concerns for respiratory distress but rather on the concern for development of worsening consciousness, hypoventilation, and airway protection. This arises from a retrospective analysis of the National Traumatic Coma Data Bank that demonstrates a greater risk for aspiration and worse clinical outcome in comatose patients (GCS <8) not endotracheally intubated.[11] Subsequent studies support this conclusion.[12] Severe brain injury is associated with decreased respiratory drive and hypoventilation, and patients likewise often have decreased muscle tone. This may increase the risk for airway obstruction and a failure to clear secretions.[13] In addition, patients with traumatic brain injury and subarachnoid hemorrhage have been shown to be at increased risk for having pulmonary edema. Indeed, as many as 30% of these patients may progress to severe acute lung injury or acute respiratory distress syndrome.[14]

Although intubation for a depressed level of consciousness is regarded as a standard of care, no definitive controlled studies are available on the subject. Recent studies dispute the requirement for intubation based on neurologic status alone. Coplin et al.[15] studied criteria used for extubation and found that neither level of consciousness nor the presence of a gag or cough reflex predicted success. In this study, 80% of patients with a GCS value of 8 or less and 90% of patients with a GCS value of 4 or less were successfully extubated. This also was the case for 88% of patients with an absent or weak gag reflex and 82% of patients with an absent or weak cough. In addition, studies have shown that the risk for ventilator-induced lung injury is increased in patients with traumatic brain injury and subarachnoid hemorrhage, and many of these patients have ventilator-associated pneumonia. This may lead to a prolonged hospital stay and increased mortality.[16,17]

Impaired consciousness requiring intubation may also occur when respiratory depression occurs secondary to sedation required to facilitate patient care. For instance, traumatically injured patients may require deep sedation and intubation to perform necessary tests and procedures. In addition, patients with status epilepticus may require deep sedation for treatment of seizures, and patients receiving high doses of benzodiazepines for treatment of alcohol withdrawal may become obtunded with therapy.

Therapeutic hyperventilation is no longer recommended for patients with traumatic brain injury because of the elevated risk of cerebral ischemia.[18-20] However, brief, target-directed hyperventilation still may be indicated in cases of acute neurologic deterioration secondary to herniation or sudden intracranial pressure elevation.[20]

WHY MIGHT ENDOTRACHEAL INTUBATION BE UNDESIRABLE?

Endotracheal intubation and mechanical ventilation are not benign procedures. The process of intubation usually requires deep sedation and usually temporary neuromuscular blockade. Sedation in an already compromised patient can lead to further deterioration, including cardiac arrest. Difficulty securing the airway may lead to hypoxemia with subsequent neurologic and cardiac sequelae. Finally, damage to anatomic structures may occur, and these mechanical complications may require additional intervention.[21]

Subsequently, even if the initial intubation is tolerated, continued sedation and mechanical ventilation may cause ICU delirium, which is associated with short- and long-term morbidity.[22]

CONCLUSION

The goal of endotracheal intubation and mechanical ventilation is to provide the delivery of the oxygen and ventilation that is primary to a patient's survival. The decision to proceed with this invasive procedure requires an understanding of the pathologic and physiologic disorders that necessitate its use. Although much information is available on the study of respiratory pathology and physiology and on the delivery and modes of mechanical ventilation, little has been written about the specific indicators for endotracheal intubation. Because of the severity of a patient's clinical condition and difficulty with study design, strong evidence and randomized controlled studies are not available on the subject. Until better clinical trials are available, one must use available clinical information in combination with specific medical knowledge and experience in making this decision.

AUTHORS' RECOMMENDATIONS

- Indications for endotracheal intubation and mechanical ventilation are commonly divided into hypoxic respiratory failure, hypercarbic ventilatory failure, and impaired consciousness requiring airway protection.
- Indications are all based on accepted practice, with few or no data available to support specific guidelines.
- Clinical assessment, combined with medical experience, is the most important tool for identifying patients requiring intubation.
- Arterial blood gas and $Paco_2$ measurements are necessary to evaluate hypercarbic ventilatory failure because pulse oximetry values can remain near normal until ventilatory collapse.

ACKNOWLEDGMENTS

The authors acknowledge the contributions of Drs. Jason Brainard and Clifford Deutschman, who authored a previous edition of this chapter.

REFERENCES

1. Marino P. Principles of mechanical ventilation. In: Marino P, ed. *The ICU Book*. Philadelphia: Lippincott, Williams & Wilkins; 2007.
2. Parke RL, McGuinness SP, Eccleston ML. A preliminary randomized controlled trial to assess effectiveness of nasal high-flow oxygen in intensive care patients. *Respir Care*. 2011;56(3):265–270.
3. Thille AW, Contou D, Fragnoli C, Córdoba-Izquierdo A, Boissier F, Brun-Buisson C. Non-invasive ventilation for acute hypoxemic respiratory failure: Intubation rate and risk factors. *Crit Care*. 2013;17(6).
4. Miguel-Montanes R, Hajage D, Messika J, et al. Use of high-flow nasal cannula oxygen therapy to prevent desaturation during tracheal intubation of intensive care patients with mild-to-moderate hypoxemia. *Crit Care Med*. 2015;43(3):574–583.
5. Keenan SP, Sinuff T, Cook DJ, Hill NS. Which patients with acute exacerbation of chronic obstructive pulmonary disease benefit from noninvasive positive-pressure ventilation? A systematic review of the literature. *Ann Intern Med*. 2003;138(11):861–870. +I827.
6. Ram FS, Picot J, Lightowler J, Wedzicha JA. Non-invasive positive pressure ventilation for treatment of respiratory failure due to exacerbations of chronic obstructive pulmonary disease. *Cochrane Database Syst Rev*. 2004;3:Cd004104.
7. Masip J, Roque M, Sánchez B, Fernández R, Subirana M, Expósito JA. Noninvasive ventilation in acute cardiogenic pulmonary edema: systematic review and meta-analysis. *J Am Med Assoc*. 2005;294(24):3124–3130.
8. Peter JV, Moran JL, Phillips-Hughes J, Graham P, Bersten AD. Effect of non-invasive positive pressure ventilation (NIPPV) on mortality in patients with acute cardiogenic pulmonary oedema: a meta-analysis. *Lancet*. 2006;367(9517):1155–1163.
9. Esteban A, Anzueto A, Alía I, et al. How is mechanical ventilation employed in the intensive care unit? An international utilization review. *Am J Respir Crit Care Med*. 2000;161(5):1450–1458.
10. Marik PE, Varon J, Trask T. Management of head trauma. *Chest*. 2002;122(2):699–711.
11. Marshall LF, Becker DP, Bowers SA, et al. The National Traumatic Coma Data Bank. Part 1: design, purpose, goals, and results. *J Neurosurg*. 1983;59(2):276–284.
12. Winchell RJ, Hoyt DB. Endotracheal intubation in the field improves survival in patients with severe head injury. *Arch Surg*. 1997;132(6):592–597.
13. Johnson VE, Huang JH, Pilcher WH. Special cases: mechanical ventilation of neurosurgical patients. *Crit Care Clin*. 2007;23(2):275–290.
14. Kahn JM, Caldwell EC, Deem S, Newell DW, Heckbert SR, Rubenfeld GD. Acute lung injury in patients with subarachnoid hemorrhage: incidence, risk factors, and outcome. *Crit Care Med*. 2006;34(1):196–202.
15. Coplin WM, Pierson DJ, Cooley KD, Newell DW, Rubenfeld GD. Implications of extubation delay in brain-injured patients meeting standard weaning criteria. *Am J Respir Crit Care Med*. 2000;161(5):1530–1536.
16. Friedman JA, Pichelmann MA, Piepgras DG, et al. Pulmonary complications of aneurysmal subarachnoid hemorrhage. *Neurosurg*. 2003;52(5):1025–1032.
17. Zygun DA, Zuege DJ, Boiteau PJE, et al. Ventilator-associated pneumonia in severe traumatic brain injury. *Neurocrit Care*. 2006;5(2):108–114.
18. Stocchetti N, Maas AI, Chieregato A, van der Plas AA. Hyperventilation in head injury: a review. *Chest*. 2005;127(5):1812–1827.
19. Muizelaar JP, Marmarou A, Ward JD, et al. Adverse effects of prolonged hyperventilation in patients with severe head injury: a randomized clinical trial. *J Neurosurg*. 1991;75(5):731–739.
20. Bratton S, Chestnut R, Ghajar J, et al. Guidelines for the management of severe traumatic brain injury. XIV. Hyperventilation. *J Neurotrauma*. 2007;24(suppl 1):S87–S90.
21. Pacheco-Lopez PC, Berkow LC, Hillel AT, Akst LM. Complications of airway management. *52nd Conference on Adult Artificial Airways and Airway Adjuncts*. 2014;59(6):1006–1021.
22. Peitz GJ, Balas MC, Olsen KM, Pun BT. Wesley Ely E. Top 10 myths regarding sedation and delirium in the ICU. *Crit Care Med*. 2013;41(9 suppl. 1):S46–S56.

What Is the Role of Noninvasive Ventilation in the Intensive Care Unit?

Felix Yu, Erik Garpestad, Nicholas S. Hill

Noninvasive ventilation (NIV) has assumed an important role in the intensive care unit (ICU), with increasing use during the past 15 years. It is now considered the ventilatory mode of first choice for such forms of acute respiratory failure (Table 7-1). Multiple randomized controlled trials have demonstrated that NIV improves outcomes in these forms of respiratory failure. Improved outcomes include avoidance of intubation and reduced morbidity and mortality compared with conventional therapy including intubation. In addition, the role of NIV is expanding as more studies are completed in other forms of respiratory failure. There are encouraging results from trials evaluating NIV use in postoperative respiratory failure and pre-oxygenation of patients with hypoxemic respiratory failure before intubation in the ICU. The results are less clear in other forms of respiratory failure such as severe asthma, pneumonia, and acute lung injury (ALI)/acute respiratory distress syndrome (ARDS) as well as in postextubation respiratory failure in patients with non–chronic obstructive pulmonary disease (COPD).

SELECTING PATIENTS FOR NONINVASIVE VENTILATION

The first question that should be addressed when selecting patients for NIV is whether the patient needs ventilatory support. Such patients usually have moderate to severe respiratory distress, signs of increased work of breathing such as tachypnea, increased use of accessory muscles, or abdominal paradox. Arterial blood gases should be obtained before starting NIV to assess the severity of the gas exchange derangement (particularly partial pressure of arterial carbon dioxide [$Paco_2$]) and to establish a baseline for comparison after the first 1 to 2 hours. Acutely ill patients should be monitored initially in an ICU or step-down unit to ensure that the patient is improving and tolerating the mask. Trials have shown that the response at the 1- to 2-hour time point is highly predictive of subsequent outcome; patients improving at this point are likely to succeed, but those failing to respond are likely to fail. Risk factors for failure after 2 hours of NIV are listed in Table 7-2.[1-3]

CONTRAINDICATIONS TO NONINVASIVE VENTILATION

When the need for ventilatory assistance is established, candidates for NIV should be screened for possible contraindications. NIV is contraindicated in patients with cardiopulmonary arrest because there is no time to place a mask and make adjustments. Any patient in shock requiring more than low doses of vasopressors is not a good candidate,[4] nor is the patient with a large acute myocardial infarction, uncontrolled arrhythmias or cardiac ischemia, or a large upper gastrointestinal bleed that is threatening the upper airway. Uncooperative and agitated patients and those with severe claustrophobia are unlikely to tolerate the mask. Patients with copious secretions, impaired swallowing, and frequent vomiting are at risk for aspiration and are poor candidates. Recent upper gastrointestinal surgery is also a relative contraindication because of the risk for abdominal distension and suture line rupture, although there have been some reports of successful use of NIV in these patients. Upper airway obstruction due to epiglottitis or angioedema is best treated with intubation to avoid progression to complete airway obstruction and the need for emergent cricothyrotomy, although upper airway obstruction due to glottic edema after extubation may respond well.[5] Impaired mental status is a relative contraindication, with one of the major concerns being the patient's inability to remove the mask in the event of vomiting. However, hypercapnic coma in patients with COPD exacerbations should not be considered a contraindication, and one trial has shown good outcomes with NIV use in these patients[6] (Table 7-3).

APPLICATIONS OF NONINVASIVE VENTILATION IN THE INTENSIVE CARE UNIT

NIV has been tried for many types of respiratory failure in the ICU. However, the evidence to support these applications varies depending on the diagnosis or circumstance. Table 7-4 lists the most common applications and the levels of evidence supporting them. In the following, we discuss the

Table 7-1 **Indications for NIV in Critically Ill Patients**

- Exacerbations of COPD
- Acute cardiogenic pulmonary edema
- Hypoxemic respiratory failure in immunocompromised patients
- Facilitating extubation in patients with COPD who fail spontaneous breathing trials

COPD, chronic obstructive pulmonary disease; *NIV*, noninvasive ventilation.

Table 7-2 **Risk Factors for Failure of NIV**

- pH < 7.25
- Relative risk > 35
- APACHE II score > 29
- ALI/ARDS
- Pneumonia
- Severe hypoxemia
- Shock
- Metabolic acidosis
- Impaired mental status

ALI, acute lung injury; *APACHE*, Acute Physiology and Chronic Health Evaluation; *ARDS*, acute respiratory distress syndrome; *NIV*, noninvasive ventilation.

Table 7-3 **Contraindications to NIV**

- Cardiopulmonary arrest, shock
- Uncontrolled cardiac ischemia or arrhythmias
- Uncooperative or agitated
- Severe upper gastrointestinal hemorrhage
- Coma, nonhypercapnic
- High aspiration risk, vomiting
- Copious secretions
- Upper airway obstruction
- Severe bulbar dysfunction
- Recent esophageal or upper airway surgery
- Multiorgan dysfunction
- Inability to fit mask because of craniofacial abnormalities

NIV, noninvasive ventilation.

Table 7-4 **Indications for NIV Use**

Strength of Recommendation*	Indication for NIV	Quality of Evidence†
Strong	COPD exacerbations	A
	Acute cardiogenic pulmonary edema	A
	Immunocompromised states	A
	Facilitating extubation in COPD	A
Intermediate	Postoperative respiratory failure	B
	Preoxygenation in hypoxemic respiratory failure	B
	Facilitation of flexible bronchoscopy	B
	Palliation in DNR/DNI patients	B
	Postextubation respiratory failure	B
Weak	ALI/ARDS	C
	Neuromuscular disease	C
	Pneumonia	C
	Status asthmaticus	C

*Strength of recommendation: strong, recommended therapy; intermediate, strongly consider in good candidates for NIV; weak, cautious trial can be performed in otherwise excellent candidates for NIV.
†Quality of evidence: *A*, multiple randomized controlled trials showing benefit with NIV; *B*, single randomized trial or nonrandomized trials showing benefit with NIV; *C*, conflicting evidence or evidence of harm with NIV.
ALI, acute lung injury; *ARDS*, acute respiratory distress syndrome; *COPD*, chronic obstructive pulmonary disease; *DNI*, do not intubate; *DNR*, do not resuscitate; *NIV*, noninvasive ventilation.

evidence supporting the various applications in more detail, starting with those supported by the strongest evidence.

First-Line Therapy

COPD Exacerbations

Multiple randomized, trials meta-analyses, and, more recently, comparative effectiveness analyses have shown decreased intubation and improved mortality rates with NIV use compared with standard medical therapy in patients with exacerbations of COPD.[7-13] Therefore NIV should be considered the standard of care in patients with COPD exacerbations requiring ventilatory support in the absence of contraindications. The physiologic rationale in these patients is that NIV unloads the inspiratory muscles and increases tidal volume, decreases the dead space-to-tidal volume ratio, lowers respiratory rate, and improves alveolar ventilation.[7] The addition of positive end-expiratory pressure (PEEP) decreases the work of breathing by decreasing the inspiratory threshold load imposed by auto-PEEP that is frequently present in these patients.[14]

Acute Cardiogenic Pulmonary Edema

Multiple randomized trials and meta-analyses have shown that either continuous positive airway pressure (CPAP) alone or NIV lowers intubation rates and mortality when compared with conventional medical therapy in patients with cardiogenic pulmonary edema.[15-25] The benefit in these patients primarily reflects an increase in intrathoracic pressure. Higher intrathoracic pressure increases functional residual capacity (FRC), recruiting flooded alveoli, improving gas exchange, and improving lung compliance. An increase in intrathoracic pressure also reduces cardiac preload and afterload, improving hemodynamics in most patients with cardiogenic pulmonary edema.[26,27] Longer term use of CPAP in stable congestive heart failure patients improved left ventricular ejection fraction, decreased mitral regurgitation, and decreased atrial natriuretic peptide levels compared with controls.[28] Whether CPAP alone or NIV (i.e., pressure support plus PEEP) is the preferred modality is unclear. An early study showed an increased rate of myocardial infarctions with NIV,[24] but subsequent trials and meta-analyses have failed to replicate this and have instead demonstrated that both modalities similarly reduce the need for intubation and lower mortality rates.[17,25] Although CPAP has been suggested as the preferred initial modality because of its greater simplicity and lower expense, most centers initially use NIV because bilevel devices are readily available and unloading of the inspiratory muscles may be achieved more quickly. In unstable patients with pulmonary edema complicating ST-elevation myocardial infarction, or in the presence of cardiogenic shock, early intubation is recommended.

Immunocompromised States

NIV decreases mortality compared with oxygen therapy alone in immunocompromised patients with hypoxemic respiratory failure. This includes patients with hematologic malignancies, patients who have had solid organ transplantation, or patients with HIV or AIDS.[29,30] The beneficial effects are attributed to the avoidance of infectious complications related to intubation. These patients are particularly vulnerable to intubation-associated pneumonias and septic complications.[31] We would recommend instituting this therapy early when there is a window of opportunity to avoid the progression to overt respiratory failure and the need for intubation. Once intubated, mortality rates among the immunocompromised may be very high,[31] although they appear to be declining.[32] In a retrospective observational study of patients with malignancy (including hematologic malignancies) and ARDS, mortality rates improved over time (89% in the first 5 years compared with 52% over the last 5 years). However, there was continued evidence of high mortality (68.5%) in patients with severe ARDS (partial pressure of arterial oxygen (Pao_2)/fraction of inspired oxygen (Fio_2) ≤ 100). Higher rates of NIV failure were observed in patients with moderate or severe ARDS and in patients experiencing NIV failure.[32]

Extubating Patients with COPD

Studies have shown decreased duration of mechanical ventilation and improved mortality when intubated COPD patients who have failed spontaneous breathing trials are extubated and supported with NIV.[33,34] However, this approach should be used with extreme caution. Patients should be excellent candidates for NIV in every other way—hemodynamically stable, cooperative, having a good cough and manageable secretions, and able to be ventilated with pressure support levels not exceeding 15 cm H_2O. Furthermore, initial intubation should not have been technically difficult because of the potential for catastrophe should these patients require emergent reintubation. The authors have found early extubation to NIV to be useful in avoiding the need for tracheostomies in such patients. However, if this approach fails and reintubation

is necessary, we usually proceed to prompt placement of a surgical airway.

OTHER INTENSIVE CARE UNIT APPLICATIONS

Preoxygenation Before Intubation

NIV can be an effective way of preoxygenating critically ill patients with hypoxemic respiratory failure before intubation.[35] In one randomized trial,[35] patients managed with NIV in preparation for intubation had improved oxygen saturations and a decreased incidence of significant desaturations during intubation. Anecdotally, we have had good success using this technique in our ICU. The beneficial effect of NIV likely is due to an increase in FRC with increased oxygen stores.

Flexible Bronchoscopy

NIV has been used during flexible bronchoscopy to avoid intubation.[36,37] This technique may be especially useful in immunocompromised patients at high risk for infectious complications from airway invasion. The technique involves passing the bronchoscope through an adapter attached to the NIV mask. In one trial, flexible bronchoscopy performed in eight immunocompromised patients with hypoxemic respiratory failure improved oxygenation compared with oxygen supplementation alone. None of these patients required intubation.[37] Because of the risk for respiratory deterioration during the procedure, clinicians should be prepared for possible emergency intubation. An alternative technique to consider in these patients is performing bronchoscopy through a supraglottic device, such as a laryngeal mask airway, but this technique requires deep sedation.

Postoperative Respiratory Failure

One randomized trial in patients with postoperative respiratory failure after lung resection surgery showed decreased intubation rates and mortality with NIV compared with standard therapy.[38] Another randomized trial found that prophylactic CPAP at 10 cm H_2O for 12 to 24 hours after thoracoabdominal aortic surgery reduced pulmonary complications and decreased hospital length of stay compared with oxygen supplementation alone.[39] Twenty-four hours of CPAP use after upper abdominal surgery was also associated with fewer intubations, a decreased occurrence of pneumonia and septic complications, and shorter ICU lengths of stay than oxygen therapy alone.[40] Similar efficacy has been reported for postgastric bypass patients.[41] One of the main reasons for the beneficial effect of CPAP or NIV in the postoperative setting is the avoidance of a sedation- or analgesic-associated reduction in the FRC and concomitant impairment of cough. These predispose to atelectasis, hypoxemia, pneumonia, and respiratory failure.

Obesity Hypoventilation Syndrome

Acute hypercapnic respiratory failure related to obesity hypoventilation is becoming more prevalent given the obesity epidemic in the general population. A single-center prospective observational study examined the use of NIV in these patients. Compared with COPD patients with acute hypercapnic respiratory failure, patients with obesity hypoventilation syndrome (OHS) were slightly older, more often female, and had similar initial arterial blood gas values. These patients also had lower late NIV failure and hospital mortality rates and better survivals at 1 year. The authors concluded that when used for acute hypercapnic respiratory failure in the ICU, NIV for OHS patients has similar efficacy and better outcomes than for COPD patients.[42]

Neuromuscular Disease

Evidence supports the use of home NIV in patients with neuromuscular disorders such as myopathies, muscular dystrophies, spinal muscular atrophy, scoliosis, and amyotrophic lateral sclerosis.[43-46] NIV reverses hypoventilation, stabilizes the upper airway, and improves obstructive sleep apnea. When these patients are admitted to the hospital, it is usually because of a respiratory infection. Aggressive management of secretion retention is paramount in avoiding respiratory catastrophe. Such patients should be managed only in an ICU where they can be monitored closely and frequently assisted with coughing. They should receive around-the-clock NIV and help with coughing using manually assisted coughing combined with mechanical insufflation and exsufflation ("cough assist") as often as necessary.[47] There is a subset of rapidly progressive neuromuscular disorders, including myasthenic crisis and Guillain-Barré syndrome, that involves "bulbar" muscles, impairing swallowing and the ability to mobilize secretions. Patients with these usually require preemptive intubation to avoid an unanticipated respiratory arrest, although a retrospective observational study[48] in patients with myasthenic crises showed that early use of NIV reduced the need for intubation and prolonged mechanical ventilation.

Palliative Care

NIV has a potential role in the treatment of patients with do-not-resuscitate/do-not-intubate (DNR/DNI) orders and end-of-life care. A study of NIV use in patients with heterogeneous respiratory failure and DNR/DNI status showed favorable outcomes in those with the types of respiratory failure expected to do well with NIV, such as COPD and cardiogenic pulmonary edema.[49] NIV can also be used for palliation of dyspnea or to extend life for a few hours to permit settling of affairs, but it should be discontinued if the mask is poorly tolerated or if dyspnea is not improved.

POSSIBLE ROLE IN THE INTENSIVE CARE UNIT

Asthma

Evidence regarding the use of NIV in severe asthma is lacking. One randomized trial in an Israeli emergency department of patients with acute asthma showed that NIV improved forced expiratory volume in 1 second more rapidly and decreased the need for hospitalization compared with sham NIV.[50] However, the patients were not in respiratory failure, and all patients had normal arterial blood gases. A Cochrane review concluded that more trials are needed before NIV can be recommended in this setting.[51] NIV can be tried cautiously in patients with asthma who fail to respond to initial bronchodilator therapy and have persistently increased work of breathing. This approach can be combined with helium-oxygen mixtures and continuous nebulization, although evidence to support this combination of therapies is lacking. However, patients with acute asthma treated with NIV must be watched closely because they can rapidly deteriorate. Emergency intubation can be dangerous if delayed too long because these patients can have profound oxygen desaturations and can also progress to hemodynamic collapse from hyperinflation and increased intrathoracic pressure.

Pneumonia

Acute pneumonia has long been considered a risk factor for NIV failure.[3] A trial evaluating NIV use in heterogeneous respiratory failure showed very poor outcome in the group of patients with pneumonia, with all such patients requiring intubation.[52] Another study evaluated NIV use in patients with hypoxemic respiratory failure and identified community-acquired pneumonia as a subcategory with a high NIV failure rate (50% intubation rate).[3] A randomized trial showed benefit of NIV in patients with severe community-acquired pneumonia but only in the subgroup with underlying COPD.[2] These data suggest that NIV should not be used routinely in patients with severe pneumonia.

Acute Lung Injury and Acute Respiratory Distress Syndrome

Similar to pneumonia, the evidence does not support the routine use of NIV in patients with ALI/ARDS. In a trial by Antonelli et al.,[3] ARDS, along with a higher Simplified Acute Physiology (SAPS) II score (>35), was identified as a risk factor for NIV failure. A recent trial evaluated NIV use in patients with ALI/ARDS and found a very high rate of failure (70%). Risk factors for NIV failure included shock (100% intubation rate), metabolic acidosis, and severe hypoxemia. The authors concluded that NIV should be used cautiously, if at all, if risk factors for failure are present.[1] A recent cohort study showed that some patients with ARDS may benefit from NIV. When used as first-line therapy for ARDS patients who are not yet undergoing intubation on admission to the ICU, NIV was able to prevent subsequent intubation in 54% of patients. A SAPS II score higher than 34 and lack of improvement in Pao_2/Fio_2 ratio to more than 175 after 1 hour of therapy were risk factors for NIV failure.[53] This latest study suggests that some patients with ALI/ARDS, especially less severely ill patients without shock, metabolic acidosis, or severe hypoxemia, may benefit from NIV. Close monitoring is essential, and if the Pao_2/Fio_2 ratio does not improve after 1 hour, then intubation and mechanical ventilation should be initiated.

Interstitial Lung Disease

ICU admissions for acute respiratory failure due to interstitial lung disease are associated with a high mortality rate. However, in selected patients, NIV may play a role in preventing intubation and improving survival. A prospective observational study[54] revealed that patients with Acute Physiology and Chronic Health Evaluation (APACHE) II scores less than 20 and mixed interstitial lung disease requiring noncontinuous NIV had a higher survival rate than those requiring continuous NIV or invasive mechanic ventilation. Likewise, a small retrospective study[55] of patients who had idiopathic pulmonary fibrosis with acute respiratory failure found a poor overall prognosis; however, for those who survived, NIV use was associated with a shorter ICU length of stay and improved 90-day survival. Interestingly, patients in this study with a higher level of the N-terminal prohormone brain natriuretic peptide (NT-proBNP) at baseline had a higher risk of NIV failure.

Postextubation Respiratory Failure

A large multicenter trial evaluated a heterogeneous group of patients with postextubation respiratory failure and randomized patients to treatment with NIV or standard therapy. Unexpectedly, the group that received NIV had an increased ICU mortality, as well as a 10-hour longer delay before reintubation.[56] These results underscore the importance of proper patient selection, with certain causes such as pneumonia and ALI/ARDS having poor outcomes. It is also clear that not delaying a needed intubation is essential. Postextubation respiratory failure can be treated with NIV if the patient is without contraindications and has a form of respiratory failure likely to respond to NIV, such as COPD or cardiogenic pulmonary edema. Again, closely evaluating the patient at the 1- to 2-hour point is critical to avoid delaying intubation.

In addition, the results of studies evaluating prophylactic NIV use after extubation to avoid reintubation have been mixed. Several meta-analyses have revealed a potential benefit to immediate NIV application postextubation.[59,60] However, most patients enrolled in these studies underwent intubation because of acute respiratory failure from COPD, in which the benefit of NIV is well established (see previously). A randomized controlled study evaluating NIV use after planned extubation in a mixed group of patients found no difference in reintubation rates between early NIV and standard medical treatment.[61] However, a further, smaller, randomized controlled trial in patients with varied causes for their acute respiratory failure did show a reduced reintubation rate benefit when NIV was used immediately after extubation.[62] Further study is clearly needed on the use of NIV after extubation.

CONCLUSION

The role of NIV in the ICU is gaining importance as the evidence supporting its use in certain forms of acute respiratory failure accumulates. Some studies support the use of NIV to preoxygenate patients with hypoxemic respiratory failure before intubation, as well as to facilitate flexible bronchoscopy in certain patients at high risk for infectious or bleeding complications from endotracheal intubation. The results of NIV or CPAP use in postoperative respiratory failure are encouraging, and this application requires further study. Data to support use in other forms of respiratory failure, including severe pneumonia, status asthmaticus, ALI/ARDS, and hypoxemic respiratory failure after extubation, are weaker, but selected patients with these conditions can be tried on NIV as long as they are closely monitored and undergo intubation promptly if they fail to improve. Recent surveys have shown that the use of NIV is increasing in critical care units throughout Europe[63] and presumably also in the United States. Patients who undergo NIV should be monitored closely in an ICU or step-down unit for mask tolerance and leaks, respiratory rate, use of accessory muscles, synchrony with the ventilator, and gas exchange. A careful assessment within 1 to 2 hours is important in determining the likelihood of success with NIV and is usually sufficient to decide to continue NIV or intubation and initiate invasive mechanic ventilation. Future studies should further define the role of NIV in the ICU and will likely expand the use of this important technology.

AUTHORS' RECOMMENDATIONS

- NIV has become an important part of the critical care ventilator armamentarium.
- Strong evidence supports the use of NIV for acute respiratory failure associated with COPD exacerbations, acute cardiogenic pulmonary edema, and immunocompromised states.
- If used, NIV should be applied with caution and in a closely monitored setting for patients with OHS, asthma, pneumonia, or ARDS.
- Patients must be carefully selected for NIV, which should be reserved for patients who require ventilatory assistance but have no contraindications.
- If patients are not improving within the first 1 or 2 hours of NIV, then intubation should be performed without further delay.

REFERENCES

1. Rana S, Hussam J, Gay P, et al. Failure of non-invasive ventilation in patients with acute lung injury: observational cohort study. *Crit Care.* 2006;10:R79.
2. Confalonieri M, Potena A, Carbone G, et al. Acute respiratory failure in patients with severe community-acquired pneumonia. *Am J Respir Crit Care Med.* 1999;160:1585–1591.
3. Antonelli M, Conti G, Moro ML, et al. Predictors of failures of noninvasive positive pressure ventilation in patients with acute hypoxemic respiratory failure: a multi-center study. *Intensive Care Med.* 2001;27:1718–1728.
4. Gray AJ, Goodacre S, Newby DE, et al. 3CPO Study Investigators. A multicentre randomised controlled trial of the use of continuous positive airway pressure and non-invasive positive pressure ventilation in the early treatment of patients presenting to the emergency department with severe acute cardiogenic pulmonary oedema: the 3CPO trial. *Health Technol Assess.* 2009;13:1–106.
5. Nava S, Gregoretti C, Fanfulla F, et al. Noninvasive ventilation to prevent respiratory failure after extubation in high-risk patients. *Crit Care Med.* 2005;33:2465–2470.
6. Gonzalez Diaz G, Carillo A, Perez P, et al. Noninvasive positive-pressure ventilation to treat hypercapnic coma secondary to respiratory failure. *Chest.* 2005;127:952–960.

7. Brochard L, Isabey D, Piquet J, et al. Reversal of acute exacerbations of chronic obstructive lung disease by inspiratory assistance with a face mask. *N Engl J Med*. 1990;323:1523–1530.

8. Bott J, Carroll MP, Conway JH, et al. Randomised controlled trial of nasal ventilation in acute ventilatory failure due to chronic obstructive airways disease. *Lancet*. 1993;341:1555–1557.

9. Kramer N, Meyer TJ, Meharg J, et al. Randomized, prospective trial of noninvasive positive pressure ventilation in acute respiratory failure. *Am J Respir Crit Care Med*. 1995;151:1799–1806.

10. Plant PK, Owen JL, Elliott MW. Early use of non-invasive ventilation for acute exacerbations of chronic obstructive pulmonary disease on general respiratory wards: a multicentre randomised controlled trial. *Lancet*. 2000;355:1931–1935.

11. Lightowler J. Noninvasive positive pressure ventilation for the treatment of respiratory failure due to exacerbations of chronic obstructive pulmonary disease (Cochrane Review). *BMJ*. 2003:185–189.

12. Keenan SP, Sinuff T, Cook DJ, et al. Which patients with acute exacerbation of chronic obstructive pulmonary disease benefit from noninvasive positive pressure ventilation? A systematic review of the literature. *Ann Intern Med*. 2003;138:861–870.

13. Lindenauer PK, Stefan MS, Shieh MS, et al. Outcomes associated with invasive and noninvasive ventilation among patients hospitalized with exacerbations of chronic obstructive pulmonary disease. *JAMA Intern Med*. 2014;174(12):1982–1993L.

14. Appendini L, Patessio A, Zanaboni S, et al. Physiologic effects of positive end-expiratory pressure and mask pressure support during exacerbations of chronic obstructive pulmonary disease. *Am J Respir Crit Care Med*. 1994;149:1069–1076.

15. Bersten AD, Holt AW, Vedig AE, et al. Treatment of severe cardiogenic pulmonary edema with continuous positive airway pressure delivered by face mask. *N Engl J Med*. 1991;325:1825–1830.

16. Lin M, Yang Y, Chiany H, et al. Reappraisal of continuous positive airway pressure therapy in acute cardiogenic pulmonary edema: short-term results and long-term follow-up. *Chest*. 1995;107:1379–1386.

17. Nava S, Carbone G, DiBattista N, et al. Noninvasive ventilation in cardiogenic pulmonary edema: a multicenter randomized trial. *Am J Respir Crit Care Med*. 2003;168:1432–1437.

18. Crane SD, Elliott MW, Gilligan P, et al. Randomised controlled comparison of continuous positive airways pressure, bilevel non-invasive ventilation, and standard treatment in emergency department patients with acute cardiogenic pulmonary oedema. *Emerg Med J*. 2004;21:155–161.

19. Pang D, Keenan SP, Cook DJ, et al. The effect of positive airway pressure on mortality and the need for intubation in cardiogenic pulmonary edema. *Chest*. 1998;114:1185–1192.

20. Rasanen J, Heikkila J, Downs J, et al. Continuous positive airway pressure by face mask in acute cardiogenic pulmonary edema. *Am J Cardiol*. 1985;55:296–300.

21. Lin M, Chiang HT. The efficacy of early continuous positive airway pressure therapy in patients with acute cardiogenic pulmonary edema. *J Formos Med Assoc*. 1991;90:736–743.

22. Masip J, Roque M, Sanchez B, et al. Noninvasive ventilation in acute cardiogenic pulmonary edema. *JAMA*. 2005;294:3124–3130.

23. Ho KM, Wong KA. Comparison of continuous and bi-level positive airway pressure non-invasive ventilation in patients with acute cardiogenic pulmonary oedema: a meta-analysis. *Crit Care*. 2006;10:R49.

24. Mehta S, Jay GD, Woolard RH, et al. Randomized prospective trial of bilevel versus continuous positive airway pressure in acute pulmonary edema. *Crit Care Med*. 1997;25:620–628.

25. Winck J, Azevedo L, Costa-Pereira A, et al. Efficacy and safety of non-invasive ventilation in the treatment of acute cardiogenic pulmonary edema: a systematic review and meta-analysis. *Crit Care*. 2006;10:R69.

26. Naughton M, Rahman M, Hara K, et al. Effect of continuous positive airway pressure on intrathoracic and left ventricular transmural pressures in patients with congestive heart failure. *Circulation*. 1995;91:1725–1731.

27. Tkacova R, Rankin F, Fitzgerald F, et al. Effects of continuous positive airway pressure on obstructive sleep apnea and left ventricular afterload in patients with heart failure. *Circulation*. 1998;98:2269–2275.

28. Tkacova R, Liu PP, Naughton MT, et al. Effect of continuous positive airway pressure on mitral regurgitant fraction and atrial natriuretic peptide in patients with heart failure. *J Am Coll Cardiol*. 1997;30:739–745.

29. Hilbert G, Gruson D, Vargas F, et al. Noninvasive ventilation in immunosuppressed patients with pulmonary infiltrates, and acute respiratory failure. *N Engl J Med*. 2001;344:481–487.

30. Antonelli M, Conti G, Bufi M, et al. Noninvasive ventilation for treatment of acute respiratory failure in patients undergoing solid organ transplantation: a randomized trial. *JAMA*. 2000;283:2239–2240.

31. Hauringa AJ, Leyva FJ, Girault SA, et al. Outcome of bone marrow transplantation patients requiring mechanical ventilation. *Crit Care Med*. 2000;28:1014–1017.

32. Azoulay E, Lemiale V, Mokart D, et al. Acute respiratory distress syndrome in patients with malignancies. *Intensive Care Med*. 2014;40:1106–1114.

33. Ferrer M, Esquinas A, Arancibia F, et al. Noninvasive ventilation during persistent weaning failure: a randomized controlled trial. *Am J Respir Crit Care Med*. 2003;168:70–76.

34. Nava S, Ambrosino N, Clini E, et al. Non-invasive mechanical ventilation in the weaning of patients with respiratory failure due to chronic obstructive pulmonary disease: a randomized study. *Ann Intern Med*. 1998;128:721–728.

35. Baillard C, Fosse JP, Sebbane M, et al. Noninvasive ventilation improves preoxygenation before intubation in hypoxic patients. *Am J Respir Crit Care Med*. 2006;174:171–177.

36. Antonelli M, Conti G, Rocco M, et al. Noninvasive positive-pressure ventilation vs. conventional oxygen supplementation in hypoxemic patients undergoing diagnostic bronchoscopy. *Chest*. 2002;121:1149–1154.

37. Antonelli M, Conti G, Riccioni L, et al. Noninvasive positive-pressure ventilation via face mask during bronchoscopy with BAL in high-risk hypoxemic patients. *Chest*. 1996;110:724–728.

38. Auriant I, Jallot A, Herve P, et al. Noninvasive ventilation reduces mortality in acute respiratory failure following lung resection. *Am J Respir Crit Care Med*. 2001;164:1231–1235.

39. Kindgen-Milles D, Muller E, Buhl R, et al. Nasal continuous positive airway pressure reduces pulmonary morbidity and length of stay following thoracoabdominal aortic surgery. *Chest*. 2005;128:821–828.

40. Squadrone V, Coha M, Cerutti E, et al. Continuous positive airway pressure for treatment of postoperative hypoxemia. *JAMA*. 2005;293:589–595.

41. Joris JL, Sottiaux TM, Chiche JD, et al. Effect of bi-level positive airway pressure (BiPAP) nasal ventilation on the postoperative pulmonary restrictive syndrome in obese patients undergoing gastroplasty. *Chest*. 1997;111:665–670.

42. Carrillo A, Ferrer M, Gonzalez-Diaz G, et al. Noninvasive ventilation in acute hypercapnic respiratory failure caused by obesity hypoventilation syndrome and chronic obstructive pulmonary disease. *Am J Respir Crit Care Med*. 2012;186:279–1285.

43. Simonds AK, Muntoni F, Heather S, et al. Impact of nasal ventilation on survival in hypercapnic Duchenne muscular dystrophy. *Thorax*. 1998;53:949–952.

44. Young HK, Lowe A, Fitzgerald DA, et al. Outcome of noninvasive ventilation in children with neuromuscular disease. *Neurology*. 2007;68:198–201.

45. Bach JR, Salstein K, Sinquee D, et al. Long-term survival in Werdnig-Hoffmann disease. *Am J Phys Med Rehabil*. 2007;86:339–345.

46. Simonds AK, Elliott MW. Outcome of domiciliary nasal intermittent positive pressure ventilation in restrictive and obstructive disorders. *Thorax*. 1995;50:604–609.

47. Tzeng AC, Bach JR. Prevention of pulmonary morbidity for patients with neuromuscular disease. *Chest*. 2000;118:1390–1396.

48. Seneviratne J, Mandrekar J, et al. Noninvasive ventilation in myasthenic crisis. *Arch Neurol*. 2008;65:54–58.

49. Levy MM, Tanios MA, Nelson D, et al. Outcomes of patients with do-not-intubate orders treated with noninvasive ventilation. *Crit Care Med*. 2004;32:2002–2007.

50. Soroksky A, Stav D, Shpirer I. A pilot prospective, randomized, placebo-controlled trial of bi-level positive airway pressure in acute asthmatic attack. *Chest*. 2003;123:1018–1025.

51. Lim 1 WJ, Mohammed Akram R, Carson KV, et al. Non-invasive positive pressure ventilation for treatment of respiratory failure due to severe acute exacerbations of asthma. *Cochrane Database Syst Rev*. 2012;12:CD004360.

52. Honrubia T, Garcia Lopez F, Franco N, et al. Noninvasive vs. conventional mechanical ventilation for acute respiratory failure. *Chest*. 2005;128:3916–3924.

53. Antonelli M, Conti G, Esquinas A, et al. A multiple-center survey on the use in clinical practice of noninvasive ventilation as a first-line intervention for acute respiratory distress syndrome. *Crit Care Med*. 2007;35:18–25.

54. Gungor G, Tatar D, et al. Why do patients with interstitial lung disease fail in the ICU? A 2-center cohort study. *Respir Care*. 2013;58:525–531.

55. Vianello A, Arcaro G, et al. Noninvasive ventilation in the event of acute respiratory failure in patients with idiopathic pulmonary fibrosis. *J Crit Care*. 2014;29:562–567.

56. Esteban A, Frutos-Vivar F, Ferguson ND, et al. Noninvasive positive-pressure ventilation for respiratory failure after extubation. *N Engl J Med*. 2004;350:2452–2460.

57. Burns K, Meade M, et al. Noninvasive ventilation as a weaning strategy for mechanical ventilation in adults with respiratory failure: a cochrane systematic review. *CMAJ*. 2014;186: E112–E122.

58. Burns K, Adhikari N, et al. Use of noninvasive ventilation to wean critically ill adults off invasive ventilation meta-analysis and systematic review. *BMJ*. 2009;338:b1574.

59. Krishna B, Sampath S, Moran JL. The role of non-invasive positive pressure ventilation in post-extubation respiratory failure: an evaluation using meta-analytic techniques. *Indian J Crit Care Med*. 2014;17:253–261.

60. Lin C, Yu H, Fan H, Li Z. The efficacy of noninvasive ventilation in managing postextubation respiratory failure: a meta-analysis. *Heart & Lung*. 2014;43:99–104.

61. Su C, Chiang L, et al. Preventative use of noninvasive ventilation after extubation: a prospective, multicenter randomized controlled trial. *Respir Care*. 2012;57:204–210.

62. Ornico S, Lobo S, Sanches H, et al. Noninvasive ventilation immediately after extubation improves weaning outcome after acute respiratory failure: a randomized controlled trial. *Crit Care*. 2013;17:R39.

63. Demoule A, Girou E, Richard JC, et al. Increased use of noninvasive ventilation in French intensive care units. *Intensive Care Med*. 2006;32:1747–1755.

8 How Does One Evaluate and Monitor Respiratory Function in the Intensive Care Unit?

Yuda Sutherasan, Lorenzo Ball, Paolo Pelosi

Over recent decades, we have seen many advancements in mechanical ventilation (MV) and respiratory monitoring, some resulting in documented decreases in mortality.[1] Nevertheless, the mortality attributable to acute respiratory distress syndrome (ARDS) and postoperative pulmonary complications remains high. Although invasive, MV is the cornerstone in the treatment of respiratory failure. MV itself can induce lung injury in both ARDS and healthy lungs (ventilator-induced lung injury [VILI]).[2,3] The main mechanisms of VILI are barotrauma due to high transpulmonary pressure (stress), volutrauma due to alveolar overdistension (strain), atelectrauma due to cyclic opening and collapsed ventilatory units, and biotrauma due to the release of inflammatory cytokines. Many studies have looked at techniques for improving outcomes in patients at risk for VILI, and to date, limiting lung stretch is the most effective strategy identified.

As part of the process of prevention, early detection, and treatment of respiratory failure and pulmonary complications, whether related to the primary disease process or to the potential harmful effects of MV, respiratory monitoring has evolved significantly in several different ways to now hold a central place in modern intensive care practice.

In this review, we highlight various methods of respiratory monitoring in the intensive care unit (ICU), with particular emphasis on implementing protective ventilatory strategies to minimize VILI, with the ultimate goal of improving outcomes.

INVASIVE AND NONINVASIVE CARBON DIOXIDE MONITORING

Capnometry is one of the simplest noninvasive tools for indirect assessment of the partial pressure of arterial carbon dioxide ($Paco_2$) and can provide information about alveolar ventilation, pulmonary perfusion, ventilator disconnection, or tube misplacement. Waveform analysis, with capnography, provides additional information, such as evidence of obstructive airway disease. The characteristic waveform of capnography is composed of three phases. The first phase, which is early expiration, represents the gas flow originated from dead space formed by airways and apparatuses, where CO_2 is virtually absent. Phase II represents the alveolar gas that is progressively emptying from alveoli. Phase III represents CO_2 removed from alveolar gas, the so-called alveolar plateau. The end-tidal CO_2 concentration (P_{ETCO_2}) is measured at the highest point in phase III (Fig. 8-1).

An immediate qualitative bedside interpretation of capnography is done by inspecting the slope of phase III, representing ventilation and perfusion heterogeneity. A steeper slope of phase II to phase III is found in patients with severe asthma or in chronic obstructive airway disease and correlates with the severity of obstruction.[4] The different characteristics of capnography are demonstrated in Figure 8-1.

Measurement of Ventilatory Dead Space

Physiologic dead space (Vd_{phy}) comprises airway dead space and alveolar dead space. The dead space (Vd) in volumetric capnography can be quantified by plotting CO_2 elimination (Vco_2) against exhaled tidal volume (V_T). The Vd_{phy}/V_T ratio can be calculated by the modified Bohr equation and equals ($Paco_2$–P_{ETCO_2})/$Paco_2$, assuming that $Paco_2$ is comparable to the alveolar partial pressure of CO_2 (Pco_2). The alveolar dead space is calculated by subtraction of airway dead space from physiologic dead space. The Douglas bag method is a more accurate but cumbersome technique that requires sampling of exhaled gases in a specific bag. Sinha et al.[5] demonstrated good agreement between dead space measured by volumetric capnography and the Douglas bag method.

Clinical Applications of Dead Space Measurement

Patients with ARDS have an increased alveolar dead space because of closed, injured alveoli: the percentage of alveolar dead space is associated with mortality in ARDS.[6] Positive end-expiratory pressure (PEEP) can both decrease and increase dead space. On the one hand, PEEP induces alveolar recruitment, and this reduces dead space. Conversely, high levels of PEEP may result in alveolar overdistension, compressing adjacent vessels and pulmonary

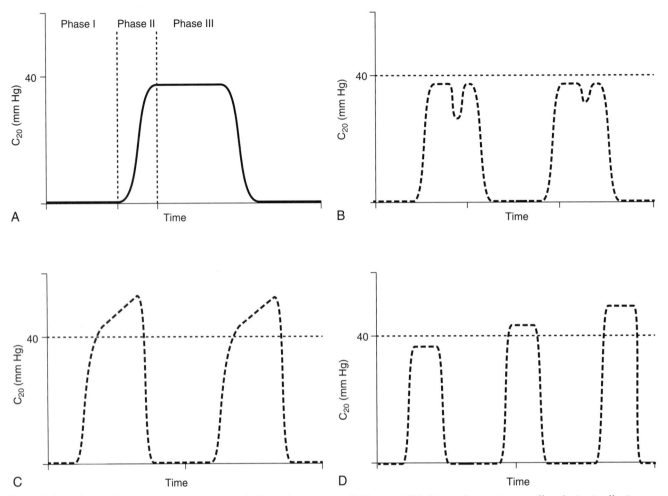

Figure 8-1. Different characteristic of capnograms, **A,** Normal capnogram. **B,** Curare cleft indicates the inspiratory effort during ineffective neuromuscular blockage. **C,** Shark fin appearance—prolongation of phase II and steep slope of phase III. **D,** Hypoventilation.

tissue, thereby increasing alveolar dead space. Blanch and colleagues observed that, in patients with respiratory failure who responded to PEEP with alveolar recruitment, a decrease of the $Paco_2$–P_{ETCO_2} gradient correlated with the PEEP level.[7,8] Another study, by the same authors, showed good correlation between severity of ARDS with parameters derived from volumetric capnography.[9]

A reduction in pulmonary artery blood flow leads to an increase in alveolar dead space. A normal alveolar dead space fraction increases the negative predictive value of routine D-dimer plasma level in ruling out pulmonary embolism (PE).[10] Alveolar dead space estimated by volumetric capnography showed good diagnostic accuracy in the emergency department, where a rapid exclusion of PE is warranted.[11] The dead space fraction may be useful for monitoring treatment response after thrombolytic therapy in patients with massive PE.[12]

Partial Rebreathing Technique of Carbon Dioxide Measurement

With the use of the indirect Fick principle, cardiac output (CO) is the ratio between Vco_2 (the elimination of arterial CO_2 content) and the difference between venous CO_2 content (C_Vco_2) and arterial CO_2 content (C_aco_2). The partial rebreathing of CO_2 measurement technique is a

noninvasive CO monitoring for mechanically ventilated patients that uses this principle. Vco_2 is derived from the difference of CO_2 concentration between inspired and expired gas, and this is then used to calculate pulmonary blood flow.[13] Several studies have found a good correlation between CO estimated by NICO and that measured by means of thermodilution methods, but they also found important limitations, especially when the patients have an intrapulmonary shunt or when $Paco_2$ is lower than 30 mm Hg.[14]

Transcutaneous Carbon Dioxide Monitoring

The standard method for direct measurement of $Paco_2$ is arterial blood gas analysis. However, continuous monitoring requires an invasive procedure that has several technical issues. Likewise, noninvasive measurement such of P_{ETCO_2} is limited to mechanically ventilated patients. Transcutaneous CO_2 monitoring TC_{CO_2} is a commercially available alternative that is applicable to nonintubated patients. Three different technologies allow TC_{CO_2} measurement: direct measurement of CO_2 gas that has diffused through the skin by sensor warming, an electrochemical measurement technique measuring pH from an electrolyte layer in contact with skin, and an optical-only CO_2 technique that uses a principle analogous to pulse oximetry.[15]

The TC_{CO_2} technique has been used in neonates, patients with sleep disorders, and critical care patients for decades, despite limited accuracy and side effects. Several studies showed the efficacy in monitoring patients with hypercapnic respiratory failure undergoing noninvasive MV.[16,17]

GAS EXCHANGE MONITORING

Critical care patients often show an increased oxygen demand caused by events such as fever, delirium, shivering, seizures, or systemic inflammatory response.

The most basic approach to gas exchange monitoring is the arterial blood gas analysis, in particular the assessment of SaO_2 (arterial oxygen saturation); more complete information can be provided by mixed venous blood gas analysis obtained from a pulmonary artery catheter, namely SvO_2 (mixed venous oxygen saturation).

The relationship between the two is described by the formula $SvO_2 = SaO_2 - VO_2/CO \times 1/Hb$, where VO_2 is the oxygen consumption, CO is cardiac output, and Hb is the hemoglobin concentration.[18]

Several studies investigated the usefulness of targeting SvO_2 above 70% as a therapeutic goal in high-risk surgical patients and septic shock, showing encouraging results,[18-20] at the cost of performing an invasive maneuver for the placement of the pulmonary artery catheter.[21]

Saturation of central venous blood, drawn from a central venous catheter, is referred to as $ScvO_2$ (central venous oxygen saturation) and is considered as a surrogate of SvO_2.[22] It is still debated whether such approximation is acceptable in patients with sepsis because of the uneven contribution of upper body and splanchnic circulation to $ScvO_2$. Devices capable of continuously monitoring either $ScvO_2$ or SvO_2 are becoming widely available, and their cost-effectiveness is under investigation.

RESPIRATORY MECHANICS

Respiratory System Compliance, Resistance, and Static Pressure-Volume Curve Analysis

The airway opening pressure (P_{AO}) is the pressure that overcomes total airway resistance and elastic recoil of the total respiratory system. To measure respiratory system mechanics during MV, one must separate the P_{AO} into two distinct components: the resistive airway pressure (P_{aw}) and the static or plateau pressure (Pplat). Importantly, for these values to be measured, patients require neuromuscular blockade and volume-controlled ventilation. During constant inspiratory flow, resistive P_{aw} can be measured, as can Pplat, if an inspiratory pause has been set.

Static lung compliance is measured to assess the effect of lung injury on lung parenchyma by various diseases, particularly ARDS. Total respiratory system compliance measurement is a better measure than lung compliance. Total respiratory system compliance is calculated by the ratio of tidal volume to plateau pressure minus total PEEP.

Low respiratory system compliance may result from high Pplat level associated with increased end-expiratory lung volume (EELV) from dynamic hyperinflation consequent of intrinsic PEEP (PEEPi). The end-expiratory occlusion technique can be used to measure PEEPi. However, the limitation of this technique is that it underestimates actual PEEPi in cases of severe narrowing of airways from the equal pressure point, creating upstream and downstream compartments, and it is unreliable when patients are not receiving controlled MV.[23]

High respiratory system resistance may be caused by either bronchospasm or obstruction of the endotracheal tube. The elastic properties of the respiratory system are the result of the complex relationship between the lung elastance and the chest wall elastic recoil. The pressure-volume (PV) curve is useful for understanding alterations in respiratory system mechanics. The standard technique to plot the PV curve is the "supersyringe" method. This involves inflation of a small volume of gas at very low flow rates during measurement and the plotting of the volume-pressure (VP) relationship. Hysteresis is the area between the inflation and deflation limb of the PV curve (PV loop). A greater area is observed in ARDS because of the high alveolar opening pressures. In ARDS, the inspiratory PV curve demonstrates the critical alveolar opening pressure, the alveolar closing pressure, and the recruitability of alveoli. The pressure at which significant alveolar recruitment begins creates a lower inflection point (LIP) on the curve. The exact method to identify the LIP, sometimes known as Pflex, is still debated. Gattinoni et al.[24] proposed Pflex as the pressure at the intersection between the extrapolated lines drawn from the portion of the PV curve at low lung volume (low compliance) and from the steep portion of the PV curve. In ARDS, an MV strategy that included setting PEEP at 2 cm H_2O above Pflex was shown to be associated with lower mortality compared with a higher stretch approach.[25] The upper inflection point (UIP) indicates the presence of alveolar strain. Therefore, when setting tidal volume and PEEP, physicians should try to avoid the presence of a UIP. This technique is mainly used in research rather than in clinical practice.[26]

Dynamic Pressure–Time and Pressure Volume Curve

Commercially available ventilators are able to display the dynamic pressure curve without interfering with the ventilation. Therefore several parameters may be used as indicators of lung recruitability and overhyperinflation, especially in ARDS. The parameters derived from the airway pressure profile such as the distension index (%E_2) or the stress index were recently proposed (Fig. 8-2).

Distension Index (Intratidal Pressure-Volume Loop)

The %E_2 (distension index) is the ratio of the compliance of the last 20% of the dynamic VP curve to the total compliance (C_{20}/C). This parameter is derived from multiple linear regression analysis of resistive P_{aw} and flow that included the nonlinearity part of the PV loop. Positive values of %E_2 indicate tidal overdistension, and negative values indicate tidal recruitment.[27] In ARDS, a %E_2 higher than 30% indicates lung overinflation[28,29] (Fig. 8-2).

Stress Index

The stress index is identified from the shape of the inspiratory pressure–time curve during constant flow in volume-controlled ventilation[30] and is calculated from the midportion of the curve. If downward concavity is present, then the stress index is less than 1 and means tidal recruitment. An upward convexity means that the stress index is greater than 1 and hyperinflation is occurring. The presence of a straight line, where the stress index equals 1, represents normal ventilation[30] (Fig. 8-2).

The use of $\%E_2$ and stress index is controversial in patients with ARDS. During low tidal volume ventilation in injured lungs, the PEEP level providing the lowest lung elastance was erroneously identified as overdistending by the stress index and $\%E_2$ in an experimental study.[31] Furthermore, Formenti and colleagues[32] demonstrated elevation of the stress index despite tidal recruitment without overinflation in a swine model of pleural effusion.

APPLICATION OF ESOPHAGEAL PRESSURE MEASUREMENT

Physiologic Background

Stress and distension indices are calculated from the pressure curve and are based on the total respiratory system compliance, which is influenced by the interaction between the lungs and the chest wall. This assumes that the disease process principally affects the lungs, and the chest wall is passive. However, many cases of ARDS derive from extrapulmonary disease (such as sepsis or pancreatitis), whereas other patients have decreased chest wall compliance from increased abdominal pressure, obesity, or pregnancy. This results in higher than normal pleural pressure. The pleural pressure can be indirectly measured with an esophageal balloon catheter. The esophagus is a passive structure adjacent to the pleural space. The pressure at the lower third of the esophagus is comparable to the pleural pressure in the upright position. In addition, with commercially available double balloon catheters, gastric pressure can be measured simultaneously, and its value approximates intra-abdominal pressure (IAP).[33] To test whether the esophageal balloon is placed in the correct position in spontaneous breathing patients, one can use the Baydur technique, and the end-expiratory occlusion maneuver can be applied. When the subjects start to inspire, the fluctuation and ratio of change of both esophageal and airway pressure should be comparable. In passively mechanically ventilated patients, the catheter should be inserted into the stomach and tested by observation of the transient increase in the balloon pressure during abdominal compression. Then the catheter is

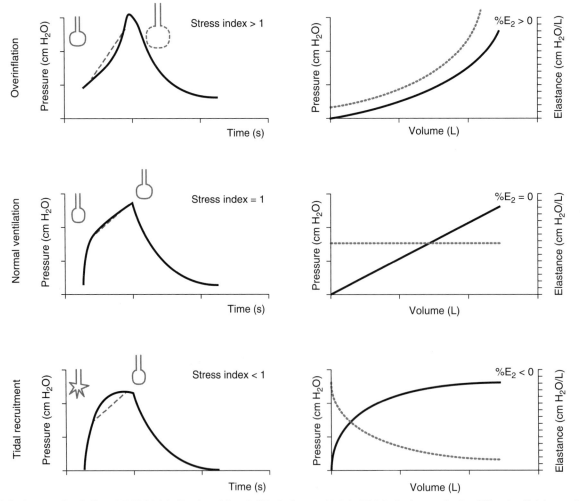

Figure 8-2. Stress index (*left*) and %E2 (*right*). (*Readapted from Ball L, Sutherasan Y, Pelosi P. Monitoring respiration: What the clinician needs to know. Best Pract Res Clin Anaesthesiol. 2013; 27:209–223 with permission*).

withdrawn proximally until the point where the cardiac pulsation can be clearly observed. External chest compression can be applied after airway occlusion. A $\Delta P_{es}/\Delta P_{aw}$ ratio (esophageal pressure/airway pressure ratio) ranging from 0.8 to 1.2 (10% to 20%) is considered to be marker of correct placement.[33,34]

Applications and Limitations

Transpulmonary pressure is a distending force of the lung, which is the difference between estimated alveolar pressure and pleural pressure. Esophageal pressure is a less accurate surrogate of pleural pressure in the supine position because of the compressive effect of the heart and because P_{es} is the pressure measured only in a mid-lung region. This may be negatively affected by raised IAP and asymmetric lung disease.

Nevertheless, in an ARDS experimental model, with high potential for recruitment, we found good correlations between the variations of invasive pleural pressure measurement and esophageal pressure regardless of the dependent, nondependent, or middle lung regions.[35] In spontaneous breathing patients, esophageal pressure in obese patients tends to be higher than in nonobese patients.[36]

Talmor and colleagues[37] demonstrated the benefit of titrating PEEP using transpulmonary pressure in ARDS. Oxygenation was improved compared with the conventional ARDSNet (ARMA study group) protocol at 72 hours. There was no statistically significant difference in mortality.

Other investigators have proposed the use of a transpulmonary lung approach based on PEEP titration to target an elastance-derived transpulmonary pressure of 26 cm H_2O (centimeters of water) according to the Gattinoni method. In an experimental ARDS canine model with a stiff chest wall, the transpulmonary pressure based on the lung approach appears to increase lung recruitment without hemodynamic disturbance.[38]

The incidence of intra-abdominal hypertension is high (>30%) in critically ill patients and is associated with elevated mortality.[29,39,40] In ARDS with IAP lower than 12 mm Hg, PEEP titration with respiratory mechanics is unaffected by IAP.[41] There is a linear correlation between IAP and chest wall elastance in patients with extrapulmonary ARDS.[42]

In anesthetized, obese patients, increases in body mass index correlate with decreases in lung volume and compliance.[43] Increases in IAP, such as by insufflation, are correlated with a further reduction of chest wall compliance.[44] This may explain why severely obese patients undergoing MV are more prone to having ARDS.[45]

In patients with ARDS, we recommend adjusting the level of PEEP with either IAP or transpulmonary pressure. These measurements are especially important when ARDS develops (1) secondary to extrapulmonary disease, (2) in high-risk postoperative abdominal surgical patients who have abdominal hypertension, and (3) in patients who are obese.

Parameters During Weaning

Work of breathing (WOB) refers to the volume of lung expansion that results from respiratory muscle contraction and is determined by total respiratory system compliance and airway resistance. Monitoring of WOB may be useful for the evaluation of difficult-to-wean patients. In assist-control ventilation, the WOB can be measured with the calculation of the pressure time product (PTP) from P_{es}. This estimates the effort made by the respiratory muscles. The PTP is calculated from the difference between P_{es} during assisted breathing and the elastic recoil pressure of the chest wall during passive ventilation in a similar volume and flow setting. However, P_{es} can be altered by artifacts induced by expiratory muscle contraction. For this problem to be resolved, intragastric pressure should be simultaneously assessed. This allows for calculation of the trans-diaphragmatic pressure, the difference between P_{es} and intragastric pressure.

The rapid shallow breathing index (RSBI) is calculated as the ratio between respiratory rate in minutes^{-1} and tidal volume in liters. It is a widely used tool to predict weaning success: if the RSBI is less than 100, then the patient is likely to wean. However, in elderly patients older than 70 years, the cutoff value should be raised to 130.[46]

Jubran and colleagues[47] have proposed a new index, the "Pes trend index," calculated by performing repeated measurements of P_{es} over time. The trend of P_{es} swing during a 9-minute spontaneous breathing trial was used for predicting weaning success, with an area under the receiver operating characteristic curve of 0.94. A high swing of P_{es} during the weaning period resulted in a higher chance of weaning failure. This index showed greater diagnostic accuracy when compared with the RSBI, but it is clearly more complex and invasive.

Airway Occlusion Pressure

The airway occlusion pressure ($P_{0.1}$) is the measurement of the negative airway pressure within 100 milliseconds (0.1 second) after inspiratory occlusion. $P_{0.1}$ is used for estimation of neural inspiratory drive. The $P_{0.1}$ is thought to correlate with WOB and predict failure to wean. In patients with chronic obstructive pulmonary disease, a $P_{0.1}$ lower than 6 cm H_2O was associated with successful weaning.[48] In postoperative patients with sepsis, during gradual decrease of pressure support, a $P_{0.1}$ higher than 2.9 cm H_2O was associated with the use of the sternocleidomastoid muscle as an accessory muscle of inspiration.[49] Therefore it may be a useful tool for optimizing the level of pressure support during weaning.

Maximal Inspiratory Pressure

Maximal inspiratory pressure (P_{Imax}) measurement is a test that reflects inspiratory muscle function, especially the diaphragm. P_{Imax} measurement is performed by occlusion of the proximal end of the endotracheal tube for 25 seconds with a one-way valve that prevents the patient from generating an inspiratory flow. The P_{Imax} is measured at end inspiration, and several studies have shown that a P_{Imax} of less than −20 to −30 cm H_2O provided high sensitivity, but low specificity, for predicting weaning success.

The combination of $P_{0.1}$ and P_{Imax}, the $P_{0.1}/P_{Imax}$ ratio, when less than 0.3, has been shown to be a sensitive predictor of weaning failure.[50]

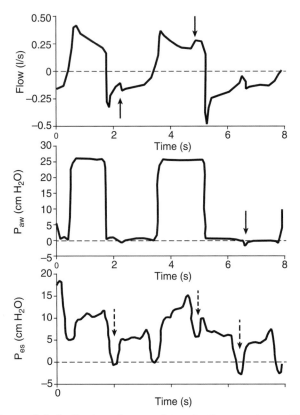

Figure 8-3. Ineffective trigger and termination asynchrony. The solid arrows show positive change during the expiratory phase and the negative deflection found in the pressure–time waveform (*middle panel*). The dashed-line arrows show negative deflection indicating nontriggering inspiratory efforts in the esophageal pressure-time waveform (*lower panel*). (*Readapted from Ball L, Sutherasan Y, Pelosi P. Monitoring respiration: What the clinician needs to know.* Best Pract Res Clin Anaesthesiol. *2013; 27:209–223 with permission*).

Asynchrony and Waveform Monitoring

Prolonged MV is associated with a high incidence of patient ventilator asynchrony.[51] Although automated detection of asynchrony would be a valuable tool, it has been infrequently studied, and the most commonly used detection method is careful visual inspection of the flow and pressure-time waveform.[52]

Ineffective triggering is the most common cause of asynchrony and usually results from PEEPi. We can detect this by identifying a sudden positive change of flow during the expiratory phase of the flow-time waveform and a negative deflection in the pressure-time waveform (Fig. 8-3).

Flow asynchrony occurs when the ventilator delivers a flow rate insufficient to match patient demand. This results in a concave distortion of the pressure-time waveform.

Asynchrony also occurs at end inspiration, particularly when the ventilator inspiratory time fails to match the neural inspiratory time. This is known as "termination asynchrony." Delayed termination of mechanical ventilator inspiration causes a pressure spike and a rapid decline of inspiratory flow at the end of inspiration. This asynchrony may coexist with ineffective triggering.[53]

Expiratory flow limitation due to collapse of small airways at a critical closing pressure results in air trapping or PEEPi. Flow-volume loop (FV loop) analysis can be used to characterize airway obstruction: a concave shape in the expiratory limb of the FV loop and the presence of a LIP on the inspiratory limb of the PV loop. Applying appropriate levels of PEEP in this setting may prevent end-expiratory airway collapse.[23,54] Conversely, where there is diffuse airway narrowing without peripheral airway collapse, PEEP might worsen lung overdistension (Fig. 8-4) and increase the WOB.

Finally, the ventilator itself may activate diaphragmatic contraction, causing air entrainment in sedated, mechanically ventilated patients. This process, which is rarely recognized, has been termed "reverse triggering."[55]

LUNG VOLUME MEASUREMENT/ FUNCTIONAL RESIDUAL CAPACITY/EELV

In nonventilated patients, the volume of gas left in the lungs at end expiration is the functional residual capacity (FRC). When a patient is mechanically ventilated with PEEP, the term EELV is used. During titration of PEEP, an increase in EELV may indicate either alveolar recruitment or alveolar overdistension. An integrated approach, including tidal compliance, oxygenation, and EELV, is helpful to guide an optimal PEEP to avoid overdistension and alveolar injury. An increase in EELV and lung compliance means alveolar recruitment, whereas an increase in EELV accompanied by a decrease in lung compliance suggests the presence of alveolar overdistension. Bikker and colleagues[56] demonstrated, in abdominal surgery and abdominal sepsis, that when PEEP was increased, there was a good correlation between changes in dynamic compliance and EELV.

The gold standard bedside technique for the measurement of EELV is the helium dilution method. A simpler alternative is the modified nitrogen washout/wash-in technique, which shows good precision in determining FRC as well as a good correlation with computed tomography (CT) scan findings and helium dilution.[57,58] The LUFU system (Dräger Medical, Lübeck, Germany) estimates FRC by oxygen washout, a variant of multiple breath nitrogen washout, with a sidestream O_2 analyzer. This is a promising automated technique that has been shown to be equally effective to the helium dilution technique in ARDS.[59]

EXTRAVASCULAR LUNG WATER MEASUREMENT

Extravascular lung water (EVLW) is the amount of water contained in the lungs outside of the pulmonary circulation. It consists of alveolar-interstitial extravasate, lymphatic fluid, and intracellular water. EVLW can be accurately estimated at the bedside by transpulmonary thermodilution.[62] This parameter, particularly when indexed for ideal body weight, may be useful in the ICU: it is an independent prognostic indicator in critically ill patients,[60] and it may help distinguish ARDS from nonexudative lung injury.[61] Lung ultrasound (LUS) has been proposed as a tool for estimating EVLW, both by visual inspection and scoring of sonographic images[63] and computer-aided automated analysis.[64]

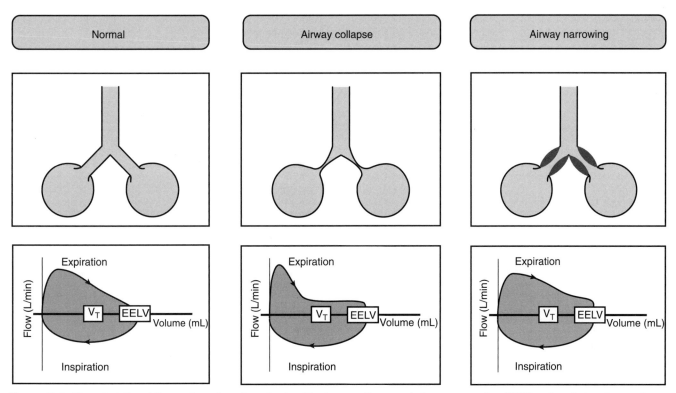

Figure 8-4. Characteristics of flow-volume loop in patients with airway collapse and airway narrowing. *EELV*, end-expiratory lung volume; *V_T*, exhaled tidal volume. *(Readapted from Ball L, Sutherasan Y, Pelosi P. Monitoring respiration: What the clinician needs to know. Best Pract Res Clin Anaesthesiol. 2013; 27:209–223 with permission).*

IMAGING

Computed Tomography

Several imaging techniques have been proposed as tools to assess lung aeration. Quantitative lung CT is currently the gold standard[64,65] and can be used to determine degrees of lung injury, aeration, and recruitability.[66] This could be a valuable tool in titrating PEEP.[67,68] However, routine CT scanning in ARDS is limited in clinical practice because of issues with transporting unstable critically ill patients, radiation exposure, and time and equipment constraints.

Lung Ultrasound

Lung ultrasound (LUS) is an increasingly used tool for lung assessment in intensive care. It has been used to estimate lung recruitability, especially when recruitment leads to volume changes greater than 600 mL.[68,69] It is also reported to be helpful in evaluating the response to diuretics and to inotropes in cardiogenic pulmonary edema,[70] during dialysis,[71] and in response to continuous positive airway pressure.[72] LUS has been shown to accurately predict postextubation distress after successful spontaneous breathing trials.[73]

Electrical Impedance Tomography

Electrical impedance tomography (EIT) is a bedside tool for the assessment of regional ventilation and respiratory monitoring.[74] EIT's major potential role in clinical practice is to evaluate lung inflation and distinguish recruitment from overdistension, thus preventing VILI. Although elegant, EIT has not been widely adopted because of cost, technical limitations,[64] and the absence of outcome data. Studies in animal models have reported that continuous EIT guidance of MV can help reduce histologic evidence of VILI.[75]

> **AUTHORS' RECOMMENDATIONS**
>
> - Monitoring respiratory function is necessary to determine individual responses to different ventilatory settings and to minimize VILI.
> - Esophageal pressure monitoring can be used to titrate and optimize airway pressure to ensure alveolar recruitment and safe end inspiratory and expiratory lung volumes. It is particularly useful in scenarios in which abnormal chest wall compliance is a major factor in respiratory failure.
> - Asynchrony can be detected by simple visual inspection of flow and pressure–time waveform.
> - EVLW measurement can be used to determine the contribution of pulmonary edema to low lung compliance.
> - LUS is increasingly used for early detection of pneumothorax, EVLW, and for the assessment of lung recruitability.

REFERENCES

1. Esteban A, Frutos-Vivar F, Muriel A, et al. Evolution of mortality over time in patients receiving mechanical ventilation. *Am J Respir Crit Care Med*. 2013;188:220–230.

2. Sutherasan Y, Vargas M, Pelosi P. Protective mechanical ventilation in the non-injured lung: review and meta-analysis. *Crit Care.* 2014;18:211.

3. Sutherasan Y, D'Antini D, Pelosi P. Advances in ventilator-associated lung injury: prevention is the target. *Expert Rev Respir Med.* 2014;8:233–248.

4. You B, Peslin R, Duvivier C, et al. Expiratory capnography in asthma: evaluation of various shape indices. *Eur Respir J.* 1994;7: 318–323.

5. Sinha P, Soni N. Comparison of volumetric capnography and mixed expired gas methods to calculate physiological dead space in mechanically ventilated ICU patients. *Intensive Care Med.* 2012;38:1712–1717.

6. Lucangelo U, Bernabe F, Vatua S, et al. Prognostic value of different dead space indices in mechanically ventilated patients with acute lung injury and ARDS. *Chest.* 2008;133:62–71.

7. Blanch L, Fernandez R, Benito S, et al. Effect of peep on the arterial minus end-tidal carbon dioxide gradient. *Chest.* 1987;92:451–454.

8. Coffey RL, Albert RK, Robertson HT. Mechanisms of physiological dead space response to peep after acute oleic acid lung injury. *J Appl Physiol.* 1983;55:1550–1557.

9. Blanch L, Lucangelo U, Lopez-Aguilar J, et al. Volumetric capnography in patients with acute lung injury: effects of positive end-expiratory pressure. *Eur Respir J.* 1999;13:1048–1054.

10. Kline JA, Israel EG, Michelson EA, et al. Diagnostic accuracy of a bedside d-dimer assay and alveolar dead-space measurement for rapid exclusion of pulmonary embolism: a multicenter study. *JAMA.* 2001;285:761–768.

11. Verschuren F, Liistro G, Coffeng R, et al. Volumetric capnography as a screening test for pulmonary embolism in the emergency department. *Chest.* 2004;125:841–850.

12. Verschuren F, Heinonen E, Clause D, et al. Volumetric capnography as a bedside monitoring of thrombolysis in major pulmonary embolism. *Intensive Care Med.* 2004;30:2129–2132.

13. Lee AJ, Cohn JH, Ranasinghe JS. Cardiac output assessed by invasive and minimally invasive techniques. *Anesthesiol Res Pract.* 2011;2011:475151.

14. Peyton PJ, Chong SW. Minimally invasive measurement of cardiac output during surgery and critical care: a meta-analysis of accuracy and precision. *Anesthesiology.* 2010;113:1220–1235.

15. Eberhard P. The design, use, and results of transcutaneous carbon dioxide analysis: current and future directions. *Anesth Analg.* 2007;105:S48–S52.

16. Lee SK, Kim DH, Choi WA, et al. The significance of transcutaneous continuous overnight CO_2 monitoring in determining initial mechanical ventilator application for patients with neuromuscular disease. *Ann Rehabil Med.* 2012;36:126–132.

17. Storre JH, Magnet FS, Dreher M, et al. Transcutaneous monitoring as a replacement for arterial PCO_2 monitoring during nocturnal non-invasive ventilation. *Respir Med.* 2011;105:143–150.

18. Gattinoni L, Brazzi L, Pelosi P, et al. A trial of goal-oriented hemodynamic therapy in critically ill patients. SVO_2 collaborative group. *N Engl J Med.* 1995;333:1025–1032.

19. Pearse R, Dawson D, Fawcett J, et al. Early goal-directed therapy after major surgery reduces complications and duration of hospital stay. A randomised, controlled trial [isrctn38797445]. *Crit Care.* 2005;9:R687–R693.

20. Pearse R, Dawson D, Fawcett J, et al. Changes in central venous saturation after major surgery, and association with outcome. *Crit Care.* 2005;9:R694–R699.

21. van Beest P, Wietasch G, Scheeren T, et al. Clinical review: use of venous oxygen saturations as a goal—a yet unfinished puzzle. *Crit Care.* 2011;15:232.

22. Teixeira C, da Silva NB, Savi A, et al. Central venous saturation is a predictor of reintubation in difficult-to-wean patients. *Crit Care Med.* 2010;38:491–496.

23. Marini JJ. Dynamic hyperinflation and auto-positive end-expiratory pressure: lessons learned over 30 years. *Am J Respir Crit Care Med.* 2011;184:756–762.

24. Gattinoni L, Pesenti A, Avalli L, et al. Pressure-volume curve of total respiratory system in acute respiratory failure. Computed tomographic scan study. *Am Rev Respir Dis.* 1987;136:730–736.

25. Amato MB, Barbas CS, Medeiros DM, et al. Effect of a protective-ventilation strategy on mortality in the acute respiratory distress syndrome. *N Engl J Med.* 1998;338:347–354.

26. Brochard L, Martin GS, Blanch L, et al. Clinical review: respiratory monitoring in the ICU - a consensus of 16. *Crit Care.* 2012;16:219.

27. Carvalho AR, Pacheco SA, de Souza Rocha PV, et al. Detection of tidal recruitment/overdistension in lung-healthy mechanically ventilated patients under general anesthesia. *Anesth Analg.* 2013;116:677–684.

28. Bersten AD. Measurement of overinflation by multiple linear regression analysis in patients with acute lung injury. *Eur Respir J.* 1998;12:526–532.

29. Ball L, Sutherasan Y, Pelosi P. Monitoring respiration: what the clinician needs to know. *Best Pract Res Clin Anaesthesiol.* 2013;27:209–223.

30. Grasso S, Terragni P, Mascia L, et al. Airway pressure-time curve profile (stress index) detects tidal recruitment/hyperinflation in experimental acute lung injury. *Crit Care Med.* 2004;32:1018–1027.

31. Carvalho AR, Spieth PM, Pelosi P, et al. Ability of dynamic airway pressure curve profile and elastance for positive end-expiratory pressure titration. *Intensive Care Med.* 2008;34:2291–2299.

32. Formenti P, Graf J, Santos A, et al. Non-pulmonary factors strongly influence the stress index. *Intensive Care Med.* 2011;37:594–600.

33. Akoumianaki E, Maggiore SM, Valenza F, et al. The application of esophageal pressure measurement in patients with respiratory failure. *Am J Respir Crit Care Med.* 2014;189:520–531.

34. Cortes GA, Marini JJ. Two steps forward in bedside monitoring of lung mechanics: transpulmonary pressure and lung volume. *Crit Care.* 2013;17:219.

35. Pelosi P, Goldner M, McKibben A, et al. Recruitment and derecruitment during acute respiratory failure: an experimental study. *Am J Respir Crit Care Med.* 2001;164:122–130.

36. Owens RL, Campana LM, Hess L, et al. Sitting and supine esophageal pressures in overweight and obese subjects. *Obesity (Silver Spring).* 2012;20:2354–2360.

37. Talmor D, Sarge T, Malhotra A, et al. Mechanical ventilation guided by esophageal pressure in acute lung injury. *N Engl J Med.* 2008;359:2095–2104.

38. Staffieri F, Stripoli T, De Monte V, et al. Physiological effects of an open lung ventilatory strategy titrated on elastance-derived end-inspiratory transpulmonary pressure: study in a pig model. *Crit Care Med.* 2012;40:2124–2131.

39. Vidal MG, Ruiz Weisser J, Gonzalez F, et al. Incidence and clinical effects of intra-abdominal hypertension in critically ill patients. *Crit Care Med.* 2008;36:1823–1831.

40. Malbrain ML, Chiumello D, Pelosi P, et al. Incidence and prognosis of intraabdominal hypertension in a mixed population of critically ill patients: a multiple-center epidemiological study. *Crit Care Med.* 2005;33:315–322.

41. Krebs J, Pelosi P, Tsagogiorgas C, et al. Effects of positive end-expiratory pressure on respiratory function and hemodynamics in patients with acute respiratory failure with and without intra-abdominal hypertension: a pilot study. *Crit Care.* 2009;13:R160.

42. Gattinoni L, Pelosi P, Suter PM, et al. Acute respiratory distress syndrome caused by pulmonary and extrapulmonary disease. Different syndromes? *Am J Respir Crit Care Med.* 1998;158:3–11.

43. Pelosi P, Croci M, Ravagnan I, et al. The effects of body mass on lung volumes, respiratory mechanics, and gas exchange during general anesthesia. *Anesth Analg.* 1998;87:654–660.

44. Pelosi P, Ravagnan I, Giurati G, et al. Positive end-expiratory pressure improves respiratory function in obese but not in normal subjects during anesthesia and paralysis. *Anesthesiology.* 1999;91:1221–1231.

45. Anzueto A, Frutos-Vivar F, Esteban A, et al. Influence of body mass index on outcome of the mechanically ventilated patients. *Thorax.* 2011;66:66–73.

46. Krieger BP, Isber J, Breitenbucher A, et al. Serial measurements of the rapid-shallow-breathing index as a predictor of weaning outcome in elderly medical patients. *Chest.* 1997;112:1029–1034.

47. Jubran A, Grant BJ, Laghi F, et al. Weaning prediction: esophageal pressure monitoring complements readiness testing. *Am J Respir Crit Care Med.* 2005;171:1252–1259.

48. Sassoon CS, Te TT, Mahutte CK, et al. Airway occlusion pressure. An important indicator for successful weaning in patients with chronic obstructive pulmonary disease. *Am Rev Respir Dis.* 1987;135:107–113.

49. Perrigault PF, Pouzeratte YH, Jaber S, et al. Changes in occlusion pressure (p0.1) and breathing pattern during pressure support ventilation. *Thorax.* 1999;54:119–123.

50. Capdevila XJ, Perrigault PF, Perey PJ, et al. Occlusion pressure and its ratio to maximum inspiratory pressure are useful predictors for successful extubation following t-piece weaning trial. *Chest*. 1995;108:482–489.
51. Thille AW, Rodriguez P, Cabello B, et al. Patient-ventilator asynchrony during assisted mechanical ventilation. *Intensive Care Med*. 2006;32:1515–1522.
52. Gutierrez G, Ballarino GJ, Turkan H, et al. Automatic detection of patient-ventilator asynchrony by spectral analysis of airway flow. *Crit Care*. 2011;15:R167.
53. Nilsestuen JO, Hargett KD. Using ventilator graphics to identify patient-ventilator asynchrony. *Respir Care*. 2005;50:202–234. discussion 232–204.
54. Jain M, Sznajder JI. Peripheral airways injury in acute lung injury/acute respiratory distress syndrome. *Curr Opin Crit Care*. 2008;14:37–43.
55. Akoumianaki E, Lyazidi A, Rey N, et al. Mechanical ventilation-induced reverse-triggered breaths: a frequently unrecognized form of neuromechanical coupling. *Chest*. 2013;143:927–938.
56. Bikker IG, van Bommel J, Reis Miranda D, et al. End-expiratory lung volume during mechanical ventilation: a comparison with reference values and the effect of positive end-expiratory pressure in intensive care unit patients with different lung conditions. *Crit Care*. 2008;12:R145.
57. Olegard C, Sondergaard S, Houltz E, et al. Estimation of functional residual capacity at the bedside using standard monitoring equipment: a modified nitrogen washout/washin technique requiring a small change of the inspired oxygen fraction. *Anesth Analg*. 2005;101:206–212.
58. Chiumello D, Cressoni M, Chierichetti M, et al. Nitrogen washout/washin, helium dilution and computed tomography in the assessment of end expiratory lung volume. *Crit Care*. 2008;12:R150.
59. Patroniti N, Saini M, Zanella A, et al. Measurement of end-expiratory lung volume by oxygen washin-washout in controlled and assisted mechanically ventilated patients. *Intensive Care Med*. 2008;34:2235–2240.
60. Sakka SG, Klein M, Reinhart K, et al. Prognostic value of extravascular lung water in critically ill patients. *Chest*. 2002;122:2080–2086.
61. Berkowitz DM, Danai PA, Eaton S, et al. Accurate characterization of extravascular lung water in acute respiratory distress syndrome. *Crit Care Med*. 2008;36:1803–1809.
62. Sakka SG, Ruhl CC, Pfeiffer UJ, et al. Assessment of cardiac preload and extravascular lung water by single transpulmonary thermodilution. *Intensive Care Med*. 2000;26:180–187.
63. Volpicelli G, Skurzak S, Boero E, et al. Lung ultrasound predicts well extravascular lung water but is of limited usefulness in the prediction of wedge pressure. *Anesthesiology*. 2014;121:320–327.
64. Corradi F, Ball L, Brusasco C, et al. Assessment of extravascular lung water by quantitative ultrasound and ct in isolated bovine lung. *Respir Physiol Neurobiol*. 2013;187:244–249.
65. Bellani G, Mauri T, Pesenti A. Imaging in acute lung injury and acute respiratory distress syndrome. *Curr Opin Crit Care*. 2012;18:29–34.
66. Gattinoni L, Caironi P, Cressoni M, et al. Lung recruitment in patients with the acute respiratory distress syndrome. *N Engl J Med*. 2006;354:1775–1786.
67. Gattinoni L, Caironi P. Refining ventilatory treatment for acute lung injury and acute respiratory distress syndrome. *JAMA*. 2008;299:691–693.
68. Luecke T, Corradi F, Pelosi P. Lung imaging for titration of mechanical ventilation. *Currt Opin Anaesthiol*. 2012;25:131–140.
69. Bouhemad B, Brisson H, Le-Guen M, et al. Bedside ultrasound assessment of positive end-expiratory pressure-induced lung recruitment. *Am J Respir Crit Care Med*. 2011;183:341–347.
70. Via G, Lichtenstein D, Mojoli F, et al. Whole lung lavage: A unique model for ultrasound assessment of lung aeration changes. *Intensive Care Med*. 2010;36:999–1007.
71. Trezzi M, Torzillo D, Ceriani E, et al. Lung ultrasonography for the assessment of rapid extravascular water variation: Evidence from hemodialysis patients. *Intern Emerg Med*. 2013;8:409–415.
72. Liteplo AS, Murray AF, Kimberly HH, et al. Real-time resolution of sonographic b-lines in a patient with pulmonary edema on continuous positive airway pressure. *Am J Emerg Med*. 2010;28(541):e545–548.
73. Soummer A, Perbet S, Brisson H, et al. Ultrasound assessment of lung aeration loss during a successful weaning trial predicts postextubation distress. *Crit Care Med*. 2012;40:2064–2072.
74. Riera J, Riu PJ, Casan P, et al. Electrical impedance tomography in acute lung injury. *Med Intensiva*. 2011;35:509–517.
75. Wolf GK, Gomez-Laberge C, Rettig JS, et al. Mechanical ventilation guided by electrical impedance tomography in experimental acute lung injury. *Crit Care Med*. 2013;41:1296–1304.

9 What Is the Optimal Approach to Weaning and Liberation from Mechanical Ventilation?

Alistair Nichol, Stephen Duff, Ville Pettila, David J. Cooper

"Weaning" refers to the transition from full mechanical ventilatory support to spontaneous ventilation with minimal support. "Liberation" refers to discontinuation of mechanical ventilation.[1] This chapter focuses on the clinical assessment of readiness to wean, the technique for conducting a spontaneous breathing trial (SBT), and the assessment of readiness of extubation. In addition, we will review the evidence supporting various ventilator strategies in the difficult-to-wean patient.

Mechanically ventilated intensive care patients may be classified as simple to wean, difficult to wean, or prolonged weaning.[2,3] Simple-to-wean patients are extubated on the first attempt, make up the vast majority of the patients in the intensive care unit (ICU; ~69%), and have a low mortality rate (~5%).[4,5] The remaining cohort of difficult-to-wean (requiring up to three attempts or up to 7 days from the onset of weaning) or prolonged-wean (over three attempts or greater than 7 days from the onset of weaning) patients require greater effort to successfully liberate from mechanical ventilation. These difficult-to-wean and prolonged-wean patients have an associated higher mortality rate (~25%).[4,5]

Prolonged mechanical ventilation is associated with increased mortality[6] and costs (mechanical ventilation costs > U.S. $2000/day).[7] It has been estimated that the 6% of patients who require prolonged mechanical ventilation consume 37% of ICU resources,[8] and 40% to 50% of the time spent undergoing mechanical ventilation occurs after this weaning process has started.[4,6,9] In part, the reason is that more severely ill patients usually require longer periods of mechanical ventilation. Prolonged weaning may result, though, from an excessive use of sedatives, the absence of weaning-liberation protocols, and myriad of organizational and cultural factors that fail to optimize weaning conditions. In general, the duration of mechanical ventilation should be minimized, and liberation from mechanical ventilation should be considered as soon as possible.

Expert consensus[2] has proposed that the weaning process be considered in the following six steps:

1. Treatment of acute respiratory failure
2. Clinical judgment that weaning may be possible
3. Assessment of the readiness to wean
4. An SBT
5. Extubation
6. Possibly re-intubation

Depending on the mechanism of acute respiratory failure—whether it is a problem of oxygenation, ventilation, or airway (or a combination)—most critically ill patients require a period in which they will require full ventilatory support after intubation. Consideration of the weaning process should begin very soon after intubation. Weaning involves several discrete logical and sequential steps. If patients fail to make sufficient progress, then a contingency plan is required. Failure to wean/liberate involves either (1) the failure of an SBT or (2) the need for re-intubation/ventilation or death within 48 hours of extubation.[2]

CLINICAL SUSPICION THAT WEANING MAY BE POSSIBLE

Because of the significant morbidity and mortality associated with prolonged mechanical ventilation, it is generally accepted that all ventilated ICU patients should be assessed for their readiness to wean at least on a daily basis. The importance of this "readiness" assessment has been highlighted by several trials that have demonstrated that weaning can be achieved in most patients after the first formal assessment of readiness[10,11] and the finding that nearly 50% of unexpected self-extubations during the weaning process did not require re-intubation.[12,13] The benefit of early weaning should be balanced against the significant morbidity and mortality associated with failed extubation. Two large prospective observational studies found a fivefold to tenfold increased mortality in patients requiring re-intubation.[13,14] It is unclear, though, how much of this effect is confounded by population and disease severity differences.[14]

ASSESSMENT OF READINESS TO WEAN

The clinical assessment of readiness to wean is a two-step process that is based on (1) the assessment of predictors of weaning and (2) the successful completion of an SBT. Both of these steps require a reliable and reproducible institutional sedation strategy that maximizes the patient's capability of being assessed and undergoing SBTs. Ventilator liberation protocols should be developed, locally, in concert with analgesia protocols.[15,16] The concept of nocturnal rest, in conjunction with daytime respiratory muscle training, is an important one for those patients whose weaning is more difficult and prolonged.

Predictors of Successful Weaning

The initial screening evaluation of readiness to wean is composed of a clinical examination and an assessment of several objective criteria (respiratory, cardiovascular, and neurologic) that aim to predict the likelihood of successfully weaning[4,5,9-11,17,18] (Table 9-1). Individually, these predictors are neither highly sensitive nor specific, but together with the clinical examination they allow the clinician to identify patients who will clearly not be suitable for weaning and who may have detrimental effects from aggressive reduction in ventilatory support. All other patients should undergo a SBT. This is an important point because (1) many patients who meet some but not all of the criteria for weaning will still successfully wean and (2) clinicians frequently underestimate the ability of patients to wean.

Individual Limitations of the Readiness-to-Wean Predictors

It is important to be aware of the individual limitations of these prediction criteria because many have been examined only retrospectively, and of those who have been studied prospectively, many have demonstrated high false-positive and false-negative rates.

A minute ventilation less than 10 L/min is only associated with a positive predictive value of 50% and a negative predictive value of 40%.[19] The *maximal inspiratory pressure*, a measure of respiratory muscle strength, was initially suggested to be a good indicator of weaning success.[20] These findings were not replicated in subsequent trials.

Static compliance (i.e., tidal volume/plateau pressure–positive end expiratory pressure) has a low positive predictive value (60%) and negative predictive value (53%).[19] *Occlusion pressure* (P0.1) is the airway pressure 0.1 second after the initiation of a spontaneous breath in a measure of respiratory drive. The results from studies determining the utility of this index have been conflicting to date.[21-23]

A reduction in central venous saturation of more than 4.5% at the thirtieth minute of an SBT in patients who had failed their first T-tube SBT was an independent predictor of re-intubation, with a sensitivity of 88% and a specificity of 95%.[24] A previous study showed that on discontinuation of the ventilator, mixed venous oxygen saturation fell progressively in the failure group ($P = .01$) whereas it did not change in the success group.[25]

A low left ventricular ejection fraction (LVEF) (36% [27 to 55] vs. 51% [43 to 55], $P = .04$), shortened deceleration time of E wave (DTE), and increased Doppler E velocity to tissue Doppler E' velocity ratio (E/E') assessed by transoesophageal echocardiography with an experienced operator were predictive of extubation failure in a prospective observational study.[26] Given the expense and limited availability of expert transthoracic echocardiogram (TTE), though, we

recommend that evidence of benefit of TTE-guided interventions should be available before its introduction into routine clinical practice.

B-type natriuretic peptide (BNP) and N-terminal pro-BNP levels either at baseline[27] or the relative change during an SBT[28-30] have been associated with extubation failure due to heart failure. There was significant heterogeneity, though, between results, which may be explained by the different populations studied, fluid balance, the use of cardioactive drugs, and underlying cardiovascular or renal dysfunction.

The rapid shallow breathing index (RSBI) (respiratory rate/tidal volume) measured over 1 minute in the spontaneously breathing patient has demonstrated a high sensitivity (97%) and a moderate specificity (65%) for predicting patients who will subsequently successfully pass an SBT

Table 9-1 **Clinical and Objective Measures of Readiness to Wean**

Clinical assessment	Resolution of acute process requiring Intubation/ventilation
	Patient awake and cooperative
	Chest wall pain controlled
	Adequate cough
	Absence of excessive tracheobronchial secretions
	Absence of
	    Nasal flaring
	    Suprasternal and intercostal recession
	    Paradoxical movement of the rib cage or abdomen

Objective measures	Respiratory stability: Oxygenation
	  SaO_2 >90% on FIO_2 ≤0.4
	  PaO_2 ≥ 50-60 mm Hg on FIO_2 ≤0.5
	  Alveolar-arterial PO_2 gradient <350 mm Hg (FIO_2 1.0)
	  PaO_2/FIO_2 ≥150
	Respiratory stability: Function
	  Respiratory rate ≤35 breath/min^{-1}
	  Maximal inspiratory pressure ≤ −20 to −25 cm H_2O
	  Tidal volume > 5 mL/kg^{-1}
	  Minute ventilation <10 L/min^{-1}
	  No significant respiratory acidosis
	  Respiratory rate/tidal volume <105 breath/min^{-1}/L^{-1} *
	  CROP index >13 mL/breath/min^{-1}†
	  Integrative index of Jabour <4 per minute^{-1}‡
	  IWI of ≥25 mL/cm H_2O breaths/min^{-1}/L^{-1}§
	Cardiovascular stability
	  Heart rate <140 beats/min^{-1}
	  Systolic blood pressure >90 and <160 mm Hg
	  Minimal inotropic/vasopressor support
	Neurologic function
	  Including normal mentation on sedation

*The respiratory rate/tidal volume ratio is also known as the RSBI.
†CROP index = [compliance (dynamic) × maximum inspiratory pressure × (arterial partial pressure of oxygen/alveolar partial pressure of oxygen)]/respiratory rate.
‡Integrative index of Jabour = pressure time product × (minute ventilation to bring the $PaCO_2$ to 40 mm Hg/tidal volume during spontaneous breathing).
§IWI = (compliance (static) × arterial oxygen saturation/(respiratory rate/tidal volume during spontaneous breathing).
CROP, Compliance, Respiratory rate, arterial Oxygenation and maximal inspiratory Pressure; *FIO₂*, fracture of inspired oxygen; *IWI*, integrative weaning index; *PaO₂*, partial pressure of arterial oxygen; *PO₂*, partial pressure of oxygen; *RSBI*, rapid shallow breathing index; *SaO₂*, arterial oxygen saturation.

compared with the other predictors.[19] The measurement of RSBI value may be affected by the airway pressure protocol. In prospective studies, RSBI values were significantly lower in patients while they were on a continuous positive airway pressure (CPAP) of 5 cm H_2O compared with T-piece (median 71 vs. 90 breaths/L/min)[31] or a spontaneously breathing room air trial without ventilator support (median 36 vs. 71 breaths/L/min).[32]

The trend rather than an individual value of RSBI may be a better predictor of weaning success. RSBI remained unchanged or decreased in successful extubation; in contrast, RSBI tended to increase in those who failed extubation in three prospective observational studies.[31,33-35] Although many clinicians use RSBI in their clinical practice, there is some controversy to its utility: one small randomized controlled trial (RCT) reported that the use of this measure prolonged weaning time and did not reduce the incidence of extubation failure or tracheostomy.[36] This trial was small, though, and there was a high likelihood of selection bias and crossover in the non-RSBI utilization arm. Results from another RCT suggested that the predictive value of RSBI may be increased using automatic tube compensation (ATC).[37]

Overall, individual "predictor" criteria should not be considered as reliable indicators to predict successful weaning. When combined with the clinical examination, though, they may assist the clinician to identify patients who will clearly *not* be suitable for weaning and who may have detrimental effects from an unnecessary SBT.

The failure of these individual indices to predict successful weaning prompted the authors to combine several individual indices in an attempt to increase specificity and sensitivity. However, these predictors (Table 9-1) are more complex and are more commonly used in clinical trials than in routine clinical practice.

A *Compliance, Respiratory rate, arterial Oxygenation and maximal inspiratory Pressure (CROP) index* (see Table 9-1) more than 13 mL/breath/min has prospectively determined a positive predictive value of 71% and a negative predictive value of 70% to predict weaning success.[19] A *Jabour pressure time product* (see Table 9-1) less than 4 per minute has been shown in a retrospective study to have a positive predictive value of 96% and a negative predictive value of 95%.[38]

An *integrative weaning index (IWI)* (see Table 9-1) of 25 mL/cm H_2O breaths/min/L or more has been shown in a prospective study to have a positive predictive value of 0.99 and a negative predictive value of 0.86 to predict weaning success ($n = 216$ in the prospective-validation group).[39] Future research is required to identify simple predictors that are sufficiently sensitive and specific to predict successful weaning. In the absence of such measures, the clinician should have a low threshold for conducting a daily SBT.

Spontaneous Breathing Trial

The initiation of the weaning process is defined as the commencement of the first SBT. There are several techniques that can be used to conduct an SBT. These include techniques such as (1) T-tube/T-piece, (2) pressure support ventilation (PSV), or (3) ATC, all of which may be

Table 9-2 **Clinical and Objective Determinants of Failure of an SBT**	

Clinical assessment	Agitation and anxiety
	Reduced level of consciousness
	Significant sweating
	Cyanosis
	Evidence of increased respiratory muscle effort
	  Increased accessory muscle usage
	  Facial signs of distress
	  Dyspnea

Objective measures	Respiratory stability: Oxygenation
	  Pao$_2$ ≤50-60 mm Hg on Fio$_2$ ≥0.5 or Sao$_2$ <90%
	Respiratory stability: Function
	  Paco$_2$ >50 mm Hg or an increase in Paco$_2$ >8 mm Hg
	  pH < 7.32 or a decrease of pH ≥ 0.07 pH units
	  Respiratory rate/tidal volume >105 breath/min^{-1}/L^{-1}*
	  Respiratory rate >35 breath/min^{-1} or increase ≥50%
	Cardiovascular stability
	  Heart rate >140 beats/min^{-1} (or increase ≥20%)
	  Systolic blood pressure >180 mm Hg (or increase ≥20%)
	  Systolic blood pressure <90 mm Hg
	  Significant cardiac arrhythmias
	Neurologic function
	  Reduced level of consciousness

*The respiratory rate/tidal volume is also known as the RSBI.
*F*io$_2$, fracture of inspired oxygen; *Paco$_2$*, partial pressure of arterial oxygen; *Pao$_2$*, partial pressure of arterial oxygen; *RSBI*, rapid shallow breathing index; *Sao$_2$*, arterial oxygen saturation; *SBT*, spontaneous breathing trial.

used with or without CPAP. Failure of an SBT is defined as the development of respiratory (function or oxygenation), cardiovascular, or neurological instability and is determined by clinical assessment and objective testing during the trial (Table 9-2).* There appears to be little predictive advantage by increasing the duration of the SBT assessment to greater than 20 to 30 minutes.[5,42] Prospective studies have demonstrated that most patients successfully pass their first SBTs and more than 60% of patients successfully wean[†] (Table 9-3). Interestingly, to date, trials have not demonstrated that any one of these techniques is superior in its ability to predict weaning success (Table 9-3). Clinicians still need to be aware of the relative advantages and disadvantages of each technique, though.

T-Tube/T-piece: This well-established method involves attaching the end of the endotracheal tube to a short piece of tubing that acts as a reservoir and a connection to the humidified fresh gas flow. There were initial concerns that the increased resistance to airflow and the increased work of breathing induced by the endotracheal tube resulted in a workload in excess of that required when the tube was removed. These studies, though, did not account for the airway inflammation and edema that frequently accompanies extubation, which results in little difference between the preextubation and postextubation workload.[45,46] Therefore many clinicians use this method because it is simple,

---

*References 2, 10, 11, 19, 40, 41.
†References 5, 10, 11, 17, 37, 43, 44.

Table 9-3 **Success of SBT and Success in Weaning from Mechanical Ventilation**

Author	Year	Number	Passed Initial SBT	Extubated at 48 hr (From All Extubated)	Method
TRIALS DESCRIBING SUCCESS RATE OF INITIAL SBT AND EXTUBATION					
Brochard	1994	456	347 (76%)	330(95%)	T-piece
Esteban	1995	546	416 (76%)	358 (86%)	T-piece
Vallverdu	1998	217	148 (68%)	125 (84%)	T-piece
Esteban	1999	526	416 (79%)	346(82%)	T-piece
TRIALS DESCRIBING SUCCESS RATE OF INITIAL SBT AND EXTUBATION WITH DIFFERING TECHNIQUES					
Esteban	1997	484	397(82%)	323(81%)	PSV/T-piece
Subgroup		236	205(86%)	167 (81%)	PSV 7 cm H_2O
Subgroup		246	192(78%)	156 (81%)	T-piece
Farias	2001	257	201 (78%)	173(86%)	PSV/T-piece
Subgroup		125	99 (79%)	79 (80%)	PSV 10 cm H_2O
Subgroup		132	102(77%)	89 (87%)	T-piece
Haberthur*	2002	90	78 (87%)	62 (79%)	ATC/PSV/T-piece
Subgroup		30	29(96%)	25 (86%)	ATC
Subgroup		30	23(77%)	18 (78%)	PSV 5 cm H_2O
Subgroup		30	24(80%)	19 (79%)	T-piece
Matić	2004	260	200 (77%)	Not specified	PSV/T-piece
Subgroup		110	80 (73%)	Not specified	T-piece
Subgroup		150	120 (80%)	Not specified	PSV
Cohen	2006	99	90 (91%)	73 (74%)	ATC/CPAP
Subgroup		51	49 (96%)	42 (82%)	ATC
Subgroup		48	41 (85%)	31 (65%)	CPAP
Cohen	2009	190	161(85%)	139(86%)	ATC/PSV
Subgroup		87	81(93%)	71(88%)	ATC
Subgroup		93	80(86%)	68(85%)	PSV
Figueroa-Casas	2010	118	108 (92%)	115 (97%)	ATC/CPAP
Subgroup		58	56 (97%)	57 (99%)	ATC
Subgroup		60	52 (87%)	58 (97%)	CPAP

* Some patients initially randomized to the T-piece/PSV groups who failed an SBT were subsequently extubated after an ATC trial.
ATC, automatic tube compensation; *CPAP*, continuous positive airway pressure; *PSV*, pressure support ventilation; *SBT*, spontaneous breathing trial.

well tested, and imposes a pulmonary workload that is comparable to that encountered after extubation.

Pressure support ventilation (PSV): PSV is becoming more common for conducting the SBT. Despite the theoretical concerns that (1) the use of PSV may not mimic the "true" postextubation workload and (2) the difficulty predicting the level of PSV necessary to completely compensate for the resistive load,[47] this does not appear problematic in practice.[9,44,48] Pressure support is typically reduced to relatively low levels (≤10 cm H_2O) so that most of its impact is dissipated because of tube resistance and the patient experiences no elevation in inspiratory pressure at the end of the endotracheal tube.[9,43,44,48] The major advantage of this technique over the T-piece is that it does not require disconnection from the ventilator, and apnea alarms and pressure monitors remain in place.

Automatic tube compensation (ATC): ATC is an automatic method by which the ventilator compensates for the degree of resistance provided by the endotracheal tube that is increasingly found on modern ventilators. Because tube resistance varies with length, girth, and secretions, this is theoretically advantageous, but literature is limited. Haberthur and colleagues reported that ATC was as effective as PSV or T-piece weaning.[44] This result was subsequently confirmed by a larger RCT comparing PSV with ATC in 190 patients.[37] Figueroa-Casas and colleagues compared ATC with CPAP during SBT.[49] There was no difference in duration of weaning, rate of unsuccessful extubation, or duration of mechanical ventilation. A bench study showed that ATC may not sufficiently compensate for the pressure-time product increase caused by tracheal secretions and higher tidal volume.[50] Because low-level PSV achieves the same goals and because most weaning patients receive some PSV either alone or in conjunction with another ventilatory mode, the potential for ATC to add any clinically relevant benefit during weaning is questionable.

Continuous positive airway pressure (CPAP): Proponents of CPAP argue that it increases functional residual capacity, maintains small airway patency, may be beneficial on left ventricular dysfunction, and has minimal harmful effects.[51] Despite the potential risk that a patient may pass the SBT but experience cardiac failure on extubation, most clinicians are comfortable using low levels of CPAP (<5 cm H_2O) in combination with the techniques mentioned earlier.

Automated weaning: Systems aim to reduce the requirement for clinician input in the weaning process and improve outcomes. The most commonly studied systems are SmartCare and Adaptive Support Ventilation (ASV).[52] ASV can automatically switch from controlled to spontaneous ventilation, but SmartCare requires clinician input to initiate this. However, SmartCare can automatically reduce pressure support based on patient demographic and ventilator feedback parameters. It will provide the patient with SBT and recommend consideration of extubation when it considers an SBT successful.

A Cochrane meta-analysis compared SmartCare with usual care and found a trend toward decreased weaning time, time to successful extubation, and length of ICU stay.[53] There were many limitations to this analysis, though. There was substantial unexplained heterogeneity ($I^2 = 68\%$), and only three of the trials included reached full recruitment. There was no reduction in time to first SBT, mortality, or adverse events, including re-intubation. Three trials used SIMV (synchronized intermittent mechanical ventilation) as a control arm—a mode known to prolong mechanical ventilation.[10,11] In the subgroup analysis, there was a greater reduction in weaning time in trials that used protocolized weaning as the control arm, suggesting that these protocols may have used more conservative criteria as opposed to expert clinician judgment. Large RCTs are needed to address these limitations before automated weaning systems should be routinely used.

SUITABILITY FOR EXTUBATION

Extubation is the final stage in successful liberation of a patient from the mechanical ventilator, but it would be unwise to extubate any patient before assessing the ability of the patient to protect and maintain a patent airway. This clinical assessment involves (1) testing for adequate level of consciousness, (2) cough strength, (3) frequency of secretions, and (4) airway patency. The likelihood of undergoing a successful extubation is significantly higher if the Glasgow Coma Score is 8 or greater.[54] In addition, although there are several objective measures of cough strength (e.g., card moistening[55] and spirometry[56]), most clinicians subjectively determine the presence of a moderate to strong cough before extubation. The presence of a weak cough, measured as a cough peak flow of 60 L/min or less, is a strong independent risk factor for extubation failure.[56-58] It is important to evaluate the volume and thickness of

secretions because the likelihood of weaning success decreases with increased secretions and reduced suctioning intervals.[18,55] Poor cough strength and greater secretions may have synergistic effects, reducing the chances of extubation success in burn and medical ICU patients.[57]

The most common test for airway patency is determination of a "cuff leak," which is neither sensitive nor specific. The presence of a "leak" after deflation of the endotracheal tube cuff is reassuring; however, the absence of a leak does not predict extubation failure.[59,60] It is unclear whether the absence of a leak predicts laryngeal edema and whether pretreatment in this scenario with corticosteroids is effective. A double-blind multicenter trial of 761 adults considered at high risk for postextubation laryngeal edema (ventilated >36 hours), were pretreated and posttreated with methylprednisolone 12 hours before and every 4 hours after planned extubation. Corticosteroid therapy reduced the incident of reintubation by 4% and laryngeal edema by 11%.[61]

VENTILATOR MANAGEMENT OF THE DIFFICULT-TO-WEAN PATIENT

The difficult-to-wean patient has already failed at least one SBT or required reintubation within 48 hours of extubation. The failure of an SBT may be accompanied by significantly increased inspiratory effort,[40] which translates to increased respiratory muscle workload.[62] This extra burden does not appear to cause long-lasting (low frequency) fatigue, but it is uncertain whether it may induce short-lasting (high frequency) fatigue.[40] Therefore after the failure of either an SBT or trial of extubation, the clinician must (1) determine the presence of exacerbating factors that reduced the success of weaning[2,63] (Table 9-4) and (2) provide ventilatory management to balance the need for adequate ventilator support (minimizing respiratory fatigue) against the need to minimize support (increase patient respiratory autonomy) to improve the chances of subsequent successful weaning.

The clinician should conduct a careful physical examination and review the patient's diagnostic tests to uncover and treat any reversible contributory factors (Table 9-4). In the absence of any obvious remedial conditions or while such conditions are being treated, the patient should "rest" on the ventilator. The most commonly used modes of ventilation are assist-control mechanical ventilation (ACV), SIMV, and PSV.

Assist-control mechanical ventilation (ACV): ACV is widely used to rest the respiratory muscles after the increased pulmonary workload during a failed weaning attempt. The diaphragm, in failure-to-wean patients, though, does not demonstrate that low-frequency muscle fatigue[41] and even short periods of ACV may induce diaphragm dysfunction and injury.[64] Weaning techniques that include respiratory muscle exercise are required to minimize respiratory muscle atrophy and dysfunction.

Synchronised intermittent mechanical ventilation (SIMV): The use of SIMV as a weaning tool involves a progressive reduction of the mechanical ventilator respiratory rate in steps of 1 to 3 breath/min, and 30 to 60 minutes later the patient is assessed for signs of failure to adapt to the

Table 9-4 **Assessment of Factors that Reduce the Success of Weaning**	
Respiratory	Increased restrictive load: bronchospasm, tube kinking, tube obstruction Increased chest wall elastic load: pleural effusion, pneumothorax, abdominal distension Increase lung elastic load: infection, edema, hyperinflation
Cardiovascular	Cardiac dysfunction either long standing or secondary to increased load
Neuromuscular	Depressed central drive: metabolic alkalosis, sedatives analgesics Neural transmission: spinal cord injury, Gullain-Bárre syndrome, myasthenia gravis, phrenic nerve injury Peripheral dysfunction: critical illness neuropathy and myopathy
Neurophysiologic	Delirium Depression Anxiety
Metabolic	Hypophosphatemia Hypomagnesemia Hypokalemia Hyperglycemia Steroid use—controversial
Nutrition	Obesity Malnutrition Overfeeding
Anemia	Hemoglobin 7.0-10.0 g/dL

increased patient load (similar to failure of breathing trial criteria; Table 9-2). Accumulated evidence suggests that SIMV is a suboptimal weaning mode.

SIMV involves three different types of breath: a volume- or pressure-controlled breath, volume- or pressure-assisted breath, and a spontaneous breath that is usually pressure supported. SIMV may contribute to respiratory muscle fatigue or prevent recovery from fatigue[11] secondary to an increased work of breathing associated with patient-ventilator dysynchrony, increased effort to activate the SIMV demand valve, inadequate gas flow,[65,66] or the inability of the respiratory center to coordinate with the intermittent nature of the support and different types of breath.[62]

A 457-patient RCT demonstrated that SIMV (with T-piece SBTs) resulted in a slightly longer duration of mechanical ventilation (9.9 ± 8.2 days) compared with a PSV strategy (9.7 ± 3.7 days).[10] This trial also found that SIMV had higher rates of weaning failure (SIMV, 42%; PSV, 23%; T-piece, 43%).[10] Esteban and colleagues looked at four different weaning approaches involving 546 patients, and they reported that a SIMV-based weaning strategy resulted in longer duration of mechanical ventilation (5 days) compared with a PSV-based strategy (4 days) and T-piece ventilation (3 days).[11]

Pressure support ventilation (PSV): PSV allows the patient to determine the depth, length, flow, and rate of breathing.[67] PSV can be used for SBTs (typically ≤ 10 cm H_2O) or,

less effectively, as a weaning tool involving the gradual reduction of pressure support by 2 to 4 cm H_2O once or twice a day as tolerated. This method results in a progressive reduction in ventilatory support over hours to days. Two large RCTs have demonstrated that PSV is superior to SIMV in reducing the duration of mechanical ventilation of difficult-to-wean patients.[10,11] Although one of these trials demonstrated that PSV weaning was more efficient than T-piece weaning,[10] the other trial demonstrated T-piece trials to be superior.[11] These potentially contradictory results may be accounted for by differences in the trial weaning protocols, though. One small, prospective RCT has suggested that pressure support weaning is superior to T-piece weaning in patients with chronic obstructive pulmonary disease (COPD).[68] Overall, progressive decrements in pressure support, as part of a challenge-to-wean protocol, should be limited to patients who fail spontaneous weaning trials.

T-Piece trials: This method is the oldest ventilator weaning technique and involves sequentially increasing the amount of time the patient spends on the T-piece.[10,11] Traditionally, many units repeatedly placed patients on T-tubes for a short period multiple times each day. The demonstration that single daily T-tube trials were as efficient, though, has significantly reduced the clinical use of this more labor-intensive practice.[11] T-piece trials are limited by the absence of apnea and volume alarms in this setting.

Non-invasive ventilation: The increasing clinical use and familiarity with noninvasive ventilation (NIV) in the critical care setting makes it an attractive tool in the difficult-to-wean patient. The potential advantages of NIV are to avoid the complications of intubation and sedation and reduce the total time of invasive mechanical ventilation. The use of NIV in weaning can be separated into (1) preventing extubation failure in selected patients, (2) being used as a rescue therapy for postextubation respiratory distress, and (3) permitting early extubation in patients who fail to meet standard extubation criteria.

1. *Preventing extubation failure in selected patients (prophylactic therapy):* Prophylactic NIV has the potential to prevent hypoxia, hypercapnia, and atelectasis and reduce the work of breathing, thereby reducing the rate of respiratory complications. RCTs have demonstrated that in high-risk postoperative patients (vascular, abdominal, and thoracicoabdominal surgery), NIV results in trends toward improved oxygenation and reduced infection rate, re-intubation rate, length of hospital stay, and mortality.[69-71]

2. *Rescue therapy to avoid reintubation for postextubation respiratory distress (rescue therapy):* NIV for patients with acute postextubation respiratory failure (in the ICU) is ineffective.[72] A meta-analysis of two RCTs that compared NIV with the standard medical therapy in patients (n=302) with postextubation respiratory failure did not demonstrate a reduction in the reintubation rate (risk ratio [RR], 1.03; 95% confidence interval [CI], 0.84 to 1.25) or ICU mortality (RR, 1.14; 95% CI, 0.43 to 3.0) in the NIV group.[73]

3. *Permitting early extubation in patients who fail to meet standard extubation criteria (facilitation therapy):* Interest

has emerged in using NIV in highly selected patients to facilitate earlier removal of the endotracheal tube while still allowing a progressive stepwise reduction of ventilator support. This strategy involves extubating the patient who has failed an SBT directly on to NIV (PSV + CPAP) compared with standard therapy (invasive mechanical ventilation). This approach clearly can only be successful for patients who have good airway protection, a strong cough, and minimal secretions; therefore they are likely to be conscious, alert patients with slowly resolving lung injury but who retain good respiratory neuromuscular function. In practice, these patients frequently have COPD. A recent meta-analysis (n = 994) suggested that mortality was significantly reduced in COPD patients weaned on noninvasive positive-pressure ventilation (NPPV) versus intermittent positive-pressure ventilation (IPPV) (RR, 0.36; 95% CI, 0.24 to 0.56). The benefit in mixed populations was much smaller (RR, 0.81; 95% CI, 0.47 to 1.40), though.[74] NIV was associated with reduced weaning failure, ventilator-associated pneumonia, total duration of ventilation, length of hospital, and ICU stay in the COPD subgroup.

Role of Tracheostomy in Weaning

The insertion of a tracheostomy tube (whether surgical or percutaneous) is an important tool in the difficult-to-wean patient. Tracheostomy is usually far less irritating to the patient than an endotracheal tube, and the decreased sedation requirements usually enable weaning strategies that would otherwise not be possible. Tracheostomy also provides a more secure airway,[75] reduces vocal cord damage, reduces the work of breathing, and facilitates airway toilet.[76,77] A meta-analysis of RCTs comparing early with late or no tracheostomy found lower all-cause mortality in the early group with moderate heterogeneity (odds ratio [OR], 0.72).[78] Ventilator-associated pneumonia was also lower (OR, 0.6), and tracheostomy complications were equivalent. Data on length of stay and long-term outcomes were deemed inadequate.

Consideration of Weaning Protocols

Several studies have reported that either lack of attention to screening for the ability to progress or the unnecessary delay in progression through the weaning steps is associated with increased morbidity and mortality[4,18,79] and that weaning protocols have resulted in reduced ventilator-associated pneumonia, self-extubation rates, tracheostomy rates, and cost.[4,9] A Cochrane review suggested that a protocolized weaning strategy may result in a shorter duration of weaning and ICU stay.[80] There was significant heterogeneity, though, between studies (I = 76%); there was low-quality evidence; and the quality of usual care provided in the control arms was unclear. The use of such protocols is controversial, with some suggesting that informed clinical judgment is superior. In an Italian multicenter study, higher levels of physician-to-patient ratios resulted in shorter weaning duration, suggesting that physician input is important to earlier weaning.[81]

AUTHORS' RECOMMENDATIONS

- Sedation reduction and use of short-acting, titratable, sedative infusions is essential to enable early and appropriate clinical assessments. Assessment of readiness to wean and reductions in sedative infusions should be considered early and frequently in critically ill patients receiving mechanical ventilation.
- Once the acute insult has resolved, clinicians should have a low threshold for conducting an SBT in all critically ill patients.
- The SBT should last more than 30 minutes and may use the following
  - A T-piece/T-tube
  - PSV (≤10 cm H_2O)
  - ATC
  - ± CPAP (≤5 cm H_2O)
- Current data support PSV as being the simplest and most effective technique.
- If the patient fails an SBT, then the clinician should do the following
  - Address all contributory causes of failure to wean
  - Not perform a repeat SBT for 24 hours
  - Support the patient with a nonfatiguing mode of ventilation (most commonly PSV)
  - Consider tracheostomy
- Weaning protocols should be considered in ICUs.

REFERENCES

1. Slutsky AS. Mechanical ventilation. American College of Chest Physicians' Consensus Conference. *Chest*. 1993;104:1833–1859.
2. Boles JM, Bion J, Connors A, et al. Weaning from mechanical ventilation. *Eur Respir J*. 2007;29:1033–1056.
3. Brochard L. Pressure support is the preferred weaning method. In: *As presented at the 5th International Concensus Conference in Intensive Care Medicine: Weaning from Mechanical Ventilation*. ; April 28–29, 2005.
4. Ely EW, Baker AM, Dunagan DP, et al. Effect on the duration of mechanical ventilation of identifying patients capable of breathing spontaneously. *N Engl J Med*. 1996;335:1864–1869.
5. Esteban A, Alia I, Tobin MJ, et al. Effect of spontaneous breathing trial duration on outcome of attempts to discontinue mechanical ventilation. Spanish Lung Failure Collaborative Group. *Am J Respir Crit Care Med*. 1999;159:512–518.
6. Esteban A, Anzueto A, Frutos F, et al. Characteristics and outcomes in adult patients receiving mechanical ventilation: a 28-day international study. *JAMA*. 2002;287:345–355.
7. Cooper LM, Linde-Zwirble WT. Medicare intensive care unit use: analysis of incidence, cost, and payment. *Crit Care Med*. 2004;32:2247–2253.
8. Wagner DP. Economics of prolonged mechanical ventilation. *Am Rev Respir Dis*. 1989;140:S14–S18.
9. Kollef MH, Shapiro SD, Silver P, et al. A randomized, controlled trial of protocol-directed versus physician-directed weaning from mechanical ventilation. *Crit Care Med*. 1997;25:567–574.
10. Brochard L, Rauss A, Benito S, et al. Comparison of three methods of gradual withdrawal from ventilatory support during weaning from mechanical ventilation. *Am J Respir Crit Care Med*. 1994;150:896–903.
11. Esteban A, Frutos F, Tobin MJ, et al. A comparison of four methods of weaning patients from mechanical ventilation. Spanish Lung Failure Collaborative Group. *N Engl J Med*. 1995;332:345–350.
12. Epstein SK, Nevins ML, Chung J. Effect of unplanned extubation on outcome of mechanical ventilation. *Am J Respir Crit Care Med*. 2000;161:1912–1916.
13. Thille AW, Harrois A, Schortgen F, Brun-Buisson C, Brochard L. Outcomes of extubation failure in medical intensive care unit patients. *Crit Care Med*. 2011;39:2612–2618.
14. Menon N, Joffe AM, Deem S, et al. Occurrence and complications of tracheal reintubation in critically ill adults. *Respir Care*. 2012;57:1555–1563.

15. Kress JP, Pohlman AS, O'Connor MF, Hall JB. Daily interruption of sedative infusions in critically ill patients undergoing mechanical ventilation. *N Engl J Med*. 2000;342:1471–1477.
16. Kress JP, Gehlbach B, Lacy M, Pliskin N, Pohlman AS, Hall JB. The long-term psychological effects of daily sedative interruption on critically ill patients. *Am J Respir Crit Care Med*. 2003;168:1457–1461.
17. Vallverdu I, Calaf N, Subirana M, Net A, Benito S, Mancebo J. Clinical characteristics, respiratory functional parameters, and outcome of a two-hour T-piece trial in patients weaning from mechanical ventilation. *Am J Respir Crit Care Med*. 1998;158:1855–1862.
18. Coplin WM, Pierson DJ, Cooley KD, Newell DW, Rubenfeld GD. Implications of extubation delay in brain-injured patients meeting standard weaning criteria. *Am J Respir Crit Care Med*. 2000;161:1530–1536.
19. Yang KL, Tobin MJ. A prospective study of indexes predicting the outcome of trials of weaning from mechanical ventilation. *N Engl J Med*. 1991;324:1445–1450.
20. Sahn SA, Lakshminarayan S. Bedside criteria for discontinuation of mechanical ventilation. *Chest*. 1973;63:1002–1005.
21. Herrera M, Blasco J, Venegas J, Barba R, Doblas A, Marquez E. Mouth occlusion pressure (P0.1) in acute respiratory failure. *Intensive Care Med*. 1985;11:134–139.
22. Capdevila XJ, Perrigault PF, Perey PJ, Roustan JP, d'Athis F. Occlusion pressure and its ratio to maximum inspiratory pressure are useful predictors for successful extubation following T-piece weaning trial. *Chest*. 1995;108:482–489.
23. Montgomery AB, Holle RH, Neagley SR, Pierson DJ, Schoene RB. Prediction of successful ventilator weaning using airway occlusion pressure and hypercapnic challenge. *Chest*. 1987;91:496–499.
24. Teixeira C, da Silva NB, Savi A, et al. Central venous saturation is a predictor of reintubation in difficult-to-wean patients. *Crit Care Med*. 2010;38:491–496.
25. Jubran A, Mathru M, Dries D, Tobin MJ. Continuous recordings of mixed venous oxygen saturation during weaning from mechanical ventilation and the ramifications thereof. *Am J Respir Crit Care Med*. 2012;158.
26. Caille V, Amiel JB, Charron C, Belliard G, Vieillard-Baron A, Vignon P. Echocardiography: a help in the weaning process. *Crit Care*. 2010;14:22.
27. Mekontso-Dessap A, De Prost N, Girou E, et al. B-type natriuretic peptide and weaning from mechanical ventilation. *Intensive Care Med*. 2006;32:1529–1536.
28. Chien J-Y, Lin M-S, Huang Y-CT, Chien Y-F, Yu C-J, Yang P-C. Changes in B-type natriuretic peptide improve weaning outcome predicted by spontaneous breathing trial. *Crit Care Med*. 2008;36:1421–1426.
29. Grasso S, Leone A, De Michele M, et al. Use of N-terminal pro-brain natriuretic peptide to detect acute cardiac dysfunction during weaning failure in difficult-to-wean patients with chronic obstructive pulmonary disease. *Crit Care Med*. 2007;35:96–105. http://dx.doi.org/10.1097/01.CCM.0000250391.89780.64.
30. Zapata L, Vera P, Roglan A, Gich I, Ordonez-Llanos J, Betbesé AJ. B-type natriuretic peptides for prediction and diagnosis of weaning failure from cardiac origin. *Intensive Care Med*. 2011;37:477–485.
31. Patel KN, Ganatra KD, Bates JH, Young MP. Variation in the rapid shallow breathing index associated with common measurement techniques and conditions. *Respir Care*. 2009;54:1462–1466.
32. El-Khatib MF, Jamaleddine GW, Khoury AR, Obeid MY. Effect of continuous positive airway pressure on the rapid shallow breathing index in patients following cardiac surgery. *Chest*. 2002;121:475–479.
33. Verceles AC, Diaz-Abad M, Geiger-Brown J, Scharf SM. Testing the prognostic value of the rapid shallow breathing index in predicting successful weaning in patients requiring prolonged mechanical ventilation. *Heart Lung*. 2012;41:546–552.
34. Adams RC, Gunter OL, Wisler JR, et al. Dynamic changes in respiratory frequency/tidal volume may predict failures of ventilatory liberation in patients on prolonged mechanical ventilation and normal preliberation respiratory frequency/tidal volume values. *Am Surg*. 2012;78:69–73.
35. Segal L, Oei E, Oppenheimer B, et al. Evolution of pattern of breathing during a spontaneous breathing trial predicts successful extubation. *Intensive Care Med*. 2010;36:487–495.
36. Tanios MA, Nevins ML, Hendra KP, et al. A randomized, controlled trial of the role of weaning predictors in clinical decision making. *Crit Care Med*. 2006;34:2530–2535.
37. Cohen J, Shapiro M, Grozovski E, Fox B, Lev S, Singer P. Prediction of extubation outcome: a randomized, controlled trial with automatic tube compensation vs. pressure support ventilation. *Crit Care*. 2009;13:R21.
38. Jabour ER, Rabil DM, Truwit JD, Rochester DF. Evaluation of a new weaning index based on ventilatory endurance and the efficiency of gas exchange. *Am Rev Respir Dis*. 1991;144:531–537.
39. Nemer SN, Barbas CS, Caldeira JB, et al. A new integrative weaning index of discontinuation from mechanical ventilation. *Crit Care*. 2009;13:R152.
40. Jubran A, Tobin MJ. Pathophysiologic basis of acute respiratory distress in patients who fail a trial of weaning from mechanical ventilation. *Am J Respir Crit Care Med*. 1997;155:906–915.
41. Laghi F, Cattapan SE, Jubran A, et al. Is weaning failure caused by low-frequency fatigue of the diaphragm? *Am J Respir Crit Care Med*. 2003;167:120–127.
42. Perren A, Domenighetti G, Mauri S, Genini F, Vizzardi N. Protocol-directed weaning from mechanical ventilation: clinical outcome in patients randomized for a 30-min or 120-min trial with pressure support ventilation. *Intensive Care Med*. 2002;28:1058–1063.
43. Farias JA, Retta A, Alia I, et al. A comparison of two methods to perform a breathing trial before extubation in pediatric intensive care patients. *Intensive Care Med*. 2001;27:1649–1654.
44. Haberthur C, Mols G, Elsasser S, Bingisser R, Stocker R, Guttmann J. Extubation after breathing trials with automatic tube compensation, T-tube, or pressure support ventilation. *Acta Anaesthesiol Scand*. 2002;46:973–979.
45. Straus C, Louis B, Isabey D, Lemaire F, Harf A, Brochard L. Contribution of the endotracheal tube and the upper airway to breathing workload. *Am J Respir Crit Care Med*. 1998;157:23–30.
46. Mehta S, Nelson DL, Klinger JR, Buczko GB, Levy MM. Prediction of post-extubation work of breathing. *Crit Care Med*. 2000;28:1341–1346.
47. Nathan SD, Ishaaya AM, Koerner SK, Belman MJ. Prediction of minimal pressure support during weaning from mechanical ventilation. *Chest*. 1993;103:1215–1219.
48. Matic I, Majeric-Kogler V. Comparison of pressure support and T-tube weaning from mechanical ventilation: randomized prospective study. *Croat Med J*. 2004;45:162–166.
49. Figueroa-Casas JB, Montoya R, Arzabala A, Connery SM. Comparison between automatic tube compensation and continuous positive airway pressure during spontaneous breathing trials. *Respir Care*. 2010;55:549–554.
50. Oto J, Imanaka H, Nakataki E, Ono R, Nishimura M. Potential inadequacy of automatic tube compensation to decrease inspiratory work load after at least 48 hours of endotracheal tube use in the clinical setting. *Respir Care*. 2012;57:697–703.
51. Hess D. Ventilator modes used in weaning. *Chest*. 2001;120:474S–476S.
52. Rose L, Cardwell C, Jouvet P, McAuley D, Blackwood B. Automated versus non-automated weaning for reducing the duration of mechanical ventilation for critically ill adults and children. *Cochrane Database Syst Rev*. 2013;7.
53. Burns KE, Lellouche F, Nisenbaum R, Lessard MR, Friedrich JO. Automated weaning and SBT systems versus non-automated weaning strategies for weaning time in invasively ventilated critically ill adults. *Cochrane Database Syst Rev*. 2014;9.
54. Namen AM, Ely EW, Tatter SB, et al. Predictors of successful extubation in neurosurgical patients. *Am J Respir Crit Care Med*. 2001;163:658–664.
55. Khamiees M, Raju P, DeGirolamo A, Amoateng-Adjepong Y, Manthous CA. Predictors of extubation outcome in patients who have successfully completed a spontaneous breathing trial. *Chest*. 2001;120:1262–1270.
56. Smina M, Salam A, Khamiees M, Gada P, Amoateng-Adjepong Y, Manthous CA. Cough peak flows and extubation outcomes. *Chest*. 2003;124:262–268.
57. Salam A, Tilluckdharry L, Amoateng-Adjepong Y, Manthous CA. Neurologic status, cough, secretions and extubation outcomes. *Intensive Care Med*. 2004;30:1334–1339.

58. Smailes ST, McVicar AJ, Martin R. Cough strength, secretions and extubation outcome in burn patients who have passed a spontaneous breathing trial. *Burns*. 2013;39:236–242.

59. Fisher MM, Raper RF. The 'cuff-leak' test for extubation. *Anaesthesia*. 1992;47:10–12.

60. Maury E, Guglielminotti J, Alzieu M, Qureshi T, Guidet B, Offenstadt G. How to identify patients with no risk for postextubation stridor? *J Crit Care*. 2004;19:23–28.

61. Francois B, Bellissant E, Gissot V, et al. 12-h pretreatment with methylprednisolone versus placebo for prevention of postextubation laryngeal oedema: a randomised double-blind trial. *Lancet*. 2007;369:1083–1089.

62. Imsand C, Feihl F, Perret C, Fitting JW. Regulation of inspiratory neuromuscular output during synchronized intermittent mechanical ventilation. *Anesthesiology*. 1994;80:13–22.

63. Alia I, Esteban A. Weaning from mechanical ventilation. *Crit Care*. 2000;4:72–80.

64. Vassilakopoulos T, Petrof BJ. Ventilator-induced diaphragmatic dysfunction. *Am J Respir Crit Care Med*. 2004;169:336–341.

65. Gherini S, Peters RM, Virgilio RW. Mechanical work on the lungs and work of breathing with positive end-expiratory pressure and continuous positive airway pressure. *Chest*. 1979;76:251–256.

66. Gibney RT, Wilson RS, Pontoppidan H. Comparison of work of breathing on high gas flow and demand valve continuous positive airway pressure systems. *Chest*. 1982;82:692–695.

67. MacIntyre NR. Respiratory function during pressure support ventilation. *Chest*. 1986;89:677–683.

68. Matic I, Danic D, Majeric-Kogler V, Jurjevic M, Mirkovic I, Mrzljak Vucinic N. Chronic obstructive pulmonary disease and weaning of difficult-to-wean patients from mechanical ventilation: randomized prospective study. *Croat Med J*. 2007;48:51–58.

69. Bohner H, Kindgen-Milles D, Grust A, et al. Prophylactic nasal continuous positive airway pressure after major vascular surgery: results of a prospective randomized trial. *Langenbecks Arch Surg*. 2002;387:21–26.

70. Squadrone V, Coha M, Cerutti E, et al. Continuous positive airway pressure for treatment of postoperative hypoxemia: a randomized controlled trial. *JAMA*. 2005;293:589–595.

71. Kindgen-Milles D, Muller E, Buhl R, et al. Nasal-continuous positive airway pressure reduces pulmonary morbidity and length of hospital stay following thoracoabdominal aortic surgery. *Chest*. 2005;128:821–828.

72. Glossop A, Shepherd N, Bryden D, Mills G. Non-invasive ventilation for weaning, avoiding reintubation after extubation and in the postoperative period: a meta-analysis. *Br J Anaesth*. 2012;109:305–314.

73. Agarwal R, Aggarwal AN, Gupta D, Jindal SK. Role of noninvasive positive-pressure ventilation in postextubation respiratory failure: a meta-analysis. *Respir Care*. 2007;52:1472–1479.

74. Burns KE, Meade MO, Premji A, Adhikari NK. Noninvasive positive-pressure ventilation as a weaning strategy for intubated adults with respiratory failure. *Cochrane Database Syst Rev*. 2013;9.

75. Stauffer JL, Olson DE, Petty TL. Complications and consequences of endotracheal intubation and tracheotomy. A prospective study of 150 critically ill adult patients. *Am J Med*. 1981;70:65–76.

76. Diehl JL, El Atrous S, Touchard D, Lemaire F, Brochard L. Changes in the work of breathing induced by tracheotomy in ventilator-dependent patients. *Am J Respir Crit Care Med*. 1999;159:383–388.

77. Davis Jr K, Campbell RS, Johannigman JA, Valente JF, Branson RD. Changes in respiratory mechanics after tracheostomy. *Arch Surg*. 1999;134:59–62.

78. Siempos II, Ntaidou TK, Filippidis FT, Choi AMK. Effect of early versus late or no tracheostomy on mortality of critically ill patients receiving mechanical ventilation: a systematic review and meta-analysis. *Lancet Respir Med*. June 2014.

79. Ely EW, Baker AM, Evans GW, Haponik EF. The prognostic significance of passing a daily screen of weaning parameters. *Intensive Care Med*. 1999;25:581–587.

80. Blackwood B, Alderdice F, Burns K, Cardwell C, Lavery G, O'Halloran P. Use of weaning protocols for reducing duration of mechanical ventilation in critically ill adult patients: Cochrane systematic review and meta-analysis. *BMJ*. 2011;342.

81. Polverino E, Nava S, Ferrer M, et al. Patients' characterization, hospital course and clinical outcomes in five Italian respiratory intensive care units. *Intensive Care Med*. 2010;36:137–142.

10 | How Does Mechanical Ventilation Damage Lungs? What Can Be Done to Prevent It?

Joshua A. Marks, Maurizio Cereda

To address the question whether ventilators damage lungs, one must first understand several commonly used related terms. Ventilator-induced lung injury (VILI) denotes acute lung damage that develops during mechanical ventilation. VILI is pathologically characterized by inflammatory-cell infiltrates, hyaline membranes, alveolar hemorrhage, increased vascular permeability, pulmonary edema, loss of functional surfactant, and ultimately alveolar collapse. Ventilator strategies designed to reduce VILI have improved outcomes among patients with acute respiratory distress syndrome (ARDS), characterized by progressive hypoxemia requiring a greater fraction of inspired oxygen to maintain an acceptable arterial oxygenation and chest imaging that demonstrates bilateral interstitial or alveolar opacities. In fact, the clinical presentation of VILI is largely indistinguishable from ARDS, highlighting the clinical importance of VILI. Alveolar overdistension, lung strain, and atelectasis are the key inciting and defining features of VILI. Overdistension reflects the presence of an elevation in transpulmonary pressure, defined as the difference between the airway pressure and the pleural pressure at the end of inspiration. Strain is the ratio of the volume of gas delivered during a tidal breath to the amount of aerated lung receiving that breath: Larger strain is matched by a higher mechanical stress on alveolar structures.[1] When there is heterogeneous consolidation or atelectasis, a disproportionate volume from a given tidal breath is delivered to the open alveoli. The result is regional alveolar overdistension and excessive strain because a normal tidal volume is selectively directed to only a portion of the lung. This process is conceptually akin to delivering a standard tidal volume to a "baby lung."[2]

Atelectrauma occurs with repetitive, cyclic opening and closing of airways and lung units during inspiration and expiration. It is magnified when focal consolidation causes heterogeneous ventilation because more alveoli are exposed to the injurious impact of neighboring alveoli that are opening and collapsing. The stretching or shear forces between aerated and atelectatic lung are greater than those in other lung regions. The relevance of intermittent atelectasis has been questioned because alveolar edema, rather than collapse, seems to dominate the pulmonary microenvironment in many conditions.[3] Recent experimental data show that air fluid levels and surfactant dysfunction cause epithelial shear and cell damage in the conducting small airways.[4,5]

Barotrauma, which grammatically should reflect ventilation with high pressures, actually results from ventilating lungs using high volumes. This process can lead to alveolar rupture, air leaks, or even pneumothoraces, pneumomediastinum, and subcutaneous emphysema. Despite the misnomer, the critical component in barotrauma is regional overdistension and not high airway pressure. Some experts have suggested the use of the term *volutrauma*, which implicates excessive volume, with alveolar lung stretching, and not airway pressure, as the determinant of injury.

Biotrauma results from the physical forces of atelectrauma, barotrauma, and volutrauma that cause the release of intracellular mediators. Cells are either directly injured by these mediators or indirectly injured through the activation of cell-signaling pathways in epithelial, endothelial, or inflammatory cells. The translocation of these mediators or bacteria from the airspaces into the systemic circulation through areas of increased alveolar-capillary permeability, as is classically seen in ARDS or as a result of volutrauma, has been touted as a contributor to multiorgan dysfunction and death.

HOW DO VENTILATORS DAMAGE THE LUNGS IN PATIENTS?

Although a clear entity, the exact mechanisms of VILI in patients, and the appropriate treatment in each individual, remain unknown. Although VILI is typically considered an independent form of secondary injury, damage by the ventilator is probably an essential contributor to the natural history and evolution of ARDS.[6] The vast majority of research in the field of optimal ventilator management has focused, with limited success, on developing new ways to treat well-established ARDS; however, relatively little attention has been paid to understanding the progression of injury, particularly in patients who do not initially have ARDS.

Moderate tidal volume (V_T; i.e., 12 mL/kg) worsens survival in patients with preexisting ARDS.[7] According to the baby lung construct, inspired gas is concentrated in a smaller, yet otherwise functional, fraction of ventilated parenchyma (i.e., lung capacity), causing overstretching.[8] In an effort to reduce inspiratory strain, clinicians prescribe V_T according to patient weight,[7] but there are two corollaries to the baby lung model that have relevant implications on clinical management.

First, the volume and the strain of the ventilated lung are variable and reflect the severity of injury.[9] Indeed, patients with small lung capacity may undergo unacceptable stretch even with a very low V_T.[10] Because it is hard to quantify overdistension and strain at the bedside (inspiratory airway pressures are notoriously inaccurate[11] and a safe threshold[12] is unknown), it is difficult to identify those patients at increased risk of VILI who might benefit from an even greater reduction in V_T.

Second, it remains unclear how ventilation affects patients without ARDS. Moderate V_T does not injure healthy lungs[13]: Clinically acceptable V_T sizes may not cause enough stress to worsen injury if the lung capacity is not significantly reduced. However, observational studies[14] and interventional trials,[15] including some conducted on intraoperative patients, have suggested that V_T reduction may improve pulmonary outcomes in patients without ARDS.[16,17] Animal studies have shown that the presence of systemic inflammation, as in sepsis, may raise the sensitivity to mechanical stress in lung tissue; that is, less deformation is required to cause injury.[18] Whether this particular mechanism is relevant to humans is unknown, but it is debatable whether it explains the beneficial effects of low V_T in patients without a severe inflammatory process. Because the key mechanism inciting VILI in the absence of severe lung injury is undefined, generalized application of low V_T in heterogeneous populations of ventilated patients may not necessarily yield the desired beneficial effects.

The role of atelectasis in ventilated humans is also unclear. Despite compelling evidence from animal experiments on atelectrauma,[19-21] clinical trials have shown only marginal effects of lung recruitment and high positive end expiratory pressure (PEEP) in established ARDS.[22-24] This discrepancy could be due to ineffective study recruitment. Indeed, studies have shown that dynamic responses to recruitment and PEEP as measured with radiological and functional instruments[25,26] better predict ARDS outcomes than one-time measurements of hypoxemia. A key characteristic of ARDS is inflammatory changes that are heterogeneously distributed throughout the lung parenchyma,[27] an aspect ignored by consensus definitions of ARDS[28] and in most study enrollment criteria.[7,29] This spatial variation may explain the inconsistent findings in many human trials. Although a specific treatment may very well improve one area of lung, it may simultaneously worsen another.[30]

Atelectasis may also generate VILI by increasing susceptibility to V_T dimensions.[31] According to accepted paradigms of VILI, atelectrauma occurs in injured, collapsible lung regions,[32,33] but recent evidence has shown limited inflammatory activation when the effects of atelectasis are separated from those of high inspiratory stretch.[34] However, atelectasis might modify the intrapulmonary distribution of mechanical stress and consequently of inflammation. Said differently, poorly recruited atelectasis may render lungs more vulnerable to moderate V_T by reciprocally increasing stretch in ventilated airspaces.[27,35,36] Mechanical stress would then be focally amplified in areas of the lung that are adjacent or interspersed with collapsed tissue.[37] A recent study showed a correlation between localized aeration heterogeneity as seen on computed tomography scan (a possible marker of elevated local stretch) and outcomes in ARDS.[38] Recruitment may decrease the amount of stretch the lungs receive from a given V_T,[37,39,40] thereby limiting the injury.

Atelectasis could contribute to generating injury in non-ARDS patients. A controlled study in ventilated intensive care unit (ICU) patients without ARDS showed improved pulmonary outcomes with the use of high and low PEEP.[41] Furthermore, two successful trials on perioperative lung protection compared low V_T in combination with aggressive lung recruitment in the treatment group to higher V_T and low PEEP in the controls.[16,17] Although this approach was designed to determine whether adequate PEEP could prevent the atelectasis associated with low V_T, avoiding atelectasis, and not PEEP per se, could be the determinant of success. Because of the design of these trials, it is not possible to separate the contributions of the two interventions. Counter to the hypothesis that atelectasis causes new injury in healthy lungs, a trial of higher and lower intraoperative PEEP—with the same low V_T in both arms of the study—failed to demonstrate benefit with higher PEEP.[42]

HOW TO MINIMIZE LUNG DAMAGE?

The ARMA trial established improved survival with the use of 6 rather than 12 mL/kg V_T.[7] As a result of this study and prior work by other authors,[43] ventilation with low V_T (i.e., low-stretch ventilation) is currently the accepted standard of care in established ARDS. Earlier studies, with less dramatic differences in V_T between the experimental and control groups, failed to improve outcome.[44,45] However, a recent observational study confirmed a dose–response relationship between V_T and ARDS mortality.[46] This study also showed that the effects of V_T selection during the ICU course extend over the long term.

The current clinical approach is to set the ventilator index V_T to predicted body weight (PBW), based on height, as a surrogate of lung size.[7] T_V is set to 4 to 6 mL/kg IBW while also ensuring that the plateau pressure is less than 30 cm H_2O and high $Paco_2$ (partial pressure of carbon dioxide in arterial blood) levels are tolerated. PEEP is adjusted according to ARDSnet nomograms to maintain a goal $Paco_2$ (partial pressure of oxygen in arterial blood) of 55 to 80 mm Hg and a SpO_2 (O_2 saturation by pulse oximetry) of 88% to 95%. Hypercapnia is limited by acceptable pH, and the effectiveness of metabolic correction remains unclear.[47] Although this strategy decreases mortality, it represents a "one size fits all" model that does not account for individual patient characteristics, such as lung capacity, recruitable atelectasis, and chest wall mechanics. As a consequence, weight-based V_T settings may leave a proportion of severely ill patients underprotected, whereas others may be treated with unnecessary aggressiveness (i.e., obese patients with low chest wall compliance). It is not clear how to personalize treatment. Although bedside measurements of lung capacity and strain remain experimental,[9] titration to transpulmonary pressure measured via esophageal manometry seems to be a promising approach. This methodology allows the clinician to correct airway pressure for the effect of chest wall mechanics and to personalize both PEEP and V_T settings to minimize peak pulmonary distension while maintaining recruitment.[48]

For patients with the highest severity illness, it is possible that even the most aggressive V_T reduction does not achieve sufficient lung protection. The use of extracorporeal lung assist methods has been implemented in select situations,[49] but its generalized use is supported only by one randomized study with important design limitations.[50] In addition, the risk/benefit assessment for this approach remains difficult and poorly understood. High-frequency oscillatory ventilation, an appealing technique for extreme V_T reduction and aggressive recruitment, has not been shown to improve outcomes.[51]

On the basis of the existing evidence, ventilator management targeted to recruitment with high PEEP ("open lung ventilation") cannot be recommended as the standard of care.[22-24] However, trials have showed some benefit in patients with the highest severity of illness.[52] Expert sources, including society guidelines, recommend the use of high PEEP in this subset of patients.[53] Future studies should use better instruments to stratify patients and monitor effectiveness. Techniques including esophageal manometry or bedside imaging tools such as electrical impedance tomography may provide more support for this approach.[48,54] Absent these data, the hypothetical benefits of the open lung approach in each individual patient should be weighed against tangible adverse effects. Similar caution should be applied to alternative ventilator modalities that augment mean airway pressures with the goal of maximizing recruitment.[55] Careful patient selection and monitoring of the effects of higher airway pressure on lung overdistension, pulmonary and systemic circulation,[56] and alveolar dead space should be used to avoid undesired responses. Worsening hemodynamics in the face of the unclear biological effects of recruitment are considered by many clinicians to be unacceptable.

Recent trials have suggested that the outcomes of early severe ARDS can be improved with the early adoption of a course of muscle relaxation.[57] A recent study suggested that by maintaining tight control of inspired strain in the early stage of severe ARDS, muscle paralysis optimizes protection from VILI. However, the design of this particular study did not clarify the effect of patient inspiratory effort.

Other usable complementary strategies of lung protection include prone positioning, which in a recent study showed dramatic positive effects on outcomes of severe ARDS.[58] Prone positioning has been studied for many years because of its ability to improve oxygenation in a large proportion of patients.[59] Placing patients in a prone position reopens collapsed dorsal lung regions and increases the homogeneity of the distribution of ventilation, thereby redistributing and attenuating regional inspiratory stress.[60] This effect likely attenuates VILI and could explain observed outcomes. In one particular study, prone positioning was used for longer periods of time and in more severe patients than in previous studies that had more ambiguous results.[61] Therefore prone positioning can be considered as an adjunct to stretch limitation and, possibly, an alternative to PEEP to improve recruitment and minimize regional stress.

Approximately 67% of ARDS cases arise after hospital admission,[62] which provides ample opportunity for preventive interventions. Clinical studies have reported a variable incidence of ARDS (8% to 25%)[14,15] in patients who undergo mechanical ventilation for other reasons. Thus, it is likely that ventilator management has a role in generating new lung injury and in worsening preexisting pulmonary lesions. However, predicting which patients are at risk for having lung injury and ARDS, as well as the potential severity of illness, remains challenging. Scoring systems have been developed to identify patients at risk, but their application has been inconsistent, and their ability to connect specific treatments with disease prevention is unconfirmed.[63]

A recent meta-analysis showed beneficial outcome effects from the use of lower and higher V_T in heterogeneous populations of non-ARDS patients in the ICU and in the operating room.[64] On the basis of this evidence, the use of low V_T seems logical in ventilated patients at risk of progression to ARDS, including victims of sepsis or trauma or those undergoing high-risk surgical procedures.[65] However, a word of caution is warranted. Many studies in patients without ARDS have shown outcome differences when comparing control and treatment V_T values that greatly differed.[66] Whether smaller differences in V_T would have produced similar results is unclear, but many practitioners have already abandoned large V_T (i.e., >10 mL/kg) in non-ARDS patients. A recent meta-analysis that included intraoperative ventilation studies showed that, relative to standard management, use of lower V_T decreased the onset of ARDS but did not demonstrate any effects on survival or ICU length of stay.[66]

Use of surrogate outcomes such as onset of ARDS to gauge the effectiveness of preventive strategies does not guarantee success in improving death or long-term functional impairment.[67] The success of low V_T ventilation in a population at high risk for mortality due to ARDS does not necessarily translate into benefits in patients who are at much lower risk, such as those ventilated in the operating room. Conversely, undesired responses, often undetected by underpowered clinical trials, may affect more patients than the beneficial ones.[68] For example, decreasing V_T in a patient without ARDS may worsen atelectasis and lead to increased lung damage and hypoxemia. Although studies to date have not reported an increased requirement for sedation when higher V_T are used,[15] sedation practices and goals vary greatly from center to center. If minimal sedation and spontaneous breathing modes, as opposed to deeper sedation and controlled ventilation, are the usual practice, then a reduction in V_T may be most relevant to patient discomfort, ventilator asynchrony, and eventually sedation usage, with all of the resultant sequelae.

AUTHORS' RECOMMENDATIONS

- Our current knowledge of alveolar mechanics and VILI is incomplete.
- The outcomes from ARDS can be improved by implementation of existing evidence and a better understanding of the pathophysiology.
- V_T settings should be dynamically adapted to individual patients' mechanical characteristics rather than to body weight alone.
- Appropriate combinations of PEEP and V_T blunt the effects of inspiration on airspace overdistension and ventilation heterogeneity, thereby decreasing injury progression.
- Regional force distribution and focal airspace deformation are major players in determining the response of lung tissue to ventilator settings and possibly other therapies, such as prone positioning.
- Our understanding of ARDS and the manner in which we currently ventilate patients' lungs have been influenced profoundly by lung imaging.
- Further ongoing research, including novel imaging modalities, will continue to enlighten us and change the way we practice.

REFERENCES

1. Protti A, Cressoni M, Santini A, Langer T, Mietto C, Febres D, et al. Lung stress and strain during mechanical ventilation: any safe threshold? *Am J Respir Crit Care Med*. May 15, 2011;183(10): 1354–1362.
2. Gattinoni L, Pesenti A. The concept of "baby lung". *Intensive Care Med*. 2005;31(6):776–784.
3. Hubmayr RD. Perspective on lung injury and recruitment: a skeptical look at the opening and collapse story. *Am J Res Crit Care Med*. 2002;165(12):1647–1653.
4. Bilek AM, Dee KC, Gaver 3rd DP. Mechanisms of surface-tension-induced epithelial cell damage in a model of pulmonary airway reopening. *J Appl Physiol*. 2003;94(2):770–783. Bethesda, Md.: 1985.
5. Glindmeyer HW, Smith BJ, Gaver 3rd DP. In situ enhancement of pulmonary surfactant function using temporary flow reversal. *J Appl Physiol*. 2012;112(1):149–158. Bethesda, Md.: 1985.
6. Slutsky AS, Ranieri VM. Ventilator-induced lung injury. *N Engl J Med*. November 28, 2013;369(22):2126–2136.
7. Ventilation with lower tidal volumes as compared with traditional tidal volumes for acute lung injury and the acute respiratory distress syndrome. The acute respiratory distress syndrome network. *N Engl J Med*. 2000;342(18):1301–1308.
8. Gattinoni L, Pesenti A, Avalli L, Rossi F, Bombino M. Pressure-volume curve of total respiratory system in acute respiratory failure. Computed tomographic scan study. *Am Rev Res Dis*. 1987;136(3):730–736.
9. Mattingley JS, Holets SR, Oeckler RA, Stroetz RW, Buck CF, Hubmayr RD. Sizing the lung of mechanically ventilated patients. *Crit Care*. 2011;15(1):R60.
10. Terragni PP, Rosboch G, Tealdi A, Corno E, Menaldo E, Davini O, et al. Tidal hyperinflation during low tidal volume ventilation in acute respiratory distress syndrome. *Am J Respir Crit Care Med*. January 15, 2007;175(2):160–166.
11. Talmor D, Sarge T, O'Donnell CR, Ritz R, Malhotra A, Lisbon A, et al. Esophageal and transpulmonary pressures in acute respiratory failure. *Crit Care Med*. May 2006;34(5):1389–1394.
12. Hager DN, Krishnan JA, Hayden DL, Brower RG, Network ACT. Tidal volume reduction in patients with acute lung injury when plateau pressures are not high. *Am J Res Crit Care Med*. 2005;172(10):1241–1245.
13. Wilson MR, Patel BV, Takata M. Ventilation with "clinically relevant" high tidal volumes does not promote stretch-induced injury in the lungs of healthy mice. *Crit Care Med*. October 2012;40(10):2850–2857.
14. Gajic O, Dara SI, Mendez JL, Adesanya AO, Festic E, Caples SM, et al. Ventilator-associated lung injury in patients without acute lung injury at the onset of mechanical ventilation. *Crit Care Med*. 2004;32(9):1817–1824.
15. Determann RM, Royakkers A, Wolthuis EK, Vlaar AP, Choi G, Paulus F, et al. Ventilation with lower tidal volumes as compared with conventional tidal volumes for patients without acute lung injury: a preventive randomized controlled trial. *Crit Care*. 2010;14(1):R1.
16. Futier E, Constantin JM, Paugam-Burtz C, Pascal J, Eurin M, Neuschwander A, et al. A trial of intraoperative low-tidal-volume ventilation in abdominal surgery. *N Eng J Med*. 2013;369(5): 428–437.
17. Severgnini P, Selmo G, Lanza C, Chiesa A, Frigerio A, Bacuzzi A, et al. Protective mechanical ventilation during general anesthesia for open abdominal surgery improves postoperative pulmonary function. *Anesthesiol*. June 2013;118(6):1307–1321.
18. Levine GK, Deutschman CS, Helfaer MA, Margulies SS. Sepsis-induced lung injury in rats increases alveolar epithelial vulnerability to stretch. *Crit Care Med*. 2006;34(6):1746–1751.
19. Tremblay L, Valenza F, Ribeiro SP, Li J, Slutsky AS. Injurious ventilatory strategies increase cytokines and c-fos m-RNA expression in an isolated rat lung model. *J Clin Invest*. March 1, 1997;99(5): 944–952.
20. Schiller HJ, McCann 2nd UG, Carney DE, Gatto LA, Steinberg JM, Nieman GF. Altered alveolar mechanics in the acutely injured lung. *Crit Care Med*. May 2001;29(5):1049–1055.
21. Muscedere JG, Mullen JB, Gan K, Slutsky AS. Tidal ventilation at low airway pressures can augment lung injury. *Am J Res Crit Care Med*. 1994;149(5):1327–1334.
22. Meade MO, Cook DJ, Guyatt GH, Slutsky AS, Arabi YM, Cooper DJ, et al. Ventilation strategy using low tidal volumes, recruitment maneuvers, and high positive end-expiratory pressure for acute lung injury and acute respiratory distress syndrome: a randomized controlled trial. *JAMA*. 2008;299(6):637–645.
23. Mercat A, Richard JC, Vielle B, Jaber S, Osman D, Diehl JL, et al. Positive end-expiratory pressure setting in adults with acute lung injury and acute respiratory distress syndrome: a randomized controlled trial. *JAMA*. 2008;299(6):646–655.
24. Brower RG, Lanken PN, MacIntyre N, Matthay MA, Morris A, Ancukiewicz M, et al. Higher versus lower positive end-expiratory pressures in patients with the acute respiratory distress syndrome. *N Engl J Med*. July 22, 2004;351(4):327–336.
25. Gattinoni L, Caironi P, Cressoni M, Chiumello D, Ranieri VM, Quintel M, et al. Lung recruitment in patients with the acute respiratory distress syndrome. *N Engl J Med*. 2006;354(17):1775–1786.
26. Goligher EC, Kavanagh BP, Rubenfeld GD, Adhikari NK, Pinto R, Fan E, et al. Oxygenation response to positive end-expiratory pressure predicts mortality in acute respiratory distress syndrome. A secondary analysis of the LOVS and ExPress trials. *Am J Respir Crit Care Med*. July 1, 2014;190(1):70–76.
27. Bellani G, Guerra L, Musch G, Zanella A, Patroniti N, Mauri T, et al. Lung regional metabolic activity and gas volume changes induced by tidal ventilation in patients with acute lung injury. *Am J Respir Crit Care Med*. 2011;183(9):1193–1199.
28. Force ADT, Ranieri VM, Rubenfeld GD, Thompson BT, Ferguson ND, Caldwell E, et al. Acute respiratory distress syndrome: the berlin definition. *JAMA*. 2012;307(23):2526–2533.
29. Brower RG, Lanken PN, MacIntyre N, Matthay MA, Morris A, Ancukiewicz M, et al. Higher versus lower positive end-expiratory pressures in patients with the acute respiratory distress syndrome. *N Engl J Med*. 2004;351(4):327–336.
30. Vieira SR, Puybasset L, Richecoeur J, Lu Q, Cluzel P, Gusman PB, et al. A lung computed tomographic assessment of positive end-expiratory pressure-induced lung overdistension. *Am J Respir Crit Care Med*. November 1998;158(5 Pt 1):1571–1577.
31. Albaiceta GM, Blanch L. Beyond volutrauma in ARDS: the critical role of lung tissue deformation. *Crit Care*. 2011;15(2):304.
32. Otto CM, Markstaller K, Kajikawa O, Karmrodt J, Syring RS, Pfeiffer B, et al. Spatial and temporal heterogeneity of ventilator-associated lung injury after surfactant depletion. (1985) *J Appl Physiol*. May 2008;104(5):1485–1494.
33. de Prost N, Costa EL, Wellman T, Musch G, Tucci MR, Winkler T, et al. Effects of ventilation strategy on distribution of lung inflammatory cell activity. *Crit Care*. 2013;17(4):R175.

34. Wakabayashi K, Wilson MR, Tatham KC, O'Dea KP, Takata M. Volutrauma, but not atelectrauma, induces systemic cytokine production by lung-marginated monocytes. *Crit Care Med.* January 2014;42(1):e49–e57.

35. Tsuchida S, Engelberts D, Peltekova V, Hopkins N, Frndova H, Babyn P, et al. Atelectasis causes alveolar injury in nonatelectatic lung regions. *Am J Respir Crit Care Med.* August 1, 2006;174(3): 279–289.

36. Retamal J, Bergamini B, Carvalho AR, Bozza FA, Borzone G, Borges J, et al. Non-lobar atelectasis generates inflammation and structural alveolar injury in the surrounding healthy tissue during mechanical ventilation. *Crit Care.* September 9, 2014;18(5):505.

37. Cereda M, Emami K, Xin Y, Kadlecek S, Kuzma NN, Mongkolwisetwara P, et al. Imaging the interaction of atelectasis and overdistension in surfactant-depleted lungs. *Crit Care Med.* 2013;41(2):527–535.

38. Cressoni M, Cadringher P, Chiurazzi C, Amini M, Gallazzi E, Marino A, et al. Lung inhomogeneity in patients with acute respiratory distress syndrome. *Am J Respir Crit Care Med.* 2014;189(2): 149–158.

39. Halter JM, Steinberg JM, Gatto LA, DiRocco JD, Pavone LA, Schiller HJ, et al. Effect of positive end-expiratory pressure and tidal volume on lung injury induced by alveolar instability. *Crit Care.* 2007;11(1):R20.

40. Seah AS, Grant KA, Aliyeva M, Allen GB, Bates JH. Quantifying the roles of tidal volume and PEEP in the pathogenesis of ventilator-induced lung injury. *Ann Biomed Eng.* May 2011;39(5): 1505–1516.

41. Manzano F, Fernandez-Mondejar E, Colmenero M, Poyatos ME, Rivera R, Machado J, et al. Positive-end expiratory pressure reduces incidence of ventilator-associated pneumonia in nonhypoxemic patients. *Crit Care Med.* 2008;36(8):2225–2231.

42. PROVE Network Investigators for the Clinical Trial Network of the European Society of Anaesthesiology, Hemmes SN, Gama de Abreu M, Pelosi P, Schultz MJ. High versus low positive end-expiratory pressure during general anaesthesia for open abdominal surgery (PROVHILO trial): a multicentre randomised controlled trial. *Lancet.* August 9, 2014;384(9942):495–503.

43. Amato MB, Barbas CS, Medeiros DM, Magaldi RB, Schettino GP, Lorenzi-Filho G, et al. Effect of a protective-ventilation strategy on mortality in the acute respiratory distress syndrome. *N Eng J Med.* 1998;338(6):347–354.

44. Brochard L, Roudot-Thoraval F, Roupie E, Delclaux C, Chastre J, Fernandez-Mondejar E, et al. Tidal volume reduction for prevention of ventilator-induced lung injury in acute respiratory distress syndrome. The multicenter trail group on tidal volume reduction in ARDS. *Am J Respir Crit Care Med.* 1998;158(6):1831–1838.

45. Stewart TE, Meade MO, Cook DJ, Granton JT, Hodder RV, Lapinsky SE, et al. Evaluation of a ventilation strategy to prevent barotrauma in patients at high risk for acute respiratory distress syndrome. Pressure- and volume-limited ventilation strategy group. *N Engl J Med.* February 5, 1998;338(6):355–361.

46. Needham DM, Colantuoni E, Mendez-Tellez PA, Dinglas VD, Sevransky JE, Dennison Himmelfarb CR, et al. Lung protective mechanical ventilation and two year survival in patients with acute lung injury: prospective cohort study. *BMJ.* 2012;344:e2124.

47. Hickling KG, Henderson SJ, Jackson R. Low mortality associated with low volume pressure limited ventilation with permissive hypercapnia in severe adult respiratory distress syndrome. *Intensive Care Med.* 1990;16(6):372–377.

48. Talmor D, Sarge T, Malhotra A, O'Donnell CR, Ritz R, Lisbon A, et al. Mechanical ventilation guided by esophageal pressure in acute lung injury. *N Engl J Med.* November 13, 2008;359(20): 2095–2104.

49. Terragni PP, Del Sorbo L, Mascia L, Urbino R, Martin EL, Birocco A, et al. Tidal volume lower than 6 ml/kg enhances lung protection: role of extracorporeal carbon dioxide removal. *Anesthesiol.* October 2009;111(4):826–835.

50. Peek GJ, Mugford M, Tiruvoipati R, Wilson A, Allen E, Thalanany MM, et al. Efficacy and economic assessment of conventional ventilatory support versus extracorporeal membrane oxygenation for severe adult respiratory failure (CESAR): a multicentre randomised controlled trial. *Lancet.* October 17, 2009;374(9698): 1351–1363.

51. Ferguson ND, Slutsky AS, Meade MO. High-frequency oscillation for ARDS. *N Engl J Med.* June 6, 2013;368(23):2233–2234.

52. Briel M, Meade M, Mercat A, Brower RG, Talmor D, Walter SD, et al. Higher vs lower positive end-expiratory pressure in patients with acute lung injury and acute respiratory distress syndrome: systematic review and meta-analysis. *JAMA.* 2010;303(9):865–873.

53. Dellinger RP, Levy MM, Rhodes A, Annane D, Gerlach H, Opal SM, et al. Surviving sepsis campaign: international guidelines for management of severe sepsis and septic shock: 2012. *Crit Care Med.* February 2013;41(2):580–637.

54. Wolf GK, Gomez-Laberge C, Rettig JS, Vargas SO, Smallwood CD, Prabhu SP, et al. Mechanical ventilation guided by electrical impedance tomography in experimental acute lung injury. *Crit Care Med.* May 2013;41(5):1296–1304.

55. Andrews PL, Shiber JR, Jaruga-Killeen E, Roy S, Sadowitz B, O'Toole RV, et al. Early application of airway pressure release ventilation may reduce mortality in high-risk trauma patients: a systematic review of observational trauma ARDS literature. *J Trauma Acute Care Surg.* October 2013;75(4):635–641.

56. Jardin F, Vieillard-Baron A. Right ventricular function and positive pressure ventilation in clinical practice: from hemodynamic subsets to respirator settings. *Intensive Care Med.* 2003;29(9): 1426–1434.

57. Papazian L, Forel JM, Gacouin A, Penot-Ragon C, Perrin G, Loundou A, et al. Neuromuscular blockers in early acute respiratory distress syndrome. *N Engl J Med.* September 16, 2010;363(12): 1107–1116.

58. Guerin C, Reignier J, Richard JC, Beuret P, Gacouin A, Boulain T, et al. Prone positioning in severe acute respiratory distress syndrome. *N Eng J Med.* 2013;368(23):2159–2168.

59. Bryan AC. Conference on the scientific basis of respiratory therapy. Pulmonary physiotherapy in the pediatric age group. Comments of a devil's advocate. *Am Rev Res Dis.* 1974;110(6 Pt 2):143–144.

60. Richter T, Bellani G, Scott Harris R, Vidal Melo MF, Winkler T, Venegas JG, et al. Effect of prone position on regional shunt, aeration, and perfusion in experimental acute lung injury. *Am J Respir Crit Care Med.* August 15, 2005;172(4):480–487.

61. Taccone P, Pesenti A, Latini R, Polli F, Vagginelli F, Mietto C, et al. Prone positioning in patients with moderate and severe acute respiratory distress syndrome: a randomized controlled trial. *JAMA.* November 11, 2009;302(18):1977–1984.

62. Shari G, Kojicic M, Li G, Cartin-Ceba R, Alvarez CT, Kashyap R, et al. Timing of the onset of acute respiratory distress syndrome: a population-based study. *Respir Care.* May 2011;56(5):576–582.

63. Gajic O, Dabbagh O, Park PK, Adesanya A, Chang SY, Hou P, et al. Early identification of patients at risk of acute lung injury: evaluation of lung injury prediction score in a multicenter cohort study. *Am J Respir Crit Care Med.* February 15, 2011;183(4):462–470.

64. Serpa Neto A, Cardoso SO, Manetta JA, Pereira VG, Esposito DC, Pasqualucci MdeO, et al. Association between use of lung-protective ventilation with lower tidal volumes and clinical outcomes among patients without acute respiratory distress syndrome: a meta-analysis. *JAMA.* October 24, 2012;308(16):1651–1659.

65. Futier E, Marret E, Jaber S. Perioperative positive pressure ventilation: an integrated approach to improve pulmonary care. *Anesthesiol.* August 2014;121(2):400–408.

66. Sutherasan Y, Vargas M, Pelosi P. Protective mechanical ventilation in the non-injured lung: review and meta-analysis. *Crit Care.* March 18, 2014;18(2):211.

67. Rubenfeld GD. Who cares about preventing ARDS? *Am J Respir Crit Care Med.* 2015;191(3):255–260.

68. Goldenberg NM, Steinberg BE, Lee WL, Wijeysundera DN, Kavanagh BP. Lung-protective ventilation in the operating room: time to implement? *Anesthesiol.* July 2014;121(1):184–188.

11 Is Extracorporeal Life Support an Evidence-Based Intervention for Critically Ill Adults with ARDS?

Eliotte Hirshberg, Fernando Zampieri, Michael Lanspa,
Kimberly S. Bennett, R. Duncan Hite, Alan H. Morris

Extracorporeal life support (ECLS) is a treatment option for patients with inadequate oxygen delivery. Inadequate oxygen delivery can result from either ineffective oxygenation from severe lung disease or ineffective cardiac output from severe circulatory failure or both. This chapter addresses the evidence supporting use of ECLS in adults with respiratory failure. We discuss limitations in ECLS clinical trial design, the importance of detailed protocols in multicenter trials, the evolution of acute respiratory distress syndrome (ARDS) management over time, and the economic feasibility of ECLS. We briefly review ECLS techniques and advances and focus on a detailed review of the highest quality ECLS evidence. We do not discuss the evidence for ECLS in children and neonates. Therefore we ask the question, "Is ECLS an evidence-based intervention for critically ill adults with ARDS?"

WHY EVIDENCE IN CRITICAL CARE IS OFTEN INSUFFICIENT

Many clinicians hold strong beliefs regarding the efficacy of ECLS for patients with severe ARDS despite a paucity of credible evidence.[1] The highest quality evidence to guide decisions about ECLS for adults with ARDS comes from four randomized controlled trials (RCTs; Table 11-1).[2-5] An actively enrolling prospective RCT (the Extracorporeal Membrane Oxygenation for Severe Acute Respiratory Distress Syndrome [EOLIA] trial) may also advance our understanding (http://www.clinicaltrials.gov/ct2/show /NCT01470703?term=eolia&rank=1; http://revaweb.org /gb/etudes.php#e2). However, current ECLS literature is dominated by observational studies, clinical experiences, clinical reports, and opinions. Observational studies and trials of ECLS with low credibility are difficult to interpret for various reasons that have not changed over the past 30 years.[6] These reasons, detailed later, are central to the controversy surrounding ECLS today.

It is generally accepted that scientifically rigorous clinical experiments provide the best foundation for the evaluation of the efficacy of clinical interventions.[7,8] Personal clinical experiences, including observational case series and case reports, provide important preliminary information that can stimulate thinking and create hypotheses, but they fall short of rigorous compelling evidence that a therapy is either effective or efficacious. Unfortunately, rigorous experiments addressing the benefit for ECLS in ARDS are uncommon. Even clinical trial evidence, our most credible source of evidence, is often of low quality.[9-12]

A persistent threat to the credibility of critical care trial results is the introduction of both random and systematic error. Systematic error (bias) is the more challenging and requires careful attention in experimental design. The belief that bias plays little role in clinical trials[13,14] is incorrect for many critical care experiments.[7] Differential (between-group) bias frequently exists because of uneven distribution of confounders, but it can also exist because of uneven distribution of the experimental intervention, especially in nonblinded (open) clinical trials. In ECLS trials, variable application of mechanical ventilation in both the intervention and control arm can be a confounder. Confounders introduced after subject assignment to the clinical trial groups are better termed "co-interventions" and should be distinguished from confounders that exist before subject allocation to the experimental groups.[15-17]

Clinical trials that test complex and multifaceted interventions such as ECLS are particularly vulnerable to confounding from management issues such as transfusion or mechanical ventilation practices that are not uniform among experimental groups. Co-interventions in clinical trials are frequently neither controlled nor measured, and this deficiency threatens the internal validity of critical care clinical trials. In nonblinded (open) scientifically rigorous critical care clinical trials, all experimental arms require well-defined protocols that contain enough detail to standardize clinician decisions about both the experimental intervention and important co-interventions.[7,18,19] In clinical studies of ECLS, between-group nonuniformity can occur in the management of the ECLS

Table 11-1 **RCTs of ECLS for ARDS in Adults**

Study, Year	Number of Subjects (Intervention/Control)	Study Design	Intervention	Control	Survival
ECMO in severe ARDS, 1979[4,102]	90 (42/48)	Prospective, nonblinded RCT	Mechanical ventilation + partial VA ECMO	Mechanical ventilation alone	9.5% ECMO; 8.3% control; no statistically significant difference
PCIRV and ECCO$_2$R for ARDS, 1994[3]	40 (21/19)	Prospective, nonblinded RCT	LFPPV + ECCO$_2$R	Conventional positive-pressure ventilation	32% ECCO$_2$R; 42% control; no statistically significant difference
CESAR, 2009 ECMO in ARDS vs conventional ventilation[5]	180	Prospective multicenter referral to expert center, nonblinded RCT	Combination of mechanical ventilation + either VA or VV ECMO	Conventional mechanical ventilation	36% ECMO; 50% control; no statistically significant difference
ECCO$_2$R + 3 mL/kg V_T in ARDS vs 6 mL/kg mechanical ventilation[2]	79	Prospective, nonblinded RCT	Low (3 mL/kg) V_T ventilation + ECCO$_2$R	Standard 6 mL/kg ventilation	Overall mortality 16.5%; no difference between groups* Primary outcome VFD–28

*Primary endpoint VFDs, not mortality.
ARDS, acute respiratory distress syndrome; *CESAR*, Conventional Ventilation or ECMO for Severe Adult Respiratory Failure; *ECCO$_2$R*, extracorporeal CO$_2$ removal; *ECLS*, extracorporeal life support; *ECMO*, extracorporeal membrane oxygenation; *LFPPV*, low-frequency positive-pressure ventilation; *PCIRV*, pressure-controlled inverse ratio ventilation; *RCT*, randomized controlled trial; *VA*, venoarterial; *VFD*, ventilator-free day; *V$_T$*, tidal volume; *VV*, veno-venous.

itself (the experimental intervention) because in the past, the methods used were commonly not replicable.[7]

Inconsistency in study subject selection is an additional cause of variability in clinical ECLS study results. Randomization cannot account for differences between the study subjects and the population of interest from which they are derived. The patients who arrive at study institutions constitute a convenience sample; even a multicenter study may be seen roughly as a conglomerate of convenience samples. The process of obtaining consent may also result in a selection bias; many critically ill patients are unable to provide their own consent. A myriad of technical and personnel ECLS aspects must be considered. Therefore the link between any given patient and the ECLS study population may vary. This variation produces questions about generalizability (external validity) with almost all clinical studies. Consequently, clinicians who try to apply study results must always ask whether the patient under consideration belongs to the subset of subjects from which the study results were obtained and whether their setting is similar to the study setting, before using a study intervention.[16,20] Guides to assess the evaluation of external validity have been published.[21]

Meta-analyses are meant to overcome some of the limitations of many clinical studies by pooling their results, but the quality of a meta-analysis depends on the quality of the clinical studies on which it is based.[19,22,23] In addition, there are several steps that must be performed to obtain reliable results through meta-analysis, but few analyses follow all the appropriate procedures.[24] Many meta-analyses may produce positive results simply because of an insufficient

sample size, without proper adjustment for multiple comparisons.[24] Scientists expect experimental results that properly describe the way the world works to be independently reproduced by other investigators. For such results to be reproduced, it is required that the methods of the experiment be replicable.[7,25-27] Unfortunately, the methods of most ECLS studies lack detail and are not replicable. Even the use of Bayesian methods (which adjust for uncertainty) would not overcome the limitations imposed by some methodological inadequacies of included studies. Therefore conclusions of meta-analysis results must be interpreted with caution.

IMPORTANCE OF ADEQUATELY EXPLICIT PROTOCOLS FOR CLINICAL TRIALS

We define an adequately explicit protocol as a protocol with enough detail to respond consistently to changing patient conditions. Adequately explicit protocols generate specific instructions (patient-specific or personalized) that do not require judgments by the clinician.[28] Although adequately explicit computerized protocols often contain the greatest detail,[7,28-31] paper-based versions can also contain enough detail to be adequately explicit.[32,33]

Most clinical study protocols are not adequately explicit. Even systematic and scholarly collections of flow diagrams commonly lack necessary detail and do not standardize clinician decisions.[34-36] Most protocols can elicit different clinical decisions from different clinicians because clinician decision makers must fill in the gaps in the insufficiently detailed protocol logic. Clinicians' judgments will vary with their backgrounds and experience, as will their choices of the rules and variables they use to fill in the gaps of inadequately explicit guidelines and protocols. This is a major contributor to unwarranted variation in clinical care.[37-39] Protocols and flow diagrams are commonly but inappropriately called algorithms.[34,36]

An algorithm in mathematics or engineering is a precise solution,[40] although its definition allows for the more liberal use common in medicine ("a set of rules for solving a problem in a finite number of steps").[41] "Solving a problem" is the operative concept—our current techniques have not solved the problem. It is important to make this distinction between adequately explicit protocols and the more common guidelines and protocols because it may help us to develop more scientifically rigorous clinical trials for ECLS.[7,18,42] Adequately explicit protocols can enable replicable clinical trial methods in multicenter trials of ECLS, thus enhancing the quality and reproducibility of future ECLS trial results.

HISTORY OF ARDS PATIENT SURVIVAL AND MANAGEMENT

ARDS therapy is usually supportive. Mechanical ventilation strategy, positive end-expiratory pressure (PEEP), inspired oxygen (O_2), and breathing mechanics play central roles. Other therapeutic interventions that should be assessed include prone positioning, neuromuscular blockade, and intravenous fluid administration.[43-47] Although diffuse, ARDS injury is not uniform, but this was not widely appreciated in early studies. The static thoracic compliance of ARDS patients appears to be directly proportional to the fraction of aerated lung, and only a small fraction of the lung appears to receive the tidal volume.[48] After this understanding, newer therapeutic approaches focused on reducing the vigor of mechanical ventilation. These included intravenous oxygenation, permissive hypercapnia, pressure-controlled inverse ratio ventilation (PCIRV), low tidal volume mechanical ventilation, high frequency oscillatory ventilation, and airway pressure release ventilation, among others.[49-53]

Survival of ARDS patients is highly variable. Survival from severe ARDS in the 1970s was as low as 10% to 15%.[4,54,55] After 1988, survival from ARDS was higher.[46,47,56] More recently, reported survival from ARDS has increased to 60% to 80%.[57-59] This secular increase in survival, combined with advances in mechanical ventilation and in ECLS technology, makes historical comparisons challenging. Changes in ARDS definitions, including the new Berlin definition, and in trial enrollment criteria also make comparison between studies difficult.[60,61] Few recent studies include clear patient criteria for ECLS therapy. Uniformly applied extracorporeal membrane oxygenation (ECMO) entry criteria, similar to those used in the 1970s trial of ECMO, could enhance replicability of subject selection in future ECLS trials.[4]

The H1N1 epidemic was associated with an increase in ARDS incidence and stimulated use of newer therapeutic approaches, including ECLS, for ARDS. Unfortunately, the observational studies examining ECLS for ARDS after H1N1 influenza have the limitations described earlier. Two national ARDS registry reports led to conflicting conclusions regarding ECLS therapy for H1N1-induced respiratory failure. A retrospective cohort study matched 80 patients with H1N1 influenza–associated ARDS who were referred to one of four ECLS centers in the United Kingdom. Patients referred to an ECLS center survived at nearly twice the rate of the group who were not referred to an ECLS center.[62] The results were consistent with three different methods of statistical matching. A major limitation to this design is the inability to control for confounders such as mechanical ventilation strategies and ECMO patient selection criteria. Patients with mechanically ventilated lungs from the ARDS Network H1N1 influenza registry were treated with lung-protective mechanical ventilation strategy (6 mL/kg predicted body weight), and some received ECLS. Survival of ARDS Network H1N1 influenza registry patients who received ECLS did not seem to differ from those who met ECLS eligibility criteria but were not treated with ECLS.[63,64] ECLS eligibility was determined by the presence of severe hypoxemia within the first 7 days of mechanical ventilation. Of 600 adult patients with H1N1 and requiring mechanical ventilation, 31 patients received ECLS and 569 did not receive ECLS. Ninety-one (16%) of these 569 were deemed eligible for ECLS. Unadjusted 60-day survival did not differ between the ECLS-eligible group (66%) and the group that actually received ECLS (52%).[63] In summary, survival of ARDS Network H1N1 registry patients who were eligible for ECLS but were treated with conventional therapy appeared similar to survival of ECLS-supported H1N1 patients in the United Kingdom and in the previously reported H1N1 patient survival in Australia and New Zealand.[62,63,65]

Lung-protective ventilation (6 mL/kg predicted body weight tidal volume strategy) with the appropriate application of PEEP is the most credible evidence-based approach for management of ARDS.[32,62,63,65-70] Theoretically, ECLS technology could allow almost complete lung rest. However, if or how total lung rest with ECLS might further increase survival remains unknown.[71] A retrospective examination of mechanical ventilation practices during ECMO suggested that the higher PEEP levels in the first 3 days of ECMO therapy were associated with increased survival. The authors of that study concluded that further research on appropriate mechanical ventilation practice during ECLS was needed.[72] More recently, researchers have described ECLS as a "super protective" mechanical ventilation strategy.[73] The ECLS organization registry and reported case series indicate that prolonged (9 to 14 days) mechanical ventilation before ECLS support is common and is associated with decreased survival in adult patients.[74-77] ECLS supporters argue that early intervention with ECLS increases survival by reducing mechanical ventilation exposure. These observations underscore the importance of both co-intervention protocols and unambiguous patient section criteria for ECLS therapy rather than reliance on clinician judgment for ventilator management or patient selection.

Unfortunately, the accuracy with which clinicians predict survival in individual patients with ARDS (compared with large groups) is frequently low.[78] Using defined fraction of inspired O_2 (FIO_2) and PEEP conditions for determining the ratio of partial pressure of arterial O_2 (Pao_2)/Fio_2 might enhance patient selection because Fio_2 and PEEP seem to predict patient outcome.[79] In fact, this selection strategy was used in the 1970s ECMO trial, the first ECLS clinical trial.[4] An important conclusion to be drawn from this discussion of variation in survival over time is that the use of historical controls for estimating ECLS efficacy is dangerous. This emphasizes the need for carefully crafted randomized controlled clinical trials.[32,33,46,56]

ECONOMIC FEASIBILITY OF ECLS IN PATIENTS WITH ARDS

There are important unresolved cost-effectiveness issues that present practical barriers to widespread ECLS use for respiratory failure. Although the prices for ECLS systems are falling, training and maintaining a center is expensive and requires significant resources. Therefore it is not surprising that ECLS access across the United States is variable.[80] Although the CESAR (Conventional Ventilation or ECMO for Severe Adult Respiratory Failure) trial authors asserted that ECLS could be cost-effective, their results should be interpreted with caution; the study design did not allow credible conclusions about the efficacy of ECLS.[5,64,81,82] The cost of ECLS-related complications must also be incorporated. Zangrillo's meta-analysis noted a 54% ECMO patient mortality with frequent complications, including renal failure, pneumonia, sepsis, and bleeding.[83] In a recent hypothetical cost-effective simulation of ECLS with Markov chain analysis, Park showed that ECLS could be associated with acceptable costs, although the analysis did not account for training and personnel costs.[84] The costs of keeping an ECLS team ready in places with low demand may be unjustified.

SOME PRINCIPLES AND OBJECTIVES OF ECLS

ECLS can support patient gas exchange (oxygenation and alveolar ventilation) and hemodynamic function with two general strategies of circulatory access: venovenous (VV) or venoarterial (VA). With VA cannulation, blood is drained from the right atrium via the central venous system and returned to the proximal arterial system. VA support bypasses both ventricles and the intervening pulmonary system, unloading the patient's natural heart and lung and providing gas exchange and hemodynamic support. In most cases, partial support is achieved, with some residual pulmonary blood flow present in the natural lung.

With VV cannulation, blood is drained and subsequently returned via the right internal jugular vein or femoral veins. VV support has its origins in the work of Kolobow, Gattinoni, and others, who introduced VV cannulation for extracorporeal CO_2 removal ($ECCO_2R$).[68,85,86] Newer cannulation techniques allow for higher blood flows and minimal recirculation and also can provide adequate support of oxygenation. Although VV support does not directly provide hemodynamic support, improved oxygen delivery may improve myocardial performance.

ECLS now includes older techniques that emphasize CO_2 removal ($ECCO_2R$) or arterial oxygenation (ECMO). Modern ECLS equipment enables both of these and blurs the distinction between them. Technologic advances have improved cannula flows and mechanics, and VV has begun to supplant the VA approach, unless concomitant cardiac failure exists. Although VA cannulation can support lung and cardiac failure, VV cannulation is often preferred for patients who have adequate intrinsic cardiac function. VV ECMO use is increasing.[87]

Patient selection criteria for ECLS vary considerably.[75,88-90] These criteria also determine the ECLS technique (e.g., VV or VA ECMO or $ECCO_2R$). $ECCO_2R$ has been used primarily in patients without refractory hypoxemia.[91,92] Different cannulations, pump systems, and complication rates are reported for the different techniques.[93] Therefore direct comparison of study results is complicated by the use of VV and VA ECLS techniques within individual published case series. This limits the ability of such case series to accurately inform readers and clinicians about the true effects, risks, and complications they may encounter if and when extracorporeal support is attempted at their local institutions.

Technical advances and extensive clinical experience have made it clear that patients with ARDS can be supported successfully with ECLS.[54,94-100] However, technical accomplishment does not equal clinical efficacy.

CLINICAL TRIAL EVIDENCE ADDRESSING THE USE OF ECLS FOR ARDS

Because randomized controlled clinical trials provide the most compelling evidence for clinical decision-making, it is pertinent to note that only four RCTs of ECLS in adult respiratory failure have been published to date (Table 11-1). ECLS enthusiasts often disregard the first two trials, noting their use of more complicated equipment, older techniques, and inexperience as the reasons for the negative trial results. They argue that current ECLS techniques save patients who are otherwise destined to die. However, Roger Bone[6] cautioned against the early adoption of ECLS and suggested the need for clear diagnostic criteria and measurement of anticipated adverse effects before the widespread use of ECLS could be justified.[6]

The first ECLS RCT in adults, the randomized multicenter trial of ECMO for ARDS, selected a subset of ARDS patients with severe disease and poor outcome—only 8 (9%) of 90 randomized patients survived[101,102] with no difference in survival between ECMO and conventional care.[4] Efforts to introduce widespread clinical use of ECMO for adults with ARDS were thereafter abandoned.

Kolobow, Gattinoni, and their colleagues subsequently introduced the concept of "lung rest." The need to ventilate the injured natural lung could be reduced in proportion to the CO_2 removed by a spiral silicone membrane ($ECCO_2R$). The $ECCO_2R$ relieved the natural lung of some of its ventilatory burden.[68,85,86] They intended to increase patient survival after reduction of the intensity of mechanical ventilation and of the consequent putative iatrogenic lung damage.[103,104] The intermediate goal of their low-frequency positive-pressure ventilation extracorporeal CO_2 removal

(LFPPV-ECCO$_2$R) was to reduce the motion of the diseased lung to a minimum with almost complete elimination of ventilation (with only 3 to 5 breaths/min). This technique has shown benefit in recent small studies of patients with chronic obstructive pulmonary disease.[105,106] The management of the natural lungs of the randomized patients in the National Institutes of Health (NIH) collaborative ECMO trial of 1974-1977[4] did not adhere to these principles of lung rest.[94] Therefore a superimposed iatrogenic lung injury due to higher end-inspiratory pressures or tidal volumes to ARDS lungs of the study subjects might have introduced enough bias to affect the ECMO trial outcome.[48,104,107]

Gattinoni et al. reported an increase in survival of ARDS patients after use of PCIRV followed by LFPPV-ECCO$_2$R, but their observational study was an uncontrolled clinical application.[19,55,107-112] In the second RCT of ECLS in adults, Morris et al.[3] subsequently observed a similar survival between a control and interventional group with an overall increased survival of all patients when compared with historical controls of the 1970s.[3] Unexpectedly, the 42% survival of their control patients supported with continuous positive-pressure ventilation was not statistically significantly different from the 33% survival of patients supported with PCIRV/LFPPV-ECCO$_2$R.[3]

A trial in which LFPPV-ECCO$_2$R was used as its primary intervention represents a significantly different intervention than the primary intervention of ECMO in the 1974-1977 trial (Table 11-1). The higher survival of ARDS patients after support with LFPPV-ECCO$_2$R is intriguing. Pulmonary blood flow is likely an important determinant of lung response to injury.[105,106,113,114] Pulmonary blood flow is preserved in VV LFPPV-ECCO$_2$R, whereas the 1974-1977 VA ECMO technique markedly reduced pulmonary blood flow to the natural lung. The preservation of natural lung blood flow, with the low natural lung ventilation, leads to a low overall ventilation-perfusion (V/Q) ratio during VV LFPPV-ECCO$_2$R. The 1974-1977 VA ECMO technique produced an oligemic natural lung with a high overall V/Q ratio.[2] On the basis of observations in animals, a high overall V/Q ratio might cause lung necrosis in patients with ARDS.[115,116] Both preserved pulmonary blood flow and lung rest are two significant differences between LFPPV-ECCO$_2$R and ECMO that may be important contributors to the difference in patient survival between the LFPPV-ECCO$_2$R[3] and the 1974-1977 ECMO clinical trials.[4] However, the high survival rate in the control group during the ECCO$_2$R trial suggests that other variables than the differences between ECCO$_2$R and ECMO contributed more significantly to the higher survival.

The highest quality randomized clinical trials of extracorporeal support for adults with ARDS enrolled only 90,[4] 40,[3] and 79 patients.[2] The power to detect a real difference between control and LFPPV-ECCO$_2$R therapy group survival depends on the number of patients studied.[16,117-119] Assuming that the observed survival rates of 42% for the control group and 33% for the LFPPV-ECCO$_2$R group represent the true survival rates of these two treatment groups, the number of study patients required to detect this difference in survival 80% of the time (power=0.8) is approximately 400 in each treatment group.[117] Only multicenter trials can provide sufficient patient enrollment to

make such studies feasible. Detailed or adequately explicit protocols could enable the multiple clinical sites, in such a multicenter trial, to function as an extended laboratory with replicable methods.[7]

The largest completed prospective ECLS trial to date, CESAR, was a multicenter trial. However, the methods of CESAR seemed to lack detailed co-intervention protocols and reproducible patient selection criteria for requiring ECLS.[128] Central to their study was the identification of "potentially reversible respiratory failure" patients.[120] Many patients randomized to the ECLS arm did not receive ECLS once transferred to the ECLS center, and several ECLS patients required VA rather than VV ECMO. However, the methods do not indicate exactly how this identification was achieved. Fundamental to the success of the CESAR trial was the trial design that included referral to a facility with ECLS expertise. The astute researchers recognized the need for ECLS-specific training, exposure, and experience.[5,120,121] Peek et al.[5,121] report an increase in 6-month disability-free survival in the ECLS group. Although some may find it reasonable to conclude from CESAR that ECLS in the hands of an experienced team poses no additional harm to adult patients with ARDS, we conclude that the trial, which was designed for effectiveness, not efficacy, does not provide adequate information to inform either regarding ECLS support for ARDS patients. There was no within-site allocation of patients into the two therapy arms. As a result, the likely substantial intersite variations of mechanical ventilation strategy could have created a design bias that significantly influenced the results. Patients treated at the ECLS referral center may have been more likely to receive standardized, lung-protective mechanical ventilation than those treated in other ICUs. Conventional care was neither protocolized nor clearly defined and was not likely the same at all referring hospitals.

In the Xtravent-study, Bein and colleagues asked if ECLS for CO$_2$ removal plus very low tidal volume would improve ventilator-free days in patients with established ARDS. In this high-quality multicenter RCT of 79 patients with ARDS and a high plateau pressure (>25 cm H$_2$O), patients were randomized to ECCO$_2$R plus 3 mL/kg tidal volume versus conventional 6 mL/kg tidal volume ventilation.[2] Clear inclusion and exclusion criteria ensured patient uniformity. Identical ventilator protocols (except for the tidal volume breaths [3 mL and 6 mL/kg]) served to standardize mechanical ventilation, an important study co-intervention. Despite the design strengths of this study, a time limitation was imposed on the investigators, and they were unable to meet their prespecified sample size. They concluded that ventilation with 3 mL/kg tidal volume and ECCO$_2$R was safe and feasible and not associated with a significant reduction in ventilator-free days at 28 days.[2]

After the 2009 H1N1 novel influenza pandemic, several institutions reported observational data suggesting ECLS increased survival compared with historical survival data.[65,122] Most of this literature comes from ECLS-positive case series and observational studies that likely include publication bias. More recently, two meta-analyses addressed ECLS for severe respiratory failure in adult patients.[123,124] Zampieri et al. used a strict evaluation score of quality and only five studies based on a potential

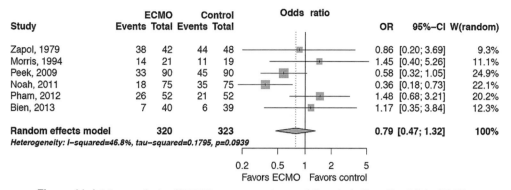

Figure 11-1 Meta-analysis of ECLS in severe respiratory failure including all published RCTs.

49 were considered for the final analysis.[124] The analysis included three studies (353 patients total) including the CEASAR RCT but excluded the older previously mentioned RCTs and included one retrospective case series and one case control analysis.[5,62,124,125] Munshi included 10 studies (RCT and observational).[123] Despite differences in conception and in study selection, both meta-analyses reached similar conclusions. More important, both were sensitive to the statistical method. A benefit of ECLS was not found in the main analysis and could only be found in subgroup or sensitivity analyses.[123,124]

We repeated Zampieri's meta-analysis with the highest quality evidence available and included the RCTs by Zapol, Morris, and Bein.[2-4] In this analysis, the data from the CESAR study were included as presented in the "intention-to-treat" analysis (therefore not all patients in fact received ECLS), and data from a study by Noah et al. were added as reported by the authors in the propensity analysis with replacement (thereby assuring that both groups would be paired for illness severity).[62] This analysis workflow maximized group balance. The random-effects model again showed no survival benefit with ECLS with an odds ratio of 0.79 (Fig. 11-1). Including the highest quality evidence (four RCTs and two case control studies), the survival benefit of ECLS for adults with severe respiratory failure remains undemonstrated.

We also performed a trial sequential analysis (TSA) to control for bias that could arise from multiple testing and to provide an estimate of the required sample size that would be needed to achieve a definitive answer. The same studies were included. RCTs were added as low risk of bias and observational studies were added as high risk of bias for this analysis. The boundaries were established to limit the global type 1 error to 5% and were calculated with the O'Brien-Fleming function, which considered a power of 80% to detect a 20% decrease in mortality with ECMO, considering a mean mortality in control patients of 50% (based on the pooling of all previous studies included). Heterogeneity correction was based on a diversity meta-analysis [D^2]. A D^2 analysis adjusts for diversity and is conceptually defined as $(vR-vF)/vR$, where vR is the total variance in the random-effects model and vF is the total variance in the fixed-effect model. We used TSA software, version 0.9 beta (http://www.ctu.dk/tsa/, Copenhagen Trial Unit, Copenhagen, Denmark) for this analysis. The information fraction was too low to assess futility; nevertheless, the TSA analysis highlighted that there is no definitive answer to this subject (the analysis is underpowered). Considering the proposed effect size estimation presented above (20% reduction in mortality, a very optimistic estimation), more than 1680 patients would be needed to be included in a controlled clinical trial to establish a robust conclusion.

The EOLIA trial at the time of this writing is a currently enrolling trial of ECLS (http://www.clinicaltrials.gov/ct2/show/NCT01470703?term=eolia&rank=1; http://revaweb.org/gb/etudes.php#e2). EOLIA is designed to determine the impact of early (immediate) initiation of ECLS with lung rest on survival. EOLIA has already randomized 172 of the 220 patients needed to reach a 90% probability of stopping the study early, according to its sequential analytical plan (Alain Combes, MD, written communication, 2015). The ECLS group will be compared with a conventional ARDS management group with lung-protective ventilation plus all possible salvage therapies, including ECLS. EOLIA will improve on prior study designs with a larger sample size and by inclusion of a detailed lung-protective mechanical ventilation control arm protocol. However, crossover from the control arm to the intervention arm by offering ECLS as salvage therapy to control-arm subjects based on clinician judgment (Alain Combes, MD, written communication, 2015) presents a methodological problem that will diminish the internal validity of the experimental results. In addition, reliance on clinician judgment to determine the need for salvage therapy is imprecise. Prediction of imminent death is imperfect with reported survival of approximately 16% of patients thought unequivocally destined to die by all clinicians participating in direct care of ICU patients.[126] Imprecise selection of patients requiring ECLS will result in systematic bias and will threaten the internal validity of the trial results. Furthermore, internal validity should generally precede external validity in study sequences that lead to credible foundations for general clinical applications.[14,16,20]

Clinical trial evidence supporting the routine use of ECLS therapy for adult patients with ARDS is lacking. The EOLIA trial will provide a step forward in helping to understand the potential impact of ECLS in the management of ARDS, but it will not be conclusive based on the methodological issues noted previously. A carefully crafted multicenter trial designed to determine important differences in outcomes other than mortality is feasible. A future efficacy trial of ECLS that uses strict patient selection criteria, possibly with some of the criteria in newly developed predictions scores for ECLS survival, such as the Respiratory Extracorporeal Membrane Oxygenation Survival Predication (RESP) score[127] or the ECMOnet score,[128] and the standardization of co-intervention management protocols is still needed before widespread adoption of ECLS for respiratory distress can be recommended.[128]

CONCLUSION

ECLS is a technically demanding set of strategies capable of supporting life in adults with severe lung failure. In the hands of skilled clinicians, ECLS has become part of routine ARDS management. Although ECLS will likely continue to be applied to adults with respiratory failure, we currently lack the ability to consistently identify those patients who should receive ECLS. Until detailed and replicable methods for conducting ECLS in either clinical care or in clinical trials have been described, investigators cannot duplicate ECLS studies. There is insufficient evidence to support the widespread use of ECLS in adult patients with ARDS. The role of ECLS in the routine care of adults with ARDS remains unknown and ill defined.

AUTHORS' RECOMMEDNATIONS

- The widespread use of ECLS in adult patients with ARDS in not supported by the evidence.
- Clear criteria to identify patients with ARDS who would benefit most from ECLS therapy are still needed.
- A robust clinical trial testing the efficacy of ELCS therapy for adults with ARDS compared with standard lung protective ventilation requires a carefully crafted multicenter trial with target enrollment near 1700 patients.

REFERENCES

1. Mitchell MD, Mikkelsen ME, Umscheid CA, Lee I, Fuchs BD, Halpern SD. A systematic review to inform institutional decisions about the use of extracorporeal membrane oxygenation during the H1N1 influenza pandemic. *Crit Care Med.* 2010;38(6):1398–1404.
2. Bein T, Weber-Carstens S, Goldmann A, et al. Lower tidal volume strategy (approximately 3 mL/kg) combined with extracorporeal CO_2 removal versus 'conventional' protective ventilation (6 mL/kg) in severe ARDS: the prospective randomized Xtravent-study. *Intensive Care Med.* 2013;39(5):847–856.
3. Morris A, Wallace C, Menlove R, et al. Randomized clinical trial of pressure-controlled inverse ratio ventilation and extracorporeal CO_2 removal for ARDS. [erratum 1994;149(3, Pt 1):838, Letters to the editor 1995;151(1):255–256, 1995;151(4):1269-1270, and 1997;156(3):1016-1017] *Am J Respir Crit Care Med.* 1994;149(2):295–305.
4. Zapol WM, Snider MT, Hill JD, et al. Extracorporeal membrane oxygenation in severe acute respiratory failure. *JAMA.* 1979;242:2193–2196.
5. Peek GJ, Mugford M, Tiruvoipati R, et al. Efficacy and economic assessment of conventional ventilatory support versus extracorporeal membrane oxygenation for severe adult respiratory failure (CESAR): a multicentre randomised controlled trial. *Lancet.* 2009;374(9698):1351–1363.
6. Bone R. Extracorporeal membrane oxygenation for acute respiratory failure (Editorial). *JAMA.* 1986;256(7):910.
7. Morris A. The importance of protocol-directed patient management for research on lung-protective ventilation. In: Dreyfuss D, Saumon G, Hubamyr R, eds. *Ventilator-Induced Lung Injury. Lung Biology in Health and Disease.* vol. 215. New York: Taylor & Francis Group; 2006:537–610.
8. Schultz S. Homeostasis, humpty dumpty, and integrative biology. *News Physiol Sci.* 1996;11:238–246.
9. Eddy DM, Billings J. The quality of medical evidence, implications for quality of care. *Health Aff (Millwood).* 1988;7:19.
10. Herbert RD, Bo K. Analysis of quality of interventions in systematic reviews. *BMJ.* 2005;331(7515):507–509.
11. Ioannidis JPA. Why most published research findings are false. *PLoS Med.* 2005;2(8):e124.
12. Morris AH, Ioannidis JPA. Limitations of medical research and evidence at the patient-clinician encounter scale. *Chest J.* 2013;143(4):1127–1135.
13. Friedman LM, Furberg CD, DeMets DL. *Fundamentals of Clinical Trials.* 3rd ed. New York: Springer-Verlag; 1998. 361 p.
14. Rothman K, Greenland S. *Modern Epidemiology.* 2nd ed. Philadelphia, Pennsylvania: Lippincott-Raven; 1998.
15. Cochrane-Collaboration. *The Cochrane Reviewer's Handbook Glossary* Version 4.1.4. ed: The Cochrane Collaboration; 2001.
16. Hulley S, Cummings S, Warren S, Grady D, Hearst N, Newman T. *Designing Clinical Research.* 2nd ed. Philadelphia: Lippincott Williams and Wilkins; 2001. 336 p.
17. Sackett D, Haynes R, Guyatt G, Tugwell P. *Clinical epidemiology: a basic science for clinical medicine.* 2nd ed. Little. Boston: Brown; 1991. 187–248 p.
18. Morris A. Developing and implementing computerized protocols for standardization of clinical decisions. *Ann Intern Med.* 2000;132:373–383.
19. Morris A, Cook D. Clinical trial issues in mechanical ventilation. In: Marini J, Slutsky A, eds. *Physiologic Basis of Ventilatory Suport. Lung Biology in Health and Disease.* New York: Marcel Dekker, Inc; 1998:1359–1398.
20. Hébert PC, Cook DJ, Wells G, Marshall J. The design of randomized clinical trials in critically ill patients. *Chest.* 2002;121(4):1290–1300.
21. Bornhoft G, Maxion-Bergemann S, Wolf U, et al. Checklist for the qualitative evaluation of clinical studies with particular focus on external validity and model validity. *BMC Med Res Methodol.* 2006;6:56.
22. Feinstein A, Horwitz R. Clinical Judgment revisited: the distraction of quantitative models. *Am J Med.* 1997;103:529–535.
23. LeLorier J, Gregoire G, Benhaddad A, Lapierre J, Derderian F. Discrepancies between meta-analyses and subsequent large randomized, controlled trials. [see comments] *N Engl J Med.* 1997;337(8):536–542.
24. Jackson D, Turner R, Rhodes K, Viechtbauer W. Methods for calculating confidence and credible intervals for the residual between-study variance in random effects meta-regression models. *BMC Med Res Methodol.* 2014;14:103.
25. Babbie E. *Observing Ourselves: Essays in Social Research.* Belmont, Cal: Wadsworth Pub. Co; 1986.
26. Campbell D, Stanley J. *Experimental and Quasi-Experimental Designs for Research (Reprinted from Handbook of Research on Teaching, 1963).* Boston: Houghton Mifflin Co.; 1966. 84 p.
27. Giancoli D. *Physics.* 3rd ed. Englewood Cliffs, NJ: Prentice Hall; 1995. 3 p.
28. Blagev DP, Hirshberg EL, Sward K, et al. The evolution of eProtocols that enable reproducible clinical research and care methods. *J Clin Monit Comput.* 2012;26(4):305–317.
29. East T, Heermann L, Bradshaw R, et al. Efficacy of computerized decision support for mechanical ventilation: results of a prospective multi-center randomized trial. *Proc AMIA Symp.* 1999:251–255.
30. East TD, Böhm SH, Wallace CJ, et al. A successful computerized protocol for clinical management of pressure control inverse ratio ventilation in ARDS patients. *Chest.* 1992;101(3):697–710.
31. Henderson S, Crapo R, Wallace C, East T, Morris A, Gardner R. Performance of computerized protocols for the management of arterial oxygenation in an intensive care unit. *Int J Clin Monit Comput.* 1992;8:271–280.
32. The Acute Respiratory Distress Syndrome Network. Ventilation with lower tidal volumes as compared with traditional tidal volumes for Acute Lung Injury and the Acute Respiratory Distress Syndrome. *N Engl J Med.* 2000;342(18):1301–1308.

33. The Acute Respiratory distress Syndrome Network. *Mechanical Ventilation Protocol (Complete)*. World Wide Web www.ardsnet.org. or NAPS Document No 05542 (Microfiche Publications, 248 Hempstead Turnpike, West Hempstead, New York 11552). 2000.

34. Armstrong R, Bullen C, Cohen S, Singer M, Webb A. *Critical Care Algorithms*. New York, NY: Oxford University Press; 1991. 100 p.

35. Don H, ed. *Decision Making in Critical Care*. Philadelphia: BC Decker Inc; 1985.

36. Karlinsky J, Lau J, Goldstein R. *Decision Making in Pulmonary Medicine*. Philadelphia: BC Decker; 1991.

37. Wennberg JE. Unwarranted variations in healthcare delivery: implications for academic medical centres. *BMJ*. 2002;325(7370): 961–964.

38. Wennberg JE. Time to tackle unwarranted variations in practice. *BMJ*. 2011;342.

39. Wennberg JE, Gittelsohn A. Small area variation analysis in health care delivery. *Science*. 1973;142:1102–1108.

40. von Bertalanffy L. *General System Theory*. New York: George Braziller; 1968. 295 p.

41. Flexner S. *The Random House Dictionary of the English Language*. 2nd ed. New York: Random House Inc.; 1987. 193–4 p.

42. Holcomb BW, Wheeler AP, Ely EW. New ways to reduce unnecessary variation and improve outcomes in the intensive care unit. *Curr Opin Crit Care*. 2001;7(4):304–311.

43. Alhazzani W, Alshahrani M, Jaeschke R, et al. Neuromuscular blocking agents in acute respiratory distress syndrome: a systematic review and meta-analysis of randomized controlled trials. *Crit Care*. 2013;17(2):R43.

44. Grissom CK, Hirshberg EL, Dickerson JB, et al. Fluid management with a simplified conservative protocol for the acute respiratory distress syndrome. *Crit Care Med*. 2015;43(2):288–295.

45. Lee JM, Bae W, Lee YJ, Cho YJ. The efficacy and safety of prone positional ventilation in acute respiratory distress syndrome: updated study-level meta-analysis of 11 randomized controlled trials. *Crit Care Med*. 2014;42(5):1252–1262.

46. The National Heart Lung and Blood Institute Acute Respiratory Distress Syndrome Clinical Trials Network. Comparison of two fluid-management strategies in acute lung injury. *N Engl J Med*. 2006;354(24):2564–2575.

47. The National Heart Lung and Blood Institute Acute Respiratory Distress Syndrome Clinical Trials Network. Pulmonary-artery versus central venous catheter to guide treatment of acute lung injury. *N Engl J Med*. 2006;354(21):2213–2224.

48. Gattinoni L, Pesenti A, Avalli L, Rossi F, Bombino M. Pressure-volume curve of total respiratory system in Acute Respiratory Failure. *Am Rev Respir Dis*. 1987;136:730–736.

49. Darioli R, Perret C. Mechanical controlled hypoventilation in status asthmaticus. *Am Rev Respir DIs*. 1984;129:385–387.

50. Dreyfuss D, Saumon G, Hubamyr R. In: Lenfant C, ed. *Ventilator-Induced Lung Injury*. New York: Taylor & Francis Group; 2006.

51. Hickling K. Low volume ventilation with permissive hypercapnia in the Adult Respiratory Distress Syndrome. *Clin Intensive Care*. 1992;3:67–78.

52. Mortensen J. An intravenacaval blood gas exchange (IVCB-GE) device: a preliminary report. *Trans Am Soc Artif Organs*. 1987;33:570–572.

53. Mortensen J. Intravascular oxygenator: a new alternative method for augmenting blood gas transfer in patients with acute respiratory failure. *Artif Organs*. 1992;16(1):75–82.

54. Bartlett RH. Extracorporeal Life Support in the Management of Severe Respiratory Failure. *Clin Chest Med*. 2000;21(3):555–561.

55. Lewandowski K, Slama K, Falke K. Approaches to improved survival in ARDS. In: Vincent J-L, ed. *Yearbook of Intensive Care and Emergency Medicine*. Berlin: Springer-Verlag; 1992:372–383.

56. Brower RG, Lanken PN, MacIntyre N, et al. Higher versus lower positive end-expiratory pressures in patients with the acute respiratory distress syndrome. *N Engl J Med*. 2004;351(4):327–336.

57. Briel M, Meade M, Mercat A, et al. Higher vs lower positive end-expiratory pressure in patients with acute lung injury and acute respiratory distress syndrome: systematic review and meta-analysis. *JAMA*. 2010;303(9):865–873.

58. Esan A, Hess DR, Raoof S, George L, Sessler CN. Severe hypoxemic respiratory failure: part 1—ventilatory strategies. *Chest*. 2010;137(5):1203–1216.

59. Raoof S, Goulet K, Esan A, Hess DR, Sessler CN. Severe hypoxemic respiratory failure: Part 2–nonventilatory strategies. *Chest*. 2010;137(6):1437–1448.

60. The A.R.D.S. definition task force. Acute respiratory distress syndrome: the berlin definition. *JAMA*. 2012;307(23):2526–2533.

61. Ferguson ND, Fan E, Camporota L, et al. The Berlin definition of ARDS: an expanded rationale, justification, and supplementary material. *Intensive Care Med*. 2012;38(10):1573–1582.

62. Noah MA, Peek GJ, Finney SJ, et al. Referral to an extracorporeal membrane oxygenation center and mortality among patients with severe 2009 influenza A(H1N1). *JAMA*. 2011;306(15): 1659–1668.

63. Miller RI, Dean N, Rice T, for the NHLBI ARDS Network, et al. ARDS Network registry 2009 pandemic influenza A(H1N1) infection patients with severe hypoxemia: outcomes in those treated with and without ECMO. *Am J Respir Crit Care Med*. 2011;183:A1638.

64. Morris AH, Hirshberg E, Miller RR, Statler KD, Hite RD. Counterpoint: efficacy of extracorporeal membrane oxygenation in 2009 influenza A(H1N1). *Chest*. 2010;138(4):778–781.

65. Davies A, Jones D, Bailey M, et al. Extracorporeal membrane oxygenation for 2009 influenza A(H1N1) Acute Respiratory Distress Syndrome. *JAMA*. 2009;302(17):1888–1895.

66. Dreyfuss D, Saumon G. Ventilator-induced lung injury: lessons from experimental studies. *Am J Respir Crit Care Med*. 1998;157(1):294–323.

67. Gajic O, Dara SI, Mendez JL, et al. Ventilator-associated lung injury in patients without acute lung injury at the onset of mechanical ventilation. *Crit Care Med*. 2004;32(9):1817–1824.

68. Gattinoni L, Kolobow T, Tomlinson T, et al. Low-frequency positive pressure ventilation with extracorporeal carbon dioxide removal (LFPPV -ECCO$_2$R): an experimental study. *Anesth Analg*. 1978;57:470–477.

69. Gattinoni L, Kolobow T, Tomlinson T, White D, Pierce J. Control of intermittent positive pressure breathing (IPPB) by extracorporeal removal of carbon dioxide. *Brit J Anaesth*. 1978;50(8):753–758.

70. Plataki M, Hubmayr RD. The physical basis of ventilator-induced lung injury. *Expert Rev Respir Med*. 2010;4(3):373–385.

71. Bellani G, Guerra L, Musch G, et al. Lung regional metabolic activity and gas volume changes induced by tidal ventilation in patients with acute lung injury. *Am J Respir Crit Care Med*. 2011;183(9):1193–1199.

72. Schmidt M, Stewart C, Bailey M, et al. Mechanical ventilation management during extracorporeal membrane oxygenation for acute respiratory distress syndrome: a retrospective international multicenter study. *Crit Care Med*. 2015;43(3):654–664.

73. Terragni P, Ranieri VM, Brazzi L. Novel approaches to minimize ventilator-induced lung injury. *Curr Opin Crit Care*. 2015;21(1):20–25.

74. Extracorporeal Life Support Organization. *The Extracorporeal Life Support Organization. ECLS Registry Report* Ann Arbor, MI, USA: 2011.

75. Fuehner T, Kuehn C, Hadem J, et al. Extracorporeal membrane oxygenation in awake patients as bridge to lung transplantation. *Am J Respir Crit Care Med*. 2012;185(7):763–768.

76. Mehta NM, Turner D, Walsh B, et al. Factors associated with survival in pediatric extracorporeal membrane oxygenation–a single-center experience. *J Pediatr Surg*. 2010;45(10):1995–2003.

77. Park YH, Hwang S, Park HW, et al. Effect of pulmonary support using extracorporeal membrane oxygenation for adult liver transplant recipients with respiratory failure. *Transplant Proc*. 2012;44(3):757–761.

78. Donahoe M, Rogers R. An anecdote is an anecdote…but a clinical trial is data. *Am J Respir Crit Care Med*. 1994;149:293–294.

79. Villar J, Perez-Mendez L, Lopez J, et al. An early PEEP/FIO2 trial identifies different degrees of lung injury in patients with acute respiratory distress syndrome. *Am J Respir Crit Care Med*. 2007;176(8):795–804.

80. Wallace DJ, Angus DC, Seymour CW, et al. Geographic access to high capability severe acute respiratory failure centers in the United States. *PLoS One*. 2014;9(4):e94057.

81. Morris AH. Exciting new ECMO technology awaits compelling scientific evidence for widespread use in adults with respiratory failure. *Intensive Care Med*. 2012;38(2):186–188.

82. Morris AH, Hirshberg E, Miller RR, Statler KD, Hite RD. Rebuttal from Dr Morris et al. *Chest*. 2010;138(4):783–784.

83. Zangrillo A, Landoni G, Biondi-Zoccai G, et al. A meta-analysis of complications and mortality of extracorporeal membrane oxygenation. *Crit Care Resusc*. 2013;15(3):172–178.

84. Park M, Mendes PV, Zampieri FG, et al. The economic effect of extracorporeal membrane oxygenation to support adults with severe respiratory failure in Brazil: a hypothetical analysis. *Rev Bras Ter Intensiva*. 2014;26(3):253–262.

85. Kolobow T, Gattinoni L, Tomlinson T, Pierce J. Control of breathing using an extracorporeal membrane lung. *Anesthesiology.* 1977;46:138–141.

86. Kolobow T, Gattinoni L, Tomlinson T, Pierce J. An alternative to breathing. *J Thorac Cardiovasc Surg.* 1978;75(2):261–266.

87. Mendiratta P, Tang X, Collins II RT, Rycus P, Brogan TV, Prodhan P. Extracorporeal membrane oxygenation for respiratory failure in the elderly: a review of the Extracorporeal Life Support Organization registry. *ASAIO J.* 2014;60(4):385–390.

88. Bonastre J, Suberviola B, Pozo JC, et al. Extracorporeal lung support in patients with severe respiratory failure secondary to the 2010-2011 winter seasonal outbreak of influenza A (H1N1) in Spain. *Med Intensiva.* 2012;36(3):193–199.

89. Ma D, Kim J, Jung S, Choo S, Chung C, Lee J. Outcomes of venovenous extracorporeal membrane oxygenation support for acute respiratory distress syndrome in adults. *Korean J Thorac Cardiovasc Surg.* 2012;45(2):91–94.

90. Wong I, Vuylsteke A. Use of extracorporeal life support to support patients with acute respiratory distress syndrome due to H1N1/2009 influenza and other respiratory infections. *Perfusion.* 2011;26(1):7–20.

91. Terragni P, Maiolo G, Ranieri VM. Role and potentials of low-flow CO(2) removal system in mechanical ventilation. *Curr Opin Criti Care.* 2012;18(1):93–98.

92. Terragni PP, Del Sorbo L, Mascia L, Urbino R, Martin EL, Birocco A, et al. Tidal volume lower than 6 ml/kg enhances lung protection: role of extracorporeal carbon dioxide removal. *Anesthesiology.* 2009;111(4):826–835.

93. Brodie D, Bacchetta M. Extracorporeal membrane oxygenation for ARDS in adults. *N Engl J Med.* 2011;365(20):1905–1914.

94. Anderson HI, Delius R, Sinard J, et al. Early experience with extracorporeal membrane oxygenation in the modern era. *Ann Thorac Surg.* 1992;53:553–563.

95. Anderson HI, Steimle C, Shapiro M, et al. Extracorporeal life support (ECLS) for adult cardiorespiratory failure. *Surgery.* 1993;114(2):161–172. discussion 72–73.

96. Anderson III HL, Snedecor SM, Otsu T, Bartlett RH. Multicenter comparison of conventional venoarterial access versus venovenous double-lumen catheter access in newborn infants undergoing extracorporeal membrane oxygenation. *J Pediatr Surg.* 1993;28(4):530–535.

97. Bartlett RH, Roloff DW, Custer JR, Younger JG, Hirschl RB. Extracorporeal life support: the University of Michigan experience. *JAMA.* 2000;283(7):904–908.

98. Bohn D. Pushing the boundaries for the use of ECMO in acute hypoxic respiratory failure. *Intensive Care Med.* 2005;31(7):896–897.

99. Custer J, Bartlett R. Recent research in extracorporeal life support for respiratory failure. *ASAIO J.* 1992;38(4):754–771.

100. Macintosh I, Butt WW, Robertson CF, Best D, Shekerdemian LS. Extending the limits of extracorporeal membrane oxygenation: lung rest for a child with non-specific interstitial pneumonia. *Intensive Care Med.* 2005;31(7):993–996.

101. Blake L. Goals and progress of the National Heart and Lung Institute collaborative extracorporeal membrane oxygenation study. In: Zapol W, Qvist J, eds. *Artificial lungs for acute respiratory failure.* New York, NY: Academic Press; 1976:513–524.

102. NHLI. *Protocol for Extracorporeal Support for Respiratory Insufficiency Collaborative Program.* Bethesda: National Heart and Lung Institute, Division of Lung Diseases; 1974.

103. Gattinoni L, Pesenti A, Rossi G, et al. Treatment of acute respiratory failure with low-frequency positive-pressure ventilation and extracorporeal removal of CO$_2$. *Lancet.* 1980;2(8189):292–294.

104. Pesenti A, Gattinon L, Kolobow T, Damia G. Extracorporeal circulation in adult respiratory failure. *Trans Am Soc Artif Intern Organs.* 1988;34:43–47.

105. Del Sorbo L, Pisani L, Filippini C, et al. Extracorporeal CO$_2$ removal in hypercapnic patients at risk of noninvasive ventilation failure: a matched cohort study with historical control. *Crit Care Med.* 2015;43(1):120–127.

106. Nava S, Ranieri VM. Extracorporeal lung support for COPD reaches a crossroad. *The Lancet Respiratory medicine.* 2014;2(5):350–352.

107. Gattinoni L, Pesenti A, Mascheroni D, et al. Low frequency positive pressure ventilation with extracorporeal CO$_2$ removal in severe acute respiratory failure. *JAMA.* 1986;256(7):881–886.

108. Brunet F, Mira J, Lanore J, et al., eds. *ECCO$_2$R-LFPPV Does Improve Arterial Oxygenation in Patients with ARDS in Whom Mechanical Ventilation (MV) Failed. 2nd European Congress on Extracorporeal Lung Support.* Marburg, Germany: Philipps-University; 1992. Department of Anaesthesiology and Intensive Care Therapy.

109. Gattinoni L, Pesenti A, Caspani M, et al. The role of total static lung compliance in the management of severe ARDS unresponsive to conventional treatment. *Intensive Care Med.* 1984;10:121–126.

110. Marini JJ, Kelsen SG. Re-targeting ventilatory objectives in adult respiratory distress syndrome (Editorial). *Am Rev Respir Dis.* 1992;146:2–3.

111. Müller E, Knoch M, Holtermann W, Wagner P, Lennartz H, eds. *Extracorporeal Support in Patients with ARDS: The Results and Experiences of the Marburg group. 2nd European Congress on Extracorporeal Lung Support.* Marburg, Germany: Philipps-University; 1992. Department of Anaesthesiology and Intensive Care Therapy.

112. Wagner P, Knoch M, Sangmeister C, Muller E, Lennartz H. Extracorporeal gas exchange in adult respiratory distress syndrome: associated morbidity and its surgical treatment. *Br J Surg.* 1990;77:1395–1398.

113. Edmunds L, Holm J. Effect of inhaled CO$_2$ on hemorrhagic consolidation due to unilateral pulmonary arterial ligation. *J Appl Physiol.* 1969;26(6):710–715.

114. Morgan T, Edmunds L. Pulmonary artery occlusion III. Biochemical alterations. *J Appl Physiol.* 1967;22:1012–1016.

115. Kolobow T, Solca M, Gattinoni L, Pesenti A. Adult respiratory distress syndrome (ARDS): why did ECMO fail? (Editorial). *Int J Artif Organs.* 1981;4(2):58–59.

116. Kolobow T, Spragg R, Pierce J. Massive pulmonary infarction during total cardiopulmonary bypass in unanesthetised spontaneously breathing lambs. *Int J Artif Organs.* 1981;4(2):76–81.

117. Cohen J. *Statistical Power Analysis for the Behavioral Sciences.* 2nd ed. Hillsdale, NJ: Lawrence Erlbaum Associates; 1988.

118. Lachin JM. Introduction to sample size determinations and power analysis for clinical trials. *Controlled Clin Trials.* 1981;2:93–113.

119. Pocock SJ. *Clinical Trials: A Practical Approach.* New York, NY: John Wiley & Sons; 1983. 266 p.

120. Peek G, Clemens F, Elbourne D, et al. CESAR: conventional ventilatory support vs extracorporeal membrane oxygenation for severe adult respiratory failure. *BMC Health Services Res.* 2006;6:163.

121. Peek GJ, Elbourne D, Mugford M, et al. Randomised controlled trial and parallel economic evaluation of conventional ventilatory support versus extracorporeal membrane oxygenation for severe adult respiratory failure (CESAR). *Health Tech Assessment.* 2010;14(35):1–46.

122. Patroniti N, Zangrillo A, Pappalardo F, et al. The Italian ECMO network experience during the 2009 influenza A(H1N1) pandemic: preparation for severe respiratory emergency outbreaks. *Intensive Care Med.* 2011;37(9):1447–1457.

123. Munshi L, Telesnicki T, Walkey A, Fan E. Extracorporeal life support for acute respiratory failure. A systematic review and meta-analysis. *Ann Am Thorac Soc.* 2014;11(5):802–810.

124. Zampieri FG, Mendes PV, Ranzani OT, et al. Extracorporeal membrane oxygenation for severe respiratory failure in adult patients: a systematic review and meta-analysis of current evidence. *J Crit Care.* 2013;28(6):998–1005.

125. Pham T, Combes A, Roze H, et al. Extracorporeal membrane oxygenation for pandemic influenza A(H1N1)-induced acute respiratory distress syndrome: a cohort study and propensity-matched analysis. *Am J Respir Crit Care Med.* 2013;187(3):276–285.

126. Meadow W, Pohlman A, Frain L, et al. Power and limitations of daily prognostications of death in the medical intensive care unit. *Crit Care Med.* 2011;39(3):474–479.

127. Schmidt M, Bailey M, Sheldrake J, et al. Predicting Survival after Extracorporeal Membrane Oxygenation for Severe Acute Respiratory Failure. The Respiratory Extracorporeal Membrane Oxygenation Survival Prediction (RESP) Score. *Am J Respir Crit Care Med.* 2014;189(11):1374–1382.

128. Pappalardo F, Pieri M, Greco T, et al. Predicting mortality risk in patients undergoing venovenous ECMO for ARDS due to influenza A (H1N1) pneumonia: the ECMOnet score. *Intensive Care Med.* 2013;39(2):275–281.

12 What Factors Predispose Patients to Acute Respiratory Distress Syndrome?

Ognjen Gajic, Alice Gallo De Moraes, Ronaldo Sevilla Berrios

Acute respiratory distress syndrome (ARDS) is a common complication of critical illness or injury associated with significant morbidity and mortality. The pathogenesis of ARDS involves mechanical and inflammatory injury to the lungs, which causes marked derangement in alveolar-capillary permeability and the passage of protein-rich edema fluid into the air spaces.[1,2] ARDS usually occurs in a context of uncontrolled response to local or systemic inflammation. The clinical pathogenesis is often multifactorial with complex interaction of risk factors and risk modifiers (Fig. 12-1).

PREDISPOSING CONDITIONS

Sepsis, pneumonia, and shock are the most common conditions predisposing to ARDS.[3,4] However, only a minority of these patients actually have ARDS (Fig. 12-2). Other typical predisposing conditions include aspiration, trauma, and massive blood product transfusion.[5,6] Atypical respiratory infections, including viral (*influenza*) and fungal (*Pneumocystis jiroveci*, *Histoplasma* spp., *Blastomyces* spp.) infections, are unusual but important causes of ARDS, especially in patients with compromised immune systems. Several emerging pathogens, such as severe acute respiratory syndrome, Middle East respiratory syndrome-coronavirus, and epidemic H1N1 influenza, also confer increased risk for ARDS.[7] Additional patient risk factors include gastroesophageal reflux disease, chronic silent aspiration, and drug exposures.[3,8]

Certain host genetic variants have been associated with development of sepsis and ARDS.[9] These abnormalities include mutations in the surfactant protein-B.[10] Genetic associations have been generally difficult to replicate, and the role of genetic predisposition in development of ARDS is presently unclear.[10]

RISK MODIFIERS

Sepsis in alcoholics is associated with a distinctly high risk of ARDS. Chronic alcohol use carries a twofold to threefold increase in ARDS development.[11,12] The exact mechanism

of this association remains unknown, but it may be related to a reduction in the antioxidant capacity of the lung.[12] In addition, acute and chronic consumption of alcohol cause an increase in the systemic levels of adenosine[13,14] and a dose-dependent reduction in alveolar fluid clearance through stimulation of the adenosine type 1 receptor, adding to the lung injury.[15,16] A recent study in trauma patients demonstrated that the risk of ARDS increased in direct proportion to the blood alcohol content.[17]

A history of tobacco exposure (including second-hand smoking) has been associated with an increased risk of ARDS in trauma patients.[18] Another study found an independent dose–response association between current cigarette smoking and subsequent development of ARDS.[19]

Hypoalbuminemia is a well-known marker of acute or chronic illness or malnutrition and poor surgical outcomes.[20,21] It was also found to be an independent risk factor for ARDS.[22] This appears to be mediated by decreases in plasma oncotic pressure with increased pulmonary permeability in the critically ill, independent of underlying cause and fluid status.[23]

Hypercapnic acidosis protects against ventilator-induced lung injury in several animal models of ARDS.[24,25] However, low pH and, in particular, metabolic acidosis have been associated with increased risk of ARDS.[26,27]

Obesity is also an independent risk factor for the development of ARDS.[28] Although the effects of body position and compression atelectasis may in part explain the observed association,[2] additional mechanisms have been proposed. These include an imbalance between proinflammatory and anti-inflammatory cytokines, which increases lung inflammation and injury through the tumor necrosis factor-α and interleukin-6 pathways.[29-32]

Diabetes mellitus seems to be associated with a lower risk of ARDS in septic shock.[33] Indeed, a recent meta-analysis that included a total of 12,794 adult patients suggested that diabetes protected against ARDS.[34] Although the exact mechanism is not known, one possible explanation is that diabetic patients have impaired activation of the inflammatory cascade in the lungs.[35]

An alternative hypothesis for ARDS pathogenesis has been proposed, suggesting that surfactant dysfunction

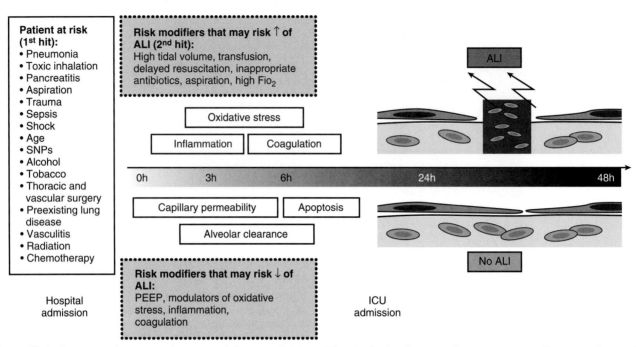

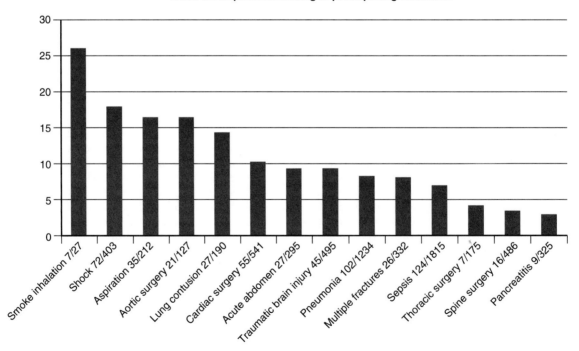

Figure 12-1 Illustration of interaction between risk factors and risk modifiers in the development of acute respiratory distress syndrome. *ALI,* acute lung injury; *Fio₂,* fraction of inspired oxygen; *ICU,* intensive care unit; *PEEP,* positive end-expiratory pressure; *SNP,* single nucleotide polymorphism.

Figure 12-2 Predisposing factors for development of acute respiratory distress syndrome. *ALI,* acute lung injury. *(With permission from Gajic O, Dabbagh O, Park PK, et al. Early identification of patients at risk of acute lung injury: evaluation of lung injury prediction score in a multicenter cohort study. Am J Respir Crit Care Med. 2011;183[4]:462–470.)*

may be a critical step in ARDS progression.[36] Both spontaneous and mechanical hyperventilation can induce surfactant dysfunction, leading to higher surface tension and atelectasis. This injury is augmented by supine position and sedation, and this effect can be particularly pronounced in obese patients.[2] However, trials administering surfactant in ARDS patients did not show a mortality benefit.[37]

RISK PREDICTION MODELS

The Lung Injury Prediction Score (LIPS) was created in 2011 with the intent to facilitate the design and conduct of ARDS prevention studies.[38] The model includes risk factors and risk modifiers present at the time of hospital admission, before ARDS occurs. It was later validated[26] and refined (Table 12-1). A simplified model, the Early Acute Lung Injury Score, predicts ARDS on the basis of oxygen requirement, respiratory rate, and presence of immunosuppression in patients with bilateral infiltrates on chest imaging.[39]

HOSPITAL-ACQUIRED EXPOSURES

Hospitalized patients are frequently exposed to various potentially harmful factors that may modify their risk of ARDS development. Compared with patients who died of other causes, ARDS decedents have a markedly higher incidence of potentially preventable adverse events (medical or surgical misadventures).[40] High tidal volume ventilation,[41-43] high oxygen concentration,[44] and plasma transfusion from multiparous female donors[45] each have been implicated as iatrogenic contributors to ARDS. In septic patients, delays in fluid resuscitation and in the initiation of antimicrobial treatment have also been associated with ARDS.[46] Although lung-protective mechanical ventilation is considered a standard of care for patients with established ARDS, recent studies suggest that its application to all mechanically ventilated patients is safe and beneficial.[41-43]

A large case-control study found iatrogenic risk factors to be significantly greater in patients with ARDS than in matched controls and deemed most of these factors to be preventable.[47] Of note, in the same study, aspirin administration appeared to be protective. The U.S. Critical Illness and Injury Trials Group is currently conducting a clinical trial that is sponsored by the National Heart, Lung, and Blood Institute of aspirin versus placebo in patients at high risk of ARDS (NCT01504867).[48]

Recent publications have suggested multiple potential strategies directed at preventing ARDS. These include early identification of "at-risk" patients, standardization of clinical practice to prevent iatrogenic injury, and early treatment of predisposing conditions.[47,49] The Checklist for Lung Injury Prevention (CLIP) has been developed to ensure compliance with evidence-based practice that may affect ARDS occurrence and is currently used in clinical trials of ARDS prevention.[48] CLIP items include lung-protective mechanical ventilation, aspiration precautions, early adequate antimicrobial therapy,

Table 12-1 LIPS Calculation Table

	LIPS Points	Examples
Predisposing conditions		(1) Patient with history of alcohol abuse with septic shock from pneumonia requiring $Fio_2 > 0.35$ in the emergency room: Sepsis + shock + pneumonia + alcohol abuse + $Fio_2 > 0.35$ $1 + 2 + 1.5 + 1 + 2 = 7.5$
Shock	2	
Aspiration	2	
Sepsis	1	
Pneumonia	1.5	
High-risk surgery*		
Orthopedic spine	1	
Acute abdomen	2	
Cardiac	2.5	
Aortic vascular	3.5	
High-risk trauma		(2) Motor vehicle accident with traumatic brain injury, lung contusion, and shock requiring $Fio_2 > 0.35$ Traumatic brain injury + lung contusion + shock + $Fio_2 > 0.35$ $2 + 1.5 + 2 + 2 = 7.5$
Traumatic brain injury	2	
Smoke inhalation	2	
Near drowning	2	
Lung contusion	1.5	
Multiple fractures	1.5	
Risk modifiers		(3) Patient with history of diabetes mellitus and urosepsis with shock $1 + 2 - 1 = 2$
Alcohol abuse	1	
Obesity (BMI > 30)	1	
Hypoalbuminemia	1	
Chemotherapy	1	
$Fio_2 > 0.35$ (> 4 L/min)	2	
Tachypnea (RR > 30)	1.5	
$SpO_2 < 95\%$	1	
Acidosis (pH < 7.35)	1.5	
Diabetes mellitus[†]	−1	

BMI, body mass index; *Fio₂*, fraction of inspired oxygen; *LIPS*, lung injury prediction score; *RR*, respiratory rate; *SpO₂*, oxygen saturation by pulse oximetry.
*Add 1.5 points if emergency surgery.
[†]Only if sepsis.
With permission from Gajic O, Dabbagh O, Park PK, et al. Early identification of patients at risk of acute lung injury: evaluation of lung injury prediction score in a multicenter cohort study. *Am J Respir Crit Care Med.* 2011;183(4):462–470.

restrictive fluid and transfusion management, and early assessment for extubation with daily awakening and breathing trials.

A population-based cohort study conducted in Olmsted County, Minnesota, reported a decrease in the incidence of ARDS from 82.4 cases per 100,000 person-years in 2001 to 38.9 cases per 100,000 person-years in 2008.[50] This decrease in ARDS incidence was observed despite a stable incidence of community-acquired ARDS and an increase in the population's severity of illness, comorbidity burden, and predisposing conditions for ARDS over the same time period. This decrease was attributed to the prevention strategies described above, including lung-protective ventilation strategies in all mechanically ventilated patients, restrictive transfusion practice, male-donor-predominant plasma, improved sepsis treatment, and more conservative fluid management.[45,50,51]

In addition to the aspirin administration mentioned previously,[48] several other pharmacologic therapies for prevention of ARDS in patients at risk are being evaluated in clinical studies. These include inhaled beta agonists,[52] inhaled heparin,[53] inhaled steroids,[54] peroxisome proliferator receptor antagonist, angiotensin inhibitors, curcumin, and vitamin D.[55,56] Of those, only inhaled beta agonists have been formally evaluated in a Phase II randomized control trial. In 362 patients undergoing esophagectomy, intraoperative administration of inhaled salmeterol reduced several biomarkers of alveolar inflammation and injury and was associated with decreased incidence of postoperative adverse events (predominantly pneumonia); however, the incidence of ARDS did not differ between the groups.[52]

In conclusion, although sepsis, pneumonia, and shock commonly predispose patients to ARDS, many risk factors are modifiable. Ongoing clinical studies are evaluating various promising preventative strategies. Meanwhile, attention to best practices and avoidance of iatrogenic exposures is a simple and powerful strategy for reducing the burden of this important complication of critical illness.

AUTHORS' RECOMMENDATIONS

- Sepsis, pneumonia, and shock are the most common conditions predisposing to ARDS.
- Certain host genetic variants have been associated with development of sepsis and ARDS.
- Abuse of alcohol and tobacco predispose to ARDS, as does malnutrition and obesity.
- The LIPS and the simplified Early Acute Lung Injury Score predicts ARDS based on clinical and investigational criteria.
- Hospital-acquired ARDS may result from medley factors of which high-tidal volume ventilation, high oxygen concentration, and plasma transfusion are most commonly implicated.
- The CLIP has been developed to ensure compliance with evidence-based practice that may affect ARDS occurrence.
- To date, no pharmacologic intervention has been shown to prevent ARDS.

REFERENCES

1. Matthay MA, Zemans RL. The acute respiratory distress syndrome: pathogenesis and treatment. *Annu Rev Pathol.* 2011;6:147–163.
2. Albert RK. The role of ventilation-induced surfactant dysfunction and atelectasis in causing acute respiratory distress syndrome. *Am J Respir Crit Care Med.* 2012;185(7):702–708.
3. Bice T, Li G, Malinchoc M, et al. Incidence and risk factors of recurrent acute lung injury. *Crit Care Med.* 2011;39(5):1069–1073.
4. Wind J, Versteegt J, Twisk J, et al. Epidemiology of acute lung injury and acute respiratory distress syndrome in The Netherlands: a survey. *Respir Med.* 2007;101(10):2091–2098.
5. Wallis JP. Transfusion-related acute lung injury (TRALI): presentation, epidemiology and treatment. *Intensive Care Med.* 2007;33(suppl 1):S12–S16.
6. Khan H, Belsher J, Yilmaz M, et al. Fresh-frozen plasma and platelet transfusions are associated with development of acute lung injury in critically ill medical patients. *Chest.* 2007;131(5):1308–1314.
7. Kojicic M, Li G, Hanson AC, et al. Risk factors for the development of acute lung injury in patients with infectious pneumonia. *Crit Care.* 2012;16(2):R46.
8. Dhokarh R, Li G, Schmickl CN, et al. Drug-associated acute lung injury: a population-based cohort study. *Chest J.* 2012;142(4):845–850.
9. Marshall RP, Webb S, Hill MR, et al. Genetic polymorphisms associated with susceptibility and outcome in ARDS. *Chest.* 2002;121(suppl 3):68S–69S.
10. Gong MN, Wei Z, Xu LL, et al. Polymorphism in the surfactant protein-B gene, gender, and the risk of direct pulmonary injury and ARDS. *Chest.* 2004;125(1):203–211.
11. Moss M, Burnham EL. Chronic alcohol abuse, acute respiratory distress syndrome, and multiple organ dysfunction. *Crit Care Med.* 2003;31(suppl 4):S207–S212.
12. Moss M, Parsons PE, Steinberg KP, et al. Chronic alcohol abuse is associated with an increased incidence of acute respiratory distress syndrome and severity of multiple organ dysfunction in patients with septic shock. *Crit Care Med.* 2003;31(3):869–877.
13. Dohrman DP, Diamond I, Gordon AS. The role of the neuromodulator adenosine in alcohol's actions. *Alcohol Health Res World.* 1997;21(2):136–143.
14. Nagy LE, Diamond I, Collier K, et al. Adenosine is required for ethanol-induced heterologous desensitization. *Mol Pharmacol.* 1989;36(5):744–748.
15. Dada L, Gonzalez AR, Urich D, et al. Alcohol worsens acute lung injury by inhibiting alveolar sodium transport through the adenosine A1 receptor. *PLoS One.* 2012;7(1):e30448.
16. Factor P, Mutlu GM, Chen L, et al. Adenosine regulation of alveolar fluid clearance. *Proc Natl Acad Sci USA.* 2007;104(10):4083–4088.
17. Afshar M, Smith GS, Terrin ML, et al. Blood alcohol content, injury severity, and adult respiratory distress syndrome. *J Trauma Acute Care Surg.* 2014;76(6):1447–1455.
18. Calfee CS, Matthay MA, Eisner MD, et al. Active and passive cigarette smoking and acute lung injury after severe blunt trauma. *Am J Respir Crit Care Med.* 2011;183(12):1660–1665.
19. Iribarren C, Jacobs Jr DR, Sidney S, et al. Cigarette smoking, alcohol consumption, and risk of ARDS: a 15-year cohort study in a managed care setting. *Chest.* 2000;117(1):163–168.
20. Buzby GP, Mullen JL, Matthews DC, et al. Prognostic nutritional index in gastrointestinal surgery. *Am J Surg.* 1980;139(1):160–167.
21. Dempsey DT, Mullen JL. Prognostic value of nutritional indices. *JPEN J Parenter Enteral Nutr.* 1987;11(suppl 5):109S–114S.
22. Mangialardi RJ, Martin GS, Bernard GR, et al. Hypoproteinemia predicts acute respiratory distress syndrome development, weight gain, and death in patients with sepsis. *Crit Care Med.* 2000;28(9):3137–3145.
23. Aman J, van der Heijden M, van Lingen A, et al. Plasma protein levels are markers of pulmonary vascular permeability and degree of lung injury in critically ill patients with or at risk for acute lung injury/acute respiratory distress syndrome. *Crit Care Med.* 2011;39(1):89–97.
24. Ijland MM, Heunks LM, van der Hoeven JG. Bench-to-bedside review: hypercapnic acidosis in lung injury–from 'permissive' to 'therapeutic'. *Crit Care.* 2010;14(6):237.
25. Wu SY, Wu CP, Kang BH, et al. Hypercapnic acidosis attenuates reperfusion injury in isolated and perfused rat lungs. *Crit Care Med.* 2012;40(2):553–559.
26. Gajic O, Dabbagh O, Park PK, et al. Early identification of patients at risk of acute lung injury: evaluation of lung injury prediction score in a multicenter cohort study. *Am J Respir Crit Care Med.* 2011;183(4):462–470.
27. Gong MN, Thompson BT, Williams P, et al. Clinical predictors of and mortality in acute respiratory distress syndrome: potential role of red cell transfusion. *Crit Care Med.* 2005;33(6):1191–1198.
28. Karnatovskaia LV, Lee AS, Bender SP, et al. Obstructive sleep apnea, obesity, and the development of acute respiratory distress syndrome. *J Clin Sleep Med.* 2014;10(6):657–662.
29. Wang C. Obesity, inflammation, and lung injury (OILI): the good. *Mediators Inflamm.* 2014;2014:978463.
30. Leal Vde O, Mafra D. Adipokines in obesity. *Clin Chim Acta.* 2013;419:87–94.
31. Mancuso P. Obesity and lung inflammation. *J Appl Physiol (1985).* 2010;108(3):722–728.
32. Simpson SQ, Casey LC. Role of tumor necrosis factor in sepsis and acute lung injury. *Crit Care Clin.* 1989;5(1):27–47.
33. Moss M, Guidot DM, Steinberg KP, et al. Diabetic patients have a decreased incidence of acute respiratory distress syndrome. *Crit Care Med.* 2000;28(7):2187–2192.
34. Gu WJ, Wan YD, Tie HT, et al. Risk of acute lung injury/acute respiratory distress syndrome in critically ill adult patients with pre-existing diabetes: a meta-analysis. *PLoS One.* 2014;9(2):e90426.
35. Filgueiras Jr LR, Martins JO, Serezani CH, et al. Sepsis-induced acute lung injury (ALI) is milder in diabetic rats and correlates with impaired NFκB activation. *PLoS One.* 2012;7(9):e44987.

36. Petty TL, Silvers GW, Paul GW, et al. Abnormalities in lung elastic properties and surfactant function in adult respiratory distress syndrome. *Chest*. 1979;75(5):571–574.

37. Kesecioglu J, Beale R, Stewart TE, et al. Exogenous natural surfactant for treatment of acute lung injury and the acute respiratory distress syndrome. *Am J Respir Crit Care Med*. 2009;180(10):989–994.

38. Trillo-Alvarez C, Cartin-Ceba R, Kor DJ, et al. Acute lung injury prediction score: derivation and validation in a population-based sample. *Eur Respir J*. 2011;37(3):604–609.

39. Levitt JE, Calfee CS, Goldstein BA, et al. Early acute lung injury: criteria for identifying lung injury prior to the need for positive pressure ventilation. *Crit Care Med*. 2013;41(8):1929–1937.

40. TenHoor T, Mannino DM, Moss M. Risk factors for ARDS in the United States: analysis of the 1993 National Mortality Followback Study. *Chest*. 2001;119(4):1179–1184.

41. Serpa Neto A, Simonis FD, Barbas CS, et al. Association between tidal volume size, duration of ventilation, and sedation needs in patients without acute respiratory distress syndrome: an individual patient data meta-analysis. *Intensive Care Med*. 2014;40(7):950–957.

42. Gajic O, Dara SI, Mendez JL, et al. Ventilator-associated lung injury in patients without acute lung injury at the onset of mechanical ventilation. *Crit Care Med*. 2004;32(9):1817–1824.

43. Neto AS, Cardoso SO, Manetta JA, et al. Association between use of lung-protective ventilation with lower tidal volumes and clinical outcomes among patients without acute respiratory distress syndrome: a meta-analysis. *JAMA*. 2012;308(16):1651–1659.

44. Rachmale S, Li G, Wilson G, et al. Practice of excessive F_1O_2 and effect on pulmonary outcomes in mechanically ventilated patients with acute lung injury. *Respir Care*. 2012;57(11):1887–1893.

45. Toy P, Gajic O, Bacchetti P, et al. Transfusion-related acute lung injury: incidence and risk factors. *Blood*. 2012;119(7):1757–1767.

46. Iscimen R, Cartin-Ceba R, Yilmaz M, et al. Risk factors for the development of acute lung injury in patients with septic shock: an observational cohort study. *Crit Care Med*. 2008;36(5):1518–1522.

47. Ahmed AH, Litell JM, Malinchoc M, et al. The role of potentially preventable hospital exposures in the development of acute respiratory distress syndrome: a population-based study. *Crit Care Med*. 2014;42(1):31–39.

48. Kor DJ, Talmor DS, Banner-Goodspeed VM, et al. Lung Injury Prevention with Aspirin (LIPS-A): a protocol for a multicentre randomised clinical trial in medical patients at high risk of acute lung injury. *BMJ Open*. 2012;2(5).

49. Litell JM, Gong MN, Talmor D, et al. Acute lung injury: prevention may be the best medicine. *Respir Care*. 2011;56(10):1546–1554.

50. Li G, Malinchoc M, Cartin-Ceba R, et al. Eight-year trend of acute respiratory distress syndrome: a population-based study in Olmsted County, Minnesota. *Am J Respir Crit Care Med*. 2011;183(1):59–66.

51. Wiedemann H, Wheeler A, Bernard G, et al. National Heart, Lung, and Blood Institute Acute Respiratory Distress Syndrome (ARDS) Clinical Trials Network: comparison of two fluid-management strategies in acute lung injury. *N Eng J Med*. 2006;354(24):2564–2575.

52. Perkins GD, McAuley DF, Thickett DR, et al. The β-Agonist Lung Injury Trial (BALTI) a randomized placebo-controlled clinical trial. *Am J Respir Crit Care Med*. 2006;173(3):281–287.

53. Dixon B, Schultz MJ, Smith R, et al. Nebulized heparin is associated with fewer days of mechanical ventilation in critically ill patients: a randomized controlled trial. *Crit Care*. 2010;14(5):R180.

54. Karnatovskaia LV, Lee AS, Gajic O, et al. The influence of prehospital systemic corticosteroid use on development of acute respiratory distress syndrome and hospital outcomes. *Crit Care Med*. 2013;41(7):1679–1685.

55. Jeng L, Yamshchikov AV, Judd SE, et al. Alterations in vitamin D status and anti-microbial peptide levels in patients in the intensive care unit with sepsis. *J Transl Med*. 2009;7:28.

56. Festic E, Kor DJ, Gajic O. Prevention of acute respiratory distress syndrome. *Curr Opin Crit Care*. 2015;21(1):82–90.

HEMODYNAMIC MANAGEMENT

13 | What Is the Role of Invasive Hemodynamic Monitoring in Critical Care?

Daniel De Backer

The main indications for hemodynamic monitoring in critical care are the identification of the type of shock, guidance of therapeutic interventions, and the cardiopulmonary evaluation of the patient with respiratory failure. Hemodynamic monitoring techniques are classified as invasive, minimally invasive, and noninvasive. Invasive monitoring includes the pulmonary artery catheter and transpulmonary thermodilution techniques. Minimally invasive approaches include noncalibrated pulse wave analysis and esophageal Doppler. Noninvasive techniques comprise bioreactance and bioimpedance techniques, noninvasive pulse contour methods, and echocardiography. Although few data are available to demonstrate outcome benefit from hemodynamic monitoring,[1] these techniques are widely used. Over the past two decades, there has been a marked trend in favor of less-invasive hemodynamic monitoring versus more traditional invasive techniques.

Echocardiography, which can be minimally invasive (transesophageal echo) or noninvasive (transthoracic echo), provides extensive hemodynamic information.[2] Echocardiography has been recommended in the initial hours for the classification of shock.[3,4] However, echocardiography outside of the operating room tends to be discontinuous and will not easily provide minute-to-minute response to fluid boluses, pressors, or inotropes during these dynamic changes. In addition, echocardiographic study evaluation requires significant bedside skills that may not be available around the clock.[5]

The information provided by noninvasive techniques is often limited to cardiac output and stroke volume variations, whereas invasive techniques provide additional information such as intravascular pressures and cardiac volumes. In general, the more invasive the technique in critical illness, the more accurate the data accrued. Accordingly, the choice of the hemodynamic monitoring technique should not be guided only on invasiveness but should also take into account the accuracy of the technique and, more importantly, the potential interest of the additionally measured variables. The selection of a hemodynamic monitoring device should clearly be individualized based on the patient's circumstances[4] and the skills available.

INVASIVE OR NONINVASIVE ARTERIAL PRESSURE MONITORING?

Arterial pressure is a key determinant of organ perfusion and is routinely measured in critically ill patients, either noninvasively or invasively. Noninvasive blood pressure measurement may be inaccurate in critical illness, particularly in patients with shock, when accuracy of measurements is particularly important.[6] As an example, an overestimation of 5 to 10 mm Hg will have minimal effect on patient management if real mean arterial pressure is 80 mm Hg, but it could have important consequences if mean arterial pressure is 55 mm Hg. Consequently, invasive arterial pressure monitoring is recommended in patients with circulatory failure.[3]

CENTRAL VENOUS PRESSURE AND CENTRAL VENOUS OXYGEN SATURATION

Central venous access is often required for the care of critically ill patients, especially when in shock, and the measurements of central venous pressure (CVP) and oxygen saturation can provide important information on the hemodynamic state.

However, CVP is an unreliable measure of cardiac function and volume status because of, among other things, changes in intrathoracic pressure. A very high CVP may reflect impaired cardiac function (biventricular or right heart), hypervolemia, or tamponade. A low CVP may suggest hypovolemia, but it can be misleading in patients with isolated left heart dysfunction. Importantly, the measured CVP is strongly affected by intrathoracic pressures; thus, it may overestimate the true CVP (transmural CVP) in patients undergoing mechanic ventilation, severely limiting the capacity of CVP to evaluate preload responsiveness and even cardiac function. Nevertheless, it does reflect the backpressure of the venous system and hence the driving force for tissue edema.

Measurement of central venous oxygen saturation (ScvO$_2$) provides information on the adequacy of oxygen transport and hence cardiac output. A low $ScvO_2$, suggestive of excessive oxygen extraction per unit blood, may represent low or inadequate cardiac output, anemia, hypoxemia, agitation, or a combination of all of these factors.

In patients with septic shock, hemodynamic optimization based on these variables has been proposed to improve outcome. In a pivotal trial, the Rivers study, early goal-directed therapy (EGDT) based on CVP and $ScvO_2$ was associated with a marked reduction in mortality.[7] Two more recent trials, ProCESS (Protocolized Care for Early Septic Shock) and ARISE (Australasian Resuscitation in Sepsis Evaluation), each including several thousand patients, failed to confirm these results.[8,9] Several factors may explain this. At inclusion, $ScvO_2$ was close to 50% in both groups in the Rivers trial, whereas, by the time of inclusion, it was already reaching the goals (70%) in ProCESS and ARISE. This likely represents lead-time bias—patients had been preresuscitated before inclusion, and if the main variable to correct is already within target values, then minimal effect is to be expected from the intervention.

In the ARISE trial, 78% of the patients reached the $ScvO_2$ goal at inclusion, and this proportion increased to only 82%,[9] illustrating that the studied interventions mostly failed to improve the monitored variable. Second, the recruitment rate was much lower in the ARISE and ProCESS trials (1 and 0.5 patients per center per month, respectively), whereas it was 8 patients/month in the single-center trial. This may have resulted in selection bias toward less severe patients, which might be reflected by the very low mortality in these trials. This does not alter the conclusions of these trials, but it does limit external validity. Finally, in ARISE and ProCESS, the control groups were essentially resuscitated by the time of inclusion as a direct consequence of care standards that evolved after the Rivers trial.[7] This is reflected by the large amount of fluid administered and short delay to receiving appropriate antibiotics, two of the pillars of the Surviving Sepsis Guidelines.[10] Implementation and compliance with these guidelines is associated with decreased mortality rates compared with more traditional standards of care.[11] Of note, several "before-and-after" trials that seemed to confirm these data suggested an outcome advantage for EGDT, and a recent meta-analysis taking into account these observational trials and one of the recent multicentric randomized trials[12] also suggested that EGDT may be associated with an improved outcome. Thus, the actual conclusions from these trials is that protocolized EGDT may not offer survival benefit in all patients with septic shock, but that hemodynamic optimization based on $ScvO_2$ may still be justified in the most severe patients presenting with an altered $ScvO_2$.

PULMONARY ARTERY CATHETER

The pulmonary artery catheter (PAC), although invasive, provides quasi-continuous information on cardiovascular status. The PAC measures three types of variables: intravascular/intrachamber pressures, cardiac output, and mixed-venous blood gases.

Measurements of pulmonary artery pressure are undoubtedly useful in cases of right ventricular dysfunction in which evaluation of the right ventricular afterload is crucial for diagnosis and therapeutics.[13] With the exception of echocardiography, none of the noninvasive techniques can determine pulmonary artery pressure at the bedside. Measurements of pulmonary artery occlusion or "wedge" pressure (PAOP [or PAWP]) may aid in the diagnosis of left ventricular dysfunction and guiding fluid management. In addition, the PAOP provides information on lung hydrostatic pressure; thus, it may be used to characterize the risk of cardiogenic pulmonary edema. Cardiac output is measured intermittently by manual injection of a cold bolus or automatically using a semicontinuous system. Several cardiac output measurements are averaged, and rapid changes cannot be detected, even with the semicontinuous method. Thermodilution reliably measures cardiac output, except in severe tricuspid regurgitation or intracardiac shunt. At high cardiac output, the precision of semicontinuous cardiac output measurements is lower than that of classic thermodilution,[14] but this has often minor consequences on patient management.

Measurement of cardiac output is useful for diagnosing the type of shock and evaluating the effect of therapies.[3] Finally, each hemodynamic evaluation can be accompanied by measurement of mixed venous oxygen saturation (SvO_2), which enables the interpretation of the cardiac output by comparing oxygen transport with oxygen consumption. Although related, SvO_2 differs from $ScvO_2$. SvO_2 represents the venous blood collected from all parts of the body, whereas $ScvO_2$ represents only the blood drained from the upper part of the body. As such, SvO_2 is a superior measure of global oxygen dynamics.

What is the impact of use of the PAC on outcome? Observational trials demonstrate that the use of the PAC allows more accurate determination of the hemodynamic state than clinic evaluation, is associated with significant changes in therapy, and may be associated with improved outcome.[15] On the other hand, several randomized studies failed to demonstrate improved outcomes associated with its use in intensive care unit (ICU) patients with various medical conditions.[16-20] Several factors may explain these findings. One argument is that the mechanic complication rate of PACs is so high that it outweighs its potential benefits. However, there were no statistically significant differences in such complications in those studies. In addition, perioperative studies of hemodynamic optimization with the PAC have demonstrated reduced perioperative complications[21] and improved survival,[22] suggesting that, in a broad context, the device is safe.

A more likely explanation is that many physicians fail to adequately interpret the data obtained in the complex situations that arise in critically ill patients,[23,24] resulting in incorrect decisions. Most of the trials with the PAC in critical care patients did not use decision-support algorithms. Interestingly, the addition of echocardiographic data does not necessarily improve the interpretation of the data,[25] suggesting that the physicians are more at fault than the monitoring device.[26] Another factor is that the patients included in these trials were highly selected. In the Fluids and Catheters Treatment Trial, the number of patients not included, because they were already monitored by a PAC at the time of screening, was twice the number of patients randomized, suggesting that the most severely ill patients (in whom information was deemed more valuable) were not included.[27] This high rate of exclusion may bias the results of these trials.[28] Investigators did not include patients with cardiogenic shock because they were sicker, were being managed with a PAC for other reasons, and had significantly higher mortality rates than the patients included in the trial.[29]

As a result of these negative trials and because of the wide availability of alternative techniques, the use of the PAC has decreased over time[30] and has probably been abandoned altogether by many clinicians. However, it is worth arguing that the PAC remains a useful device in select patients in the ICU, and medical and nursing staff should be familiar with insertion, setup, and monitoring techniques.

TRANSPULMONARY THERMODILUTION AND PULSE WAVE ANALYSIS

A widely used alternative to the PAC is the transpulmonary thermodilution technique coupled with pulse wave analysis (peripherally inserted continuous cardiac output). This is a minimally invasive technique that still requires placement of arterial and central venous lines. Transpulmonary thermodilution is used principally for the calibration of pulse-wave-derived continuous cardiac output measurement.

Stroke volume can be estimated from an arterial pressure waveform. Calibration with transpulmonary thermodilution is used to capture differences in arterial compliance and vascular tone from one patient to another and from one time to another in a given patient.[31,32] The accuracy of pulse wave analysis is highly dependent on the delay between two calibrations. Any change in vascular tone can significantly alter the precision of these devices[33] and should prompt recalibration. Devices that use autocalibration now allow reliable measurements even in patients with septic shock,[14] but they still lack the additional cardiac function and volumetric measurements.

Transpulmonary thermodilution requires the use of a modified arterial catheter equipped with a thermistor. This catheter is inserted in the femoral artery. The thermodilution curve can be determined using a modified proprietary algorithm. Cardiac output is determined by the area under the curve as in standard thermodilution. Transpulmonary thermodilution is slightly less sensitive to valvular regurgitation than right-sided thermodilution.

A further useful aspect of transpulmonary thermodilution is that it also allows the measurement of extravascular lung water (EVLWI) and of the volumes of cardiac chambers (global end-diastolic volume index [GEDVI]) on the basis of the curve characteristics and loss of thermal indicator. GEDVI is an index of preload. Volumetric indices may perform better than pressures in patients with raised intrathoracic or intra-abdominal pressures or with decreased left ventricular compliance. EVLWI reflects the degree of pulmonary edema, whatever its cause, and may predict adverse outcomes.[34] Both indices are useful in establishing the diagnosis and to guide fluid management. Given the additional value of volumetric measurements, transpulmonary thermodilution should be considered as an integral part of hemodynamic assessment (diagnostic purposes as well as evaluation of response to therapy).

Cardiac function index (CFI) is a derived parameter calculated as cardiac index divided by GEDVI. In patients with cardiogenic shock, CFI reflects left ventricular ejection fraction,[35,36] provided that right ventricular function is maintained.[36] It has been proposed as a substitute to the PAC to identify myocardial depression in septic patients.[35]

Complications related to hemodynamic monitoring with transpulmonary thermodilution are relatively minor and related to arterial and central venous catheterization (local bleeding and infections).[37] To date, no study has compared vascular complications from PAC with that of transpulmonary thermodilution and pulse wave analysis (TTPWA).

HEMODYNAMIC OPTIMIZATION WITH PULMONARY ARTERY CATHETERS OR TRANSPULMONARY THERMODILUTION

On the basis of the principles of determination of adequacy of cardiac output, preload responsiveness, and cardiac function, several trials have evaluated the effect of hemodynamic optimization on outcome.[22,38-41] In general, these devices perform better in the controlled perioperative arena, rather than in the chaotic intensive care setting.

Perioperative optimization with the PAC resulted in decreased perioperative complications[21] and improved survival rate.[22] Transpulmonary thermodilution can also be used for this purpose, also resulting in a decreased incidence of perioperative complications.[38,42]

In critical illness, there is little evidence that measurement of transpulmonary thermodilution improves outcome. In patients with cardiogenic shock after cardiac arrest, hemodynamic monitoring with transpulmonary thermodilution was associated with higher fluid intake in the first 24 hours and resulted in a lower incidence of acute kidney injury compared with CVP and arterial pressure monitoring.[41] In patients with Tako Tsubo cardiomyopathy related to subarachnoid hemorrhage, a CFI below 4.2 per minute was predictive of an impaired ejection fraction and impaired 3-month neurologic outcome.[39] Patients with poor neurologic outcome also had high values of EVLWI. In a randomized trial, these authors reported that hemodynamic resuscitation targeted on transpulmonary thermodilution indices was associated with better long-term neurologic outcome in patients with high-grade subarachnoid hemorrhage.[40]

There are few data comparing PAC and TTPWA. A small-sized randomized trial directly comparing the two techniques, pressure-guided resuscitation compared with volumetric variables, resulted in a shorter duration of mechanic ventilation in shock patients with impaired cardiac function, but not in patients with preserved cardiac function, whereas survival rate was not affected in either group.[43]

CONCLUSION

Invasive hemodynamic evaluation is widely used in critically ill patients. The PAC and TTPWA are probably the most widely used devices. No large-scale trial has demonstrated improved outcomes with these techniques in critical care. Basic hemodynamic monitoring may be sufficient in simple cases, but invasive monitoring may be of value in complex cases.

AUTHORS' RECOMMENDATIONS

- The use of invasive hemodynamic monitoring with PAC or transpulmonary thermodilution provides important information on the hemodynamic condition of the patient, on the type of shock, and on the response to therapy.
- Large-scale randomized trials failed to demonstrate benefit with the use of invasive hemodynamic monitoring in critical care.
- Trials of pulmonary artery catheterization did not use specific protocols for hemodynamic management or ensure that physicians using these devices were appropriately trained in their use.
- Trials show that pulmonary artery catheterization is safe.
- The use of invasive techniques should be limited to selected patients, especially in those with comorbidities, complex hemodynamic conditions, or multiple organ dysfunction.

REFERENCES

1. Ospina-Tascon GA, Cordioli RL, Vincent JL. What type of monitoring has been shown to improve outcomes in acutely ill patients? *Intensive Care Med*. 2008;34:800–820.
2. De Backer D, Cholley BP, Slama M, Vieillard-Baron A, Vignon P. *Hemodynamic monitoring using echocardiography in the critically ill*. Heidelberg Dordrecht London New York: Springer; 2011. 1-311.
3. Cecconi M, De Backer D, Antonelli M, et al. Consensus on circulatory shock and hemodynamic monitoring. Task force of the European Society of Intensive Care Medicine. *Intensive Care Med*, 2014;40:1795-1815.
4. Vincent JL, De Backer D. Circulatory shock. *N Engl J Med*. 2013;369:1726–1734.
5. Expert Round Table on Echocardiography in ICU. International consensus statement on training standards for advanced critical care echocardiography. *Intensive Care Med*. 2014;40:654–666.
6. Monnet X, Picard F, Lidzborski E, et al. The estimation of cardiac output by the Nexfin device is of poor reliability for tracking the effects of a fluid challenge. *Crit Care*. 2012;16:R212.
7. Rivers E, Nguyen B, Havstadt S, et al. Early goal-directed therapy in the treatment of severe sepsis and septic shock. *N Engl J Med*. 2001;345:1368–1377.
8. Yealy DM, Kellum JA, Huang DT, et al. A randomized trial of protocol-based care for early septic shock. *N Engl J Med*. 2014;370:1683–1693.
9. Peake SL, Delaney A, Bailey M, et al. Goal-directed resuscitation for patients with early septic shock. *N Engl J Med*. 2014;371:1496–1506.
10. Dellinger RP, Levy MM, Rhodes A, et al. Surviving Sepsis Campaign: international guidelines for management of severe sepsis and septic shock, 2012. *Intensive Care Med*. 2013;39:165–228.
11. Levy MM, Rhodes A, Phillips GS, et al. Surviving Sepsis Campaign: association between performance metrics and outcomes in a 7.5-year study. *Intensive Care Med*. 2014;40:1623–1633.
12. Gu WJ, Wang F, Bakker J, et al. The effect of goal-directed therapy on mortality in patients with sepsis – earlier is better: a meta-analysis of randomized controlled trials. *Crit Care*. 2014;18:570.
13. Ventetuolo CE, Klinger JR. Management of acute right ventricular failure in the intensive care unit. *Ann Am Thorac Soc*. 2014;11:811–822.
14. De Backer D, Marx G, Tan A, et al. Arterial pressure-based cardiac output monitoring: a multicenter validation of the third-generation software in septic patients. *Intensive Care Med*. 2011;37:233–240.
15. Mimoz O, Rauss A, Rekik N, et al. Pulmonary artery catheterization in critically ill patients: a prospective analysis of outcome changes associated with catheter-prompted changes in therapy. *Crit Care Med*. 1994;22:573–579.
16. Wheeler AP, Bernard GR, Thompson BT, et al. Pulmonary-artery versus central venous catheter to guide treatment of acute lung injury. *N Engl J Med*. 2006;354:2213–2224.
17. Richard C, Warszawski J, Anguel N, et al. Early use of the pulmonary artery catheter and outcomes in patients with shock and acute respiratory distress syndrome: a randomized controlled trial. *JAMA*. 2003;290:2713–2720.
18. Sandham JD, Hull RD, Brant RF, et al. A randomized, controlled trial of the use of pulmonary-artery catheters in high-risk surgical patients. *N Engl J Med*. 2003;348:5–14.
19. Binanay C, Califf RM, Hasselblad V, et al. Evaluation study of congestive heart failure and pulmonary artery catheterization effectiveness: the ESCAPE trial. *JAMA*. 2005;294:1625–1633.
20. Rajaram SS, Desai NK, Kalra A, et al. Pulmonary artery catheters for adult patients in intensive care. *Cochrane Database Syst Rev*. 2013;2:CD003408.
21. Polonen P, Ruokonen E, Hippelainen M, et al. A prospective, randomized study of goal-oriented hemodynamic therapy in cardiac surgical patients. *Anesth Analg*. 2000;90:1052–1059.
22. Wilson J, Woods I, Fawcett J, et al. Reducing the risk of major elective surgery: randomised controlled trial of preoperative optimisation of oxygen delivery. *BMJ*. 1999;318:1099–1103.
23. Gnaegi A, Feihl F, Perret C. Intensive care physicians' insufficient knowledge of right-heart catheterization at the bedside: time to act? *Crit Care Med*. 1997;25:213–220.
24. Iberti TJ, Fischer EP, Leibowitz AB, et al. A multicenter study of physicians' knowledge of the pulmonary artery catheter. Pulmonary Artery Catheter Study Group. *JAMA*. 1990;264:2928–2932.
25. Jain M, Canham M, Upadhyay D, et al. Variability in interventions with pulmonary artery catheter data. *Intensive Care Med*. 2003;29:2059–2062.
26. De Backer D. Hemodynamic assessment: the technique or the physician at fault? *Intensive Care Med*. 2003;29:1865–1867.
27. Wiedemann HP, Wheeler AP, Bernard GR, et al. Comparison of two fluid-management strategies in acute lung injury. *N Engl J Med*. 2006;354:2564–2575.
28. De Backer D, Schortgen F. Physicians declining patient enrollment in clinical trials: what are the implications? *Intensive Care Med*. 2014;40:117–119.
29. Allen LA, Rogers JG, Warnica JW, et al. High mortality without ESCAPE: the registry of heart failure patients receiving pulmonary artery catheters without randomization. *J Card Fail*. 2008;14:661–669.
30. Koo KK, Sun JC, Zhou Q, et al. Pulmonary artery catheters: evolving rates and reasons for use. *Crit Care Med*. 2011;39:1613–1618.
31. van Lieshout JJ, Wesseling KH. Continuous cardiac output by pulse contour analysis? *Br J Anaesth*. 2001;86:467–469.
32. Michard F. Pulse contour analysis: fairy tale or new reality? *Crit Care Med*. 2007;35:1791–1792.
33. Hamzaoui O, Monnet X, Richard C, et al. Effects of changes in vascular tone on the agreement between pulse contour and transpulmonary thermodilution cardiac output measurements within an up to 6-hour calibration-free period. *Crit Care Med*. 2008;36:434–440.
34. Jozwiak M, Silva S, Persichini R, et al. Extravascular lung water is an independent prognostic factor in patients with acute respiratory distress syndrome. *Crit Care Med*. 2013;42:472–480.
35. Ritter S, Rudiger A, Maggiorini M. Transpulmonary thermodilution-derived cardiac function index identifies cardiac dysfunction in acute heart failure and septic patients: an observational study. *Crit Care*. 2009;13:R133.
36. Perny J, Kimmoun A, Perez P, et al. Evaluation of cardiac function index as measured by transpulmonary thermodilution as an indicator of left ventricular ejection fraction in cardiogenic shock. *Biomed Res Int*. 2014;2014:598029.
37. Belda FJ, Aguilar G, Teboul JL, et al. Complications related to less-invasive haemodynamic monitoring. *Br J Anaesth*. 2011;106:482–486.
38. Goepfert MS, Reuter DA, Akyol D, et al. Goal-directed fluid management reduces vasopressor and catecholamine use in cardiac surgery patients. *Intensive Care Med*. 2007;33:96–103.

39. Mutoh T, Kazumata K, Terasaka S, et al. Impact of transpulmonary thermodilution-based cardiac contractility and extravascular lung water measurements on clinical outcome of patients with Takotsubo cardiomyopathy after subarachnoid hemorrhage: a retrospective observational study. *Crit Care*. 2014;18:482.

40. Mutoh T, Kazumata K, Terasaka S, et al. Early intensive versus minimally invasive approach to postoperative hemodynamic management after subarachnoid hemorrhage. *Stroke*. 2014;45:1280–1284.

41. Adler C, Reuter H, Seck C, et al. Fluid therapy and acute kidney injury in cardiogenic shock after cardiac arrest. *Resuscitation*. 2013;84:194–199.

42. Salzwedel C, Puig J, Carstens A, et al. Perioperative goal-directed hemodynamic therapy based on radial arterial pulse pressure variation and continuous cardiac index trending reduces postoperative complications after major abdominal surgery: a multicenter, prospective, randomized study. *Crit Care*. 2013;17:R191.

43. Trof RJ, Beishuizen A, Cornet AD, et al. Volume-limited versus pressure-limited hemodynamic management in septic and nonseptic shock. *Crit Care Med*. 2012;40:1177–1185.

14 Does the Use of Echocardiography Aid in the Management of the Critically Ill?

Sara Nikravan, Andrew J. Patterson

Rapidly identifying causes of hemodynamic instability is essential during the care of critically ill patients. Central venous pressure catheters, pulse pressure variability devices, and transesophageal echocardiograms are commonly used in the intensive care unit (ICU) for evaluation of hemodynamic status.[1,2] During the past 5 years, focused bedside transthoracic echocardiography (F-TTE) has emerged as an alternative. A primary advantage of F-TTE is that it can be easily performed by noncardiologists.[1-3] The purpose of this chapter is to highlight the evidence supporting its utility.

HISTORY

The first F-TTE examination for use by noncardiologists was proposed in 1989.[4] Described as the Focused Assessed Transthoracic Echocardiography (FATE) examination, it was intended to quickly answer specific clinic questions about cardiopulmonary status[1,3,5] and exclude obvious disease. Emphasis was placed on ventricle wall thickness and chamber dimensions, ventricle contractility, and visualization of the pleura on both sides.[4] Initially, four scanning positions were highlighted: the subcostal view, the apical view, the parasternal views (both long and short), and a pleural view. The FATE examination evolved to include five basic views: parasternal long axis, parasternal short axis (across the aortic valve, mitral valve, and left ventricle at the level of the papillary muscles), apical four chamber, subcostal four chamber, and subcostal inferior vena cava (IVC).[6]

When used to answer specific questions about potential cardiac causes of nontraumatic symptomatic hypotension, F-TTE performed by noncardiologists has demonstrated utility in the ICU.[7,8] The speed with which assessments can be made and the diagnostic accuracy compared with more invasive techniques are two recognized benefits.[7,9-11] F-TTE has also been shown to be useful in the diagnosis and management of pulmonary embolism, septic cardiomyopathy, cardiac tamponade, myocardial infarction, global left ventricular (LV) dysfunction, aortic root dilation and dissection, right ventricular (RV) dysfunction and dilation, and valvular disease.[1,4,5,12-15]

Three consensus statements with regard to the use of F-TTE by noncardiologists have been published by (1) the American College of Chest Physicians (ACCP), (2) the American Society of Echocardiography (ASE), and (3) the American College of Emergency Physicians (ACEP).[5,16] Both the ASE and ACEP define the role of F-TTE as a time-sensitive assessment tool for the symptomatic patient, primarily for evaluation of global cardiac function, relative chamber size, volume status, and assessment of pericardial effusion. They emphasize that although other pathologic conditions (e.g., regional wall motion abnormalities, aortic dissection, cardiac masses or thrombus, valvulopathies) may be visualized, formal echocardiography or cardiology consultation should be obtained if these abnormalities are suspected.[3,5]

F-TTE DURING CARDIOPULMONARY ARREST

F-TTE may be of value during the management of cardiac arrest for diagnosis, treatment, and prognostication. For instance, Oren-Grinberg and colleagues[1] published a case reporting visualization of a large clot in transit with handheld echocardiography during a cardiac arrest. This finding informed the clinicians with regard to the cause of hemodynamic instability in their patient and prompted administration of thrombolytics. Clinicians have described the effectiveness of F-TTE in differentiating between true pulseless electric activity (PEA) and pseudo-PEA. In addition to helping to guide management, this differentiation can ultimately assist in outcome prognostication because patients with pseudo-PEA tend to have a higher survival rate than those in true PEA.[12,17] Consequently, F-TTE in resuscitation examination has been incorporated into the adult advanced life support algorithm during pulse checks, thus minimizing interruptions in chest compressions.[12]

F-TTE IN TRAUMA AND THE SURGICAL ICU

Rapid volume assessment and goal-directed resuscitation are essential elements in the initial management of trauma patients. The BEAT (Bedside Echocardiographic Assessment in Trauma/Critical Care) examination was developed in 2008. It has been validated for the assessment of cardiac function and preload during trauma care.[18] During this examination, an IVC collapsibility index is used to distinguish patients who will likely respond to fluid resuscitation from those who will not. BEAT has been shown to be most effective at the extremes of volume status.[2,19,20]

Obtaining adequate subcostal views of the IVC can be challenging in trauma patients because of abdominal injuries, drains, tubes, and/or bandages.[2,18] Tissue-Doppler imaging of the tricuspid valve from the apical four-chamber view with F-TTE shows promise as an alternative method for volume assessment in the patient with such barriers.[13]

The utility of F-TTE has also been demonstrated in patients with penetrating and blunt trauma, improving outcomes by decreasing the time required to accurately diagnose and treat traumatic cardiac and thoracic injury.[5,21,22]

F-TTE IN THE POSTCARDIAC SURGERY PATIENT

F-TTE has not been shown to be consistently helpful in the postcardiac surgery patient population. These patients typically have chest incisions, bandages, and chest tubes that make examinations technically difficult. For example, Price and colleagues[23] reviewed prospectively collected data on postoperative patients after cardiac surgery for the diagnosis of tamponade with F-TTE. They found that when cardiac tamponade occurred less than 72 hours after surgery, F-TTE failed to visualize up to 60% of the pericardial fluid collections. They noted that when occurring so acutely after surgery, these pericardial effusions were small and localized and did not result in the typical echocardiographic findings of "tamponade." F-TTE was more effective in the diagnosis of late tamponade (>72 hours).

Handheld bedside ultrasound may be of some utility in the cardiac surgery patient population for the early diagnosis of pleural effusions, facilitating interventions at a lower cost and without reexposure to radiation.[24] In addition, when pleural or pericardial effusions have been diagnosed, ultrasound is helpful in guiding emergency interventions at the bedside.[5,25]

TRAINING

No formalized program has been uniformly accepted for the training of noncardiologists in F-TTE. Numerous studies have corroborated that the learning curve is steep and that with a combination of didactics and hands-on exercises, the noncardiologist can become proficient.[5,6,26] For instance, Beraud and colleagues[6] published an assessment of proficiency among critical care medicine fellows, at Stanford University, after implementation of a structured handheld ultrasound curriculum. All of the trainees had completed a residency in anesthesiology, internal medicine, emergency medicine, or both internal and emergency medicine before fellowship. With an average of 8 hours of didactics, 15 hours of bedside instruction, and 30 proctored examinations, the fellows at Stanford were able to obtain adequate imaging and accurately diagnose asystole, LV dysfunction, RV dilation and dysfunction, pericardial effusion, and a normal heart in a patient with poor thoracic windows in less than 2 minutes as compared with experts who reached a diagnosis in less than 30 seconds.

THE FUTURE

There is now an abundance of data supporting the use of F-TTE by noncardiologists in high-acuity clinic settings, including the emergency room and the ICU. However, to date, no randomized controlled trial has compared F-TTE with alternative approaches. It is likely that F-TTE will be embraced into critical care in the belief that additional information will translate into improved outcomes, as was the case with the previous generation of monitoring devices. In the future, training standards are likely to be formalized and certifications of proficiency offered by national societies and boards. In addition, medical schools are likely to incorporate ultrasound training into their curricula. The optimal blend of didactic, bedside, and problem-based learning may depend on the education level of trainees and the intended purpose for the use of F-TTE.

CASE SCENARIOS

Below are examples of how F-TTE findings can be used to guide therapy.

Case Stem

A 68-year-old male is admitted to the ICU for persistent hypotension despite 3 L intravenous fluids and escalating doses of dopamine. His wife reports a past medical history positive for hypertension and prostate cancer. He underwent prostatectomy 5 years ago.

Vital Signs: Blood pressure 82/38 mm Hg, heart rate 121 beats/min, hemoglobin saturation in blood (SpO_2) 95% on 5 L nasal cannula O_2, temperature 38.3°C.

Electrocardiogram: Sinus tachycardia, no evidence of ST or T wave abnormalities.

Urinalysis (UA): 2 + leukocyte esterase, 0 nitrites, 6 to 10 white blood cells, moderate bacteria.

Renal function abnormal with creatinine elevated from baseline. Broad-spectrum antibiotics have been administered for presumed urosepsis and septic shock.

Scenario 1

The ICU physician performs F-TTE on the patient's arrival to the ICU and observes the following (Fig. 14-1):

Scenario 2

The ICU physician performs F-TTE upon the patient's arrival to the ICU and observes the following (Fig. 14-2):

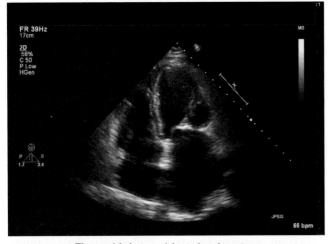

Figure 14-1 Apical four-chamber view.

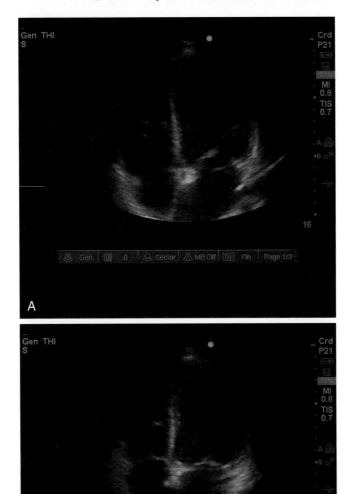

Figure 14-2 **A,** Apical four-chamber view in diastole. **B,** Apical four-chamber view in systole.

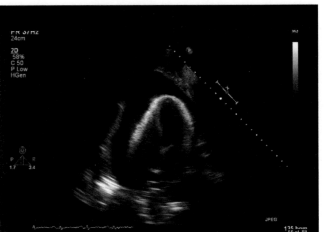

Figure 14-3 Apical four-chamber view.

Scenario 3

The ICU physician performs F-TTE on the patient's arrival to the ICU and observes the following (Fig. 14-3):

In the first scenario, a calcified and stenotic mitral valve is visualized. The correct interventions would be to discontinue dopamine, initiate norepinephrine for blood pressure support, continue intravenous fluid resuscitation, and await formal echocardiography for confirmation.

In the second scenario, septic cardiomyopathy is noted with both LV and RV dysfunction. The correct intervention would be to change the dopamine infusion to epinephrine to provide greater inotropic support.

In the third scenario, a large pericardial effusion is noted. Closer evaluation reveals collapse of the right atrium during diastole, an echocardiographic sign suggesting tamponade physiology. Given the clinic presentation and F-TTE findings, the clinical team should administer intravenous fluids, discontinue dopamine, and perform pericardial drainage. The ultrasound probe could be used to guide the pericardiocentesis.

AUTHORS' RECOMMENDATIONS

- F-TTE is a valuable tool in the assessment of hypotension in medical and surgical ICUs.
- F-TTE is less effective immediately after cardiac surgery.
- F-TTE may be of value during cardiac arrest to distinguish between PEA and pseudo-PEA.
- F-TTE should be a core competence for graduates of critical care training programs.

REFERENCES

1. Oren-Grinberg A, Gulati G, Fuchs L, Pinto DS. Hand-held echocardiography in the management of cardiac arrest. *Anesth Analg.* 2012;115(5):1038–1041.
2. Stawicki SP, Braslow BM, Panebianco NL, et al. Intensivist use of hand-carried ultrasonography to measure IVC collapsibility in estimating intravascular volume status: correlations with CVP. *J Am Coll Surg.* 2009;209(1):55–61.

3. Manasia AR, Nagaraj HM, Kodali RB, et al. Feasibility and potential clinical utility of goal-directed transthoracic echocardiography performed by noncardiologist intensivists using a small hand-carried device (SonoHeart) in critically ill patients. *J Cardiothorac Vasc Anesth*. 2005;19(2):155–159.

4. Jensen M, Sloth E, Larsen K, Schmidt M. Transthoracic echocardiography for cardiopulmonary monitoring in intensive care. *J Anaesthesiol*. 2004;21(9):700–707.

5. Labovitz AJ, Noble VE, Bierig M, et al. Focused cardiac ultrasound in the emergent setting: a consensus statement of the American Society of Echocardiography and American College of Emergency Physicians. *J Am Soc Echocardiogr Off Publ Am Soc Echocardiogr*. 2010;23(12):1225–1230.

6. Beraud A-S, Rizk NW, Pearl RG, Liang DH, Patterson AJ. Focused transthoracic echocardiography during critical care medicine training: curriculum implementation and evaluation of proficiency. *Crit Care Med*. 2013;41(8):e179–81.

7. Marcelino PA, Marum SM, Fernandes APM, Germano N, Lopes MG. Routine transthoracic echocardiography in a general Intensive Care Unit: an 18 month survey in 704 patients. *Eur J Intern Med*. 2009;20(3):e37–42.

8. Jones AE, Tayal VS, Sullivan DM, Kline JA. Randomized, controlled trial of immediate versus delayed goal-directed ultrasound to identify the cause of nontraumatic hypotension in emergency department patients. *Crit Care Med*. 2004;32(8):1703–1708.

9. Willenheimer RB, Israelsson BA, Cline CMJ, Erhardt LR. Simplified Echocardiography in the Diagnosis of Heart Failure. *Scand Cardiovasc J*. 1, 1997;31(1):9–16.

10. Moore CL, Rose GA, Tayal VS, Sullivan DM, Arrowood JA, Kline JA. Determination of left ventricular function by emergency physician echocardiography of hypotensive patients. *Acad Emerg Med Off J Soc Acad Emerg Med*. 2002;9(3):186–193.

11. Kimura BJ, Pezeshki B, Frack SA, DeMaria AN. Feasibility of "limited" echo imaging: characterization of incidental findings. *J Am Soc Echocardiogr Off Publ Am Soc Echocardiogr*. 1998;11(7):746–750.

12. Breitkreutz R, Walcher F, Seeger FH. Focused echocardiographic evaluation in resuscitation management: concept of an advanced life support-conformed algorithm. *Crit Care Med*. 2007;35(suppl 5):S150–S161.

13. Arbo JE, Maslove DM, Beraud A-S. Bedside assessment of right atrial pressure in critically ill septic patients using tissue Doppler ultrasonography. *J Crit Care*. 2013;28(6):1112.e1–1112.e5.

14. Mansencal N, Redheuil A, Joseph T, et al. Use of transthoracic echocardiography combined with venous ultrasonography in patients with pulmonary embolism. *Int J Cardiol*. 2004;96(1):59–63.

15. Mazraeshahi RM, Farmer JC, Porembka DT. A suggested curriculum in echocardiography for critical care physicians. *Crit Care Med*. 2007;35(suppl 8):S431–S433.

16. Mayo PH, Beaulieu Y, Doelken P, et al. American College of Chest Physicians/La Société de Réanimation de Langue Française statement on competence in critical care ultrasonography. *Chest*. 2009;135(4):1050–1060.

17. Salen P, Melniker L, Chooljian C, et al. Does the presence or absence of sonographically identified cardiac activity predict resuscitation outcomes of cardiac arrest patients? *Am J Emerg Med*. 2005;23(4):459–462.

18. Gunst M, Ghaemmaghami V, Sperry J, et al. Accuracy of cardiac function and volume status estimates using the bedside echocardiographic assessment in trauma/critical care. *J Trauma*. 2008;65(3):509–516.

19. Feissel M, Michard F, Faller J-P, Teboul J-L. The respiratory variation in inferior vena cava diameter as a guide to fluid therapy. *Intensive Care Med*. 2004;30(9):1834–1837.

20. Bendjelid K, Romand J-A, Walder B, Suter PM, Fournier G. Correlation between measured inferior vena cava diameter and right atrial pressure depends on the echocardiographic method used in patients who are mechanically ventilated. *J Am Soc Echocardiogr Off Publ Am Soc Echocardiogr*. 2002;15(9):944–949.

21. Rozycki GS, Feliciano DV, Ochsner MG, et al. The role of ultrasound in patients with possible penetrating cardiac wounds: a prospective multicenter study. *J Trauma*. 1999;46(4):543–551. discussion 551–2.

22. Rozycki GS, Feliciano DV, Schmidt JA, et al. The role of surgeon-performed ultrasound in patients with possible cardiac wounds. *Ann Surg*. 1996;223(6):737–746.

23. Price S, Prout J, Jaggar SI, Gibson DG, Pepper JR. "Tamponade" following cardiac surgery: terminology and echocardiography may both mislead. *Eur J Cardio-Thorac Surg Off J Eur Assoc Cardio-Thorac Surg*. 2004;26(6):1156–1160.

24. Piccoli M, Trambaiolo P, Salustri A, et al. Bedside diagnosis and follow-up of patients with pleural effusion by a hand-carried ultrasound device early after cardiac surgery. *Chest*. 2005;128(5):3413–3420.

25. Vayre F, Lardoux H, Pezzano M, Bourdarias JP, Dubourg O. Subxiphoid pericardiocentesis guided by contrast two-dimensional echocardiography in cardiac tamponade: experience of 110 consecutive patients. *Eur J Echocardiogr J Work Group Echocardiogr Eur Soc Cardiol*. 2000;1(1):66–71.

26. Jones AE, Tayal VS, Kline JA. Focused training of emergency medicine residents in goal-directed echocardiography: a prospective study. *Acad Emerg Med Off J Soc Acad Emerg Med*. 2003;10(10):1054–1058.

15 How Do I Manage Hemodynamic Decompensation in a Critically Ill Patient?

Allison Dalton, Michael O'Connor

The ability to evaluate and manage a critically ill patient is one of the most important skills any intensivist brings to the bedside. Patients already resident in the intensive care unit (ICU) can decompensate because of any of several causes; thus, the differential diagnosis is broader than it is in less complex patients. Appropriate management is dependent on correct identification of the cause or causes of decompensation. The classes of shock are cardiogenic, hypovolemic (e.g., hemorrhagic), vasodilatory (e.g., septic, adrenal insufficiency, anaphylaxis), or obstructive (e.g., tension pneumothorax, cardiac tamponade).[1]

The goal of evaluating circulation is ultimately to determine whether the patient has adequate end-organ perfusion. Clinically, mental status and urine output are widely accepted as the most reliable indicators of adequate end-organ perfusion, but they may not be readily assessed in a substantial percentage of critically ill patients. Signs of hypoperfusion may include tachycardia, tachypnea, low mean blood pressure, and low urine output. Encephalopathy, a marker for cerebral perfusion, is also a predictor for higher mortality when associated with hemodynamic instability.[2]

TARGETS OF TREATMENT

Mean arterial blood pressure is a primary indicator of hemodynamic instability. End-organ perfusion is maintained over a wide range of mean arterial pressures (MAPs) because of autoregulation.[3] In patients with chronic hypertension, the autoregulation curve is shifted to the right, indicating that these patients require higher MAPs to achieve adequate end-organ perfusion.[4] Because of its close association with sufficient perfusion, MAP goals become a target for the initial resuscitation efforts in shock. Recent literature suggests that a MAP of 65 mm Hg is sufficient for patients with septic shock and is generally associated with good outcomes in critically ill patients.[5,6]

Mixed venous or central venous oxygen saturation or content can be reliably used to make inferences about the balance of oxygen delivery to the peripheral tissues and oxygen uptake by them. Mixed venous oxygen saturation (SvO_2) is measured from the pulmonary arterial port of a pulmonary artery catheter. For patients without pulmonary artery access, central venous oxygen saturation ($ScvO_2$) is often used as an alternative. $ScvO_2$ is typically measured from a central line placed within the superior vena cava. Multiple studies have revealed variable correlation between SvO_2 and $ScvO_2$.[7-9] However, Chawla et al.[10] found that $ScvO_2$ drawn from a port within the right atrium had good correlation with SvO_2, although there was a bias toward $ScvO_2$ being 5.2% higher than the SvO_2. This difference can be explained by the addition of blood from the coronary sinus, which drains the high oxygen extraction system of the heart, into the measurement of SvO_2 but not the $ScvO_2$. Multiple studies focused in goal-directed resuscitation have used $ScvO_2$ to determine if fluid administration is sufficient.[11-13] A $ScvO_2$ greater than 70%[14] is common in resuscitation algorithms and may improve outcomes.[12,13]

IS THIS HYPOVOLEMIA? IS THE PATIENT VOLUME RESPONSIVE?

Hypovolemic shock, when recognized, is readily treatable, which makes recognition imperative. Because only approximately 50% of patients in shock will respond to a volume challenge, it is important to determine which patients will benefit from volume infusion.[15] Hemodynamic parameters may be used to predict fluid responsiveness. There is essentially no evidence that traditional measures, such as central venous pressure (CVP) and pulmonary artery occlusion pressure predict volume responsiveness.[15-18]

Systolic Pressure Variation and Pulse Pressure Variation

Dynamic parameters, namely systolic pressure variation (SPV) and pulse pressure variation (PPV), are superior to all alternatives in making inference about volume responsiveness.[17-20] These methods assess the variation in the blood pressure components caused by cyclic increases in intrathoracic pressure by positive pressure mechanic ventilation. Increased intrathoracic pressure will cause increase in stroke volume as well as systolic and pulse pressures early in mechanic inspiration secondary to a transient increase in left ventricular (LV) end diastolic volume, decrease in afterload, and decrease in right ventricular (RV) volume.[21] This increase in systolic pressure is termed delta up (dUp). Immediately after, the sustained intrathoracic pressure decreases RV preload, and increased transpulmonary pressures during this phase of mechanic inspiration result in elevated RV afterload.[17] The combination of reduction in RV preload and increase in RV afterload leads to decreased RV stroke volume, which leads to decreased LV preload and stroke volume.[17] This decrease in systolic pressure is termed delta down (dDown). SPV is defined as the difference between dUp and dDown within one mechanic breath.[22] dDown has independently been shown to predict whether a patient will be volume responsive.[23,24]

There are disadvantages to the use of SPV and PPV. The patient must be in sinus rhythm to interpret the dynamic data.[25] Although PPV and LV stroke volume are tightly coupled in mechanically ventilated patients, PPV has been regarded as less reliable in spontaneously breathing patients.[26,27] Recent literature suggests that PPV and SPV may also be of value in predicting volume responsiveness in spontaneously breathing patients and are likely superior to all other techniques. Hong et al.[28] studied a group of nonintubated adult patients undergoing elective thoracic surgery. The patients were instructed to breathe in a pattern of forced inspiration followed by slow, passive expiration. The authors found that forced inspiration during spontaneous breathing can predict fluid responsiveness with a PPV threshold of 13.7% with an area under the curve of 0.910 (95% confidence interval 0.806–0.969, $P < 0.0001$).[28] In comparison, PPV in tidal breathing failed to accurately predict volume responsiveness in these patients.

Inferior Vena Cava Collapsibility on Ultrasound

Bedside ultrasound of the inferior vena cava (IVC) is an alternative means for assessing volume responsiveness. The advantages of bedside ultrasound include its noninvasive nature and easy availability.[29,30] Measurement of the dynamic change in the diameter of the IVC with the respiratory cycle has been shown to be a means to determining whether a patient will respond to a fluid challenge.[31,32] Because the IVC does not have the same compensatory vasoconstriction to volume loss, it may better reflect a patient's volume status than arterial measures such as blood pressure, pulse rate, and aortic diameter.[33] Although the performance of IVC ultrasound is better in mechanically ventilated patients than in spontaneously breathing patients, its performance in either context is adequate (sensitivity 0.81 vs. 0.7 and specificity 0.87 vs. 0.85, respectively).[32] Similar to the PPV/SPV literature, it is likely that uncontrolled spontaneous ventilation may result in variable and inconsistent changes in intrathoracic pressure, leading to less consistent changes in IVC diameter.[32] In a meta-analysis of spontaneously breathing patients, Dipti et al.[33] found that the maximal IVC diameter during exhalation was significantly lower in those who were hypovolemic as compared with those who were determined to be euvolemic.

Passive Leg Raise

Passive leg raise predicts the volume responsiveness of patients with shock. For this maneuver to be performed, the patient is placed in the supine position and bilateral lower extremities are raised to a 45-degree angle. Passive leg raise is correlated with increases in pulmonary artery occlusion pressure and end-diastolic dimension.[34,35] Monnet et al.[36] revealed passive leg raise to be the equivalent of a 500-cc fluid challenge. Importantly, passive leg raise is effective in determining fluid responsiveness in cardiac arrhythmias and in patients who are spontaneously breathing.[36] An algorithm for assessing volume responsiveness appears in Figure 15-1.

In recent years, a series of studies have been published that have measured the mean systemic pressure in hypotensive patients, and they have shown that it reliably predicts volume responsiveness. If these observations are replicated and instruments that can be used to measure this become available in clinic practice, then it is possible that determination of the mean systemic pressure may become the gold standard for making inferences about volume status and volume responsiveness.[37,38]

Treating Hypovolemic Shock

There is no consensus on what fluids should be used to treat hypovolemic shock, although there is growing consensus that lower-sodium crystalloid solutions are superior to normal saline.[39-42] The surviving sepsis guidelines recommend initial resuscitation with crystalloid because it is less expensive than albumin.[43] More recent analysis suggests that resuscitation with albumin may have some outcome benefit in sepsis,[44] particularly in its most severe form (Albios Study, supplementary material).[45] Hydroxyethyl

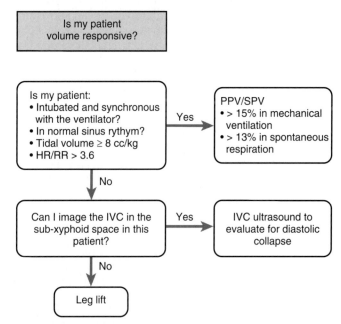

Figure 15-1. An algorithm for determining volume responsiveness in the shock state: PPV/SPV[17-20]; PPV/SPV[28]; IVC ultrasound[31,32]; and leg lift[34-36]. *HR*, heart rate; *IVC*, inferior vena cava; *PPV*, pulse pressure variation; *RR*, respiratory rate; *SPV*, systolic pressure variation.

starches should be avoided because of a link to increased need for renal replacement therapy and mortality when used in septic shock.[46,47] Although many experts continue to recommend volume resuscitation to a CVP endpoint, clinic endpoints (mental status, urine volume), MAP, lactate levels, and mixed/central venous saturations are likely more valid endpoints.[15,43]

IS THIS SEPTIC SHOCK?

Septic shock is caused by infection/inflammation and manifests as decreased vascular tone, resulting in hypotension and redistribution of blood flow. Surviving sepsis guidelines recommend a protocol driven by early resuscitation at the earliest sign of hypoperfusion.[43,48] Because elevated lactate is an independent marker of morbidity and mortality,[49-51] experts also recommend normalization of lactate levels as a marker of normalization of tissue perfusion. Jansen et al.[12] incorporated a normalization of lactate algorithm for the management of patients with sepsis. Jansen's study, protocol-driven normalization of lactate, resulted in a significant reduction in ICU length of stay and ICU and hospital mortality in the treatment group.[12]

Prompt administration of appropriate antibiotics after the diagnosis of septic shock is imperative to improving outcomes. Broad-spectrum empiric antibiotics should be given within the first hour of recognition of sepsis or septic shock.[43] Every hour of delay in administration of antibiotics increases mortality in septic shock.[52,53] Empirically administered antibiotics should provide coverage for infection with gram-positive, gram-negative, and anaerobic bacteria, and it may include fungal and viral coverage in some patients.[52] Source control with diagnosis of a specific infectious source and subsequent intervention should be performed.

Septic patients who have been adequately volume resuscitated may require therapy with vasoactive drugs to achieve adequate blood pressure and vital organ perfusion. The goal of the addition of vasopressors (e.g., norepinephrine) is not solely to increase MAP to a target of 65 mm Hg but also to obtain acceptable end-organ perfusion.

Norepinephrine and vasopressin can be used to support the circulation of septic patients.[54] The VASST (Vasopressin and Septic Shock Trial) demonstrated a survival benefit in a subgroup of patients requiring less than 15 μg/min of norepinephrine with the addition of vasopressin.[54] If end-organ perfusion remains insufficient despite sufficient volume resuscitation and adequate MAP, then inotropes (i.e., dobutamine) may be added to increase cardiac output.[55]

IS THIS OBSTRUCTIVE SHOCK?

The evaluation of a patient for cardiogenic or obstructive shock requires the concurrent or sequential completion of several diagnostic evaluations in short order. These include the inspection of ventilator flow waveforms for the presence of auto-positive end-expiratory pressure (PEEP), chest radiography or ultrasonography to assess for the presence of tension pneumothorax, measurement of bladder pressures in patients with a tense or distended abdomen to evaluate for abdominal compartment syndrome, and finally the performance of echocardiography (e.g., FOCUS [focused cardiac ultrasound] examination or FATE [focused assessed transthoracic echocardiography]) to evaluate the patient for cardiogenic shock and tamponade.

Abdominal Compartment Syndrome

Cardiogenic and obstructive shock are important causes of hypotension, and patients who have neither hypovolemic nor septic shock will need to be evaluated for these. Obstructive shock can be pericardial, thoracic, or abdominal in origin. Intra-abdominal hypertension is the result of diminished abdominal wall compliance, increased intraluminal contents, increased intra-abdominal contents, or capillary leak/fluid resuscitation. Intra-abdominal hypertension progresses to abdominal compartment syndrome when the compartment pressure is greater than 25 mm Hg, at which point the transmitted pressure affects cardiac, pulmonary, and renal functions as well as cerebrospinal pressure.[56,57] Patients in the intensive care setting have multiple risk factors for the development of intra-abdominal hypertension, including abdominal surgery, trauma, burns, ileus, acute pancreatitis, intra-abdominal infections/abscesses, intraperitoneal fluid (ascites, hemoperitoneum), sepsis, acidosis, and massive fluid resuscitation. High peak airway pressures on the ventilator can be a trigger to consider increased abdominal pressures. At present, assessment of bladder pressures is the gold standard of measurement for abdominal compartment syndrome.[58] If abdominal compartment syndrome is suspected, then the World Society for Abdominal Compartment Syndrome recommends various medical and surgical interventions that include decompressive laparotomy.[58]

Auto-PEEP

Additional causes of obstructive shock arise from the thorax. Auto-PEEP is the process by which the respiratory system is unable to return to functional residual capacity at the end of the expiratory phase of ventilation. Auto-PEEP impairs venous return to the heart, increases risk of barotrauma to the lungs, and can increase the patient's work of breathing while impeding their ability to trigger the ventilator.[1] Short respiratory cycles, high minute volumes, and obstructive lung disease predispose a patient to auto-PEEP. It is diagnosed on ventilator waveforms by persistence of flow at end expiration. Management of auto-PEEP includes decreasing respiratory rate and/or decreasing the I:E ratio to allow for more expiratory time.[59]

Tension Pneumothorax

Tension pneumothorax occurs when air is able to enter the chest via a one-way valve type of mechanism causing increased intrapleural pressure.[1] As intrathoracic pressure increases, there is mediastinal shift, which results in ventilatory compromise, compression of the vena cava at both the thoracic inlet in the neck and at the diaphragm leading to decreased venous return to the heart, and direct compression of the heart. In the hands of experienced intensivists, thoracic ultrasound is at least comparable to and likely superior to the gold standard of chest radiography in diagnosing pneumothorax.[60] Management includes needle thoracostomy followed by chest tube placement.

Cardiac Tamponade

Pericardial effusion can produce cardiac tamponade physiology by compressing cardiac chambers (especially right-sided structures), causing decreased LV preload and decreased cardiac output. In some instances (e.g., patients with a right ventricular assist device [RVAD]), mediastinal fluid can compress the great veins of the thorax and obstruct venous return without directly impinging on the pump itself. Pulsus paradoxus and electric alternans accompanying tachycardia and hypotension can often signal the presence of tamponade physiology. Bedside echocardiography can reveal pericardial effusion and collapse of right-sided cardiac chambers.[61] Prompt needle decompression with or without ultrasound guidance is the definitive treatment of hemodynamically significant pericardial effusions.

IS THIS CARDIOGENIC SHOCK?

Decreased cardiac output secondary to decreased contractility, increased diastolic stiffness, increased afterload, valvular abnormalities, and abnormal heart rates/rhythms lead to ventricular dysfunction and cardiogenic shock.[1] Acute myocardial ischemia and infarction are the most common causes of cardiogenic shock arising from the left ventricle.[62] LV shock as a result of systolic dysfunction manifests as decreased stroke volume and decreased cardiac output. Diastolic dysfunction leads to decreased cardiac output secondary to decreased end-diastolic filling and proportionate reduction in stroke volumes. Declining cardiac output leads to hypoperfusion and low SvO_2 and $ScvO_2$.

Acute RV shock is most often the result of elevated pulmonary vascular resistance (e.g., pulmonary embolus). In the modern era, RV infarction is a relatively less frequent and less important cause of RV failure. Elevated right-sided pressures (including CVP) with low cardiac output and no echocardiographic evidence of LV shock help to identify isolated RV shock. Symptoms are similar to those of cardiac tamponade and constrictive pericarditis; hence, these conditions must be excluded.[1]

Echocardiography is the gold standard in the evaluation of cardiogenic causes of shock. Echocardiography was once limited to cardiologists, but now intensivists and other noncardiologists are trained in basic emergency ultrasound. After completion of as little as a 10-hour training course, intensivists can perform a limited transthoracic echocardiogram with 84% accuracy in their interpretation.[63] Bedside evaluation with echocardiography has changed management in 37% of patients.[63] The American Society of Echocardiography and the American College of Emergency Physicians developed a consensus statement regarding the FOCUS transthoracic echocardiography examination as a concise way in which to rule in or rule out various diagnoses in patients with shock.[64] FOCUS consists of evaluation for presence of pericardial effusion, assessment of global cardiac systolic function, existence of ventricular enlargement, and estimation of intravascular volume.[65]

Treating Cardiogenic Shock

Identifying right-versus left-sided cardiogenic shock is imperative because treatment strategies differ, and to avoid potentially dangerous management, the origin of the cardiogenic shock must be elucidated. Management of patients with LV shock focuses on optimizing preload (as ejection fraction has fallen) and afterload and by increasing contractility by means of vasopressors (to increase diastolic pressure and, hence, perfusion of the coronary arteries), inotropes, and mechanical support such as intra-aortic balloon counterpulsation.[1] Excluding circumstances in which a patient presents with pulmonary edema, patients in LV shock should receive gentle fluid resuscitation.

Management of right-sided shock includes maintaining arterial pressure with vasoconstrictors, cardiac contractility with beta-1 agonists, and selective pulmonary vasodilation. Excess fluid infusion may further impair RV function by causing right-to-left intraventricular septal shift, which limits LV filling.[67] Right-sided volume overload may be managed with diuretics, splanchnic vasodilators (e.g., nitroglycerin), or hemofiltration. In patients with pulmonary embolism, treatment with anticoagulation, thrombolytics, and/or surgical embolectomy can improve underlying right heart failure.[1,68] Right heart shock arising from elevated pulmonary vascular resistance can be treated with pulmonary vasodilation using inspired oxygen, inhaled nitric oxide, or prostaglandin E1.[1] An algorithm for the management of a patient with narrow-pulse pressure shock unresponsive to volume is presented in Figure 15-2.

Unidentified, untreated shock is associated with high morbidity and mortality.[7] Appropriate treatment relies on recognition of a shock state as well as determining the type of shock from which the patient is suffering. As outlined previously, different forms of shock have specific management goals. With the use of basic history, physical examination, laboratory results, and additional tools (PPV, ultrasonography, bladder pressures, and ventilator waveforms), diagnosis can be made and treatment enacted.

AUTHORS' RECOMMENDATIONS

- When approaching a patient in shock, consider the four classes of shock: hypovolemic, vasodilatory, cardiogenic, and obstructive.
- Dynamic hemodynamic parameters are more accurate than static measurements in the assessment of volume status and fluid responsiveness.
- Echocardiography is a useful tool for assessment of intravascular volume and fluid responsiveness but also for cardiogenic and obstructive causes of shock.

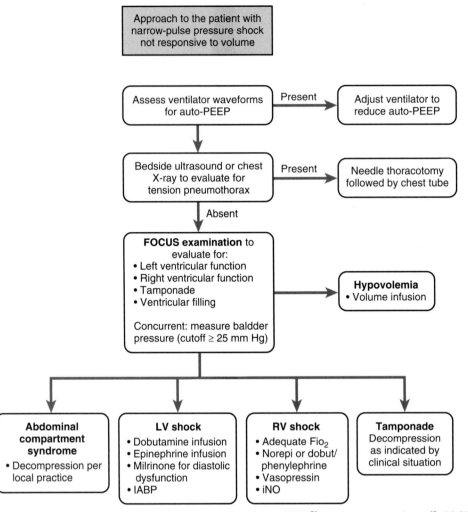

Figure 15-2. An approach to the patient with narrow-pulse pressure shock: Auto-PEEP[59]; tension pneumothorax[60]; FOCUS examination[64,65]; abdominal compartment syndrome[58]; tamponade[61]; LV shock[1]; and RV shock.[1,67,68] F_{IO_2}, fraction of inspired oxygen; *FOCUS,* focused cardiac ultrasound; *IABP,* intra-aortic balloon pump; *iNO,* inhaled nitric oxide; *PEEP,* positive end-expiratory pressure.

REFERENCES

1. Hall J, Schmidt G, Wood L. *Principles of Critical Care.* New York: McGraw-Hill; 2005. 249–265.
2. Sprung C, Peduzzi P, Shatney C, et al. Impact of encephalopathy on mortality in the sepsis syndrome. *Crit Care Med.* 1990;18: 801–806.
3. Marik P, Varon J, Trask T. Management of head trauma. *Chest.* 2002;122:699–711.
4. Peterson E, Wang Z, Britz G. Regulation of cerebral blood flow. *Int J Vasc Med.* 2011:1–8.
5. Asfar P, Meziani F, Hamel J, et al. High versus low blood-pressure target in patients with septic shock. *N Eng J Med.* 2014;370: 1583–1593.
6. Lehman L, Saeed M, Talmor D, et al. Method of blood pressure measurement in the ICU. *Crit Care Med.* 2013;41:34–40.
7. Kopterides P, Bonovas S, Mavrou I, et al. Venous oxygen saturation and lactate gradient from superior vena cava to pulmonary artery in patients with septic shock. *Shock.* 2009;31:561–567.
8. Varpula M, Karlsson S, Ruokonen E, et al. Mixed venous oxygen saturation cannot be estimated by central venous oxygen saturation in septic shock. *Intensive Care Med.* 2006;32:1336–1343.
9. Sander M, Spies C, Foer A, et al. Agreement of central venous saturation and mixed venous saturation in cardiac surgery patients. *Intensive Care Med.* 2007; 33: 1719-1725.
10. Chawla L, Zia H, Gutierrez G, et al. Lack of evidence between central and mixed venous oxygen saturation. *Chest.* 2004;126: 1891–1896.
11. Rivers E, Nguyen B, Havstad S, et al. Early goal-directed therapy in the treatment of severe sepsis and septic shock. *N Eng J Med.* 2001;345:1368–1377.
12. Jansen T, von Bommel J, Schoonderbeek F, et al. Early lactate-guided therapy in intensive care unit patients. *Am J Crit Care Med.* 2010;182:752–761.
13. Yealy D, Kellum J, Huang D, et al. A randomized trial of protocol-based care for early septic shock. *N Eng J Med.* 2014;370: 1683–1693.
14. Reinhart K, Rudolph T, Bredle D, et al. Comparison of central-venous to mixed-venous oxygen saturation during changes in oxygen supply/demand. *Chest.* 1989;95:1216–1221.
15. Marik P, Baram M, Vahid B. Does the central venous pressure predict fluid responsiveness? A systematic review of the literature and the tale of seven mares. *Chest.* 2008;134:172–178.
16. Osman D, Ridel C, Ray P, et al. Cardiac filling pressures are not appropriate to predict hemodynamic response to volume challenge. *Crit Care Med.* 2007;1:64–68.
17. Michard F, Teboul J. Using heart-lung interactions to assess fluid responsiveness during mechanical ventilation. *Crit Care Med.* 2000;4:282–289.
18. Marik P, Monnet X, Teboul J. Hemodynamic parameters to guide fluid therapy. *Ann Intensive Care.* 2011;1:1–9.

19. Preisman S, Kogan S, Berkenstadt H, et al. Predicting fluid responsiveness in patients undergoing cardiac surgery: functional haemodynamic parameters including Respiratory Systolic Variation Test and static preload indicators. *Br J Anaesth.* 2005;95: 746–755.

20. Huang C, Fu J, Hu H, et al. Prediction of fluid responsiveness in acute respiratory distress syndrome patients ventilated with low tidal volume and high positive end-expiratory pressure. *Crit Care Med.* 2008;36:2810–2816.

21. Tavanier B, Makhotine O, Lebuffe G, et al. Systolic pressure variation as a guide to fluid therapy in patients with sepsis-induced hypotension. *Anesthesiology.* 1998;89:1313–1321.

22. Perel A, Pizov R, Gotev S. Systolic blood pressure variation is a sensitive indicator of hypovolemia in ventilated dogs subjected to graded hemorrhage. *Anesthesiology.* 1987;67:498–502.

23. Coriat P, Vrillon M, Perel A, et al. A comparison of systolicblood pressure variations and echocardiographic estimates of end-diastolic left ventricular size in patients after aortic surgery. *Anesth Analg.* 1994;78:46–53.

24. Rooke G, Schwid H, Shapita Y. The effect of graded hemorrhage and intravascular volume replacement on systolic pressure variation in humans during mechanical and spontaneous ventilation. *Anesth Analg.* 1995;80:925–932.

25. Michard F, Teboul J. Predicting Fluid Responsiveness in ICU Patients: A Critical Analysis of the Evidence. *Chest.* 2002;121: 2000–2008.

26. Mesquida J, Kim H, Pinsky M. Effect of tidal volume, intrathoracic pressure, and cardiac contractility on variations in pulse pressure, stroke volume, and intrathoracic blood volume. *Intensive Care Med.* 2011;37:1672–1679.

27. Coudray A, Romand J, Treggiari M, et al. Fluid responsiveness in spontaneously breathing patients: A review of indexes used in intensive care. *Critical Care Med.* 2005;33:2757–2762.

28. Hong D, Lee J, Seo J, et al. Pulse pressure variation to predict fluid responsiveness in spontaneously breathing patients: tidal vs forced inspiratory breathing. *Anaesthesia.* 2014;69:717–722.

29. Au S, Vieillard-Baron A. Bedside echocardiography in critically ill patients: a true hemodynamic monitoring tool. *J Clin Monit Comput.* 2012;26:355–360.

30. Royce C, Canty D, Faris J, et al. Core review: physician-performed ultrasound: the time has come for routine use in acute care medicine. *Anesth Analg.* 2012;115:1007–1028.

31. Muller L, Bobbia X, Toumi M, et al. Respiratory variations of inferior vena cava diameter to predict fluid responsiveness in spontaneously breathing patients with acute circulatory failure: need for a cautious use. *Crit Care.* 2012;16:188–200.

32. Zhang Z, Xiao X, Ye S, et al. Ultrasonographic measurement of the respiratory variation in the inferior vena cava diameter is predictive of fluid responsiveness in critically ill patients: systemic review and meta-analysis. *Ultrasound Med Biol.* 2014;40:845–853.

33. Dipti A, Soucy Z, Surana A, et al. Role of inferior vena cava diameter in assessment of volume status: a meta-analysis. *Am J Emerg Med.* 2012;30:1414–1419.

34. Bendjelid K, Romand J. Fluid responsiveness in mechanically ventilated patients: a review of indices used in intensive care. *Intensive Care Med.* 2003;29:352–360.

35. Boulain T, Archard J, Teboul J, et al. Changes in BP induced by passive leg raising predict response to fluid loading in critically ill patients. *Chest.* 2002;121:1245–1252.

36. Monnet X, Rienzo M, Osman D, et al. Passive leg raising predicts fluid responsiveness in the critically ill. *Crit Care Med.* 2006;34:1402–1407.

37. Maas J, Geerts B, van den Berg P, et al. Assessment of venous return curve and mean systemic filling pressure in postoperative cardiac surgery patients. *Crit Care Med.* 2009;37:912–918.

38. Maas J, Pinsky M, Aarts L, et al. Bedside assessment of total systemic vascular compliance, stressed volume, and cardiac function curves in intensive care unit patients. *Anesth Analg.* 2012;115: 880–887.

39. Kiraly L, Differding J, Enomoto T, et al. Resuscitation with normal saline (NS) vs. lactated ringers (LR) modulates hypercoagulability and leads to increased blood loss in an uncontrolled hemorrhagic shock swine model. *J Trauma.* 2006;64:901–908.

40. Raghunathan K, Shaw A, Nathanson B, et al. Association between the choice of IV crystalloid and in-hospital mortality among critically ill adults with sepsis. *Crit Care Med.* 2014;42:1585–1591.

41. Shaw A, Bagshaw S, Goldstein S, et al. Major complications, mortality, and resource utilization after open abdominal surgery. *Ann Surg.* 2012;255:821–829.

42. Young J, Utter G, Schermer C, et al. Saline versus plasma-lyte A in initial resuscitation of trauma patients: a randomized trial. *Ann Surg.* 2013;00:1–8.

43. Dellinger R, Levy M, Rhodes A, et al. Surviving Sepsis Campaign: international guidelines for management of severe sepsis and septic shock. *Crit Care Med.* 2012;2013(41):580–637.

44. Finfer S, McEvoy S, Bellomo R, et al. Impact of albumin compared to saline on organ function and mortality of patients with severe sepsis. *Intensive Care Med.* 2011;37:86–96.

45. P1 C, Tognoni G, et al. Albumin replacement in patients with severe sepsis or septic shock. *N Engl J Med.* April 10, 2014;370(15): 1412–1421.

46. Myburgh J, Finfer S, Bellomo R, et al. Hydroxyethyl starch or saline for fluid resuscitation in intensive care. *N Eng J Med.* 2012;367:1901–1911.

47. Perner A, Haase N, Guttormsen A, et al. Hydroxyethyl starch 130/0.42 versus Ringer's acetate in severe sepsis. *N Eng J Med.* 2012;367:124–134.

48. Rivers E, Nguyen B, Havstad S, et al. Early goal-directed therapy in the treatment of severe sepsis and septic shock. *N Eng J Med.* 2001;345:1368–1377.

49. Kompanje E, Jansen T, van der Hoven B, et al. The first demonstration of lactic acid in human blood in shock by Johann Joseph Scherer (1814-1869) in January 1843. *Intensive Care Med.* 2007;33:1967–1971.

50. Bakker J. Lactate: may I have your votes please? *Intensive Care Med.* 2001;27:6–11.

51. Mikkelsen M, Miltiades A, Gaieski D, et al. Serum lactate is associated with mortality in severe sepsis independent of organ failure and shock. *Critical Care Med.* 2009;37:1670–1677.

52. Kumar A, Roberts D, Wood K, et al. Duration of hypotension before initiation of effective antimicrobial therapy is the critical determinant of survival in human septic shock. *Critical Care Med.* 2006;34:1589–1596.

53. Morrell M, Fraser V, Kollef M. Delaying the empiric treatment of candida bloodstream infection until positive blood culture results are obtained: a potential risk factor for hospital mortality. *Antimicrob Agents Chemother.* 2005;49:3640–3645.

54. Russell J, Walley K, Singer J, et al. VASST investigators: vasopressin versus norepinephrine infusion in patients with septic shock. *N Eng J Med.* 2008;358:877–887.

55. Ruokonen E, Parvianen I, Uusaro A. Treatment of impaired perfusion in septic shock. *Ann Med.* 2002;34:590–597.

56. Schein M, Ivatury R. Intra-abdominal hypertension and the abdominal compartment syndrome. *Br J Surg.* 1998;85:1027–1028.

57. Malbrain M, De laet I, De Waele J, et al. Abdominal hypertension: definitions, monitoring, interpretation and management. *Best Pract Res Clin Anaesthesiol.* 2013;27:249–270.

58. Kirkpatrick A, Roberts D, de Waele J, et al. Intra-abdominal hypertension and the abdominal compartment syndrome: updated consensus definitions and clinical practice guidelines from the World Society of the Abdominal Compartment Syndrome. *Intensive Care Med.* 2013;39:1190–1206.

59. Pepe P, Marini J. Occult positive end-expiratory pressure in mechanically ventilated patients with airflow obstruction: the auto-PEEP effect. *Am Rev Respir Dis.* 1982;126:166–170.

60. Ashton-Cleary D. Is thoracic ultrasound a viable alternative to conventional imaging in the critical care setting? *Br J Anaesth.* 2013;111:152–160.

61. Beaulieu Y. Bedside echocardiography in the assessment of the critically ill. *Crit Care Med.* 2007;35:S235–S249.

62. Page D, Caulfield J, Kastor J, et al. Myocardial changes associated with cardiogenic shock. *N Eng J Med.* 1971;285:133–137.

63. Manasia A, Nagaraj H, Kodali R, et al. Feasibility and potential clinical utility of goal-directed transthoracic echocardiography performed by noncardiologist intensivists using a small hand-carried device (SonoHeart) in critically ill patients. *J Cardiothorac Vasc Anesth.* 2005;19:155–159.

64. Spencer K, Kimura B, Korcarz C, et al. Focused cardiac ultrasound: recommendations from the American Society of Echocardiography. *J Am Soc Echocardiogr*. 2013;26:567–581.

65. Labovitz A, Noble V, Bierig M, et al. Focused cardiac ultrasound in the emergent setting: a consensus statement of the American Society of Echocardiography and American College of Emergency Physicians. *J Am Soc Echocardiogr*. 2010;23:1225–1230.

66. Deleted in review.

67. Jacobs A, Leopold J, Bates E, et al. Cardiogenic shock cause by right ventricular infarction: A report from the SHOCK registry. *J Am Coll Cardiol*. 2003;41:1273–1279.

68. Konstantinides S, Geibel A, Heusel G, et al. Prognosis of Pulmonary Embolism-3 Trial I. Heparin plus alteplase compared with heparin alone in patients with submassive pulmonary embolism. *N Eng J Med*. 2002;347:1143–1150.

16 What Are the Best Tools to Optimize the Circulation?

Xavier Monnet, Michael R. Pinsky

Implicit in any attempt to optimize the circulation are two key issues. First, it is important to identify those measures or parameters that constitute the most appropriate treatment options. Second, it is essential to define the actual goals that will drive resuscitation. Thus, we first define measures that identify volume responsiveness and circulatory failure. We then define the goals of resuscitation that these measures will be used to achieve.

HEMODYNAMIC MONITORING-DEFINED ASSESSMENT OF THE CIRCULATION

In acute circulatory failure, volume expansion is most often the first therapeutic choice. Fluid administration can be expected to increase cardiac output and oxygen delivery. Nevertheless, improvement can occur only if changes in cardiac preload result in significant changes in cardiac output (i.e., if both ventricles are preload dependent[1]; Fig. 16-1). If no test is used to predict preload dependence a priori, then volume expansion often will not result in the expected increase in cardiac output.[2] Thus preload dependence should be tested before fluid is administered. This approach will help avoid fluid overload, which is an independent predictor of mortality in patients with septic shock[3] or acute respiratory distress syndrome (ARDS).[4] Several indices and tests have been developed to test volume responsiveness.

Ability of Static Indices of Cardiac Preload to Predict Volume Responsiveness

Static markers of cardiac preload, such as the central venous pressure (CVP), do not reliably predict fluid responsiveness.[5,6] This failure can be explained by basic physiology. The slope of the cardiac function curve depends on the cardiac systolic function (Fig. 16-1). Because this slope is unknown in a given patient at any given moment, an absolute "static" value of any measure of preload could correspond to a point on any number of curves and thus to preload dependence and preload independence. Only extreme values can inform on the presence of fluid responsiveness. Furthermore, the measurement of any static marker is subject to error. For instance, the measurement of CVP requires a precise positioning of the pressure

transducer with respect to the right atrium. The measurement must also be made at end expiration and should account for the transmission of intrathoracic pressure to the right atrium. Likewise, the pulmonary artery occlusion pressure suffers from many possible errors in its measurement and interpretation.[7,8]

To address the shortcomings of static indices, dynamic alternatives have been developed to predict preload responsiveness within an overall concept of functional hemodynamic monitoring.[9] Dynamic measures involve altering cardiac preload via mechanical ventilation, postural changes, or administration of small amounts of fluid and measuring the resultant change of cardiac output or stroke volume.[10]

Dynamic Parameters to Predict Volume Responsiveness

Several tests have been developed to detect volume responsiveness before administering fluid. The appropriate approach is most often determined by the clinical setting and the patient's condition. These tests allow the practitioner to avoid administering fluid if it is not hemodynamically effective.

Variations of Stroke Volume Induced by Mechanical Ventilation

During mechanical ventilation, insufflation increases the intrathoracic pressure and, as a result, decreases venous return. Furthermore, increased right ventricular afterload decreases right ventricular outflow and thus left ventricular preload. In conventional ventilation, these changes should occur at expiration. If the left ventricle is preload dependent, then the left ventricular stroke volume transiently decreases at expiration. Hence, a cyclic variation of stroke volume under mechanical ventilation indicates the preload dependence of either ventricle.[9]

Several surrogates or estimations of stroke volume have been used to quantify its respiratory variations. These include the systemic arterial pulse pressure,[11] which is proportional to stroke volume. Indeed, studies have demonstrated that pulse pressure variation (PPV) is a valuable indicator of fluid responsiveness, provided that the conditions of its validity are fulfilled.[12] Overall, variation greater than 13% is significantly associated with fluid

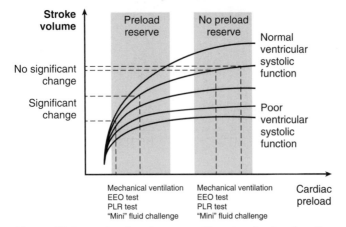

Figure 16-1. Cardiac function curve. There is a family of cardiac function curves depending on the ventricular contractility. If the ventricles are functioning on the steep part of cardiac function curve, then changes in cardiac preload induced by mechanical ventilation, end-expiratory occlusion (*EEO*), passive leg raising (*PLR*) or mini fluid challenge result in significant changes in stroke volume. This is not the case if the ventricles are functioning on the steep part of the cardiac function curve.

responsiveness. Of course, as for many tests, this is not a strict cutoff. The farther from 13% the PPV value, the higher its diagnostic value.

Other parameters used to estimate stroke volume responses to respiratory variation include pulse contour analysis, subaortic blood flow measured by descending echocardiography, aortic blood flow measured with esophageal Doppler monitoring, and amplitude of the plethysmography signal with pulse oximetry.[1] These indices—in particular, those of PPV—are solidly evidence based.[12] Indeed, several commonly used bedside monitors can measure PPV.

The respiratory variation of stroke volume as a marker of preload responsiveness is not valid under several conditions that are not uncommon. First, during spontaneous breathing, stroke volume variations relate more to the respiratory irregularity than to preload dependence.[13,14] Second, arrhythmias directly affect stroke volume variability within the respiratory cycles, a response likely related to arrhythmia rather than heart-lung interactions. The third important limitation relates to ARDS. In such a case, the low tidal volume[15] and/or the low lung compliance[16] will reduce the transmission of changes in alveolar pressure to the intrathoracic structures; both diminish the amplitude of the ventilation-induced changes of intravascular pressure. The net result would be false-negative responses to PPV. Open chest surgery, a low ratio of heart rate over respiratory rate (corresponding in fact to respiratory rates at ≥40 breaths/min), or intra-abdominal hypertension also reduce the ability of PPV measurements to predict fluid responsiveness.[10] Overall, the limitations to the use of PPV are much more frequently encountered in the intensive care unit than in the operating room.

Respiratory Variation of Vena Caval Diameter

Mechanical ventilation can alter the diameter of vena cava, an effect that is exaggerated in hypovolemia. The magnitude of this change in the inferior vena cava (IVC) at the diaphragmatic inlet, as well as collapse of the superior vena cava (SVC), reliably predicted fluid responsiveness.[17,18]

The most important limitation of these methods is that they become unreliable during spontaneous breathing activity because respiratory efforts are variable and lack homogeneity. Mechanically ventilating poorly compliant lungs with a low tidal volume should minimize the effect of ventilation on the vena cava diameter and thus invalidate the method. Conversely, this approach is valuable in patients with cardiac arrhythmias.

Respiratory variation in the IVC can be measured with transthoracic echocardiography. This approach may be particularly valuable during the early phase of care, before arterial cannulation. The collapsibility of the SVC has been validated only in a single study and requires transesophageal echocardiography. In a patient equipped with an arterial catheter, it is easier to use PPV than SVC collapsibility.

End-Expiratory Occlusion Test

As stated previously, inspiration under mechanical ventilation cyclically reduces cardiac preload. Briefly holding mechanical ventilation at end expiration interrupts this cyclic decrease and induces a transient increase in cardiac preload. If the right ventricle is preload dependent, then the end-expiratory occlusion (EEO) test will increase right ventricular output and, if sufficient to increase flow into the pulmonary circulation, left ventricular preload. A preload-dependent patient will respond to EEO with an increase in cardiac output (Fig. 16-1) . Some studies have shown that cardiac output increases of more than 5% during a 15-second EEO test reliably predict volume responsiveness.[16,19]

Beyond its simplicity, the EEO test is useful during cardiac arrhythmias because it exerts its effects over the course of several cardiac cycles[19] (Fig. 16-2). The EEO test can be used in patients who are not fully paralyzed or deeply sedated unless respiratory triggering interrupts the 15-second occlusion. The EEO test is also much easier to use with a real-time measurement of cardiac output, such as pulse contour analysis. The increase in arterial pulse pressure during EEO is also indicative of fluid responsiveness, but it requires a large-scale display of the arterial pressure curve.[19] The EEO test also appears to be independent of the magnitude of positive end-expiratory pressure.[20]

Fluid Challenge

The most intuitive way to test fluid responsiveness is to administer a small volume of fluid, observe its effects on cardiac output, and expect that a larger volume expansion will exert similar effects (Fig. 16-1). However, in the "classic" fluid challenge, infusing 300 to 500 mL of fluid is too large to be negligible.[21] In the early phase of shock, it may be necessary to perform several fluid challenges a day, inevitably leading to a total volume of fluid that can contribute to fluid overload.

In studying an alternative approach, the "mini fluid challenge," Muller and colleagues found that the use of a 100-mL colloid bolus predicted the echocardiographic response equal to that of a 500-mL crystalloid infusion.[22] However, it is not clear that echocardiography is precise enough to be used by nonexperts. Thus, the need for more precise measurements of cardiac output must be determined.

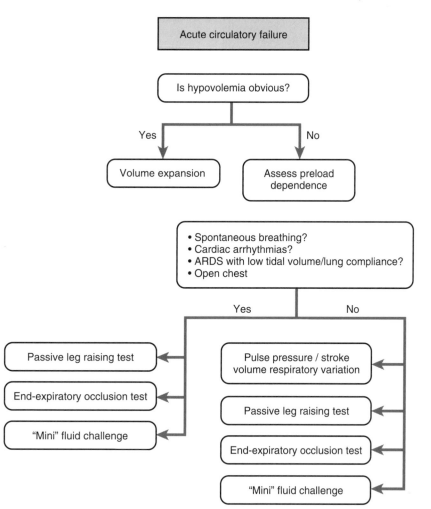

Figure 16-2. Decision-making algorithm of fluid administration. *ARDS*, acute respiratory distress syndrome.

Passive Leg Raising Test

In a patient lying in the semirecumbent position, elevating the legs at 45 degrees and lowering the trunk induces a transfer of venous blood from the lower part of the body toward the cardiac cavities. The passive leg raising (PLR) test increases right and left cardiac preload and acts as a transient and reversible volume challenge[23] (Fig. 16-1). Several studies and a subsequent meta-analysis have indicated that a 10% increase in cardiac output induced by PLR is a reliable test of preload responsiveness.[14,24]

Because its hemodynamic effects occur over a long period of time, PLR remains valid in the presence of both cardiac arrhythmias and spontaneous breathing and is independent of mechanical ventilation. Thus, the PLR test can be used in conjunction with low tidal volume, low lung compliance, and very high respiratory rates (Fig. 16-2).

Proper performance of PLR is important. The test should start from the semirecumbent and not from the horizontal supine position because lowering the trunk is associated with a transfer of venous blood from the large splanchnic compartment to the cardiac chambers, enhancing the hemodynamic effect.[23,25] Furthermore, PLR-induced hemodynamic changes cannot be assessed by simply observing the simple arterial pressure, an approach associated with

a significant number of false negatives.[14,23] Rather, a technique that directly measures cardiac output is mandatory.[26] In addition, PLR must be assessed with a real-time measurement of cardiac output because the maximal effect usually occurs within 1 minute.[14] In patients with a profound vasodilatation and capillary leak, the effects of PLR progressively vanish over a few minutes. Thus, pulmonary or transpulmonary thermodilution techniques, which require repeat cold fluid boluses, are not suitable. More suitable techniques include the use of esophageal Doppler or pulse-contour analysis to measure changes in aortic blood flow and thus cardiac output, cardiac output measured by bioreactance and endotracheal bioimpedance cardiography, subaortic blood velocity measured by echocardiography, and ascending aortic velocity measured by suprasternal Doppler monitoring.[23] Interestingly, in patients undergoing mechanical ventilation with perfectly regular ventilation, the PLR-induced changes in cardiac output can be simply and noninvasively estimated by the changes in end-tidal carbon dioxide, allowing the use of PLR without measuring cardiac output.[27]

Intra-abdominal hypertension could reduce the validity of the PLR test, perhaps by interfering with the transfer of blood from the lower limbs toward the cardiac chambers

Table 16-1 **Markers of Tissue Hypoperfusion**
Hyperlactatemia
Metabolic acidosis
Anion gap acidosis
Delayed capillary refill
Mottled skin
Altered sensorium
Decreased urine output
Ileus
Decreased mixed venous and central venous oxygen saturation
Increased veno-arterial carbon dioxide gap

through the IVC.[28] One study suggested that the PLR test was not reliable if the intra-abdominal pressure was higher than 16 mm Hg.[29] Nevertheless, this study did not measure the intra-abdominal pressure during PLR. Thus, this possible limitation of the PLR test requires confirmation.

AUTHORS' RECOMMENDATIONS

- In patients with circulatory shock, the initial therapy should be to target a minimal mean arterial pressure of 65 mm Hg, and then volume status, blood flow, and organ perfusion should be assessed.
- Resuscitation therapy should be targeted to individual patient responsiveness as measured by estimates of organ perfusion adequacy (e.g., lactate, v-a Pco_2 [venous-arterial partial pressure of carbon dioxide] difference, urine output, sensorium, skin perfusion; Table 16-1).
- Optimal fluid management improves patient outcome by avoiding both hypovolemia and hypervolemia.
- Assess both volume status and volume responsiveness.
- Commonly used measures of preload (e.g., CVP, global end-diastolic volume) alone should not be used to guide resuscitation therapy.
- Dynamic measure of fluid responsiveness (e.g., PPV, stroke volume variation, change in cardiac output with PLR) should be used if available and are preferable to static measures of preload.

REFERENCES

1. Monnet X, Teboul JL. Assessment of volume responsiveness during mechanical ventilation: recent advances. *Crit Care.* 2013;17:217.
2. Michard F, Teboul JL. Predicting fluid responsiveness in ICU patients: a critical analysis of the evidence. *Chest.* 2002;121:2000–2008.
3. Vincent JL, Sakr Y, Sprung CL, et al. Sepsis in European intensive care units: results of the SOAP study. *Crit Care Med.* 2006;34:344–353.
4. Jozwiak M, Silva S, Persichini R, et al. Extravascular lung water is an independent prognostic factor in patients with acute respiratory distress syndrome. *Crit Care Med.* 2013;41:472–480.
5. Marik PE, Baram M, Vahid B. Does central venous pressure predict fluid responsiveness? A systematic review of the literature and the tale of seven mares. *Chest.* 2008;134:172–178.
6. Marik PE, Cavallazzi R. Does the central venous pressure predict fluid responsiveness? An updated meta-analysis and a plea for some common sense. *Crit Care Med.* 2013;41:1774–1781.
7. Pinsky MR. Pulmonary artery occlusion pressure. *Intensive Care Med.* 2003;29:19–22.
8. Richard C, Monnet X, Teboul JL. Pulmonary artery catheter monitoring in 2011. *Curr Opin Crit Care.* 2011;17:296–302.
9. Garcia X, Pinsky MR. Clinical applicability of functional hemodynamic monitoring. *Ann Intensive Care.* 2011;1:35.
10. Marik PE, Monnet X, Teboul JL. Hemodynamic parameters to guide fluid therapy. *Ann Intensive Care.* 2011;1:1.
11. Michard F, Boussat S, Chemla D, et al. Relation between respiratory changes in arterial pulse pressure and fluid responsiveness in septic patients with acute circulatory failure. *Am J Respir Crit Care Med.* 2000;162:134–138.
12. Marik PE, Cavallazzi R, Vasu T, et al. Dynamic changes in arterial waveform derived variables and fluid responsiveness in mechanically ventilated patients: a systematic review of the literature. *Crit Care Med.* 2009;37:2642–2647.
13. Heenen S, De Backer D, Vincent JL. How can the response to volume expansion in patients with spontaneous respiratory movements be predicted? *Crit Care.* 2006;10:R102.
14. Monnet X, Rienzo M, Osman D, et al. Passive leg raising predicts fluid responsiveness in the critically ill. *Crit Care Med.* 2006;34:1402–1407.
15. De Backer D, Heenen S, Piagnerelli M, et al. Pulse pressure variations to predict fluid responsiveness: influence of tidal volume. *Intensive Care Med.* 2005;31:517–523.
16. Monnet X, Bleibtreu A, Ferré A, et al. Passive leg raising and end-expiratory occlusion tests perform better than pulse pressure variation in patients with low respiratory system compliance. *Crit Care Med.* 2012;40:152–157.
17. Feissel M, Michard F, Faller JP, et al. The respiratory variation in inferior vena cava diameter as a guide to fluid therapy. *Intensive Care Med.* 2004;30:1834–1837.
18. Vieillard-Baron A, Chergui K, Rabiller A, et al. Superior vena caval collapsibility as a gauge of volume status in ventilated septic patients. *Intensive Care Med.* 2004;30:1734–1739.
19. Monnet X, Osman D, Ridel C, et al. Predicting volume responsiveness by using the end-expiratory occlusion in mechanically ventilated intensive care unit patients. *Crit Care Med.* 2009;37:951–956.
20. Silva S, Jozwiak M, Teboul JL, et al. End-expiratory occlusion test predicts preload responsiveness independently of positive end-expiratory pressure during acute respiratory distress syndrome. *Crit Care Med.* 2013;41:1692–1701.
21. Vincent JL, Weil MH. Fluid challenge revisited. *Crit Care Med.* 2006;34:1333–1337.
22. Muller L, Toumi M, Bousquet PJ, et al. An increase in aortic blood flow after an infusion of 100 ml colloid over 1 minute can predict fluid responsiveness: the mini-fluid challenge study. *Anesthesiol.* 2011;115:541–547.
23. Monnet X, Teboul JL. Passive leg raising. *Intensive Care Med.* 2008;34:659–663.
24. Cavallaro F, Sandroni C, Marano C, et al. Diagnostic accuracy of passive leg raising for prediction of fluid responsiveness in adults: systematic review and meta-analysis of clinical studies. *Intensive Care Med.* 2010;36:1475–1483.
25. Jabot J, Teboul JL, Richard C, et al. Passive leg raising for predicting fluid responsiveness: importance of the postural change. *Intensive Care Med.* 2009;35:85–90.
26. De Backer D, Pinsky MR. Can one predict fluid responsiveness in spontaneously breathing patients? *Intensive Care Med.* 2007;33:1111–1113.
27. Monnet X, Bataille A, Magalhaes E, et al. End-tidal carbon dioxide is better than arterial pressure for predicting volume responsiveness by the passive leg raising test. *Intensive Care Med.* 2013;39:93–100.
28. Malbrain ML, Reuter DA. Assessing fluid responsiveness with the passive leg raising maneuver in patients with increased intra-abdominal pressure: be aware that not all blood returns!. *Crit Care Med.* 2010;38:1912–1915.
29. Mahjoub Y, Touzeau J, Airapetian N, et al. The passive leg-raising maneuver cannot accurately predict fluid responsiveness in patients with intra-abdominal hypertension. *Crit Care Med.* 2010;38:1824–1829.

GENERAL CRITICAL CARE MANAGEMENT

17 What Strategies Can Be Used to Optimize Antibiotic Use in the Critically Ill?

Cheston B. Cunha, Steven M. Opal

Septic patients in the intensive care unit (ICU) represent some of the sickest patients in the hospital, and optimal initial antibiotic selection is paramount to their survival. In this patient population, the key is to select an empiric regimen that maximizes antibiotic effect but also limits the development of resistance.[1,2] Within each antibiotic class are drugs that may have a high or low resistance potential. The precise mechanism by which the difference arises is unknown. "Low resistance potential" antibiotics are antimicrobials that rarely induce resistance among bacteria, even when used frequently and for extended periods of time. In addition to selecting antibiotics that have a low resistance potential, consideration should be given toward selecting an agent with favorable pharmacokinetics (PK) and pharmacodynamics (PD).[3] Essentially, septic patients should be treated urgently with the highest tolerable/nontoxic antimicrobial dose of a drug with low resistance potential to maximize microbial killing while minimizing the risk of selecting out drug-resistant mutants.[4-7]

ANTIBIOTIC PHARMACOKINETIC AND PHARMACODYNAMIC CONSIDERATIONS TO MINIMIZE RESISTANCE AND OPTIMIZE EFFECTIVENESS

PK define the fate of an antibiotic within the body (i.e., absorption, volume of distribution, blood and tissue levels, hepatic metabolism/excretion, and renal excretion). Antibiotic PK describe the effects of the antibiotic on both the host and the infecting microorganism. Both parameters are essential to consider in choosing an antimicrobial regimen for critically ill patients with serious infections. The inhibitory/cidal effect of antibiotics on bacteria can be categorized as demonstrating concentration-dependent killing, time-dependent killing, or a combination of both and depends on the antibiotic and the targeted pathogen. Concentration-dependent killing kinetics describe the increased bacterial killing that occurs as antibiotic concentrations increase above the minimal inhibitory concentration (MIC) and are expressed as the maximum serum antibiotic concentration (C_{max}) to the MIC ratio (C_{max}/MIC).[8,9] The fluoroquinolones—aminoglycosides, metronidazole, and daptomycin—all exhibit concentration-dependent killing. When selecting these antibiotics, the dose must be maximized for optimal effect. The higher the dose used, the more potent the antibiotic killing. Achieving a high concentration is particularly important when selecting an antibiotic with a relatively wide toxic-to-therapeutic ratio (i.e., aminoglycosides), making once daily dosing highly desirable. There are two benefits to this dosing strategy. Giving a high dose of the antibiotic only once per day generates a very high, but rapidly cleared, peak serum concentration, providing optimal and rapid bacterial killing. As the drug concentration subsequently falls, tissue levels rapidly diminish, preventing accumulation and decreasing the risk of toxicity.[10] Adding to the optimized killing provided by the single daily peak level is the prolonged postantibiotic effect (PAE) characteristic of aminoglycosides. The PAE extends antimicrobial capacity well after the serum concentrations have fallen below the MIC for the pathogenic microorganism (up to 8 to 12 hours).

Antibiotics that display time-dependent killing kinetics include the β-lactams, carbapenems, macrolides, and linezolid. In these compounds, an increase in the serum concentration above 4–5× MIC does not increase killing. Thus the key to antimicrobial activity lies in keeping the blood level close to this point for as long as possible—the time of drug concentration above the MIC for the dosing period (T>MIC).[8] Therefore, even when antibiotics that demonstrate time-dependent killing are used, there is little downside with high doses of the drug, particularly in critically ill patients with infection.[9] The killing kinetics of other antimicrobials may have more complex PD that better fit an integration of the time over MIC, expressed as the area under the concentration curve over the MIC (AUC_{0-24}: MIC).[10-12]

Some antimicrobials, such as doxycycline or vancomycin, exhibit kinetics that are dependent on time and concentration, reflecting the MIC of the pathogen.[13] When gram-positive cocci with an MIC of less than 1 µg/mL are exposed to vancomycin, the drug functions with time-dependent killing kinetics. However, when the MIC is greater than 1 µg/mL, the kinetics are dependent on concentration. The aminoglycosides and quinolones also demonstrate this duality with some pathogens (i.e., concentration-dependent kinetics [C_{max}/MIC ratio]) as well as AUC_{0-24}/MIC ratio[14] (Table 17-1).

Table 17-1 Antibiotic Dosing: PK/PD Considerations

Antibiotic PK/PD Parameters	Optimal Dosing Strategies
CONCENTRATION-DEPENDENT ANTIBIOTICS (C_{MAX}:MIC)	
• Quinolones • Aminoglycosides • Vancomycin if MIC ≥ 1 µg/mL • Tigecycline • Colistin • Doxycycline	**Use highest effective dose** (without toxicity)
TIME-DEPENDENT ANTIBIOTICS (T > MIC)	
• PCN concentrations > MIC for 70% of the dosing interval • β-Lactam concentrations > MIC for 60% of the dosing interval • Carbapenems concentrations > MIC for 40% of the dosing interval	
Vancomycin if MIC ≤ 1 µg/mL	**Use high doses** (which increase serum concentrations and increase T > MIC for more of the dosing interval)
OTHER ANTIBIOTICS (C_{MAX}:MIC/T > MIC AND/OR AUC_{0-24}/MIC)	
Quinolones	
>125 (effective)	
>250 (more effective)	**Use highest effective dose** (without toxicity)

Adapted from: Roberts JA, Pharm B, Lipman J. Pharmacokinetic issues for antibiotics in the critically ill patient. *Crit Care Med*. 2009;37:840-851; Roberts JA, Lipman J. Optimizing use of beta-lactam antibiotics in the critically ill. *Semin Respir Crit Care Med*. 2007;28:579-585; Roberts JA, Pharm B, Kruger P, Paterson DL, Lipman J. Antibiotic resistance—What's dosing got to do with it? *Crit Care Med*. 2008;36:2433-2440.
AUC, area under the concentration curve; *C_{max}*, peak serum concentrations; *MIC*, minimal inhibitory concentration; *PAE*, postantibotic effect; *PCN*, penicillin; *PD*, pharmacodynamic; *PK*, pharmacokinetic; *T*, time.

PK principles dictate the concentration and distribution of each antibiotic in serum and body fluids over time. The overall concentrations of drug in the serum are affected by the antibiotic's peak serum concentrations, volume of distribution, serum half-life ($t_{1/2}$), protein binding, and renal or hepatic function. Peak serum concentration, protein binding, and volume of distribution (V_d) will directly determine the tissue concentrations of an antibiotic in the tissue where the pathogen resides[8,10-12,15] (Table 17-2).

For the most part, antibiotics that exhibit time-dependent killing are bacteriostatic whereas those with concentration-dependent kinetics are bactericidal. Exceptions to this are the penicillins, carbapenems, and monobactams, which are bactericidal despite relying on time-dependent kinetics[16] (Tables 17-3 and 17-4). In addition, certain antibiotics may exhibit both types of killing kinetics depending on how they are used; for example,

doxycycline, which uses time-dependent kinetics and is usually bacteriostatic, is bactericidal at high concentrations, a characteristic usually reserved for concentration-dependent antibiotics.[13] In addition to these factors, antibiotics that exhibit concentration-dependent kinetics tend to have prolonged PAE, but there are some antibiotics that are dependent on time (e.g., doxycycline) that also have a PAE.[8,15]

ANTIBIOTIC SUSCEPTIBILITY TESTING AND RESISTANCE

A discussion on maximizing the dosing of antimicrobials would not be complete without consideration of antibiotic resistance. Resistant organisms are becoming more prevalent worldwide and pose a significant problem for clinicians and ICUs. Despite this fact, there is no international agreement on the definitions of the terms "resistant" or "susceptible."[17,18] The breakpoints used in susceptibility testing are based on achievable serum concentrations using the recommended doses of antibiotics for bloodstream infections. Interpretation of susceptibility reports on nonbloodstream isolates must be carefully performed. Infections are difficult to treat when the chosen antibiotic does not adequately penetrate the target tissues (e.g., the prostate or the central nervous system). The clinician must extrapolate likely tissue concentrations at the infection site from achievable serum concentration. Failure to consider this issue may result in clinical failure to eradicate infection despite laboratory reports indicating that the organism in question is susceptible.[19] It is critical to remember that with certain organisms (e.g., methicillin-resistant *Staphylococcus aureus* [MRSA]), in vitro susceptibility testing does not predict in vivo clinical effectiveness.[20] The source of discordance may lie in patient physiology that differs from in vitro conditions (e.g., the media used for testing).[21,22] Local acidosis and hypoxia may also decrease the activity of some antibiotics.[23]

Even without these confounding factors, inherent differences between in vitro susceptibility and in vivo efficacy must be taken into account. As an example, treating MRSA with trimethoprim-sulfamethoxyzole (TMP-SMX), doxycycline, or clindamycin, which are often reported as effective on in vitro testing, may not be successful.[20,21] Instead, anti-MRSA antibiotics such as minocycline, linezolid, daptomycin, or vancomycin, with proven clinical effectiveness against MRSA, provide a greater chance of eradicating the infection. *Listeria monocytogenes* appears susceptible to cephalosporins, but clinical experience indicates that this β-lactam class of antibiotics does not work in vivo for meningitis, for example (Table 17-5).

Resistance potential (high vs. low) is an inherent property of an antibiotic (Table 17-6). With high resistance potential antibiotics (e.g., macrolides, TMP-SMX, ampicillin), loss of efficacy is also a function of frequency and duration of use. Low resistance potential antibiotics (e.g., doxycycline, ceftriaxone, amikacin) are less affected by extensive/prolonged use. All other factors being equal, resistance is more likely to develop when tissue concentrations are subtherapeutic in difficult-to-penetrate tissue spaces (e.g., chronic prostatitis, abscesses, biofilm-associated device infections). Relative resistance, such as that as seen with

Table 17-2 Antibiotics: Relevant PK Characteristics in the ICU

Antibiotic PK Parameters	Sepsis ↑ with Capillary Permeability* (Intravascular → Interstitial Fluid Shifts)	Suggested Dosing Recommendations
WATER-SOLUBLE ANTIBIOTICS (LOW V_d WATER SOLUBLE)		
• Renally eliminated • High serum concentrations • Limited tissue penetration	• ↑ V_d → ↓ serum concentrations	• ↑ Dose of hydrophilic antibiotic • Change to a lipid-soluble antibiotic
LIPID-SOLUBLE ANTIBIOTICS (HIGH V_d → LIPID SOLUBLE)		
• Hepatically eliminated • High tissue penetration • Good serum concentration		• No change in V_d → no change in serum or tissue concentrations • No change needed

*Also with mechanical ventilation, burns, and hypoalbuminemia.
ICU, intensive care unit; *PK,* pharmacodynamics; *Vd,* volume of distribution.
Adapted from: Roberts JA, Pharm B, Lipman J. Pharmacokinetic issues for antibiotics in the critically ill patient. *Crit Care Med.* 2009;37:840-851.

Table 17-3 Inherent Resistance Potential of Selected Antibiotics

High Resistance Potential Antibiotics	Usual Resistant Organisms for Each Antibiotic	Preferred Low Resistance Potential Antibiotic Alternatives
AMINOGLYCOSIDES		
Gentamicin/ tobramycin	*P. aeruginosa*	Amikacin
CEPHALOSPORINS		
Ceftazidime	*P. aeruginosa*	Cefepime
TETRACYCLINES		
Tetracycline	*S. pneumoniae* *S. aureus*	Doxycycline or Minocycline
QUINOLONES		
Ciprofloxacin	*S. pneumoniae*	Levofloxacin or Moxifloxacin
Ciprofloxacin	*P. aeruginosa*	Levofloxacin
GLYCOPEPTIDES		
Vancomycin	MSSA MRSA	Linezolid or Daptomycin or Minocycline
CARBAPENEMS		
Imipenem	*P. aeruginosa*	Meropenem or Doripenem
MACROLIDES		
Azithromycin	*S. pneumoniae*	No other macrolide Alternatives include doxycycline, levofloxacin, or moxifloxacin
DIHYDROFOLATE REDUCTASE INHIBITORS		
TMP-SMX	*S. pneumoniae*	Doxycycline

MRSA, methicillin-resistant *S. aureus; MSSA,* methicillin-sensitive *S. aureus; TMP-SMX,* trimethoprim-sulfamethoxazole.

antibiotics such as aminoglycosides, may be overcome if antibiotic tissue concentrations are higher than the organism's MIC (Table 17-3). It is always beneficial to use the highest nontoxic dose possible to treat serious infections in ICU patients.

SPECIFIC ANTIBIOTIC CLASSES

β-Lactams

β-Lactam antibiotics use time-dependent killing and are bactericidal. Although they exert a short but measurable PAE on gram-positive organisms, they have no PAE when used against gram-negative organisms. Maximum bacterial killing occurs when drug concentrations are 5× the MIC of the target organism, but no additional benefit is conferred by raising concentrations above this level.[24,25] Thus the goal should be to maintain a serum concentration greater than the MIC for the longest duration possible—at least 60% (penicillins) to 70% (cephalosporins) of the dosing interval. Strategies to achieve this PD effect include increasing the dosing frequency, giving β-lactams with a long serum half-life, or giving the drug as a continuous infusion.[23,24,26-28] Ultimately, when β-lactams are used in the ICU, combining higher doses with increased frequency of administrations will maximize antibiotic effect without increasing the risk of developing resistance.[24,25] Among cephalosporins, cefepime has good activity against *Pseudomonas aeruginosa*. This drug is typically used for systemic *P. aeruginosa* infections and febrile neutropenia as monotherapy or in combination with an aminoglycoside (e.g., amikacin). In extended spectrum β-lactamase–producing organisms, multidrug-resistant organisms (MDROs; with MICs=4 to 8 µg/mL), and *P. aeruginosa* infection, a "high dose" of cefepime should be used.[29-31]

Carbapenems

Structurally similar to β-lactam antibiotics, carbapenems also rely on time-dependent killing. Concentrations should be targeted to remain at 5× the MIC for more than 40% or longer of the dosing interval, which can best be achieved by using high doses or long-acting agents (e.g., ertapenem for susceptible organisms).[24,25,32,33]

Quinolones

As described previously, the fluoroquinolones exhibit both time- and concentration-dependent killing. AUC_{0-24}/MIC ratios directly correlate with clinical outcomes; that is, an

Table 17-4 Empiric Antibiotic Coverage for Common ICU Infections

Infection Type/Site	Usual Pathogen at Site	Usual Nonpathogens at Site	Preferred Empiric Therapy with Low Resistance Potential Antibiotics	Penicillin Allergy
CVC-ASSOCIATED BACTEREMIA*				
	MSSA MRSA CoNS GNBs (aerobic) VSE	*B. fragilis* Non-Group D streptococci	Meropenem plus either vancomycin (if MRSA likely) or linezolid (if VRE likely)	Meropenem plus either vancomycin (if MRSA likely) or linezolid (if VRE likely)
INTRA-ABDOMINAL SEPSIS				
Cholecystitis/cholangitis	*E. coli* *K. pneumoniae* VSE	*B. fragilis*	Levofloxacin or moxifloxacin	Levofloxacin or moxifloxacin
Peritonitis/colon perforation	*B. fragilis* GNBs (aerobic)	Non-Group D streptococci	Ertapenem or piperacillin/ tazobactam or moxifloxacin or tigecycline	Ertapenem or moxifloxacin or tigecycline
VAP/NP	*P. aeruginosa* GNBs (aerobic)	*B. fragilis* MSSA/MRSA VSE/VRE *Burkholderia cepacia* *A. baumannii* *S. maltophilia*	Meropenem or doripenem or levofloxacin (750 mg) or cefepime	Meropenem or doripenem or levofloxacin (750 mg)
UROSEPSIS				
Community acquired	GNBs (aerobic) VSE	*B. fragilis* MSSA/MRSA	Piperacillin/tazobactam or meropenem	Meropenem
Nosocomial	*P. aeruginosa* GNBs (aerobic)	*B. fragilis* MSSA/MRSA	Piperacillin/tazobactam or meropenem	Meropenem
SKIN AND SOFT TISSUE INFECTIONS				
Cellulitis	Group A, B, C, G streptococci	MSSA/MRSA	Ceftriaxone or cefazolin	Vancomycin or clindamycin
Abscess	MSSA/MRSA	Group A, B, C, G streptococci	Ceftaroline or minocycline or Vancomycin or linezolid	Vancomycin or linezolid or minocycline

Adapted from: Cunha BA, ed. *Antibiotic Essentials.* 12th ed. Sudbury, MA: Jones & Bartlett; 2013: 17–151.

*Remove/replace CVC as soon as possible.

CoNS, coagulase negative staphylococci; *CVC,* central venous catheter; *GNB,* gram-negative bacilli; *ICU,* intensive care unit; *MRSA,* methicillin-resistant *S. aureus; MSSA,* methicillin-sensitive *S. aureus; NP,* nosocomial pneumonia; *VAP,* ventilator-associated pneumonia; *VRE,* vancomycin-resistant enterococci; *VSE,* vancomycin-sensitive enterococci.

AUC_{0-24}/MIC ratio of greater than 125 is usually considered predictive of efficacy in gram-negative infections. Using the highest doses of quinolones, though, to achieve an AUC_{0-24}/MIC ratio of more than 250 may be superior and will help reduce the development of resistance.[24] This dosing strategy also confers the benefits of maximizing the C_{max}/MIC ratio.[34-36]

Vancomycin

The PD of vancomycin vary depending on the MICs of the staphylococcal pathogen causing the infection. In cases in which the MICs are greater than 1, vancomycin acts in a concentration-dependent killing manner, whereas in the setting of MICs of less than 1, its kinetics demonstrate time-dependent killing. Because concerns about the nephrotoxicity of vancomycin are largely unfounded, care should be taken to utilize the highest possible dose to maximize efficacy. Using inadequate doses of vancomycin has been associated with the development of resistance; therefore a preferred dosing strategy would be to use high-dose vancomycin (e.g., 60 mg/kg intravenously [IV] every 24 hours [q24h]) with doses appropriately adjusted for kidney function.[23]

Linezolid

Linezolid demonstrates bacteriostatic activity against staphylococci and enterococci, but it exhibits bactericidal activity against non-Group D streptococci. Linezolid exhibits time-dependent killing kinetics. Despite its bacteriostatic activity against staphylococci, linezolid can be successfully used to treat acute bacterial endocarditis when compared with bactericidal agents.[23] Dosing of linezolid does not need to be adjusted for renal/hepatic dysfunction.

Table 17-5 **Difficulties with the Interpretation of Antibiotic Susceptibility Testing Data**

1. The cultured isolate is *not* necessarily the pathogen (e.g., skin colonizers, colonizers of body/fluid secretions).

2. Treating "colonizers" from fluid/body secretions from nonsterile sites often misses the true pathogens at the site of infection.

3. An antibiotic selected based on the cultured "colonizer" is often misleading.

4. Selection of an antibiotic based on susceptibility testing does not guarantee antibiotic effectiveness.

5. Isolates reported to be "resistant" are not always resistant; in fact, such isolates are often nonsusceptible or only relatively resistant (i.e., easily susceptible with high-dose therapy).

IN VITRO SUSCEPTIBILITY VS. IN VIVO EFFECTIVENESS

1. Interpretation (breakpoints of resistance) not universally agreed upon (U.S. [Clinical Laboratory Standards Institute] vs. Europe [European Committee on Antimicrobial Susceptibility Testing]).

2. In vitro susceptibility not always predictive of in vivo effectiveness.
   Examples:
   - MRSA reported as "susceptible" to doxycycline and TMP-SMX may not be clinically effective.
   - MRSA reported as "susceptible" in vitro to quinolones or cephalosporins (except ceftaroline) are not effective in vivo.
   - Klebsiella pneumoniae reported as "susceptible" in vitro to TMP-SMX is not effective in vivo.
   - Streptococci (Groups A–D) reported as "susceptible" in vitro to aminoglycosides are not effective in vivo.
   - L. monocytogenes appears susceptible in vitro but is not effective in vivo.

3. Nonsusceptible isolates in vitro may be susceptible in vivo with full/high doses if the MIC can be exceeded.

MIC, minimal inhibitory concentration; *MRSA,* methicillin-resistant *S. aureus; TMP-SMX,* trimethoprim-sulfamethoxazole.
Adapted from: Cunha BA, ed. *Antibiotic Essentials.* 12th ed. Sudbury, MA: Jones & Bartlett; 2013: 2-10.

Daptomycin

Daptomycin exhibits concentration-dependent killing and is bactericidal with dual PD characteristics (i.e., C_{max}/MIC as well as AUC_{0-24}/MIC ratio). It also has a prolonged PAE. Dosing of daptomycin depends on the site of infection. Lower doses are needed for skin and soft tissue infections whereas larger doses are required to treat bacteremia.[23] Relative or complete resistance may be present when patients with prior exposure to vancomycin are treated for staphylococcal infection, reflecting thickening of the cell wall.[9] In cases in which relatively resistant organisms are suspected, high-dose daptomycin (10 to 12 mg/kg [IV] q24h) has been successfully used.[37,38] Daptomycin should be avoided in cases of pneumonia because the calcium present in surfactant inactivates the antibiotic.

Tigecycline

Tigecycline, a derivative of minocycline that is structurally similar to the tetracyclines, exhibits time-dependent

Table 17-6 **Effective Approaches to Minimize Resistance**

1. **Avoid "covering" colonizers** that rarely, if ever, cause infection at the infection site being treated.

2. **Select a low resistance potential antibiotic effective against the usual site-determined pathogens.**

3. **Always consider the penetration potential of the antibiotic selected** to be sure of therapeutic concentrations at the site of infection.

4. **Use a loading dose or high dose for the first 3 days** to eliminate selecting out potentially resistant mutants.

5. **Use the shortest effective duration of therapy**, taking into account host factors, inoculation size, and pathogen virulence.

INEFFECTIVE APPROACHES TO MINIMIZE RESISTANCE

6. Switching from broad-spectrum to narrow-spectrum antibiotics is less relevant if using appropriate low resistance potential antibiotics.

7. Combination therapy does not prevent resistance.

8. Antibiotic "cycling" does not prevent resistance.

9. De-escalation decreases unnecessary/excessive antibiotic use, but does not, per se, decrease resistance.

10. Decreasing "antibiotic tonnage" or volume decreases costs and *Clostridium difficile* rates, but not resistance.

11. Avoid prolonged/low-dose antibiotic therapy.

Adapted from: Cunha BA. Antibiotic Resistance: Effective Control Strategies. *Lancet* 357:1307-1308 and 1101, 2001; Roberts JA, Pharm B, Kruger P, Paterson DL, Lipman J. Antibiotic resistance—What's dosing got to do with it? *Crit Care Med.* 2008;36:2433-2440.

killing. Concerns in the literature about the potential therapeutic failures of tigecycline relate to treating organisms that are innately resistant to tigecycline (e.g., *P. aeruginosa*) or to inadequate dosing. When tigecycline is administered, a loading dose, typically twice the maintenance dose, should be given, but the optimal tigecycline dosing strategy has not yet been determined. Given the high volume of distribution (V_d) of the drug (8 L/kg), the initial dose may not be sufficient to achieve therapeutic serum concentrations. A higher loading dose may be necessary when treating relatively resistant gram-negative bacilli.[39,40] The half-life of tigecycline is so long ($t_{1/2}$=42 hours) that after the initial loading dose of tigecycline, the maintenance dose (half of the loading dose) should instead be dosed every 24 hours.[39]

Aminoglycosides

Aminoglycosides demonstrate concentration-dependent killing kinetics. Amikacin, the aminoglycoside with the highest anti-*P. aeruginosa* activity, achieves much higher serum/MIC ratios than other aminoglycosides and is preferred in the critically ill. This drug may be used as monotherapy for gram-negative bacteremia and used as part of combination therapy to either increase coverage (e.g., tigecycline plus amikacin) or for possible synergy (e.g., levofloxacin plus amikacin). One-time daily dosing

Table 17-7 Summary of Optimal Empiric Antibiotic Use in the ICU

1. Base empiric coverage on likely pathogens at site of infection (lungs, not respiratory secretion isolates)

2. Avoid "covering" only cultured organism (colonization) from nonsterile sites
   - Respiratory secretions in intubated patients
   - Urine in patients with Foley catheters
   - Wounds with a nonpurulent discharge

3. Select antibiotic with high degree activity (and low resistance potential) against the usual pathogens at infection site
   - VAP/NP: *P. aeruginosa* and aerobic GNBs (not MSSA/MRSA)
   - Urosepsis: aerobic GNBs and enterococci (not MSSA/MRSA or *B. fragilis*)
   - Intra-abdominal sepsis: *B. fragilis* and aerobic GNBs (not MSSA/MRSA)

4. Minimize resistance by preferentially using low resistance potential (vs. high resistance potential) antibiotics with a spectrum appropriate for the infection site

5. Use full dose/highest dose (nontoxic) possible to maximize effectiveness and minimize the emergence of resistant organisms

6. Use strict infection control precautions to minimize spread of MDROs in ICU and the hospital

GNB, gram-negative bacilli; *ICU,* intensive care unit; *MDRO,* multidrug-resistant organism; *MRSA,* methicillin-resistant S. aureus; *MSSA,* methicillin-sensitive S. aureus; *NP,* nosocomial pneumonia; *VAP,* ventilator-associated pneumonia.

Table 17-8 Consequences of Suboptimal Antibiotic Therapy

1. **Therapeutic failure**
   Consequences
   - Wasted resources (drug costs of unsuccessful therapy)
   - Cost of re-treatment with another effective antibiotic (sometimes more expensive/toxic)
   - Costs of tests and consultants to evaluate and or re-treat therapeutic failure
   - Covering/chasing colonizers often means missing or not optimally treating the pathogens at the infection site
   - ↑ Length of stay
   - Legal implications of therapeutic failure

2. **Antibiotic resistance**
   Causes
   - Failure to select low resistance potential antibiotics (vs. high resistance potential antibiotics)
   - Failure to use full/highest tolerable dosing without toxicity (vs. low dose/prolonged treatment duration)
   - Failure to penetrate the target site of infection in therapeutic concentration results in subtherapeutic concentrations at the infection site → therapeutic failure/resistance
   - All other things being equal, subtherapeutic/low antibiotic concentrations likely to promote resistance
   Consequences
   - Cost of cohorting MDRO patients (impairs patient flow/bed utilization)
   - Risk of spread of MDROs within the ICU, hospital, and community
   - Compromised hospital reputation and or public image

ICU, intensive care unit; *MDRO,* multidrug-resistant organism.

optimizes amikacin PK/PD advantages and limits the risk of nephrotoxicity and ototoxicity.[41-43]

Colistin

Colistin is primarily used for serious infection due to MDRO *Acinetobacter* sp. or *P. aeruginosa* resistant to other antibiotics. Acquired resistance to colistin is rare, but many common gram-negative microorganisms are intrinsically resistant (*Proteus, Morganella, Serratia, Burkholderia* spp.). The limiting factor with colistin use is the potential for nephrotoxicity. Recent studies suggest that colistin, when properly dosed, is less nephrotoxic than was once thought.[44] Colistin should be given with a loading dose and then given in a maintenance dose of 1.7 mg/kg (IV) every 8 hours. Renal function should be monitored because renal failure may increase the serum half-life from 3.5 hours up to as long as 48 to 72 hours.[45,46] Colistin should be considered the drug of last resort. It is the only antibiotic active against MDRO *Acinetobacter* spp. and *P. aeruginosa.*

CONCLUSION

When selecting an empiric antibiotic for the septic ICU patient, clinicians must take into account the spectrum of activity, delivery of the drug to the site where the pathogen is located, resistance potential, optimized dosing based on PK/PD, and duration of treatment needed to eradicate the infection. The goal should be to use the highest dose of an antibiotic but avoid toxicity, in situations in which there is relative resistance (e.g., penicillin-resistant pneumococci). It is important to resist the temptation to treat isolates that represent colonization rather than true infection because this increases the risk of developing antibiotic resistance.[4] Empiric antibiotic therapy should be reserved for patients with true infection and not used in patients with infectious mimics or otherwise unexplained fever or leukocytosis (Table 17-4).

Ultimately, when using antibiotics in the ICU setting, it is critical to select an agent with a low resistance potential and give the drug at the highest dose without causing toxicity for the shortest amount of time necessary to cure the infection (Tables 17-7 and 17-8). In this way, clinicians will gain the maximum benefit from antimicrobials with the fewest adverse effects.

AUTHORS' RECOMMENDATIONS

- When selecting an empiric antibiotic for the septic ICU patient, clinicians must take into account spectrum of activity, delivery of the drug to the site where the pathogen is located, resistance potential, optimized dosing based on PK/PD, and duration of treatment needed to eradicate the infection.
- The goal should be to use the highest dose of an antibiotic, yet avoid toxicity.
- Antibiotics should not be administered to treat isolates that represent colonization rather than true infection, or infectious mimics such as unexplained fever or leukocytosis.
- The selected agent should be administered for the shortest duration necessary to cure the infection.

REFERENCES

1. Vincent JL, Opal SM, Marshall JC, Tracey KJ. Sepsis definitions: time for change. *Lancet.* 2013;381:774–775.
2. Dellinger RP, Levy MM, Rodes A, Annane D, Gerlach H, Opal SM, et al. Surviving Sepsis Campaign: international guidelines for management of severe sepsis and septic shock: 2012. *CCM Journal.* 2013;41:580–637.
3. Hurford A, Morris AM, FIsman DN, Wu J. Linking antimicrobial prescribing to antimicrobial resistance in the ICU: before and after an antimicrobial stewardship program. *Epidemics.* 2012;4:203–210.
4. Cunha CB, Varughese CA, Mylonakis E. Antimicrobial stewardship programs (ASPs): the devil is in the details. *Virulence.* 2013;4:147–149.
5. Rimawi RH, Mazer MA, Siraj DS, Gooch M, Cook PP. Impact of regular collaboration between infectious diseases and critical care practitioners on antimicrobial utilization and patient outcome. *Crit Care Med.* 2013;41:2099–2107.
6. Njoku JA, Hermsen ED. Antimicrobial stewardship in the intensive care unit: a focus of potential pitfalls. *J Pharm Pract.* 2010;23:50–60.
7. Amer MR, Akhras NS, Mahmood WA, Al-Jazairi AS. Antimicrobial stewardship program implementation in a medical intensive care unit at a tertiary care hospital in Saudi Arabia. *Ann Saudi Med.* 2013;33:547–554.
8. Roberts JA, Pharm B, Lipman J. Pharmacokinetic issues for antibiotics in the critically ill patient. *Crit Care Med.* 2009;37:840–851.
9. Cunha BA. Vancomycin revisited: a reappraisal of clinical use. *Crit Care Clin.* 2008;24:393–420.
10. Drusano GL. Antimicrobial pharmacodynamics: critical interactions of "bug and drug.". *Nat Rev Microbiol.* 2004;2:289–300.
11. Owens Jr RC, Shorr AF. Rational dosing of antimicrobial agents: pharmacokinetic and pharmacodynamic strategies. *Am J Health Syst Pharm.* 2009;66:S23–S30.
12. Winterboer TM, Lecci KA, Olsen KM. Continuing education: alternative approaches to optimizing antimicrobial pharmacodynamics in critically ill patients. *J Pharm Pract.* 2010;23:6–18.
13. Cunha BA, Domenico P, Cunha CB. Pharmacodynamics of doxycycline. *Clin Microbiol Infect.* 2000;6:270–273.
14. Bailey TC, Little JR, Littenberg B, et al. A meta-analysis of extended-interval dosing versus multiple daily dosing of aminoglycosides. *Clin Infect Dis.* 1997;24:786–795.
15. Ambrose PG, Owens Jr RC, Quintiliani R, Yeston N, Crowe HM, Cunha BA, Nightingale CH. Antibiotic use in the critical care unit. *Crit Care Clin.* 1998;14:283–308.
16. Goff DA, Nicolau DP. When pharmacodynamics trump costs: an antimicrobial stewardship program's approach to selecting optimal antimicrobial agents. *Clin Ther.* 2013;35:766–771.
17. Kahlmeter G. Defining antibiotic resistance-towards international harmonization. *Ups J Med Sci.* 2014;119:78–86.
18. Turnidge J, Paterson DL. Setting and revising antibacterial susceptibility breakpoints. *Clin Microbiol Infect.* 2007;20:391–408.
19. Lodise TP, Butterfield J. Use of pharmacodynamic principles to inform β-lactam dosing: "S" does not always mean success. *J Hosp Med.* 2011;6:S16–S23.
20. Cunha BA. Minocycline versus doxycycline for meticillin-resistant Staphylococcus aureus (MRSA): in vitro susceptibility versus in vivo effectiveness. *Int J Antimicrob Agents.* 2010;35:517–518.
21. Domenico P, O'Leary R, Cunha BA. Differential effects of bismuth and salicylate salts on the antibiotic susceptibility of Pseudomonas aeruginosa. *Eur J Clin Microbiol Infect Dis.* 1992;11:170–175.
22. Cunha BA. Problems arising in antimicrobial therapy due to false susceptibility testing. *J Chemother.* 1997;1:25–35.
23. Cunha BA, ed. *Antibiotic Essentials.* 12th ed. Sudbury, Massachusetts: Jones & Bartlett; 2013.
24. Roberts JA, Pharm B, Kruger P, Paterson DL, Lipman J. Antibiotic resistance – What's dosing got to do with it? *Crit Care Med.* 2008;36:2433–2440.
25. Roberts JA, Lipman J. Optimizing use of beta-lactam antibiotics in the critically ill. *Semin Respir Crit Care Med.* 2007;28:579–585.
26. McKinnon PS, Paladine JA, Schentag JJ. Evaluation of area under the inhibitory curve (AUIC) and time above the minimum inhibitory concentration (T>MIC) as predictors of outcome for cefepime and ceftazidime in serious bacterial infections. *Int J Anti Agents.* 2008;31:345–351.
27. Roberts JA, Paratz J, Paratz E, et al. Continuous infusion of beta-lactam antibiotics in severe infections: a review of its role. *Int J Antimicrob Agents.* 2007;30:111–118.
28. Roberts JA, Boots R, Rickard CM, et al. Is continuous infusion ceftriaxone better than once-a- day dosing in intensive care? A randomized controlled pilot study. *J Antimicrob Chemother.* 2006;59:285–291.
29. Altshuler J. Treatment of extended-spectrum beta-lactamase Enterobacteriaceae with cefepime: the dose matters, too. *Clin Infect Dis.* 2013;57:915–916.
30. Tamma PD, Girdwood SCT, Gopaul R, et al. The use of cefepime for treating AmpC β-lactamase-producing Enterobacteriaceae. *Clin Infect Dis.* 2013;57:781–788.
31. Yahave D, Paul M, Fraser A, et al. Efficacy and safety of cefepime: a systematic review and meta-analysis. *Lancet Infect Dis.* 2007;7:338–348.
32. Ogutlu A, Guclu E, Karabay O, Utku AC, Tuna N, Yahyaoglu M. Effects of Carbapenem consumption on the prevalence of Acinetobacter infection in intensive care unit patients. *Ann Clin Microbiol Anti.* 2014;13:7.
33. Palmore TN, Henderson DK. Carbapenem-resistant Enterobacteriaceae: a call for cultural change. *Ann Int Med.* 2014;160:567–570.
34. Noreddin AM, Elkhatib WF. Levofloxacin in the treatment of community-acquired pneumonia. *Expert Rev Anti Infect Ther.* 2010;8:505–514.
35. Gous A, Lipman J, Scibante J, et al. Fluid shifts have no influence on ciprofloxacin pharmacokinetics in intensive care patients with intra-abdominal sepsis. *Int J Antimicrob Agents.* 2005;26:50–55.
36. Zelenitsky SA, Ariano RE. Support for higher ciprofloxacin AUC_{24}/MIC targets in treating Enterobacteriaceae bloodstream infection. *J Anti Chemo.* 2010;65:1725–1732.
37. Cunha BA, Eisenstein LE. Hamid NS Pacemaker-induced Staphylococcus aureus mitral valve acute bacterial endocarditis complicated by persistent bacteremia from a coronary stent: cure with prolonged/high-dose daptomycin without toxicity. *Heart Lung.* 2006;35:207–211.
38. Cunha BA, Mickail N, Eisenstein LE. Faecalis vancomycin-sensitive enterococcal bacteremia unresponsive to a vancomycin tolerant strain successfully treated with high-dose daptomycin. *Heart Lung.* 2007;36:456–461.
39. Cunha BA. Once-daily tigecycline therapy of multidrug-resistant and non-multidrug-resistant gram-negative bacteremias. *J Chemother.* 2007;19:232–233.
40. Cunha BA. Pharmacokinetic considerations regarding tigecycline for multidrug-resistant (MDR) *Klebsiella pneumoniae* or MDR Acinetobacter baumannii urosepsis. *J Clin Microbiol.* 2009;47:1613.
41. Layeux B, Taccone FS, Fagnoul D, et al. Amikacin monotherapy for sepsis caused by panresistant *Pseudomonas aeruginosa*. *Antimicrob Agents Chemother.* 2010;54:4939–4941.
42. Le J, McKee B, Srisupha-Olarn W, Burgess D. In vitro activity of carbapenems alone and in combination with amikacin against KPC-producing *Klebsiella pneumoniae*. *J Clin Med Res.* 2011;3:106–110.
43. Taccone FS. Optimizing amikacin regimens in septic patients. *Int J Antimicrob Agents.* 2012;39:264–265.
44. Cheng CY, Sheng WH, Want JT, et al. Safety and efficacy of intravenous colistin (colistin methanesulphonate) for severe multidrug-resistant Gram-negative bacteria infections. *Int J Antimicrob Agents.* 2010;35:297–300.
45. Couet W, Gregoire N, Marchan S, et al. Colistin pharmacokinetics: the fog is lifting. *Clin Microbiol Infect.* 2012;18:30–39.
46. Daikos GL, Skiada A, Pavleas J, et al. Serum bactericidal activity of three different dosing regimens of colistin with implications for optimum clinical use. *J Chemother.* 2010;22:175–178.

18 Is Prophylaxis for Stress Ulceration Useful?

Eimhin Dunne, Ivan Hayes, Brian Marsh

First described in the 1970s,[1,2] stress-related mucosal damage (SMRD) was once considered a common complication of critical illness. However, it is now questionable whether the early descriptive work on the epidemiology and pathophysiology of stress ulceration remains applicable to the modern-day intensive care patient. Early endoscopic studies reported gastroduodenal abnormalities in most patients admitted to an intensive care unit (ICU), with more than 20% experiencing a gastrointestinal bleed significant enough to warrant blood transfusion.[3] With the evolution of critical care, a decade later, the number experiencing a clinically significant bleed had dramatically fallen.[4-6] Although infrequent now, clinically significant bleeding (CSB) remains associated with significant increased mortality and excess length of ICU stay estimated at 4 to 5 days.[7] However, preventative measures to reduce stress ulceration have no effect on mortality or length of stay.[8]

The management of SMRD in critically ill patients remains a contentious issue for intensivists. The potential benefit of prophylactic treatment must be weighed against the adverse risks and cost associated with treatment. If the decision to treat is made, then there is further uncertainty about the choice and formulation of agent. Undoubtedly, certain subsets of critically ill patients are at greater risk, and the identification and treatment of this group are likely to result in safe, cost-effective therapy.

DEFINITIONS

SRMD represents upper gastrointestinal damage ranging from asymptomatic superficial subepithelial lesions through to deeper lesions and ulceration extending into the submucosa and muscularis propria, causing occult bleeding, overt bleeding, or CSB.

Overt bleeding manifests as hematemesis, gross blood, or coffee-ground-like material in the nasogastric aspirate, hematochezia, or melena. CSB is overt bleeding complicated by hemodynamic changes (hypotension, tachycardia, or orthostasis) or by the need for blood transfusion or surgery.

PATHOPHYSIOLOGY

The pathophysiology of SRMD is complex, and uncertainty remains regarding the exact mechanisms. However,

it is likely that it arises from an altered balance of adequate mucosal protection and gastric acid production. The synthesis of the protective barrier is weakened when gut perfusion is compromised. Its protective effect is impaired by the presence of bile salts and uremic toxins, all common findings in critically ill patients.[9] Interestingly, intraluminal gastric hyperacidity has not been identified as a major contributor to the development of SMRD outside of head trauma and burn patients.[10]

Under normal physiologic circumstances, defense mechanisms prevent the erosion of the upper gastrointestinal mucosal lining by the acidic intraluminal contents. A glycoprotein mucous layer lines the stomach and forms a physical barrier to hydrogen ion back-diffusion (Fig. 18-1, A). Bicarbonate is trapped in this protective layer and neutralizes hydrogen ions before they reach the gastric epithelial layer. Adequate perfusion and oxygen delivery maintain intramural pH and prostaglandin synthesis, which is necessary for maintenance of the protective barrier layer.

Shock is common in critically ill patients, and septic shock is the most frequent cause of death in intensive care.[11] Early in the systemic inflammatory response, splanchnic blood flow is reduced, resulting in gastric intestinal mucosal hypoperfusion. This is exacerbated by absolute or relative hypovolemia and arterial hypotension. The combination of hypovolemia, redistribution of cardiac output, and intense splanchnic microvascular vasoconstriction results in hypoperfusion and tissue hypoxia. Hypoxia leads to uncoupling of oxidative phosphorylation. Energy is derived from anaerobic glycolysis resulting in regional lactic acidosis and a decrease in tissue pH.

Hypoperfusion initially causes an ischemic mucosal injury. Accumulation of oxygen-free radicals contributes to tissue inflammation and cell death. A reduction in prostaglandin synthesis results in breakdown in the protective mucosal barrier; the epithelial layer is exposed to hydrochloric acid and pepsin, and erosions ensue (Fig. 18-1, B).

In the severely physiologically stressed critically ill patient, the combination of hypovolemia, activation of the sympathetic nervous system, global and regional hypoperfusion, endogenous and exogenous vasoactive agents, the release of proinflammatory cytokines, and activation of coagulation create a milieu that favors gastrointestinal ulceration and impairs protective and healing mechanisms.

Gastric intraluminal acidity (pH < 4) is necessary for the generation of stress ulceration. Fasting and prolonged gastric transit times may contribute to a more acidic upper gastrointestinal tract. This increased duration and intensity of acid exposure may increase the likelihood of erosions and ulceration.

EPIDEMIOLOGY

SMRD was once considered an unavoidable complication of critical illness.[12,13] Early endoscopic evidence based on 40 patients reported gastroduodenal abnormalities in almost 75% of patients admitted to an ICU, with more than 20% (9 of 40) of patients experiencing a gastrointestinal bleed significant enough to warrant blood transfusion.[3] With the evolution of critical care, a decade later, the number experiencing a clinically significant bleed had fallen to 2 to 4%.[4-6] Nonetheless, on the basis of the early endoscopic studies and the fact that CSB remains associated with significant morbidity and mortality, stress ulcer prophylaxis (SUP) has become a standard of care in patients admitted to the ICU, with the intervention endorsed by many professional bodies.[14] It has been reported that 90% of ICU patients will receive some form of SUP.[15] Consequently, it is difficult to ascertain the true incidence of SMRD in the modern-day intensive care patient not receiving SUP.

A recently published large cohort study involving more than 35,000 patients in more than 70 hospitals between 2003 and 2008 reported the risk of gastrointestinal hemorrhage at 4%.[16] A meta-analysis from 2010 based on 17 studies performed between 1980 and 2004 estimates the risk of CSB from stress ulceration at 1% in ICU patients.[14] The variation in prevalence likely relates to the clinical endpoints studied and how the conditions of overt bleeding and CSB are defined.

The downward trajectory in the prevalence of CSB as a result of SMRD is due, at least in part, to improvements in the overall management of the intensive care patient. The decline in prevalence is widely attributed to the development of early goal-directed therapy with rapid restoration of intravascular volume and organ perfusion pressure, the use of lung-protective ventilatory strategies with a shorter duration of mechanical ventilation, the institution of Surviving Sepsis Campaign guidelines, and early enteral nutrition.[8,14,17]

RISK FACTORS

Not all critically ill patients are at equal risk for having gastrointestinal hemorrhage. In the prospective multicenter cohort study of 2252 intensive care patients by Cook and associates,[4] two independent risk factors for CSB were identified: respiratory failure (requiring mechanical ventilation for >48 hours; odds ratio [OR] 15.6) and coagulopathy (platelets <50,000; international normalized ratio >1.5 or activated partial thromboplastin time >2 times the control; OR, 4.3).

There was a trend toward increased bleeding in patients with hypotension (OR, 3.7), sepsis (OR, 2.0), renal failure (OR, 1.6), and glucocorticoid use (OR, 1.5), but these did not reach statistical significance.[4] In a later study of 1077 critically ill mechanically ventilated patients, using a multivariable analysis, the same group[18] demonstrated that renal failure (OR, 1.16) was independently associated with CSB, whereas enteral nutrition (OR, 0.3) and prophylaxis with ranitidine (OR, 0.39) conferred significantly lower bleeding rates. Two factors that appear to be independently predictive of stress ulcer bleeding in trauma patients are severe injury, as defined by an Injury Severity Score greater than 16, and injuries to the central nervous system (brain and spinal cord).[19] In an observational study by Maury and coworkers,[20] *Helicobacter pylori* infection was found to be associated with a 20% absolute increase in risk in critically ill patients who developed upper gastrointestinal hemorrhage (36% vs. 16%; *P* = .04; Table 18-1).

MANAGEMENT

The prevention or limitation of SRMD and stress ulceration begins with restoration of splanchnic perfusion and prompt effective treatment of the underlying condition. Early goal-directed therapy with fluid and catecholamine resuscitation has been shown to reduce mortality and multiorgan dysfunction in patients with severe sepsis and septic shock.[21] In shocked patients with splanchnic hypoperfusion, adequate volume loading is likely to be the most important initial intervention. The types of fluids, resuscitation endpoints, and monitoring techniques remain controversial. These issues are covered elsewhere in this book.

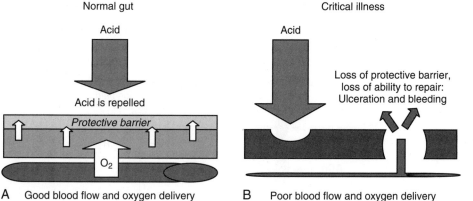

Figure 18-1. Development of stress ulcers: gastric mucosa. **A,** Normal mucosal barrier function. **B,** In critical illness, normal cytoprotective mechanisms are lost, and hypoperfused mucosa is exposed to gastric acid.

SPECIFIC STRESS ULCER PROPHYLAXIS

Although CSB from SRMD occurs infrequently, the associated morbidity and mortality warrant a preventative approach in at-risk patients. Specific pharmacologic anti-stress ulcer therapies can be broadly divided into four groups: antacids, cytoprotectants, H_2-receptor antagonists, and proton pump inhibitors (PPIs) (Fig. 18-2).

Antacids act locally by directly neutralizing gastric acid and transiently increasing intraluminal pH. Frequent oral administration is required. Adverse effects include vomiting, constipation, metabolic alkalosis, and a range of electrolyte disturbances. Antacids are less efficacious than H_2-receptor antagonists and PPIs in reducing gastric acidity, and they are currently not recommended as prophylaxis.

Sucralfate is the most extensively studied of the cytoprotectant agents. It is a sulfated polysaccharide complexed with aluminum hydroxide, which adheres to epithelial cells to form a physical protective gel layer on the gastric mucosa, reducing direct acid contact. Sucralfate is administered orally or by nasogastric tube. It does not significantly alter intraluminal pH; this may confer benefit in terms of gastric bacterial colonization. Other proposed benefits of sucralfate include (1) stimulation of mucous and bicarbonate secretion, (2) stimulation of epidermal growth factor, and (3) improved mucosal blood flow and enhanced prostaglandin release. Adverse effects are reduced absorption of enteral feed and some medications (quinolones, theophylline, phenytoin, ranitidine, ketoconazole, digoxin).[22] There is also the potential for bezoar formation, clogging of nasogastric tubes, need for feeding breaks, and increased serum aluminum levels in patients receiving renal replacement therapy. Because sucralfate acts directly on the stomach, administration distal to the pylorus is ineffective. Sucralfate is more effective than placebo but inferior to H_2-receptor antagonists.[23]

Gastric acid secretion is an active, energy-demanding process. Agents such as H_2-receptor antagonists and PPIs, by diminishing energy-demanding gastric acid secretion, may protect against the development of stress ulcers related to hypoperfusion.

H_2-receptor antagonists act by reversible competitive inhibition of histamine-stimulated acid production and decrease overall gastric secretions. Enteral and parenteral formulations are available. These agents require frequent dosing, and there is some evidence to suggest that continuous infusions of the intravenous formulations may achieve better pH control than bolus administration.[24,25] The phenomenon of tachyphylaxis, displayed by H_2-receptor antagonists, raises concerns about their suitability for longer term use in the critically ill. Seventy percent of patients will achieve a gastric intraluminal pH of more than 4 within 24 hours, but this falls to just 26% by day 3.[26,27] Adverse effects include central nervous system disturbances, especially in elderly patients with intravenous administration. In rare instances, hematologic disorders such as thrombocytopenia have been associated with H_2-receptor antagonists. Cimetidine and ranitidine cause inhibition of cytochrome P-450 metabolism that reduces the clearance of many drugs (e.g., warfarin and phenytoin). H_2-receptor antagonists reduce the risk of CSB when compared with placebo.[23]

PPIs are substituted benzimidazoles that inhibit the H^+/K^+ ATPase (gastric hydrogen potassium adenosine triphosphate) enzyme on the parietal cell. This inhibits histamine-induced and vagally mediated acid secretion, making PPIs the most potent agents in raising the pH of gastric contents. PPIs irreversibly bind to the proton pump, and subsequent secretion of acid can only occur with the synthesis of new enzyme.[28] There are enteral and intravenous formulations available. Patients do not have tolerance to the antacid effects of PPIs, with 100% of patients maintaining a

Table 18-1 **Risk Factors for Stress Ulceration**
Mechanical ventilation*
Coagulopathy*
Acute renal failure[†]
Major trauma (Injury Severity Score >16)
Hypotension
Sepsis
Shock
Organ dysfunction
Liver failure
Cardiac arrest
Brain or spinal cord injury
Thermal injury (>35% total-body surface area)
High-dose glucocorticoids
Organ transplantation
Anticoagulation
After major surgery, with or without nasogastric tube
History of gastritis, peptic ulcer disease, gastrointestinal bleeding

*Independent risk factors.
[†]Independent risk factor in mechanically ventilated patient.

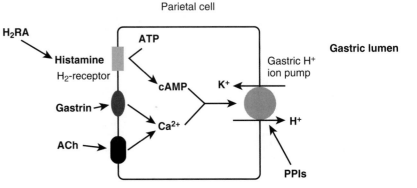

Parietal cell

Figure 18-2. Gastric acid production and the effect of acid reduction therapy. *ACh*, acetylcholine; *ATP*, adenosine triphosphate; *Ca²⁺*, calcium ion; *cAMP*, cyclic adenosine monophosphate; *H⁺*, hydrogen ion; *H₂RA*, H_2-receptor antagonist; *K⁺*, potassium chloride; *PPI*, proton pump inhibitor.

gastric intraluminal pH of more than 4 at day 3.[26] However, rebound acid hypersecretion is common after discontinuation. Adverse effects are generally mild (e.g., gastrointestinal upset or headache), but an association with *Clostridium difficile* diarrhea has been reported.[29] PPIs are metabolized by the cytochrome P-450 enzyme system; therefore there is potential for drug interaction. Omeprazole interferes with metabolism of cyclosporine, diazepam, phenytoin, and warfarin and increases the metabolism of several antipsychotic drugs and theophylline.[30] Pantoprazole undergoes dual-pathway metabolism in the liver to inactive metabolites through the cytochrome P-450 system and sulfate conjugation. This results in fewer drug interactions that make pantoprazole particularly useful in critically ill patients, who typically are on numerous medications. A meta-analysis performed by Alhazzani and colleagues in 2013 concluded that PPIs provide the most reliable and sustained control of gastric acidity, making them more effective than H_2-receptor antagonists at reducing clinically significant and overt upper gastrointestinal bleeding.[17] However, the investigators observed no corresponding reduction in mortality rates or length of hospital stay. An earlier large-scale cohort study performed between 2003 and 2008 involving more than 35,000 patients found a greater risk of gastrointestinal bleeding when PPIs were used compared with H_2-receptor antagonists,[16] but the validity of this trial was questioned because the authors did not differentiate between overt and clinically significant gastrointestinal bleeding. The Surviving Sepsis Campaign recommends the use of PPIs over H_2-receptor antagonists for SUP.[31]

In patients with bleeding peptic ulcers, who require a higher gastric pH to maintain clot stability, the results of two trials suggest that omeprazole infusion can maintain the intragastric pH higher than 6 for several days, whereas the initial effectiveness of the H_2-receptor antagonists in keeping the pH above 6 is quickly lost, most likely as a result of tolerance.[27,32] A meta-analysis of 11 trials compared the efficacy of PPIs and H_2-receptor antagonists in reducing the rate of rebleeding in patients with bleeding peptic ulcer disease.[33] PPIs were found to be more effective in preventing persistent or recurrent bleeding, but there was no significant difference in the need for surgery or mortality rate.[33] Blood clot integrity is dependent on a pH higher than 6, which is only reliably achieved with PPIs. Questions remain outstanding regarding the appropriate PPI dosing regimen for patients with bleeding peptic ulcers. An intragastric pH higher than 6 during most of the 24-hour periods is a prerequisite for the control of bleeding in patients with active bleeding ulcers because platelet aggregation will not occur below a pH of 5.9 and is optimal at a pH of 7 to 8.[34] In a crossover trial in 10 patients taking omeprazole, a 40-mg intravenous bolus was compared with an 80-mg bolus plus 8-mg-per-hour infusion with the outcome measure of mean intragastric pH. The two regimens were equivalent for the first 12 hours. When the time with an intragastric pH above 6 during the first 24 hours was considered, the 80-mg bolus and 8-mg-per-hour infusion were superior.[35] A more recent trial involving more than 230 patients with bleeding ulcers comparing continuous infusion of PPI with twice-daily dosing of intravenous PPI failed to show a difference in rebleeding rates, need for surgical intervention, blood transfusion requirements, or mortality.[36]

When CSB occurs, the patient should be hemodynamically assessed and appropriate volume resuscitation instituted. Early multidisciplinary involvement is recommended with angiographic embolization, endoscopic intervention, and surgical control of bleeding vessels all options for definitive treatment in patients with gastrointestinal bleeding.

ENTERAL NUTRITION

The recognition of the importance of establishing enteral nutrition as soon as possible in the critically ill patient may have contributed to the decline in SMRD-related bleeding over the last 30 years.[8] Enteral feeding may reduce the incidence of overt gastrointestinal bleeding due to stress ulceration,[4,18,37] but there are conflicting data,[38] and most studies are now outdated, having been performed over two decades ago. A subgroup analysis in a large meta-analysis investigating H_2-receptor antagonists and placebo reported a potential increased risk of pneumonia and mortality without reducing the risk of gastrointestinal bleeding in patients receiving SUP.[14] The suggestion that enteral nutrition may provide adequate protection in non–high-risk patients without the need for additional therapy needs further investigation in larger-scale prospective studies.

Is Prophylaxis for Stress Ulceration Harmful?

Infectious Complications

1. *Ventilator-Associated Pneumonia*

In the European Prevalence of Infection in Intensive Care (EPIC) study,[39] pneumonia (46.9%) and lower respiratory tract infection (17.8%) were found to be the most common ICU-acquired infections. SUP was one of seven risk factors identified for ICU-acquired infection.[39] Bacterial colonization of the aerodigestive tract and the aspiration of contaminated secretions into the lower airways are believed to contribute to the pathogenesis of ventilator-associated pneumonia (VAP).[40] Concerns have been raised that the administration of pH-altering drugs (antacids, H_2-receptor antagonists, and PPIs) increase gastric intraluminal pH, facilitating bacterial proliferation, predisposing to tracheal colonization, and increasing the risk of nosocomial pneumonia.[41,42] However, data relating intragastric pH to nosocomial pneumonia are weak and conflicting. A randomized controlled trial of 244 patients found that patients treated with sucralfate had a lower median gastric pH, less frequent gastric colonization, and a reduced incidence of late-onset nosocomial pneumonia,[43] supporting the importance of gastric acidity. A trial of acidified enteral feed (pH < 3.5) to maintain gastric acidity and reduce bacterial colonization, in 120 critically ill patients,[42] demonstrated reduced levels of gram-negative bacterial growth in tracheal suction. However, this did not translate into a reduction in frequency of nosocomial pneumonia.

A prospective randomized controlled trial compared the use of antacids, continuous intravenous cimetidine, or sucralfate in critically ill trauma patients to determine the role of gastric colonization in the development of pneumonia.[38] The authors concluded that the gastric biology of the three groups was nearly identical, and stress ulcer prophylactic agents that elevate gastric pH did not increase the incidence of pneumonia.

Overall, there is no clear evidence that antacid therapy increases the risk of ventilator-associated infections. It is biologically plausible that the rate of VAP is likely to be greater with PPI use, compared with sucralfate or H_2-receptor antagonists, because of the greater acid suppression achieved for longer duration by PPIs and consequential greater bacterial colonization. Furthermore, some studies have suggested that PPIs can diminish cell immunity and leukocyte function through acidification of the phagolysosome and an inhibition of phagocytosis.[44]

2. C. difficile Infection

Some studies have reported a link between acid-reducing therapy and C. difficile infection.[44] Pathophysiologic explanations include a weakened physical barrier to ingested bacteria due to the altered pH and the facilitation of bacterial proliferation.[44] In a recent retrospective analysis of more than 3000 medical ICU patients, the use of PPIs for SUP was identified as a strong independent risk factor for the development of C. difficile–associated diarrhea.[45] In addition, there was an increased risk of death in the cohort that had C. difficile–associated diarrhea (30.9%), compared with those patients who did not (21.9%), and an excess length of ICU stay of up to 8 days.[45]

Inappropriate Continuation

There is no clear recommendation on when to discontinue SUP in the critically ill, which probably explains the results of a recent observational study showing that one third of patients were discharged home with a PPI with no clear indication for their continued use.[46]

There are no published data on late CSB in the critical care population. Consideration should be made of the continued presence of risk factors, such as persistent mechanical ventilation, catabolism, and coagulation disorders. Given the low incidence of CSB in patients without specific risk factors and the cost implications, it seems reasonable to discontinue prophylaxis when the original indication has subsided, and probably when the patient is discharged from ICU. Chronic therapy with PPIs has been linked to the development of osteoporosis and fractures.[47]

AUTHORS' RECOMMENDATIONS

- CSB from stress ulceration occurs infrequently.
- When CSB occurs, it is associated with increased hospital costs, greater length of stay, and higher patient morbidity and mortality.
- Early restoration of intravascular volume and organ perfusion may limit SMRD and progression to stress ulceration.
- Pharmacologic SUP is not necessary in all ICU patients but is recommended for those with established risk factors.
- The debate continues on which agent should be used as first-line therapy. The choice should be based on the potential for drug interactions, the risk of adverse effects, and local policy and resources.
- Acute therapies that increase gastric pH may increase the rate of ventilator-associated infections and C. difficile colitis, both of which are associated with increased patient morbidity and mortality.
- Prophylactic therapy should be discontinued at the earliest possible opportunity, when the original indication has resolved.

REFERENCES

1. Skillman JJ, Silen W. Acute gastroduodenal "stress" ulceration: barrier disruption of varied pathogenesis? *Gastroenterology.* 1970;59:478–482.
2. Lucas CE, Sugawa C, Riddle J, et al. Natural history and surgical dilemma of "stress" gastric bleeding. *Arch Surg.* 1971;102:266–273.
3. Peura DA, Johnson LF. Cimetidine for prevention and treatment of gastroduodenal mucosal lesions in patients in an ICUs. *Ann Intern Med.* 1985;103:173–177.
4. Cook DJ, Fuller HD, Guyatt GH, Marshall J, et al. Risk factors for gastrointestinal bleeding in critically ill patients. Canadian Critical Care Trials Group. *N Engl J Med.* 1994;330:377–381.
5. Cook D, Guyatt G, Marshall J, et al. A comparison of sucralfate and ranitidine for the prevention of upper gastrointestinal bleeding in patients requiring mechanical ventilation: Canadian Critical Care Trials Group. *N Engl J Med.* 1998;338:791–797.
6. Zandstra DF, Stoutenbeek CP. The virtual absence of stress-ulceration related bleeding in ICU patients receiving prolonged mechanical ventilation without any prophylaxis: a prospective cohort study. *Intensive Care Med.* 1994;20:335–340.
7. Cook DJ, Griffith LE, Walter SD, et al. Canadian Critical Care Trials Group: the attributable mortality and length of intensive care unit stay of clinically important gastrointestinal bleeding in critically ill patients. *Crit Care.* 2001;5:368–375.
8. Faisy C, Guerot E, Diehl JL, et al. Clinically significant gastrointestinal bleeding in critically ill patients with and without stress-ulcer prophylaxis. *Intensive Care Med.* 2003;29:1306–1313.
9. Schindlbeck N, Lippert M, Heinrich C, Müller-Lissner S. Intragastric bile acid concentrations in critically ill, artificially ventilated patients. *Am J Gastroenterol.* 1989;84(6):624–628.
10. Mutlu GM, Mutlu EA, Factor P. GI complications in patients receiving mechanical ventilation. *Chest.* 2001;119:1222–1241.
11. Angus DC, Linde-Zwirble WT, Lidicker J, et al. Epidemiology of severe sepsis in the United States: analysis of incidence, outcome, and associated costs of care. *Crit Care Med.* 2001;29:1303–1310.
12. Reilly J, Fennerty MB. Stress ulcer prophylaxis: the prevention of gastrointestinal bleeding and the development of nosocomial infections in critically ill patients. *J Pharm Pract.* 1998;11:418–432.
13. Eddleson JM, Pearson RC, Holland J, et al. Prospective endoscopic study of stress erosions and ulcers in critically ill adult patients treated with either sucralfate or placebo. *Crit Care Med.* 1994;22:1949–1954.
14. Marik PE, Vasu T, Hirani A, et al. Stress ulcer prophylaxis in the new millennium: a systematic review and meta-analysis. *Crit Care Med.* 2010;38:2222–2228.
15. Daley RJ, Rebuck JA, Welage LS, et al. Prevention of stress ulceration: current trends in critical care. *Crit Care Med.* 2004;32:2008–2013.
16. MacLaren R, Reynolds P, Allen R. Histamine-2-receptor antagonists vs proton pump inhibitors on gastrointestinal tract hemorrhage and infectious complications in the intensive care unit. *JAMA Intern Med.* 2014;174(4):564–574.
17. Alhazzani W, Alenezi F, Jaeschke R, et al. Proton pump inhibitors versus histamine 2 receptor antagonists for stress ulcer prophylaxis in critically ill patients: a systematic review and meta-analysis. *Crit Care Med.* 2013;41:693–705.
18. Cook D, Heyland D, Griffith L, et al. Risk factors for clinically important upper gastrointestinal bleeding in patients requiring mechanical ventilation. *Crit Care Med.* 1999;27:2812–2817.
19. Simons RK, Hoyt DB, Winchel RJ, et al. A risk analysis of stress ulceration after trauma. *J Trauma.* 1995;39:289–294.
20. Maury E, Tankovic J, Ebel A, Offenstadt G. An observational study of upper gastrointestinal bleeding in intensive care units: Is Helicobacter pylori the culprit. *Crit Care Med.* 2005;33:1513.
21. Rivers E, Nguyen B, Havstad S, et al. Early goal-directed therapy in the treatment of severe sepsis and septic shock. *N Engl J Med.* 2001;345:1368–1377.
22. Daley RJ, Rebuck JA, Welage LS, Rogers FB. Prevention of stress ulceration: current trends in critical care. *Crit Care Med.* 2004;32:2008–2013.
23. Cook DJ, Reeve BK, Guyatt GH, et al. Stress ulcer prophylaxia in critically ill patients. Recolving discordant meta-analyses. *JAMA.* 1996;275:308–314.

24. Baghaie AA, Mojtahedzadeh M, Levine RL, et al. Comparison of the effect of intermittent administration and continuous infusion of famotidine on gastric pH in critically ill patients: results of a prospective randomized, crossover study. *Crit Care Med.* 1995;23:687.

25. Ballesteros MA, Hogan DL, Koss MA, Isenberg JI. Bolus or intravenous infusion of ranitidine: effects on gastric pH and acid secretion. *Ann Intern Med.* 1990;112:334.

26. Netzer P, Gaia C, Sandoz M, et al. Effect of repeated injection and continuous infusion of omeprazole and ranitidine on intragastric pH over 72 hours. *Am J Gastroenterol.* 1999;94:351–357.

27. Merki HS, Wilder-Smith CH. Do continuous omeprazole and ranitidine retain their effect with prolonged dosing? *Gastroenterology.* 1994;106:60–64.

28. Pisengna JR. Pharmacology of acid suppression in the hospital setting: focus on proton pump inhibition. *Crit Care Med.* 2002; 30(suppl).

29. Dial S, Alrassadi K, Manoukian C, et al. Risk of Clostridium difficile diarrhea among hospital inpatients prescribed proton pump inhibitors: cohort and case control studies. *CMAJ.* 2004;171:33–38.

30. Spirt MJ. Stress related mucosal disease: risk factors and prophylactic therapy. *Clin Ther.* 2004;26:197–213.

31. Dellinger RP, Levy MM, Rhodes A, et al. Surviving Sepsis Campaign: international guidelines for management of severe sepsis and septic shock: 2012. *Crit Care Med.* 2013;41:580–637.

32. Labenz J, Peiz U, Leusing C, et al. Efficacy of primed infusions with high dose ranitidine and omeprazole to maintain high intragastric pH in patients with peptic ulcer bleeding: a prospective randomised controlled study. *Gut.* 1997;40:36–41.

33. Gisbert JP, Gonzalez L, Calvet X, et al. Proton pump inhibitors versus H2-antagonists: a meta-analysis of their efficacy in treating bleeding peptic ulcer. *Aliment Pharmacol Ther.* 2002;3:645–646.

34. Green FW, Kaplan MM, Curtis LE, et al. Effect of acid and pepsin on blood coagulation and platelet aggregation. *Gastroenterology.* 1978;74:38–43.

35. Laterre PF, Horsmans Y. Intravenous omeprazole in critically ill patients: a randomized, crossover study comparing 40 with 80 mg plus 8 mg/hour on intragastric pH. *Crit Care Med.* 2001;29:1931–1935.

36. Andriulli A, Loperfido S, Focareta R, et al. High- versus low-dose proton pump inhibitors after endoscopic hemostasis in patients with peptic ulcer bleeding: a multicentre, randomized study. *Am J Gastroenterol.* 2008;103(12):3011.

37. Gramlich L, Kichian K, Pinilla J, et al. Does enteral nutrition compared to parenteral nutrition result in better outcomes in critically ill adult patients? A systematic review of the literature. *Nutrition.* 2004;20:843–848.

38. Simms H, DeMaria E, McDonald L, et al. Role of gastric colonization in the development of pneumonia in critically ill trauma patients: results of a prospective randomized trial. *J Trauma.* 1991;31:531–536.

39. Vincent JL, Bihari DJ, Suter PM, et al. The prevalence of nosocomial infection in intensive care units in Europe. Results of the European Prevalence of Infection in Intensive care (EPIC) study. EPIC International Advisory Committee. *JAMA.* 1995;274:639–644.

40. du Moulin GC, Paterson DG, Hedley-White J, Lisbon A. Aspiration of gastric bacteria in antacid treated patients: a frequent cause of postoperative colonization of the airway. *Lancet.* 1982;1:242–245.

41. Apte NM, Karnad DR, Medhekar TP, et al. Gastric colonization and pneumonia in intubated critically ill patients receiving stress ulcer prophylaxis: a randomized, controlled trial. *Crit Care Med.* 1992;20:590–593.

42. Heyland DK, Cook DJ, Schoenfeld PS, et al. The effect of acidified enteral feeds on gastric colonization in critically ill patients: results of a multicenter randomized trial. Canadian Critical Care Trials Group. *Crit Care Med.* 1999;27:2399–2406.

43. Prod'hom G, Leuenberger P, Koerfer J, et al. Nosocomial pneumonia in mechanically ventilated patients receiving antacid, ranitidine, or sucralfate as prophylaxis for stress ulcer: a randomized controlled trial. *Ann Intern Med.* 1994;120:653–662.

44. Howell MD, Novack V, Grgurich P, et al. Iatrogenic gastric acid suppression and the risk of nosocomial Clostridium difficile infection. *Arch Intern Med.* 2010;170:784–790.

45. Buendgens L, Bruensing J, Matthes M, et al. Administration of proton pump inhibitors in critically ill medical patients is associated with increased risk of developing Clotridium difficile-associated diarrhea. *J Crit Care.* 2014;29: 696.e11–e15.

46. Farley KJ, Barned KL, Crozier TM. Inappropriate continuation of stress ulcer prophylaxis beyond the intensive care setting. *Crit Care Resusc.* 2013;15:147–151.

47. Khalili H, Huang ES, Jacobson BC, Camargo Jr CA, Feskanich D, Chan AT. Use of proton pump inhibitors and risk of hip fractures in relation to dietary and lifestyle factors: a prospective cohort study. *BMJ.* 2012;344:e372.

19 Should Fever Be Treated?

Taka-Aki Nakada, Waka Takahashi, James A. Russell

Body temperature is a fundamental physiologic parameter that is altered by several pathologic processes. Abnormal or altered body temperature is a key to aid in diagnosis and is often a component of therapeutic strategy.[1] Fever is particularly common in critically ill patients who are admitted to the intensive care unit (ICU).[2-5]

However, it is unclear if alterations in temperature are themselves pathologic or if they represent an adaptive response to pathology. Thus, before reviewing the evidence and making recommendations for fever control in the critically ill, it is fundamentally important to understand the mechanisms of temperature control and fever generation.

Infection such as that induced by gram-negative bacteria induces several important changes in host physiology by generating pathogen-associated molecular patterns (PAMPs) that bind to pattern recognition receptors (PRRs) such as toll-like receptor 4 (TLR-4).[6] This process activates host fixed-tissue macrophages to release circulating substances such as prostanoids that alter activity in thermoregulatory regions of the preoptic area (POA) of the rostral hypothalamus[7-10] (Fig. 19-1). Inflammatory cytokines released from immune cells also induce expression of prostaglandin E_2 (PGE_2) in endothelial cells around the POA that further signal the hypothalamic temperature control center.[11,12] PGE_2 reduces cyclic adenosine monophosphate (cAMP) levels in the POA, and reduced activity of cAMP causes fever. Thus, temperature and generation of fever are controlled predominantly via a PGE_2–dependent pathway; however, it is possible that cytokines or the hepatic branch of the vagus contribute to fever, although such suggestions are controversial.[9,10,13]

Data suggest that fever accompanies infection or sterile noninfective inflammation (postoperative patients, pancreatitis, trauma, inflammatory disorders such as lupus) and drug reactions.[2,14] In infection, fever may modulate the host defense response,[4,13] affecting cellular innate immunity, CD4 T cells, or B cells.[15] Fever also decreases inflammatory cytokines such as tumor necrosis factor-α[15,16] and delays expression of interferon-γ expression,[16] rapidly increases expression of cytoprotective heat shock proteins,[4,13,17-19] and inhibits nuclear factor-κB. These changes can limit the deleterious effects of infection, reducing organ dysfunction and improving survival.[18,20,21] Fever may also affect the pathogen by inhibiting growth[22] or increasing antibiotic susceptibility.[23] These effects suggest that fever is adaptive.

Conversely, an elevated body temperature has several detrimental effects that need to be considered. Fever increases energy expenditure and oxygen demand and decreases vascular tone, resulting in an imbalance between oxygen demand and supply. Thus, controlling fever may decrease (1) global oxygen demand when oxygen supply is limited[24]; (2) the risk of oxygen supply/demand mismatch; (3) the metabolic rate, and with it catabolism; and (4) the risk of septic encephalopathy, thereby decreasing the need for sedatives and antipsychotic drugs. These possibilities provide a rationale for treating fever.[4,13]

The association between fever and the clinical outcome of critically ill patients has been assessed in several observational cohort studies.[3,24-32] A retrospective observational cohort study of 24,204 adult patients in medical-surgical ICUs demonstrated that the presence of fever greater than 39.5°C was associated with significantly increased mortality rates.[25] The effect of fever on outcome may be particularly critical in patients with neurologic disorders.[33-35] A prospective cohort study of patients emergently admitted to a neurological ICU revealed that elevated body temperature was independently associated with increased length of ICU stay, increased mortality, and worse hospital disposition.[36] Controlling body temperature to avoid fever in patients who had cardiac arrest outside of the hospital has been widely studied and appears to improve neurologic outcomes and reduce mortality[37-40] (Table 19-1), but a randomized controlled trial (RCT) showed that hypothermia in severe bacterial meningitis did not improve outcome and may even have been harmful[41] (Table 19-1).

The benefits of actively preventing fever in ICU patients who do not have a neurologic disorder are unknown.[2,4,13,42-48] As such, guidelines generated by the American College of Critical Care Medicine (ACCM) and the Infectious Diseases Society of America (IDSA) make no recommendations regarding temperature management in adult patients.[1] We therefore review recent evidence from RCTs.

EVIDENCE FROM RANDOMIZED CONTROLLED TRIALS

The mechanism of cooling to control fever is likely important. Interventions to control fever that were assessed in RCTs include external cooling and nonsteroidal anti-inflammatory drugs (NSAIDs) such as ibuprofen and acetaminophen (paracetamol).

Although fever is inconsistently defined, a core body temperature of 38.3°C or greater is most commonly used in the literature and in the ACCM/IDSA guidelines for fever in critically ill adult patients.[1] These

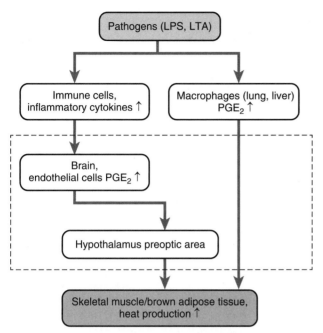

Figure 19-1. Lipopolysaccharide (*LPS*), a main component of the outer membrane of gram-negative bacteria, is a pathogen-associated molecular pattern that is recognized by pattern recognition receipters such as toll-like receptor 4 on immune cells. In lung and liver, prostaglandin E$_2$ (*PGE$_2$*), synthesized by activated macrophages, is released into the circulation and circulates to the preoptic area (POA) in the rostral pole of the hypothalamus, the brain's thermoregulatory center. In addition to the PGE$_2$ from the lung and liver, PGE$_2$ is also expressed by local brain endothelial cells. Inflammatory cytokines released from immune cells induce expression of PGE$_2$ in such endothelial cells around the POA. PGE$_2$ diffuses into the parenchyma and signals the hypothalamic temperature control center. PGE$_2$ reduces cyclic adenosine monophosphate (cAMP) levels in the POA, and reduced activity of cAMP causes fever. Thus temperature and generation of fever are controlled predominantly via a PGE$_2$-dependent pathway. *LTA,* lipoteichoic acid.

guidelines recommended that an intravascular, esophageal, or bladder thermistor most accurately measures temperature. In addition, the guidelines state that oral or infrared ear thermometry are accurate and acceptable for use in the ICU,[49] whereas temporal artery, axillary, or chemical dot temperatures are not.[1]

External Cooling

There have been two RCTs of external cooling for non-neurologic critically ill patients[50,51] (Table 19-2). The first RCT (n=38) assessed the efficacy of external cooling in febrile patients admitted to a surgical ICU without neurologic factors, and it failed to demonstrate a significant effect on length of hospital stay or mortality.[50] This study was limited by a sample size that left it severely underpowered and ineffective external cooling—patients who received external cooling had similar body temperature compared with the control group. The second RCT was conducted to evaluate the safety and efficacy of fever control by external cooling in febrile patients who had septic shock.[51] This RCT enrolled 200 critically ill patients who had infection with a core body temperature greater than 38.3°C and required vasopressor infusion, ventilator support, and sedation. The intervention group (n=101) had external cooling to

normothermia for 48 hours whereas controls (n=99) had usual care without cooling. Because there was no difference in adverse events between the two groups, fever control by the external cooling was demonstrated to be safe. This study successfully attained rapid, significant fever control by external cooling. However, the primary outcome variable, the number of patients reaching a 50% decrease in the dose of vasopressors within 48 hours, was not significantly different between the two groups. The patients who had external cooling required significantly lower vasopressor dosage at 12 hours and had significantly decreased 14-day mortality compared with patients without external cooling (19% vs. 34 %; *P*=.013). External cooling can cause shivering and thus increase the need for sedation and even neuromuscular paralysis. Although the use of sedation and neuromuscular paralysis was similar between groups, it is unclear if sedation of neuromuscular blockade was managed by a protocol. Importantly, the groups differed at baseline; initial vasopressor doses in patients without external cooling were higher than the patients with external coolings. The adjusted analyses confirmed the efficacy of cooling; nonetheless, post hoc statistical adjustment of baseline differences in the primary outcome variable (vasopressor dose) between study groups is always a concern in the interpretation of RCTs.

Although additional trials need to be performed, external cooling is simple, easily implemented, and lacks some of the potential adverse effects of antipyretics. Subsequent validation in larger RCTs is required; however, we suggest that cooling of febrile patients who have septic shock should be considered in patients who are on high doses of vasopressor, who require inotropic agents (e.g., dobutamine), or who have marked tachycardia.[52]

Ibuprofen

A large (n=450) RCT funded by the National Institutes of Health published in 1997 compared ibuprofen, an NSAID, with placebo in patients with severe sepsis.[53] Ibuprofen significantly decreased core temperature, heart rate, oxygen consumption, and lactate level. In addition, potential drug-induced adverse events, including renal dysfunction and gastrointestinal bleeding, did not differ between the two groups. There was, however, no significant difference in organ failure or 30-day mortality between study groups (ibuprofen vs. placebo, 37% vs. 40%, respectively).

A smaller RCT (n=53) evaluated the efficacy and safety of intravenous ibuprofen (100, 200, or 400 milligrams every 4 hours for six doses) in critically ill patients with fever. Intravenous ibuprofen effectively controlled fever and was not associated with an increase in adverse events, but there was no difference in mortality between ibuprofen and placebo.[54] This was a very small RCT, though, that was not even close to being of adequate power for mortality assessment. Taken together, ibuprofen can safely reduce fever in critically ill patients, but there is no reported evidence to support a beneficial effect on clinical outcomes.

Acetaminophen (Paracetamol)

To our knowledge, there are no RCTs of acetaminophen (paracetamol) for fever control in sepsis or septic shock.

Table 19-1 Fever Control in Neurologic Critically Ill Patients

Study, Year	Setting	Population	Patients (n)	Intervention	Primary Outcome	Main Findings
Bernard, 2002[37]	RCT	Out-of-hospital cardiac arrest	77	Target temperature 33°C within 2 hours after the ROSC and maintained for 12 hours	Survival to hospital discharge with good neurologic function	Patients treated with hypothermia had a good outcome compared with those with normothermia (49% vs. 26%, P = .046).
Hypothermia After Cardiac Arrest study group, 2002[38]	RCT	Postcardiac arrest	136	Target temperature 32 to 34°C for 24 hours	Favorable neurologic outcome within 6 months after cardiac arrest	Patients in the hypothermia group had a favorable neurologic outcome compared with the normothermia group (55% vs. 39%, RR 1.40, 95% CI 1.08-1.81).
Nielsen, 2013[39]	RCT	Out-of-hospital cardiac arrest	939	Targeted temperature 33 or 36°C	Mortality	There were no significant differences between the two groups in neurologic function or death at 180 days.
Mourvillier, 2013[41]	RCT	Severe bacterial meningitis	130	Targeted temperature 32 to 34°C for 48 hours using cold IV fluids	Glasgow outcome scale score at 3 months	Moderate hypothermia did not improve outcome in patients with severe bacterial meningitis (unfavorable outcome, 86% (hypothermia) vs. 74% (control), RR, 2.17, 95% CI, 0.78–6.01, P = 0.13).

CI, confidence interval; *IV,* intravenous; *RCT,* randomized controlled trial; *ROSC,* return of spontaneous circulation; *RR,* relative risk.

Table 19-2 RCTs of Fever Control in Nonneurologic Critically Ill Patients

Study, Year	Setting	Population	Patients (n)	Intervention	Duration	Main Findings
Gozzoli, 2001[50]	Surgical ICU	Postoperative	38	External cooling	24 hours	Treatment of fever had no effect on length of ICU stay, duration of hospital stay, and ICU mortality
Schortgen, 2012[51]	Medical ICUs	Septic shock	200	External cooling	48 hours	Decreased vasopressor requirement and decreased mortality at 14 days
Bernard, 1997[53]	Surgical, trauma, and medical centers	Severe sepsis	455	IV ibuprofen	Every 6 hours for 48 hours	No significant improvement of mortality rate at 30 days
Morris, 2010[54]	Medical hospitals	Critically ill	53	IV ibuprofen	Every 4 hours for 24 hours	No significant differences in renal function, bleeding, or mortality
Schulman, 2005[55]	Trauma ICU	Trauma	82	Enteral acetaminophen (paracetamol) every 6 hours for >38.5°C External cooling added for >39.5°C	Febrile episode	Terminated early because of strong trend to higher mortality rate (P = .06) in intervention group

ICU, intensive care unit; *IV,* intravenous; *RCT,* randomized controlled trial.

Table 19-3 **Large-Scale Observational Studies Assessing Fever in Critically Ill Patients**

Study, Year	Study Design	Population	Patients, n (Infected %)	Timing of Fever Record	Primary Outcome	Infected Group	Noninfected Group
Young, 2012[26]	Retrospective	ICU	636,051 (20.8%)	First 24 hours in ICU	Hospital mortality	Increased peak temperature was associated with decreased mortality.	Peak temperature >39.0°C was associated with increased mortality.
Lee, 2012[32]	Prospective	ICU stay >48 hours	1425 (42.5%)	ICU stay	28-day mortality	Fever was not associated with mortality. NSAID or acetaminophen (paracetamol) use was associated with increased mortality.	High fever (>39.5°C) was associated with mortality. NSAIDs or acetaminophen (paracetamol) use was not associated with mortality.
Kushimoto, 2013[31]	Prospective	Severe sepsis	624 (100%)	Initial day of severe sepsis	28-day mortality	Hypothermia (<36.5) was associated with increased mortality and organ failure.	-

ICU, intensive care unit; *NSAID,* nonsteroidal anti-inflammatory drug.

One small RCT (Table 19-2) compared enteral acetaminophen (paracetamol) (650 mg every 6 hours for the febrile episode) for temperatures greater than 38.5°C with additional external cooling for temperatures greater than 40°C to a specified fever control regimen in 82 trauma patients without traumatic brain injury. There were no significant differences in infections between the two groups; however, a trend to increased mortality in the aggressive fever control group (mortality: aggressive vs. permissive, 16% vs. 3%; *P* = .06) resulted in premature termination of the RCT at an interim analysis.[55]

LARGE-SCALE OBSERVATIONAL STUDIES AND ONGOING RCTS

The association of fever and mortality may be different in critically ill patients who have infection compared with those who do not have infection. Two separate, relevant large-scale observational studies were published in 2012.

A large retrospective study using two independent cohorts (Australia and New Zealand, n=269,078; United Kingdom, n=366,973) tested whether peak temperature in the first 24 hours after ICU admission was associated with altered hospital mortality. In critically ill patients with infection, increased peak body temperature in the first 24 hours after ICU admission was associated with decreased hospital mortality compared with patients with normal body temperature (36.5 to 36.9°C), resulting in the hypothesis that fever control in patients with infection may be harmful. On the other hand, analysis of the patients without infection revealed that body temperature above 40.0°C was associated with increased hospital mortality[26] (Table 19-3). The inability to assess cause and effect limits the value of

this study. Fever could simply identify sicker patients with a poorer prognosis.

Consistent with the finding of harmful effects of fever in patients without infection, another prospective observational cohort study of critically ill patients in Korea and Japan (n=1425) demonstrated that noninfectious critically ill patients who had maximum body temperature above 39.5°C during their ICU stay had increased 28-day mortality compared with patients who had normal body temperature (36.5 to 37.4°C)[32] (Table 19-3). The study also demonstrated that mortality in septic patients receiving acetaminophen (paracetamol) or NSAIDs was increased compared with patients who did not receive fever control. This finding was not present in the nonseptic patient group. When patients were stratified by temperature, 28-day mortality was lower in patients with low-grade fever (body temperature 37.5 to 38.4°C) as compared with patients with normal body temperature (36.5 to 37.4°C) (16.9% vs. 24.5%; odds ratio 0.45; 95% confidence interval 0.24 to –0.85; *P* = .014). The 28-day mortality of patients with medium-grade fever (38.5 to 39.4°C) was 23.8% and that of high-grade fever (39.4°C) was 30.5%, not significantly different from the normal body temperature group. Conversely, a prospective observational study that enrolled 624 critically ill patients with severe sepsis (Table 19-3) demonstrated that hypothermia (≤36.5°C) was associated with increased 28-day mortality compared with nonhypothermia (28-day mortality, 38.1% vs. 17.9%; odds ratio, 2.78; 95% confidence interval, 1.56 to 4.97; *P* < .001).[31] These three inconsistent results from the observational study of critically ill patients with infection emphasize the need for future RCTs on fever control.

Fortunately, there are several ongoing RCTs of fever control in the critically ill[56] (Table 19-4). A Phase IIb RCT (the Permissive Hyperthermia Through Avoidance of

Table 19-4 **Ongoing RCT Assessing Fever in Critically Ill Patients**					
Trial Name	Population	Patients (n)	Intervention	Control	Primary Endpoint
HEAT[57]	Critically ill patients with infection	700	Intravenous paracetamol	Placebo (5% dextrose)	Days alive and free of ICU support out of 28 days
CASS[58]	Septic shock	560	Mild hypothermia (cooling to 32 to 34°C)	No intervention for fever	30-day mortality
FACE II	Febrile patients in ICU (≧38.0)	310	Fever control ≤38.0°C (cooling or medications)	Fever control ≤39.5°C (cooling or medications)	Days alive and free of ICU support out of 28 days

CASS, The Cooling And Surviving Septic Shock; *FACE II*, Fever and Antipyretic in Critically Ill Evaluation Phase II randomized controlled trial; *HEAT*, Permissive Hyperthermia Through Avoidance of Paracetamol in Known or Suspected Infection in ICU; *ICU*, intensive care unit.

Paracetamol in Known or Suspected Infection in ICU [HEAT] trial) is evaluating the safety and efficacy of intravenous acetaminophen (paracetamol) (1 gram every 6 hours during antimicrobial therapy in the ICU) in febrile critically ill patients with infection. It is being conducted at 22 ICUs in Australia and New Zealand (sample size = 700 patients; primary outcome variable = ICU support-free survival at 28 days).[57]

In addition, a Phase III RCT (the Cooling and Surviving Septic Shock [CASS] study, NCT01455116) evaluating the efficacy and safety of mild induced hypothermia (targeting temperature 32 to 34°C for 24 hours followed by 48 hours of fever control at 36 to 38°C for 72 hours) in 560 severe sepsis patients is being conducted in seven Danish ICUs.[58] There are to be 280 patients in the mild induced hypothermia group (targeting temperature 32 to 34°C for 24 hours followed by 48 hours of fever control at 36 to 38°C for 72 hours using either an internal or external cooling system) and 280 patients in the normothermia for 24 hours group; the primary outcome variable is 30-day mortality.

CONCLUSION

Further randomized controlled study trials are needed to determine if fever control in critically ill patients with severe sepsis/septic shock is of value and to identify the patients who are most likely to benefit. Cooling is simple, safe and easily implemented. Cooling should be considered for patients in septic shock, in particular those who are receiving high-dose vasopressors or inotropes, those who have marked tachycardia, and those who have progressive secondary organ dysfunction. However, this approach represents opinion and is not supported by data.

AUTHORS' RECOMMENDATIONS

- There is substantial evidence that fever control has beneficial clinical effects in neurologic critically ill patients.
- One RCT shows beneficial effects of external cooling on outcomes in septic shock and suggests that cooling of febrile patients who have septic shock should be considered. Significant methodological concerns, though, limit the extrapolation of these findings.
- In large-scale trials, the associations between mortality in critically ill patients with infection and body temperature are inconsistent.
- There are several ongoing RCTs of fever control in critically ill patients.

REFERENCES

1. O'Grady NP, Barie PS, Bartlett JG, et al. American College of Critical Care M, Infectious Diseases Society of A. Guidelines for evaluation of new fever in critically ill adult patients: 2008 update from the American college of critical care medicine and the infectious diseases society of America. *Crit Care Med.* 2008;36:1330–1349.
2. Niven DJ, Leger C, Stelfox HT, Laupland KB. Fever in the critically ill: a review of epidemiology, immunology, and management. *J Intensive Care Med.* 2012;27:290–297.
3. Circiumaru B, Baldock G, Cohen J. A prospective study of fever in the intensive care unit. *Intensive Care Med.* 1999;25:668–673.
4. Schortgen F. Fever in sepsis. *Minerva Anestesiol.* 2012;78:1254–1264.
5. Niven DJ, Stelfox HT, Shahpori R, Laupland KB. Fever in adult ICUs: an interrupted time series analysis. *Crit Care Med.* 2013;41:1863–1869.
6. Kawai T, Akira S. The role of pattern-recognition receptors in innate immunity: update on toll-like receptors. *Nature Immunol.* 2010;11:373–384.
7. Ivanov AI, Pero RS, Scheck AC, Romanovsky AA. Prostaglandin e(2)-synthesizing enzymes in fever: differential transcriptional regulation. *Am J Physiol Regul Integr Comp Physiol.* 2002;283:R1104–R1117.
8. Steiner AA, Ivanov AI, Serrats J, et al. Cellular and molecular bases of the initiation of fever. *PLoS Biol.* 2006;4:e284.
9. Nakamura K. Central circuitries for body temperature regulation and fever. *Am J Physiol Regul Integr Comp Physiol.* 2011;301: R1207–R1228.
10. Hasday JD, Thompson C, Singh IS. Fever, immunity, and molecular adaptations. *Compr Physiol.* 2014;4:109–148.
11. Matsumura K, Cao C, Ozaki M, Morii H, Nakadate K, Watanabe Y. Brain endothelial cells express cyclooxygenase-2 during lipopolysaccharide-induced fever: light and electron microscopic immunocytochemical studies. *J Neurosci.* 1998;18:6279–6289.
12. Yamagata K, Matsumura K, Inoue W, et al. Coexpression of microsomal-type prostaglandin e synthase with cyclooxygenase-2 in brain endothelial cells of rats during endotoxin-induced fever. *J Neurosci.* 2001;21:2669–2677.
13. Launey Y, Nesseler N, Malledant Y, Seguin P. Clinical review: fever in septic ICU patients–friend or foe? *Crit Care.* 2011;15:222.
14. Laupland KB. Fever in the critically ill medical patient. *Crit Care Med.* 2009;37:S273–S278.
15. Ozveri ES, Bekraki A, Cingi A, et al. The effect of hyperthermic preconditioning on the immune system in rat peritonitis. *Intensive Care Med.* 1999;25:1155–1159.
16. Jiang Q, Cross AS, Singh IS, Chen TT, Viscardi RM, Hasday JD. Febrile core temperature is essential for optimal host defense in bacterial peritonitis. *Infection Immun.* 2000;68:1265–1270.
17. Murapa P, Ward MR, Gandhapudi SK, Woodward JG, D'Orazio SE. Heat shock factor 1 protects mice from rapid death during listeria monocytogenes infection by regulating expression of tumor necrosis factor alpha during fever. *Infection Immun.* 2011;79: 177–184.
18. Hasday JD, Singh IS. Fever and the heat shock response: distinct, partially overlapping processes. *Cell Stress Chaperones.* 2000;5: 471–480.

19. Sucker C, Zacharowski K, Thielmann M, Hartmann M. Heat shock inhibits lipopolysaccharide-induced tissue factor activity in human whole blood. *Thromb J.* 2007;5:13.

20. Villar J, Ribeiro SP, Mullen JB, Kuliszewski M, Post M, Slutsky AS. Induction of the heat shock response reduces mortality rate and organ damage in a sepsis-induced acute lung injury model. *Crit Care Med.* 1994;22:914–921.

21. Sun Z, Andersson R. Nf-kappab activation and inhibition: a review. *Shock.* 2002;18:99–106.

22. Small PM, Tauber MG, Hackbarth CJ, Sande MA. Influence of body temperature on bacterial growth rates in experimental pneumococcal meningitis in rabbits. *Infection Immun.* 1986;52:484–487.

23. Mackowiak PA, Marling-Cason M, Cohen RL. Effects of temperature on antimicrobial susceptibility of bacteria. *J Infect Dis.* 1982;145:550–553.

24. Manthous CA, Hall JB, Olson D, et al. Effect of cooling on oxygen consumption in febrile critically ill patients. *Am J Respir Crit Care Med.* 1995;151:10–14.

25. Laupland KB, Shahpori R, Kirkpatrick AW, Ross T, Gregson DB, Stelfox HT. Occurrence and outcome of fever in critically ill adults. *Crit Care Med.* 2008;36:1531–1535.

26. Young PJ, Saxena M, Beasley R, et al. Early peak temperature and mortality in critically ill patients with or without infection. *Intensive Care Med.* January 31, 2012. [Epub head of print].

27. Barie PS, Hydo LJ, Eachempati SR. Causes and consequences of fever complicating critical surgical illness. *Surg Infect.* 2004;5:145–159.

28. Pittet D, Thievent B, Wenzel RP, Li N, Auckenthaler R, Suter PM. Bedside prediction of mortality from bacteremic sepsis. A dynamic analysis of ICU patients. *Am J Respir Crit Care Med.* 1996;153:684–693.

29. Osmon S, Warren D, Seiler SM, Shannon W, Fraser VJ, Kollef MH. The influence of infection on hospital mortality for patients requiring > 48 h of intensive care. *Chest.* 2003;124:1021–1029.

30. Peres Bota D, Lopes Ferreira F, Melot C, Vincent JL. Body temperature alterations in the critically ill. *Intensive Care Med.* 2004;30:811–816.

31. Kushimoto S, Gando S, Saitoh D, et al. The impact of body temperature abnormalities on the disease severity and outcome in patients with severe sepsis: an analysis from a multicenter, prospective survey of severe sepsis. *Crit Care.* 2013;17:R271.

32. Lee BH, Inui D, Suh GY, et al. Fever, Antipyretic in Critically ill patients Evaluation Study G. Association of body temperature and antipyretic treatments with mortality of critically ill patients with and without sepsis: multi-centered prospective observational study. *Crit Care.* 2012;16:R33.

33. Polderman KH. Induced hypothermia and fever control for prevention and treatment of neurological injuries. *Lancet.* 2008;371:1955–1969.

34. Saini M, Saqqur M, Kamruzzaman A, Lees KR, Shuaib A, Investigators V. Effect of hyperthermia on prognosis after acute ischemic stroke. *Stroke.* 2009;40:3051–3059.

35. Hajat C, Hajat S, Sharma P. Effects of poststroke pyrexia on stroke outcome: a meta-analysis of studies in patients. *Stroke.* 2000;31:410–414.

36. Diringer MN, Reaven NL, Funk SE, Uman GC. Elevated body temperature independently contributes to increased length of stay in neurologic intensive care unit patients. *Crit Care Med.* 2004;32:1489–1495.

37. Bernard SA, Gray TW, Buist MD, et al. Treatment of comatose survivors of out-of-hospital cardiac arrest with induced hypothermia. *N Eng J Med.* 2002;346:557–563.

38. Hypothermia after Cardiac Arrest Study Group. Mild therapeutic hypothermia to improve the neurologic outcome after cardiac arrest. *N Eng J Med.* 2002;346:549–556.

39. Nielsen N, Wetterslev J, Cronberg T, et al. Targeted temperature management at 33°C versus 36°C after cardiac arrest. *N Eng J Med.* 2013;369:2197–2206.

40. Rittenberger JC, Callaway CW. Temperature management and modern post-cardiac arrest care. *N Eng J Med.* 2013;369:2262–2263.

41. Mourvillier B, Tubach F, van de Beek D, et al. Induced hypothermia in severe bacterial meningitis: a randomized clinical trial. *JAMA.* 2013;310:2174–2183.

42. Shann F. Antipyretics in severe sepsis. *Lancet.* 1995;345:338.

43. Eyers S, Weatherall M, Shirtcliffe P, Perrin K, Beasley R. The effect on mortality of antipyretics in the treatment of influenza infection: systematic review and meta-analysis. *J R Soc Med.* 2010;103:403–411.

44. Haupt MT, Jastremski MS, Clemmer TP, Metz CA, Goris GB. Effect of ibuprofen in patients with severe sepsis: a randomized, double-blind, multicenter study. The ibuprofen study group. *Crit Care Med.* 1991;19:1339–1347.

45. Geurts M, Macleod MR, Kollmar R, Kremer PH, van der Worp HB. Therapeutic hypothermia and the risk of infection: a systematic review and meta-analysis. *Crit Care Med.* 2014;42:231–242.

46. dRehman T. Deboisblanc BP. Persistent fever in the ICU. *Chest.* 2014;145:158–165.

47. Egi M. Fever and antipyretic therapy in critically ill patients. *J Jpn Soc Intensive Care Med.* 2011;18.

48. Arons MM, Wheeler AP, Bernard GR, et al. Effects of ibuprofen on the physiology and survival of hypothermic sepsis. Ibuprofen in sepsis study group. *Crit Care Med.* 1999;27:699–707.

49. Lefrant JY, Muller L, de La Coussaye JE, et al. Temperature measurement in intensive care patients: comparison of urinary bladder, oesophageal, rectal, axillary, and inguinal methods versus pulmonary artery core method. *Intensive Care Med.* 2003;29:414–418.

50. Gozzoli V, Schottker P, Suter PM, Ricou B. Is it worth treating fever in intensive care unit patients? Preliminary results from a randomized trial of the effect of external cooling. *Arch Intern Med.* 2001;161:121–123.

51. Schortgen F, Clabault K, Katsahian S, et al. Fever control using external cooling in septic shock: a randomized controlled trial. *Am J Respir Crit Care Med.* 2012;185:1088–1095.

52. Russell JA. Control of fever in septic shock: Should we care or intervene? *Am J Respir Crit Care Med.* 2012;185:1040–1041.

53. Bernard GR, Wheeler AP, Russell JA, et al. The effects of ibuprofen on the physiology and survival of patients with sepsis. The ibuprofen in sepsis study group. *N Eng J Med.* 1997;336:912–918.

54. Morris PE, Promes JT, Guntupalli KK, Wright PE, Arons MM. A multi-center, randomized, double-blind, parallel, placebo-controlled trial to evaluate the efficacy, safety, and pharmacokinetics of intravenous ibuprofen for the treatment of fever in critically ill and non-critically ill adults. *Crit Care.* 2010;14:R125.

55. Schulman CI, Namias N, Doherty J, et al. The effect of antipyretic therapy upon outcomes in critically ill patients: a randomized, prospective study. *Surg Infect.* 2005;6:369–375.

56. Taccone FS, Saxena M, Schortgen F. What's new with fever control in the ICU. *Intensive Care Med.* 2014;40:1147–1150.

57. Young PJ, Saxena MK, Bellomo R, et al. The heat trial: a protocol for a multicentre randomised placebo-controlled trial of iv paracetamol in ICU patients with fever and infection. *Crit Care Resusc.* 2012;14:290–296.

58. The Cooling in Septic Shock (CASS) study. Danish Procalcitonin Study Group. NCT01455116.

20 | What Fluids Should I Give to the Critically Ill Patient? What Fluids Should I Avoid?

Anders Perner

Many critically ill patients are hypovolemic, which may result in impaired cardiac output and organ perfusion, leading to poor outcome. Therefore fluid therapy is a mainstay in the resuscitation of critically ill patients, and fluid is one of the most frequently used interventions. Thus, one third of all patients in intensive care units (ICUs) worldwide receive fluid for resuscitation each day.[1] Therefore differences in patient outcomes among different types of fluids will affect global health, and differences in direct and related costs will affect health-care expenditure.

When deciding what fluid to give a critically ill patient, clinicians may choose between colloid and crystalloid solutions, and if the latter is chosen between saline and balanced salt solutions. Blood products may be considered for resuscitation of hemorrhagic shock for their oxygen carrying and hemostatic properties and for their colloidal effects.

CRYSTALLOIDS

Crystalloids are salt solutions used for intravenous infusion. Presently, none of the commercially available solutions contains electrolyte and buffer concentrations comparable to those of plasma; in particular, bicarbonate is very rarely found in these solutions.

Isotonic saline (0.9% sodium chloride) is still frequently used despite concentrations of sodium and chloride (154 mmol/L) well above those found in plasma. Alternatively, so-called balanced salt solutions include Ringer's lactate (or Hartmann solution) and Ringer's acetate. The concentrations of electrolytes in these solutions better resemble those of plasma, and most preparations include sodium, chloride, potassium, and calcium. However, bicarbonate is normally not included because bicarbonate-containing fluids, particularly those in plastic containers, have a shorter shelf-life. Instead, the balanced solutions are buffered with lactate or different combinations of acetate, gluconate, and malate.

COLLOIDS

Colloid solutions contain large molecules that prolong the time the fluid remains in the circulation. The molecules used to obtain the colloidal and thereby volume expansion are human albumin or synthetically modified sugars or collagens. The most frequently used synthetic colloid solutions are hydroxyethyl starch (HES), gelatin, and dextrans.

Colloid solutions have been extensively administered for volume expansion in critically ill patients, but clinical practice has varied, mainly because of regional differences in the types of colloid solutions available.[1] Moreover, in recent years, results of large trials have examined the effects and side effects of colloids in critically ill patients.[2-4] These trials raise questions regarding the clinical efficacy of colloids and have clearly demonstrated some harmful effects in groups of critically ill patients.

In the following section, I describe what fluids to give to critically ill patients and what fluids to avoid. My recommendations are based on the results of recently updated high-quality systematic reviews and recently conducted high-quality randomized trials. These findings allow evidence-based choices to be made and are likely to improve care and outcome and reduce costs.

IN GENERAL ICU PATIENTS, WHAT FLUIDS SHOULD I GIVE AND WHAT SHOULD I AVOID?

The short answer is to give crystalloids and avoid the synthetic colloids (HES, gelatins, and dextrans). The systematic review of the Cochrane Collaboration comparing crystalloid with colloid solutions showed that crystalloids were associated with improved mortality compared with HES solutions, whereas there were no differences in mortality between crystalloids and the other colloid solutions analyzed (albumin, gelatins, and dextrans).[5] The increased mortality with the use of HES is most likely mediated through impaired kidney function and hemostasis, resulting in an increased use of renal replacement therapy and increased bleeding (Table 20-1). A recently published large randomized trial, the CRISTAL (Colloids Versus Crystalloids for the Resuscitation of the Critically Ill) trial,[6] was not included in the Cochrane analysis. The CRISTAL trial compared any crystalloid to any colloid solution in ICU patients with shock. The results indicated that colloids (mainly HES) versus crystalloids (mainly saline) improved 90-day mortality, which was a secondary outcome measure. The primary outcome measure, 28-day mortality, did not differ between the groups, and the trial had high risk of bias in several domains (unblinded, uncertain allocation concealment, and baseline imbalance).[7] Moreover, the results differed from those of the high-quality trials,[2-4] and the editor argued in an accompanying editorial for cautious interpretation of these findings and advocated that crystalloids should be the first-line fluid in patients with shock.[8]

The interpretation of the Cochrane meta-analyses on crystalloid versus gelatin and dextran solutions was hampered by low-quality trial data and few patients and events and therefore wide confidence intervals on the point estimates.[5] Because gelatins and dextrans have registered side effects that are similar to those observed with HES, these synthetic colloids should be avoided in critically ill patients. This recommendation is substantiated by the fact that no patient group in any high-quality trial has been shown to benefit from any colloid solution, including the trial using human albumin (Table 20-1), although the latter showed that albumin is safe to administer to critically ill patients, excluding those with trauma.[2] As a blood product fractionated from human plasma, albumin is an expensive and limited resource; thus it is of limited value in many health-care systems. The same may be said of red blood cells, plasma, and platelets, but these products have a larger potential for harm than albumin, and their safety has not been ensured in large trials in the critically ill. Liberal transfusion of red blood cells may even increase the mortality of general ICU patients, as observed in the Transfusion Requirement in Critical Care (TRICC) trial.[9] Thus blood products should only be used for patients with severe anemia or bleeding or as a prophylactic in high-risk patients with severely impaired hemostasis.

Overall, the recommendations of the European Society of Intensive Care Medicine Task Force on colloids support the notion that crystalloid solutions should be preferred over colloids in the vast majority of critically ill patients.[10]

The choice between the different crystalloid solutions is more difficult because there are no data from high-quality trials supporting this decision. Saline may be preferred in patients at risk of brain edema because the high plasma concentrations of sodium may reduce brain swelling and intracranial pressure. Conversely, severe acidosis may be worsened by saline-induced hyperchloremia. A balanced crystalloid solution may be the better choice in these patients. Observations in cohort studies have suggested that the use of balanced crystalloids reduces the risk of acute kidney injury and even mortality as compared with the use of saline.[11,12] These results need to be confirmed in randomized trials before implementing them into clinical practice because of the high risk of bias in observational studies of critically ill patients.

IN PATIENTS WITH SEPSIS, WHAT FLUIDS SHOULD I GIVE AND WHAT SHOULD I AVOID?

Again, the short answer is give crystalloids and avoid the synthetic colloids (HES, gelatins, and dextrans). There are high-quality data to guide clinicians on choice of fluids in patients with sepsis. An updated systematic review showed that crystalloids are superior to HES with respect to mortality, use of renal replacement therapy and blood products, and adverse reactions.[13] There are no high-quality data on the other synthetic colloids, but they have the

Table 20-1 Characteristics and Results of the Trials with Low Risk of Bias Randomizing Critically Ill Patients to Colloids versus Crystalloids

Trial	The SAFE Trial[2]	The 6S Trial[3]	The CHEST[4]
Colloid solution	4% Albumin	6% Tetrastarch in Ringer's acetate	6% Tetrastarch in saline
Crystalloid comparator	Saline	Ringer's acetate	Saline
Patients	Adult ICU patients	Adult ICU patients with severe sepsis	Adult ICU patients
Number of patients randomized	7000	805	7000
Outcomes	**Relative Risks (95% confidence intervals)**		
Mortality	0.99 (0.91-1.09)	1.17 (1.01-1.36)	1.06 (0.96-1.18)
Renal replacement therapy	Similar duration of therapy in the two groups	1.35 (1.01-1.80)	1.21 (1.00-1.45)
Bleeding	—	1.55 (1.16-2.08)	—
Use of blood transfusion	Higher volume of red blood cells given in the albumin vs. the saline group	1.28 (1.12-1.47)	Higher volume of red blood cells given in the HES vs. the saline group
Adverse reactions*		1.56 (0.97-2.53)	1.86 (1.46-2.38)

*The definitions of adverse reactions differed between trials.
CHEST, Crystalloid versus Hydroxyethyl Starch Trial; *HES,* hydroxyethyl starch; *ICU,* intensive care unit; *SAFE,* Saline versus Albumin Fluid Evaluation; *6S,* Scandinavian Starch for Severe Sepsis/Septic Shock.

same registered side effects as HES; therefore they should be avoided in sepsis.

Regarding albumin, there are now two large trials comparing albumin with crystalloids in patients with sepsis: the subgroup analysis of the SAFE (Saline versus Albumin Fluid Evaluation) trial and the recent ALBIOS (Albumin Italian Outcome Sepsis) trial.[2,14] Neither showed significantly improved mortality, use of life support, or length of ICU or hospital stay with albumin as compared with saline. The lack of benefit is supported by a recently updated systematic review that included trials of patients with sepsis regardless of severity.[15] Extensive subgroup and sensitivity analysis was applied to challenge the overall result; the conclusions remained unchanged. Because albumin is an expensive and limited resource, it may be reasonable to avoid its use in patients with sepsis before we have identified subgroups of patients (e.g., early shock) who will benefit from albumin.

IN PATIENTS WITH TRAUMA, WHAT FLUIDS SHOULD I GIVE AND WHAT SHOULD I AVOID?

Saline or isotonic balanced salt solutions should be used in patients with trauma, in particular those with obvious traumatic brain injury, whereas colloids should be avoided. The latter is particular true for albumin. All of the balanced crystalloids have concentrations of sodium below that of saline, and Ringer's lactate and Hartmann solutions are hypotonic, which may worsen brain edema.

The best evidence on the choice of fluid in trauma comes from the predefined subgroup analysis of the 1186 patients with trauma in the SAFE study.[2] Albumin increased 28-day mortality in these patients, an effect that may have been mediated by increased intracranial pressure in those with traumatic brain injury.[16,17] If this is an effect caused by albumin crossing a leaky blood–brain barrier, then the same may apply for the synthetic colloid solutions. In addition, the synthetic colloids directly impair coagulation, and HES as compared with saline was shown to increase the use of blood products in patients with blunt trauma.[18] In the latter trial, there were no data on bleeding, but a nonsignificant 86% relative risk increase in mortality with HES was observed.[19] In addition, HES has been shown to increase bleeding in patients with severe sepsis and those undergoing surgery.[20,21] There are presently not enough high-quality data to support that any of the synthetic colloids can be used safely in trauma; therefore all synthetic colloids (HES, gelatins, and dextrans) should be avoided in these patients.

IN PATIENTS WITH HEMORRHAGIC SHOCK, WHAT FLUIDS SHOULD I GIVE AND WHAT SHOULD I AVOID?

A crystalloid solution should be used in patients with life-threatening bleeding, and blood products, including red blood cells, plasma, and platelets, should be considered early. Synthetic colloids (HES, gelatins, and dextrans) should be avoided because they impair hemostasis and increase bleeding. The synthetic colloids induce coagulopathy, and HES and gelatin have been shown to increase bleeding compared with crystalloids in patients undergoing surgery.[21,22] Furthermore, HES has been shown to increase bleeding in severe sepsis.[20] Balanced blood component therapy mimicking full blood should be considered early in patients with hemorrhagic shock, including those with trauma,[23] but there are still no high-quality data supporting this approach.

IN PATIENTS WITH BURN INJURY, WHAT FLUIDS SHOULD I GIVE AND WHAT SHOULD I AVOID?

There are no data from high-quality trials that can inform us on the choice of fluids in patients with burn injury. Patients with burn injury likely represent a specific entity because of the massive leak of fluids in the burned areas. These patients receive high volumes of fluid, and Ringer's lactate solution has traditionally been used. There are no updated systematic reviews comparing crystalloid and colloid therapy for these patients, but there are at least three smaller randomized trials, two comparing Ringer's lactate solution with albumin[24,25] and one comparing Ringer's lactate solution with HES.[26] Taken together, the trial results do not support the use of colloids for patients with burn injury, but the quality of the evidence is low. Therefore it is difficult to give firm recommendations, but high fluid volumes are often needed, and these patients are at increased risk of dysnatremias and acidosis. Thus high volume saline resuscitation should probably be avoided.

CONCLUSION

Updated systematic reviews, including data from recent high-quality trials, show that crystalloid solutions should be used for the vast majority of critically ill patients. No critically ill patients should be given HES, and gelatins and dextrans should be avoided because of lack of safety data and concerns about harmful side effects. Patients with traumatic brain injury should not be given albumin. However, there are no high-quality data showing an overall benefit of albumin, which is an expensive and limited resource.

AUTHOR'S RECOMMENDATIONS

- Crystalloid solutions should be used for critically ill patients.
- No high-quality data have shown a benefit of colloid solutions.
- HES should not be given because of its life-threatening side effects.
- The safety of gelatins and dextrans has not been adequately assessed.
- Albumin is an expensive and limited resource without apparent benefit for patients.

REFERENCES

1. Finfer S, Liu B, Taylor C, et al. Resuscitation fluid use in critically ill adults: an international cross-sectional study in 391 intensive care units. *Crit Care*. 2010;14:R185.
2. Finfer S, Bellomo R, Boyce N, French J, Myburgh J, Norton R. A comparison of albumin and saline for fluid resuscitation in the intensive care unit. *N Engl J Med*. 2004;350:2247–2256.
3. Perner A, Haase N, Guttormsen AB, et al. Hydroxyethyl starch 130/0.42 versus Ringer's acetate in severe sepsis. *N Engl J Med*. 2012;367:124–134.
4. Myburgh JA, Finfer S, Bellomo R, et al. Hydroxyethyl starch or saline for fluid resuscitation in intensive care. *N Engl J Med*. 2012;367:1901–1911.
5. Perel P, Roberts I, Ker K. Colloids versus crystalloids for fluid resuscitation in critically ill patients. *Cochrane Database Syst Rev*. 2013;2:CD000567.
6. Annane D, Siami S, Jaber S, et al. Effects of fluid resuscitation with colloids vs crystalloids on mortality in critically ill patients presenting with hypovolemic shock: the CRISTAL randomized trial. *JAMA*. 2013;310:1809–1817.
7. Perner A, Haase N, Wetterslev J. Mortality in patients with hypovolemic shock treated with colloids or crystalloids. *JAMA*. 2014;311:1067.
8. Seymour CW, Angus DC. Making a pragmatic choice for fluid resuscitation in critically ill patients. *JAMA*. 2013;310:1803–1804.
9. Hebert PC, Wells G, Blajchman MA, et al. A multicenter, randomized, controlled clinical trial of transfusion requirements in critical care. *N Engl J Med*. 1999;340:409–417.
10. Reinhart K, Perner A, Sprung CL, et al. Consensus statement of the ESICM task force on colloid volume therapy in critically ill patients. *Intensive Care Med*. 2012;38:368–383.
11. Yunos NM, Bellomo R, Hegarty C, Story D, Ho L, Bailey M. Association between a chloride-liberal vs chloride-restrictive intravenous fluid administration strategy and kidney injury in critically ill adults. *JAMA*. 2012;308:1566–1572.
12. Raghunathan K, Shaw A, Nathanson B, et al. Association between the choice of IV crystalloid and in-hospital mortality among critically ill adults with sepsis. *Crit Care Med*. 2014;42:1585–1591.
13. Haase N, Perner A, Hennings LI, et al. Hydroxyethyl starch 130/0.38–0.45 versus crystalloid or albumin in patients with sepsis: systematic review with meta-analysis and trial sequential analysis. *BMJ*. 2013;346:f839.
14. Caironi P, Tognoni G, Masson S, et al. Albumin replacement in patients with severe sepsis or septic shock. *N Engl J Med*. 2014;370:1412–1421.
15. Patel A, Laffan MA, Waheed U, Brett SJ. Randomised trials of human albumin for adults with sepsis: systematic review and meta-analysis with trial sequential analysis of all-cause mortality. *BMJ*. 2014;349:g4561.
16. Myburgh J, Cooper DJ, Finfer S, et al. Saline or albumin for fluid resuscitation in patients with traumatic brain injury. *N Engl J Med*. 2007;357:874–884.
17. Cooper DJ, Myburgh J, Heritier S, et al. Albumin resuscitation for traumatic brain injury: is intracranial hypertension the cause of increased mortality? *J Neurotrauma*. 2013;30:512–518.
18. James MF, Michell WL, Joubert IA, Nicol AJ, Navsaria PH, Gillespie RS. Resuscitation with hydroxyethyl starch improves renal function and lactate clearance in penetrating trauma in a randomized controlled study: the FIRST trial (Fluids in Resuscitation of Severe Trauma). *Br J Anaesth*. 2011;107:693–702.
19. James MFM, Michell WL, Joubert IA, Nicol AJ, Navsaria PH, Gillespie RS. Reply from the authors. *Br J Anaesth*. 2012;108:160–161.
20. Haase N, Wetterslev J, Winkel P, Perner A. Bleeding and risk of death with hydroxyethyl starch in severe sepsis: post hoc analyses of a randomized clinical trial. *Intensive Care Med*. 2013;39:2126–2134.
21. Rasmussen KC, Johansson PI, Hojskov M, et al. Hydroxyethyl starch reduces coagulation competence and increases blood loss during major surgery: results from a randomized controlled trial. *Ann Surg*. 2014;259:249–254.
22. Mittermayr M, Streif W, Haas T, et al. Hemostatic changes after crystalloid or colloid fluid administration during major orthopedic surgery: the role of fibrinogen administration. *Anesth Analg*. 2007;105:905–917.
23. Johansson PI, Sorensen AM, Larsen CF, et al. Low hemorrhage-related mortality in trauma patients in a Level I trauma center employing transfusion packages and early thromboelastography-directed hemostatic resuscitation with plasma and platelets. *Transfusion*. 2013;53:3088–3099.
24. Goodwin CW, Dorethy J, Lam V, Pruitt Jr BA. Randomized trial of efficacy of crystalloid and colloid resuscitation on hemodynamic response and lung water following thermal injury. *Ann Surg*. 1983;197:520–531.
25. Cooper AB, Cohn SM, Zhang HS, Hanna K, Stewart TE, Slutsky AS. Five percent albumin for adult burn shock resuscitation: lack of effect on daily multiple organ dysfunction score. *Transfusion*. 2006;46:80–89.
26. Bechir M, Puhan MA, Fasshauer M, Schuepbach RA, Stocker R, Neff TA. Early fluid resuscitation with hydroxyethyl starch 130/0.4 (6%) in severe burn injury: a randomized, controlled, double-blind clinical trial. *Crit Care*. 2013;17:R299.

21 Should Blood Glucose Be Tightly Controlled in the Intensive Care Unit?

Jean-Charles Preiser, Aurelie Thooft

Before 2001, the hyperglycemia found in most critically ill patients was considered to be a component of the stress response. Current understanding was completely changed by the publication of the seminal study by van den Berghe et al. in 2001.[1] This investigation compared an intensive insulin regimen targeting a blood glucose level between 80 and 110 mg/dL with a "conventional" management cohort in which blood glucose was treated only when above 200 mg/dL. The authors of the study demonstrated a 4% decrease in the absolute mortality of critically ill patients randomized to intensive insulin therapy. These unexpectedly impressive results triggered a huge wave of enthusiasm. Recommendations to implement tight glucose control in intensive care units (ICUs) were rapidly issued by several health-care agencies (Joint Commission on Accreditation of Healthcare Organization, the Institute for Healthcare Improvement, and the Volunteer Hospital Organization). Simultaneously, several different teams tried to reproduce the results and to examine the underlying mechanisms of the findings of the Leuven team. Overall, the results of the first Leuven study have not been reproduced. Nonetheless, these follow-up studies have given rise to several controversies and raised important but as yet unanswered questions for the physicians taking care of critically ill patients: What is the optimal value of blood glucose? What are the risks associated with hypoglycemia? What categories of patient might benefit from tight glucose control by intensive insulin therapy?

PATHOPHYSIOLOGY AND MECHANISM OF ACTION

It has long been recognized that critically ill patients tend to be hyperglycemic.[2] For many years, this was attributed to stress and was thought to be a part of the host response to critical illness. The Leuven studies started with the hypothesis that hyperglycemia was not just a biomarker. Rather, these investigators postulated that elevations in serum glucose contributed to the pathophysiology of critical illness. This proposal spawned the current field of investigation. The initial question might be reframed as, "What is the optimal blood glucose concentration in the critically ill patient?" Further exploration and investigation of this question are warranted.

The physiology behind "stress hyperglycemia" is complex. The elaboration of glucose, primarily by the liver, is known to be an essential component of the host's response. Gluconeogenesis reflects the energy demand that results from injury, ischemia, or other deleterious processes. White blood cells, the main effectors of the inflammatory response, are more or less obligate glucose users. Because the blood supply to injured tissue often has been interrupted or diminished, delivery is primarily through mass action across the intracellular matrix. Increases in concentration facilitate this movement. Gluconeogenesis, the process by which the liver synthesizes glucose, is driven primarily by the direct action of glucagon and epinephrine on hepatocytes. This is enhanced by cortisol and perhaps by inflammatory cytokines. In addition, these hormones, and the cytokines to some degree, limit the peripheral response to insulin. This latter effect has been termed *insulin resistance*, although there are no data in nonseptic patients or animals to indicate that the direct responses of the insulin signaling pathway are impaired. At some point, the process becomes maladaptive in the critically ill patient. This is especially true in sepsis and multiple-organ dysfunction. Thus the previously asked question must be expanded to examine the time course of stress hyperglycemia and the actual glucose concentration.

In experimental conditions, concentrations of glucose higher than 300 mg/dL are clearly deleterious.[3] Furthermore, new insights into the cellular mechanisms of glucose toxicity suggest a link among glucose, cytopathic hypoxia, and the production of reactive oxygen and nitrogen species.[4,5] However, it is essential to recognize that only clinical data can be used to define the optimal value for tight glucose control. Indeed, the ultimate proof that hyperglycemia is an independent risk factor for poor outcome in critically ill patients is lacking.[6] Importantly, insulin exerts effects other than the promotion of glucose metabolism and utilization. These include vasodilatory, anti-inflammatory, and antiapoptotic activities most easily viewed as homeostatic control mechanisms that limit some of the processes that occur in inflammation and other potentially injurious responses. Such a role for insulin might explain some of the beneficial but unexpected effects of intensive insulin therapy.

PRESENTATION OF AVAILABLE DATA BASED ON SYSTEMATIC REVIEW

It has been difficult to replicate the results of the Leuven study.[1] This inability leaves several practical questions unanswered. First, it is unclear just what constitutes "normoglycemia" in critical illness.[7] Retrospective data and the two Leuven studies[1,8] clearly indicate that a blood glucose higher than 180 mg/dL cannot be considered acceptable. However, the optimal target for blood glucose concentration remains unknown. Interestingly, several retrospective trials[9,10] found that patients in whom blood glucose was below 150 mg/dL had a better outcome than those with higher levels.

To solve the issues of the external validity of the Leuven study and the optimal blood glucose target, large single-center and multicenter prospective trials of tight glucose control using intensive insulin therapy comparing two ranges of blood glucose were launched. The designs of these trials (Table 21-1) were similar. All aimed to compare the effects of insulin therapy titrated to restore and maintain blood glucose between 80 and 110 mg/dL for adult studies and between 72 and 126 mg/dL for one study conducted in several mixed pediatric ICUs.[11] They differed in the target range of blood glucose for the control (nonintensive insulin therapy) group. The Normoglycemia in Intensive Care Evaluation—Survival Using Glucose Algorithm Regulation (NICE-SUGAR)[12] and GluControl trials[13] used a target value of 140 to 180 mg/dL. Both of the Leuven studies,[1,8] the VISEP (Efficacy of Volume Substitution and Insulin Therapy in Severe Sepsis) study,[14] and two other single-center large-scale trials[15,16] used a target value of 180 to 200 mg/dL. The CGAO-REA (Computerized Glucose Control in Critically Ill Patients) study[17] used a target value of less than 180 mg/dL, and the pediatric study has a target of 180 and 215 mg/dL.

The results of these trials are summarized in Table 21-1. Basically, there were no significant differences in the vital outcomes between the two groups, with the notable exceptions of the Leuven I study[1] and the NICE-SUGAR study, in opposite directions. Not surprisingly, tight glucose control by intensive insulin therapy is associated with a fourfold to sixfold increase in the incidence of hypoglycemia. This represents the major concern when starting intensive insulin therapy and leads to a major increase in the workload placed on the ICU care team.[18] A post hoc analysis of the NICE-SUGAR study revealed a strong, dose-dependent association between the risk of death and moderate (41 to 70 mg/dL) and severe (<40 mg/dL) hypoglycemia.[19] Although Macrae and associates[11] were unable to demonstrate an improvement of the primary outcome (number of days alive and free from mechanical ventilation at 30 days), they found a shortening of the length of stay and a decrease in health-care costs. In the VISEP and GluControl studies, the rate of hypoglycemia and the mortality in the patients who experienced at least one such episode (defined as blood glucose <40 mg/dL) were higher than in patients who did not experience hypoglycemia.[13,14] In contrast, in both Leuven studies,[1,8] patients with hypoglycemia had no detectable differences in outcome compared with patients who had no hypoglycemic episodes. This does not exclude the possibility that long-lasting hypoglycemia, with consequent decreases in glucose availability for tissues that are glucose dependent, may be deleterious or even life threatening. An accurate understanding of the consequences of hypoglycemia in critically ill patients clearly requires further investigation.

Systematic reviews and meta-analyses including data on glucose control recorded in the ICU and in other patients are also available. The design and main results of the seven meta-analyses[20-26] are summarized in Table 21-2. These analyses yielded different results, including the overall effects on mortality. The meta-analyses by Pittas and colleagues[20]

Table 21-1 Summary of the Prospective Large-Scale Randomized Controlled Trials of Tight Glucose Control by Intensive Insulin Therapy

	Study	No. of Subjects (Intervention/No Intervention)	Study Design	Intervention (Blood Glucose Target)	Control (Blood Glucose Target)	Primary Outcome Variable
Single center	van der Bergeh et al. (Leuven I), 2001	765/783	Single-blind	80–110 mg/dL	180–200 mg/dL	ICU mortality
	van der Bergeh et al. (Leuven II), 2006	595/605	Single-blind	80–110 mg/dL	180–200 mg/dL	ICU mortality
	Arabi, 2008	266/257	Single-blind	80–110 mg/dL	180–200 mg/dL	ICU mortality
	De La Rosa	254/250	Single-blind	80–110 mg/dL	180–200 mg/dL	28-day mortality
Multicenter	Brunkhorst et al., 2008 (VISEP)	247/289	Single-blind	80–110 mg/dL	180–200 mg/dL	28-day mortality and SOFA
	Finfer et al., 2009 (NICE-SUGAR)	3054/3050	Single-blind	80–110 mg/dL	140–180 mg/dL	90-day mortality
	Preiser et al., 2009 (GluControl)	542/536	Single-blind	80–110 mg/dL	140–180 mg/dL	ICU mortality
	Kaflon et al., 2014	1336/1312	Single-blind	80–110 mg/dL	<180 mg/dL	90-day mortality
	Macrae et al., 2014	694/675	Single-blind	72–126 mg/dL	180–215 mg/dL	Number of days alive and free

ICU, intensive care unit, *NICE-SUGAR,* Normoglycemia in Intensive Care Evaluation—Survival Using Glucose Algorithm Regulation; *SOFA,* Sequential Organ Failure Assessment.

and Gandhi and associates[21] revealed decreased short-term mortality (respective relative risks [95% confidence interval] of 0.85 [0.75 to 0.97] and 0.69 [0.51 to 0.94]). In contrast, the five other studies[22-26] showed no significant effect on mortality and an increased risk of hypoglycemia.

INTERPRETATION OF DATA

The results of the different large-scale individual trials can be summarized as follows: In critically ill patients staying in an ICU, tight glucose control by intensive insulin therapy improved survival only in one proof-of-concept study (Leuven I[1]). There are multiple potential explanations for the discrepant results. These include differences in the study population and in the treatment protocol, especially with regard to the amount of intravenous glucose, which was higher in Leuven I than in the other settings. Another possible explanatory factor is the quality of glucose control. Unfortunately, at the present time, there is no agreement on the best index to assess and compare this variable.[27] Finally, the statistical power of each of these individual studies is probably too low. The rate of hypoglycemia in virtually all studies is increased fivefold.[22] Most hypoglycemic episodes are classified as a nonserious adverse event. However, this interpretation may be questioned after the recent publication of data from a retrospective cohort of 102 patients with at least one episode of severe hypoglycemia (<40 mg/dL) matched with 306 control patients from a cohort of 5365 patients.[28] In this study, hypoglycemia was found to be an independent risk predictor of mortality, possibly related to neuroglycopenia.

In contrast to studies that included patients who were not critically ill,[20,21] the meta-analysis that focused on critically ill patients[22] did not demonstrate an advantage of tight glucose control. The meta-analysis of Pittas and colleagues[20]

included patients with stroke, acute myocardial infarction, and diabetes. The results of the large trials on the effects of glucose-insulin-potassium (GIK) after acute myocardial infarction in patients with diabetes, a different intervention than tight glucose control, were included and substantially influenced the overall results. Incidentally, most large trials of GIK during myocardial ischemia were conducted before the 1990s and involved populations with diabetes and acute myocardial infarction. The positive results of some of these studies in all probability reflect the metabolic effects of insulin. This includes the ability to promote the use of glucose as a primary myocardial energy substrate. In myocytes, insulin increases glycolytic substrate and enhances adenosine triphosphate (ATP) synthesis, particularly during ischemia. These effects are independent of glycemic control.

The meta-analysis by Gandhi and associates[21] focused on perioperative glucose control. Most of the included studies involved coronary artery bypass surgery and patients who were not critically ill. The authors of this meta-analysis acknowledged that the available mortality data represent only 40% of the optimal information size required to reliably detect a treatment effect. Furthermore, methodological and reporting biases may weaken inferences.[21]

In the meta-analysis of Wiener,[22] only studies performed in ICUs and aiming to reach a predefined blood glucose level were included. However, this analysis included studies of various sizes that targeted different blood glucose levels. When evaluating the data from the largest individual prospective studies that used a 80- to 110-mg/dL blood glucose target in the intensive treatment arm,[1,8,12,15,16] the Leuven I study still appears as the outlier (see Table 21-1). The aggregation of individual data from participants in each of these prospective studies could solve the remaining

Table 21-2 Summary of Meta-Analyses on Insulin Therapy

Study	Number of Trials Included/Retrieved	Number of Subjects (Intervention/No Intervention)	Intervention	Control	Outcomes
Pittas et al., 2004	35/941	Not indicated: total of 8432	Insulin therapy	No insulin	Short-term or hospital mortality
Gandhi et al., 2008	34/445	2192/2163	Intravenous perioperative insulin	Higher blood glucose target	Mortality and 11 outcome variables
Wiener et al., 2008	29/1358	4127/4188	Tight glucose control	Usual care	Short-term mortality, septicemia, new need for dialysis, hypoglycemia
Griesdale et al., 2009	26/54	Not indicated: total of 13567	Intensive insulin therapy	Conventional glycemic control	Mortality risk and hypoglycemia risk
Marik et al., 2010	7/59	Not indicated: total of 11412	Intensive insulin therapy	Less strict glucose control	28-day mortality
Song et al., 2014	12/26	2094/2006	Tight glucose control	Higher blood glucose target	28- and 90-day ICU and hospital mortality
Srinivasan et al., 2014	4/33	Not indicated: total of 3288	Intensive insulin therapy	Conventional glycemic control	30-day mortality

questions.[29] Griesdale and associates[23] analyzed this point in their meta-analysis. When they looked at the effect of intensive insulin therapy according to the type of ICU, they demonstrated a possible benefit among the surgical ICU patients, although they did not find any effect on the overall risk of death. The lower mortality rate of surgical patients in comparison with that of the other patients demonstrates that this is a distinct group and makes it difficult for an extrapolation to whole ICU patients.

Marik et al.[24] raised the question of any variables that would differ between the Leuven study and the others. They identified route of administration of calories and attributed a positive effect to intensive insulin therapy when the large amount of calories are intravenously administered.

Song et al.[25] performed a meta-analysis on a subcohort containing only septic patients. This group has an insulin-resistant state with an important metabolic modification and an unfavorable prognosis when hyperglycemic.[30] However, the authors failed to demonstrate a positive effect of insulin in these patients. The recommendations of the Surviving Sepsis Campaign currently are to treat the hyperglycemia to maintain a level less than 180 mg/dL. No minimum value is recommended other than avoiding hypoglycemia, in agreement with other protocol recommendations.[31-33] In a pediatric population, the meta-analysis of Srinivasan[26] showed the same conclusions in terms of mortality and hypoglycemia rate.

CONCLUSION

Intensive insulin therapy titrated to restore and maintain blood glucose between 80 and 110 mg/dL improved the survival of critically ill patients in one pioneering proof-of-concept study performed in a surgical ICU.[1] This result was not confirmed in any of the subsequent trials.[8,12-16] The underlying reasons for this discrepancy are currently under investigation and could be linked to the fact that this study analyzed a particular subgroup of patients. Studies using intensive insulin therapy reveal a high rate of hypoglycemia that may alter outcome.[34] The effects of severe hyperglycemia (>180 mg/dL) are well documented. The choice of intermediate target appears logical to minimize the risks for hypoglycemia. A blood glucose target less than 180 mg/dL is presently recommended by the Surviving Sepsis Campaign.[35]

AUTHOR'S RECOMMENDATIONS

- Severe hyperglycemia is harmful.
- Intensive insulin therapy titrated to achieve a blood glucose level between 80 and 110 mg/dL was found to improve survival in one study.
- Intensive insulin therapy is labor intensive and increases the risk for hypoglycemia.
- Particularities of the case mix, usual care, and quality of glucose control in the unit where intensive insulin therapy was found to be beneficial compared with other ICUs might explain the differences in the effects of intensive insulin therapy.

REFERENCES

1. Van den Berghe G, Wouters P, Weekers F, et al. Intensive insulin therapy in the critically ill patients. *N Engl J Med.* 2001;345:1359–1367.
2. Dungan KM, Braithwaite SS, Preiser JC, et al. Stress hyperglycemia. *Lancet.* 2009;373:1798–1807.
3. Brownlee M. Biochemistry and molecular cell biology of diabetic complications. *Nature.* 2001;414:813–820.
4. Szabo C, Biser A, Benko R, et al. Poly(ADP-Ribose) polymerase inhibitors ameliorate nephropathy of type 2 diabetic Leprdb/db mice. *Diabetes.* 2006;55:3004–3012.
5. Ceriello A. Oxidative stress and diabetes-associated complications. *Endocr Pract.* 2006;12:60–62.
6. Corstjens AM, van der Horst IC, Zijlstra JG, et al. Hyperglycaemia in critically ill patients: marker or mediator of mortality? *Crit Care.* 2006;10:216.
7. Preiser JC. Restoring normoglycemia: not so harmless. *Crit Care.* 2008;12:116.
8. Van den Berghe G, Wilmer A, Hermans G, et al. Intensive insulin therapy in the medical ICU. *N Engl J Med.* 2006;35:449–461.
9. Krinsley JS. Effect of an intensive glucose management protocol on the mortality of critically ill adult patients. *Mayo Clin Proc.* 2004;79:992–1000.
10. Finney SJ, Zekveld C, Elia A, Evans TW. Glucose control and mortality in critically ill patients. *JAMA.* 2003;290:2041–2047.
11. Macrae D, Grieve R, Allen E, et al. A randomized trial of hyperglycemic control in pediatric intensive care. *N Engl J Med.* 2014;370:107–118.
12. Finfer S, Chittock DR, Su SY, for the NICE-SUGAR Study Investigators, et al. Intensive versus conventional glucose control in critically ill patients. *N Engl J Med.* 2009;360:1346–1349.
13. Preiser JC, Devos P, Ruiz-Santana S, et al. A prospective randomised multi-centre controlled trial on tight glucose control by intensive insulin therapy in adult intensive care units: the GluControl study. *Intensive Care Med.* 2009;36:2316–2321.
14. Brunkhorst FM, Engel C, Bloos F, et al. Intensive insulin therapy and pentastarch resuscitation in severe sepsis. *N Engl J Med.* 2008;358:125–139.
15. De La Rosa GD, Donado JH, Restrepo AH, et al. Strict glycaemic control in patients hospitalised in a mixed medical and surgical intensive care unit: a randomised clinical trial. *Crit Care.* 2008;12:R120.
16. Arabi YM, Dabbagh OC, Tamim HM, et al. Intensive versus conventional insulin therapy: a randomized controlled trial in medical and surgical critically ill patients. *Crit Care Med.* 2008;36:3190–3197.
17. Kalfon P, Giraudeau B, Ichai C, et al. Tight computerized versus conventional glucose control in the ICU: a randomized controlled trial. *Intensive Care Med.* 2014;40:171–181.
18. Aragon D. Evaluation of nursing work effort and perceptions about blood glucose testing in tight glycemic control. *Am J Crit Care.* 2006;15:370–377.
19. Finfer S, Liu B, Chittock DR, et al. Hypoglycemia and risk of death in critically ill patients. *N Engl J Med.* 2012;367:1108–1118.
20. Pittas A, Siegel RD, Lau J. Insulin therapy for critically ill hospitalized patients: a meta-analysis of randomized controlled trials. *Arch Intern Med.* 2004;164:2005–2011.
21. Gandhi GY, Murad MH, Flynn DN, et al. Effect of perioperative insulin infusion on surgical morbidity and mortality: systematic review and meta-analysis of randomized trials. *Mayo Clin Proc.* 2008;83:418–430.
22. Wiener RS, Wiener DC, Larson RJ. Benefits and risks of tight glucose control in critically ill adults: a meta-analysis. *JAMA.* 2008;300:933–944.
23. Griesdale DE, de Souza RJ, van Dam RM, et al. Intensive insulin therapy and mortality among critically ill patients: a meta-analysis including NICE-SUGAR study data. *CMAJ.* 2009;180:821–827.
24. Marik PE, Preiser JC. Toward understanding tight glycemic control in the ICU: a systematic review and meta-analysis. *Chest.* 2010;137:544–551.
25. Song F, Zhong LJ, Han L, et al. Intensive insulin therapy for septic patients: a meta-analysis of randomized controlled trials. *Biomed Res Int.* 2014;2014:698265.

26. Srinivasan V, Agus MS, et al. Tight glucose control in critically ill children—a systematic review and meta-analysis. *Pediatr Diabetes.* 2014;15:75–83.

27. Eslami S, de Keizer NF, Schultz MJ, et al. A systematic review on quality indicators for tight glycaemic control in critically ill patients: need for an unambiguous indicator reference subset. *Crit Care.* 2008;12:R139.

28. Krinsley JS, Grover A. Severe hypoglycemia in critically ill patients: risk factors and outcomes. *Crit Care Med.* 2007;35:2262.

29. Stewart LA, Tierney JF. To IPD or not to IPD? Advantages and disadvantages of systematic reviews using individual patient data. *Eval Health Prof.* 2002;25:76–97.

30. Leonidou L, Michalaki M, Leonardou A, et al. Stress-induced hyperglycemia in patients with severe sepsis: a compromising factor for survival. *Am J Med Sci.* 2008;336:467–471.

31. Ichai C, Preiser JC. International recommendations for glucose control in adult non diabetic critically ill patients. *Crit Care.* 2010;14:R166.

32. Qaseem A, Humphrey LL, Chou R, et al. Use of intensive insulin therapy for the management of glycemic control in hospitalized patients: a clinical practice guideline from the American College of Physicians. *Ann Intern Med.* 2011;154:260–267.

33. Jacobi J, Bricher N, Krinsley J, et al. Guidelines for the use of an insulin infusion for the management of hyperglycemia in critically ill patients. *Crit Care Med.* 2012;40:3251–3276.

34. Krinsley JS, Preiser JC. Moving beyond tight glucose control to safe effective glucose control. *Crit Care.* 2008;12:149.

35. Dellinger RP, Levy MM, Rhodes A, et al. Surviving Sepsis Campaign: international guidelines for management of severe sepsis and septic shock: 2012. *Crit Care Med.* 2012;41:580–637.

22 Is Hypothermia Useful in Managing Critically Ill Patients? Which Ones? Under What Conditions?

Tomas Drabek, Patrick M. Kochanek

There has been a dramatic reawakening of interest in therapeutic hypothermia (TH) since the dawn of the twenty-first century as a consequence of the publication of a series of clinical trials that appeared to demonstrate improved clinical outcomes. The major attraction of TH is the combination of low cost, reproducibility, and simplicity. A multitude of animal studies have suggested that TH may be beneficial in clinical conditions that may result in neurologic injury.[1]

Several mechanisms that mediate the protective effects of hypothermia have been identified. However, the overall response probably results from a combination of multiple mechanisms that vary with the level and duration of hypothermia. Thus the level of hypothermia to be used in different settings may vary widely: deep hypothermia (15 to 22 °C) is used in cardiac surgery to enable circulatory arrest while mild hypothermia (32 to 34 °C) is used to improve outcome after cardiac arrest (CA) and other ischemia/reperfusion events. Hypothermia can be induced simply, with surface cooling or with sophisticated techniques with specially designed catheters and blankets. The almost universal ability to induce hypothermia makes it a widely applicable, highly attractive approach.

Despite its long history, the widespread clinical application of hypothermia is a relatively new phenomenon. Two seminal clinical trials published in 2002 demonstrated the benefit of therapeutic hypothermia after CA.[2,3] Recent findings suggest that even mild hypothermia (36 °C) may have favorable physiologic effects and that avoidance of hyperthermia may be a desirable clinical goal. In this chapter, we focus on mild to moderate hypothermia that does not require the use of cardiopulmonary bypass and can be accomplished in an intensive care unit (ICU).

TEMPERATURE MONITORING

The normal body temperature in healthy individuals (measured in the oral cavity) is 36.8 ± 0.4 °C with normal diurnal variations of 0.5 °C. Rectal temperatures are usually 0.4 °C higher than oral readings.[4] Lower-esophageal temperature closely reflects the core temperature, as well as rectal temperature and bladder temperature. The temperature measured with pulmonary artery catheters most closely correlates with brain temperature during rapid cooling.[5] Clinically, tympanic temperature, which measures radiating heat from the tympanic membrane, is often used as a surrogate for deep brain temperature. On the basis of the method of cooling, the difference in temperature between various monitoring sites could be significant. In addition, there is no generally accepted, clearly defined range for various levels of hypothermia. In clinical practice, temperatures of 33 to 36 °C are usually referred to as mild hypothermia, 28 to 32 °C as moderate hypothermia, and below 28 °C as deep hypothermia.[6]

COOLING METHODS

Traditionally, external cooling with ice packs applied over great vessels or ice-water soaked cloth blankets has been used to treat hyperthermia and, eventually, induce hypothermia. Gastric, peritoneal, or pulmonary lavage was used to rewarm drowning victims, and this approach could be used in reverse for cooling. Recently, cooling with a rapid intravenous (IV) infusion of ice-cold solutions gained popularity for its ease, general availability, and considerable lack of adverse effects even in CA victims. Bernard et al. used large volumes (30 mL/kg) of ice-cold (4 °C) IV fluid in CA victims and was able to decrease the core temperature from 35.5 to 33.8 °C within 30 minutes.[2] Using a similar approach, Kim et al. achieved a 1.5 °C temperature decrease over 30 minutes. Most important, they did not observe any clinically important changes in vital signs, electrolytes, arterial blood gases, or coagulation parameters.[7] Although IV fluids can initiate cooling effectively, they are not effective for maintaining hypothermia.[8] Cooling blankets with circulating water offer fairly rapid cooling but require attaching a bulky control console to the patient. Similar limitations apply to intravascular cooling catheters. However, both contemporary surface cooling devices and intravascular cooling catheters are able to maintain hypothermia precisely. Kliegel et al. successfully combined the rapid induction of hypothermia with IV fluids and subsequent cooling with an intravascular catheter.[9] Submersion in ice water represents the fastest cooling method (0.11 to 0.25 °C/min). This approach may be useful in heat stroke victims but is unlikely to be feasible in the ICU. An effort to eliminate the potential complications associated with whole-body hypothermia led to the development of devices to induce selective brain hypothermia. Cooling helmets have been used in multiple trials in both pediatric and adult populations.[10-12] Other techniques that might provide more rapid cooling are being explored. Such techniques include nasopharyngeal cooling,[13] neck cooling,[14,15] and direct cooling of blood in the carotid arteries. Cooling with extracorporeal circulation is extremely effective, but its use is logistically limited.

COMPLICATIONS ASSOCIATED WITH THERAPEUTIC HYPOTHERMIA

Hypothermia initiates multiple physiologic changes in the circulatory, respiratory, neurologic, immunologic, and coagulation systems. It also has profound metabolic effects. These changes are temperature dependent. Mild hypothermia most often induces sinus tachycardia. More dangerous cardiovascular complications usually are seen at temperatures below 30 °C. These include atrial fibrillation, bradycardia, and terminal ventricular fibrillation (VF) at approximately 25 °C. The mild hypothermia currently used in clinical practice is hemodynamically well tolerated, with an approximately 25% decrease in cardiac output and an increase in systemic vascular resistance and central venous pressure. In healthy subjects, mild hypothermia increased myocardial perfusion.[16] Hypothermia also induces the release of endogenous catecholamines with a fourfold to sevenfold increase in norepinephrine levels even with minimal temperature changes (0.7 to 1.2 °C).[17] This adrenergic response is associated with an increase in blood pressure, vascular tone, and oxygen consumption that could be detrimental in patients with marginal cardiac reserve.

The impact of hypothermia on coagulation is a result of platelet depletion or dysfunction and clotting factor depletion. The magnitude of changes is often difficult to assess because clinical laboratories adjust the temperatures of all samples to a standard 37 °C. The effects of hypothermia on coagulation thus may be undetected.[18] Reed and colleagues cooled plasma containing clotting factors equivalent to 100% of normal to 35, 33, and 31 °C. Partial thromboplastin time (PTT) in these samples was prolonged as if factor IX had been depleted to 39%, 16%, and 2.5% of normal, respectively. Factor activity is also severely impaired below 30 °C; for example, at 25 °C clotting activity ranges from 0% (factor VIII and factor IX) to 5% (factor II and factor VII).[19] This suggests that factors are dysfunctional, not depleted, because the changes were observed despite 100% or greater factor concentrations measured in the studied samples. Thromboelastography (TEG) may be a useful tool in the setting of TH.[20] TEG from hypothermic swine (32 °C) showed prolonged initial clotting time (R time) and decreased clotting rapidity (alpha angle). These changes suggest a deficit in thrombin availability and/or delay in thrombin generation or activation but not a decrease in clot strength or an increase in clot lysis.[21] Other TEG-based studies suggest that clot firmness is decreased in temperatures less than 30 °C.[22] Bleeding time, one indicator of platelet function, was prolonged 2.5-fold in a sample from a cold (32 °C) versus warm (37 °C) extremity in baboons.[23] In a similar experiment in human volunteers, clotting times were three times longer at 22 °C than at 37 °C.[24] Concurrent acidosis and hypothermia further impaired coagulation.[25] These effects should be taken into consideration when resuscitating trauma victims with ongoing bleeding. Systemic and local normothermia is essential for coagulation. However, trials indicate that neither mild nor moderate therapeutic hypothermia is associated with bleeding complications in patients with severe traumatic brain injury (TBI).[26,27] In patients after CA, there was a trend toward higher bleeding in patients treated with hypothermia (relative risk [RR], 1.30; 95% confidence interval [CI], 0.97 to 1.74), which did not reach significance ($P = .085$).[28]

Hypothermia may lead to leukopenia and an increased risk of infection. Several studies in patients after CA, TBI, or acute stroke showed an increased risk of pneumonia, especially when the duration of hypothermia was prolonged (>48 to 72 hours).[29-31] Shorter hypothermic periods (<24 hours) appear to be safer.[2,3,27] Recent meta-analysis confirms increased risk for pneumonia and sepsis (RR 1.44 [95% CI, 1.10 to 1.90]; 1.80 [95% CI, 1.04 to 3.10], respectively), but the prevalence of all infections was not increased (rate ratio, 1.21 [95% CI, 0.95 to 1.54]).[32] Obviously, the trade off of increased infection rate may be worthwhile if greater neuroprotection can be achieved.

Electrolyte disorders, although common in TH, are usually minor and can be treated easily in a critical care setting. The most commonly observed abnormalities are hypernatremia and hypokalemia, as well as hypomagnesemia, hypophosphatemia, and hypocalcemia.[33,34] Magnesium supplementation may be especially important given its known protective role in neuronal and myocardial injury.[33,35-37]

Hypothermia-induced decreases in insulin sensitivity may lead to hyperglycemia. This could enhance the susceptibility to infection and also might exacerbate secondary brain injury.[38-40] Tight glycemic control may be warranted, although work by Vespa et al. suggests caution and use of insulin at a higher glucose target level of probably more than 150 mg/dL (8 mmol/L).[41]

Drug metabolism is profoundly altered by hypothermia. Some drugs are affected more than others. Mild to moderate hypothermia decreases systemic clearance of cytochrome P450-metabolized drugs by approximately 7% to 22% per degree Celsius below 37 °C.[42] Hypothermia decreases the potency and efficacy of certain drugs.[42]

MECHANISM OF ACTION OF HYPOTHERMIA

Cerebral metabolic rate is decreased by 5% to 7% for each degree decrease in body temperature.[43] However, this observation does not explain the ability of even small temperature changes to affect physiology and provide neuroprotection. Protection by hypothermia in experimental central nervous system (CNS) injury might involve a myriad of mechanisms: maintenance of physiologic adenosine triphosphate (ATP) concentrations, suppression of glutamate release, attenuation of oxidative or nitrative stress, blunting of the inflammatory response, prevention of energy failure, limitation of cytoskeletal damage, increased levels of neurotrophins, prevention of anoxic depolarization, regulation of gene expression, attenuation of apoptosis or limitation of blood-brain barrier injury, and vasogenic edema. In TBI or ischemic stroke, TH reduces intracranial pressure (ICP).[44,45] However, direct neuroprotection has been more difficult to demonstrate outside of the laboratory.

Various combinations of those mechanisms could be responsible for the different outcome in the wide variety of CNS injuries, with hypothermia being beneficial in only selected settings.

HYPOTHERMIA IN CARDIAC ARREST

It has been known for decades that patients who undergo accidental hypothermia, such as near drowning in cold water, survive a much longer period of CA than would be expected if the accident happened at ambient temperature. The initial case series of therapeutic hypothermia applied to victims of CA of various origin (e.g., respiratory failure, trauma) was published in 1958. The target temperatures and duration of cooling were 30 to 34 °C for 24 to 72 hours. In 1959, Benson and colleagues reported the first case series of in-hospital CA patients. Their data revealed favorable neurologic recovery in 50% in the hypothermic group versus 14% in the normothermic group. Despite these early promising results, the clinical use of hypothermia was abandoned, for unclear reasons, until the late 1990s. It is possible that the complications associated with deeper levels of hypothermia (<30 °C) and prolonged use, as observed in animal studies, played a role.[46,47] Laboratory studies in the 1980s explored the potential of mild hypothermia to protect while limiting complications. Busto and colleagues found that small increments in intraischemic temperatures (33, 34, 36, and 39 °C) translate into large differences in neuronal loss in a rat model.[48] Safar's group followed that work showing benefit in experimental CA.[49] These studies provided evidence that even mild hypothermia could significantly improve outcome in CA.

Timing of hypothermia induction also is critical. Initiating hypothermia during the insult yields the best outcome but is rarely clinically feasible. Delayed hypothermia is beneficial in the early postinsult period, but the effect declined over time.[50] On the basis of studies by Colbourne and colleagues in gerbils, minimal delay and longer duration are of utmost importance to fully benefit from hypothermia.[51-53] Prehospital initiation of cooling in the clinical setting is feasible,[54-56] and decreased time to target temperature surprisingly was not beneficial,[57,58] possibly because it was associated with higher incidence of complications linked to IV cooling with fluids.[59]

Several randomized human trials assessed the efficacy of hypothermia after CA. After a small study by Hachimi-Idrissi et al.,[60] two studies published in 2002 clearly established the value of hypothermia in CA. Bernard et al. in Australia studied 77 patients after CA from VF. The patients assigned to hypothermia were cooled to 33 °C over 12 hours with ice packs. A total of 21 (49%) of 43 patients in the hypothermic group survived with good neurologic outcome, whereas this was noted in only 9 (26%) of 34 patients who were not cooled ($P = .046$). The odds ratio (OR) for a good outcome with hypothermia was 5.25 (95% CI, 1.47 to 18.76; $P = .011$).[2] In the European multicenter Hypothermia After Cardiac Arrest (HACA) trial, patients resuscitated after CA from VF or ventricular tachycardia (VT) were randomly assigned to hypothermia (32 to 34 °C for 24 hours, cooling with cold air) or to normothermia. In the hypothermia group, 75 (55%) of 136 patients showed favorable neurologic outcome compared with 54 (39%) of 137 in the normothermic group (RR, 1.68; 95% CI, 1.29 to 2.07; number needed to treat [NNT] = 6).[3] Hypothermia appeared effective despite a relative delay in initiation and slow onset. Three questions arose after publication of these trials: (1) Were these studies of hypothermia versus hyperthermia, rather than normothermia (fever was a frequent complication in the control groups)? (2) Is it necessary to cool the patient below 34 °C, with associated problems such as shivering and the requirement for deep sedation, to have a beneficial effect? (3) Is TH effective for CA caused from events other than VF/VT?

As TH began to be used routinely, several registries for follow-up were established. Arrich et al. evaluated the data from 650 patients from 19 centers entered into the European Resuscitation Council Hypothermia After CA Registry. Of all patients, 462 (79%) received TH, 347 (59%) were cooled with an endovascular device, and 114 (19%) received other cooling methods such as ice packs, cooling blankets, or cold fluids. The rate of adverse events was lower (hemorrhage, 3%; arrhythmia, 6%), and the cooling rate was faster than in published clinical trials.[61]

Lopez-de-Sa et al. compared hypothermia at 32 °C versus 34 °C, concluding that lower temperature was associated with more favorable outcomes, and lower incidence of clinical seizures (1/18 vs. 11/18; $P = .0002$) in patients with shockable rhythms.[62]

As a result of these studies the International Liaison Committee on Resuscitation recommended that, "Unconscious adult patients with spontaneous circulation after out-of-hospital CA should be cooled to 32 °C to 34 °C for 12 to 24 hours when the initial rhythm was VF. Cooling to 32 °C to 34 °C for 12 to 24 hours may be considered for unconscious adult patients with spontaneous circulation after out-of-hospital CA from any other rhythm or CA in hospital."[63,64]

Oksanen et al. reviewed the data from CA survivors admitted to Finnish ICUs between 2004 and 2005. Almost all ICUs used hypothermia (19 of 20), but it seemed to be implemented only in selected groups of patients (4% in 2004, 28% in 2005). Survival rate at 6 months was 55%.[65] It was estimated that if physicians in the United States were to use TH in all eligible patients, 2298 additional patients per year might achieve a good neurologic outcome.[66]

However, not all studies have reported improved outcomes with TH.[67,68] Tiainen et al. studied cognitive and neurophysiologic outcome in a cohort of 70 patients randomly assigned to hypothermia (33 °C for 24 hours) or normothermia. Three months after CA, 28 of 36 patients in the hypothermic group compared with 22 of 34 in the normothermic group were alive (P=.226). There was no difference in cognitive decline or neurophysiologic deficits.[68]

Although TH has been widely adopted in ICUs worldwide, with anecdotal reports of improved outcomes, there remained the problems of selection bias, temperature control, and study size in the Bernard and HACA studies.[69] Nielsen and colleagues undertook a large multicenter trial that randomized CA patients to targeted temperature management (TTM) at 33 or 36 °C[70,71] for 24 hours, with gradual rewarming at temperature control to 37 °C for up to 72 hours. The primary endpoint of the study was survival at 180 days after inclusion. At 72 hours, 50% of the patients in the 33 °C group (235 of 473 patients) had died, compared with 48% of the patients in the 36 °C group (225 of 466 patients) (OR with a temperature of 33 °C, 1.06; 95% CI, 0.89 to 1.28; P=.51). At the end of the 180-day follow-up period, 54% of the patients in the 33 °C group had died or had poor neurologic outcome, compared with 52% of patients in the 36 °C group (OR, 1.02; 95% CI, 0.88 to 1.16; P=.78). There was no benefit to cooling below 36 °C. There was no evidence that early versus late cardiopulmonary resuscitation (CPR), duration of CPR, or time to hospital admission had any discernable impact on outcomes. On the basis of these findings, current guidelines suggest TTM at 32 to 36 °C (mild hypothermia).[71a]

It remains for future trials to determine if the benefits conferred by TTM or mild to moderate hypothermia can be extended to other settings. Recent meta-analysis of patients presenting with nonshockable rhythms documented reduced in-hospital mortality with hypothermia, but the quality of studies was low.[72] Several additional studies that were not included in that meta-analysis supported this observation.[73,74] A review of low-quality trials in a pediatric population demonstrated no difference in mortality, but no recommendations were drawn.[75] A strict control of the temperature avoiding hyperthermia (>37.5 °C) and severe hypothermia (<32 °C) is recommended in children.[75a] Data from in-hospital CA are emerging,[76,77] but the initial results are not compelling.[78-80] The optimal selection of patient population is being debated.[81-83] Multiple trials are underway. Prognostication of outcome of both adult[84,85] and pediatric[86,87] patients treated with hypothermia after CA remains challenging.[88]

THERAPEUTIC HYPOTHERMIA IN ISCHEMIC STROKE

In animal models of focal brain ischemia, hypothermia has been shown to reduce lesion size by up to 90%.[89,90] These data resulted in interest in the use of TH in patients with ischemic stroke. Brain temperatures in stroke patients exceed core temperature by at least 1 °C (1.0 to 2.1 °C).[91,92] A large cohort trial of 3790 patients demonstrated that the avoidance of hyperthermia in stroke patients improved outcome.[93] However, a pharmacologic-based strategy to induce hypothermia with acetaminophen (paracetamol) resulted in a body temperature decrease of only 0.22 °C.[94] Schwab et al. conducted two noncontrolled trials in patients who underwent acute ischemic stroke to evaluate the effect of hypothermia (33 °C for 24 to 72 hours). In the first study, hypothermia was initiated in 25 patients 14 hours after first symptoms (range, 4 to 24 hours). Target temperature was

achieved after 3 to 6 hours. Passive rewarming was achieved over 18 hours (range, 17 to 24 hours). ICP decreased in all patients during hypothermia, but significant increases in ICP were observed during rewarming. Pneumonia was observed in 40% of patients.[45] In the second study, 50 patients were subjected to hypothermia in a manner similar to that in the previous study. ICP decreased from 20±14 to 12±5 mm Hg during hypothermia. Shorter rewarming periods (<16 hours) were associated with a marked ICP increase and higher mortality when compared with longer rewarming periods.[31] Mortality in this study was 38%, which compares favorably with outcomes of other studies with similar patient populations without hypothermia having mortality rates of 78% to 79%,[95,96] although Hawthorne effects and selection bias should be considered.

Kammersgaard et al. used hypothermia (35.5 °C for 6 to 17 hours) in 17 awake stroke patients and compared the outcome data with matched subjects from the Copenhagen registry. Neurologic impairment as assessed by the Scandinavian Stroke Scale at 6 months was similar (42±14 vs. 48±11, respectively; P=.21).[97]

De Georgia and colleagues conducted a feasibility trial of 40 patients randomized to intravascular cooling (33 °C for 24 hours) or control therapy after ischemic stroke. Clinical outcomes and lesion size at one month were similar in both groups. No adverse side effects were observed.[98]

Hemicraniectomy represents the most invasive approach to treat ischemic stroke. Georgiadis et al. randomized 36 patients to either hemicraniectomy or hypothermia. Mortality was 12% in hemicraniectomy compared with 47% in hypothermia. The latter also was associated with a higher complication rate.[99] Els et al. compared hypothermia with hemicraniectomy (HH) (n=12) to hemicraniectomy alone (HA) (n=13), with a trend toward better outcome in the HH at 6 months (P<.08).[100]

Thus there currently are no robust data to support the use of induced hypothermia in patients with ischemic stroke. Recent meta-analysis of seven small clinical trials did not show any benefit on mortality or stroke severity.[101] However, some trials report benefits on incidence and severity of complications associated with stroke and on outcome.[102-104] Given that several small trials suggested benefit, additional larger trials are planned[105] or underway.[106]

HYPOTHERMIA FOR SPINAL CORD INJURY

There are a limited number of studies addressing the use of hypothermia after traumatic spinal cord injury (SCI). The results from the animal studies are mixed but overall suggest beneficial effects.[107] However, the models are varied. Several case series using whole-body hypothermia for SCI have been published, documenting feasibility.[108-110] Regional cooling of spinal cord is a viable alternative.[111] This approach, reviewed by Kwon et al., was assessed in small case series in 1970s and 1980s.[112] Despite some encouraging results, the authors of all respective studies acknowledge the limitations (e.g., small number of patients, differences in clinical assessment of deficits, and lack of controls) and the need for larger controlled studies.[113,114] A large multicenter prospective study (ARCTIC [Acute Rapid Cooling Trial for Injuries of the Spinal Cord]) is currently proposed.

Currently, there is emerging evidence suggesting that hypothermia might be beneficial after traumatic SCI but definitive studies are still lacking.[114a] Preventive induction of regional hypothermia for major vascular procedures with or without additional measures including systemic hypothermia has not been validated in a large prospective randomized study.

HYPOTHERMIA FOR TRAUMATIC BRAIN INJURY

Current diagnostic and therapeutic approaches to patients with TBI vary widely between institutions. Treatments are generally targeted at maintaining cerebral perfusion pressure, minimizing ICP, or reducing overall brain metabolic activity. In TBI, neuronal death is biphasic: early, due to the injury itself, and late, a consequence of hypoxic-ischemic and inflammatory damage.[115]

Many experimental studies in animals have suggested benefit with the use of TH after TBI. Multiple RCTs have been conducted, investigating the use of hypothermia after TBI in both pediatric and adult populations. Be aware: the pathophysiology of TBI in pediatric and adult patients has distinct features[116] that could contribute to different outcomes. The depth and duration of hypothermia applied have varied widely, as have the use of other therapeutic modalities (e.g., cerebrospinal fluid [CSF] drainage, osmotic therapy, and sedation). Better results were achieved in centers with expertise in applied hypothermia. Several published meta-analyses reported conflicting results (Table 22-1): some indicated improved neurologic outcome and mortality when hypothermia was used,[117,118] but others did not support that observation.[119] No improvement in outcome with hypothermia was seen in the five pediatric studies. Varied results were reported in 14 studies on adult patients, 2 of which reported a tendency of higher mortality and worse neurologic outcome, 4 reported lower mortality, and 9 reported favorable neurologic outcome with hypothermia. The quality of several trials was low.[120] More favorable results were observed in Asian populations versus American populations.[121] Recent meta-analysis of pediatric patients with TBI documented increased mortality and increased incidence of cardiac arrhythmias with hypothermia.[122]

Hypothermia is effective in reducing increased ICP; however, rewarming needs to be very slow to prevent rebound intracranial hypertension. Patients who are hypothermic on admission should be kept hypothermic or very slowly rewarmed. Reductions in ICP do not necessarily translate to improved neurologic outcomes.[123]

In an international multicenter trial led by Hutchison et al., TH did not improve the neurologic outcome in TBI and may have increased mortality. This study has been criticized because of apparently delayed commencement of hypothermia and the relatively short duration of therapy. This may have resulted in rewarming occurring during the anticipated period of peak edema.[124] A large multicenter study exploring very early hypothermia was terminated for futility.[125] In the study by Maekawa and colleagues, prolonged TH (32 to 34 °C) compared with TTM (35.5 to 37 °C) did not improve neurologic outcome or mortality after severe TBI.[126]

In conclusion, TH has not, to date, been convincingly shown to improve outcomes in TBI. If TH or TTM is to be used, early initiation, therapy for greater than 48 hours, and slow rewarming, with tight monitoring of ICP, appear important.

HYPOTHERMIA FOR MYOCARDIAL INFARCTION

It is possible that hypothermia could limit myocardial injury in acute myocardial infarction (AMI). In a multicenter but small study, Dixon et al. randomized 42 patients with AMI to primary percutaneous coronary intervention (PCI) with or without endovascular cooling (33 °C for 3 hours). There was no statistically significant difference in the median infarct size.[127] The feasibility of endovascular cooling in awake patients undergoing PCI was confirmed in a nonrandomized study (LOWTEMP trial).[128] Wolfrum et al. found that compared with historic controls, the initiation of hypothermia did not delay other interventions.[129] In a nonrandomized study, Hovdenes et al. reported that PCI could be performed on CA patients who had AMI, including some who required an intraaortic balloon pump.[130] Hypothermia also improved hemodynamics in patients after CA in cardiogenic shock.[131] A retrospective Danish study in 68 patients after CA documented safety of PCI treatment under hypothermia.[132]

In summary, these data suggest that hypothermia is feasible in hemodynamically unstable CA patients who require hemodynamic support, and the initiation of hypothermia protocol does not delay further interventions. Coronary angiography should be performed as soon as possible (less than 2 hours), in particular in hemodynamically unstable patients.[133] However, TH does not currently have a role in AMI patients without CA.

HYPOTHERMIA FOR HYPOXIC-ISCHEMIC ENCEPHALOPATHY

Hypoxic-ischemic encephalopathy (HIE) from asphyxial insults is associated with high mortality and long-term neurodevelopmental disability in survivors. This is especially true in infants and children. The injury is two staged. A certain amount of damage results from acute, primary neuronal death. This often is followed by a second, delayed period of neuronal loss. This secondary injury provides a therapeutic window in which further damage might be prevented. Logically, hypothermia might be of value during this time.

Selective head cooling has been tested primarily in infants. However, body core temperature must be decreased to achieve cooling of deep brain structures.[134]

The data from 11 randomized controlled trials (RCTs) comprising 1505 near-term infants were summarized in a recent Cochrane review. TH resulted in a statistically significant and clinically important reduction in the combined outcome of mortality or major neurodevelopmental disability to 18 months of age with NNT for an additional beneficial outcome (NNTB) 7 (95% CI, 5 to 10) (8 studies, 1344 infants). Cooling also resulted in statistically significant reductions in mortality NNTB = 11 [8 to 25] (11 studies, 1468 infants) and in neurodevelopmental disability in survivors NNTB = 8 [5 to 14] (8 studies, 917 infants). Some

Table 22-1 **Summary of Meta-Analyses on Therapeutic Hypothermia**

Study, Year	Number of Trials	Number of Subjects (Intervention/No Intervention)	Intervention	Control	Outcomes
CARDIAC ARREST					
Holzer, 2005	3	195/198	Hypothermia	Standard care	Improved survival with favorable neurologic recovery—RR = 1.68 (1.29-2.07)
Cheung, 2006	4	231/203	Hypothermia	Standard care	Reduced mortality—RR = 0.75 (0.62-0.92), Reduced poor neurologic outcome—RR = 0.72 (0.62-0.84)
Nielsen, 2011	5	254/224	Hypothermia	Standard care	Nonsignificant reduction in mortality—RR = 0.84 (0.70-1.01) and reduction in poor neurologic outcome—RR = 0.78 (0.64-0.95)
Arrich, 2012	5	253/226	Hypothermia	Standard care	Hypothermia improved good neurologic outcome—RR = 1.55 (1.22-1.96) and survival—RR = 1.35 (1.10-1.65)
TRAUMATIC BRAIN INJURY IN ADULTS					
Harris, 2002	7	254/245	Hypothermia	Standard care	Nonsignificant improvement in GOS—OR = 0.61 (0.26-1.46, $P = .3$); decrease of ICP—OR = −2.98 (−7.58-1.61; $P = .2$); significant prolongation of PTT—OR = 2.22 (1.73-2.71; $P < .001$)
Henderson, 2003	8	748 total	Hypothermia	Normothermia	Nonsignificant reduction of mortality—OR 0.81 (0.59-1.13), strong trend for reduction of poor neurologic outcome—OR 0.75 (0.56-1.01; $P = .06$); reduced risk of pneumonia in normothermic group OR—0.42 (0.25-0.70; $P = .001$)
McIntyre, 2003	12	543/526	Hypothermia	Normothermia	Reduced mortality—RR = 0.70 (0.56-0.87) and reduced poor neurologic outcome—RR = 0.65 (0.48-0.89)
Alderson, 2004	14	540/523	Hypothermia	Open or normothermia	Nonsignificant reduction in mortality—OR = 0.80 (0.61-1.04); nonsignificant reduction of mortality or severe disability—OR = 0.75 (0.56-1.00); increase risk of pneumonia—OR = 1.95 (1.18-3.23)
Brain Trauma Foundation, 2007	6	354/340	Hypothermia	Normothermia	All-cause mortality not significantly different—RR = 0.76 (0.55-1.05; $P = .16$); increased chance of good outcome—RR = 1.46 (1.12-1.92); cooling >48 hr associated with reduction of mortality—RR = 0.51 (0.24-0.78)
Peterson, 2008	8	407/374	Hypothermia	Normothermia	Reduction in mortality—RR = 0.51 (0.33-0.79) and favorable neurologic outcome—RR = 1.91 (1.28-2.85) when hypothermia used for >48 hr; increased risk of pneumonia—RR = 2.37 (1.37-4.10); no benefit for cooling <48 hr
Sydenham, 2009	23	803/784	Hypothermia	Normothermia	No reduction in mortality—OR = 0.85 (0.68-1.06); hypothermia associated with less likely unfavorable outcome—OR = 0.77 (0.62-0.94)
Georgiu, 2013	18	917/910	Hypothermia	Normothermia	Reduction in mortality—RR = 0.84 (0.72-0.98] and of poor neurologic outcome—RR = 0.81 (0.73-0.89)

Table 22-1 Summary of Meta-Analyses on Therapeutic Hypothermia—cont'd

Study, Year	Number of Trials	Number of Subjects (Intervention/No Intervention)	Intervention	Control	Outcomes
Li, 2014	13	591/561	Hypothermia	Normothermia	Trend to reduction in mortality—RR=0.86 (0.73-1.01; P=.06) and unfavorable clinical neurologic outcomes—RR=1.21 (0.95-1.53; P=.12); significant reduction of mortality with hypothermia in an Asian population—RR=0.60 (0.44-0.83, P=.002)
Crossley, 2014	20	863/976	Hypothermia	Normothermia	Reduction in mortality—RR=1.31 (1.13, 1.52; P=.0004); reduction in poor outcome—RR=1.49 (1.27, 1.74; P<.00001)
TRAUMATIC BRAIN INJURY IN CHILDREN					
Ma, 2013	6	366 total	Hypothermia	Normothermia	Increased mortality with hypothermia—RR=1.73 (1.06-2.84)
HYPOXIC ISCHEMIC ENCEPHALOPATHY IN NEWBORNS					
Jacobs, 2008	8	255/251	Hypothermia	Normothermia	Reduced risk of death or major disability—RR=0.76 (0.65-0.89)
Jacobs, 2013	11	688/612	Hypothermia	Normothermia	Reduction in mortality—RR=0.75 (0.64-0.88); reduction in neurodevelopmental disability in survivors—RR=0.77 (0.63-0.94)
Pauliah, 2013	7	301/266	Hypothermia	Standard care	Data from low- and middle-income countries; no reduction in neonatal mortality—RR=0.74 (0.44-1.25); data on morbidity and long-term neurologic outcomes were insufficient
INTRACRANIAL ANEURYSM					
Milani, 2011	4	605/611	Hypothermia	Normothermia	No difference in outcome or complications
Li, 2012		577/581	Hypothermia	Normothermia	No effect on mortality—RR=0.82 (0.62-1.09)
Zhao, 2012	3	575/584	Hypothermia	Normothermia	No difference in outcome or complications
STROKE					
Lakhan, 2012	7	131/127	Hypothermia	Normothermia	No difference in mortality or stroke severity

ICP, intracranial pressure; *GOS*, Glasgow Outcome Scale; *OR*, odds ratio; *PTT*, partial thromboplastin time; *RR*, relative risk.

adverse effects of hypothermia included an increased sinus bradycardia and a significant thrombocytopenia.[135] TH appears to be beneficial in the treatment of HIE in infants and should be instituted in term and late preterm infants with moderate-to-severe HIE if identified before 6 hours of age.[136] Unfortunately, these benefits were not seen in a meta-analysis of seven trials from low- and middle-income countries.[137]

HYPOTHERMIA IN OTHER CLINICAL SCENARIOS

Other clinical scenarios when TH could be useful were considered. TH did not improve outcome in comatose patients with severe bacterial meningitis and may even be harmful.[138] However, other small-size trial showed significant benefits of TH in community-acquired bacterial meningitis with a reduction in mortality (OR = 0.059 [0.017-0.211]) and risk of adverse neurologic outcome (OR = 0.209 [0.082-0.534]).[139]

In a large multicenter trial (IHAST), intraoperative hypothermia did not improve the neurologic outcome after craniotomy among good-grade patients with aneurysmal subarachnoid hemorrhage.[140] These disappointing results were later confirmed by a meta-analysis showing no effect intraoperative hypothermia on mortality (RR = 0.82 [0.62, 1.09]).[141]

In a small pilot trial, hypothermia prevented the development of perihemorrhagic edema after large intracranial hemorrhage and its complications. Side effects included namely pneumonia.[142,143] Larger multicenter studies are currently underway.[144]

Low grade evidence exists to support the use of TH to control seizures in patients in refractory status epilepticus.[145]

CONCLUSION

Therapeutic hypothermia remains an area of intense interest in critical care. However, promising data from animal studies have failed to translate into improved clinical outcomes for the majority of injuries, such as TBI, stroke, and MI. Enthusiasm for aggressive TH in CA has cooled; current data support TTM at 36 °C and avoidance of hyperthermia. The most compelling data for TH are in cardiac arrest and HIE in term newborns.

AUTHORS' RECOMMENDATIONS

- Targeted temperature management at 32 to 36 °C is neuroprotective in comatose patients who survive out of hospital CA and suggested in patients after in-hospital CA irrespective of the presenting rhythm. A strict control of the temperature must be maintained to avoid hyperthermia (>37.5 °C) and severe hypothermia (<32 °C) in children.
- In clinical conditions where neurologic injury is to be anticipated (e.g., stroke, SCI, TBI, subarachnoid hemorrhage is to be anticipated, data do not support TH, but hyperthermia should be avoided.
- TH is an accepted treatment of term newborns suffering hypoxic-ischemic insults in the perinatal period.
- Optimization of cooling methods, duration and depth of hypothermia, approach to rewarming, and minimization and management of side effects are needed to maximize the therapeutic potential of hypothermia.

REFERENCES

1. Nagel S, Papadakis M, Hoyte L, Buchan AM. Therapeutic hypothermia in experimental models of focal and global cerebral ischemia and intracerebral hemorrhage. *Expert Rev Neurother.* 2008;8:1255–1268.
2. Bernard SA, Gray TW, Buist MD, et al. Treatment of comatose survivors of out-of-hospital cardiac arrest with induced hypothermia. *N Engl J Med.* 2002;346:557–563.
3. Mild therapeutic hypothermia to improve the neurologic outcome after cardiac arrest. *N Engl J Med.* 2002;346:549–556.
4. Fauci AS, Braunwald E, Kasper DL, et al. *Alterations in Body Temperature. Harrison's Principles of Internal Medicine.* New York: McGraw-Hill; 2008. 117–121.
5. Janata A, Weihs W, Bayegan K, et al. Therapeutic hypothermia with a novel surface cooling device improves neurologic outcome after prolonged cardiac arrest in swine. *Crit Care Med.* 2008;36:895–902.
6. Safar PJ, Kochanek PM. Therapeutic hypothermia after cardiac arrest. *N Engl J Med.* 2002;346:612–613.
7. Kim F, Olsufka M, Carlbom D, et al. Pilot study of rapid infusion of 2 L of 4 degrees C normal saline for induction of mild hypothermia in hospitalized, comatose survivors of out-of-hospital cardiac arrest. *Circulation.* 2005;112:715–719.
8. Kliegel A, Janata A, Wandaller C, et al. Cold infusions alone are effective for induction of therapeutic hypothermia but do not keep patients cool after cardiac arrest. *Resuscitation.* 2007;73:46–53.
9. Kliegel A, Losert H, Sterz F, et al. Cold simple intravenous infusions preceding special endovascular cooling for faster induction of mild hypothermia after cardiac arrest–a feasibility study. *Resuscitation.* 2005;64:347–351.
10. Wang H, Olivero W, Lanzino G, et al. Rapid and selective cerebral hypothermia achieved using a cooling helmet. *J Neurosurg.* 2004;100:272–277.
11. Horn AR, Woods DL, Thompson C, Eis I, Kroon M. Selective cerebral hypothermia for post-hypoxic neuroprotection in neonates using a solid ice cap. *S Afr Med J.* 2006;96:976–981.
12. Battin MR, Penrice J, Gunn TR, Gunn AJ. Treatment of term infants with head cooling and mild systemic hypothermia (35.0 degrees C and 34.5 degrees C) after perinatal asphyxia. *Pediatrics.* 2003;111:244–251.
13. Lyon RM, Van Antwerp J, Henderson C, Weaver A, Davies G, Lockey D. Prehospital intranasal evaporative cooling for out-of-hospital cardiac arrest: a pilot, feasibility study. *Eur J Emerg Med.* 2014;21:368–370.
14. Poli S, Purrucker J, Priglinger M, et al. Induction of cooling with a passive head and neck cooling device: effects on brain temperature after stroke. *Stroke.* 2013;44:708–713.
15. Covaciu L, Weis J, Bengtsson C, et al. Brain temperature in volunteers subjected to intranasal cooling. *Intensive Care Med.* 2011;37:1277–1284.
16. Frank SM, Satitpunwaycha P, Bruce SR, Herscovitch P, Goldstein DS. Increased myocardial perfusion and sympathoadrenal activation during mild core hypothermia in awake humans. *Clin Sci (Lond).* 2003;104:503–508.
17. Frank SM, Higgins MS, Fleisher LA, Sitzmann JV, Raff H, Breslow MJ. Adrenergic, respiratory, and cardiovascular effects of core cooling in humans. *Am J Physiol.* 1997;272:R557–R562.
18. Brinkman AC, Ten Tusscher BL, de Waard MC, de Man FR, Girbes AR, Beishuizen A. Minimal effects on ex vivo coagulation during mild therapeutic hypothermia in post cardiac arrest patients. *Resuscitation.* 2014;85:1359–1363.
19. Johnston TD, Chen Y, Reed 2nd RL. Functional equivalence of hypothermia to specific clotting factor deficiencies. *J Trauma.* 1994;37:413–417.
20. Martini WZ, Cortez DS, Dubick MA, Park MS, Holcomb JB. Thrombelastography is better than pt, aptt, and activated clotting time in detecting clinically relevant clotting abnormalities after hypothermia, hemorrhagic shock and resuscitation in pigs. *J Trauma.* 2008;65:535–543.
21. Martini WZ. The effects of hypothermia on fibrinogen metabolism and coagulation function in swine. *Metabolism.* 2007;56:214–221.
22. Rundgren M, Engstrom M. A thromboelastometric evaluation of the effects of hypothermia on the coagulation system. *Anesth Analg.* 2008;107:1465–1468.
23. Watts DD, Trask A, Soeken K, Perdue P, Dols S, Kaufmann C. Hypothermic coagulopathy in trauma: effect of varying levels of hypothermia on enzyme speed, platelet function, and fibrinolytic activity. *J Trauma.* 1998;44:846–854.
24. Valeri CR, MacGregor H, Cassidy G, Tinney R, Pompei F. Effects of temperature on bleeding time and clotting time in normal male and female volunteers. *Crit Care Med.* 1995;23:698–704.
25. Dirkmann D, Hanke AA, Gorlinger K, Peters J. Hypothermia and acidosis synergistically impair coagulation in human whole blood. *Anesth Analg.* 2008;106:1627–1632.
26. Clifton GL, Miller ER, Choi SC, et al. Lack of effect of induction of hypothermia after acute brain injury. *N Engl J Med.* 2001;344:556–563.
27. Marion DW, Penrod LE, Kelsey SF, et al. Treatment of traumatic brain injury with moderate hypothermia. *N Engl J Med.* 1997;336:540–546.
28. Stockmann H, Krannich A, Schroeder T, Storm C. Therapeutic temperature management after cardiac arrest and the risk of bleeding: systematic review and meta-analysis. *Resuscitation.* 2014;85:1494–1503.
29. Yanagawa Y, Ishihara S, Norio H, et al. Preliminary clinical outcome study of mild resuscitative hypothermia after out-of-hospital cardiopulmonary arrest. *Resuscitation.* 1998;39:61–66.
30. Shiozaki T, Hayakata T, Taneda M, et al. A multicenter prospective randomized controlled trial of the efficacy of mild hypothermia for severely head injured patients with low intracranial pressure. Mild hypothermia study group in Japan. *J Neurosurg.* 2001;94:50–54.
31. Schwab S, Georgiadis D, Berrouschot J, Schellinger PD, Graffagnino C, Mayer SA. Feasibility and safety of moderate hypothermia after massive hemispheric infarction. *Stroke.* 2001;32:2033–2035.
32. Geurts M, Macleod MR, Kollmar R, Kremer PH, van der Worp HB. Therapeutic hypothermia and the risk of infection: a systematic review and meta-analysis. *Crit Care Med.* 2014;42:231–242.
33. Polderman KH, Peerdeman SM, Girbes AR. Hypophosphatemia and hypomagnesemia induced by cooling in patients with severe head injury. *J Neurosurg.* 2001;94:697–705.
34. Aibiki M, Kawaguchi S, Maekawa N. Reversible hypophosphatemia during moderate hypothermia therapy for brain-injured patients. *Crit Care Med.* 2001;29:1726–1730.

35. Polderman KH, Bloemers FW, Peerdeman SM, Girbes AR. Hypomagnesemia and hypophosphatemia at admission in patients with severe head injury. *Crit Care Med*. 2000;28:2022–2025.

36. Shechter M, Hod H, Rabinowitz B, Boyko V, Chouraqui P. Long-term outcome of intravenous magnesium therapy in thrombolysis-ineligible acute myocardial infarction patients. *Cardiology*. 2003;99:205–210.

37. McIntosh TK, Vink R, Yamakami I, Faden AI. Magnesium protects against neurological deficit after brain injury. *Brain Res*. 1989;482:252–260.

38. Cochran A, Scaife ER, Hansen KW, Downey EC. Hyperglycemia and outcomes from pediatric traumatic brain injury. *J Trauma*. 2003;55:1035–1038.

39. Rovlias A, Kotsou S. The influence of hyperglycemia on neurological outcome in patients with severe head injury. *Neurosurgery*. 2000;46:335–342. discussion 342–333.

40. Cherian L, Hannay HJ, Vagner G, Goodman JC, Contant CF, Robertson CS. Hyperglycemia increases neurological damage and behavioral deficits from post-traumatic secondary ischemic insults. *J Neurotrauma*. 1998;15:307–321.

41. Vespa P, Boonyaputthikul R, McArthur DL, Miller C, Etchepare M, Bergsneider M, et al. Intensive insulin therapy reduces microdialysis glucose values without altering glucose utilization or improving the lactate/pyruvate ratio after traumatic brain injury. *Crit Care Med*. 2006;34:850–856.

42. Tortorici MA, Kochanek PM, Poloyac SM. Effects of hypothermia on drug disposition, metabolism, and response: A focus of hypothermia-mediated alterations on the cytochrome p450 enzyme system. *Crit Care Med*. 2007;35:2196–2204.

43. Rosomoff HL, Holaday DA. Cerebral blood flow and cerebral oxygen consumption during hypothermia. *Am J Physiol*. 1954;179:85–88.

44. Polderman KH. Induced hypothermia and fever control for prevention and treatment of neurological injuries. *Lancet*. 2008;371:1955–1969.

45. Schwab S, Schwarz S, Spranger M, Keller E, Bertram M, Hacke W. Moderate hypothermia in the treatment of patients with severe middle cerebral artery infarction. *Stroke*. 1998;29:2461–2466.

46. Steen PA, Soule EH, Michenfelder JD. Deterimental effect of prolonged hypothermia in cats and monkeys with and without regional cerebral ischemia. *Stroke*. 1979;10:522–529.

47. Steen PA, Milde JH, Michenfelder JD. The detrimental effects of prolonged hypothermia and rewarming in the dog. *Anesthesiology*. 1980;52:224–230.

48. Morikawa E, Ginsberg MD, Dietrich WD, et al. The significance of brain temperature in focal cerebral ischemia: Histopathological consequences of middle cerebral artery occlusion in the rat. *J Cereb Blood Flow Metab*. 1992;12:380–389.

49. Safar P, Tisherman SA, Behringer W, et al. Suspended animation for delayed resuscitation from prolonged cardiac arrest that is unresuscitable by standard cardiopulmonary-cerebral resuscitation. *Crit Care Med*. 2000;28:N214–N218.

50. Colbourne F, Corbett D. Delayed and prolonged post-ischemic hypothermia is neuroprotective in the gerbil. *Brain Res*. 1994;654:265–272.

51. Clark DL, Penner M, Orellana-Jordan IM, Colbourne F. Comparison of 12, 24 and 48 h of systemic hypothermia on outcome after permanent focal ischemia in rat. *Exp Neurol*. 2008;212:386–392.

52. Corbett D, Nurse S, Colbourne F. Hypothermic neuroprotection. A global ischemia study using 18- to 20-month-old gerbils. *Stroke*. 1997;28:2238–2242. discussion 2243.

53. Colbourne F, Corbett D. Delayed postischemic hypothermia: A six month survival study using behavioral and histological assessments of neuroprotection. *J Neurosci*. 1995;15:7250–7260.

54. Kim F, Olsufka M, Longstreth Jr WT, et al. Pilot randomized clinical trial of prehospital induction of mild hypothermia in out-of-hospital cardiac arrest patients with a rapid infusion of 4 degrees C normal saline. *Circulation*. 2007;115:3064–3070.

55. Bernard SA, Smith K, Cameron P, Rapid infusion of Cold Hartmanns Investigators, et al. Induction of prehospital therapeutic hypothermia after resuscitation from nonventricular fibrillation cardiac arrest. *Crit Care Med*. 2012;40:747–753.

56. Skulec R, Truhlar A, Seblova J, Dostal P, Cerny V. Pre-hospital cooling of patients following cardiac arrest is effective using even low volumes of cold saline. *Crit Care*. 2010;14:R231.

57. Hunter BR, O'Donnell DP, Allgood KL, Seupaul RA. No benefit to prehospital initiation of therapeutic hypothermia in out-of-hospital cardiac arrest: a systematic review and meta-analysis. *Acad Emerg Med*. 2014;21:355–364.

58. Diao M, Huang F, Guan J, et al. Prehospital therapeutic hypothermia after cardiac arrest: a systematic review and meta-analysis of randomized controlled trials. *Resuscitation*. 2013;84:1021–1028.

59. Kim F, Nichol G, Maynard C, et al. Effect of prehospital induction of mild hypothermia on survival and neurological status among adults with cardiac arrest: a randomized clinical trial. *JAMA*. 2014;311:45–52.

60. Hachimi-Idrissi S, Corne L, Ebinger G, Michotte Y, Huyghens L. Mild hypothermia induced by a helmet device: a clinical feasibility study. *Resuscitation*. 2001;51:275–281.

61. Arrich J. Clinical application of mild therapeutic hypothermia after cardiac arrest. *Crit Care Med*. 2007;35:1041–1047.

62. Lopez-de-Sa E, Rey JR, Armada E, et al. Hypothermia in comatose survivors from out-of-hospital cardiac arrest: pilot trial comparing 2 levels of target temperature. *Circulation*. 2012;126:2826–2833.

63. Part 4: Advanced life support. *Circulation*. 2005;112(III):25–54.

64. Deakin CD, Morrison LJ, Morley PT, Advanced life support chapter Collaborators, et al. Part 8: Advanced life support: 2010 international consensus on cardiopulmonary resuscitation and emergency cardiovascular care science with treatment recommendations. *Resuscitation*. 2010;81(suppl 1):e93–e174.

65. Oksanen T, Pettila V, Hynynen M, Varpula T. Therapeutic hypothermia after cardiac arrest: implementation and outcome in finnish intensive care units. *Acta Anaesthesiol Scand*. 2007;51:866–871.

66. Majersik JJ, Silbergleit R, Meurer WJ, Brown DL, Lisabeth LD, Morgenstern LB. Public health impact of full implementation of therapeutic hypothermia after cardiac arrest. *Resuscitation*. 2008;77:189–194.

67. Pfeifer R, Jung C, Purle S, et al. Survival does not improve when therapeutic hypothermia is added to post-cardiac arrest care. *Resuscitation*. 2011;82:1168–1173.

68. Tiainen M, Poutiainen E, Kovala T, Takkunen O, Happola O, Roine RO. Cognitive and neurophysiological outcome of cardiac arrest survivors treated with therapeutic hypothermia. *Stroke*. 2007;38:2303–2308.

69. Nielsen N, Friberg H, Gluud C, Herlitz J, Wetterslev J. Hypothermia after cardiac arrest should be further evaluated–a systematic review of randomised trials with meta-analysis and trial sequential analysis. *Int J Cardiol*. 2011;151:333–341.

70. Nielsen N, Winkel P, Cronberg T, et al. Detailed statistical analysis plan for the target temperature management after out-of-hospital cardiac arrest trial. *Trials*. 2013;14:300.

71. Nielsen N, Wetterslev J, Cronberg T, et al. Targeted temperature management at 33 degrees C versus 36 degrees C after cardiac arrest. *N Engl J Med*. 2013;369:2197–2206.

71a. Nolan JP, Soar J, Cariou A, et al. European resuscitation council and European society of intensive care medicine guidelines for post-resuscitation care 2015: section 5 of the European resuscitation council guidelines for resuscitation 2015. *Resuscitation*. 2015;95:202–222.

72. Kim YM, Yim HW, Jeong SH, Klem ML, Callaway CW. Does therapeutic hypothermia benefit adult cardiac arrest patients presenting with non-shockable initial rhythms?: a systematic review and meta-analysis of randomized and non-randomized studies. *Resuscitation*. 2012;83:188–196.

73. Lundbye JB, Rai M, Ramu B, et al. Therapeutic hypothermia is associated with improved neurologic outcome and survival in cardiac arrest survivors of non-shockable rhythms. *Resuscitation*. 2012;83:202–207.

74. Testori C, Sterz F, Behringer W, et al. Mild therapeutic hypothermia is associated with favourable outcome in patients after cardiac arrest with non-shockable rhythms. *Resuscitation*. 2011;82:1162–1167.

75. Scholefield B, Duncan H, Davies P, et al. Hypothermia for neuroprotection in children after cardiopulmonary arrest. *Cochrane Database Syst Rev*. 2013;2:CD009442.

75a. Maconochie IK, de Caen AR, Aickin R, Pediatric basic life support and pediatric advanced life support chapter Collaborators, et al. Part 6: Pediatric basic life support and pediatric advanced life support: 2015 international consensus on cardiopulmonary resuscitation and emergency cardiovascular care science with treatment recommendations. *Resuscitation*. 2015;95:e147–e168.

76. Dankiewicz J, Schmidbauer S, Nielsen N, et al. Safety, feasibility, and outcomes of induced hypothermia therapy following in-hospital cardiac arrest-evaluation of a large prospective registry. *Crit Care Med.* 2014;42:2537–2545.

77. Mikkelsen ME, Christie JD, Abella BS, American Heart Association's Get With the Guidelines-Resuscitation Investigators, et al. Use of therapeutic hypothermia after in-hospital cardiac arrest. *Crit Care Med.* 2013;41:1385–1395.

78. Nichol G, Huszti E, Kim F, American Heart Association Get With the Guideline-Resuscitation Investigators, et al. Does induction of hypothermia improve outcomes after in-hospital cardiac arrest? *Resuscitation.* 2013;84:620–625.

79. Kory P, Fukunaga M, Mathew JP, et al. Outcomes of mild therapeutic hypothermia after in-hospital cardiac arrest. *Neurocrit Care.* 2012;16:406–412.

80. Sandroni C, Nolan J, Cavallaro F, Antonelli M. In-hospital cardiac arrest: incidence, prognosis and possible measures to improve survival. *Intensive Care Med.* 2007;33:237–245.

81. Hessel 2nd EA. Therapeutic hypothermia after in-hospital cardiac arrest: a critique. *J Cardiothorac Vasc Anesth.* 2014;28:789–799.

82. Abella BS. Pro: The case for using therapeutic hypothermia after in-hospital cardiac arrest. *J Cardiothorac Vasc Anesth.* 2011;25:362–364.

83. Do R, Kim F. Con: Therapeutic hypothermia should not be applied to all victims of cardiac arrest. *J Cardiothorac Vasc Anesth.* 2011;25:365–367.

84. Oddo M, Rossetti AO. Early multimodal outcome prediction after cardiac arrest in patients treated with hypothermia. *Crit Care Med.* 2014;42:1340–1347.

85. Fugate JE, Wijdicks EF, Mandrekar J, et al. Predictors of neurologic outcome in hypothermia after cardiac arrest. *Ann Neurol.* 2010;68:907–914.

86. Abend NS, Topjian AA, Kessler SK, et al. Outcome prediction by motor and pupillary responses in children treated with therapeutic hypothermia after cardiac arrest. *Pediatr Crit Care Med.* 2012;13:32–38.

87. Fink EL, Berger RP, Clark RS, et al. Serum biomarkers of brain injury to classify outcome after pediatric cardiac arrest. *Crit Care Med.* 2014;42:664–674.

88. Kamps MJ, Horn J, Oddo M, et al. Prognostication of neurologic outcome in cardiac arrest patients after mild therapeutic hypothermia: a meta-analysis of the current literature. *Intensive Care Med.* 2013;39:1671–1682.

89. Xue D, Huang ZG, Smith KE, Buchan AM. Immediate or delayed mild hypothermia prevents focal cerebral infarction. *Brain Res.* 1992;587:66–72.

90. Maier CM, Ahern K, Cheng ML, Lee JE, Yenari MA, Steinberg GK. Optimal depth and duration of mild hypothermia in a focal model of transient cerebral ischemia: effects on neurologic outcome, infarct size, apoptosis, and inflammation. *Stroke.* 1998;29:2171–2180.

91. Schwab S, Schwarz S, Aschoff A, Keller E, Hacke W. Moderate hypothermia and brain temperature in patients with severe middle cerebral artery infarction. *Acta Neurochir Suppl.* 1998;71:131–134.

92. Schwab S, Spranger M, Aschoff A, Steiner T, Hacke W. Brain temperature monitoring and modulation in patients with severe MCA infarction. *Neurology.* 1997;48:762–767.

93. Hajat C, Hajat S, Sharma P. Effects of poststroke pyrexia on stroke outcome : a meta-analysis of studies in patients. *Stroke.* 2000;31:410–414.

94. Kasner SE, Wein T, Piriyawat P, et al. Acetaminophen for altering body temperature in acute stroke: a randomized clinical trial. *Stroke.* 2002;33:130–134.

95. Hacke W, Schwab S, Horn M, Spranger M, De Georgia M, von Kummer R. 'Malignant' middle cerebral artery territory infarction: clinical course and prognostic signs. *Arch Neurol.* 1996;53:309–315.

96. Berrouschot J, Sterker M, Bettin S, Koster J, Schneider D. Mortality of space-occupying ('malignant') middle cerebral artery infarction under conservative intensive care. *Intensive Care Med.* 1998;24:620–623.

97. Kammersgaard LP, Rasmussen BH, Jorgensen HS, Reith J, Weber U, Olsen TS. Feasibility and safety of inducing modest hypothermia in awake patients with acute stroke through surface cooling: A case-control study: the Copenhagen Stroke Study. *Stroke.* 2000;31:2251–2256.

98. De Georgia MA, Krieger DW, Abou-Chebl A, et al. Cooling for Acute Ischemic Brain Damage (COOL AID): a feasibility trial of endovascular cooling. *Neurology.* 2004;63:312–317.

99. Georgiadis D, Schwarz S, Aschoff A, Schwab S. Hemicraniectomy and moderate hypothermia in patients with severe ischemic stroke. *Stroke.* 2002;33:1584–1588.

100. Els T, Oehm E, Voigt S, Klisch J, Hetzel A, Kassubek J. Safety and therapeutical benefit of hemicraniectomy combined with mild hypothermia in comparison with hemicraniectomy alone in patients with malignant ischemic stroke. *Cerebrovasc Dis.* 2006;21:79–85.

101. Lakhan SE, Pamplona F. Application of mild therapeutic hypothermia on stroke: a systematic review and meta-analysis. *Stroke Res Treat.* 2012;2012:295906.

102. Hong JM, Lee JS, Song HJ, Jeong HS, Choi HA, Lee K. Therapeutic hypothermia after recanalization in patients with acute ischemic stroke. *Stroke.* 2014;45:134–140.

103. Piironen K, Tiainen M, Mustanoja S, et al. Mild hypothermia after intravenous thrombolysis in patients with acute stroke: a randomized controlled trial. *Stroke.* 2014;45:486–491.

104. Horn CM, Sun CH, Nogueira RG, et al. Endovascular reperfusion and cooling in cerebral acute ischemia (ReCCLAIM I). *J Neurointerv Surg.* 2014;6:91–95.

105. Lyden PD, Hemmen TM, Grotta J, Rapp K, Raman R. Endovascular therapeutic hypothermia for acute ischemic stroke: ICTuS 2/3 protocol. *Int J Stroke.* 2014;9:117–125.

106. van der Worp HB, Macleod MR, Bath PM, Euro HYP-1 Investigators, et al. Eurohyp-1: European multicenter, randomized, phase III clinical trial of therapeutic hypothermia plus best medical treatment vs. Best medical treatment alone for acute ischemic stroke. *Int J Stroke.* 2014;9:642–645.

107. Batchelor PE, Skeers P, Antonic A, et al. Systematic review and meta-analysis of therapeutic hypothermia in animal models of spinal cord injury. *PLoS One.* 2013;8:e71317.

108. Levi AD, Green BA, Wang MY, et al. Clinical application of modest hypothermia after spinal cord injury. *J Neurotrauma.* 2009;26:407–415.

109. Levi AD, Casella G, Green BA, et al. Clinical outcomes using modest intravascular hypothermia after acute cervical spinal cord injury. *Neurosurgery.* 2010;66:670–677.

110. Dididze M, Green BA, Dietrich WD, Vanni S, Wang MY, Levi AD. Systemic hypothermia in acute cervical spinal cord injury: a case-controlled study. *Spinal Cord.* 2013;51:395–400.

111. Hansebout RR, Hansebout CR. Local cooling for traumatic spinal cord injury: outcomes in 20 patients and review of the literature. *J Neurosurg Spine.* 2014;20:550–561.

112. Kwon BK, Mann C, Sohn HM, et al. Hypothermia for spinal cord injury. *Spine J.* 2008;8:859–874.

113. Dietrich WD, Levi AD, Wang M, Green BA. Hypothermic treatment for acute spinal cord injury. *Neurotherapeutics.* 2011;8:229–239.

114. Dietrich WD, Cappuccino A, Cappuccino H. Systemic hypothermia for the treatment of acute cervical spinal cord injury in sports. *Curr Sports Med Rep.* 2011;10:50–54.

114a.Alkabie S, Boileau AJ. The role of therapeutic hypothermia after traumatic spinal cord injury—a systematic review. *World Neurosurgery.* 2015 Sep 30. pii: S1878–8750(15)01247-4. doi: 10.1016/j.wneu.2015.09.079. [Epub ahead of print]

115. Berger RP, Adelson PD, Richichi R, Kochanek PM. Serum biomarkers after traumatic and hypoxemic brain injuries: Insight into the biochemical response of the pediatric brain to inflicted brain injury. *Dev Neurosci.* 2006;28:327–335.

116. Adelson PD. Hypothermia following pediatric traumatic brain injury. *J Neurotrauma.* 2009;26:429–436.

117. Crossley S, Reid J, McLatchie R, et al. A systematic review of therapeutic hypothermia for adult patients following traumatic brain injury. *Crit Care.* 2014;18:R75.

118. Georgiou AP, Manara AR. Role of therapeutic hypothermia in improving outcome after traumatic brain injury: a systematic review. *Br J Anaesth.* 2013;110:357–367.

119. Sydenham E, Roberts I, Alderson P. Hypothermia for traumatic head injury. *Cochrane Database Syst Rev.* 2009:CD001048.

120. Sandestig A, Romner B, Grande PO. Therapeutic hypothermia in children and adults with severe traumatic brain injury. *Ther Hypothermia Temp Manag.* 2014;4:10–20.

121. Li P, Yang C. Moderate hypothermia treatment in adult patients with severe traumatic brain injury: a meta-analysis. *Brain Inj.* 2014;28:1036–1041.

122. Ma C, He X, Wang L, et al. Is therapeutic hypothermia beneficial for pediatric patients with traumatic brain injury? A meta-analysis. *Child's Nerv Syst.* 2013;29:979–984.

123. Adelson PD, Ragheb J, Kanev P, et al. Phase II clinical trial of moderate hypothermia after severe traumatic brain injury in children. *Neurosurgery.* 2005;56:740–754. discussion 740–754.

124. Hutchison JS, Ward RE, Lacroix J, et al. Hypothermia therapy after traumatic brain injury in children. *N Engl J Med.* 2008;358: 2447–2456.

125. Clifton GL, Valadka A, Zygun D, et al. Very early hypothermia induction in patients with severe brain injury (the National Acute Brain Injury Study: Hypothermia II): a randomised trial. *Lancet Neurol.* 2011;10:131–139.

126. Maekawa T, Yamashita S, Nagao S, Hayashi N, Ohashi Y. Prolonged mild therapeutic hypothermia versus fever control with tight hemodynamic monitoring and slow rewarming in patients with severe traumatic brain injury: a randomized controlled trial. *J Neurotrauma.* 2014;32:422–429.

127. Dixon SR, Whitbourn RJ, Dae MW, et al. Induction of mild systemic hypothermia with endovascular cooling during primary percutaneous coronary intervention for acute myocardial infarction. *J Am Coll Cardiol.* 2002;40:1928–1934.

128. Kandzari DE, Chu A, Brodie BR, et al. Feasibility of endovascular cooling as an adjunct to primary percutaneous coronary intervention (results of the LOWTEMP pilot study). *Am J Cardiol.* 2004;93:636–639.

129. Wolfrum S, Pierau C, Radke PW, Schunkert H, Kurowski V. Mild therapeutic hypothermia in patients after out-of-hospital cardiac arrest due to acute ST-segment elevation myocardial infarction undergoing immediate percutaneous coronary intervention. *Crit Care Med.* 2008;36:1780–1786.

130. Hovdenes J, Laake JH, Aaberge L, Haugaa H, Bugge JF. Therapeutic hypothermia after out-of-hospital cardiac arrest: experiences with patients treated with percutaneous coronary intervention and cardiogenic shock. *Acta Anaesthesiol Scand.* 2007;51:137–142.

131. Zobel C, Adler C, Kranz A, Seck C, et al. Mild therapeutic hypothermia in cardiogenic shock syndrome. *Crit Care Med.* 2012;40:1715–1723.

132. Chisholm GE, Grejs A, Thim T, et al. Safety of therapeutic hypothermia combined with primary percutaneous coronary intervention after out-of-hospital cardiac arrest. *Eur Heart J Acute Cardiovasc Care.* 2015;4:60–63.

133. Noc M, Fajadet J, Lassen JF, et al. Invasive coronary treatment strategies for out-of-hospital cardiac arrest: A consensus statement from the European association for percutaneous cardiovascular interventions (EAPCI)/stent for life (SFL) groups. *EuroIntervention.* 2014;10:31–37.

134. Van Leeuwen GM, Hand JW, Lagendijk JJ, Azzopardi DV, Edwards AD. Numerical modeling of temperature distributions within the neonatal head. *Pediatr Res.* 2000;48:351–356.

135. Jacobs SE, Berg M, Hunt R, Tarnow-Mordi WO, Inder TE, Davis PG. Cooling for newborns with hypoxic ischaemic encephalopathy. *Cochrane Database Syst Rev.* 2013;1. CD003311.

136. Jacobs S, Hunt R, Tarnow-Mordi W, Inder T, Davis P. Cooling for newborns with hypoxic ischaemic encephalopathy. *Cochrane Database Syst Rev.* 2007:CD003311.

137. Pauliah SS, Shankaran S, Wade A, Cady EB, Thayyil S. Therapeutic hypothermia for neonatal encephalopathy in low- and middle-income countries: a systematic review and meta-analysis. *PLoS One.* 2013;8:e58834.

138. Mourvillier B, Tubach F, van de Beek D, et al. Induced hypothermia in severe bacterial meningitis: a randomized clinical trial. *JAMA.* 2013;310:2174–2183.

139. Kutlesa M, Lepur D, Barsic B. Therapeutic hypothermia for adult community-acquired bacterial meningitis-historical control study. *Clin Neurol Neurosurg.* 2014;123:181–186.

140. Todd MM, Hindman BJ, Clarke WR, Torner JC, Intraoperative Hypothermia for Aneurysm Surgery Trial Iinvestigators. Mild intraoperative hypothermia during surgery for intracranial aneurysm. *N Engl J Med.* 2005;352:135–145.

141. Li LR, You C, Chaudhary B. Intraoperative mild hypothermia for postoperative neurological deficits in intracranial aneurysm patients. *Cochrane Database Syst Rev.* 2012;2:CD008445.

142. Staykov D, Wagner I, Volbers B, Doerfler A, Schwab S, Kollmar R. Mild prolonged hypothermia for large intracerebral hemorrhage. *Neurocrit Care.* 2013;18:178–183.

143. Kollmar R, Staykov D, Dorfler A, Schellinger PD, Schwab S, Bardutzky J. Hypothermia reduces perihemorrhagic edema after intracerebral hemorrhage. *Stroke.* 2010;41:1684–1689.

144. Kollmar R, Juettler E, Huttner HB, Investigators CINCH, et al. Cooling in intracerebral hemorrhage (CINCH) trial: Protocol of a randomized German-Austrian clinical trial. *Int J Stroke.* 2012;7:168–172.

145. Zeiler FA, Zeiler KJ, Teitelbaum J, et al. Therapeutic hypothermia for refractory status epilepticus. *Can J Neurol Sci.* 2015;42: 221–229.

23 What Are the Special Considerations in the Management of Morbidly Obese Patients in the Intensive Care Unit?

Ali A. El Solh

Obesity is a chronic metabolic condition with important public health implications. It has been linked to increased morbidity and mortality from acute and chronic medical problems including hypertension, cardiovascular diseases, dyslipidemia, diabetes mellitus, arthritis, sleep apnea, and certain forms of cancer.

Although far from being ideal, the most convenient method of quantifying and defining the degree of obesity is with the body mass index (BMI), which is the ratio of a person's weight (in kilograms) to height (in meters) squared.[1] In 1998, the World Health Organization committee and the National Institutes of Health (NIH) put forward a classification that became the worldwide standard for comparison of obesity rates within and across populations. The consensus defined "morbid obesity" (MO)—also termed *clinically severe obesity*—as a BMI of 40 kg/m^2 or more or a BMI of more than 35 kg/m^2 and significant comorbidities.[2]

Although the U.S. prevalence of obesity has leveled in the last decade, compared with some European countries, the prevalence of obesity in the United States is three times higher than that in France and 1.5 times higher than that in the United Kingdom. According to the latest National Health and Nutrition Examination Survey (NHANES), the age-adjusted obesity prevalence was 35.7% in the United States in 2010 with no sex differences. Extreme obesity has more than doubled since the 1988-1994 NHANES, shifting from 2.9% to 6.3% in 2010 for grade 3 (severe) obesity and reaching 15.2% for grade 2 obesity.[3] The age-adjusted prevalence of overweight and obesity combined (BMI ≥25 kg/m^2) was 68.8% in 2010 with a mean BMI of 28.7 kg/m^2 in the U.S. population.[3] With such a global epidemic, it is not surprising that an increasing number of morbidly obese patients are admitted to the intensive care unit (ICU). Hence, what are the special considerations in the management of morbidly obese patients in the ICU?

Critically ill obese patients present intensive care physicians with unique challenges that only a thorough knowledge of the peculiar pathophysiologic changes that occur in this population will allow for anticipation of complications and effective delivery of care.

Airway Management

MO has been considered one of the risk factors for difficult intubation.[4] However, the reader should be aware that MO, as defined by BMI, does not necessarily indicate increased fat deposits in and around the airway: Many patients have a gynecoid pattern of obesity. In two series of morbidly obese patients undergoing upper abdominal surgery, the incidence of difficult intubation was estimated at 13% and 24%, respectively.[5,6] More recently, the magnitude of this risk was challenged. A study of more than 90,000 Danish patients undergoing intubation for surgery put the frequency of difficult intubation closer to 6.4% in those with a BMI of 35 kg/m^2 or more compared with 5.2% in the overall population.[7] In the Australian Incident Monitoring Study, limited neck mobility and mouth opening accounted for most cases of difficult intubation in obese subjects.[8] Other studies added to the preceding list a short sternomental distance, a receding mandible, a large neck circumference, and a Mallampati score of 3 or greater as predictors of difficult intubation.[9,10] Although these multivariate predictive models have yet to be tested in an ICU setting, neither obesity nor BMI predicted problems with tracheal intubation.[10,11] One of the reasons for the observed differences among these studies is the lack of consensus on the definition of the term *difficult intubation*.[12] Nonetheless, the increased bulk of soft tissues in the upper airway make the morbidly obese, particularly those with obstructive sleep apnea, prone to partial obstruction. Hiremath et al.[13] found that 8 of 15 individuals with Cormack and Lehane grade 4 laryngoscopic views had apnea-hypopnea indices consistent with previously undiagnosed sleep apnea syndrome whereas only 2 matched controls without a difficult

144

laryngoscopic view had similar scores. Within this context, the American Society of Anesthesiology recommends that awake intubation be considered in the morbidly obese patient if difficult mask ventilation and difficult intubation are anticipated.[14]

Emergency airway management of the critically ill morbidly obese patient is frequently complicated by the patient's limited physiologic reserve. Morbidly obese patients are more prone to hypoxemia because of reductions in expiratory reserve volume, functional residual capacity (FRC), and maximum voluntary ventilation.[15] Severely obese patients undergoing surgery have significantly lower nadir SpO_2 (oxygen saturation by pulse oximetry) during intubation compared with normal and overweight patients despite similar preoxygenation duration and baseline SpO_2 readings.[16] Moreover, the increased intra-abdominal pressure is thought to place the obese patient at a higher risk of aspiration of gastric content.[17] These levels are traditionally considered to be a risk factor in the adult obese patient for aspiration pneumonitis. Given these physiologic changes, a rapid sequence induction (RSI) has been advocated.[18] However, the use of RSI in fasted patients with no risk factors for aspiration other than obesity is debatable. Obese patients without symptoms of gastroesophageal reflux have a resistance gradient between the stomach and the gastroesophageal junction similar to that in nonobese subjects.[19] In addition, there are drawbacks for RSI that could prove deleterious in these patients. First, although cricoid pressure may or may not decrease the risk of aspiration,[20] there is evidence that it may worsen the quality of laryngeal exposure.[21] Second, the application of cricoid pressure can lead to a complete airway occlusion, occurring between 6% and 11% of the time.[22]

In short, the degree of obesity or neck size that justifies advanced interventions for intubation remains unknown. The experience and ability of the laryngoscopist are probably the most important determinants for establishing an airway in the morbidly obese patient.

In patients who require tracheostomy, morbidly obese patients with increased submental and anterior cervical adipose tissue present a unique surgical challenge. The initial goal of securing a stable airway can be compromised by the size discrepancy and curvature mismatch between a standard-size tracheostomy tube and the increased distance between the skin and trachea. Standard tracheostomy tubes are typically too short and too curved. One study of 427 critically ill morbidly obese patients undergoing surgical tracheostomy reported a complication rate of 25%; most complications were minor.[23] Life-threatening complications occurred in 10% and were related to tube obstruction and extratracheal tube placement. Some surgeons advocate performing a Bjork flap at the time of surgery to prevent tube misplacement in the pretracheal fascia.[24] Others favor a cervical lipectomy in combination with tracheostomy.[24] There are no studies that prove that these interventions are effective.

Percutaneous dilational tracheostomy (PDT) remains controversial for these patients. Obese patients with large and thick necks were traditionally considered poor candidates for PDT.[25] However, PDT has been performed in these patients with low rates of complications.[26] A large retrospective study of more than 3000 cases of PDT in which 16% of patients had a BMI of 35 kg/m^2 or greater appears to confirm the safety of this procedure in this high-risk group. The authors postulated that the introduction of extra-long tracheostomy tubes in obese patients may have contributed to the low complication rate in this high-risk group.[27] There was likely selection bias in this study because high BMI does not necessarily translate into airway disease and the best "obese" candidates were likely selected for PDT. In the absence of large randomized trials, no recommendation could be made regarding PDT in this population. The outcome of PDT depends largely on the skills and the experience of the operator.

Despite substantial investigation, the optimal timing of tracheotomy for critically ill obese patients requiring mechanical ventilation (MV) continues to be debated between those who support early intervention, citing the benefits of early liberation from MV, and those who argue against this approach because of a lack of supportive evidence. To date, no randomized trial of tracheotomy time has been completed in morbidly obese patients. One retrospective study of 102 morbidly obese patients requiring artificial ventilation did suggest a reduced duration of MV and ICU length of stay and a lower incidence of nosocomial pneumonia in those who underwent early tracheostomy (≤9 days) compared with late tracheostomy.[28] However, no difference in hospital mortality was observed. Because of the possibility of selection bias in retrospective designs, a consensus on when a tracheostomy should be performed in these patients awaits a randomized clinical trial.

Respiratory

The most prominent pulmonary function test abnormalities associated with obesity are decreased expiratory reserve volume and FRC, whereas the vital capacity and total lung capacity are essentially unchanged.[15,29] Relative to nonobese subjects, the total respiratory system compliance is decreased because of the greater degree of chest wall compression and cephalad displacement of the diaphragm. In the supine and Trendelenburg positions, FRC may fall below the closing capacity, leading to small airway collapse, atelectasis, ventilation perfusion mismatch, and hypoxemia.[30] As lung volumes are reduced and airway resistance is increased, a tidal volume based on a patient's actual body weight is likely to result in high airway pressures, alveolar overdistention, and barotrauma. The current consensus would favor that the initial tidal volume be calculated according to ideal body weight (IBW), on the basis of the patient's height, and then adjusted according to the desired plateau pressure and systemic arterial blood gases.[31]

The role of positive end-expiratory pressure (PEEP) on respiratory mechanics and blood gases in postoperative mechanically ventilated morbidly obese subjects has been tested by several studies. Pelosi et al.[32] applied a PEEP of 10 cm H_2O to nine anesthetized-paralyzed morbidly obese subjects after abdominal surgery and found a significant reduction in respiratory system elastance and resistance. This reduction was attributed to alveolar recruitment or to the re-opening of closed airways. The authors also found a small but significant improvement in arterial oxygenation, which was correlated with the amount of recruited volume. In a similar group of subjects, Koutsoukou and colleagues[33] found that the PEEP used (4 to 16 cm) caused a significant reduction in elastance and resistance of the respiratory system. However, PEEP had no significant effect on gas exchange. In both studies, oxygenation remained markedly abnormal even after the application of PEEP, probably reflecting residual atelectasis. Indeed, the extent of atelectasis, which was correlated with the amount of venous admixture, was not reduced by inflation of the lungs with conventional tidal volume, or even with a doubled tidal volume.[34]

In patients with acute respiratory distress syndrome (ARDS), prone positioning is known to improve gas exchange and outcomes (see Chapter 32). With the weight of the mediastinal structures, particularly the heart, supported by the sternum, less pulmonary tissue is compressed. The delivered tidal volume and peak pressure are dispersed to more alveoli, decreasing the risk of further alveolar injury from stretch and strain forces. Proning reduces $\dot{V}/\dot{Q}$ (ventilation-perfusion) mismatch, reduces right-to-left shunt, and improves oxygenation.[35] One case control study with morbidly obese patients (BMI ≥35 kg/m^2) and ARDS (Pao$_2$ [partial pressure of oxygen, arterial]/Fio$_2$ [fraction of inspired oxygen] ratio ≤200 mm Hg) documented improvement in oxygenation and decreased 90-day mortality without significant increase in duration of MV, length of stay, or incidence of nosocomial pneumonia.[36] However, abdominally obese patients (with sagittal abdominal diameter ≥26 cm) were at higher risk of renal failure and hypoxic hepatitis.[37] It is speculated that the increased intra-abdominal pressure from prone positioning might have been the culprit. Given the limited data specific to prone positioning in morbidly obese patients, the feasibility and effect of proning in morbidly patients with ARDS will likely be affected by the degree of familiarity of nurses and physicians with proning and the availability of the appropriate resources.

The rate of reintubation after extubation in severely obese patients has been reported at 8% to 14% among patients undergoing MV for more than 48 hours.[38,39] Earlier investigations suggested that the prophylactic use of noninvasive ventilation (NIV) in morbidly obese patients during the first 24 hours postoperatively reduced pulmonary dysfunction after gastroplasty and accelerated reestablishment of preoperative pulmonary function. Joris and colleagues[40] demonstrated that the application of bilevel positive airway pressure set at 12 and 4 cm H$_2$O significantly improved the peak expiratory flow rate, the forced vital capacity, and the oxygen saturation on the first postoperative day. This improvement was attributed to a combined effect of improved lung inflation, prevention of alveolar collapse, and reduced inspiratory threshold load. In a parallel study of 50 morbidly obese patients admitted to a medical ICU with acute respiratory failure, patients who were successfully treated with NIV had a shorter hospital stay and a lower mortality.[41] The reduction in the rate of respiratory failure was more pronounced when NIV was immediately instituted afterextubation.[42] Subgroup analysis of patients with hypercapnia showed reduced hospital mortality in the NIV group compared with controls. In contrast, patients who failed a trial of NIV and those who required invasive

MV demonstrated a longer ICU and hospital length of stay and higher mortality (31%).[41]

Deep Venous Thrombosis Prophylaxis

MO is a risk factor for venous thromboembolic disease (VTE)[43,44] because of increased venous stasis, decreased mobility, and a possibly a hypercoagulable state.[45] Unfortunately, limited data exist on effective prophylactic regimens of anticoagulation in critically ill morbidly obese patients. These patients are typically excluded from trials because of the equivocal results of the diagnostic tests used to confirm or exclude thromboembolic disease.

Studies in which the effectiveness of VTE prophylaxis in obese hospitalized patients is evaluated are listed in Table 23-1.[46-60] Despite the absence of well-designed randomized controlled trials in critically ill morbidly obese patients, the use of prophylaxis is indicated. Pharmacokinetic and epidemiologic studies suggest that the standard fixed doses of thromboprophylaxis are suboptimal in this population. A retrospective study demonstrated that high-dose thromboprophylaxis (heparin 7500 U 3 times a day instead of standard dosing of 5000 U 2 to 3 times a day or enoxaparin 40 mg twice a day [instead of 40 mg once a day]) approximately halved the odds of symptomatic VTE in patients with weight greater than 100 kg or BMI greater than 40 kg/m^2, with no increased risk of bleeding.[49] Although this would appear to be a reasonable starting point, there is no universal consensus on the optimal regimens (mechanical or pharmacologic) and duration of VTE prophylaxis in these patients.

Pharmacotherapy

Several factors underlie the rate and extent of drug distribution in the morbidly obese patient, including degree of tissue perfusion, binding of drugs to plasma proteins, and permeability of tissue membranes. In general, the extent to which obesity influences the volume of distribution of a drug depends on its lipid solubility.[61] Early work with barbiturates clearly demonstrated the close correlation between lipid solubility and drug distribution. However, lipophilic compounds do not always have larger volumes of distribution. For example, the volume of distribution of digoxin is not significantly influenced by obesity despite its relatively high lipid partition coefficient. Conversely, the volume of distribution for some hydrophilic drugs in adipose tissue may be only a fraction of the volume of distribution in other tissues. The reason is that the water content in adipose tissue is 20% to 50% of that in other tissues.[62] Hence, distribution of these drugs may warrant adjusting the dose in proportion to the excess in body weight with the use of a dosing weight correction factor (DWCF).

$$\text{Adjusted weight (AW)} = \text{DWCF (TBW} - \text{IBW)} + \text{IBW}$$

In the case of the least liposoluble drugs (atracurium, H$_2$ blockers) and specific lipophilic drugs (methylprednisolone), distribution is restricted to lean mass, and loading is usually based on IBW.

The influence of pathophysiologic and histologic changes associated with obesity on hepatic and renal metabolism has yet to be fully elucidated. Previous evidence has suggested

Table 23-1 Evidence of Efficacy of VTE Prophylaxis in Hospitalized Obese Patients

Author, Year	Study Design	Intervention	Outcome
Samama, 1999	Randomized, controlled trial	738 hospitalized medical patients > 40 years old, including 20% of obese patients randomized to enoxaparin 40 mg/day or placebo	RR, 0.37 (97.6% CI, 0.22-0.63) with enoxaparin 40 mg/day. Major hemorrhage in 1.7% vs. 1.1% in the placebo group.
Kalfarentzos, 2001	Randomized, controlled trial	60 patients undergoing bariatric surgery, randomized to 5700 or 9500 IU of nadroparin	No incidence of DVT in both groups receiving nadroparin. Major hemorrhage reported in 6.7% in the group receiving higher dose of nadroparin.
Scholten, 2002	Prospective noncontrolled study	481 patients undergoing bariatric surgery receiving prophylaxis with 30 mg SC q12h or 40 mg q12h of enoxaparin	Incidence of symptomatic VTE of 5.4% with enoxaparin 30 mg q12h, and of 0.6% with 40 mg q12h. Major hemorrhage in 1.0% and 0.25% in the two groups of enoxaparin, respectively.
Gonzalez, 2004	Prospective noncontrolled study	380 patients undergoing bariatric surgery with SCD	Incidence of symptomatic DVT of 0.26%. No PE reported.
Alikhan, 2003	Randomized, controlled trial	866 hospitalized obese medical patients > 40 years old randomized to enoxaparin 40 mg/day or placebo	RR, 0.49 (95% CI, 0.18-1.36) with enoxaparin 40 mg/day.
Shepherd, 2003	Prospective noncontrolled study	700 patients undergoing bariatric surgery receiving prophylaxis with continuous intravenous UH during the perioperative period	Incidence of DVT and symptomatic PE of 0% and 0.4%, respectively. Postoperative hemorrhage in 2.3%.
Miller, 2004	Retrospective cohort	255 patients undergoing bariatric surgery receiving prophylaxis with LDUH 5000 or 7500 IU q8h	Overall incidence of VTE of 1.2%. Prospective hemorrhage in 2.4%.
Shepherd, 2004	Prospective noncontrolled study	19 patients undergoing bariatric surgery receiving prophylaxis with continuous intravenous UH during the perioperative period	No symptomatic VTE confirmed. Major hemorrhage in 10.5%.
Leizorovicz, 2004	Randomized, controlled trial	3706 hospitalized medical patients > 40 years, including 30% of obese patients randomized to dalteparin 5000 IU/day or placebo	RR, 0.55 (95% CI, 0.38-0.80) with dalteparin 5000 IU/day. Major hemorrhage in 0.49% vs 0.16% in the placebo group.
Kucher, 2005	Subgroup analysis of randomized, controlled trial	1118 hospitalized obese medical patients > 40 years randomized to dalteparin 5000 IU/day or placebo	VTE occurred in 2.8% of the dalteparin and 4.3% of the placebo group. RR, 0.64 (95% CI, 0.32-1.28) with dalteparin 5000 IU/day.
Hamad, 2005	Multicentric retrospective cohort	668 patients undergoing bariatric surgery receiving prophylaxis with enoxaparin 30 mg (daily or q12h) or 40 mg (daily or q12h) or no prophylaxis	Overall incidence of objectively confirmed symptomatic PE of 0.9%, and DVT of 0.1%; highest incidence without prophylaxis. Major hemorrhage in 0.9%.
Quebbemann, 2005	Prospective noncontrolled study	822 patients undergoing bariatric surgery receiving prophylaxis with continuous intravenous UH at 400 U/hr from the preoperative period until discharge	Overall incidence of objectively confirmed symptomatic VTE of 0.1%. Major hemorrhage in 1.3%.
Cossu, 2007	Retrospective cohort	151 patients underwent surgery for morbid obesity. In the first 65 cases, prophylaxis consisted in a single intravenous injection of heparin sodium (2500-5000 IU) at the time of induction of anesthesia. Later cases (86 cases) adjusted according to PT, TT, and aPTT.	Two cases of VTE in the first group and one in the second group. Major bleeding occurred in 2.33%.
Raftopoulos, 2008	Retrospective cohort	Group A: Enoxaparin 1 hour before surgery followed by enoxaparin 30 mg SC twice a day until discharge from hospital. Group B: No preoperative heparin, then enoxaparin 30 mg SC twice a day followed by a 10-day course of enoxaparin 40 mg SC once a day at home after hospital discharge.	VTE event occurred in Group A (1.14%) vs. Group B (0%). The incidence of significant bleeding was lower in Group B (Group A [5.3%] vs. Group B [0.56%], $P = 0.02$).

Table 23-1 **Evidence of Efficacy of VTE Prophylaxis in Hospitalized Obese Patients—cont'd**

Author, Year	Study Design	Intervention	Outcome
Borkgren-Okonek, 2008	Prospective open trial	223 undergoing Roux-en-Y gastric bypass assigned to receive enoxaparin 40 mg (BMI < 50 kg/m²) or 60 mg (BMI > 50 kg/m²) every 12 hours during hospitalization and once daily for 10 days after discharge.	One patient had nonfatal venous thrombo-embolism (0.45%). Four patients required transfusion (1.79%).
Wang, 2014	Retrospective cohort	9241 inpatients with weight > 100 kg comparing high-dose thromboprophylaxis (heparin 7500 U three times daily or enoxaparin 40 mg twice daily) to standard doses (heparin 5000 U two or three times daily or enoxaparin 40 mg once daily).	The rate of VTE was 1.48% of those who received standard doses compared with 0.77% in those who received high doses. High-dose thromboprophylaxis did not increase bleeding (OR, 0.84; 95% CI, 0.66-1.07; $P = 0.15$).

aPTT, activated partial thromboplastin time; *BMI,* body mass index; *CI,* confidence interval; *DVT,* deep vein thrombosis; *LDUH,* low-dose unfractionated heparin; *OR,* odds ratio; *PE,* pulmonary embolism; *PT,* prothrombin time; *RR,* relative risk; *SC,* subcutaneous; *SCD,* sequential compression device; *TT,* thrombin time; *UH,* unfractionated heparin; *VTE,* venous thromboembolic disease.

that hepatic oxidative metabolism is not different from lean individuals but more recent investigasuggested suggested that hepatic oxidative metabolism is not different from lean individuals, but more recent investigations pointed to an increased activity of cytochrome P450 enzymes. Kotlyar and Carson[63] have provided strong evidence that the condition of obesity significantly increases hepatic CYP2E1 activity while decreasing hepatic CYP3A4 activities. The use of the creatinine clearance equations to assess renal function in the morbidly obese can be misleading. In a study involving 12 men and 31 women who weighed more than 195% of their IBW, creatinine clearance was overestimated by 51 to 61 mL/min/1.73 m² when total body weight (TBW) was used and underestimated by 36 to 40 mL/min/1.73 m² when IBW was used.[64] Salazar and Corcoran[65] proposed alternative formulas based on animal models for creatinine clearance in obese subjects. However, these equations have not been validated in critically ill morbidly obese patients. A recent formula derived from the Modification of Diet in Renal Disease (MDRD) Study group[66] [GFR = 170 × (serum creatinine)$^{-0.999}$ × (age, years)$^{-0.176}$ × 0.762 (if female) × 1.18 (if Black) × (blood urea nitrogen)$^{-0.17}$ × (albumin)$^{+0.318}$] has the advantage of predicting glomerular filtration rate (GFR) rather than creatinine clearance. Data obtained in an ICU from a morbidly obese patient with 51-chromium–labeled ethylenediamine tetra-acetic acid clearance as the gold standard suggest close estimation of the MDRD formula to the actual GFR.[67] A comprehensive review of this topic has been published elsewhere,[62,68] but what follows are details about some of the commonly used drugs.

Sedatives and Analgesics

There are no established guidelines for the optimal drug of choice for sedation in critically ill morbidly obese patients. Midazolam, lorazepam, propofol, and dexmedetomidine are currently the four sedatives most commonly administered in the ICU. Propofol is a hypnotic agent with a rapid onset and offset. Volume of distribution and clearance are increased in obese patients and correlate with adjusted body weight (ABW).[69] Because propofol is emulsified in a soybean base, it may increase carbon dioxide (CO_2) production.

The lipophilic benzodiazepines demonstrate increased volume of distribution and increased elimination half-life in obese patients.[70] Midazolam has the shortest half-life among benzodiazepines, but its sedative effect might be prolonged in morbidly obese individuals because of its accumulation in adipose tissue. When combined with propofol or fentanyl, its clearance might decrease because of competitive inhibition of CYP3A4.[67] The combination of haloperidol and midazolam can decrease the dose required to produce sedation and minimize the risk of respiratory depression. Dose calculations for continuous benzodiazepine infusion in obese patients should follow IBW because clearance is not significantly different from nonobese patients. Nonetheless, daily discontinuation with retitration to a target sedation endpoint is advocated to reduce the duration of MV and ICU length of stay.

The synthetic opioids (remifentanil, fentanyl, and alfentanil) are lipophilic compounds with a rapid onset of action and minimal histamine-related vasodilation. Their cardiovascular responses to endotracheal intubation in morbidly obese patients are comparable.[71] Significantly less expensive than the other synthetic opioids, fentanyl is often the preferred analgesic agent for critically ill patients with hemodynamic instability or morphine allergy. Similar pharmacokinetics of fentanyl in obese and nonobese patients was documented, suggesting dosing on the basis of IBW. A more recent investigation observed that the relationship between TBW and the fentanyl doses required to achieve and maintain postoperative analgesic endpoints had a nonlinear profile[72] (Table 23-2). In contrast, pharmacokinetic data suggest that remifentanil should be based on IBW.[73] As for morphine dosing, a tenfold variation in dosing requirement was reported that was unrelated to age, gender, or body surface area.[74,75]

Neuromuscular Blockade

Atracurium and vecuronium have limited volume of distribution, but although vecuronium, rocuronium, and cisatracurium dosing is based on IBW, the hyposensitivity to atracurium observed in obese individuals necessitates calculation of the dose on the basis of TBW.[62] There are no studies demonstrating a reduction in neuromuscular complications when intermittent dosing techniques are used instead of continuous infusions. Periodic monitoring with the train of four should be conducted routinely to adjust the rate of infusion. However, increased adiposity around the wrist may require more milliamperes to produce the desired result.

Table 23-2 **Proposed Dosing of Commonly Used Drugs in Obese Patients**		
Drug	**Initial**	**Maintenance**
Lidocaine	TBW	IBW
Digoxin	IBW	IBW
Beta-blockers	IBW	IBW
Aminoglycosides	AW	AW
Vancomycin	AW	AW
Atracurium	TBW	TBW
Vencuronium	IBW	IBW
Fentanyl	$52/(1 + [196.4 \times e^{-0.025 TBW} - 53.66]/100)$	
Phenytoin	TBW	IBW
Corticosteroids	IBW	IBW
Cyclosporine	IBW	IBW
Aminophylline	IBW	IBW
Heparin*	ABW	–
Enoxaparin*	TBW	TBW
Drotrecogin alfa	ABW	ABW

*Dosing for treatment of venous thromboembolism.
Male: IBW = 50 kg + 2.3 kg per inch of height >5 ft.
Female: IBW = 45.5 kg + 2.3 kg per inch of height >5 ft.
AW = IBW + 0.4 (TBW − IBW).
ABW, adjusted body weight, *AW,* adjusted weight; *IBW,* ideal body weight, TBW, total body weight.

Anticoagulants

MO has little to no effect on the weight-based heparin dosing protocols that use TBW in systemic anticoagulation.[76] As alluded to previously, large studies evaluating the safety and efficacy of using weight-based dosing of low molecular weight heparins (LMWHs) for the treatment of venous thromboembolism in these critically ill morbidly obese patients are limited. Pharmacokinetic studies suggest that body mass does not appear to have a significant effect on the response to LMWHs in obese patients with normal renal function.[77] Nonetheless, monitoring of anti–factor Xa activity (anti-Xa) should be considered. Although the timing of the blood sampling in relation to the dose and the optimal range of values has yet to be clearly defined, a peak anti-Xa level drawn 4 hours after a dose is given is considered the most useful.[78] For twice-daily administration, a target of anti-Xa level of 0.6 to 1.0 IU/mL has been recommended. The range at 4 hours for those treated with a once-daily dose is less certain, but a level of 1.0 to 2.0 IU/mL is suggested.

Anticoagulant treatment options have been significantly expanded by the addition of an oral direct thrombin inhibitor and two Xa-inhibitors. Unfortunately, there are few data focusing on dosing in obesity. Dabigatran is approved in the United States for prevention of stroke and systemic embolism in nonvalvular atrial fibrillation (AF).[79] The RE-LY (Randomized Evaluation of Long-term Anticoagulation Therapy) trial noted a 20% decrease in trough concentrations in patients weighing more than 100 kg; however, dose adjustments have not been recommended.[80] Rivaroxaban is approved for prevention of stroke and systemic embolism in nonvalvular AF, treatment of deep vein thrombosis (DVT) and pulmonary embolism (PE), and DVT prophylaxis after knee and hip surgery.[81-83] A Phase II study demonstrated that a TBW more than 120 kg was not associated with clinically significant changes in pharmacokinetic or pharmacodynamics parameters; thus dose adjustments are not warranted.[84] Studies with rivaroxaban have included a small proportion of patients with a BMI of 28 kg/m^2 or more or weights exceeding 100 kg; subgroup analyses have shown that dose modifications are unnecessary.[81,85]

Apixaban is the most recent agent to be approved for prevention of stroke and systemic embolism in nonvalvular AF.[86] One study found that a 10-mg dose of apixaban yielded a 20% decrease in peak concentration in patients weighing more than 120 kg. The authors concluded that these alterations were not clinically significant and no dose alteration is needed.[87]

Nutritional Care

There is a paucity of data for any specific feeding strategy of critically ill morbidly obese patients. In general, the energy expenditure of morbidly obese patients is increased because of an increase in lean body mass.[88] Inadequate nutritional intake combined with elevated basal insulin concentrations suppresses lipid mobilization from body stores, causing accelerated proteolysis, which in turn forces rapid loss of muscle mass and early deconditioning. Conversely, aggressively high caloric formulas have been associated with increased CO_2 production,[89] which increases the work of breathing and may prolong the need for MV. It is wrong to assume that morbidly obese patients can tolerate prolonged periods of fasting; if tolerated, then enteral nutritional support should be commenced within 48 hours after admission to an ICU.[90]

The most challenging question is how to assess the energy requirements of morbidly obese patients. Several predictive equations have been developed to estimate energy requirements, but adapting these formulas for morbidly obese patients is problematic. Estimates of energy expenditure in the critically ill have been derived traditionally from the Harris-Benedict equation, but clinicians and investigators are unclear whether IBW or actual body weight should be used.[91] In morbidly obese individuals, indirect calorimetry is considered the method of choice to determine energy expenditure if the inspired oxygen is less than 60%.[90] Whether any of these measures translate into improved outcome cannot be determined in the absence of randomized clinical trials.[92]

Hypocaloric, high-protein enteral or parenteral nutrition is thought to achieve net protein anabolism and avoid overfeeding complications such as hyperglycemia. This involves the administration of no more than 60% to 70% of requirements or administration of 11 to 14 kcal/kg current body weight/day or 22 to 25 kcal/kg ideal weight/day, with 2 to 2.5 g/kg ideal weight/day of proteins.[93] Several studies evaluated the use of hypocaloric high-protein nutritional support in critically ill obese patients.[94] Overall, these studies showed a preserved nitrogen balance and decreased morbidity, but studies were small, and there was no mortality benefit. The hypocaloric high-protein diet has not been evaluated in patients with renal or liver disease; therefore the use of hypocaloric nutritional support in obese patients should be used with caution in patients with these conditions.

Diagnostic Imaging

Diagnostic imaging is a core component of diagnosis and response to therapeutics in modern medicine. However, studies that are readily available to normal weight patients may prove difficult and hazardous to morbidly obese critically ill patients.

Radiography can be limited by X-ray beam attenuation, which results in decreased image contrast and amplification of noise and an increase in exposure time resulting in motion artifacts. Raising kilovolt (peak) and milliampere-second helps in improving the image quality.[95] The use of multiple cassettes may be needed to cover the entire chest or abdomen.

Ultrasound image quality is affected by fat to a greater degree than any other imaging modality.[95] The ultrasound beam is attenuated by fat at a rate of 0.63 dB/cm. Use of the lowest frequency transducer (1.5 to 2.0 MHz) may partially overcome the increased image attenuation. For fluoroscopy, computed tomography, and magnetic resonance imaging (MRI), the weight and aperture diameter limitations of the imaging modality should be obtained before these patients are transported out of the ICU (Table 23-3). MRI scanners with a high signal-to-noise ratio and strong gradients (≥1.5 T) cannot accommodate patients weighing 350 lb (159 kg). A vertical-field open MRI system is needed for patients who weigh up to 550 lb (250 kg) and can offer a range of vertical apertures from 40 to 55 cm.

Intravenous Access

MO poses a particular challenge for intravenous access. Possible explanations for complications related to central venous catheter placement in obese patients include loss of anatomic landmarks, increased depth of insertion, need for multiple needle passes, increased duration of cannulation, and difficulty in maintaining proper angle during insertion. An increased risk of blood stream infection has also been suggested when femoral placement was attempted in this population.[96] The use of

Table 23-3 Weight and Aperture Diameter Limitations per Imaging Modality

Imaging Modality	Maximum Aperture Diameter (cm)	Weight Limit (lb)
Fluoroscopy	63	700
Vertical-field MRI	55	550
Cylindrical-bore MRI	70	550

MRI, magnetic resonance imaging.

two-dimensional ultrasound guidance for cannulation of the internal jugular veins unequivocally decreases the risk of failed catheter placement, improves first-pass success, and facilitates faster placement compared with the landmark method.[97]

Outcomes of Critically Ill Obese Patients

Since 2001, there have been numerous reports trying to elucidate the relationship between BMI and critical care outcome. Earlier studies of morbidly obese patients in the critical care setting (BMI > 40 kg/m^2) reported higher mean length of stay in the ICU and longer duration of MV compared with nonobese patients (BMI < 30 kg/m^2).[98-100] There was also a higher in-hospital mortality of the obese versus the nonobese patients.

Recently, these dire prognostications for critically obese patients have been subsequently challenged by parallel investigations.[101-103] More contemporary studies have demonstrated that the relation between BMI and mortality appears to reflect a U-shaped curve, with underweight and severely obese patients having significantly higher adjusted mortality across all age groups and moderately overweight and less severely obese patients having comparatively improved mortality.[104] The NIH ARDS-Net study databases are a useful source of outcome data on different types of critically ill patients. A secondary analysis of pooled data from three studies revealed that the unadjusted outcomes across BMI groups did not differ significantly for any of the dependent variables (28-day mortality, achievement of unassisted ventilation, 180-day mortality rate, or ventilator-free days).[102] The authors acknowledged that improved outcomes in the study population could have been the result of increased intensity of care of the study population and standardized weaning procedures that were used. In line with these findings, three systematic reviews concluded that obesity was associated with comparable or lower risk of death compared with normal weight.[105-107] Potential hypotheses have been advanced to explain this "obesity paradox." It is important to note that patients with a BMI less than 40 kg/m^2 appeared to have better than expected outcomes in the ICU; as such, overweight and obesity may represent enhanced physiologic reserve. Alternatively, specific hormonal mechanisms could play a role in the relation between obesity and mortality. Bornstein and colleagues[108] reported a positive association between leptin concentrations and survival of septic patients, suggesting that leptin could play a role in the adaptive response to critical illness.

Against this improved outlook of obesity outcome in predominantly medical ICUs, morbidly obese patients requiring admission to surgical or trauma units had more adverse events than their counterparts. MO was reported as an independent risk factor for death in surgical patients who required 4 days or more of ICU stay, indicating that complications of health-care processes may be the key to improved outcomes in this cohort. The increased mortality was attributed to organ failures, need of more vasopressors, and failed extubation.[109] However, these complications were not higher in obese cardiac patients who required bypass graft surgery than nonobese, although the risks of sternal wound infection were substantially increased in the obese and severely obese.[110,111]

In trauma patients, obesity seems to be associated with poorer outcomes.[112-114] In blunt trauma, obese patients sustain different types of injuries than lean patients, with higher frequency of thoracoabdominal wounds and less traumatic brain injuries. Moreover, obese trauma patients had a more than twofold increase in risk of acquiring a bloodstream, urinary tract, or respiratory tract infection after hospital admission,[115] including sepsis, ventilator-associated pneumonia, and catheter-associated bacteremia.[116] Further studies are needed to clarify whether obesity is deleterious in this population or not and to assess the possible differences in outcome between various surgical interventions.

CONCLUSION

The treatment of the critically ill morbidly obese patient remains a daunting task for critical care practitioners. Despite the growing global obesity epidemic, the management approach for the morbidly obese in intensive care settings is based mostly on expert opinion. Future randomized controlled trials are needed to guide clinicians in providing care to this unique population.

AUTHOR'S RECOMMENDATIONS

- Raised BMI does not necessarily translate into difficult airway or intubation. Android pattern obesity and large neck circumference predict difficult intubation and may alert the clinician to the need for advanced airway equipment. Management results not from failure of intubation but from failure of ventilation.
- Morbidly obese patients have reduced FRC, leading to increased airway closure, atelectasis, and ventilation perfusion mismatch—particularly in the supine position.
- Airway resistance is also increased.
- Higher levels of PEEP may be required because of increased chest wall elastance.
- Tidal volumes should be calculated based on height rather than weight.
- NIV immediately after extubation might reduce the rate of respiratory failure and decrease mortality in patients with hypercarbia.
- When unfractionated heparin/LMWH is used to prevent or treat DVT or PE in obese patients, higher doses than normal are required.
- Enteral feeding should be started early, and there is a strong argument to use a hypocaloric approach: 11 to 14 kcal/kg ABW per day and protein intake of 2.0 to 2.5 g/kg IBW per day.
- Before transport for diagnostic imaging studies, a discussion with the radiology department regarding the patient's weight and body diameter is recommended.
- Peripheral and central intravenous access may be difficult: ultrasound guidance is recommended.
- Critically ill overweight and obese patients are not at elevated risk for adverse outcomes. However, as weight escalates above a BMI of 40 kg/m^2, outcomes deteriorate, particularly in surgical and trauma patients. Overall, the effect of MO on critical care outcome remains controversial, with the worst outcome reported in obese trauma patients.

REFERENCES

1. Kral JG, Heymsfield S. Morbid obesity: definitions, epidemiology, and methodological problems. *Gastroenterol Clin North Am.* 1987;16(2):197–205.
2. Gastrointestinal surgery for severe obesity: National Institutes of Health Consensus Development Conference Statement. *Am J Clin Nutr.* 1992;55(suppl 2):615S–619S.
3. Flegal KM, Carroll MD, Kit BK, Ogden CL. Prevalence of obesity and trends in the distribution of body mass index among US adults, 1999–2010. *JAMA.* 2012;307(5):491–497.
4. el-Ganzouri AR, McCarthy RJ, Tuman KJ, Tanck EN, Ivankovich AD. Preoperative airway assessment: predictive value of a multivariate risk index. *Anesth Analg.* 1996;82(6):1197–1204.
5. Buckley FP, Robinson NB, Simonowitz DA, Dellinger EP. Anaesthesia in the morbidly obese. A comparison of anaesthetic and analgesic regimens for upper abdominal surgery. *Anaesthesia.* 1983;38(9):840–851.
6. Dominguez-Cherit G, Gonzalez R, Borunda D, Pedroza J, Gonzalez-Barranco J, Herrera MF. Anesthesia for morbidly obese patients. *World J Surg.* 1998;22(9):969–973.
7. Lundstrom LH, Moller AM, Rosenstock C, Astrup G, Wetterslev J. High body mass index is a weak predictor for difficult and failed tracheal intubation: a cohort study of 91,332 consecutive patients scheduled for direct laryngoscopy registered in the Danish Anesthesia Database. *Anesthesiology.* 2009;110(2):266–274.
8. Williamson JA, Webb RK, Van der Walt JH, Runciman WB. The Australian Incident Monitoring Study. Pneumothorax: an analysis of 2000 incident reports. *Anaesth Intensive Care.* 1993;21(5):642–645.
9. Naguib M, Malabarey T, AlSatli RA, Al Damegh S, Samarkandi AH. Predictive models for difficult laryngoscopy and intubation. A clinical, radiologic and three-dimensional computer imaging study. *Can J Anaesth.* 1999;46(8):748–759.
10. Brodsky JB, Lemmens HJ, Brock-Utne JG, Vierra M, Saidman LJ. Morbid obesity and tracheal intubation. *Anesth Analg.* 2002;94(3):732–736. table of contents.
11. Gaszynski T. Standard clinical tests for predicting difficult intubation are not useful among morbidly obese patients. *Anesth Analg.* 2004;99(3):956.
12. Collins JS, Lemmens HJ, Brodsky JB. Obesity and difficult intubation: where is the evidence? *Anesthesiology.* 2006;104(3):617, author reply 618–619.
13. Hiremath AS, Hillman DR, James AL, Noffsinger WJ, Platt PR, Singer SL. Relationship between difficult tracheal intubation and obstructive sleep apnoea. *Br J Anaesth.* 1998;80(5):606–611.
14. Apfelbaum JL, Hagberg CA, Caplan RA, et al. Practice guidelines for management of the difficult airway: an updated report by the American Society of Anesthesiologists Task Force on Management of the Difficult Airway. *Anesthesiology.* 2013;118(2):251–270.
15. Salome CM, King GG, Berend N. Physiology of obesity and effects on lung function. *J Appl Physiol.* 2010;108(1):206–211.
16. Juvin P, Lavaut E, Dupont H, et al. Difficult tracheal intubation is more common in obese than in lean patients. *Anesth Analg.* 2003;97(2):595–600. table of contents.
17. Dority J, Hassan ZU, Chau D. Anesthetic implications of obesity in the surgical patient. *Clin Colon Rectal Surg.* 2011;24(4):222–228.
18. Freid EB. The rapid sequence induction revisited: obesity and sleep apnea syndrome. *Anesthesiol Clin North Am.* 2005;23(3):551–564. viii.
19. Zacchi P, Mearin F, Humbert P, Formiguera X, Malagelada JR. Effect of obesity on gastroesophageal resistance to flow in man. *Dig Dis Sci.* 1991;36(10):1473–1480.
20. Butler J, Sen A. Best evidence topic report. Cricoid pressure in emergency rapid sequence induction. *EMJ.* 2005;22(11):815–816.
21. Haslam N, Parker L, Duggan JE. Effect of cricoid pressure on the view at laryngoscopy. *Anaesthesia.* 2005;60(1):41–47.
22. Allman KG. The effect of cricoid pressure application on airway patency. *J Clin Anesth.* 1995;7(3):197–199.
23. El Solh AA, Jaafar W. A comparative study of the complications of surgical tracheostomy in morbidly obese critically ill patients. *Crit Care.* 2007;11(1):R3.
24. Gross ND, Cohen JI, Andersen PE, Wax MK. 'Defatting' tracheotomy in morbidly obese patients. *Laryngoscope.* 2002;112(11): 1940–1944.
25. Byhahn C, Lischke V, Meininger D, Halbig S, Westphal K. Perioperative complications during percutaneous tracheostomy in obese patients. *Anaesthesia.* 2005;60(1):12–15.

26. Mansharamani NG, Koziel H, Garland R, LoCicero III J, Critchlow J, Ernst A. Safety of bedside percutaneous dilatational tracheostomy in obese patients in the ICU. *Chest*. 2000;117(5):1426–1429.

27. Dennis BM, Eckert MJ, Gunter OL, Morris Jr JA, May AK. Safety of bedside percutaneous tracheostomy in the critically ill: evaluation of more than 3000 procedures. *J Am Coll Surg*. 2013;216(4):858–865. discussion 865–857.

28. Alhajhusain AA, Ali AW, Najmuddin A, Hussain K, Aqeel M, El Solh A. Timing of tracheotomy in mechanically ventilated critically ill morbidly obese patients. *Crit Care Res Pract* 2014:840638.

29. Jones RL, Nzekwu MM. The effects of body mass index on lung volumes. *Chest*. 2006;130(3):827–833.

30. Holley HS, Milic-Emili J, Becklake MR, Bates DV. Regional distribution of pulmonary ventilation and perfusion in obesity. *J Clin Invest*. 1967;46(4):475–481.

31. El-Solh AA. Clinical approach to the critically ill, morbidly obese patient. *Am J Respir Crit Care Med*. 2004;169(5):557–561.

32. Pelosi P, Ravagnan I, Giurati G, et al. Positive end-expiratory pressure improves respiratory function in obese but not in normal subjects during anesthesia and paralysis. *Anesthesiology*. 1999;91(5):1221–1231.

33. Koutsoukou A, Koulouris N, Bekos B, et al. Expiratory flow limitation in morbidly obese postoperative mechanically ventilated patients. *Acta Anaesthesiol Scand*. 2004;48(9):1080–1088.

34. Rothen HU, Sporre B, Engberg G, Wegenius G, Hedenstierna G. Re-expansion of atelectasis during general anaesthesia: a computed tomography study. *Br J Anaesth*. 1993;71(6):788–795.

35. Fernandez R, Trenchs X, Klamburg J, et al. Prone positioning in acute respiratory distress syndrome: a multicenter randomized clinical trial. *Intensive Care Med*. 2008;34(8):1487–1491.

36. De Jong A, Molinari N, Sebbane M, et al. Feasibility and effectiveness of prone position in morbidly obese patients with ARDS: a case-control clinical study. *Chest*. 2013;143(6):1554–1561.

37. Weig T, Janitza S, Zoller M, et al. Influence of abdominal obesity on multiorgan dysfunction and mortality in acute respiratory distress syndrome patients treated with prone positioning. *J Crit Care*. 2014;29(4):557–561.

38. Blouw EL, Rudolph AD, Narr BJ, Sarr MG. The frequency of respiratory failure in patients with morbid obesity undergoing gastric bypass. *AANA J*. 2003;71(1):45–50.

39. Gaszynski TG,W, Strzelczyj J. Critical respiratory events in morbidly obese. *Twoj Magazyn Medyczny Chirurgia*. 2003;3:55–58.

40. Joris JL, Sottiaux TM, Chiche JD, Desaive CJ, Lamy ML. Effect of bi-level positive airway pressure (BiPAP) nasal ventilation on the postoperative pulmonary restrictive syndrome in obese patients undergoing gastroplasty. *Chest*. 1997;111(3):665–670.

41. Duarte AG, Justino E, Bigler T, Grady J. Outcomes of morbidly obese patients requiring mechanical ventilation for acute respiratory failure. *Crit Care Med*. 2007;35(3):732–737.

42. El-Solh AA, Aquilina A, Pineda L, Dhanvantri V, Grant B, Bouquin P. Noninvasive ventilation for prevention of post-extubation respiratory failure in obese patients. *Eur Respir J*. 2006;28(3):588–595.

43. Rocha AT, de Vasconcellos AG, da Luz Neto ER, Araujo DM, Alves ES, Lopes AA. Risk of venous thromboembolism and efficacy of thromboprophylaxis in hospitalized obese medical patients and in obese patients undergoing bariatric surgery. *Obes Surg*. 2006;16(12):1645–1655.

44. Eichinger S, Hron G, Bialonczyk C, et al. Overweight, obesity, and the risk of recurrent venous thromboembolism. *Arch Intern Med*. 2008;168(15):1678–1683.

45. Overby DW, Kohn GP, Cahan MA, et al. Prevalence of thrombophilias in patients presenting for bariatric surgery. *Obes Surg*. 2009;19(9):1278–1285.

46. Cossu ML, Pilo L, Piseddu G, Tilocca PL, Cossu F, Noya G. Prophylaxis of venous thromboembolism in bariatric surgery. *Chir Ital*. 2007;59(3):331–335.

47. Borkgren-Okonek MJ, Hart RW, Pantano JE, et al. Enoxaparin thromboprophylaxis in gastric bypass patients: extended duration, dose stratification, and antifactor Xa activity. *Surg Obes Relat Dis: Off J Am Soc Bariat Surg*. 2008;4(5):625–631.

48. Raftopoulos I, Martindale C, Cronin A, Steinberg J. The effect of extended post-discharge chemical thromboprophylaxis on venous thromboembolism rates after bariatric surgery: a prospective comparison trial. *Surg Endoscopy*. 2008;22(11):2384–2391.

49. Wang TF, Milligan PE, Wong CA, Deal EN, Thoelke MS, Gage BF. Efficacy and safety of high-dose thromboprophylaxis in morbidly obese inpatients. *Thromb Haemost*. 2014;111(1):88–93.

50. Samama MM, Cohen AT, Darmon JY, et al. A comparison of enoxaparin with placebo for the prevention of venous thromboembolism in acutely ill medical patients. Prophylaxis in Medical Patients with Enoxaparin Study Group. *N Engl J Med*. 1999;341(11):793–800.

51. Kalfarentzos F, Stavropoulou F, Yarmenitis S, et al. Prophylaxis of venous thromboembolism using two different doses of low-molecular-weight heparin (nadroparin) in bariatric surgery: a prospective randomized trial. *Obes Surg*. 2001;11(6):670–676.

52. Scholten DJ, Hoedema RM, Scholten SE. A comparison of two different prophylactic dose regimens of low molecular weight heparin in bariatric surgery. *Obes Surg*. 2002;12(1):19–24.

53. Gonzalez QH, Tishler DS, Plata-Munoz JJ, et al. Incidence of clinically evident deep venous thrombosis after laparoscopic Roux-en-Y gastric bypass. *Surg Endoscopy*. 2004;18(7):1082–1084.

54. Alikhan R, Cohen AT, Combe S, et al. Prevention of venous thromboembolism in medical patients with enoxaparin: a subgroup analysis of the MEDENOX study. *Blood Coagulation Fibrinolysis: Int J Haemostasis Thromb*. 2003;14(4):341–346.

55. Shepherd MF, Rosborough TK, Schwartz ML. Heparin thromboprophylaxis in gastric bypass surgery. *Obes Surg*. 2003;13(2):249–253.

56. Miller MT, Rovito PF. An approach to venous thromboembolism prophylaxis in laparoscopic Roux-en-Y gastric bypass surgery. *Obes Surg*. 2004;14(6):731–737.

57. FS M, Rosborough TK, Schwartz ML. Unfractionated heparin infusion for thromboprophylaxis in highest risk gastric bypass surgery. *Obes Surg*. 2004;14(5):601–605.

58. Kucher N, Leizorovicz A, Vaitkus PT, et al. Efficacy and safety of fixed low-dose dalteparin in preventing venous thromboembolism among obese or elderly hospitalized patients: a subgroup analysis of the PREVENT trial. *Arch Intern Med*. 2005;165(3):341–345.

59. Hamad GG, Choban PS. Enoxaparin for thromboprophylaxis in morbidly obese patients undergoing bariatric surgery: findings of the prophylaxis against VTE outcomes in bariatric surgery patients receiving enoxaparin (PROBE) study. *Obes Surg*. 2005;15(10):1368–1374.

60. Quebbemann B, Akhondzadeh M, Dallal R. Continuous intravenous heparin infusion prevents peri-operative thromboembolic events in bariatric surgery patients. *Obes Surg*. 2005;15(9):1221–1224.

61. Ritschel WA, Kaul S. Prediction of apparent volume of distribution in obesity. *Methods Find Exp Clin Pharmacol*. 1986;8(4):239–247.

62. Erstad B. Drug dosing in the critically ill obese patient. In: El Solh AA, ed. *Critical Care Management of the Obese Management*. 1st ed. West Sussex, UK: Wiley-Blackwell; 2012:197–207.

63. Kotlyar M, Carson SW. Effects of obesity on the cytochrome P450 enzyme system. *Int J Clin Pharmacol Ther*. 1999;37(1):8–19.

64. Dionne RE, Bauer LA, Gibson GA, Griffen Jr WO, Blouin RA. Estimating creatinine clearance in morbidity obese patients. *Am J Hosp Pharm*. 1981;38(6):841–844.

65. Salazar DE, Corcoran GB. Predicting creatinine clearance and renal drug clearance in obese patients from estimated fat-free body mass. *Am J Med*. 1988;84(6):1053–1060.

66. Levey AS, Bosch JP, Lewis JB, Greene T, Rogers N, Roth D. A more accurate method to estimate glomerular filtration rate from serum creatinine: a new prediction equation. Modification of Diet in Renal Disease Study Group *Ann Intern Med*. 1999;130(6):461–470.

67. Oda Y, Mizutani K, Hase I, Nakamoto T, Hamaoka N, Asada A. Fentanyl inhibits metabolism of midazolam: competitive inhibition of CYP3A4 in vitro. *Br J Anaesth*. 1999;82(6):900–903.

68. Medico CJ, Walsh P. Pharmacotherapy in the critically ill obese patient. *Crit Care Clin*. 2010;26(4):679–688.

69. Servin F, Farinotti R, Haberer JP, Desmonts JM. Propofol infusion for maintenance of anesthesia in morbidly obese patients receiving nitrous oxide. A clinical and pharmacokinetic study. *Anesthesiology*. 1993;78(4):657–665.

70. Greenblatt DJ, Abernethy DR, Locniskar A, Harmatz JS, Limjuco RA, Shader RI. Effect of age, gender, and obesity on midazolam kinetics. *Anesthesiology*. 1984;61(1):27–35.

71. Salihoglu Z, Demiroluk S, Demirkiran, Kose Y. Comparison of effects of remifentanil, alfentanil and fentanyl on cardiovascular responses to tracheal intubation in morbidly obese patients. *Eur J Anaesthesiol*. 2002;19(2):125–128.

72. Shibutani K, Inchiosa Jr MA, Sawada K, Bairamian M. Pharmacokinetic mass of fentanyl for postoperative analgesia in lean and obese patients. *Br J Anaesth*. 2005;95(3):377–383.

73. Egan TD, Huizinga B, Gupta SK, et al. Remifentanil pharmacokinetics in obese versus lean patients. *Anesthesiology.* 1998;89(3):562–573.

74. Bennett R, Batenhorst R, Graves DA, Foster TS, Griffen WO, Wright BD. Variation in postoperative analgesic requirements in the morbidly obese following gastric bypass surgery. *Pharmacotherapy.* 1982;2(1):50–53.

75. Rand CS, Kuldau JM, Yost RL. Obesity and post-operative pain. *J Psychosom Res.* 1985;29(1):43–48.

76. Spruill WJ, Wade WE, Huckaby WG, Leslie RB. Achievement of anticoagulation by using a weight-based heparin dosing protocol for obese and nonobese patients. *Am J Health-Syst Pharm.* 2001;58(22):2143–2146.

77. Nutescu EA, Spinler SA, Wittkowsky A, Dager WE. Low-molecular-weight heparins in renal impairment and obesity: available evidence and clinical practice recommendations across medical and surgical settings. *Ann Pharmacother.* 2009;43(6): 1064–1083.

78. Duplaga BA, Rivers CW, Nutescu E. Dosing and monitoring of low-molecular-weight heparins in special populations. *Pharmacotherapy.* 2001;21(2):218–234.

79. Faria R, Spackman E, Burch J, et al. Dabigatran for the prevention of stroke and systemic embolism in atrial fibrillation: a NICE single technology appraisal. *Pharmacoeconomics.* 2013;31(7):551–562.

80. Connolly SJ, Ezekowitz MD, Yusuf S, et al. Dabigatran versus warfarin in patients with atrial fibrillation. *N Engl J Med.* 2009;361(12):1139–1151.

81. Patel MR, Mahaffey KW, Garg J, et al. Rivaroxaban versus warfarin in nonvalvular atrial fibrillation. *N Engl J Med.* 2011;365(10):883–891.

82. Lassen MR, Ageno W, Borris LC, et al. Rivaroxaban versus enoxaparin for thromboprophylaxis after total knee arthroplasty. *N Engl J Med.* 2008;358(26):2776–2786.

83. Eriksson BI, Borris LC, Friedman RJ, et al. Rivaroxaban versus enoxaparin for thromboprophylaxis after hip arthroplasty. *N Engl J Med.* 2008;358(26):2765–2775.

84. Kubitza D, Becka M, Zuehlsdorf M, Mueck W. Body weight has limited influence on the safety, tolerability, pharmacokinetics, or pharmacodynamics of rivaroxaban (BAY 59-7939) in healthy subjects. *J Clin Pharmacol.* 2007;47(2):218–226.

85. Turpie AG, Lassen MR, Eriksson BI, et al. Rivaroxaban for the prevention of venous thromboembolism after hip or knee arthroplasty. Pooled analysis of four studies. *Thromb Haemost.* 2011;105(3):444–453.

86. Lopes RD, Alexander JH, Al-Khatib SM, et al. Apixaban for reduction in stroke and other ThromboemboLic events in atrial fibrillation (ARISTOTLE) trial: design and rationale. *Am Heart J.* 2010;159(3):331–339.

87. Upreti VV, Wang J, Barrett YC, et al. Effect of extremes of body weight on the pharmacokinetics, pharmacodynamics, safety and tolerability of apixaban in healthy subjects. *Brit J Clin Pharmacol.* 2013;76(6):908–916.

88. Breen HB, Ireton-Jones CS. Predicting energy needs in obese patients. *Nutr Clin Pract: Off Publ Am Soc Parenter Enteral Nutr.* 2004;19(3):284–289.

89. Dickerson RN. Specialized nutrition support in the hospitalized obese patient. *Nutr Clin Pract: Off Publ Am Soc Parenter Enteral Nutr.* 2004;19(3):245–254.

90. Choban P, Dickerson R, Malone A, et al. A.S.P.E.N. Clinical guidelines: nutrition support of hospitalized adult patients with obesity. *JPEN.* 2013;37(6):714–744.

91. Ireton-Jones CS, Turner Jr WW. Actual or ideal body weight: which should be used to predict energy expenditure? *J Am Diet Assoc.* 1991;91(2):193–195.

92. Frankenfield DC, Coleman A, Alam S, Cooney RN. Analysis of estimation methods for resting metabolic rate in critically ill adults. *JPEN.* 2009;33(1):27–36.

93. Mesejo A, Vaquerizo Alonso C, Acosta Escribano J, et al. Guidelines for specialized nutritional and metabolic support in the critically-ill patient. Update. Consensus of the Spanish Society of Intensive Care Medicine and Coronary Units-Spanish Society of Parenteral and Enteral Nutrition (SEMICYUC-SENPE): introduction and methodology. *Medicina intensiva/ Sociedad Espanola de Medicina Intensiva y Unidades Coronarias.* 2011;35(suppl 1):1–6.

94. Dickerson RN, Medling TL, Smith AC, et al. Hypocaloric, high-protein nutrition therapy in older vs younger critically ill patients with obesity. *JPEN.* 2013;37(3):342–351.

95. Uppot RN. Impact of obesity on radiology. *Radiol Clin North Am.* 2007;45(2):231–246.

96. Parienti JJ, Thirion M, Megarbane B, et al. Femoral vs jugular venous catheterization and risk of nosocomial events in adults requiring acute renal replacement therapy: a randomized controlled trial. *JAMA.* 2008;299(20):2413–2422.

97. Hind D, Calvert N, McWilliams R, et al. Ultrasonic locating devices for central venous cannulation: meta-analysis. *BMJ.* 2003;327(7411):361.

98. El-Solh A, Sikka P, Bozkanat E, Jaafar W, Davies J. Morbid obesity in the medical ICU. *Chest.* 2001;120(6):1989–1997.

99. Bercault N, Boulain T, Kuteifan K, Wolf M, Runge I, Fleury JC. Obesity-related excess mortality rate in an adult intensive care unit: a risk-adjusted matched cohort study. *Crit Care Med.* 2004;32(4):998–1003.

100. Goulenok C, Monchi M, Chiche JD, Mira JP, Dhainaut JF, Cariou A. Influence of overweight on ICU mortality: a prospective study. *Chest.* 2004;125(4):1441–1445.

101. Ray DE, Matchett SC, Baker K, Wasser T, Young MJ. The effect of body mass index on patient outcomes in a medical ICU. *Chest.* 2005;127(6):2125–2131.

102. O'Brien Jr JM, Welsh CH, Fish RH, et al. Excess body weight is not independently associated with outcome in mechanically ventilated patients with acute lung injury. *Ann Intern Med.* 2004;140(5):338–345.

103. Prescott HC, Chang VW, O'Brien Jr JM, Langa KM, Iwashyna TJ. Obesity and 1-year outcomes in older Americans with severe sepsis. *Crit Care Med.* 2014;42(8):1766–1774.

104. Tremblay A, Bandi V. Impact of body mass index on outcomes following critical care. *Chest.* 2003;123(4):1202–1207.

105. Akinnusi ME, Pineda LA, El Solh AA. Effect of obesity on intensive care morbidity and mortality: a meta-analysis. *Crit Care Med.* 2008;36(1):151–158.

106. Hogue Jr CW, Stearns JD, Colantuoni E, et al. The impact of obesity on outcomes after critical illness: a meta-analysis. *Intensive Care Med.* 2009;35(7):1152–1170.

107. Oliveros H, Villamor E. Obesity and mortality in critically ill adults: a systematic review and meta-analysis. *Obesity.* 2008;16(3):515–521.

108. Bornstein SR, Licinio J, Tauchnitz R, et al. Plasma leptin levels are increased in survivors of acute sepsis: associated loss of diurnal rhythm, in cortisol and leptin secretion. *J Clin Endocrinol Metab.* 1998;83(1):280–283.

109. Nasraway Jr SA, Albert M, Donnelly AM, Ruthazer R, Shikora SA, Saltzman E. Morbid obesity is an independent determinant of death among surgical critically ill patients. *Crit Care Med.* 2006;34(4):964–970; quiz 971.

110. Birkmeyer NJ, Charlesworth DC, Hernandez F, et al. Obesity and risk of adverse outcomes associated with coronary artery bypass surgery. Northern New England Cardiovascular Disease Study Group *Circulation.* 1998;97(17):1689–1694.

111. Moulton MJ, Creswell LL, Mackey ME, Cox JL, Rosenbloom M. Obesity is not a risk factor for significant adverse outcomes after cardiac surgery. *Circulation.* 1996;94(suppl 9):II87–92.

112. Brown CV, Neville AL, Rhee P, Salim A, Velmahos GC, Demetriades D. The impact of obesity on the outcomes of 1153 critically injured blunt trauma patients. *J Trauma.* 2005;59(5):1048–1051. discussion 1051.

113. Neville AL, Brown CV, Weng J, Demetriades D, Velmahos GC. Obesity is an independent risk factor of mortality in severely injured blunt trauma patients. *Arch Surg.* 2004;139(9):983–987.

114. Byrnes MC, McDaniel MD, Moore MB, Helmer SD, Smith RS. The effect of obesity on outcomes among injured patients. *J Trauma.* 2005;58(2):232–237.

115. Bochicchio GV, Joshi M, Bochicchio K, Nehman S, Tracy JK, Scalea TM. Impact of obesity in the critically ill trauma patient: a prospective study. *J Am Coll Surg.* 2006;203(4):533–538.

116. Yaegashi M, Jean R, Zuriqat M, Noack S, Homel P. Outcome of morbid obesity in the intensive care unit. *J Intensive Care Med.* 2005;20(3):147–154.

24 How Do I Transport the Critically Ill Patient?

David Cosgrave, John Chandler, John Bates

The provision of intensive care during transport to and from the intensive care unit (ICU) presents a major challenge. Available data[1,2] suggest that critical care transport is becoming increasingly common, driven by the centralization of specialties and an expanding number of diagnostic and therapeutic options outside of the ICU. The bulk of critical care transports happen within the hospital itself. Observational data[1,3,4] suggest that critical care transport is a high-risk but worthwhile activity and that this risk can be minimized by adequate planning, proper equipment, and appropriate staffing. Prehospital transport of the critically ill patient presents more problems because prior planning is more difficult.

Clinical data on transport of the critically ill patient are derived mainly from cohort trials and can provide guidelines in terms of personnel (physicians, nurses, and paramedics), mode of transport (air or road), and specific treatments (prehospital tracheal intubation and advanced life support).

INTRAHOSPITAL TRANSPORT OF THE CRITICALLY ILL

Adverse Effects

Several observational studies suggest that significant physiologic disturbances (large variations in heart rate, blood pressure [BP], or oxygen saturation) occur during 53% to 68% of intrahospital transports.[5-7] Physiologic variability is also common in stationary critically ill patients, occurring in 60% of such patients in a study by Hurst and colleagues[6] compared with 66% in transported patients. Many of these physiologic changes can be safely managed by an appropriately trained transport team, but serious adverse events do occur. Prospective observational studies have found an adverse event rate of 36% to 45.8%.[8,9] A large multicenter cohort study showed an odds ratio (OR) for the occurrence of adverse events in intrahospital transports of 1.9. These events included pneumothorax, ventilator-associated pneumonia, and atelectasis. Increased length of stay was noted in the same study but not a difference in mortality[10] Damm and colleagues[11] found a cardiac arrest rate of 1.6% in a prospective observational study of 123 intrahospital transports. Waydhas and colleagues[12] found that a reduction in the Pao_2/Fio_2 (partial pressure of oxygen, arterial/fraction of inspired oxygen) ratio occurred in 83.7% of patients when transported with a transport ventilator and that this was severe (>20% reduction from baseline) in 42.8%. Furthermore, the changes persisted for more than 24 hours in 20.4% of transports. Two large cohort studies in which logistic regression analysis[13,14] was used found out-of-unit transport to be an independent risk factor for ventilator-associated pneumonia (ORs of 3.1[13] and 3.8[14]). Intrahospital transport is also one of the factors associated with unplanned extubation.[15]

When compared with APACHE (Acute Physiology and Chronic Health Evaluation) II and III matched controls, patients requiring intrahospital transport were found to have a higher mortality (28.6% vs 11.4%) and a longer ICU length of stay.[16] None of the excess mortality was directly attributable to complications of the transport, and the authors concluded that the findings reflected a higher severity of illness in patients who required transportation. However, serious adverse events did occur in 5.9% of transports.

PREDICTING ADVERSE EVENTS DURING INTRAHOSPITAL TRANSPORT

Factors associated with an increased risk for adverse events during transport include pretransport secondary insults in head-injured patients, high injury severity score,[17] and high Therapeutic Interventions Severity Score (TISS) but not APACHE II score.[18] Age older than 43 years and an Fio_2 higher than 0.5 are predictive of respiratory deterioration on transport.[19]

The number of intravenous pumps and infusions, as well as the time spent outside of the unit, has been shown to correlate with the number of technical mishaps.[20] The Australian ICU Incident Monitoring study[21] found that 39% of transport problems were related to equipment, with 61% relating to patient or staff management issues. Factors limiting harm were rechecking of the patient and equipment, skilled assistance, and prior experience.

Hemodynamic variability is more frequent in patients being transferred to the ICU from the operating room than in those transported for diagnostic procedures outside of the ICU. This is probably related to emergence from anesthesia.[22]

RISK-TO-BENEFIT RATIO OF INTRAHOSPITAL TRANSPORT

Observational studies suggest that the therapeutic yield for intrahospital transport is high. Hurst and colleagues[6] found that the results of diagnostic testing facilitated by the transport resulted in a change in treatment in 39% of patients. Out-of-unit radiologic studies in ICU patients tend to be high yield. For instance, computed tomography scanning of the thorax has been shown in observational studies to change the clinical course in 26% to 57% of cases.[23,24]

MANAGEMENT OF THE TRANSPORT

A cohort study has found that transport ventilators reduce variability in blood gas parameters when compared with manual bagging.[25] Although several older studies found manual ventilation to be as good or better than use of a transport ventilator,[26-28] the performance characteristics of transport ventilators has improved significantly over time,[29-31] and the performance of many modern transport ventilators is comparable to that of ICU ventilators.[32] Changes in blood gas parameters have been shown to correlate with hemodynamic disturbances (arrhythmias, hypotension).[25]

Capnometry (end tidal carbon dioxide [$ETCO_2$]) monitoring reduces the variability $Paco_2$ (partial pressure of CO_2, arterial) in adults.[33] In children, manual ventilation without $ETCO_2$ monitoring resulted in only 31% of readings falling within the intended range.[34]

A single randomized controlled trial (RCT) found that hypothermia was common in trauma patients undergoing intrahospital transport (average temperature on return to the unit was 34.7° C) and that this was prevented by active warming during transport.[35]

Who should accompany the critically ill patient during transport? Specialized transport teams have been found to have a lower rate of complications than historic controls.[36,37] Interestingly, physician attendance was not clearly correlated with a reduced risk for mishap in an observational study of 125 transports.[18] The implementation of a pretransport checklist has been found to reduce the rate of serious adverse events from 9.1% to 5.2%[38]

INTERHOSPITAL TRANSFER

The number of interhospital transfers of critically ill patients is increasing[1,2] because of a reduction in the number of hospitals, centralization of specialist services, and reconfiguration of health-care services between acute and elective medicine.[4] Approximately 4.5% of critical care stays are associated with an interhospital transfer.[39] The benefits of transport to the patient need to be weighed against the not inconsiderable risks of the transport process.[3,19,40-44] There are few RCTs on this subject,

and conclusions have to be drawn from nonrandomized, cohort, or uncontrolled studies.

ADVERSE EFFECTS

Various published audits and descriptive studies have shown that the interhospital transport of critically ill patients is associated with an increased morbidity and mortality during and after the journey.[3,19,40-43,45] Even with specialist mobile intensive care teams, mortality before and during transport is substantial (2.5%) despite a low incidence of preventable deaths during transport (0.02% to 0.04%).[45] Singh and colleagues[46] reported an in-transit mortality of 0.1% among 19,228 interhospital transfers in Canada. Other authors have reported higher interhospital transport mortality and have found that 24% to 70% of incidents are avoidable.[40,43]

Critical events occur in 4% to 17.1% of interhospital transfers.[2,44,46] In adults, these events are mainly cardiovascular (e.g., new hypotension, arrhythmia, hypertension) or respiratory (e.g., arterial desaturation, inadvertent extubation, respiratory arrest).[2,44,46] The most common complications observed during pediatric and neonatal transportation are hypothermia, respiratory complications, and loss of intravenous access.[41,42]

DOES INTERHOSPITAL TRANSPORT CONTRIBUTE TO MORTALITY?

The long-term outlook for critically ill patients who require interhospital transport is worse than for those who do not require transport. Four cohort studies have found that transported patients have a higher ICU mortality and longer ICU stays than controls.[47-50] In three of these four studies, this difference in mortality was not significant after adjustment for severity of illness.[47,49,50] A systematic review of the impact of transfer on outcome for trauma patients found no significant association between transfer status and in-hospital mortality.[51]

PREDICTION OF ADVERSE EVENTS

The APACHE II, TISS, and Rapid Acute Physiology scoring systems do not correlate with critical events during transport in adults,[18,19,52] and the PRISM (Pediatric Risk of Mortality) score has proved to be similarly unreliable in children.[53] Independent predictors of critical events during transport include female sex, older age, higher Fio_2, multiple injury, assisted ventilation, hemodynamic instability, inadequate stabilization before transport, transport in a fixed-wing aircraft, and increased duration of transport.[19,46,54] Patients undergoing interhospital transport after cardiac arrest have a re-arrest rate of 6% during the transfer.[55]

PLANNING OF THE TRANSPORT

The importance of planning and preparing for interhospital transport cannot be overstated because poor planning has been shown to lead to an increased incidence of adverse events and mortality.[54] In an audit of transfers to a neurosurgical center, 43% were found to have inadequate injury assessment, and 24% received inadequate resuscitation. Deficiencies in assessment and resuscitation before transfer were identified in all patients who died.[54] Guidelines have been developed to address this issue in many jurisdictions, but inadequate assessment and resuscitation remain as problems. Price and colleagues[56] found that the development of national guidelines led to only modest improvements in patient care.

SELECTION OF PERSONNEL

It is recommended that a minimum of two people, in addition to the vehicle operators, accompany a critically ill patient during transport. The team leader can be a nurse or physician depending on clinical and local circumstances. It is imperative that the team leader has adequate training in transport medicine and advanced life support. Adequately trained nurses have been shown to be as safe at transporting critically ill children as doctors.[57,58] Appropriately staffed and equipped specialist retrieval teams have been shown to be superior to occasional teams at transferring critically ill adults[59] and children.[60] In an observational study, Vos and colleagues[60] demonstrated an 80% reduction in critical incidents during pediatric interhospital transport undertaken by a specialist retrieval team.

In a cohort study, Orr and colleagues[61] found an increase in mortality (23% vs 9%) among children transported by a nonspecialized team. This difference remained after adjustment for severity of illness.

MODE OF TRANSPORT

The choice between the three options of road, helicopter, and fixed-wing transport are affected by three main factors: distance, patient status, and weather conditions. Three observational studies have addressed the effect of air versus road transfer on mortality. A retrospective review of 1234 adult transfers has shown no difference in mortality or morbidity between patients transferred by air versus road,[62] whereas the other two studies found an increase in survival in patients transported by air.[63,64] Brown and colleagues[64] conducted a logistic regression analysis on 74,779 patient transfers and found an OR for survival of 1.09 among patients with a TISS greater than 15 who were transferred by air. A prospective cohort study has demonstrated that air transport is faster than ground transport, and for transfers of less than 225 km, helicopter transport is faster than fixed-wing transport.[65]

EQUIPMENT AND MONITORING

Comprehensive lists of equipment and medications needed for transport of critically ill patients are available elsewhere and are beyond the scope of this chapter.[66] It is generally accepted that the standard of organ support

and monitoring available in the ICU should be continued during the transport to the greatest extent possible. An RCT of near-continuous noninvasive BP monitoring compared with intermittent BP monitoring during interhospital transport of critically ill children found less organ dysfunction and a shorter ICU stay in the intervention group.[67] Uncontrolled observational studies have shown that point-of-care blood gas analysis during interhospital transfer allows early identification and treatment of changes in gas exchange and metabolic parameters.[68,69] Interfacility transport of patients receiving extracorporeal membrane oxygenation has been shown to be feasible and safe with good survival outcomes.[70] A retrospective study of transports of infants being transferred for therapeutic hypothermia has found that the use of a purpose-built cooling machine was associated with better temperature control and faster time to achieving target temperature than passive cooling.[71]

PREHOSPITAL TRANSPORT

Most research in the area of prehospital transport has focused on trauma patients because of the potential for early appropriate intervention to improve outcome.

RETRIEVAL SYSTEMS

The following are the four main infrastructural factors that have been addressed in clinical studies:

1. Mode of transport
2. Prehospital personnel
3. Prehospital time
4. Receiving care facility

Mode of Transport

The comparison between road and helicopter transport has been the focus of several large cohort studies in recent years.[72-77] Four of these five studies demonstrated a survival advantage for severely injured patients transported by helicopter[72,74-77] with an OR of death of 0.41 to 0.68.[72,74,76] The reason for the survival advantage is less clear. In one study, a survival advantage was demonstrated despite longer transport times in the helicopter group,[74] but patients in the helicopter group were more intensively managed in the prehospital phase. It has been suggested that patients retrieved by helicopter may be more likely to be brought to a level I or II trauma center, and this may partly explain the survival advantage.[73]

Prehospital Personnel

One RCT[78] and a systematic review of controlled nonrandomized studies[79] have addressed the issue of physician- versus paramedic-delivered prehospital care. The RCT found a 35% reduction in mortality in the physician-treated group. In the systematic review, 9 of 19 studies involving trauma patients and 4 of 5 studies involving patients who experienced out-of-hospital cardiac arrest also demonstrated a reduction in mortality in the physician-treated group.[79] The largest of these controlled studies involved 14,702 trauma patients and showed an OR for death of 0.7 in the physician-treated group.[80] The evidence indicates that physicians tend to treat patients more aggressively and have fewer prehospital tracheal intubation failures[81] than paramedics.

Prehospital Time

Severely injured patients have been shown in cohort trials to have an increased mortality,[82] length of stay, and complications[83] with prehospital times of more than 60 minutes. Time from injury to arrival at definitive care may not be as important in highly developed trauma systems with the capability to provide aggressive care in the prehospital phase.[74,84]

Receiving Care Facility

Several large cohort studies have found a reduction in mortality for severely injured trauma patients when they are transferred directly to a level I trauma center.[85-87] The largest of these included more than 6000 patients from 15 regions in the United States. Patients treated primarily in level I trauma centers had a lower in-hospital (OR, 0.8; confidence interval [CI], 0.66 to 0.98) and 1-year mortality (OR, 0.75; CI, 0.60 to 0.95). Subgroup analysis suggested that the mortality benefit was primarily confined to more severely injured patients.[87]

SPECIFIC INTERVENTIONS IN THE PREHOSPITAL SETTING

Whether advanced life support (ALS) measures (e.g., endotracheal intubation, intravenous cannulation, and fluid and drug administration) delivered at the scene and in transit are of benefit to patients when compared with basic life support (BLS) is unclear.[88] Three before and after studies of ALS compared with BLS (the Ontario Prehospital Advanced Life Support studies) looked at the effect of the institution of ALS in prehospital care in patients with out-of-hospital cardiac arrest,[89] respiratory distress,[90] and major trauma.[91] No improvement in mortality was observed among the patients with cardiac arrest or trauma, and among trauma patients with a Glasgow Coma Scale (GCS) less than 9, mortality was increased in the ALS phase. There was a small mortality benefit in patients with respiratory distress.

Similarly, a meta-analysis[88] of 15 observational and cohort studies comparing ALS with BLS for trauma patients demonstrated an increased mortality in ALS patients (OR, 2.59). The same authors subsequently published a large observational study comparing different prehospital systems in Canada. After correction for confounders using logistic regression analysis, they found a 21% increase in mortality for patients treated with onsite ALS ($P = 0.01$).[92]

One RCT and several observational studies have looked specifically at the effect of prehospital tracheal intubation on outcome. The RCT compared prehospital rapid sequence induction (RSI) by intensive care paramedics versus intubation in hospital for patients (n = 312) with traumatic brain injury (GCS < 9).[93] The authors found an improvement in neurologic outcome at 6 months (risk ratio for good outcome of 1.28 in the intervention group). In contrast, several observational studies have found an increase in mortality with prehospital intubation.[94-96]

A prospective observational study of 1320 trauma patients who underwent airway interventions by an anesthesiologist on arrival in a level I trauma center found that 31% of those who had undergone tracheal intubation met the criteria for failed intubation, with 12% having unrecognized esophageal intubation on arrival.[97] A prospective observational study found a decrease in the rate of unrecognized misplaced intubations from 9% to 0% after the introduction of continuous $ETCO_2$ monitoring in the prehospital setting.[98] A meta-analysis of the success rate of prehospital tracheal intubation has found that physicians have a better success rate than nonphysicians (success rate, 0.991 vs 0.849) but that the success rate of nonphysicians is better (0.967) if muscle relaxants are available.[81] Prehospital tracheal intubation is a complex intervention and its value is likely related to many factors, including the skill of the provider, patient population, access to drugs to facilitate the intervention, and other aspects of the prehospital trauma system.

AUTHORS' RECOMMENDATIONS

- Transport of the critically ill patient is a necessary and important part of clinical practice. It is often overlooked.
- The risk to the patient of the transport itself can be reduced by appropriate planning and training of personnel and attention to pretransport stabilization of the patient.
- Transport of critically ill patients is best undertaken by experienced specialist transport teams wherever possible. This is especially true for pediatric critical care transports.
- The prehospital interventions that are associated with improved outcome are as follows:
  - Helicopter transport of severely injured trauma patients
  - Presence of a physician on the prehospital transport team
  - Transfer directly to a level I trauma center
  - The use of continuous $ETCO_2$ monitoring for prehospital endotracheal intubation
  - The use of prehospital RSI by trained prehospital crews for patients who have traumatic brain injury with a GCS less than 9

REFERENCES

1. Mackenzie PA, Smith EA, Wallace PG. Transfer of adults between intensive care units in the United Kingdom: postal survey. *BMJ*. 1997;314:1455–1456.
2. Fried MJ, Bruce J, Colquhoun R, Smith G. Inter-hospital transfers of acutely ill adults in Scotland. *Anaesthesia*. 2010;65:136–144.
3. Gentleman D, Jennett B. Audit of transfer of unconscious head-injured patients to a neurosurgical unit. *Lancet*. 1990;335:330–334.
4. Koppenberg J, Taeger K. Interhospital transport: transport of critically ill patients. *Curr Opin Anaesthesiol*. 2002;15:211–215.
5. Evans A, Winslow EH. Oxygen saturation and hemodynamic response in critically ill, mechanically ventilated adults during intrahospital transport. *Am J Crit Care*. 1995;4:106–111.
6. Hurst JM, Davis Jr K, Johnson DJ, Branson RD, Campbell RS, Branson PS. Cost and complications during in-hospital transport of critically ill patients: a prospective cohort study. *J Trauma*. 1992;33:582–585.

7. Indeck M, Peterson S, Smith J, Brotman S. Risk, cost, and benefit of transporting ICU patients for special studies. *J Trauma.* 1988;28:1020–1025.

8. Picetti E. Intra-hospital transport of brain-injured patients: a prospective, observational study. *Neurocrit Care.* 2013;18:298–304.

9. Parmentier-Decrucq. Adverse events during intrahospital transport of critically ill patients: incidence and risk factors. *Ann Intensive Care.* 2013;3.

10. Schwebel C, Clec'h C, Magne S, et al. Safety of intrahospital transport in ventilated critically ill patients: a multicenter cohort study*. *Crit Care Med.* 2013;41:1919–1928.

11. Damm C, Vandelet P, Petit J, et al. Complications during the intrahospital transport in critically ill patients. *Ann Fr Anesth Reanim.* 2005;24:24–30.

12. Waydhas C, Schneck G, Duswald KH. Deterioration of respiratory function after intra-hospital transport of critically ill surgical patients. *Intensive Care Med.* 1995;21:784–789.

13. Bercault N, Wolf M, Runge I, Fleury JC, Boulain T. Intrahospital transport of critically ill ventilated patients: a risk factor for ventilator-associated pneumonia–a matched cohort study. *Crit Care Med.* 2005;33:2471–2478.

14. Kollef MH, Von Harz B, Prentice D, et al. Patient transport from intensive care increases the risk of developing ventilator-associated pneumonia. *Chest.* 1997;112:765–773.

15. Christie JM, Dethlefsen M, Cane RD. Unplanned endotracheal extubation in the intensive care unit. *J Clin Anesth.* 1996;8:289–293.

16. Szem JW, Hydo LJ, Fischer E, Kapur S, Klemperer J, Barie PS. High-risk intrahospital transport of critically ill patients: safety and outcome of the necessary "road trip". *Crit Care Med.* 1995;23:1660–1666.

17. Andrews PJ, Piper IR, Dearden NM, Miller JD. Secondary insults during intrahospital transport of head-injured patients. *Lancet.* 1990;335:327–330.

18. Smith I, Fleming S, Cernaianu A. Mishaps during transport from the intensive care unit. *Crit Care Med.* 1990;18:278–281.

19. Marx G, Vangerow B, Hecker H, et al. Predictors of respiratory function deterioration after transfer of critically ill patients. *Intensive Care Med.* 1998;24:1157–1162.

20. Doring BL, Kerr ME, Lovasik DA, Thayer T. Factors that contribute to complications during intrahospital transport of the critically ill. *J Neurosci Nurs.* 1999;31:80–86.

21. Beckmann U, Gillies DM, Berenholtz SM, Wu AW, Pronovost P. Incidents relating to the intra-hospital transfer of critically ill patients. An analysis of the reports submitted to the Australian Incident Monitoring Study in Intensive Care. *Intensive Care Med.* 2004;30:1579–1585.

22. Insel J, Weissman C, Kemper M, Askanazi J, Hyman AI. Cardiovascular changes during transport of critically ill and postoperative patients. *Crit Care Med.* 1986;14:539–542.

23. Roddy LH, Unger KM, Miller WC. Thoracic computed tomography in the critically ill patient. *Crit Care Med.* 1981;9:515–518.

24. Voggenreiter G, Aufmkolk M, Majetschak M, et al. Efficiency of chest computed tomography in critically ill patients with multiple traumas. *Crit Care Med.* 2000;28:1033–1039.

25. Braman SS, Dunn SM, Amico CA, Millman RP. Complications of intrahospital transport in critically ill patients. *Ann Intern wrMed.* 1987;107:469–473.

26. Gervais HW, Eberle B, Konietzke D, Hennes HJ, Dick W. Comparison of blood gases of ventilated patients during transport. *Crit Care Med.* 1987;15:761–763.

27. Weg JG, Haas CF. Safe intrahospital transport of critically ill ventilator-dependent patients. *Chest.* 1989;96:631–635.

28. Dockery WK, Futterman C, Keller SR, Sheridan MJ, Akl BF. A comparison of manual and mechanical ventilation during pediatric transport. *Crit Care Med.* 1999;27:802–806.

29. Zanetta G, Robert D, Guerin C. Evaluation of ventilators used during transport of ICU patients – a bench study. *Intensive Care Med.* 2002;28:443–451.

30. Chipman D. Performance comparison of 15 transport ventilators. *Respir Care.* 2007;52:740–751.

31. Blakeman T. Inter- and intra-hospital transport of the critically ill. *Respir Care.* 2013;58:1008–1021.

32. Boussen S. Evaluation of ventilators used during transport of critically ill patients: a bench study. *Respir Care.* 2013;58:1911–1922.

33. Palmon SC, Liu M, Moore LE, Kirsch JR. Capnography facilitates tight control of ventilation during transport. *Crit Care Med.* 1996;24:608–611.

34. Tobias JD, Lynch A, Garrett J. Alterations of end-tidal carbon dioxide during the intrahospital transport of children. *Pediatr Emerg Care.* 1996;12:249–251.

35. Scheck T, Kober A, Bertalanffy P, et al. Active warming of critically ill trauma patients during intrahospital transfer: a prospective, randomized trial. *Wien Klin Wochenschr.* 2004;116:94–97.

36. Stearley HE. Patients' outcomes: intrahospital transportation and monitoring of critically ill patients by a specially trained ICU nursing staff. *Am J Crit Care.* 1998;7:282–287.

37. Kue R, Brown P. Adverse clinical events during intrahospital transport by a specialized team: a preliminary report. *Am J Crit Care.* 2011;20:153–162.

38. Choi A. Before- and after-intervention trial for reducing unexpected events during the intrahospital transport of emergency patients. *Am J Emerg Med.* 2012;30:1433–1440.

39. Iwashyna TJ, Christie JD, Moody J, Kahn JM, Asch DA. The structure of critical care transfer networks. *Med Care.* 2009;47:787–793.

40. Henning R, McNamara V. Difficulties encountered in transport of the critically ill child. *Pediatr Emerg Care.* 1991;7:133–137.

41. Kanter RK, Boeing NM, Hannan WP, Kanter DL. Excess morbidity associated with interhospital transport. *Pediatrics.* 1992;90:893–898.

42. Lang A, Brun H, Kaaresen PI, Klingenberg C. A population based 10-year study of neonatal air transport in North Norway. *Acta Paediatr.* 2007;96:995–999.

43. Ligtenberg JJ, Arnold LG, Stienstra Y, et al. Quality of interhospital transport of critically ill patients: a prospective audit. *Crit Care.* 2005;9:R446–R451.

44. Singh JM, Ferguson ND, MacDonald RD, Stewart TE, Schull MJ. Ventilation practices and critical events during transport of ventilated patients outside of hospital: a retrospective cohort study. *Prehosp Emerg Care.* 2009;13:316–323.

45. Gilligan JE, Griggs WM, Jelly MT, et al. Mobile intensive care services in rural South Australia. *Med J Aust.* 1999;171:617–620.

46. Singh JM, MacDonald RD, Bronskill SE, Schull MJ. Incidence and predictors of critical events during urgent air-medical transport. *CMAJ.* 2009;181:579–584.

47. Duke GJ, Green JV. Outcome of critically ill patients undergoing interhospital transfer. *Med J Aust.* 2001;174:122–125.

48. Durairaj L, Will JG, Torner JC, Doebbeling BN. Prognostic factors for mortality following interhospital transfers to the medical intensive care unit of a tertiary referral center. *Crit Care Med.* 2003;31:1981–1986.

49. Odetola FO, Clark SJ, Gurney JG, Dechert RE, Shanley TP, Freed GL. Effect of interhospital transfer on resource utilization and outcomes at a tertiary pediatric intensive care unit. *J Crit Care.* 2009;24:379–386.

50. Golestanian E, Scruggs JE, Gangnon RE, Mak RP, Wood KE. Effect of interhospital transfer on resource utilization and outcomes at a tertiary care referral center. *Crit Care Med.* 2007;35:1470–1476.

51. Hill AD, Fowler RA, Nathens AB. Impact of interhospital transfer on outcomes for trauma patients: a systematic review. *J Trauma.* 2011;71:1885–1900. discussion 901.

52. Rhee KJ, Mackenzie JR, Burney RE, et al. Rapid acute physiology scoring in transport systems. *Crit Care Med.* 1990;18:1119–1123.

53. Orr RA, Venkataraman ST, Cinoman MI, Hogue BL, Singleton CA, McCloskey KA. Pretransport Pediatric Risk of Mortality (PRISM) score underestimates the requirement for intensive care or major interventions during interhospital transport. *Crit Care Med.* 1994;22:101–107.

54. Lambert SM, Willett K. Transfer of multiply-injured patients for neurosurgical opinion: a study of the adequacy of assessment and resuscitation. *Injury.* 1993;24:333–336.

55. Hartke A, Mumma BE, Rittenberger JC, Callaway CW, Guyette FX. Incidence of re-arrest and critical events during prolonged transport of post-cardiac arrest patients. *Resuscitation.* 2010;81:938–942.

56. Price SJ, Suttner N, Aspoas AR. Have ATLS and national transfer guidelines improved the quality of resuscitation and transfer of head-injured patients? A prospective survey from a Regional Neurosurgical Unit. *Injury.* 2003;34:834–838.

57. Beyer 3rd AJ, Land G, Zaritsky A. Nonphysician transport of intubated pediatric patients: a system evaluation. *Crit Care Med.* 1992;20:961–966.

58. King BR, King TM, Foster RL, McCans KM. Pediatric and neonatal transport teams with and without a physician: a comparison of outcomes and interventions. *Pediatr Emerg Care.* 2007;23:77–82.

59. Gebremichael M, Borg U, Habashi NM, et al. Interhospital transport of the extremely ill patient: the mobile intensive care unit. *Crit Care Med.* 2000;28:79–85.

60. Vos GD, Nissen AC, Nieman FH, et al. Comparison of interhospital pediatric intensive care transport accompanied by a referring specialist or a specialist retrieval team. *Intensive Care Med.* 2004;30:302–308.

61. Orr RA, Felmet KA, Han Y, et al. Pediatric specialized transport teams are associated with improved outcomes. *Pediatrics.* 2009;124:40–48.

62. Arfken CL, Shapiro MJ, Bessey PQ, Littenberg B. Effectiveness of helicopter versus ground ambulance services for interfacility transport. *J Trauma.* 1998;45:785–790.

63. Moylan JA, Fitzpatrick KT, Beyer 3rd AJ, Georgiade GS. Factors improving survival in multisystem trauma patients. *Ann Surg.* 1988;207:679–685.

64. Brown JB, Stassen NA, Bankey PE, Sangosanya AT, Cheng JD, Gestring ML. Helicopters improve survival in seriously injured patients requiring interfacility transfer for definitive care. *J Trauma.* 2011;70:310–314.

65. Goldstein L, Doig CJ, Bates S, Rink S, Kortbeek JB. Adopting the pre-hospital index for interfacility helicopter transport: a proposal. *Injury.* 2003;34:3–11.

66. Barillo DJ, Renz E, Broger K, Moak B, Wright G, Holcomb JB. An emergency medical bag set for long-range aeromedical transportation. *Am J Disaster Med.* 2008;3:79–86.

67. Stroud MH, Prodhan P, Moss M, Fiser R, Schexnayder S, Anand K. Enhanced monitoring improves pediatric transport outcomes: a randomized controlled trial. *Pediatrics.* 2011;127:42–48.

68. Kill C, Barwing J, Lennartz H. Blood gas analysis in interhospital transfer–a useful extension of respiratory monitoring? *Anasthesiol Intensivmed Notfallmed Schmerzther.* 1999;34:10–16.

69. Vos G, Engel M, Ramsay G, van Waardenburg D. Point-of-care blood analyzer during the interhospital transport of critically ill children. *Eur J Emerg Med.* 2006;13:304–307.

70. Bryner B, Cooley E, Copenhaver W, et al. Two decades' experience with interfacility transport on extracorporeal membrane oxygenation. *Ann Thorac Surg.* 2014;98:1363–1370.

71. O'Reilly KM, Tooley J, Winterbottom S. Therapeutic hypothermia during neonatal transport. *Acta Paediatr.* 2011;100:1084–1086. discussion e49.

72. Hannay RS, Wyrzykowski AD, Ball CG, Laupland K, Feliciano DV. Retrospective review of injury severity, interventions and outcomes among helicopter and nonhelicopter transport patients at a Level 1 urban trauma centre. *Can J Surg.* 2014;57:49–54.

73. Rose MK, Cummings GR, Rodning CB, Brevard SB, Gonzalez RP. Is helicopter evacuation effective in rural trauma transport? *Am Surg.* 2012;78:794–797.

74. Desmettre T, Yeguiayan JM, Coadou H, et al. Impact of emergency medical helicopter transport directly to a university hospital trauma center on mortality of severe blunt trauma patients until discharge. *Crit Care.* 2012;16:R170.

75. Galvagno Jr SM, Haut ER, Zafar SN, et al. Association between helicopter vs ground emergency medical services and survival for adults with major trauma. *JAMA.* 2012;307:1602–1610.

76. Sullivent EE, Faul M, Wald MM. Reduced mortality in injured adults transported by helicopter emergency medical services. *Prehosp Emerg Care.* 2011;15:295–302.

77. Brown JB, Stassen NA, Bankey PE, Sangosanya AT, Cheng JD, Gestring ML. Helicopters and the civilian trauma system: national utilization patterns demonstrate improved outcomes after traumatic injury. *J Trauma.* 2010;69:1030–1034. discussion 4–6.

78. Baxt WG, Moody P. The impact of a physician as part of the aeromedical prehospital team in patients with blunt trauma. *JAMA.* 1987;257:3246–3250.

79. Botker MT, Bakke SA, Christensen EF. A systematic review of controlled studies: do physicians increase survival with prehospital treatment? *Scand J Trauma Resus Emerg Med.* 2009;17:12.

80. Roudsari BS, Nathens AB, Cameron P, et al. International comparison of prehospital trauma care systems. *Injury.* 2007;38:993–1000.

81. Lossius HM, Roislien J, Lockey DJ. Patient safety in pre-hospital emergency tracheal intubation: a comprehensive meta-analysis of the intubation success rates of EMS providers. *Crit Care.* 2012;16:R24.

82. Sampalis JS, Lavoie A, Williams JI, Mulder DS, Kalina M. Impact of on-site care, prehospital time, and level of in-hospital care on survival in severely injured patients. *J Trauma.* 1993;34:252–261.

83. Baez AA, Lane PL, Sorondo B, Giraldez EM. Predictive effect of out-of-hospital time in outcomes of severely injured young adult and elderly patients. *Prehosp Disaster Med.* 2006;21:427–430.

84. Ingalls N, Zonies D, Bailey JA, et al. A review of the first 10 years of critical care aeromedical transport during operation Iraqi freedom and operation enduring freedom: the importance of evacuation timing. *JAMA Surg.* 2014;149:807–813.

85. Hartl R, Gerber LM, Iacono L, Ni Q, Lyons K, Ghajar J. Direct transport within an organized state trauma system reduces mortality in patients with severe traumatic brain injury. *J Trauma.* 2006;60:1250–1256. discussion 6.

86. Sampalis JS, Denis R, Frechette P, Brown R, Fleiszer D, Mulder D. Direct transport to tertiary trauma centers versus transfer from lower level facilities: impact on mortality and morbidity among patients with major trauma. *J Trauma.* 1997;43:288–295. discussion 95–6.

87. MacKenzie EJ, Rivara FP, Jurkovich GJ, et al. A national evaluation of the effect of trauma-center care on mortality. *N Engl J Med.* 2006;354:366–378.

88. Liberman M, Mulder D, Sampalis J. Advanced or basic life support for trauma: meta-analysis and critical review of the literature. *J Trauma.* 2000;49:584–599.

89. Stiell IG, Wells GA, Field B, et al. Advanced cardiac life support in out-of-hospital cardiac arrest. *N Engl J Med.* 2004;351:647–656.

90. Stiell IG, Spaite DW, Field B, et al. Advanced life support for out-of-hospital respiratory distress. *N Engl J Med.* 2007;356:2156–2164.

91. Stiell IG, Nesbitt LP, Pickett W, et al. The OPALS Major Trauma Study: impact of advanced life-support on survival and morbidity. *CMAJ.* 2008;178:1141–1152.

92. Liberman M, Mulder D, Lavoie A, Denis R, Sampalis JS. Multicenter Canadian study of prehospital trauma care. *Ann Surg.* 2003;237:153–160.

93. Bernard SA, Nguyen V, Cameron P, et al. Prehospital rapid sequence intubation improves functional outcome for patients with severe traumatic brain injury: a randomized controlled trial. *Ann Surg.* 2010;252:959–965.

94. Eckstein M, Chan L, Schneir A, Palmer R. Effect of prehospital advanced life support on outcomes of major trauma patients. *J Trauma.* 2000;48:643–648.

95. Stockinger ZT, McSwain Jr NE. Prehospital endotracheal intubation for trauma does not improve survival over bag-valve-mask ventilation. *J Trauma.* 2004;56:531–536.

96. Wang HE, Peitzman AB, Cassidy LD, Adelson PD, Yealy DM. Out-of-hospital endotracheal intubation and outcome after traumatic brain injury. *Ann Emerg Med.* 2004;44:439–450.

97. Cobas MA, De la Pena MA, Manning R, Candiotti K, Varon AJ. Prehospital intubations and mortality: a level 1 trauma center perspective. *Anesth Analg.* 2009;109:489–493.

98. Silvestri S, Ralls GA, Krauss B, et al. The effectiveness of out-of-hospital use of continuous end-tidal carbon dioxide monitoring on the rate of unrecognized misplaced intubation within a regional emergency medical services system. *Ann Emerg Med.* 2005;45:497–503.

25 Are Computerized Algorithms Useful in Managing the Critically Ill Patient?

Bruce A. McKinley, R. Matthew Sailors

In mathematics and computer science, an algorithm is a step-by-step procedure for solving a problem. Algorithms are used for calculation, data processing, and automated reasoning. Expressed as a finite list of well-defined instructions and starting from an initial state and initial "input," an algorithm, when executed, proceeds through a finite number of well-defined successive states, eventually producing an "output" and terminating at a final end state.

Algorithms have been used to develop, describe, and present logical processes of patient care. Since the early 1990s, processes of care designed as computer algorithms have been used to direct the care of critically ill patients. To be logical, a process of care needs to be described as a sequence of measurements, observations, or decisions. To be "computerized," the process of care must be explicit and comprehensive.

For practical use in clinical medicine, algorithms have been a logical set of rules that precisely defines a sequence of decisions and specifies interventions. Commonly, the term *protocol* is used to refer to a specific clinical process of care, and a protocol may incorporate multiple algorithms. The concept of computerized algorithms to guide bedside clinical care has been developed and used for critically ill patients. Implemented as computerized protocols, their use has been associated with improved care relative to contemporaneous clinical standards.

Computer technology is now an integral part of the U.S. health-care system. Electronic medical record (EMR) technology is used to document patient measurements and interventions; to record clinician diagnoses, interpretations, and bedside presence; and to associate these data with established codes for billing, diagnosis, and treatment. Direct use by physicians is now mandatory, and government and commercial insurance agencies require computerized record submissions for reimbursement. How well the use of computerized medical record technology improves the efficacy of medical care and the efficiency of its delivery has been a poorly analyzed and unreported aspect of EMR technology.

Apart from the advent of the EMR, computerized medical protocol technology has evolved during the past 25 years. The term *computerized protocol* implies computer technology providing information to guide patient-specific care at bedside in real time. The problem of variability of patient care among clinicians derives from individualized, subjective decision making in complex clinical circumstances. Computerized protocol technology has been successfully used to implement protocols for complex processes that require standardized decision making to decrease variability in the care of critically ill patients and offers a powerful method for implementing a broad range of evidence-based guidelines. This technology is a desirable option for the intensive care community to establish and maintain the intensivist's essential role in specifying and implementing best practices.

COMPUTER TECHNOLOGY TO ADVISE PHYSICIANS: MEDICAL INFORMATICS AND DECISION SUPPORT

Fifty years ago, Ledley and Lusted[1-3] hypothesized that medical reasoning could be mathematically modeled. In 1964, the National Library of Medicine created the Medical Literature Analysis and Retrieval System (MEDLARS), and in 1971, Medical Literature Analysis and Retrieval System Online (Medline) was initiated.[4] The National Library of Medicine developed searchable online libraries containing reference information, and the Unified Medical Language System (UMLS) research and development program, initiated in 1986, continues to provide national and international vocabularies and classifications.[5] Since the 1970s, development of government and, more recently, commercial systems has led to computer technologies that provide information to advise physicians. These include online search systems, systems to provide diagnostic assistance,[6-17] clinical data interpretation,[18-20] and expert systems to guide patient-specific care.[21,22] Information search and reference systems are now ubiquitous by means of the Internet.

Development of computer, communication, and network technology and its use in medicine during the 1970s initiated the development of medical informatics as an academic discipline and enabled optimization of acquisition, storage, retrieval, and application of medical information. Medical informatics incorporates computer science, clinical guidelines, medical terminologies, and information and communication systems with an overall goal of promoting patient care that is safe, effective, equitable, efficient, timely, and individualized. Examples of medical informatics include expert systems such as Mycin, a rule based yes/no query system to diagnose bacterial infections and recommend drug therapy,[22] and Internist-I, a ranking algorithm system to diagnose disease;[23] MUMPS (Massachusetts General Hospital Utility Multi Programming System), (http://en.wikipedia.org/wiki/MUMPS, now also known as *M*), a commonly used language specification and programming language for clinical applications that is the basis of the largest enterprise-wide EMR, VistA (Veterans Health Information Systems and Technology Architecture) and its graphic user interface, CPRS (Computerized Patient Record System), which enable health-care providers to review and update a Veterans Administration (VA) patient's electronic medical record at any VA facility (http://en.wikipedia.org/wiki/VistA); and LDS Hospital's (Intermountain Healthcare Corp, Salt Lake City, Utah) HELP (Health Evaluation through Logical Processing) system, one of the first EMR systems, designed to assist clinician decision making and operational for nearly 40 years.

Decision support tools to advise physicians are not new. For decades, physicians have used pocket editions of texts, antibiotic therapy guides, diagnostic algorithms, and protocol handbooks at the point of care (point of decision making). Computerized decision support tools, such as computerized algorithms and protocols, provide new attributes that include bedside application, incorporation of sufficient detail to be explicit, and reproducible electronic acquisition and storage of time- stamped patient measurements to permit identification of temporal changes, consistency, and reproducibility for use in algorithm logic. When explicit computerized algorithms or protocols are driven by patient measurements, the protocol output (instructions) is patient specific, at once providing individualized treatment and standardizing clinical decisions. This nonintuitive property has proved desirable among clinicians and has improved patient care outcomes.[24]

Currently, the principal role for computer technology in medicine is to record and recall data, including in-hospital patient data, patient-specific medical care payment data, and non–patient-specific publications of medical science and clinical experience. Key to the advance of medical informatics and computer technology is widely available, clinically up-to-date computerized algorithms that can be used to effect immediate decisions for immediate care.

COMPUTERIZED ALGORITHMS AS MODELS OF MEDICAL REASONING

The concept of models of medical reasoning advanced 50 years ago has been successfully demonstrated in many computerized protocols implemented during the past 25 years. The algorithms to specify clinical care processes were developed by local working groups of clinicians and informaticists to ensure safe, optimized care and to decrease variability of care (see Fig. 25-1). The rule-based expert system, comprising explicit rules that facilitate decision making in a logical, workflow-compatible sequence, has been used most extensively to model complex care processes. Rule-based expert systems have been used with long-term success. At patient bedside (point of care; point of decision making), specific, clinically current measurements are used to derive clinical decisions in a sequence that directs incremental interventions as needed to obtain and maintain a specific, measureable

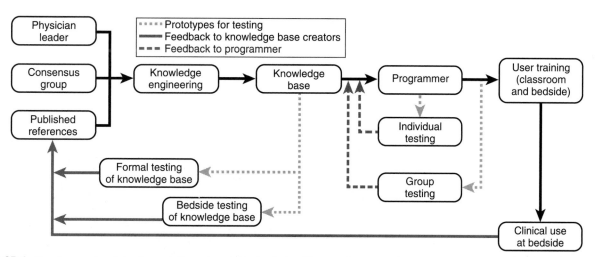

Figure 25-1. Development and implementation of computerized algorithms and a protocol system are an iterative build–test–refine process based on a consensus working group. For an intensive care process, the consensus group comprises physicians, clinical staff, especially bedside nurses, and programmer-informaticist expertise. A physician leader identifies and guides development of the clinical care process, derives consensus, and motivates review and update.

effect.[24] This type of expert system has been applicable to many aspects of intensive care. Computerized protocols comprising multiple algorithms driven by readily available, repeatable measurements, which were originally devised and refined by LDS Hospital clinicians and informacists.[26-28] This technology has been adopted by others to effectively standardize clinical decision making at bedside and provide timely, patient-specific intervention for selected aspects of critical care.

COMPUTERIZED ALGORITHMS AND PROTOCOLS: CLINICAL EXPERIENCE

The first computerized algorithms and protocol systems to guide complex processes of intensive care were developed in the late 1980s. Computerized protocol technology has since been used to implement bedside protocols to direct care processes for durations of hours to weeks.[23-32] Protocols are developed by multidisciplinary groups incorporating best available evidence and clinical experience (Fig. 25-1).

Successful implementation of a protocol for mechanical ventilatory support of patients with acute respiratory distress syndrome (ARDS) was reported in 1993.[33] Algorithms were developed through local expert consensus to standardize bedside decision making. Component algorithms provided point-of-care instructions for adjustment of the fraction of inspired oxygen, positive end-expiratory pressure, tidal volume (TV), and respiratory rate in response to threshold rules and measurement of variables directly affecting oxygenation and ventilation. The protocol comprised 30 algorithms and guided the entire process, from intubation through weaning and extubation.[33-35] Additional algorithms were developed to enable use of pulse oximetry to accurately assess arterial oxygen partial pressure (Pao_2) with noninvasive arterial hemoglobin oxygen saturation (SpO_2).[34]

Use of this first computerized protocol was associated with a dramatic increase in the survival of patients with ARDS.[25] Bedside clinicians accepted more than 90% of ARDS management protocol generated instructions.[26] The acceptance rate of computer- generated instructions from most other computerized protocol systems implemented since the early 1990s, nearly all in ICUs, has been 90% or greater, indicating detailed understanding of care process and comprehensive design of the care process model. This system was patient dedicated with the protocol logic program continuously "on" and with the user interface at bedside. Explicit criteria based on current measurements to establish a diagnosis of ARDS were required.[36] Another important principle is requirement for the bedside clinician's judgment to accept or decline all computerized protocol instructions for therapy intervention, referred to as an "open loop" control. When implemented continuously, a computerized protocol guidance system in a medical or surgical trauma intensive care unit (ICU) proved to be practical and safe, providing standardized decision making and individualized interventions for management of mechanical ventilatory support of ARDS.[33]

This protocol system, with algorithms modified to enable 6 mL/kg breaths, was used in a randomized controlled trial (RCT) in which conventional and "small" TVs were compared in the management of ARDS. The RCT, conducted between 1993 and 1998 at 10 different centers, used a bedside program with available desktop computers and user interface.[37] The protocol system was used for 32,055 hours (15 staff person years, 3.7 patient years); was active for 96% of ventilator time; and generated 38,546 instructions, 94% of which were followed. Similar results at a single participating center were documented in patients with trauma-induced ARDS (Shock Trauma ICU, Memorial Hermann Hospital, Houston, Tex.) in which the computerized system was in use 96% of the time with 95% compliance.[38] The trial demonstrated efficacy of computerized algorithms implemented as a protocol that directed permissive hypercapnia with small tidal volume compared with then conventional large tidal volume strategies. Importantly, the trial demonstrated that care that was used with a computerized protocol system for mechanical ventilatory support could be directly transferred to other clinical sites and significantly improve care. This computerized protocol-based prospective RCT provided convincing evidence and generated new knowledge that predated work of the ARDS-Net.[39]

A Houston-based team effort followed to develop a computerized protocol for management of intracranial pressure (ICP) after traumatic brain injury. A cohort study demonstrated that use of the six explicit therapeutic algorithms significantly improved compliance with established guidelines,[40] limiting untoward changes in ICP and cerebral perfusion pressure despite fewer interventions.[30] A prototype computerized protocol system using the algorithms was subsequently developed and successfully tested.[41]

Computerized protocol technology has been developed to guide fluid resuscitation of shocked trauma patients during their first ICU day.[30,38,42-47] The program was based on management principles developed by the LDS hospital group,[24,31] and used oxygen delivery (Do_2) as a quantitative measurement of hemodynamic performance.[49-51] The oxygen delivery goal was to be greater than or equal to 600 mL/O_2/min. This "shock resuscitation protocol" was used to guide the treatment of more than 400 patients during 2000-2006 and was implemented with bedside mobile computer workstations. A series of protocol modifications were made through ongoing consensus group review (see Fig. 25-1) and accrued data analysis.[27-29] This demonstrated the "process control" impact of computerized algorithms in a clinical process previously known to be variable and often chaotic.[30] Use of this protocol confirmed the relationship between the volume of resuscitation fluid administered and the development and timing of abdominal compartment syndrome[53-57] and persistent coagulopathy.[58]

The use of computerized protocol technology improved the implementation of sepsis management guidelines, when compared with conventional guideline approaches.[59,60] The Houston team constructed a comprehensive sepsis management protocol system, using Surviving Sepsis Campaign, other guidelines, and local expert consensus (see Fig. 25-2). The system standardized decision making

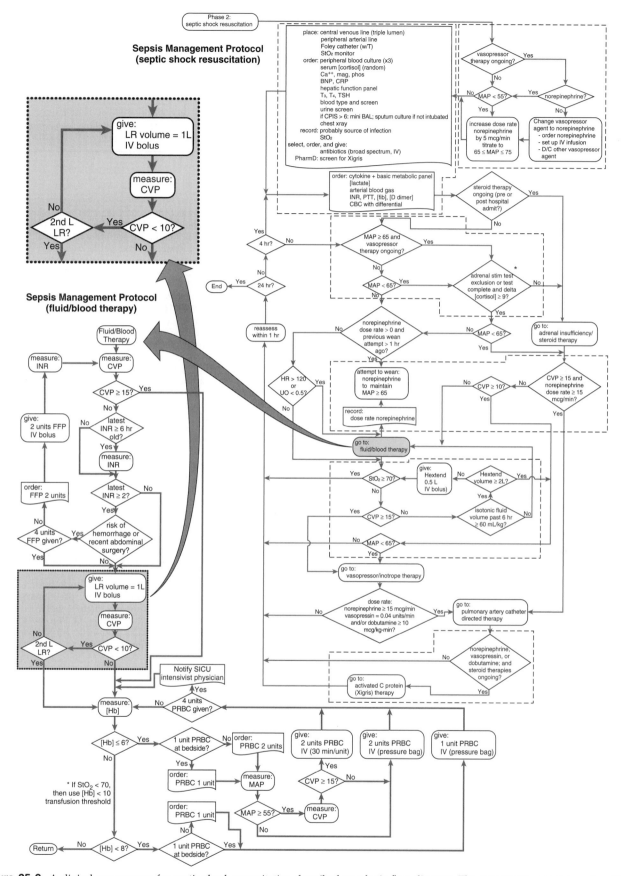

Figure 25-2. A clinical care process for septic shock resuscitation described as a logic flow diagram. The care process comprises algorithms, including an incremental process for intravenous fluid administration to effect a change in central venous pressure (*CVP*). The logic flow diagram is a format able to be interpreted and discussed by nontechnologist clinicians and is useful for specifying processes and prioritizing protocol goals logically and for encoding a knowledge base. *BAL,* bronchoalveolar lavage; *BNP,* brain natriuretic peptide; *Ca++,* calcium ion; *CBC,* complete blood cell count; *CPIS,* clinical pulmonary infection score; *CRP,* C-reactive protein; D/C; *FFP,* fresh frozen plasma; *Hb,* hemoglobin; *HR,* heart rate; *INR,* international normalized ratio; *IV,* intravenous; *LR,* lactated Ringer's solution; mag, magnesium; *MAP,* mean arterial pressure; phos, phosphorous; PRBC, packed red blood cell; *PTT,* partial thromboplastin time; *SICU,* surgical intensive care unit; *StO2,* tissue oxygenation saturation; *T3,* triiodo-thyronine; *T4,* thyroxine; *TSH,* thyroid-stimulating hormone; *UO,* urine output.

among surgical intensivists, resident physicians, and nurse practitioners. Antibiotic agents were administered within 1 hour of protocol initiation and moderate volumes of intravenous fluid were administered (2.0 ± 0.2 L during 24-hour protocol). The hospital mortality rate was much lower than that reported by the Surviving Sepsis Campaign guideline initiative (14% vs. 31%).[59] The acceptance rate for computerized protocol-generated instructions was 90%. This compared favorably with the Surviving Sepsis Campaign "bundle" compliance rate of 36%,[62] although it should be considered that the "bundle" at that time contained some highly controversial interventions (subsequently removed) and compliance required administration of the entire bundle. A similar system designed and implemented at a second site (University of Florida Health surgical ICUs, Gainesville, Fla.) had very similar results: 14% hospital mortality rate and 91% acceptance rate of computerized protocol-generated instructions.[60] At the second site, recognition of sepsis occurred earlier after onset of infection with implementation of a computerized sepsis surveillance and diagnosis system, providing a start state for the computerized protocol process, and analogous to specific criteria that had been used to diagnose ARDS or shock due to major torso trauma.

Other algorithms have been developed and are being used to optimize care. Management of blood glucose concentration with insulin therapy is a process implemented with many protocol and guideline approaches because precise glycemic control in ICU patients is thought to improve outcomes.[63-65] The protocols instruct clinicians to measure glucose concentration and administer intravenous insulin by infusion to maintain blood glucose concentration within a specified target range.[66-70] A proprietary computerized algorithm system was commercialized in 2008 and is currently used by many U.S. hospitals.[71]

In 1996, Pestotnik et al. published results of implementing antibiotic practice guidelines in a large community hospital.[72] These locally derived consensus guidelines were implemented as a rule based system for inpatient prophylactic, empiric, and therapeutic uses of antibiotics. The use of these guidelines over a 7-year period demonstrated a 23% decrease in antibiotic use, resulting in a 25% reduction in acquisition costs. Today, this system is now in use in over 200 institutions, having been commercialized in 2003.

Computerized algorithms to implement guidelines for transfusion in medical, surgical and mixed ICUs at two academic medical centers resulted in improved survival and reduced cost.[73] Burn resuscitation guided by computerized algorithms was associated with a decrease in the volume of fluid administered and improved survival.[74] On the basis of proprietary algorithms, the system has been commercially available since 2013 (http://www.arcosmedical.com/).

AUTHORS' RECOMMENDATIONS

- Computerized algorithm technology has been successfully used to implement protocols for complex critical care interventions.
- Advantages include bedside implementation and standardized decision making.
- Modern systems allow for individualization of patient care, while simultaneously restraining variability.
- The technology offers a powerful method for implementing guidelines for many aspects of care.
- Physician leadership in the future will accelerate development, and implementation of such systems will likely result in significant improvements in patient outcomes.

REFERENCES

1. Ledley RS. Digital electronic computers in biomedical science. *Science.* 1959;130(3384):1225–1234.
2. Ledley RS, Lusted LB. Reasoning foundations of medical diagnosis: symbolic logic, probability, and value theory aid our understanding of how physicians reason. *Science.* 1959;130(3366):9–21.
3. Ledley RS, Lusted LB. Computers in medical data processing. *Oper Res.* 1960:299–310.
4. Miles WD. *A History of the National Library of Medicine.* Bethesda, MD: US Department Of Health & Human Services; 1982.
5. Lindberg DA, Humphreys BL, McCray AT. The unified medical language system. *Methods Inf Med.* 1993;32(4):281–291.
6. Barnett GO, Cimino JJ, Hupp JA, Hoffer EP. DXplain. An evolving diagnostic decision-support system. *JAMA.* 1987;258(1):67–74.
7. DXplain on the internet. In: Barnett GO, Famiglietti KT, Kim RJ, Hoffer EP, Feldman MJ, eds. *Proc AMIA Symp.* ; 1998.
8. Barnett GO, Hoffer EP, Packer MS. DXplain-demonstration and discussion of a diagnostic decision support system. *Proc Annu Symp Comput Appl Med Care.* 1992:822.
9. de Dombal FT, Leaper DJ, Staniland JR, McCann AP, Horrocks JC. Computer-aided diagnosis of acute abdominal pain. *BMJ.* 1972;2(5804):9–13.
10. Integrating DXplain into a clinical information system using the World Wide Web. In: Elhanan G, Socratous SA, Cimino JJ, eds. *Proc AMIA Annu Fall Symp.* 1996.
11. Feldman MJ, Barnett GO. An approach to evaluating the accuracy of DXplain. *Comput Methods Programs Biomed.* 1991;35(4):261–266.
12. Ramnarayan P, Roberts GC, Coren M. Assessment of the potential impact of a reminder system on the reduction of diagnostic errors: a quasi-experimental study. *BMC Med Inform Decis Mak.* 2006;6(1):22.
13. Ramnarayan P, Tomlinson A, Kulkarni G, Rao A, Britto J. A novel diagnostic aid (ISABEL): development and preliminary evaluation of clinical performance. *Medinfo.* 2004:1091–1095.
14. Ramnarayan P, Tomlinson A, Rao A, Coren M, Winrow A, Britto J. ISABEL: a web-based differential diagnostic aid for paediatrics: results from an initial performance evaluation. *Arch Dis Child.* 2003;88(5):408–413.
15. Warner HR, Bouhaddou O. Innovation review: Iliad–a medical diagnostic support program. *Top Health Inf Manage.* 1994;14(4):51–58.
16. Warner HR, Haugh PJ, Bouhaddou O, et al. Iliad as an expert consultant to teach differential diagnosis. *Symp Comput Appl Med Care.* 1988;12:371–376.
17. Warner HR, Toronto AF, Veasey LG. A mathematical approach to medical diagnosis: application to congenital heart disease. *JAMA.* 1961;177:75–81.
18. Gardner RM, Cannon GH, Morris AH. Computerized blood gas interpretation and reporting system. *Respir Care.* 1985;30:695–700.
19. Pryor TA. Development of decision support systems. In: Shabot MM, Gardner RM, eds. *Decision Support Systems in Critical Care.* New York: Springer-Verlag; 1994:61–73.
20. Pryor TA, Lyndsay AE, England W. Computer analysis of serial electrocardiograms. *Comput Biomed Res.* 1973;6:228–234.
21. Shortliffe EH. Update on ONCOCIN: a chemotherapy advisor for clinical oncology. *Med Inform.* 1986;11:19–21.
22. Shortliffe EH, Davis R, Axline SG. Computer-based consultations in clinical therapeutics: explanation and rule acquisition capabilities of the MYCIN system. *Comput Biomed Res.* 1975;8:303–320.
23. Miller RA, Pople HE, Myers JD. Internist-1, an experimental computer-based diagnostic consultant for general internal medicine. *N Engl J Med.* 1982;307(8):468–476.

24. Morris AH. Decision support and safety of clinical environments. *Qual Saf Health Care.* 2002;11(1):69–75. Epub 2002/06/25.

25. Morris AH. Protocol management of adult respiratory distress syndrome. *New Horiz.* 1993;1(4):593–602. Epub 1993/11/01.

26. East TD, Bohm SH, Wallace CJ, et al. A successful computerized protocol for clinical management of pressure control inverse ratio ventilation in ARDS patients. *Chest.* 1992;101(3):697–710. Epub 1992/03/11.

27. East TD, Morris AH, Wallace CJ, et al. A strategy for development of computerized critical care decision support systems. *Int J Clin Monit Comput.* 1991;8(4):263–269. Epub 1991/01/11.

28. McKinley BA, Marvin RG, Cocanour CS, Marquez A, Ware DN, Moore FA. Blunt trauma resuscitation: the old can respond. *Arch Surg.* 2000;135(6):688–693. discussion 94-5. Epub 2000/06/08.

29. McKinley BA, Marvin RG, Cocanour CS, Pousman RM, Ware DN, Moore FA. Nitroprusside in resuscitation of major torso trauma. *J Trauma.* 2000;49(6):1089–1095.

30. McKinley BA, Parmley CL, Tonnesen AS. Standardized management of intracranial pressure: a preliminary clinical trial. *J Trauma.* 1999;46(2):271–279.

31. Morris AH. Algorithm based decision making. In: Tobin MJ, ed. *Principles and Practice of Intensive Care Monitoring.* New York: McGraw-Hill; 1997:1355–1381.

32. Morris AH. Computerized protocols and bedside decision support. *Crit Care Clin.* 1999;15(3):523–545. vi. Epub 1999/08/12.

33. Thomsen GE, Pope D, East TD, et al. Clinical performance of a rule-based decision support system for mechanical ventilation of ARDS patients. *Proc Annu Symp Comput Appl Med Care.* 1993: 339–343.

34. Sailors RM, East TD, Wallace CJ, Morris AH. A successful protocol for the use of pulse oximetry to classify arterial oxygenation into four fuzzy categories. *Proc Annu Symp Comput Appl Med Care.* 1995:248–252. Epub 1995/01/01.

35. Morris AH. Adult respiratory distress syndrome and new modes of mechanical ventilation: reducing the complications of high volume and high pressure. *New Horiz.* 1994;2(1):19–33.

36. Bernard GR, Artigas A, Brigham KL, et al. The American-European Consensus Conference on ARDS: definitions, mechanisms, relevant outcomes, and clinical trial coordination. *Am J Respir Crit Care Med.* 1994;149:818–824.

37. East TD, Heermann LK, Bradshaw RL, et al. Efficacy of computerized decision support for mechanical ventilation: results of a prospective multi-center randomized trial. *Proc AMIA Symp.* 1999:251–255. Epub 1999/11/24.

38. McKinley BA, Moore FA, Sailors RM, et al. Computerized decision support for mechanical ventilation of trauma induced ARDS: results of a randomized clinical trial. *J Trauma.* 2001;50(3):415–424.

39. Ventilation with lower tidal volumes as compared with traditional tidal volumes for acute lung injury and the acute respiratory distress syndrome. The Acute Respiratory Distress Syndrome Network. *N Engl J Med.* 2000;342(18):1301–1308.

40. Guidelines for the management of severe head injury. Brain Trauma Foundation, American Association of Neurological Surgeons, Joint Section on Neurotrauma and Critical Care. *J Neurotrauma.* 1996;13(11):641–734.

41. Nerlikar A. *Automated Protocol for Management of Intracranial Pressure Following Severe Closed Head Injury.* Houston: University of Houston; 1996.

42. McKinley BA, Kozar RA, Cocanour CS, et al. Trauma resuscitation: female hearts respond better. *Arch Surg.* 2002;137(5):578–584.

43. McKinley BA, Kozar RA, Cocanour CS, et al. Normal versus supranormal O_2 delivery goals in shock resuscitation: the response is the same. *J Trauma.* 2002;53(5):825–842.

44. McKinley BA, Marvin RG, Cocanour CS, Ware DN, Moore FA. Blunt trauma resuscitation: the old can respond. *Arch Surg.* 2000;48(4):637–642.

45. McKinley BA, Sailors RM, Glorsky SL, et al. Computer directed resuscitation of major torso trauma. *Shock.* 2001;15 (suppl): 46.

46. McKinley BA, Valdivia A, Moore FA. Goal-oriented shock resuscitation for major torso trauma. *Curr Opin Crit Care.* 2003;9:292–299.

47. McKinley BA, Sucher JF, Todd SR, et al. Central venous pressure versus pulmonary artery catheter-directed shock resuscitation. *Shock.* 2009;32(5):463–470. Epub 2009/10/16.

48. Moore FA, Moore EE, Sauaia A. Blood transfusion. An independent risk factor for postinjury multiple organ failure. *Arch Surg.* 1997;132(6):620–624.

49. Sauaia A, Moore FA, Moore EE, Haenel JB, Read RA, Lezotte DC. Early predictors of postinjury multiple organ failure. *Arch Surg.* 1994;129(1):39–45.

50. Sauaia A, Moore FA, Moore EE, Norris JM, Lezotte DC, Hamman RF. Multiple organ failure can be predicted as early as 12 hours after injury. *J Trauma.* 1998;45(2):291–301. discussion -3. Epub 1998/08/26.

51. Marr AB, Moore FA, Sailors RM, et al. 'Starling curve' generation during shock resuscitation: can it be done? *Shock.* 2004;21(4): 300–305.

52. McKinley BA, Kozar RA, Cocanour CS, et al. Normal versus supranormal oxygen delivery goals in shock resuscitation: the response is the same. *J Trauma.* 2002;53(5):825–832. Epub 2002/11/19.

53. Balogh Z, McKinley BA, Cocanour CS, Kozar RA, Cox CS, Moore FA. Patients with impending abdominal compartment syndrome do not respond to early volume loading. *Am J Surg.* 2003;186(6):602–608.

54. Balogh Z, McKinley BA, Cocanour CS, et al. Secondary abdominal compartment syndrome is an elusive early complication of traumatic shock resuscitation. *Am J Surg.* 2002;184(6):538–543.

55. Balogh Z, McKinley BA, Cocanour CS, et al. Supra-normal trauma resuscitation causes more cases of abdominal compartment syndrome. *Arch Surg.* 2003;138(6):637–643.

56. Balogh Z, McKinley BA, Cox CS, et al. Abdominal compartment syndrome: the cause or effect multiple organ failure? *Shock.* 2003;20:483–492.

57. Balogh Z, McKinley BA, Holcomb JB, et al. Both primary and secondary abdominal compartment syndrome can be predicted early and are harbingers of bad outcome. *J Trauma.* 2003;54: 848–861.

58. Gonzalez EA, Moore FA, Holcomb JB, et al. Fresh frozen plasma should be given earlier to patients requiring massive transfusion. *J Trauma.* 2007;62(1):112–119.

59. McKinley BA, Moore LJ, Sucher JF, et al. Computer protocol facilitates evidence-based care of sepsis in the surgical intensive care unit. *J Trauma.* 2011;70(5):1153–1167.

60. Croft CA, Moore FA, Efron PA, et al. Computer versus paper system for recognition and management of sepsis in surgical intensive care. *J Trauma Acute Care Surg.* 2014;76(2):311–317.

61. Deleted in proofs.

62. Levy MM, Dellinger RP, Townsend SR, et al. The Surviving Sepsis Campaign: results of an international guideline-based performance improvement program targeting severe sepsis. *Crit Care Med.* 2010;38(2):367–374.

63. van den Berghe G, Wouters P, Weekers F, et al. Intensive insulin therapy in critically ill patients. *N Engl J Med.* 2001;345(19):1359–1367.

64. Chase JG, Shaw GM, Hann CE, et al. Clinical validation of a model-based glycaemic control design approach and comparison to other clinical protocols. *Conf Proc IEEE Eng Med Biol Soc.* 2006;1:59–62.

65. Nasraway SA. Hyperglycemia during critical illness. *J Parenter Enteral Nutr.* 2006;3:254–258.

66. Morris AH, Orme Jr J, Truwit JD, et al. A replicable method for blood glucose control in critically ill patients. *Crit Care Med.* 2008;36(6):1787–1795. Epub 2008/06/04.

67. Vogelzang M, Zijlstra F, Nijsten MW. Design and implementation of GRIP: a computerized glucose control system at a surgical intensive care unit. *BMC Med Inform Decis Mak.* 2005;5:38.

68. Hoekstra M, Schoorl MA, van der Horst ICC, et al. Computer-assisted glucose regulation during rapid step-wise increases of parenteral nutrition in critically ill patients: a proof of concept study. *J Parenter Enteral Nutr.* 2010;34:549–553.

69. Morris AH. Multicenter validation of a computer-based clinical decision support tool for glucose control in adult and pediatric intensive care units. *J Diabetes Sci Technol.* 2008;2(3):357–368.

70. Lanspa MJ, Dickerson J, Morris AH, Orme JF, Holmen J, Hirshberg EL. Coefficient of glucose variation is independently associated with mortality in critically ill patients receiving intravenous insulin. *Crit Care.* 2014;18:R86.

71. Fogel SL, Baker CC. Effects of computerized decision support systems on blood glucose regulation in critically ill surgical patients. *J Am Coll Surg*. 2013;216:828–835.

72. Pestotnik SL, Classen DC, Evans RS, Burke JP. Implementing antibiotic practice guidelines through computer-assisted decision support: clinical and financial outcomes. *Ann Intern Med*. 1996;124(10):884–890.

73. Rana R, Afessa B, Keegan MT, et al. Evidence-based red cell transfusion in the critically ill: quality improvement using computerized physician order entry. *Crit Care Med*. 2006;34(7):1892–1897.

74. Salinas J, Chung KK, Mann EA, et al. Computerized decision support system improves fluid resuscitation following severe burns: an original study. *Crit Care Med*. 2011;39(9):2031–2038.

NON-ARDS AND NONINFECTIOUS RESPIRATORY DISORDERS

26 How Do I Diagnose and Treat Pulmonary Embolism?

Jacob T. Gutsche, Anita K. Malhotra

Pulmonary embolism (PE) is a common clinical problem characterized by the deposition and embolization of a venous clot. Collectively, deep vein thrombosis (DVT) and PE are referred to as venous thromboembolism (VTE). Patients with PE typically have symptoms related to ventilation-perfusion mismatch and increased pulmonary artery pressures. These abnormalities can lead to hypoxemia and right ventricular strain/failure. Because of the high potential for associated mortality, the diagnosis of PE should be considered by the intensivist confronted with acute pulmonary or cardiovascular failure.

EPIDEMIOLOGY AND NATURAL HISTORY

The annual estimated incidence of PE in the United States is 112 per 100,000 adults.[1] The incidence is significantly higher in men, and incidence and mortality increase with advancing age.[2] Mortality rates for PE remain high; data from the International Cooperative Pulmonary Embolism Registry indicate a mortality rate approaching 15% among hemodynamically stable patients and 60% in hemodynamically unstable patients.[3]

Most often, PE arises from DVTs that embolize after 3 to 7 days. In approximately 70% of patients with PE, DVT can be found in the lower limbs.[4,5] The initial studies on the natural history of VTE were intraoperative assessment during orthopedic surgery. In this setting, DVT of the calf or more proximal venous system was found in approximately 30% of patients. DVT resolved spontaneously after a few days in approximately one third of patients and did not extend in approximately 40%. However, in 25%, the clot evolved into proximal DVT and PE.[6] Major risk factors for the development of VTE are listed in Table 26-1. Even temporary immobilization for 1 to 2 days will significantly increase the risk of DVT.

PE presents with shock or hypotension in 5% to 10% of patients. In some patients without shock, there are signs of right ventricular dysfunction or injury. This abnormality is associated with poorer prognosis.

PE is difficult to diagnose because of the nonspecific clinical presentation or complete lack of symptoms. Among patients with proximal DVT who have lung scans, approximately 50% will have associated, usually clinically asymptomatic, PE.

PATHOPHYSIOLOGY

The initial clinical consequences of acute PE are primarily hemodynamic and become apparent when more than 30% to 50% of the pulmonary arterial bed is occluded by thromboemboli.[7] Large or multiple emboli can acutely increase pulmonary vascular resistance. The resultant increased afterload often cannot be overcome by the right ventricle (RV) because a nonpreconditioned, thin-walled RV cannot generate mean pulmonary arterial pressures exceeding approximately 40 mm Hg.[7] Resultant underfilling of the left ventricle (LV) decreases blood pressure and coronary blood flow. The combination of increased RV myocardial workload and a decreased RV coronary perfusion gradient (decreased systemic diastolic pressure – increased intraventricular pressure) contributes to RV ischemia. This ischemia worsens RV dysfunction and may initiate a vicious cycle that can ultimately result in pulseless electrical activity and sudden cardiac death.[8]

In up to one third of patients, right-to-left shunt through a patent foramen ovale may contribute to severe hypoxemia and will also increase the risk for systemic embolization. Ventilation-perfusion mismatch occurs in most cases. Vasoactive mediators such as serotonin released from ischemic lung tissue may exacerbate ventilation perfusion mismatch.

Diagnosis

Evaluating the likelihood of PE in an individual patient on the basis of the clinical presentation is the first and most important step to select an appropriate diagnostic strategy and interpret diagnostic test results.

CLINICAL PRESENTATION

Suspicion of PE should accompany clinical symptoms such as dyspnea, chest pain, or syncope. These abnormalities are present in more than 90% of patients with PE.[9,10] The likelihood of PE increases with the number of risk factors present. However, in approximately 30% of cases, PE occurs in the absence of any risk factor. Individual clinical signs and symptoms are not usually helpful because they are neither sensitive nor specific.

Table 26-1 Major Risk Factors for VTE

- Spinal cord injury
- Major general surgery
- Major trauma
- Major orthopedic surgery
- Pelvis, hip, and long-bone fracture
- Malignancy
- Myocardial infarction
- Congestive heart or respiratory failure

Modified from Anderson FA Jr., Spencer FA. Risk factors for venous thromboembolism. *Circulation.* 2003;107(suppl 1):9-16.

Other symptoms include cough and blood-tinged sputum. Signs include fever, tachycardia, tachypnea, cyanosis, and coarse breath sounds. PE is generally associated with hypoxemia. However, up to 20% of patients with PE have a normal arterial oxygen pressure (Pao$_2$ [partial pressure of oxygen, arterial]) and a normal alveolar-arterial oxygen gradient.[11] Auscultation may reveal a new fourth heart sound or accentuation of the pulmonic component of the second heart sound.

Electrocardiography may reveal new evidence of right ventricular strain, tachycardia, or atrial fibrillation. Electrocardiographic signs of RV strain include inversion of T waves in leads V$_1$ to V$_4$, a QR pattern of the classic S$_1$Q$_3$T$_3$ type in the lead V$_1$, and an incomplete or complete right bundle-branch block.[12] Electrocardiographic changes are generally associated with the more severe forms of PE, and lack of electrocardiographic changes does not exclude PE.

The chest radiograph is usually abnormal, with the most frequently encountered findings (platelike atelectasis, pleural effusion, or elevation of a hemidiaphragm) being nonspecific.[12] However, the chest radiograph is useful in excluding other causes of dyspnea and chest pain.

On the basis of clinical presentation or lack thereof, PE can be divided into three groups: hemodynamically unstable, hemodynamically stable and symptomatic, and asymptomatic and silent with incidental finding.

Hemodynamically Unstable Group

This group includes patients with shock or severe hypotension associated with RV dysfunction and injury. These patients require rapid, specific diagnosis and therapy because of the high mortality risk (short-term mortality >15%).[3,13]

Any intensive care unit (ICU) patient who is at risk for PE and is hemodynamically unstable should be evaluated for acute right ventricle failure and thrombus in the right ventricle or main pulmonary artery. Acute heart failure is not specific for PE; therefore other causes must be considered. The main therapeutic goal is to rapidly restore flow through the pulmonary circulation.

Hemodynamically Stable and Symptomatic Group

This group of patients can be divided into intermediate- and low-risk subgroups. Intermediate-risk PE is diagnosed when the patient has either RV dysfunction or myocardial

injury. Indicators of RV dysfunction include (1) elevated right ventricular pressures and RV dilation, (2) hypokinesis, or (3) pressure overload on echocardiography. Elevations of cardiac troponin T or I indicate RV injury. Initial therapy is aimed at the prevention of further pulmonary thromboembolism.

Asymptomatic and Silent Group with Incidental Finding

Mild, untreated PEs carry a lower immediate mortality than recurrent PEs. Because of the intrinsic fibrinolytic activity of the lung, small PEs usually resolve spontaneously. Withholding anticoagulation treatment in nonmassive PE is an acceptable strategy for patients who have an indeterminate ventilation-perfusion study, negative serial lower extremity venous examination results, adequate cardiopulmonary reserve, and relative-to-absolute contraindications to anticoagulation treatment.[11] The rationale for this approach is based on synthesis of the results of several studies. The optimal management of patients with asymptomatic PE has not been prospectively studied.

DIAGNOSIS

Clinical prediction scores have been widely used, but they do not have the necessary sensitivity and specificity to be used without diagnostic tools.[14] Several modalities are available for confirmation or exclusion of the diagnosis of PE. Laboratory studies, including arterial blood gas measurements, are nonspecific and generally unreliable.[15] Often, but not always, the arterial blood gas will demonstrate hypoxemia and respiratory alkalosis. In one study, the average Pao$_2$ in patients with PE was 72 ± 16 mm Hg, as opposed to patients without PE, for whom the Pao$_2$ was 70 ± 18 mm Hg.[11] In addition, up to 20% of patients with PE had a Pao$_2$ in the normal range, and the alveolar to arterial oxygen gradient was not found to be helpful because there was an average difference of only 2 mm Hg.[11]

Although a negative serum D dimer may be used to rule out PE, the results of this test are often of limited utility in the intensive care population. Patients with malignancy, those who are hospitalized, and pregnant women demonstrate reduced specificity with D-dimer testing.[16] Patients with either low or moderate pretest probability and a negative D dimer have no need to undergo any further testing.[17,18] However, those with positive tests or high clinical probability will require further investigation because a negative D dimer does not exclude PE in more than 15% of patients with high clinical probability.[17,18] Furthermore, D dimer is neither sensitive nor specific in the postoperative period.

The use of troponins and brain natriuretic peptide (BNP), often elevated in moderate or large PE, may be useful prognostic tests. In one study, normal levels of BNP had a 100% negative predictive value for hemodynamically stable patients.[19] Elevation of troponins are generally associated with right ventricular dysfunction and ischemia; therefore they are associated with worse outcome.

Diagnostic Tools

Because chest radiography is neither sensitive nor specific, the literature describes two modalities used in the diagnosis of PE: perfusion lung scans (V/Q scans) and computed tomography (CT) pulmonary angiography. The ease and speed of acquiring a CT scan make it the most widely used diagnostic tool for patients with suspected PE.

V/Q scans have been used to detect the presence of perfusion defects within the patient's pulmonary circulation. The major advantage of V/Q scans is the avoidance of nephrotoxic radiographic contrast. In the PIOPED (Prospective Investigation of Pulmonary Embolism Diagnosis) study, 755 patients underwent V/Q scans and selective pulmonary angiography within 24 hours of the symptoms that suggested PE.[20] Thirty-three percent of the patients had angiographic evidence of PE.[20] Almost all patients with PE (98%) had abnormal V/Q scan findings. Thus, V/Q scans are highly sensitive for acute PE. However, although PE was documented by angiography in 88%, only 41% of the patients with PE had a high-probability scan. Most patients with PE (75%) had an intermediate- or low-probability scan. Thus, specificity was low. In postoperative patients with significant atelectasis, consolidation, or PE, the negative predictive value is low. The V/Q scan is the study of choice for pregnant patients to avoid unnecessary radiation exposure.

High-resolution multidetector computed tomography (MDCT) has replaced the V/Q scan as the study of choice to diagnose PE. CT scanning is widely available, can be performed rapidly, and provides clear anatomic and pathologic lung images (so that the clinician often obtains a diagnosis despite negative results from an angiographic examination) and the ability to concurrently evaluate potential embolic sources in the legs or pelvis. Four-slice MDCT scans have an increased sensitivity for subsegmental PE. In two studies comprising approximately 100 patients, sensitivities for the detection of PE with four-slice CT angiography were reported to be 96%[21] and 100%,[22] with respective specificities of 98% and 89%. The combination of arterial-phase and venous-phase CT angiography appears more sensitive (90%) and specific (96%) than the arterial phase alone.[22] Postoperative patients with high clinical suspicion of PE and a negative MDCT scan should undergo lower extremity ultrasonography. Patients with impaired renal function should undergo hydration before administration of contrast and preferably receive nonionic contrast. Alternatively, these patients may undergo pulmonary scintigraphy, venous ultrasound, or magnetic resonance imaging.

However, if hemodynamic instability is present, echocardiography should be performed to evaluate right ventricular function. Right ventricular dysfunction is associated with increased mortality, especially in patients with hemodynamic instability.[23,24] During the diagnostic and treatment phase, echocardiography may assist clinical decision-making, although only 30% to 40% of patients have any echocardiographic abnormalities.[25] Evidence of right ventricular failure, such as severe hypokinesis, dilatation, or the McConnell sign (severe hypokinesis of the free wall with preserved apical function), may prompt an immediate surgical or catheter-based thrombectomy. Increased tricuspid regurgitation, chamber dilatation, and septal shift are suggestive of volume-pressure overload. If transesophageal echo is performed, then emboli may be seen in the main pulmonary arteries.

TREATMENT

The immediate priority is stabilization of the patient who is compromised by hemodynamic or respiratory instability. In some cases, severe hypoxemia and respiratory failure may require supplemental oxygen or mechanical ventilation.

Without treatment, mortality from hemodynamically unstable PE approaches 30%.[26] In treated patients, the overall mortality decreases to 15%.[3] The treatment of PE in the postoperative patient is complicated by the inherent potential for bleeding with therapeutic anticoagulation (TAC) and thrombolytics.

For acute PE, the options for treatment include TAC, inferior vena cava (IVC) filter placement to prevent continued embolization from the lower extremities, clot thrombolysis, and surgical or catheter embolectomy. Hemodynamically stable patients diagnosed with PE should receive TAC with intravenous unfractionated heparin (UFH) or subcutaneous low-molecular-weight heparin (LMWH). The risk of major bleeding from initiation of TAC is less than 3%.[27] Meta-analyses have shown that LMWH treatment, when adjusted to body weight, is at least as effective and safe as dose-adjusted UFH.[28] However, in postoperative and critically ill patients and in patients in whom epidural catheters have been placed, the shorter half-life and reversibility of intravenous UFH provides a safety buffer over LMWH. Furthermore, LMWH should be avoided in patients with a creatinine clearance less than 30 mL/min because of renal excretion. Therefore, despite the absence of randomized prospective trials, when there is a risk for clinically significant bleeding, UFH may be safer. In patients with moderate clinical suspicion, TAC should be started if the diagnostic evaluation is expected to exceed 4 hours; if suspicion is low, then TAC should be started if evaluation delay is greater than 24 hours.[27] As described previously, heparin should be adjusted to the goal activated partial thromboplastin time (aPTT), and anti–factor Xa levels should be checked if the patient requires large doses of UFH without achieving therapeutic aPTT. Treatment duration with anticoagulation is often a minimum of 3 months ranging to indefinite depending on the risk factors. Patients who have had PE are at high risk of recurrence, especially those with hypercoagulable states such as malignancy or inherited thrombophilic disorders such as protein C and S deficiency. Traditionally, patients with VTE have been transitioned to vitamin K antagonists, but newer anticoagulants, such as direct thrombin inhibitors and factor Xa inhibitors, are currently under investigation for use in long-term anticoagulation. The safety of these agents in the immediate postoperative period is unclear. The advantage of these agents includes a stable dosing regimen with reliable anticoagulation.

Patients who cannot undergo anticoagulation (such as those with intracranial bleeding) commonly have an IVC filter placed as soon as possible to prevent further embolization. Again, although this approach is logical, IVC filters have not been shown to increase overall survival.[29]

After the success of thrombolytics in the management of acute myocardial infarction, thrombolysis has been proposed as therapy for massive PE. Commonly used thrombolytic agents include tissue plasminogen activator, streptokinase, and urokinase. Alternative thrombolytic agents include lanoteplase, tenecteplase, and reteplase. These agents all convert plasminogen to plasmin, which in turn breaks down fibrin and promotes clot lysis. A recent meta-analysis comprising 16 randomized trials including 2115 patients reported a lower mortality in patients treated with thrombolytics (2.2% vs 3.9%).[30] Unfortunately, major bleeding rates (9.2% vs 3.4%) and intracranial hemorrhage (1.5% vs 0.2%) were significantly higher in patients receiving thrombolytic therapy when compared with TAC. Unfortunately, this meta-analysis pooled trials with different thrombolytic agents and dosing regimens, making it difficult to conclude which agent or dose should be used. Almost half of the patients in the meta-analysis came from a large multicenter trial (PEITHO [Pulmonary Embolism Thrombolysis]) comparing thrombolytics and heparin with placebo and heparin for intermediate-risk PE in normotensive patients with evidence of RV dysfunction. Despite a reduction in 7-day mortality in the thrombolytics group, the difference in 30-day mortality did not reach statistical significance.[31] Furthermore, the incidence of intracranial and major hemorrhage (11.5% vs 2.4%) was significantly higher in patients receiving thrombolysis. Until further evidence emerges, thrombolytics should be reserved for hemodynamically unstable patients who will not tolerate thrombectomy. Moreover, thrombolysis cannot be recommended for patients with recent major surgery, intracranial lesions, or traumatic injury. Relative contraindications include recent major bleeding, pregnancy, and uncontrolled hypertension.[27]

Pulmonary embolectomy has been performed in patients with massive PE, in those who are hemodynamically unstable despite heparin and fluid resuscitation, and in poor candidates for thrombolysis. Patients with life-threatening PEs may be placed on extracorporeal membrane oxygenation for stabilization and taken to the operating room for open thrombus extraction. No prospective clinical trials have evaluated outcomes from surgical embolectomy. All available data consist of case report and case series. The largest series of pulmonary embolectomies at one institution was reported by Meyer and colleagues in Paris in 1991.[32] During a 20-year period from 1968 to 1998, 96 (3%) of 3000 patients with confirmed PE underwent pulmonary embolectomy under cardiopulmonary bypass. The overall hospital mortality rate was 37.5%. A recent series comparing surgical thrombectomy to thrombolytics reported an early mortality rate of 3.6% in 28 surgical patients, but patients undergoing surgical embolectomy after failed thrombolysis had a mortality rate of 27%. In general, embolectomy is considered a therapy of last resort and should not be considered for most patients with PE.

Several catheter-based embolectomy techniques are available and can be categorized as thrombus fragmentation with pigtail or balloon catheter, rheolytic embolectomy with a hydrodynamic catheter, suction embolectomy with an aspiration catheter, and rotational thrombectomy. None of these techniques have been compared in randomized controlled trials (RCTs) to surgical thrombectomy or thrombolytics. Catheter-based embolectomy should be considered in patients failing thrombolysis as an alternative to surgical thrombectomy as dictated by experience and available expertise.

ACUTE RIGHT VENTRICULAR DYSFUNCTION MANAGEMENT

RV systolic function is determined by contractility, afterload, preload, rhythm, synchrony of ventricular contraction, and ventricular interdependence in the setting of acute pressure and volume overload. Acute dilation of the RV shifts the interventricular septum toward the left, alters LV geometry and function, and contributes to low cardiac output state.

Volume loading should be carefully performed. The absence of hemodynamic improvement with an initial fluid challenge suggests ventricular interdependence physiology. Logic would mandate cessation of fluid administration. Bedside echocardiography may be indicated in this case. Aggressive treatment of arrhythmias, atrioventricular dyssynchrony, and high-degree atrioventricular block in the acutely dilated RV are required to prevent further decomposition.

Every effort should be made to avoid hypotension, which may lead to a vicious cycle of RV subendocardial ischemia and further hypotension.[33] This may require the use of multiple vasogenic amine or phosphodiesterase inhibitor infusions. There are no data to support the use of any one medication or specific combinations.

The RV is much more sensitive to increased afterload than the LV. This may make pulmonary vascular dilators useful and may limit the value of agents that constrict.

Inhaled pulmonary vasodilators, inhaled nitric oxide, inhaled prostacyclin, iloprost, and milrinone may help to decrease pulmonary vascular resistance and improve RV function. Echocardiography is helpful in the diagnosis and management of acute RV dysfunction. In patients in low-flow states, the absence of echocardiographic evidence of pressure-overloaded RV most likely eliminates PE as a cause. Conversely, severe hypokinesis of the RV mid-free wall, with preserved contraction of the apical segment (McConnell sign), may be specific for PE.[34] RV dilation with tricuspid regurgitation and septal shift suggest volume-pressure overload, and further volume loading should be avoided.

PROPHYLAXIS

Data clearly indicate that critically ill patients are at high risk for developing DVTs,[35] and the consequences of a PE in patients with cerebrovascular compromise are severe.[36] Therefore prophylaxis is important, especially given that prevention is usually effective, as documented by nine placebo-controlled RCTs and several meta-analyses.[37-47] It is less clear how prophylaxis should be provided. A comparison of UFH (5000 IU twice daily) to LMWH (dalteparin, 5000 IU once per day and a second placebo injection to ensure parallel-group equivalence) was conducted by the Canadian Critical Care Trials Group.[48] The study did not demonstrate a statistically significant difference in asymptomatic DVTs between the two groups (hazard ratio, 0.92; 95% confidence interval [CI], 0.68 to 1.23; $P=0.57$), but LMWH was more effective in preventing PE (hazard ratio, 0.51; 95% CI, 0.30 to 0.88; $P=0.01$). Unfortunately, other LMWHs and the use of UFH 3 times daily were not assessed. Likewise, a meta-analysis of acutely ill, general medical patients comparing UFH twice and thrice daily demonstrated that the latter regimen was more effective at preventing VTE, but twice-daily dosing produced less bleeding.[49] Thus, given that there are no data comparing LMWH to thrice-daily UFH, LMWH (dalteparin) would seem to be the prophylactic regimen of choice. When anticoagulation is contraindicated, mechanical methods such as intermittent compression devices and graduated compression stockings may be used.[50-52] The Cochrane library used meta-analysis to assess 11 studies in patients who were not critically ill. The analysis included six RCTs and concluded that combining pharmacologic and mechanical prophylaxis provided the most effective prophylaxis.[53] LMWH is preferred over UFH.[48] These recommendations are consistent with those developed by the American College of Chest Physicians.[54] Finally, a study by the Canadian Critical Care Trials Group indicates that, in patients with renal impairment, dalteparin, which has minimal accumulation, should be used.[55]

AUTHORS' RECOMMENDATIONS

- VTE is a common problem in the ICU. PE is the extreme end of the disease.
- PE signs and symptoms are neither sensitive nor specific. Therefore, PE should be considered in any ICU patient with acute pulmonary or cardiovascular dysfunction.
- The diagnostic strategy and initial management is based on hemodynamic instability. The main therapeutic goal for the hemodynamically unstable patient is restoration of flow through the pulmonary artery. Hypotension should be aggressively treated with careful volume loading and vasopressors.
- Perfusion lung scanning and CT pulmonary angiography are the modalities most often used to diagnose PE.
- Anticoagulation should be initiated immediately in any patient with a confirmed PE or high clinical suspicion. Anticoagulation should be initiated early in patients with low to moderate suspicion if diagnostic workup is delayed.
- The use of thrombolysis in ICU patients should be reserved for hemodynamically unstable patients unresponsive to pharmacologic support. Unstable patients with contraindications to thrombolysis should be considered for surgical or catheter-based thrombectomy.
- Extracorporeal membrane oxygenation should be considered as a bridge to treatment in severely unstable patients.
- Prophylaxis with LMWH should be instituted in all critically ill patients without specific contraindications.

REFERENCES

1. Wiener RS, Schwartz LM, Woloshin S. Time trends in pulmonary embolism in the United States: evidence of overdiagnosis. *Arch Intern Med.* 2011;171:831–837.
2. Horlander KT, Mannino DM, Leeper KV. Pulmonary embolism mortality in the United States, 1979-1998: an analysis using multiple-cause mortality data. *Arch Intern Med.* 2003;163:1711–1717.
3. Goldhaber SZ, Visani L, De Rosa M. Acute pulmonary embolism: clinical outcomes in the International Cooperative Pulmonary Embolism Registry (ICOPER). *Lancet.* 1999;353:1386–1389.
4. Dalen JE. Pulmonary embolism: what have we learned since Virchow? Natural history, pathophysiology, and diagnosis. *Chest.* 2002;122:1440–1456.
5. Kearon C. Natural history of venous thromboembolism. *Circulation.* 2003;107:I22–I30.
6. Kakkar VV, Howe CT, Flanc C, Clarke MB. Natural history of postoperative deep-vein thrombosis. *Lancet.* 1969;2:230–232.
7. McIntyre KM, Sasahara AA. The hemodynamic response to pulmonary embolism in patients without prior cardiopulmonary disease. *Am J Cardiol.* 1971;28:288–294.
8. Wiedemann HP, Matthay RA. Acute right heart failure. *Crit Care Clin.* 1985;1:631–661.
9. Miniati M, Prediletto R, Formichi B, et al. Accuracy of clinical assessment in the diagnosis of pulmonary embolism. *Am J Respir Crit Care Med.* 1999;159:864–871.
10. Wells PS, Ginsberg JS, Anderson DR, et al. Use of a clinical model for safe management of patients with suspected pulmonary embolism. *Ann Intern Med.* 1998;129:997–1005.
11. Stein PD, Terrin ML, Hales CA, et al. Clinical, laboratory, roentgenographic, and electrocardiographic findings in patients with acute pulmonary embolism and no pre-existing cardiac or pulmonary disease. *Chest.* 1991;100:598–603.
12. Elliott CG, Goldhaber SZ, Visani L, DeRosa M. Chest radiographs in acute pulmonary embolism. Results from the International Cooperative Pulmonary Embolism Registry. *Chest.* 2000;118:33–38.
13. Kasper W, Konstantinides S, Geibel A, et al. Management strategies and determinants of outcome in acute major pulmonary embolism: results of a multicenter registry. *J Am Coll Cardiol.* 1997;30:1165–1171.
14. Lucassen W, Geersing GJ, Erkens PM, et al. Clinical decision rules for excluding pulmonary embolism: a meta-analysis. *Ann Intern Med.* 2011;155:448–460.
15. Rodger MA, Carrier M, Jones GN, et al. Diagnostic value of arterial blood gas measurement in suspected pulmonary embolism. *Am J Respir Crit Care Med.* 2000;162:2105–2108.
16. Bruinstroop E, van de Ree MA, Huisman MV. The use of D-dimer in specific clinical conditions: a narrative review. *Euro J Intern Med.* 2009;20:441–446.
17. Stein PD, Fowler SE, Goodman LR, et al. Multidetector computed tomography for acute pulmonary embolism. *N Engl J Med.* 2006;354:2317–2327.
18. Stein PD, Woodard PK, Weg JG, et al. Diagnostic pathways in acute pulmonary embolism: recommendations of the PIOPED II investigators. *Am J Med.* 2006;119:1048–1055.
19. Klok FA, Mos IC, Huisman MV. Brain-type natriuretic peptide levels in the prediction of adverse outcome in patients with pulmonary embolism: a systematic review and meta-analysis. *Am J Respir Crit Care Med.* 2008;178:425–430.
20. PIOPED Investigators. Value of the ventilation/perfusion scan in acute pulmonary embolism. Results of the prospective investigation of pulmonary embolism diagnosis (PIOPED). *JAMA.* 1990;263:2753–2759.
21. Coche E, Verschuren F, Keyeux A, et al. Diagnosis of acute pulmonary embolism in outpatients: comparison of thin-collimation multi-detector row spiral CT and planar ventilation-perfusion scintigraphy. *Radiology.* 2003;229:757–765.
22. Winer-Muram HT, Rydberg J, Johnson MS, et al. Suspected acute pulmonary embolism: evaluation with multi-detector row CT versus digital subtraction pulmonary arteriography. *Radiology.* 2004;233:806–815.
23. Grifoni S, Olivotto I, Cecchini P, et al. Short-term clinical outcome of patients with acute pulmonary embolism, normal blood pressure, and echocardiographic right ventricular dysfunction. *Circulation.* 2000;101:2817–2822.
24. ten Wolde M, Sohne M, Quak E, Mac Gillavry MR, Buller HR. Prognostic value of echocardiographically assessed right ventricular dysfunction in patients with pulmonary embolism. *Arch Intern Med.* 2004;164:1685–1689.
25. Kucher N, Rossi E, De Rosa M, Goldhaber SZ. Prognostic role of echocardiography among patients with acute pulmonary embolism and a systolic arterial pressure of 90 mm Hg or higher. *Arch Intern Med.* 2005;165:1777–1781.
26. Hills NH, Pflug JJ, Jeyasingh K, Boardman L, Calnan JS. Prevention of deep vein thrombosis by intermittent pneumatic compression of calf. *Brit Med J.* 1972;1:131–135.

27. Kearon C, Akl EA, Comerota AJ, American College of Chest P, et al. Antithrombotic therapy for VTE disease: Antithrombotic Therapy and Prevention of Thrombosis, 9th ed: American College of Chest Physicians Evidence-Based Clinical Practice Guidelines. *Chest.* 2012;141:e419S–e494S.

28. Dolovich LR, Ginsberg JS, Douketis JD, Holbrook AM, Cheah G. A meta-analysis comparing low-molecular-weight heparins with unfractionated heparin in the treatment of venous thromboembolism: examining some unanswered questions regarding location of treatment, product type, and dosing frequency. *Arch Intern Med.* 2000;160:181–188.

29. Decousus H, Leizorovicz A, Parent F, et al. A clinical trial of vena caval filters in the prevention of pulmonary embolism in patients with proximal deep-vein thrombosis. Prevention du Risque d'Embolie Pulmonaire par Interruption Cave Study Group. *N Engl J Med.* 1998;338:409–415.

30. Chatterjee S, Chakraborty A, Weinberg I, et al. Thrombolysis for pulmonary embolism and risk of all-cause mortality, major bleeding, and intracranial hemorrhage: a meta-analysis. *JAMA.* 2014;311:2414–2421.

31. Meyer G, Vicaut E, Danays T, et al. Fibrinolysis for patients with intermediate-risk pulmonary embolism. *N Engl J Med.* 2014;370:1402–1411.

32. Meyer G, Tamisier D, Sors H, et al. Pulmonary embolectomy: a 20-year experience at one center. *Ann Thorac Surg.* 1991;51:232–236.

33. Kucher N, Goldhaber SZ. Management of massive pulmonary embolism. *Circulation.* 2005;112:e28–32.

34. McConnell MV, Solomon SD, Rayan ME, Come PC, Goldhaber SZ, Lee RT. Regional right ventricular dysfunction detected by echocardiography in acute pulmonary embolism. *Am J Cardiol.* 1996;78:469–473.

35. Cade JF. High risk of the critically ill for venous thromboembolism. *Crit Care Med.* 1982;10:448–450.

36. Dellinger RP, Levy MM, Rhodes A, et al. Surviving Sepsis Campaign Guidelines Committee including the Pediatric S. Surviving sepsis campaign: international guidelines for management of severe sepsis and septic shock: 2012. *Crit Care Med.* 2013;41:580–637.

37. Halkin H, Goldberg J, Modan M, et al. Reduction of mortality in general medical in-patients by low-dose heparin prophylaxis. *Ann Intern Med.* 1982;96:561–565.

38. Pingleton SK, Bone RC, Pingleton WW, et al. Prevention of pulmonary emboli in a respiratory intensive care unit: efficacy of low-dose heparin. *Chest.* 1981;79:647–650.

39. Belch JJ, Lowe GD, Ward AG, et al. Prevention of deep vein thrombosis in medical patients by low-dose heparin. *Scott Med J.* 1981;26:115–117.

40. Gärdlund B. Randomised, controlled trial of low-dose heparin for prevention of fatal pulmonary embolism in patients with infectious diseases. The Heparin Prophylaxis Study Group. *Lancet.* 1996;347:1357–1361.

41. Samama MM, Cohen AT, Darmon JY, et al. A comparison of enoxaparin with placebo for the prevention of venous thromboembolism in acutely ill medical patients. Prophylaxis in Medical Patients with Enoxaparin Study Group. *N Engl J Med.* 1999;341:793–800.

42. Dahan R, Houlbert D, Caulin C, et al. Prevention of deep vein thrombosis in elderly medical in-patients by a low molecular weight heparin: a randomized double-blind trial. *Haemostasis.* 1986;16:159–164.

43. Hirsh DR, Ingenito EP, Goldhaber SZ. Prevalence of deep venous thrombosis among patients in medical intensive care. *JAMA.* 1995;274:335–337.

44. Fraisse F, Holzapfel L, Couland JM, et al. Nadroparin in the prevention of deep vein thrombosis in acute decompensated COPD. The Association of Non-University Affiliated Intensive Care Specialist Physicians of France. *Am J Respir Crit Care Med.* 2000;161 (4 Pt 1):1109–1114.

45. Kupfer Y, Anwar J, Seneviratne C, et al. Prophylaxis with subcutaneous heparin significantly reduces the incidence of deep venous thrombophlebitis in the critically ill. *Abstr. Am J Crit Care Med.* 1999;159(suppl):A519.

46. Geerts W, Cook D, Selby R, et al. Venous thromboembolism and its prevention in critical care. *J Crit Care.* 2002;17:95–104.

47. Attia J, Ray JG, Cook DJ, et al. Deep vein thrombosis and its prevention in critically ill adults. *Arch Intern Med.* 2001;161:1268–1279.

48. Protect Investigatiors for the Canadian Crtical Care Trials Group and the Australian and New Zealand Intensive Care Society Clinical Trials Group, Cook D, Meade M, Guyatt G, et al. Dalteparin versus unfractionated heparin in critically ill patients. *N Engl J Med.* 2011;364:1305–1314.

49. King CS, Holley AB, Jackson JL, et al. Twice vs three times daily heparin dosing for thromboembolism prophylaxis in the general medical population: a meta analysis. *Chest.* 2007;131:507–516.

50. Vanek VW. Meta-analysis of effectiveness of intermittent pneumatic compression devices with a comparison of thigh-high to knee-high sleeves. *Am Surg.* 1998;64:1050–1058.

51. Turpie AG, Hirsh J, Gent M, et al. Prevention of deep vein thrombosis in potential neurosurgical patients. A randomized trial comparing graduated compression stockings alone or graduated compression stockings plus intermittent pneumatic compression with control. *Arch Intern Med.* 1989;149:679–681.

52. Agu O, Hamilton G, Baker D. Graduated compression stockings in the prevention of venous thromboembolism. *Br J Surg.* 1999;86:992–1004.

53. Kakkos SK, Caprini JA, Geroulakos G, et al. Combined intermittent pneumatic leg compression and pharmacological prophylaxis for prevention of venous thromboembolism in high-risk patients. *Cochrane Database Syst Rev.* 2008;4:CD005258.

54. Guyatt GH, Akl EA, Crowther M, et al. Executive summary: antithrombotic therapy and prevention of thrombosis, 9th ed: American College of Chest Physicians Evidence-Based Clinical Practice Guidelines. *Chest.* 2012;141(suppl 2):7S–47S.

55. Douketis J, Cook D, Meade M, Canadian Critical Care Trials G, et al. Prophylaxis against deep vein thrombosis in critically ill patients with severe renal insufficiency with the low-molecular-weight heparin dalteparin: an assessment of safety and pharmacodynamics: the DIRECT study. *Arch Intern Med.* 2008;168:1805–1812.

27 Should Exacerbations of COPD Be Managed in the Intensive Care Unit?

Anthony O'Regan, Imran J. Meurling

CHRONIC OBSTRUCTIVE PULMONARY DISEASE PREVALENCE

It is estimated that 80 million people worldwide and up to 10% of the U.S. population have chronic obstructive pulmonary disease (COPD) (World Health Organization [WHO][1]). It is the fifth leading cause of death and chronic morbidity in the United States and accounted for 5% of total deaths worldwide in 2005 (WHO). Prevalence and mortality are increasing and are likely to continue to do so because of continued high smoking prevalence. Significantly, COPD is the only leading cause of death that is rising, and it is predicted to be the third leading cause of mortality by 2030.

Acute episodes of respiratory failure in patients with COPD are estimated to account for between 5% and 10% of acute emergency hospital admissions. Failure of first-line medical treatment is a common source of intensive care unit (ICU) referrals, accounting for 2% to 3% of non-surgical ICU admissions.[2] In a cohort of 1016 patients who were hospitalized for acute exacerbations, half of whom required intensive care, the in-hospital mortality was 11%.[3] The 6-month and 1-year mortality were 33% and 43%, respectively. Those who survived the first hospitalization had a 50% rate of rehospitalization within 6 months after discharge.

RESPIRATORY FAILURE

The pathophysiology of acute respiratory failure in COPD is incompletely understood, but it may be precipitated by any condition that increases the work of breathing or, less commonly, decreases the respiratory drive. Respiratory failure may be predominantly hypoxic (type 1) or hypercapnic (type 2). The mechanism of hypercapnea in COPD is not clear, but it is no longer thought to reflect problems with respiratory drive as suggested by the concept of "pink puffer/blue bloaters." Gas exchange abnormalities appear to predominantly reflect ventilation-perfusion mismatching due to airflow limitation, and progressive respiratory failure reflects a combination of severe airflow obstruction,

hyperinflation, and respiratory muscle fatigue. Regardless of the cause, hypercapnea and the need to assist ventilation identify patients with high initial (up to 27%) and 12-month mortality (up to 50%).[4]

Clinical Precipitants of Respiratory Failure

It has been shown that viral and bacterial infections account for between 50% and 70% of acute exacerbations and by inference a large proportion of cases of acute respiratory failure in COPD.[5,6] Numerous viral and bacterial agents have been implicated, but rhinoviruses, respiratory syncytial virus, *Haemophilus influenzae*, *Moraxella catarrhalis*, and *Streptococcus pneumoniae* are the frequent pathogens.[7-9] *Pseudomonas aeruginosa*, Enterobacteriaceae spp., and *Stenotrophomonas* spp. are also isolated, particularly from patients with severe COPD and those requiring mechanical ventilation.[10] Therefore, although still uncommon, clinicians should consider more resistant gram-negative organisms in patients requiring ICU care with COPD exacerbations. The prevalence of atypical organisms such as *Mycoplasma* and *Chlamydia* is less well defined.

Up to 10% of COPD flares are caused by environmental pollution and airway irritants such as smoke or fumes. For the remainder of cases, the etiology is not always clear. Medical conditions can mimic or cause COPD exacerbations, and patients with COPD have higher rates of comorbid illnesses, in part reflecting exposure to cigarette smoke. This is supported by results from the Toward a Revolution in COPD Health (TORCH) trial[11]; only 35% of deaths were adjudicated as due to pulmonary causes, with cardiovascular disease being the other major cause of death at 27% and cancer third at 21%.

Important differential diagnoses for patients with COPD who have increased respiratory symptoms and decreased lung function include the following:

- *Cardiovascular disease*: myocardial ischemia, heart failure, pulmonary embolism
- *Central nervous system depression*: head trauma or injudicious use of sedatives, opioids, tranquilizers, or oxygen (O_2) therapy

- *Endocrine and metabolic disorders*: myxedema or metabolic alkalosis
- *Thoracic abnormalities*: chest trauma, pneumothorax, or thoracic or abdominal surgery

Pulmonary embolism can be an occult cause of acute respiratory failure in COPD. A prospective cohort study in 2006 reported that 22% of patients with a severe COPD exacerbation of unknown etiology had coexisting pulmonary emboli.[12] A subsequent study of all patients in the emergency department with COPD exacerbations found the overall prevalence of clinically unsuspected pulmonary embolism to be relatively low at 1.3%,[13] suggesting that systematic examination for those with uncomplicated presentations is probably not useful but that a high index of suspicion is warranted in those without other apparent precipitants.

Prognostic Indicators in Patients with Acute Exacerbations of COPD

There are several potential prognostic indicators that should be considered when admitting a patient to the ICU with an acute exacerbation of COPD. The DECAF score has been developed to predict mortality. It is based on the five strongest predictors of mortality in a study from the United Kingdom in 2012: Dyspnea, Eosinophilia, Consolidation, Acidemia, and Atrial Fibrillation.[14] As a combined score, this has been shown to be a stronger predictor of mortality than the CURB-65 (Confusion of new onset, blood Urea nitrogen, Respiratory rate, Blood pressure, age 65 or older) score in patients with COPD and pneumonia, and as such it is a useful triage tool. Other factors commonly cited in literature would include a patient's age, the patient's forced expiratory volume in 1 second (FEV_1), the degree of hypoxemia or hypercapnea, the presence of other comorbidities such as cardiovascular disease, or a history of prior or frequent exacerbations. Frequent exacerbations accelerate disease progression and mortality, leading to a faster decline in lung function and quality of life.[15] The 2-year mortality after a COPD exacerbation is approximately 50%. Finally, a patient who has failed adequate treatment for a COPD exacerbation over 3 to 5 days ("late failure") has a very poor prognosis in the setting of escalation to mechanical ventilation.

Patients with chronic hypercapneic respiratory failure are particularly high risk, and, as a result, noninvasive ventilation (NIV) at home is being increasingly used. Base excess, which represents a metabolic response to chronic hypercapnea (increased bicarbonate, reduced chloride) was found to be one of the strongest prognostic indicators in this setting, as reported in a study published in 2007 by Budweiser and colleagues.[16] They also found that in a cohort of COPD patients sent home from the hospital and undergoing NIV, the 5-year survival rate was 26.4%, with deaths predominantly from respiratory causes (73.8%).

MANAGEMENT OF COPD

The treatment guidelines for management of acute exacerbations of COPD requiring admission to the ICU are broadly similar to those principles used in patients without respiratory failure, although significantly more attention must be paid to safe and appropriate gas exchange. Addressing the issue of poor respiratory mechanics due to dynamic hyperinflation, loss of alveolar volume, and impaired ventilation is fundamental to COPD management. Clinically compensated chronic respiratory failure can rapidly become decompensated respiratory failure because of poor chest wall mechanics, suboptimal respiratory muscle function, malnutrition, obesity, and myopathy. Reducing the work of breathing with noninvasive positive pressure ventilation (NIPPV) to improve oxygenation, improve rest muscles, and manage hyperinflation has become key in the management of COPD.

Indications for referral to ICU include dyspnea that does not respond to emergency treatment; changes in mental status (e.g., confusion, drowsiness, or coma); persistent or worsening hypoxemia; and/or severe or worsening hypercapnia, acidosis, or hemodynamic instability.[1]

Corticosteroids

Several randomized controlled trials have shown that for patients hospitalized with acute exacerbations of COPD, systemic corticosteroids administered for up to 2 weeks are helpful.[17] Treatment of an exacerbation of COPD with oral or parenteral corticosteroids increases the rate of improvement in lung function and dyspnea over the first 72 hours.[18] Corticosteroids also reduce the duration of hospital stay.[19] The optimal dose and need for tapering, route of administration, and length of treatment are uncertain.

Most recent guidelines suggest that intravenous corticosteroids should be given to patients who have a severe exacerbation, including all those requiring ICU admission or those who may have impaired absorption due to decreased splanchnic perfusion (e.g., patients in shock or congestive heart failure). Nonetheless, if tolerated, oral corticosteroid administration is equally effective as intravenous administration.[20] There appears to be no benefit to prolonged treatment beyond 2 weeks.[21] There is a significant side effect profile, the most common being hyperglycemia occurring in approximately 15%.[21] Studies have shown that nebulized steroid therapy is superior to placebo but not better than parenteral therapy.[22]

Bronchodilators

Inhaled short-acting β-adrenergic agonists are the mainstay of therapy for an acute exacerbation of COPD because of their rapid onset of action and efficacy in producing bronchodilation. Several randomized control trials have consistently demonstrated their efficacy.[17] Parenteral or subcutaneous injection of short-acting β-adrenergic agonists is reserved for situations in which inhaled administration is not possible. Parenteral use of these agents results in greater inotropic and chronotropic effects, which may cause arrhythmias or myocardial ischemia in susceptible individuals and is not generally recommended. These medications may be administered with a nebulizer or a metered dose inhaler with a spacer device; however, despite evidence that neither method has been shown to be superior, physicians tend to favor the nebulized route because of the ease of administration. Patients should revert to appropriate inhaled preparations as soon as possible.

Anticholinergic bronchodilators, such as ipratropium, are equally efficacious,[23] and some studies have found that combination therapy with inhaled beta agonists provides better bronchodilation than either alone.[24] The array of inhalers available for use in stable COPD patients is widening, and newer combination inhalers include a long-acting beta agonist with a long-acting anticholinergic, such as indacaterol and glycopyrronium. These dual bronchodilators have been shown to improve symptoms and lung function in COPD patients in which single bronchodilators may be insufficient,[25] but there is no proven efficacy for their use in acute exacerbations.

Methylxanthines have a long history in the treatment of COPD; however, despite widespread clinical use, their role in the acute setting is controversial. Current guidelines based on a meta-analysis of four randomized control trials recommend that theophylline should not be used in the acute setting because efficacy beyond that induced by an inhaled bronchodilator and glucocorticoid therapy has not been demonstrated. In addition to a lack of efficacy, methylxanthines caused significantly more nausea and vomiting than placebo and trended toward more frequent tremors, palpitations, and arrhythmias.[26]

Antibiotics

In patients with severe exacerbations requiring mechanical ventilation, antibiotic therapy is beneficial and has been shown to significantly decrease mortality (4% vs. 22%), the need for additional courses of antibiotics, the duration of mechanical ventilation, and the duration of hospital stay.[27] This does not suggest that bacterial etiology is actually present, and the clinical decision to withhold antibiotics is difficult in hospitalized patients. Early investigations using inflammatory markers, such as procalcitonin, to distinguish bacterial infections from other causes are encouraging.[8]

Current guidelines suggest use of antimicrobials with a spectrum of activity to cover β-lactamase–producing organisms. Although choice is somewhat dependent on the local streptococcal resistance patterns, amoxicillin–clavulanic acid, second-generation cephalosporin, or macrolides are all acceptable. Three to seven days of treatment is recommended (*Global Initiative for Chronic Obstructive Lung Disease* [GOLD]).[27] Wider spectrum antibiotics such as fluoroquinolones or β-lactam with antipseudomonal activity should be used in those at risk of resistant gram-negative infections such as *Pseudomonas* (e.g., recent hospitalization, previous colonization, previous severe exacerbation, or >4 exacerbations per year).

OXYGEN THERAPY

Adequate oxygenation can be achieved in most patients with acute exacerbations of COPD. Ventilation-perfusion mismatch is usually improved by 24% to 28% oxygen. There appears to be a tendency to develop CO_2 retention at a fraction of inspired oxygen (FIO_2) greater than 30%. The mechanism is more likely to reflect a combination of ventilation-perfusion mismatching and the Haldane effect rather than any effect on hypoxic drive for ventilation. Nevertheless, controlled oxygen therapy is recommended.

In critical care, the use of high-flow facemasks or nasal devices provides better titration of oxygen therapy compared with simple facemasks or nasal cannulae, venture masks, or other variable performance devices.

ASSISTED VENTILATION

Recognition of the need for assisted ventilation is often a clinical judgment as patients fail to improve on initial treatment. NIV is indicated after initial treatment if the pH remains less than 7.32. Studies have shown that pH and degree of hypercapnia are better predictors of need for mechanical ventilation than hypoxia.[28] The following are several absolute and relative contraindications to NIPPV:

- Respiratory arrest
- Impaired level of consciousness
- Cardiovascular collapse
- Profound hypoxemia (acute respiratory distress syndrome)
- Vomiting or very high aspiration risk due to excessive secretions
- Uncooperative patient
- Extreme obesity
- Recent facial surgery
- Burns

Several randomized control trials have validated the use of NIV in the setting of acute hypercapnic respiratory failure in COPD[29]; indeed, several studies have demonstrated the superiority of NIV over tracheal intubation and mechanical ventilation. NIV reduces intubation by up to 42%[10] and appears to reduce nosocomial complications and mortality.[30,31] Some studies have also found that patients with COPD who were randomly assigned to NIV had a shorter stay in the ICU. Use of NIV has certainly improved care for many patients with COPD and allowed some to undergo a more intense level of treatment than perhaps may have been previously available to them.

NIV on respiratory care wards and intermediate care settings is highly efficacious, with a reported failure rate of 5% to 20%. However, when patients are admitted to intensive care, presumably in a worse clinical condition, the failure rate is up to 60%.[32,33] This is particularly problematic in patients who present late with advanced respiratory failure, and mortality is higher than in patients who receive NIV at an earlier stage.[3] There are a medley of reasons for failing NIV, which include patient intolerance, inadequate augmentation of tidal volume, and problems with triggering.

The response to NIV treatment needs to be closely monitored with arterial blood gases, respiratory rate, hemodynamics, and overall degree of respiratory distress. Those who respond within 1 to 4 hours are consistently shown to have better outcomes.[32] An initial reduction in respiratory rate is generally a good indicator of a positive response to NIV. Failure of NIV, contraindications, or imminent cardiorespiratory arrest should prompt endotracheal intubation and mechanical ventilation. This should ideally be performed in the controlled setting of an ICU because intubation can precipitate a cardiovascular collapse.[2]

Once intubation has been performed, hypoxemia can be corrected, usually with modest FIO_2. After this, respiratory acidosis is corrected slowly with low rates and tidal volumes guided by air pressures and the expiratory phase. This approach is to limit auto-positive end-expiratory pressure (auto-PEEP) from air trapping, which can result in significant hemodynamic compromise and can be difficult to detect.[34]

In the first 12 to 24 hours, paralysis may be required to prevent ventilator dyssynchrony, which can increase airway resistance and decrease alveolar ventilation. Airway resistance and hyperinflation can both contribute to a need for high inflation pressures to achieve tidal volume. High mean airway pressures may lead to several serious problems, including circulatory collapse, pneumothorax, or barotrauma. It is unclear whether pressure-controlled or pressure-limited ventilation is safer than volume control. Irrespective efforts should be made to minimize auto-PEEP and end inspiratory stretch.[34]

Weaning can pose problems in ventilated COPD patients, with 20% to 30% of those meeting the traditional extubation criteria failing a trial of weaning.[2] Failure to wean raises the risks of the complications associated with prolonged ventilation. There is some evidence that expiratory flow limitation may predict successful extubation.[35] Nava and colleagues randomly assigned patients with COPD who were intubated for 48 hours to extubation and NIV or to continued invasive ventilation and conventional liberation after an unsuccessful initial spontaneous breathing trial.[36] The study demonstrated improved outcomes as measured by the percentage of patients in whom assisted ventilation could be discontinued, the duration of assisted ventilation, survival, the length of stay in the ICU, and the incidence of ventilator-associated pneumonia. More recently, this was validated by Ornico et al.,[37] who showed a significant reduction of re-intubation rates and in-hospital mortality when nasal NIV was commenced after planned extubation as compared with continuous oxygen therapy. Risk factors for postextubation respiratory failure include an age older than 65, cardiac failure as a cause for respiratory distress, an APACHE (Acute Physiology and Chronic Health Evaluation) score of 12 or greater at the time of extubation, the diagnosis of an acute exacerbation of COPD, or the presence of chronic respiratory disease with more than 48 hours of mechanical ventilation and hypercapnea during a spontaneous breathing trial. If patients do have postextubation respiratory distress, then they should undergo reintubation because persisting with NIV in this setting may worsen outcomes.[38]

PROGNOSIS AND OUTCOMES

Despite reasonable survival to hospital discharge, the decision to admit to the ICU in advanced cases is difficult, and there is no consensus. One has to take into account expected prognosis and comorbidities and estimate likely quality of life assuming survival to hospital discharge. Factors affecting the decision to ventilate include cultural attitudes toward disability, the perceived effect of treatment, financial resources, the availability of ICU and long-term ventilator beds, local medical practice, and patient wishes.

Past perception has been that survival after ICU admission was poor, especially in those deemed to have severe or end-stage disease. However, short-term survival after invasive mechanical ventilation ranges from 63% to 86%, more than would be expected in unplanned medical admissions.[33,39] In addition, survival after mechanical ventilation has been shown to be better in the absence of a major precipitating cause for acute deterioration, perhaps because shorter periods of assisted ventilation are required and thus length of ICU stay and associated complications are lessened.[40]

However, a difficulty still remains in identifying those patients most likely to derive benefit from aggressive management. Long-term survival rates are not as encouraging as survival-to-discharge figures. Rates of 52%, 42%, and 37% at 1, 2, and 3 years, respectively, were reported in one U.K. study,[40] and similar numbers have been reported from other centers.

Poor prognostic indicators include the following:

- Increased age
- Presence of severe respiratory disease
- Increased length of stay in hospital before ICU admission
- Cardiopulmonary resuscitation within 24 hours before admission
- Intubation status in the first 24 hours in the CMP (Case Mix Programme) unit
- Low pH
- Low partial pressure of arterial oxygen/FIO_2 gradient
- Hypercapnea
- Low serum albumin
- Low body mass index
- Cardiovascular, neurologic, and renal organ failure

Although all of these factors have been associated with increased in-hospital mortality[4] (SUPPORT [Surfactant, Positive Pressure, and Oxygenation Randomized Trial]), there is currently no reliable or definitive method for identifying patients at high risk of inpatient or 6-month mortality. Therefore these parameters should not influence decisions about instituting, continuing, or withdrawing life-sustaining treatment.

A small 2001 study of 166 COPD patients requiring mechanical ventilation found that absence of comorbid condition more than halved the in-hospital mortality rate (28% vs. 12%).[33] A higher mortality among those patients who required more than 72 hours of mechanical ventilation (37% vs. 16%), those without previous episodes of mechanical ventilation (33% vs. 11%), and those with a failed extubation attempt (36% vs. 11%) was also noted. Further larger studies would be helpful to assist in decision making.

Although the previous material can guide us in treatment decisions, patient preference also represents an essential component of our assessment. A prospective cohort study performed in 92 ICUs and 3 respiratory high-dependency units in the United Kingdom examined outcomes in patients with COPD admitted to the ICU for decompensated type 2 respiratory failure, including survival and quality of life at 180 days.[41] Of the survivors, 73% considered their quality of life to be the same as or better than it had been in the stable period before they were admitted, and 96% would choose similar treatment again.

Taking all of this into account, current treatment guidelines suggest that failure of NIV in most cases should be followed by a short trial of mechanical ventilation. Early reevaluation is then recommended. Patient wishes play an important role in this decision, and advanced directives based on discussion, ideally occurring during a medically stable period, regarding risks and complications of invasive ventilation are advocated.

End-of-Life Decisions in Severe COPD

In the severe and end-stage COPD patient population, decisions regarding end-of-life care and palliation should be addressed. Factors that may lead to an end-of-life discussion include the following[42]:

- FEV$_1$ below 30% predicted
- Oxygen dependence
- Requirement of domiciliary NIPPV
- One or more hospital admissions in the past year with an acute exacerbation of COPD
- Weight loss or cachexia
- Decreased functional status/decreased independence
- Age older than 70 years
- Patients receiving maximal medical management

A retrospective study performed in the Mayo Clinic[43] involving 591 patients admitted to the ICU with an acute exacerbation of COPD found that the factors most associated with a poor 1-year mortality were age and length of hospital stay. These patients may benefit from early communication regarding end of life and palliation before their next hospital admission.

Because COPD is a chronic progressive disease, there is opportunity to have the discussion early, with the knowledge that in severe and end-stage COPD patients, they will likely require more aggressive care (e.g., ventilation), with a possibly fatal outcome in an unpredictably acute setting. Given the opportunity, the following three primary end-of-life topics can be discussed[44]:

- Their disease course and likely prognosis
- Establishment of a ceiling of care
- Symptom management and control

Knowing their own disease course allows patients to participate in their management strategy and provides context for the acute decisions made during an exacerbation. When discussed early in the course of the disease, it may improve compliance with therapy, and toward more end-stage disease it allows them to know what to expect and make informed end-of-life decisions, including establishing the ceiling of care and choosing to be admitted to intensive care for ventilation. In a French study regarding patients with COPD admitted to intensive care, only 56% of patients had discussed intensive care as a possibility with their physician.[45]

A ceiling of care can be established by considering the patients comorbidities and prognosis, but it is also important to consider the patients' quality of life, the functionality of activities of daily living, and their wishes with regard to their treatment. In particular, it should be established, if possible, whether the patient should undergo mechanical ventilation in an ICU or undergo a trial of NIV. The SUPPORT published in 2000 compared patients who had stage III and IV lung cancer with patients who had severe COPD and found that 60% of patients in each group wanted comfort-focused care.[46]

AUTHORS' RECOMMENDATIONS

- COPD accounts for a large proportion of medical ICU admissions; 25% of COPD patients will require a stay in an ICU at some stage in their disease. Half of those will not survive 1 year.
- Most acute exacerbations of COPD are associated with viral or bacterial infection.
- The DECAF score may be used to predict mortality.
- Oxygen therapy, corticosteroids, β-adrenergic agonists, and anticholinergic agents continue to be the mainstay of therapy. Methylxanthines are likely ineffective.
- NIV is effective and economical in moderate to severe cases and is associated with reduced mortality, reduced invasive ventilation, and nosocomial complications.
- In severe cases, intubation is necessary, and extreme care is required to control dyssynchrony, auto-PEEP, and end-inspiratory lung stretch.
- Weaning and liberation can be difficult. Extubation to NIV may shorten duration of ICU and hospital stay.
- Advanced age, low body weight, cardiovascular disease, and multiple previous ICU admissions predict poor outcomes in patients with COPD, although no specific scoring system exists. Advanced directives and treatment limitation planning should be undertaken.

REFERENCES

1. *Gold Report*. 2008. Available at: http://www.goldcopd.com.
2. Davidson AC. The pulmonary physician in critical care: the critical care management of acute respiratory failure from COPD. *Thorax*. 2002;57:1079–1084.
3. Chandra D, Stamm JA, Taylor B, et al. Outcomes of noninvasive ventilation for acute exacerbations of chronic obstructive pulmonary disease in the United States, 1998–2008. *Am J Respir Crit Care Med*. January 15, 2012;185(2):152–159.
4. Wildman MJ, Harrison DA, Brady AR, Rowan K. Case mix and outcomes for admissions to UK adult, general critical care units with chronic obstructive pulmonary disease: a secondary analysis of the ICNARC Case Mix Programme Database. *Crit Care*. 2005;9(suppl 3):S38–S48.
5. Sapey E, Stockley RA. COPD exacerbations. 2. Aetiology. *Thorax*. 2006;61:250–258.
6. Papi A, Bellettato CM, Braccioni F, et al. Infections and airway inflammation in chronic obstructive pulmonary disease severe exacerbations. *Am J Respir Crit Care Med*. 2006;173:1114–1121.
7. Seemungal T, Harper-Owen R, Bhowmik A, et al. Respiratory viruses, symptoms, and inflammatory markers in acute exacerbations and stable chronic obstructive pulmonary disease. *Am J Respir Crit Care Med*. 2001;164:1618–1623.
8. Nseir S, Cavestri B, Di Pompeo C, et al. Factors predicting bacterial involvement in severe acute exacerbations of chronic obstructive pulmonary disease. *Respiration*. 2008;76:253–260.
9. Monso E, Ruiz J, Rosell A, et al. Bacterial infection in chronic obstructive pulmonary disease: a study of stable and exacerbated outpatients using the protected specimen brush. *Am J Respir Crit Care Med*. 1995;152:1316.
10. Soler N, Torres A, Ewig S, et al. Bronchial microbial patterns in severe exacerbations of chronic obstructive pulmonary disease (COPD) requiring mechanical ventilation. *Am J Respir Crit Care Med*. 1998;157:1498–1505.
11. Calverley PMA, Anderson JA, Celli B, et al. Salmeterol and fluticasone propionate and survival in chronic obstructive pulmonary disease. *N Engl J Med*. 2007;356:775–789. for the TORCH Investigators.
12. Tillie-Leblond I, Marquette CH, Perez T, et al. Pulmonary embolism in patients with unexplained exacerbation of chronic obstructive pulmonary disease: prevalence and risk factors. *Ann Intern Med*. 2006;144:390–393.
13. Rutschmann OT, Cornuz J, Poletti PA, et al. Should pulmonary embolism be suspected in exacerbation of chronic obstructive pulmonary disease? *Thorax*. 2007;62:103–104.

14. Steer J1, Gibson J, Bourke SC. The DECAF Score: predicting hospital mortality in exacerbations of chronic obstructive pulmonary disease. *Thorax*. November 2012;67(11):970–976. http://dx.doi.org/10.1136/thoraxjnl-2012-202103.

15. Anzueto A. Impact of exacerbations on COPD. *Eur Respir Rev*. June 1. 2010;19(116):113–118.

16. Budweiser S, Jörres RA, Riedl T, et al. Predictors of survival in COPD patients with chronic hypercapnic respiratory failure receiving non-invasive home ventilation. *Chest*. June 2007;131(6):1650–1658.

17. Snow V, Lascher S, Mottur-Pilson C. Evidence base for management of acute exacerbations of chronic obstructive pulmonary disease. *Ann Intern Med*. 2001;134:595–599.

18. Wood-Baker RR, Gibson PG, Hannay M, et al. Systemic corticosteroids for acute exacerbations of chronic obstructive airway disease. *Cochrane Database Syst Rev*. 2005;1:CD001288.

19. Niewoehner DE, Erbland ML, Deupree RH, et al. Effect of systemic glucocorticoids on exacerbations of chronic obstructive pulmonary disease. Department of Veterans Affairs Cooperative Study Group *N Engl J Med*. 1999;340:1941–1947.

20. de Jong YP, Uil SM, Grotjohan HP, et al. Oral or IV prednisolone in the treatment of COPD exacerbations: a randomized, controlled, double-blind study. *Chest*. 2007;132:1741–1747.

21. Singh JM, Palda VA, Stanbrook MB, Chapman KR. Corticosteroid therapy for patients with acute exacerbation of chronic obstructive pulmonary disease: a systematic review. *Arch Intern Med*. 2002;162:2527–2536.

22. Maltais F, Ostinelli J, Borbeau J, et al. Comparison of nebulised budesonide and oral prednisolone with placebo in the treatment of acute exacerbation of COPD: a randomized control trial. *Am J Respir Crit Care Med*. 2002;165:698–703.

23. COMBIVENT Inhalation Aerosol Study Group. In chronic obstructive pulmonary disease, a combination of ipratropium and albuterol is more effective than either agent alone: an 85-day multicenter trial. *Chest*. 1994;105:1411–1419.

24. Karpel JP. Bronchodilator responses to anticholinergic and beta-adrenergic agents in acute and stable COPD. *Chest*. 1991;99:871–876.

25. Bateman E, Ferguson Gary T, Barnes N, et al. Benefits of dual bronchodilation with QVA149 once daily versus indacaterol, glycopyrronium, tiotropium and placebo in patients with COPD: the SHINE study. *Eur Respir J*. December 2013;42(6):1484–1494.

26. Barr RG, Rowe BH, Camargo Jr CA. Methylxanthines for exacerbations of chronic obstructive pulmonary disease: meta-analysis of randomized trials. *BMJ*. 2003;327:643.

27. Falagas ME, Avgeri SG, Matthaiou DK, et al. Short- versus long-duration antimicrobial treatment for exacerbations of chronic bronchitis: a meta-analysis. *J Antimicrob Chemother*. 2008;62:442–448.

28. Plant PK, Owen JL, Elliott MW. Early use of non-invasive ventilation for acute exacerbations of chronic obstructive pulmonary disease on general respiratory wards: a multicentre randomized controlled trial. *Lancet*. 2000;355:1931–1935.

29. Truwit JD, Bernard GR. Noninvasive ventilation: Don't push too hard. *N Engl J Med*. 2004;350:2512–2515.

30. Scala R, Nava S, Conti G, et al. Non invasive ventilation versus conventional ventilation to treat hypercapnic encephalopathy in COPD. *Intensive Care Med*. 2007;33:2101–2108.

31. Moretti M, Cilione C, Tampieri A, et al. Incidence and causes of non-invasive mechanical ventilation failure after initial success. *Thorax*. 2000;55:819–825.

32. Plant PK, Elliott MW. Chronic obstructive pulmonary disease. 9. Management of ventilatory failure in COPD [review]. *Thorax*. 2003;58:537–542.

33. Nevins ML, Epstein SK. Predictors of outcome for patients with COPD requiring invasive mechanical ventilation. *Chest*. 2001;119:1840–1849.

34. Feihl F, Perret C. Permissive hypercapnia. How permissive should we be? *Am J Respir Crit Care Med*. 1994;150:1722–1737.

35. Alvesi V. Time course of expiratory flow limitation in COPD patients during acute respiratory failure requiring mechanical ventilation. *Chest*. 2003;123:1625–1632.

36. Nava S, Ambrosino N, Clini E, et al. Noninvasive mechanical ventilation in the weaning of patients with respiratory failure due to chronic obstructive pulmonary disease. A randomized, controlled trial. *Ann Intern Med*. 1998;128:721–728.

37. Ornico SR, Lobo SM, Sanches HS, et al. *Crit Care*. March 4, 2013;17(2):R39.

38. Esteban A, Frutos-Vivar F, Ferguson ND, et al. Noninvasive positive-pressure ventilation for respiratory failure after extubation. *N Engl J Med*. June 10, 2004;350(24):2452–2460.

39. Hudson LD. Survival data in patients with acute or chronic lung disease requiring mechanical ventilation. *Am Rev Respir Dis*. 1989;140:519–524.

40. Breen D, Churches T, Hawker F, et al. Acute respiratory failure secondary to chronic obstructive pulmonary disease treated in the intensive care unit: a long term follow up study. *Thorax*. 2002;57:29–33.

41. Wildman MJ, Sanderson CF, Groves J, et al. Survival and quality of life for patients with COPD or asthma admitted to intensive care in a UK multicentre cohort: the COPD and Asthma Outcome Study (CAOS). *Thorax*. February 2009;64(2):128–132.

42. Patel K, Janssen DJA, Curtis JR. Advance care planning in COPD. *Respirology*. 2012;17:72–78. http://dx.doi.org/10.1111/j.1440-1843.2011.02087.x.

43. Batzlaff CM, Karpman C, Afessa B, Benzo RP. Predicting 1-year mortality rate for patients admitted with an acute exacerbation of chronic obstructive pulmonary disease to an intensive care unit: an opportunity for palliative care. *Mayo Clin Proc*. May 2014;89(5): 638–643. http://dx.doi.org/10.1016/j.mayocp.2013.12.004. Epub 2014 March 19.

44. Dean MM. End-of-life care for COPD patients. *Prim Care Respir J*. March 2008;17(1):46–50. http://dx.doi.org/10.3132/pcrj.2008.00007.

45. Schmidt M, Demoule A, Deslandes-Boutmy E, et al. Intensive care unit admission in chronic obstructive pulmonary disease: patient information and the physicians decision-making process. *Crit Care*. 2014;18:R115.

46. Claessens MT, Lynn J, Zhong Z, et al. Dying with lung cancer or chronic obstructive pulmonary disease: insights from SUPPORT. Study to understand prognoses and preferences for outcomes and risks of treatments. *J Am Geriatr Soc*. 2000;48:S146–S153.

ARDS

28 What Is the Clinical Definition of ARDS?

Jeremy R. Beitler, Andrés Esteban, José Angel Lorente, B. Taylor Thompson

Acute respiratory distress syndrome (ARDS) is an acute, diffuse, inflammatory injury to the alveolar epithelium and pulmonary vascular endothelium that leads to nonhydrostatic pulmonary edema and impaired pulmonary gas exchange.[1] ARDS is difficult to define clinically because it represents a constellation of individually nonspecific findings triggered by a wide range of precipitating insults to the lung.[2] Still, a reproducible definition of ARDS is essential to consistently identify patients with a similar phenotype for research and clinical care.[1]

In clinical trials and other studies, a homogeneous population sample minimizes pathophysiologic variability; this minimization is important because distinct subphenotypes may carry different prognoses and respond differently to therapies. It also allows for comparison of research findings and epidemiologic data across studies. For patient care, a standardized definition promotes evidence-based management and prognostication by allowing comparison of each patient to research study participants.

Although ARDS was first described by Ashbaugh et al. in 1967,[3] no consensus definition existed until the 1994 American-European Consensus Conference (AECC) on ARDS.[4] The updated consensus Berlin definition was put forth in 2012.[1] Although the Berlin definition performs better in several respects, recent evidence suggests that substantial biological, pathologic, and clinical heterogeneity remains within this broad definition of ARDS.

FIVE DECADES OF DEFINING ARDS

Recognizing ARDS as a Clinical Entity

Five decades ago, Ashbaugh and colleagues[3] first identified ARDS as a common lung injury response to various insults—multiple trauma, lung contusion, pancreatitis, toxic ingestion, and pneumonia—that did not respond to usual respiratory support. Their series of 12 patients established the salient features of ARDS that have served as the foundation for all subsequent definitions: the acute onset of hypoxemia and bilateral infiltrates on chest radiograph that are not entirely due to heart failure.

Decreased respiratory system compliance (C_{RS}) was common to all included patients. Postmortem histologic examination demonstrated intra-alveolar edema and hyaline membranes in most patients who died early in their course and diffuse interstitial inflammation and fibrosis in patients who died after a protracted course.

After the seminal article by Ashbaugh et al., ARDS gained widespread recognition as an important clinical entity. However, a specific consensus definition remained elusive. In 1988, Murray and colleagues[2] proposed perhaps the most widely recognized diagnostic criteria for ARDS before a consensus definition. Their Lung Injury Score awards points for severity of derangement in four clinical factors: hypoxemia (partial pressure of oxygen in arterial blood [Pao_2]/fraction of inspired oxygen [Fio_2]), chest radiographic opacities (number of quadrants), positive end-expiratory pressure (PEEP) level, and C_{RS}. A numeric cutoff was proposed to define ARDS. Importantly, Murray and colleagues also recommended expanding their score-based definition to describe the time course since ARDS onset (acute or chronic phase) and underlying risk factor(s) (e.g., aspiration, sepsis). Both additions informally addressed prognostic and treatment implications of different phases and causes of ARDS.[5]

Achieving Consensus on Defining ARDS

The 1994 AECC definition represented the first international consensus on how to define ARDS.[4] Under the auspices of the American Thoracic Society and the European Society of Intensive Care Medicine, an expert panel was convened to establish diagnostic criteria for ARDS with the primary stated intent of enhancing research coordination and collaboration to more efficiently advance therapeutic investigation.

The expert panel considered timing of onset, oxygenation, chest radiograph findings, and absence of hydrostatic pulmonary edema as the defining features of ARDS.[4] Specifically, they defined ARDS as the acute onset of impaired oxygenation with a Pao_2/Fio_2 of 200 mm Hg or less accompanied by bilateral infiltrates on frontal chest radiograph and a pulmonary artery wedge pressure (PAWP) of 18 mm Hg or less (if measured) or no clinical evidence of left atrial hypertension. The AECC separately defined acute lung injury (ALI) as having a Pao_2/Fio_2 of 300 mm Hg or less while meeting all other criteria for ARDS. That is, ALI represented a broader spectrum of lung injury that included ARDS on the severe end of the spectrum. The decision to distinguish ARDS as the severe form of ALI stemmed from concern that processes other than ARDS that are associated with impaired gas exchange were likelier to be included under a more liberal threshold.

In addition to the benefits of consensus per se, the AECC definition offered several strengths. The definition was applicable to the research, epidemiology, and individual patient care settings, aiding cross-study comparison and translation of study findings to clinical practice. In addition, specific criteria for oxygenation (Pao_2/Fio_2) and radiographic findings were established, attempting to address substantial sources of heterogeneity in the literature at the time. The expert panel also recognized that lung injury occurs on a continuum of oxygenation and chest radiographic abnormalities, acknowledging that the specific thresholds chosen were in a sense arbitrary.

However, important limitations to the AECC definition became increasingly evident on its widespread adoption. Acuity of onset was not explicitly defined.[6] Oxygenation criteria did not address the impact of PEEP, Fio_2, and other ventilator settings on Pao_2/Fio_2.[7-11] Even among expert intensivists and radiologists, poor interobserver agreement in applying the AECC radiographic criteria for ARDS was demonstrated.[12,13] Finally, without accounting for the substantial variation in duration and intensity of exposure to lung injury triggers, the resultant heterogeneous patient population may exhibit a range of prognoses and responses to therapy. Perhaps because of these issues, clinical diagnosis of ARDS applying the AECC definition was shown to have only moderate sensitivity and specificity in the identification of diffuse alveolar damage on pathologic examination.[14] An updated definition was sought so that these limitations could be addressed and an advanced understanding of ARDS pathophysiology could be incorporated.

2012 BERLIN DEFINITION

The European Society of Intensive Care Medicine, with the endorsement of the American Thoracic Society and Society of Critical Care Medicine, convened an international expert panel to revise the previous AECC definition by incorporating the wealth of evidence that accumulated after the AECC definition (Table 28-1). The Berlin consensus conference updated each of the elements included from the AECC definition: timing, chest radiographic findings, origin of edema, and oxygenation. It also systematically evaluated other variables proposed to predict clinical outcomes in ARDS in an attempt to establish predictive validity. Individual patient-level meta-analysis of 4188 patients pooled from four multicenter and three single-center datasets of patients with ARDS was used to consider ancillary variables for inclusion in the updated definition to determine if these variables enhanced predictive validity without adding unnecessary complexity or jeopardizing feasibility.

Table 28-1 Berlin Definition of ARDS[1]	
Timing	Within 1 week of a known clinical insult or new or worsening respiratory symptoms
Chest imaging	Bilateral opacities not fully explained by effusions, lobar/lung collapse, or nodules
Origin of edema	Respiratory failure not fully explained by cardiac failure or fluid overload Need objective assessment (e.g., echocardiography) to exclude hydrostatic edema if no risk factor present
OXYGENATION	
Mild	200 mm Hg < Pao_2/Fio_2 ≤ 300 mm Hg with PEEP or CPAP ≥ 5 cm H_2O
Moderate	100 mm Hg < Pao_2/Fio_2 ≤ 200 mm Hg with PEEP ≥ 5 cm H_2O
Severe	Pao_2/Fio_2 ≤ 100 mm Hg with PEEP ≥ 5 cm H_2O

CPAP, continuous positive airway pressure; *Fio_2*, fraction of inspired oxygen; *Pao_2*, partial pressure of oxygen in arterial blood; *PEEP*, positive end-expiratory pressure.
Reproduced from The ARDS Definition Task Force[1] with permission.

Acuity of Onset

The AECC definition lacked specific criteria to describe acuity of onset. Several epidemiologic studies have shown that most cases of ARDS develop within the first 72 hours of hospitalization when a predisposing condition is present on admission.[15-19] In a 22-hospital cohort of 5584 patients at risk of ARDS on hospital admission, Gajic et al.[16] found that ARDS developed a median of 2 days after hospitalization (interquartile range, 1 to 4 days). Other studies have found that over half of ARDS cases occur within 24 hours of hospitalization when a risk factor is present on admission.[17,18] Virtually all cases occur within 7 days after an identifiable risk factor occurs, regardless of the mechanism.[15,16] To incorporate these findings, the Berlin definition newly requires that timing of onset be within 1 week of a known clinical insult or new or worsening respiratory symptoms.[1]

Oxygenation

For the confusion around the related AECC definitions of ALI and ARDS to be addressed, the term *ALI* was removed from the updated Berlin definition.[1] In turn, ARDS was classified into three categories depending on severity of impaired oxygenation: mild (Pao_2/Fio_2 201 to 300 mm Hg with PEEP or continuous positive airway pressure [CPAP] ≥5 cm H_2O), moderate (Pao_2/Fio_2 101 to 200 mm Hg with PEEP ≥5 cm H_2O), and severe (Pao_2/Fio_2 ≤100 mm Hg with PEEP ≥5 cm H_2O). The inclusion of a separate category for severe ARDS was influenced by recent clinical trials that tested interventions only in the subset of patients with more severe ARDS.[20,21] The prognostic utility of Pao_2/Fio_2 thresholds for mild, moderate, and severe ARDS was confirmed by individual patient-level meta-analysis: mortality was 27% (95% confidence interval [CI], 24% to 30%) for mild, 32% (95% CI, 29% to 34%) for moderate, and 45% (95% CI, 42% to 48%) for severe ARDS ($P < 0.001$).[1]

The oxygen saturation by pulse oximetry (SpO_2)/Fio_2 correlates with Pao_2/Fio_2 in patients with ARDS[22] and was considered as an alternative for oxygenation criteria in the revised definition. Concerns regarding misclassification of ARDS severity when SpO_2 was 100% led its exclusion from the revised definition.[23]

The inclusion of minimum PEEP levels in the Berlin definition was intended to address concerns regarding the influence of PEEP titration on Pao_2/Fio_2. Severity of oxygenation impairment, important for the diagnosis of ARDS and classification of disease severity, may fluctuate with PEEP and Fio_2 titration.[7-9,11] Moreover, PEEP-responsive patients appear to have a more favorable prognosis.[24] The Berlin expert panel evaluated whether a higher PEEP threshold of 10 cm H_2O or greater for severe ARDS improved prognostic performance with an individual patient-level meta-analysis. No change in prognostic performance was found; thus a PEEP threshold of 5 cm H_2O was retained irrespective of ARDS severity in the final definition.[1,23] However, PEEP titration was not standardized, and oxygenation responsiveness to PEEP titration was not assessed in the cohort used to examine the Berlin Pao_2/Fio_2 thresholds. Both may have prognostic utility[24] and are discussed in greater detail later in this chapter.

Chest Radiographic Findings

Interobserver agreement on radiographic interpretation with the AECC definition was remarkably poor. In a sample of 21 experts reviewing 28 randomly selected chest radiographs from patients with a Pao_2/Fio_2 less than 300 mm Hg, the percentage of radiographs interpreted as consistent with ARDS ranged from 36% to 71%.[12] Fewer than half of radiographs (43%) had near-complete agreement (agreement by 20 of 21 experts), and fully one third had at least five dissenting interpretations. A subsequent study evaluating whether consensus training improved interobserver agreement demonstrated improved agreement on radiographic diagnosis when two interpreters received training (88% to 94% of all pairwise interpretations).[13] However, when one of the two interpreters did not receive training, interobserver agreement remained moderately poor (68% to 78% of all pairwise interpretations). To address this issue, the Berlin definition explicitly requires that opacities on chest imaging not be fully explained by effusions, lobar collapse, or nodules. In addition, the Berlin expert panel provided 12 sample radiographs with accompanying interpretations as consistent, inconsistent, or equivocal for diagnosis of ARDS.[23]

The Berlin expert panel also considered quantifying radiographic opacities by number of involved quadrants. In a study of organ donors whose lungs were not used for transplantation, Ware and colleagues[25] compared excised lung weight with a score quantifying the degree of pulmonary edema within each quadrant on frontal radiograph. They found good correlation between radiographic assessment and lung weight ($r=0.61$, $P<0.0001$) that improved when radiographs with atelectasis were excluded ($r=0.79$, $P<0.0001$). Likewise, detailed assessment of chest computed tomography found that increased lung attenuation and the proportion of nonaerated lung predict mortality in patients with ARDS.[26] In an individual patient-level meta-analysis by the Berlin expert panel, prognostic performance of the severe ARDS classification was not improved with the additional requirement of three or more involved

quadrants; thus the number of quadrants with radiographic infiltrates was not included in the final definition. Still, detailed radiographic interpretation better quantifying the extent of pulmonary edema may yield additional prognostic information if interobserver agreement can be improved.

Origin of Edema

The AECC definition required a PAWP of 18 mm Hg or less when measured or that there be no clinical evidence of left atrial hypertension. This aspect of the definition, as for definitions that preceded it, precluded the diagnosis of ARDS in patients with coincident ARDS and left atrial hypertension. Subsequent to the AECC definition, a multicenter study of 71 patients with ARDS and pulmonary artery catheters found that 82% of patients had at least one PAWP greater than 18 mm Hg when measured serially every 8 hours for the duration of catheter placement.[27] In more than half of patients, PAWP exceeded 18 mm Hg on at least 30% of measurements. In the National Heart, Lung, and Blood Institute (NHLBI) ARDS Network Fluid and Catheter Treatment Trial,[28] 29% of 513 enrolled ARDS patients randomized to receive a pulmonary artery catheter had an initial PAWP greater than 18 mm Hg, 97% of whom also had a normal or high cardiac index that made systolic heart failure an unlikely explanation for the high PAWP.

Recognizing that patients with heart failure are also vulnerable to lung injury and the development of ARDS, the Berlin definition explicitly allows for both hydrostatic and nonhydrostatic pulmonary edema to be present, requiring only that hydrostatic edema not be the primary cause of respiratory failure. Because pulmonary artery catheter use has substantially declined[29] and judgment is necessary to determine the primary cause of respiratory failure, illustrative clinical vignettes were provided in the supplementary material for the Berlin definition. In addition, the Berlin definition stipulates that if no ARDS risk factor can be identified, objective assessment to exclude hydrostatic edema, such as by echocardiography, is required.[1]

Ancillary Variables Considered

Static C_{RS} and dead-space fraction were thought by the Berlin expert panel to have sufficient supporting data to warrant consideration in the definition. Decreased C_{RS} has been recognized as a key feature since the original description of ARDS by Ashbaugh and colleagues.[3] However, chest wall mechanics independent of lung injury often contribute substantially and unpredictably to global respiratory system mechanics,[30] potentially limiting the prognostic utility of C_{RS} in ARDS. In an individual patient-level meta-analysis, the Berlin expert panel found that including C_{RS} of 40 mL/cm H_2O or less in the diagnostic criteria for severe ARDS did not improve prognostic performance; thus it was excluded from the final definition.[23]

Pulmonary dead-space fraction has been identified repeatedly as an independent predictor of mortality in epidemiologic studies of ARDS.[31-34] However, dead-space fraction may fluctuate with changes in ventilator settings[35,36] analogous to issues surrounding Pao_2/Fio_2. Because the dead-space fraction is not routinely measured in most ARDS clinical trials or in clinical practice, the Berlin expert panel considered corrected minute ventilation (minute ventilation × partial pressure of carbon dioxide in arterial blood [$Paco_2$]/40) as a surrogate.[37] Including corrected minute ventilation greater than 10 L/min as a criterion for severe ARDS did not improve prognostic performance in the Berlin individual patient-level meta-analysis[1]; thus it was also excluded from the final definition. However, corrected minute ventilation has not previously been validated as a surrogate for dead-space fraction. Other thresholds for C_{RS} and corrected minute ventilation were not considered in formulating the Berlin definition.

PERFORMANCE OF THE BERLIN DEFINITION

The 2012 Berlin definition addresses several issues from the AECC definition: (1) establishing an explicit timing of onset, (2) removing the term *ALI* in favor of mutually exclusive categories of ARDS severity to avoid confusion, (3) facilitating interobserver agreement on chest imaging interpretation through sample radiographs, (4) allowing for the coexistence of hydrostatic and nonhydrostatic pulmonary edema, and (5) incorporating ARDS risk factors to improve reliability and face and content validity.

Thille and colleagues[38] found that increasing ARDS severity under the Berlin definition correlated with diffuse alveolar damage on postmortem examination. In an autopsy study of 356 patients with clinical diagnosis of ARDS, diffuse alveolar damage was found in 45% of patients. In those with mild, moderate, and severe ARDS, diffuse alveolar damage was found in 12%, 40%, and 58% of patients, respectively. In patients who met clinical criteria for severe ARDS for at least 72 hours, diffuse alveolar damage was found in 69% of cases. Pneumonia was the most common finding (49% of cases) on histopathologic examination among patients who met clinical criteria for ARDS but did not have diffuse alveolar damage.

Thus the Berlin definition fails to identify patients with what many consider to be the pathologic hallmark of the syndrome (i.e., diffuse alveolar damage). However, whether patients with diffuse alveolar damage at histologic examination have a different clinical phenotype than patients with other pathologic changes is not yet known.

Despite these improvements, the Berlin definition had only slightly better predictive validity for mortality than the AECC definition (c-statistic 0.577 vs. 0.536, $P < 0.001$).[1] Key residual issues in the Berlin definition may contribute to this limited gain in prognostic performance and are discussed in Table 28-2.

Table 28-2 **Limitations and Redressals in the AECC and Berlin Definitions**				
	AECC Definition	**AECC Limitations**	**Berlin Definition Redressal**	**Berlin Definition Limitations**
Timing	Acute onset	Acute time frame not specified	Acute time frame specified as 1 week	Onset typically more rapid than 1 week,[16-18] potentially increasing the risk of false-positive diagnosis
Chest imaging	Bilateral infiltrates	Poor interobserver agreement on radiograph interpretation[12,13]	Imaging criteria more explicit; sample radiographs provided	Interobserver agreement may remain problematic[12,13]; fails to capture prognostic information that may exist in imaging with better quantification of edema severity[25,26]
Origin of edema	Excludes patients with left atrial hypertension	Many patients incidentally found to have high PAWP[27,28]	Allows coincident ARDS and hydrostatic edema if risk factor present and latter is not primary cause of respiratory failure	Primary cause of respiratory failure remains subjective, and the physical examination is unreliable
Oxygenation	$Pao_2/Fio_2 \leq 200$ (ARDS) or ≤ 300 (ALI) regardless of PEEP	Ignores effects of PEEP, Fio_2, and other ventilator settings on Pao_2/Fio_2[7,9,11]	Minimum PEEP levels added to subgroups	Changes to PEEP, Fio_2, and other settings still may influence Pao_2/Fio_2 and change severity classification; no standardized assessment (e.g., standardized ventilator settings or use of OI); no stabilization period to exclude transient Pao_2/Fio_2 changes
	ALI category for $Pao_2/Fio_2 \leq 300$	Confusion regarding ALI versus ARDS	Three mutually exclusive subgroups; ALI term removed	Recent major clinical trials[20,21] defined severe ARDS as $Pao_2/Fio_2 < 150$, risking further confusion
Subphenotypes	Classify by risk factor according to direct vs. indirect injury	Prognostic utility not well validated; many patients have both direct and indirect risk factors	Removed from consensus document	Biologically distinct subphenotypes may exist[46] and may respond differently to particular therapies and/or hold different prognoses; ignores risk factors proven to have more favorable prognosis (e.g., trauma, TRALI)[44]

AECC, American-European Consensus Conference; *ALI,* acute lung injury; *ARDS,* acute respiratory distress syndrome; *Fio_2,* fraction of inspired oxygen; *Pao_2,* partial pressure of oxygen in arterial blood; *PAWP,* pulmonary artery wedge pressure; *PEEP,* positive end-expiratory pressure; *TRALI,* transfusion-related acute lung injury.

Standardized Assessment of Oxygenation

Lack of standardized assessment of oxygenation almost certainly contributes to heterogeneity among patients diagnosed clinically with ARDS. Pao_2/Fio_2 varies with key ventilator settings, including tidal volume, PEEP, and Fio_2.[7-9,11,39] Two potential remedies have been proposed that were not considered in formulating the Berlin definition: standardized ventilator settings and the oxygenation index (OI).

Several studies have confirmed that standardized ventilator settings affect Pao_2/Fio_2 criteria in evaluating for ARDS. Ferguson and colleagues[7] placed 41 patients who initially met criteria for moderate-severe ARDS on standardized ventilator settings (tidal volume, 7 to 8 mL/kg predicted body weight; PEEP, 10 cm H_2O; and Fio_2, 1.0). After just 30 minutes, 59% of patients no longer met Pao_2/Fio_2 for moderate-severe ARDS, and those same patients had substantially lower mortality (12.5% vs 52.9% for transient vs. persistent $Pao_2/Fio_2 \leq 200$ mm Hg). Villar and colleagues have shown in several studies[8,9,11] that a 24-hour trial of standardized ventilator settings reclassifies ARDS severity and results in some patients no longer meeting diagnostic criteria for ARDS. They similarly found lower mortality for patients only transiently meeting oxygenation criteria for ARDS. With these findings incorporated,, investigators involved in recent multicenter clinical trials studying high-frequency oscillatory ventilation[40] and prone positioning[20] required standardized ventilator settings and a stabilization period before randomization.

However, reclassification after a 24-hour waiting period conflates the effects of standardized settings with disease progression (or rapid resolution) and makes early intervention trials difficult if not impossible. A stabilization period may help identify a subset of patients with ARDS who are not rapidly improving and have higher mortality, for whom treatments with a marginal risk-benefit profile may still offer net benefit. Furthermore, the optimal standardized ventilator settings for diagnostic assessment and interval time on those settings before reassessment remain to be determined. Requiring standardized ventilator settings would hinder observational studies by requiring changes from usual care settings and may make comparison with existing literature difficult.

The OI (= mean airway pressure $\times Fio_2 \times 100 \div Pao_2$) is routinely used to assess disease severity in neonatal and pediatric respiratory failure[41] and has been used in adults with ARDS. Inclusion of mean airway pressure may account for oxygenation effects attributable to tidal volume and PEEP, in addition to Fio_2. Monchi et al.[42] and Seeley et al.,[43] in separate ARDS studies involving 259 and 149 patients, respectively, found that the OI was superior to Pao_2/Fio_2 in predicting mortality. Mean airway pressure is typically reported on the display of most modern ventilators, supporting widespread feasibility of adoption. With OI, concerns regarding the feasibility of standardized ventilator settings would be avoided, although variable documentation of OI in existing datasets and medical records may limit retrospective and epidemiologic studies. Still, the OI warrants further consideration as a potentially better-performing prognostic assessment of oxygenation.

Recognition of ARDS Subphenotypes

ARDS by definition is a clinical phenotype triggered by a diverse array of underlying precipitants of lung injury. Differences in insults precipitating ARDS and how each individual responds to these insults inevitably contribute to a diversity of biology within the patient population labeled as having ARDS. Different subphenotypes may carry distinct prognoses and respond uniquely to therapeutic interventions. For instance, even the original description of ARDS by Ashbaugh and colleagues[3] suggested that ARDS due to trauma may carry a more favorable prognosis compared with other causes. This finding was subsequently confirmed by Calfee and coworkers,[44] who also observed lower concentrations of lung epithelial and endothelial biomarkers of injury in patients with ARDS due to trauma compared with nontraumatic causes.

The AECC expert panel proposed classifying ARDS according to direct (alveolar epithelial) or indirect (pulmonary vascular endothelial) injury to the lung.[4] Recent evidence suggests that this classification identifies two biologically distinct subphenotypes, which may prove useful for clinical trial enrichment when testing therapies that target alveolar epithelial or vascular endothelial mechanisms.[45] Prognostic utility of this approach has not been well validated, in part because of differences in both the magnitude and duration of the insult to the lungs that are not adequately captured by this approach.[2] For instance, such risk factors as lung contusion (direct) and transfusion (indirect) are both transient insults that carry comparatively favorable prognoses with faster resolution of lung injury. By contrast, pneumonia (direct) and sepsis (indirect) occur in a sustained fashion over several days, resulting in prolonged exposure to the proinjurious event and consequently carrying a less favorable prognosis.

In the most concerted effort to date to identify biologically distinct subphenotypes of ARDS, Calfee and colleagues[46] performed latent subclass analyses of clinical data and biomarkers collected in the NHLBI ARDS Network low tidal volume and PEEP titration trials.[39,47] They identified two distinct subphenotypes of ARDS and replicated this finding in a second cohort. One subphenotype was characterized by high concentrations of inflammatory biomarkers (IL-6 and IL-8, tumor necrosis factor α), metabolic acidosis, and shock, whereas the other phenotype had less severe inflammation and shock. In both clinical trial cohorts, the proinflammatory subphenotype had roughly double the mortality rate of the other phenotype. Importantly, the PEEP strategy assigned had opposite effects on mortality in the two subphenotypes: the proinflammatory subphenotype exhibited a favorable response to higher PEEP (42% mortality with higher PEEP vs. 51% with lower PEEP), whereas the less inflamed subphenotype had an unfavorable response (24% mortality with higher PEEP vs. 16% with lower PEEP; $P = 0.049$ for interaction). These hypothesis-generating results encourage further investigation into identification of clinical-biological subphenotypes that may predict response to therapy. Identification of biomarkers or biomarker panels with better performance characteristics will aid in further distinguishing between subphenotypes.

CONCLUSION

The Berlin definition of ARDS applies to the clinical and research settings and offers several advances over the 1994 AECC definition. However, remaining issues surrounding nonstandardized assessment of oxygenation and heterogeneity of patients included in the Berlin definition limit improvement in prognostic performance over the AECC definition. In addition, the Berlin definition fails to identify patients with diffuse alveolar damage. Additional work is needed to define biologically distinct subphenotypes meeting the clinical diagnosis of ARDS to improve prognostic assessment and identify subgroups more likely to respond to therapies, new and old.

AUTHORS' RECOMMENDATIONS

- The 2012 Berlin definition is recommended for epidemiologic studies and selected clinical trials; the severity stratification by Pao_2/Fio_2 is helpful for selecting supportive therapies such as higher PEEP, prone ventilation, and neuromuscular blockade.
- Standardized assessment of Pao_2/Fio_2 should be considered in higher risk clinical studies to reduce heterogeneity of enrolled patients and enrich for a higher mortality subset; the optimal method remains to be determined.
- Future research is needed to define biologically distinct subphenotypes of ARDS that may carry different prognoses, respond differently to therapies, and may better predict the presence of diffuse alveolar damage.

REFERENCES

1. ARDS Definition Task Force, Ranieri VM, Rubenfeld GD, et al. Acute respiratory distress syndrome: the Berlin definition. *JAMA*. 2012;307(23):2526–2533.
2. Murray JF, Matthay MA, Luce JM, Flick MR. An expanded definition of the adult respiratory distress syndrome. *Am Rev Respir Dis*. 1988;138(3):720–723.
3. Ashbaugh DG, Bigelow DB, Petty TL, Levine BE. Acute respiratory distress in adults. *Lancet*. 1967;2(7511):319–323.
4. Bernard GR, Artigas A, Brigham KL, et al. The American-European Consensus Conference on ARDS. Definitions, mechanisms, relevant outcomes, and clinical trial coordination. *Am J Respir Crit Care Med*. 1994;149(3 Pt 1):818–824.
5. Thille AW, Esteban A, Fernández-Segoviano P, et al. Chronology of histological lesions in acute respiratory distress syndrome with diffuse alveolar damage: a prospective cohort study of clinical autopsies. *Lancet Respir Med*. 2013;1(5):395–401.
6. Phua J, Stewart TE, Ferguson ND. Acute respiratory distress syndrome 40 years later: time to revisit its definition. *Crit Care Med*. 2008;36(10):2912–2921.
7. Ferguson ND, Kacmarek RM, Chiche JD, et al. Screening of ARDS patients using standardized ventilator settings: influence on enrollment in a clinical trial. *Intensive Care Med*. 2004;30(6):1111–1116.
8. Villar J, Pérez-Méndez L, López J, et al. An early PEEP/FIO2 trial identifies different degrees of lung injury in patients with acute respiratory distress syndrome. *Am J Respir Crit Care Med*. 2007;176(8):795–804.
9. Villar J, Pérez-Méndez L, Blanco J, et al. A universal definition of ARDS: the PaO2/FIO2 ratio under a standard ventilatory setting–a prospective, multicenter validation study. *Intensive Care Med*. 2013;39(4):583–592.
10. Britos M, Smoot E, Liu KD, et al. The value of positive end-expiratory pressure and FiO2 criteria in the definition of the acute respiratory distress syndrome. *Crit Care Med*. 2011;39(9):2025–2030.
11. Villar J, Pérez-Méndez L, Kacmarek RM. Current definitions of acute lung injury and the acute respiratory distress syndrome do not reflect their true severity and outcome. *Intensive Care Med*. 1999;25(9):930–935.
12. Rubenfeld GD, Caldwell E, Granton J, Hudson LD, Matthay MA. Interobserver variability in applying a radiographic definition for ARDS. *Chest*. 1999;116(5):1347–1353.
13. Meade MO, Cook RJ, Guyatt GH, et al. Interobserver variation in interpreting chest radiographs for the diagnosis of acute respiratory distress syndrome. *Am J Respir Crit Care Med*. 2000;161(1):85–90.
14. Esteban A, Fernández-Segoviano P, Frutos-Vivar F, et al. Comparison of clinical criteria for the acute respiratory distress syndrome with autopsy findings. *Ann Intern Med*. 2004;141(6):440–445.
15. Hudson LD, Milberg JA, Anardi D, Maunder RJ. Clinical risks for development of the acute respiratory distress syndrome. *Am J Respir Crit Care Med*. 1995;151(2):293–301.
16. Gajic O, Dabbagh O, Park PK, et al. Early identification of patients at risk of acute lung injury: evaluation of lung injury prediction score in a multicenter cohort study. *Am J Respir Crit Care Med*. 2011;183(4):462–470.
17. Ferguson ND, Frutos-Vivar F, Esteban A, et al. Clinical risk conditions for acute lung injury in the intensive care unit and hospital ward: a prospective observational study. *Crit Care*. 2007;11(5):R96.
18. Levitt JE, Bedi H, Calfee CS, Gould MK, Matthay MA. Identification of early acute lung injury at initial evaluation in an acute care setting prior to the onset of respiratory failure. *Chest*. 2009;135(4):936–943.
19. Gong MN, Thompson BT, Williams P, Pothier L, Boyce PD, Christiani DC. Clinical predictors of and mortality in acute respiratory distress syndrome: potential role of red cell transfusion. *Crit Care Med*. 2005;33(6):1191–1198.
20. Guerin C, Reignier J, Richard JC, et al. Prone positioning in severe acute respiratory distress syndrome. *N Engl J Med*. 2013;368(23):2159–2168.
21. Papazian L, Forel JM, Gacouin A, et al. Neuromuscular blockers in early acute respiratory distress syndrome. *N Engl J Med*. 2010;363(12):1107–1116.
22. Rice TW, Wheeler AP, Bernard GR, et al. Comparison of the SpO2/FiO2 ratio and the PaO2/FiO2 ratio in patients with acute lung injury or ARDS. *Chest*. 2007;132(2):410–417.
23. Ferguson ND, Fan E, Camporota L, et al. The Berlin definition of ARDS: an expanded rationale, justification, and supplementary material. *Intensive Care Med*. 2012;38(10):1573–1582.
24. Goligher EC, Kavanagh BP, Rubenfeld GD, et al. Oxygenation response to positive end-expiratory pressure predicts mortality in acute respiratory distress syndrome: a secondary analysis of the LOVS and ExPress Trials. *Am J Respir Crit Care Med*. 2014;190(1):70–76.
25. Ware LB, Neyrinck A, O'Neal HR, et al. Comparison of chest radiograph scoring to lung weight as a quantitative index of pulmonary edema in organ donors. *Clin Transplant*. 2012;26(5):665–671.
26. Rouby JJ, Puybasset L, Cluzel P, Richecoeur J, Lu Q, Grenier P. Regional distribution of gas and tissue in acute respiratory distress syndrome. II. Physiological correlations and definition of an ARDS Severity Score. CT Scan ARDS Study Group. *Intensive Care Med*. 2000;26(8):1046–1056.
27. Ferguson ND, Meade MO, Hallett DC, Stewart TE. High values of the pulmonary artery wedge pressure in patients with acute lung injury and acute respiratory distress syndrome. *Intensive Care Med*. 2002;28(8):1073–1077.
28. Wheeler AP, Bernard GR, Thompson BT, et al. Pulmonary-artery versus central venous catheter to guide treatment of acute lung injury. *N Engl J Med*. 2006;354(21):2213–2224.
29. Wiener RS, Welch HG. Trends in the use of the pulmonary artery catheter in the United States, 1993-2004. *JAMA*. 2007;298(4):423–429.
30. Talmor D, Sarge T, O'Donnell CR, et al. Esophageal and transpulmonary pressures in acute respiratory failure. *Crit Care Med*. 2006;34(5):1389–1394.
31. Nuckton TJ, Alonso JA, Kallet RH, et al. Pulmonary dead-space fraction as a risk factor for death in the acute respiratory distress syndrome. *N Engl J Med*. 2002;346(17):1281–1286.
32. Cepkova M, Kapur V, Ren X, et al. Pulmonary dead space fraction and pulmonary artery systolic pressure as early predictors of clinical outcome in acute lung injury. *Chest*. 2007;132(3):836–842.

33. Kallet RH, Alonso JA, Pittet JF, Matthay MA. Prognostic value of the pulmonary dead-space fraction during the first 6 days of acute respiratory distress syndrome. *Respir Care.* 2004;49(9):1008–1014.

34. Raurich JM, Vilar M, Colomar A, et al. Prognostic value of the pulmonary dead-space fraction during the early and intermediate phases of acute respiratory distress syndrome. *Respir Care.* 2010;55(3):282–287.

35. Kiiski R, Takala J, Kari A, Milic-Emili J. Effect of tidal volume on gas exchange and oxygen transport in the adult respiratory distress syndrome. *Am Rev Respir Dis.* 1992;146(5 Pt 1):1131–1135.

36. Kiiski R, Kaitainen S, Karppi R, Takala J. Physiological effects of reduced tidal volume at constant minute ventilation and inspiratory flow rate in acute respiratory distress syndrome. *Intensive Care Med.* 1996;22(3):192–198.

37. Wexler HR, Lok P. A simple formula for adjusting arterial carbon dioxide tension. *Can Anaesth Soc J.* 1981;28(4):370–372.

38. Thille AW, Esteban A, Fernández-Segoviano P, et al. Comparison of the Berlin definition for acute respiratory distress syndrome with autopsy. *Am J Respir Crit Care Med.* 2013;187(7):761–767.

39. Acute Respiratory Distress Syndrome Network. Ventilation with lower tidal volumes as compared with traditional tidal volumes for acute lung injury and the acute respiratory distress syndrome. *N Engl J Med.* 2000;342(18):1301–1308.

40. Ferguson ND, Cook DJ, Guyatt GH, et al. High-frequency oscillation in early acute respiratory distress syndrome. *N Engl J Med.* 2013;368(9):795–805.

41. Trachsel D, McCrindle BW, Nakagawa S, Bohn D. Oxygenation index predicts outcome in children with acute hypoxemic respiratory failure. *Am J Respir Crit Care Med.* 2005;172(2):206–211.

42. Monchi M, Bellenfant F, Cariou A, et al. Early predictive factors of survival in the acute respiratory distress syndrome. A multivariate analysis. *Am J Respir Crit Care Med.* 1998;158(4):1076–1081.

43. Seeley E, McAuley DF, Eisner M, Miletin M, Matthay MA, Kallet RH. Predictors of mortality in acute lung injury during the era of lung protective ventilation. *Thorax.* 2008;63(11):994–998.

44. Calfee CS, Eisner MD, Ware LB, et al. Trauma-associated lung injury differs clinically and biologically from acute lung injury due to other clinical disorders. *Crit Care Med.* 2007;35(10):2243–2250.

45. Calfee CS, Janz DR, Bernard GR, et al. Biomarkers of lung epithelial and endothelial injury differentiate between direct and indirect ARDS in single and multi-center studies. *Am J Respir Crit Care Med.* 2014;189:A5091.

46. Calfee CS, Delucchi K, Parsons PE, et al. Subphenotypes in acute respiratory distress syndrome: latent class analysis of data from two randomised controlled trials. *Lancet Respir Med.* 2014;2(8):611–620.

47. National Heart, Lung, and Blood Institute ARDS Clinical Trials Network. Higher versus lower positive end-expiratory pressures in patients with the acute respiratory distress syndrome. *N Engl J Med.* 2004;351(4):327–336.

29 What Are the Pathologic and Pathophysiologic Changes That Accompany Acute Lung Injury and ARDS?

Michael Lava, Greg S. Martin

Diverse inciting events lead to acute respiratory distress syndrome (ARDS), including pneumonia, sepsis, pancreatitis, and trauma.[1-3] These are generally divided into events that directly injure the lung (e.g., pneumonia) or those that indirectly injury the lung (e.g., pancreatitis).[1,4,5] Although the method of injury varies, there is a complex and interrelated series of physiologic responses that follow a common pathway to underpin this disease. Inflammatory mediators[5] and direct injury to the alveolar capillary unit lead to increased vascular permeability and protein-rich pulmonary edema, the central finding of ARDS.[1,3,6]

PATHOPHYSIOLOGIC CHANGES

Inflammatory Injury

The role of the neutrophil is essential in the pathogenesis of ARDS. The centrality of neutrophils in the pathogenesis of ARDS is suggested in multiple ways. Biopsy and bronchoalveolar lavage (BAL) fluid studies show a significant increase in the volume of neutrophils, and labeled neutrophils transfused into an ARDS patient show a predilection for the lung.[6,7] The mechanism for neutrophil sequestration in the lung is subject to debate. Only limited evidence supports a significant role for interaction between the neutrophil and the endothelium that is mediated by cell surface adhesion molecules.[8] An alternative theory holds that neutrophil deformability is central. Under normal circumstances, the neutrophil must change shape to transit the pulmonary capillaries and exit the lung vasculature. In ARDS the local inflammatory milieu stiffens the neutrophil, leaving it unable to pass through the vasculature. This physical structural change is thought to be the primary cause of sequestration.[8]

In addition to neutrophil sequestration and inflammatory mediator release in the lung during ARDS, there is evidence that activity is effectively prolonged in ARDS. Normally, the effect of neutrophils is limited by apoptosis. In ARDS, however, BAL fluid studies have demonstrated decreased apoptosis.[9,10] Further, BAL fluid from ARDS patients can actually inhibit neutrophil apoptosis ex vivo.[9]

The neutrophil acts on both the epithelium and the endothelium, creating a vicious inflammatory cycle. After either direct injury to the lung or systemic inflammation, neutrophils in the pulmonary capillaries are activated.[11] The cells then release proteases, various cytokines, and reactive oxygen species that are cytotoxic. The resultant endothelial damage leads to the breakdown in the capillary wall, allowing adherent platelets to interact directly with neutrophils,[11-13] further exacerbating cytokine release[14] and recruiting additional neutrophils, thus initiating inflammatory lung injury.[11] Furthermore, platelet activation leads to release of additional inflammatory cytokines and promotes fibrin formation.[5]

It is important to note, however, that while neutrophils play a significant role in ARDS, they are not necessarily essential.[15] The inflammatory cycle of ARDS is complex, with multiple interrelated signalers. Among the hallmarks of ARDS is an early increase in the appearance of immature alveolar macrophages whose influx, in turn, correlates with the severity of ARDS.[16] Stressed fibroblasts, epithelial cells, endothelial cells, and local inflammatory cells release an array of inflammatory products.[17] Both direct and indirect insults to the lung lead monocytes and macrophages to produce tumor necrosis factor α (TNF-α) and interleukin-1 (IL-1) (75).[6] These cytokines act locally and lead to production of IL-8. This leads to both neutrophil recruitment and propagation of a local inflammatory environment.[18] In addition, stressed macrophages, as well as endothelial and epithelial cells, release reactive oxygen and nitrogen species that can directly injure lung tissue. Another precipitant in the cycle of inflammation is the coagulation cascade. In ARDS, activation of this process is enhanced, while the fibrinolytic cascade is downregulated.[19-21] As a result, an intravascular clot forms, precipitating microthrombosis.[6] Both thrombin and fibrin production independently lead to further exacerbation of the neutrophil-mediated inflammatory cascade.[22]

Alveolar-Capillary Barrier Dysfunction

Injury to both the alveolar epithelium and the capillary endothelium are necessary in ARDS.[6,11] The result is dysfunction in the alveolar-capillary barrier, leading to movement of intravascular proteins into the alveolar space. This "leakage" is the defining pathophysiologic feature of ARDS.

The alveolar-capillary membrane has the essential role of regulating the volume and movement of proteins and fluid into and out of the alveolar space and thus maintaining surface area for gas transport. Individual type I pulmonary epithelial cells are connected by tight junctions and form a barrier that opposes the movement of proteins into the alveolus. These cells have a characteristic NA,K-ATPase (sodium-potassium adenosine triphosphatase) transporter on their basolateral surface that removes fluid from the alveolus.[23] The inflammatory mediators released by neutrophils[11] damage endothelial cells, disrupt tight junctions, and accelerate apoptosis of both type 1 and type 2 pneumocytes.[11,24] Reactive oxygen species and elastases are expressed, leading to the formation of paracellular gaps that further impair already tenuous epithelial membranes.[25] In experimental models, these gaps form within minutes to hours of the initiating insult.[6] The damage allows protein-rich fluid to enter the alveolar space.[26] The destruction of types 1 and 2 pneumocytes occurs through both apoptosis and necrosis.[23] The loss of the Na,K-ATPase on type 1 cells, as well as a reduction in surfactant production by type 2 cells, contributes to the progressive damage.[11]

Experimentally, BAL fluid from ARDS patients induces apoptosis in cultured epithelial cells.[23] In addition, radiotracer studies show an increase in the flux of protein across the capillary[6] and in the protein concentration within the alveolar space.[27]

Other inflammatory mediators also damage the alveolar-capillary membrane. Production of reactive oxygen species leads to fatty acid damage on the endothelial and epithelial wall, leading to increased permeability edema.[7,28]

Permeability Pulmonary Edema

Movement of fluid into and out of the alveolus is primarily determined by Starling's law. In essence, the net movement of fluid through a semipermeable membrane is dependent on hydrostatic pressure, colloid osmotic pressure (COP), and the permeability of the membrane.[29,30]

The capillary endothelium is relatively permeable, allowing protein-rich fluid into the interstitium under physiologic conditions. The density of fluid in the interstitium, however, is only two thirds of that normally contained in the capillary. This high COP favors movement of fluid out of the interstitium and into the capillary, an essential mechanism to protect against the pulmonary edema.

Alveolar epithelium, on the other hand, is impermeable to large molecules. Type 1 pneumocytes, which compose 90% of the cells of the epithelium, facilitate gas exchange and are sensitive to damage.[6] They are interconnected via tight junctions that support this impermeable membrane.[31] When fluid does enter the alveolar space, it is removed with a basolateral Na,K-ATPase–dependent pump on the surface of pneumocytes. An osmotic gradient is created, and water flows into the interstitium.[11]

In ARDS, COP is diminished by the increased permeability of the endothelium, allowing egress of plasma proteins from the capillary to the interstitium. The effect of this diminution in COP is dramatic: a 50% decrease in COP increases lymphatic fluid removal fourfold.[32] In addition, for any given hydrostatic pressure gradient change, a similar decrease in COP leads to a doubling in fluid flux away from the capillary.[29] Even with increased permeability of the endothelial membrane, this decreased gradient is central to initiating and maintaining permeability pulmonary edema.[29,32,33] This state is exacerbated by the low oncotic pressure common to the critically ill.[29,33,34] Experimentally, pulmonary edema is found to develop more rapidly in low protein states and becomes especially pronounced with administration of crystalloid.[32] Under normal conditions, the pulmonary lymphatics drain fluid from the interstitium via the right lymphatic duct, preventing the development of pulmonary edema.[30] In ARDS, the lymphatic flow can increase tenfold but may still remove only 25% of the edema fluid.[29]

The combination of increased permeability and diminution of the protective clearance mechanisms may lead to overwhelming permeability pulmonary edema. At the same time, the ability of the lung to remove this fluid is hampered. When the removal mechanisms of the lung are overwhelmed, clinically apparent pulmonary edema develops.

Iatrogenic Injury

In ARDS, positive pressure ventilation is almost universally employed. Although lifesaving and necessary, this form of support both worsens preexisting lung injury and creates new injury in healthy lungs.[35] The mechanism of injury, in the end, is very similar to the inflammatory cascade induced by any other form of damage causing ARDS.[36] During ARDS, lung aeration is heterogeneous. Some alveoli are collapsed and do not participate in air exchange, whereas other segments are patent and receive more volume than intended.[35] This dichotomy allows multiple mechanisms of lung injury to occur with mechanical ventilation.

Volutrauma is damage caused by ventilation with large tidal volumes that may induce pulmonary edema and hypoxia via alveolar rupture.[35] Several experiments suggest that it is the volume, which was initially thought to be an effect of pressure, and not the pressure that causes these changes.[37] Atelectrauma is an effect of ventilating at low lung volumes or insufficient end expiratory pressure and is caused by the repeated opening of collapsed alveoli. Pathologically, this process leads to epithelial sloughing, hyaline membrane formation, and pulmonary edema.[35] Atelectrauma causes further diminution in surfactant[38,39] and creates regional hypoxia.[35] This effect is magnified by the regional differences in alveolar collapse.[35]

Both volutrauma and atelectrauma cause biotrauma, the release of inflammatory mediators. Implicated mediators include neutrophils, IL-6 and IL-8, and TNF.[35,40] In addition, the damage to the epithelial wall by the aforementioned mechanical forces may lead to bacterial translocation[41] into the capillary space and from there into the circulation.[42] It was once thought that translocation was an important precipitant of systemic inflammation and the multiple organ dysfunction syndrome,[40] but this theory is evoked only rarely in current discussions of pathophysiology.

PATHOPHYSIOLOGIC CONSEQUENCES

Clinically, ARDS manifests as refractory hypoxia, difficulty in ventilation caused by pulmonary hypertension (PH), and a significant reduction in pulmonary compliance.

Ventilation-Perfusion Mismatch and Shunt

Hypoxemia results from several important physiologic derangements: ventilation-perfusion ($\dot{V}/\dot{Q}$) mismatch causing shunt and decreased diffusion of gas across the alveolar membrane. $\dot{V}/\dot{Q}$ mismatch occurs because of the deposition of fibrous tissue and the development of infiltrate in the alveolus (discussed later in the pathology section), pulmonary edema, and significant regional atelectasis.[43] Atelectasis is in part due to the destruction of surfactant-producing type 2 pneumocytes in the alveolar epithelium and atelectotrauma.[11,38,39] Surfactant is responsible for decreasing surface tension of the alveoli, thus contributing to patent alveoli. BAL studies show that the composition of surfactant changes early in ARDS, contributing to increased surface tension and atelectasis. Evidence implicates the destruction of type 2 pneumocytes, decreased biosynthesis of surfactant and surfactant proteins by injured but intact type 2 cells, and flooding of the alveoli with protein-rich edema fluid. Atelectasis leads to a decrease in compliance, increased hypoxia, and edema that further impairs the ability of type 2 pneumocytes to produce functional surfactant[44] and increases the shunt fraction.[45]

Decreased diffusion develops because of a widened alveolar septum, widened alveolar epithelium, and as a consequence, increased distance between the alveolar and the epithelial membranes.[43]

Decreased Compliance

The alveolar capillary injury with rampant acute inflammation and accumulation of proteinaceous edema fluid in the alveolar spaces results in very stiff, noncompliant lungs. In the early stages of ARDS, pulmonary edema also contributes. As the syndrome progresses, however, fibrosis develops, and compliance may decrease even in the absence of pulmonary edema or active inflammation.[43] Fibrosis will be discussed more fully later.

Dead Space/Pulmonary Hypertension

The development of PH is common in ARDS and contributes to pulmonary insufficiency by increasing dead space ventilation and hypercarbia.[43] In the era preceding lung protective ventilation, 61% of ARDS patients had evidence of cor pulmonale by transthoracic echocardiography,[46] and nearly all patients had elevated pulmonary artery pressures by pulmonary artery catheter measurement.[47]

Early on in ARDS, PH develops due to hypoxic pulmonary vasoconstriction, VTE, and edema.[43,47] Edema contributes to PH by compressing vessels, thus increasing resistance.[47] Local production of vasoconstrictors, such as endothelin-1 and thromboxane a₂, has also been implicated.[47,48] ARDS also leads to subacute arterial, venous, and lymphatic remodeling, with intima being replaced by collagen and fibrin. This process decreases the cross section of the lumen and contributes to PH.[47] As ARDS progresses, fibrous

replacement of the microcirculation is seen, and increased muscularization of arterioles develops. As a result, PH worsens and pathologic changes become more pronounced. In addition, both microthrombi and macrothrombi are common during ARDS and have been reported to be present in 95% and 86%, respectively, of autopsy specimens.[43] It is unclear if these thrombi result from local coagulation abnormalities or embolic phenomena. Regardless, they lead to further vascular remodeling and worsening PH.[43,47]

The resulting PH causes right ventricular dysfunction and thus reduced cardiac output (CO). The development of cor pulmonale and decreased CO leads to end organ hypoperfusion and further hypoxia.[47]

PATHOLOGIC CHANGES

The classic pathologic characteristic of clinical ARDS is diffuse alveolar damage (DAD).[43,49] Three phases of evolution have been described: exudative, organizing, and fibrotic.[43,49] These stages are nearly universal and occur independent of the inciting cause of lung injury.[43] Although these changes occur sequentially, there is significant overlap between phases.[50] In fact, multiple stages can be seen in the same biopsy specimen, and although the stages are unique, the timing or progression between phases is not clinically predictable.[51] Thus, although these stages provide a useful pathologic construct, they do not represent clinical evolution.

In the exudative phase, the pathologic changes tend to be uniform.[49] The predominant finding is a hyaline membrane lining the alveolar surface. Hyaline membranes consist of cellular debris from destruction of type 1 pneumocytes,[51] plasma proteins, and surfactant.

During the exudative phase, inflammatory cell involvement reflects the accumulation and activation of lymphocytes, plasma cells, and macrophages.[50] Microthrombi, found throughout the evolution of DAD, first appear in the exudative phase.[49] The alveolar septa are thickened by protein-rich edema, and fibroblast/myofibroblast formation begins. Early in this phase, a significant loss of the epithelial coverage of much of the alveolar basement membrane contributes to hypoxia. Toward the end of this phase, epithelial regeneration is seen, with cell hyperplasia, atypia, and mitosis that can be mistaken for malignancy on open biopsy and BAL (Fig. 29-1, *A*).[52-54]

In the organizing stage (Fig. 29-1, *B*), granulation tissue begins to form in the alveolar space. During this time, the intra-alveolar and interstitial exudates begin to organize.[43] The hyaline membrane starts to disappear and is incorporated into the alveolar septum.[43,49,50] The defining feature of this stage is the evolution of organized granulation tissue, an attempt at repair. Fibroblasts and myofibroblasts migrate via breaks in the alveolar basement membrane, forming granulation tissue in the alveolar space. Type 2 pneumocytes proliferate and follow, transforming this intra-alveolar granulation tissue into septal granulation tissue. This process, the beginning of the reparative process, is termed *fibrosis by accretion*.[43,49] The end result is dense septal deposits of granulation tissue, leading to the fibrosis seen on imaging, along with dilated alveoli and alveolar ducts. During this period, there is hyperplasia of type 2 pneumocytes, as well as cytologic changes, which again can easily be mistaken for malignancy.[43,49,55] In nearly all samples, thrombi are seen on

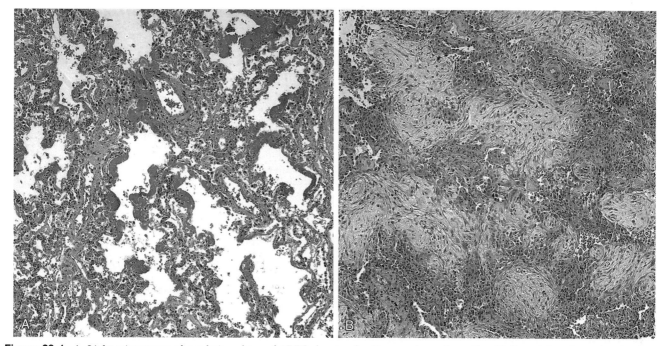

Figure 29-1. A, Light microscopy of exudative phase of ARDS showing hyaline membrane formation. **B,** Organizing phase showing intra-alveolar granulation tissue. (*Courtesy Anthony Gal, MD, Department of Pathology, Emory University School of Medicine.*)

gross examination and microscopically.[49] Although some cases of DAD go on to histologic recovery at this stage, in many, more extensive damage occurs.[50]

The final stage in the evolution of DAD is the fibrotic stage. It is generally seen only after several weeks of syndrome progression and mechanical ventilation.[43] Substantial fibrosis has occurred at this point as the dense granulation tissue seen in the organizing stage has been transformed into collagen. Fibrosis is relatively uniform, although with varying degrees of honeycombing.[49]

Although about two thirds of ARDS patients have DAD on biopsy, other patterns are common.[56] Abnormalities include acute fibrinous and/or organizing pneumonia, in which the alveolar space is filled with fibrin instead of the classic hyaline membrane, eosinophilic pneumonia, and diffuse alveolar hemorrhage.[50]

AUTHORS' RECOMMENDATIONS

- The inflammatory cycle of ARDS is complex, with multiple interrelated signalers that include neutrophils, macrophages, fibroblasts, epithelial cells, endothelial cells, and local inflammatory cells.
- These release an array of inflammatory products of which TNF-α, IL-1, and IL-8 are the most important.
- There is activation of coagulation, with microvascular thrombosis that results in further inflammation.
- The alveolar capillary interface breaks down, and protein rich exudate enters the interstitium and alveolar space. There is overwhelming permeability pulmonary edema whose clearance is hampered by reduced lymphatic clearance.
- Profound hypoxemia results in pulmonary hypertension, right ventricular dysfunction, and reduced cardiac output.
- The classic pathologic characteristic of clinical ARDS is diffuse alveolar damage (DAD).
- Three phases of evolution have been described: exudative, organizing, and fibrotic.

REFERENCES

1. Ware LB, Matthay MA. The acute respiratory distress syndrome. *N Engl J Med.* 2000;342(18):1334–1349.
2. Hudson LD, Milberg JA, Anardi D, Maunder RJ. Clinical risks for development of the acute respiratory distress syndrome. *Am J Respir Crit Care Med.* 1995;151(2):293–301, 1995/02/01.
3. Matthay MA, Ware LB, Zimmerman GA. The acute respiratory distress syndrome. *J Clin Invest.* August 1, 2012;122(8):2731–2740.
4. Reiss LK, Uhlig U, Uhlig S. Models and mechanisms of acute lung injury caused by direct insults. *Eur J Cell Biol.* June–July 2012; 91(6-7):590–601.
5. Matthay MA, Zimmerman GA. Acute lung injury and the acute respiratory distress syndrome: four decades of inquiry into pathogenesis and rational management. *Am J Respir Cell Mol Biol.* October 2005;33(4):319–327.
6. Ware LB. Pathophysiology of acute lung injury and the acute respiratory distress syndrome. *Semin Respir Crit Care Med.* August 2006;27(4):337–349.
7. Pittet JF, Mackersie RC, Martin TR, Matthay MA. Biological markers of acute lung injury: prognostic and pathogenetic significance. *Am J Respir Crit Care Med.* 1997;155(4):1187–1205.
8. Doerschuk CM. Mechanisms of leukocyte sequestration in inflamed lungs. *Microcirculation.* 2001;8(2):71–88.
9. Matute-Bello G, Liles WC, Radella 2nd F, et al. Neutrophil apoptosis in the acute respiratory distress syndrome. *Am J Respir Crit Care Med.* December 1997;156(6):1969–1977.
10. Lesur O, Kokis A, Hermans C, Fulop T, Bernard A, Lane D. Interleukin-2 involvement in early acute respiratory distress syndrome: relationship with polymorphonuclear neutrophil apoptosis and patient survival. *Crit Care Med.* December 2000;28(12): 3814–3822.
11. Matthay MA, Zemans RL. The acute respiratory distress syndrome: pathogenesis and treatment. *Annu Rev Pathol.* 2011;6: 147.
12. Scheiermann C, Kunisaki Y, Jang JE, Frenette PS. Neutrophil microdomains: linking heterocellular interactions with vascular injury. *Curr Opin Hematol.* January 2010;17(1):25–30.
13. Bozza FA, Shah AM, Weyrich AS, Zimmerman GA. Amicus or adversary: platelets in lung biology, acute injury, and inflammation. *Am J Respir Cell Mol Biol.* February 2009;40(2):123–134.
14. Zimmerman GA, Albertine KH, Carveth HJ, et al. Endothelial activation in ARDS. *Chest.* July 1999;116(suppl 1):18s–24s.

15. Laufe MD, Simon RH, Flint A, Keller JB. Adult respiratory distress syndrome in neutropenic patients. *Am J Med*. June 1986;80(6):1022–1026.

16. Rosseau S, Hammerl P, Maus U, et al. Phenotypic characterization of alveolar monocyte recruitment in acute respiratory distress syndrome. *Am J Physiol Lung Cell Mol Physiol*. July 2000;279(1):L25–L35.

17. Goodman RB, Pugin J, Lee JS, Matthay MA. Cytokine-mediated inflammation in acute lung injury. *Cytokine Growth Factor Rev*. December 2003;14(6):523–535.

18. Puneet P, Moochhala S, Bhatia M. Chemokines in acute respiratory distress syndrome. *Am J Physiol Lung Cell Mol Physiol*. January 2005;288(1):L3–L15.

19. Ware LB, Bastarache JA, Wang L. Coagulation and fibrinolysis in human acute lung injury–new therapeutic targets? *Keio J Med*. September 2005;54(3):142–149.

20. Idell S. Anticoagulants for acute respiratory distress syndrome: can they work? *Am J Respir Crit Care Med*. August 15, 2001;164(4):517–520.

21. Abraham E. Coagulation abnormalities in acute lung injury and sepsis. *Am J Respir Cell Mol Biol*. April 2000;22(4):401–404.

22. Lo SK, Lai L, Cooper JA, Malik AB. Thrombin-induced generation of neutrophil activating factors in blood. *Am J Pathol*. January 1988;130(1):22–32.

23. Budinger GR, Sznajder JI. The alveolar-epithelial barrier: a target for potential therapy. *Clin Chest Med*. December 2006;27(4):655–669. abstract ix.

24. Albertine KH, Soulier MF, Wang Z, et al. Fas and fas ligand are up-regulated in pulmonary edema fluid and lung tissue of patients with acute lung injury and the acute respiratory distress syndrome. *Am J Pathol*. November 2002;161(5):1783–1796.

25. Moraes TJ, Zurawska JH, Downey GP. Neutrophil granule contents in the pathogenesis of lung injury. *Curr Opin Hematol*. January 2006;13(1):21–27.

26. Suzuki T, Moraes TJ, Vachon E, et al. Proteinase-activated receptor-1 mediates elastase-induced apoptosis of human lung epithelial cells. *Am J Respir Cell Mol Biol*. September 2005;33(3):231–247.

27. Ware LB, Matthay MA. Alveolar fluid clearance is impaired in the majority of patients with acute lung injury and the acute respiratory distress syndrome. *Am J Respir Crit Care Med*. May 2001;163(6):1376–1383.

28. Lum H, Roebuck KA. Oxidant stress and endothelial cell dysfunction. *Am J Physiol Cell Physiol*. April 2001;280(4):C719–C741.

29. Cribbs SK, Martin GS. Fluid balance and colloid osmotic pressure in acute respiratory failure: optimizing therapy. *Expert Rev Respir Med*. December 2009;3(6):651–662.

30. Martin GS, Brigham KL. Fluid flux and clearance in acute lung injury. Compr Physiol. 2012;2:2471–2480.

31. Boitano S, Safdar Z, Welsh DG, Bhattacharya J, Koval M. Cell-cell interactions in regulating lung function. *Am J Physiol Lung Cell Mol Physiol*. September 2004;287(3):L455–L459.

32. Evidence-based colloid use in the critically ill: American Thoracic Society Consensus Statement. *Am J Respir Crit Care Med*. December 1, 2004;170(11):1247–1259.

33. Mangialardi RJ, Martin GS, Bernard GR, et al. Hypoproteinemia predicts acute respiratory distress syndrome development, weight gain, and death in patients with sepsis. Ibuprofen in Sepsis Study Group. *Crit Care Med*. September 2000;28(9):3137–3145.

34. Arif SK, Verheij J, Groeneveld AB, Raijmakers PG. Hypoproteinemia as a marker of acute respiratory distress syndrome in critically ill patients with pulmonary edema. *Intensive Care Med*. March 2002;28(3):310–317.

35. Slutsky AS, Ranieri VM. Ventilator-induced lung injury. *N Engl J Med*. November 28, 2013;369(22):2126–2136.

36. Tremblay L, Valenza F, Ribeiro SP, Li J, Slutsky AS. Injurious ventilatory strategies increase cytokines and c-fos m-RNA expression in an isolated rat lung model. *J Clin Invest*. March 1, 1997;99(5):944–952.

37. Dreyfuss D, Soler P, Basset G, Saumon G. High inflation pressure pulmonary edema. Respective effects of high airway pressure, high tidal volume, and positive end-expiratory pressure. *Am Rev Respir Dis*. May 1988;137(5):1159–1164.

38. Albert RK. The role of ventilation-induced surfactant dysfunction and atelectasis in causing acute respiratory distress syndrome. *Am J Respir Crit Care Med*. April 1, 2012;185(7):702–708.

39. Maruscak AA, Vockeroth DW, Girardi B, et al. Alterations to surfactant precede physiological deterioration during high tidal volume ventilation. *Am J Physiol Lung Cell Mol Physiol*. May 2008;294(5):L974–L983.

40. Slutsky AS, Tremblay LN. Multiple system organ failure. Is mechanical ventilation a contributing factor? *Am J Respir Crit Care Med*. June 1998;157(6 Pt 1):1721–1725.

41. Nahum A, Hoyt J, Schmitz L, Moody J, Shapiro R, Marini JJ. Effect of mechanical ventilation strategy on dissemination of intratracheally instilled *Escherichia coli* in dogs. *Crit Care Med*. October 1997;25(10):1733–1743.

42. Murphy DB, Cregg N, Tremblay L, et al. Adverse ventilatory strategy causes pulmonary-to-systemic translocation of endotoxin. *Am J Respir Crit Care Med*. July 2000;162(1):27–33.

43. Tomashefski Jr JF. Pulmonary pathology of acute respiratory distress syndrome. *Clin Chest Med*. September 2000;21(3):435–466.

44. Suratt BT, Parsons PE. Mechanisms of acute lung injury/acute respiratory distress syndrome. *Clin Chest Med*. December 2006;27(4):579–589. abstract viii.

45. Cressoni M, Caironi P, Polli F, et al. Anatomical and functional intrapulmonary shunt in acute respiratory distress syndrome. *Crit Care Med*. March 2008;36(3):669–675.

46. Vieillard-Baron A, Schmitt JM, Augarde R, et al. Acute cor pulmonale in acute respiratory distress syndrome submitted to protective ventilation: incidence, clinical implications, and prognosis. *Crit Care Med*. August 2001;29(8):1551–1555.

47. Moloney ED, Evans TW. Pathophysiology and pharmacological treatment of pulmonary hypertension in acute respiratory distress syndrome. *Eur Respir J*. April 2003;21(4):720–727.

48. Cornet AD, Hofstra JJ, Swart EL, Girbes AR, Juffermans NP. Sildenafil attenuates pulmonary arterial pressure but does not improve oxygenation during ARDS. *Intensive Care Med*. May 2010;36(5):758–764.

49. Castro CY. ARDS and diffuse alveolar damage: a pathologist's perspective. *Semin Thorac Cardiovasc Surg*. Spring 2006;18(1):13–19.

50. Beasley MB. The pathologist's approach to acute lung injury. *Arch Pathol Lab Med*. 2010;134(5):719–727.

51. Penuelas O, Aramburu JA, Frutos-Vivar F, Esteban A. Pathology of acute lung injury and acute respiratory distress syndrome: a clinical-pathological correlation. *Clin Chest Med*. December 2006;27(4):571–578. abstract vii-viii.

52. Bromberg Z, Raj N, Goloubinoff P, Deutschman CS, Weiss YG. Enhanced expression of 70-kilodalton heat shock protein limits cell division in a sepsis-induced model of acute respiratory distress syndrome. *Crit Care Med*. January 2008;36(1):246–255.

53. Beskow CO, Drachenberg CB, Bourquin PM, et al. Diffuse alveolar damage. Morphologic features in bronchoalveolar lavage fluid. *Acta Cytol*. July–August 2000;44(4):640–646.

54. Ogino S, Franks TJ, Yong M, Koss MN. Extensive squamous metaplasia with cytologic atypia in diffuse alveolar damage mimicking squamous cell carcinoma: a report of 2 cases. *Human Pathol*. October 2002;33(10):1052–1054.

55. Bromberg Z, Raj N, Goloubinoff P, Deutschman CS, Weiss YG. Enhanced expression of 70-kilodalton heat shock protein limits cell division in a sepsis-induced model of acute respiratory distress syndrome. *Crit Care Med*. January 2008;36(1):246–255.

56. Esteban A, Fernandez-Segoviano P, Frutos-Vivar F, et al. Comparison of clinical criteria for the acute respiratory distress syndrome with autopsy findings. *Ann Intern Med*. September 21, 2004;141(6):440–445.

30 What Is the Best Mechanical Ventilation Strategy in ARDS?

Margaret Doherty, Andrew C. Steel, Niall D. Ferguson

The term *acute respiratory distress syndrome* (ARDS) describes acute inflammatory lung injury caused by a wide variety of insults, resulting in severe hypoxemic respiratory failure. ARDS has been recognized as a clinical entity in adults for 50 years[1] and affects more than 100,000 adults in the United States each year.[2] Reported mortality rates in observational studies persist at between 30% and 60%—depending on severity of illness and organ function. In survivors, long-term disability is a major problem.[3,4] Data accumulated since the early 1990s have confirmed that a careful approach to mechanical ventilation can significantly improve outcomes and shorten the duration of illness. This chapter reviews current mechanical ventilation strategies and proven supportive interventions in ARDS.

STRATEGIES FOR THE MANAGEMENT OF ARDS

Although ARDS arises from a wide variety of injuries and differing pathophysiology, mechanical ventilation is usually required to sustain life. Poor application of mechanical ventilation may worsen lung injury and increase mortality. There is no specific therapy for ARDS beyond treating the underlying disease process (e.g., infection) and supportive care. Therefore the focus of respiratory support by mechanical ventilation in patients with ARDS is to provide acceptable gas exchange while simultaneously minimizing further injury to the lung.

VENTILATOR-INDUCED LUNG INJURY

Until the 1990s mechanical ventilation (MV) strategy involved the use of relatively high tidal volumes (to reduce atelectasis) in the range of 10 to 15 mL per kilogram of body weight, which was usually estimated. Depending on local preference this could be delivered by volume assist-control, synchronized intermittent mechanical ventilation, or pressure assist-control. The application of positive end-expiratory pressure (PEEP) was variable, and there were periods where both high and low levels of PEEP were fashionable. MV as a therapy targeted normalized blood gases.

An end-inspiratory airway pressure of less than 50 cm H_2O was considered acceptable in the absence of pneumothorax or surgical emphysema.[23]

In the 1970s, Webb and Tierney published data demonstrating that high peak inflation pressures severely damaged the lung in rats, revealing the existence of ventilator-induced lung injury (VILI), a process that could be attenuated by judicious use of PEEP.[24] In the 1980s computed tomography (CT) showed that consolidation in lungs affected by ARDS was not as uniform as suggested by the plain radiograph,[25] and that a multilayered topography of pathology was present (Fig. 30-1). Effectively the lung is divided into three zones: a nonrecruitable zone, in the bases, an injured but recruitable midzone, and a spared though potentially overdistended zone in the apices. In the acutely injured lung, less than 50% of the lung may contribute to gas exchange. The anterior apical segments of the lungs are relatively disease free and, being more compliant, are vulnerable to stretch injury. These observations led to the description of the "baby lung" as a functional entity.[26] The concept conveniently illustrates that healthy regions of lung parenchyma bear more stress and strain than the collapsed and consolidated regions. Repeated overdistension of this smaller and vulnerable lung tissue during tidal ventilation results in VILI. Key developments in the field of ARDS ventilation are summarized in Table 30-1.

Modern mechanical ventilation strategy is as focused to preventing VILI as it is to normalization of blood gases. This involves the following:

- Lung protection: Ventilation with low tidal volume (V_t) and low airway plateau pressure (P_{plat}; surrogate of alveolar pressure), using "permissive hypercapnia" where necessary.
- Lung recruitment: The use of appropriate levels of end-expiratory pressures (PEEP) to recruit collapsed alveolar units and avoid further injury to the lung associated with high alveolar volume swings (volutrauma) and shearing injury associated with recurrent opening and closing of collapsed lung units (atelectrauma). This general concept is known as the "open lung" approach to mechanical ventilation. Application of very high levels of PEEP for short periods of time has been proposed as a method for achieving further recruitment (recruitment maneuvers [RMs]).

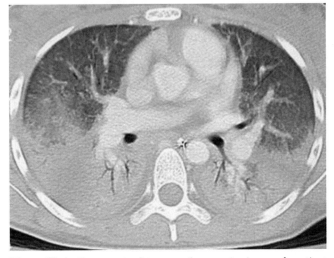

Figure 30-1. Computerized tomography scanning image of a patient with acute respiratory distress syndrome showing regional differences in lung parenchyma involvement.

Table 30-1 Key Research Landmarks in Acute Respiratory Distress Syndrome

Study	Key Development
Ashbaugh et al. (1967)[1]	The "original description" of ARDS suggesting a common pathway of lung injury irrespective of the initial injury.
Webb and Tierney (1974)[6]	An animal study illustrating the relationship among inflation pressure, PEEP, lung histology, and gas exchange. Confirmed the existence of ventilator-induced lung injury.
Gattinoni et al. (1987)[7]	The use of CT scanning in ARDS patients showed the heterogenicity of the lung injury.
Dreyfuss et al. (1988)[40]	Illustrated that inflation volume in mechanical ventilation may cause greater damage than airway pressure in itself.
Hickling et al. (1990)[47]	Advocated adopting pressure-limited ventilation and permissive hypercapnia strategies in ARDS management.
Bernard et al. (1994)[14]	American European consensus conference on ARDS. Publication of the current definition of ARDS and ALI.
Tremblay et al. (1997)[38]	Introduction of the concept of biotrauma: High tidal volume ventilation without PEEP releases proinflammatory cytokines from lung tissue.
Amato et al. (1998)[12]	Small RCT showing a decrease in mortality associated with low tidal volume ventilation and PEEP.
NIH/ARDSnet (2000)[13]	Large trial confirming reduced mortality in ARDS patients ventilated with low tidal volumes. It concluded the debate raised by earlier conflicting smaller trials.

ALI, acute lung injury; ARDS, acute respiratory distress syndrome; CT, computed tomography; PEEP, positive end-expiration pressure; RCT, randomized controlled trial.

"LOW STRETCH" APPROACH

Mechanical ventilation with tidal volumes restricted to 6 mL/kg predicted body weight, resulting in limited transpulmonary pressure, is associated with a decrease in mortality compared with higher tidal volumes and airway pressures.

Clinical research studies conducted in the mid-1990s into VILI by Brochard et al.,[9] Stewart et al.,[10] and Brower et al.[11] were underpowered, suffered design flaws, and failed to deliver anticipated outcome benefits for low stretch strategies. In an "open lung" study, Amato[12] did, however, demonstrate staggering outcome benefits (mortality rate 30% intervention group compared with 71% conventional group, $P < .001$), albeit with higher than expected mortality in the control group. The NIH/ARDSnet ARMA trial, published in 2000, eventually resolved the issue. The study overcame the problems of the previous trials by comparing patients who received tidal volumes of 6 mL/kg and plateau pressures (P_{plat}) less than 30 cm H_2O with 12 mL/kg and P_{plat} <50 cm H_2O.[13] Patients received volume assist-control ventilation, and oxygen therapy and PEEP were adjusted with a stepped protocol. Tidal volume was based on predicted (derived from height), rather than actual, body weight.

The intervention group had a mortality rate of 31%, compared with 39.8% in the high tidal volume group, absolute risk reduction (ARR) 8.8%, number needed to treat (NNT) 11 ($P < .05$). Volumes could be adjusted between 4 and 8 mL/kg to maintain the plateau pressure below 30 cm H_2O, and hypercapnia could ensue, although a pH above 7.30 was targeted. A number of issues remain unresolved from this study, in particular: (1) As minute ventilation was the same in each group, did the patients in the intervention group have more auto-PEEP as a consequence of a more rapid respiratory rate? (2) Is there a difference between 6 and 8 mL/kg if the P_{plat} is <30 cm H_2O?

Table 30-2 summarizes the data from the original low stretch studies. Although many studies have been performed subsequently, the ARMA trial remains the only large multicenter randomized controlled trial that has demonstrated a mortality benefit from a specific mechanical ventilator maneuver in ARDS.[13]

In conclusion, the current standard for mechanical ventilation care for most patients with ARDS involves setting tidal volumes at <6 mL/kg and plateau pressure below 30 cm H_2O.

OPEN LUNG APPROACH

Four mechanisms have been proposed to explain the beneficial effect of PEEP in the injured lung: (1) increased end-expiratory lung volume, thereby improving gas exchange; (2) redistribution of alveolar lung water; (3) improved ventilation-perfusion matching; and (4) stabilization of recruited lung. The use of PEEP is also thought to be protective in preventing the cyclical collapse of alveoli with tidal ventilation, splinting open alveoli throughout the respiratory cycle and avoiding atelectrauma. Although there is general agreement among experts that some amount of PEEP is beneficial, an assertion supported by observational data,[14]

Table 30-2 **Overview of Study Design and Findings of Major Randomized Controlled Trials Involving Comparison of Mechanical Ventilation with Low versus High Tidal Volume in ARDS/ALI**					
Authors	**n**	**Tidal Volume (mL/kg PBW)**	**PEEP (cm H_2O)**	**Mortality (%)**	***P* Value**
Amato et al. (1998)[12]					
Conventional	24	12	8.7 ± 0.4	72	—
Protective	29	<6	16.4 ± 0.4	38	<.001
Stewart et al. (1998)[10]					
Conventional	60	10.7 ± 1.4	7.2 ± 3.3	47	—
Protective	60	7.0 ± 0.7	8.6 ± 3.0	50	n.s.
Brochard et al. (1998)[9]					
Conventional	58	10.3 ± 7.7	10.7 ± 2.3	38	—
Protective	58	7.1 ± 1.3	10.7 ± 2.9	47	n.s.
Brower et al. (1999)[11]					
Conventional	26	10.2 ± 0.1	—	46	—
Protective	26	7.3 ± 0.1	—	50	n.s.
ARDS network (2000)[13]					
Conventional	429	11.8 ± 0.8	8.6 ± 3.6	40	—
Protective	432	6.2 ± 0.9	9.4 ± 3.6	31	0.007

ALI, acute lung injury; ARDS, acute respiratory distress syndrome; conventional study group receiving mechanical ventilation with higher tidal volume; protective, study group receiving mechanical ventilation with low tidal volume; n.s., differences not statistically significant; PEEP, positive end-expiratory pressure; PBW, predicted body weight.

exactly what level of PEEP should be used has remained a contentious issue for decades.

Open lung studies by Amato et al.[12] and Villar et al.[15] used the lower inflection point of the volume–pressure curve to estimate the critical opening pressure of the lung; this point was used to determine the best PEEP (Table 30-3). Although higher PEEP was administered in their study groups than in their controls (13.2 vs. 9.3 cm H_2O, and 14.1 vs. 9.0 cm H_2O, respectively), there was also significant variance in tidal volumes, and outcome benefits may have derived from low stretch rather than higher PEEP. Three large multicenter randomized controlled trials (RCTs) addressed the question of high versus low PEEP in the setting of a low stretch ventilation strategy (Table 30-3).[16-18] In both the ALVEOLI (Assessment of Low Tidal Volume and Elevated End-Expiratory Volume to Obviate Lung Injury) trial[16] and the Lung Open Ventilation Study (LOVS),[17] PEEP was determined according to higher and lower PEEP-FIO_2 (fraction of inspired oxygen) tables, whereas the ExPress trial compared lower levels of PEEP (5 to 9 cm H_2O) with higher levels set to achieve a plateau pressure of 28 cm H_2O.[18] In keeping with the original open-lung approach, the LOVS trial also used RMs.

The ALVEOLI and ExPress trials were stopped early because of a perceived low likelihood of achieving nominal statistical significance (futility). Outcomes in ALVEOLI were significantly better than expected, and it is likely that overrecruitment of patients with less severe ARDS (or atelectasis) may have resulted in an underpowered study. Although there were no mortality benefits reported, principally because rescue therapy was used in refractory hypoxemia in LOVS and ExPress, secondary data—such as number of ventilator-free days and duration of hospital stay—favored the high PEEP approach. These data were

subsequently systematically reviewed by Briel and colleagues,[19] who showed that, among patients with "moderate to severe ARDS," higher PEEP was associated with a clinically and statistically significant reduction in mortality (hazard ratio [95% confidence interval] of 0.85 [0.73 to 99], $P = .03$). Rates of pneumothorax and vasopressor use were similar. Although the numbers were too small to achieve statistical significance, higher PEEP in patients without ARDS (n = 404) may have resulted in excess hospital deaths.

A Cochrane Collaborative Systematic Review[19a] evaluated seven studies that compared high versus low levels of PEEP (2565 patients). In five of the studies, in most patients (2417), high versus low PEEP levels were used with the same tidal volumes. Only three studies were considered suitable for meta-analysis. There was no difference in hospital mortality outcomes (relative risk [RR] 0.9; confidence interval [CI], 0.81 to 1.01), barotrauma, or the number of ventilator-free days. Oxygenation was better in patients with higher levels of PEEP.

In conclusion, PEEP is an essential component of a mechanical ventilation strategy in ARDS. There is no widely accepted method of achieving optimal PEEP. Studies to date have used a FIO_2-PEEP stepladder or the supersyringe method to set PEEP. To date, no large randomized controlled trial that compared high versus low PEEP with a low stretch tidal volume approach has demonstrated improved outcomes. We recommend a conservative (low to moderate) PEEP strategy in ARDS.

LUNG RECRUITMENT MANEUVERS

An RM refers to the dynamic process of reopening collapsed alveoli through an intentional transient increase

Table 30-3 Randomized Trials of Open Lung Strategies (No Confounding Interventions)

A. SUMMARY OF STUDY PATIENTS AND INTERVENTIONS

Study	n	Patients	PEEP	Mode	RMs	P_{plat}
ALVEOLI[16]	549	$Pao_2/Fio_2 < 300$				
Open lung			High (PEEP/Fio_2 chart)	AC	No	≤30 cm H_2O
Control			low (PEEP/Fio_2 chart)	AC	No	≤30 cm H_2O
LOVS[35]	983	$Pao_2/Fio_2 < 250$				
Open lung			High (PEEP/Fio_2 chart)	PC	Yes	≤40 cm H_2O
Control			low (PEEP/Fio_2 chart)	AC	No	≤30 cm H_2O
ExPress[36]	767	$Pao_2/Fio_2 < 300$				
Open lung			To keep P_{plat} 30 cm H_2O	AC	No	28-32 cm H_2O
Control			5-12 cm H_2O	AC	No	≤32 cm H_2O

B. SUMMARY OF METHODOLOGICAL FEATURES

Study	Random Intentionization	Baseline Stopped Differences	SIMILARITY IN OTHER Aspects of Care	To Treat	Early
ALVEOLI	Central	Age, by 5.5 years	V_t 6 mL/kg PBW	Yes	Yes
	Automated	(Lower control group)	Weaning		
LOVS	Central	Age, by 2 years	V_t 6 mL/kg PBW	Yes	No
	Automated	(Higher control group)	Weaning		
ExPress	Central	None	V_t 6 mL/kg PBW	Yes	Yes
	Automated		Weaning		

C. MORTALITY

Study Timing	Group Rates	Unadjusted RR (95% CI)	Adjusted RR (95% CI)
ALVEOLI			
Open lung Hospital	27.5%	1.11	0.91
Control	24.9%	(0.84-1.46)	(0.69-1.20)
LOVS			
Open lung Hospital	36.4%	0.90	0,97
Control	40.4%	(0.77-1.05)	(0.84-1.12)
EXPRESS			
Open lung 28 days	27.8%	0.89	N/A
Control	31.2%	(0.72-111)	

AC, assist control; CI, cardiac index; Fio_2, fraction of inspired oxygen; N/A, not applicable; Pao_2, partial pressure of arterial oxygen; PBW, predicted body weight; PC, pressure control; PEEP, positive end-expiratory pressure; Pplat, plateau pressure; RM, recruitment maneuver; RR, relative risk; V_t, low tidal volume.

in transpulmonary pressure. This recruitment effect can be achieved through a variety of methods, the most common of which is probably the sustained inspiratory hold at 30 to 45 cm H_2O for 30 to 40 seconds. An RM may also be performed with a stepwise increase in PEEP with low levels of controlled ventilation in a sedated and paralyzed patient. Decreasing PEEP in a titrated fashion can maintain lung opening and identify the point of derecruitment by the change in compliance or oxygenation. RMs appear to improve oxygenation at least in the short term in most patients and are regarded as an essential part of rescue strategies for refractory hypoxemia. However the optimal pressure, duration, and frequency of such RMs are yet to be determined.[20-22] It is important to note that adverse events such as transient hypotension, barotrauma, and dysrrhythmia are well described, and care should be taken in patients with unilateral lung injury.[27] A Cochrane Systematic Review, in 2009[26] showed no difference in outcomes, either positive or negative, associated with RMs.

No clinical trial has demonstrated that routine use of RMs, independent of mechanical ventilation strategy, improves outcomes. However, in specific patients, whose lungs may derecruit after, for example, ventilator disconnection, airway plugging, and coughing, RMs improve oxygenation and ventilation.[28-30] Indeed, in moderate to severe ARDS meta-analysis has suggested a reduction in hospital mortality of 6% in patients who received routine RMs.[29] There are currently no data that RMs reduce the duration of mechanical ventilation, length of stay, or rate of barotrauma. A number of trials are currently underway that may resolve the issue of the use of RMs. The PHARLAP (Permissive Hypercapnia, Alveolar Recruitment and Limited Airway Pressure) trial has published a pilot study of its first 20 patients.[31] This study combines an open lung strategy with staircase recruitment maneuvers. PEEP is adjusted to a maximum of 40 cm H_2O during pressure-controlled ventilation. After recruitment, PEEP is slowly lowered by 2.5 cm H_2O decrements from 25 cm H_2O. This decreasing PEEP trial is performed to determine optimal PEEP—with the derecruitment point being identified by the surrogate: a decrease of SpO_2 (oxygen saturation by pulse oximetry). The lung is then rerecruited with a pressure of 40 cm H_2O, and the PEEP is set at the identified optimum. Hypercapnia is tolerated to a pH of 7.15. This pilot study has demonstrated a reduction in the amount of systemic cytokines and an increase in lung compliance using this strategy. A larger phase 2 trial is now underway (http://clinicaltrials.gov/ct2/show/NCT01667146).

Another trial in progress is the ART trial, which also uses a method of stepwise alveolar recruitment.[32] The maximum target PEEP is 40 cm H_2O and maximum peak airway pressure is 60 cm H_2O. The optimal PEEP is determined by static compliance measurement during decreasing PEEP titration. The control arm is managed with the protective ventilation strategy and PEEP table of the original ARDS Network trial.[13] Preliminary findings report that the strategy is feasible, and both groups have similar adverse event profiles. The results of these studies may determine the use of ARM in the future and influence the way we determine PEEP settings.

In conclusion, the routine use of RMs is not supported by clinical evidence. RMs should only be used in situations of potentially catastrophic hypoxemia.

PRESSURE VERSUS VOLUME-CONTROLLED VENTILATION IN ARDS

To date, most multicenter trials that have addressed mechanical ventilation strategies in ARDS have used volume-controlled (though pressure limited) ventilation (VCV). Outside of randomized trials, many centers use pressure-controlled ventilation (PCV) or one of its offshoots, such as bilevel CPAP (continuous positive airway pressure) (with or without spontaneous breathing), inverse ratio ventilation, or pressure-regulated volume control.[30,31] The choice of mechanical ventilation mode is physician dependent, and the literature offers us little guidance as to which mode, if any, is superior. It is known that lower driving pressures (ΔP) are associated with better outcomes in ARDS; the onus on the clinician, using pressure control, is to reduce the ΔP as compliance improves.[32] This is not required in VCV. A 2015 Cochrane collaboration systematic review[33] of VCV versus PCV included only three RCTs that included a total of 1089 patients.[33] Data on barotrauma and mortality were included. One study looked at 28-day mortality, and there was no evidence any specific ventilatory mode reduced mortality at 28 days (RR, 0.88; 95% CI, 0.73 to 1.06; 983 participants; moderate-quality evidence). With regard to in hospital mortality, the RR with PCV compared with VCV was 0.83 (95% CI, 0.67 to 1.02; not significant). Where intensive care unit (ICU) mortality was reported (two trials, 1062 patients), the RR with PCV compared with VCV was 0.84 (95% CI, 0.71 to 0.99; not significant).

It is unlikely that a difference exists in outcomes between PCV and VCV. It is essential that clinicians understand that a low stretch mechanical ventilation strategy involves both volume and pressure limitations. Volume-limited modes risk excessive plateau pressure; pressure-limited modes risk excessive tidal volumes. It is likely that rigorous attention to detail is more important than the mode of ventilation used. For example, two trials, conducted principally in the United Kingdom more than a decade after the publication of the ARDSNet ARMA trial, revealed baseline tidal volumes of >8 mL/kg in both treatment groups.[34,36] Failure to adhere to tidal volume targets appears to be endemic, even in the best academic medical centers. A prospective cohort trial of 520 patients with acute hypoxic respiratory failure at 12 ICUs in four University Medical Centers in Baltimore, between 2004 and 2007, evaluated mechanical ventilation strategy twice daily during the acute phase and followed up patients for 2 years.[35] In total, 485 patients contributed data. Of these patients, 311 (64%) died within 2 years. After several adjustments were made, each additional ventilator setting adherent to lung protective ventilation was associated with a 3% decrease in the risk of mortality over 2 years (hazard ratio, 0.97, 95% confidence interval, 0.95 to 0.99, $P = .002$). Thirty-seven percent of patients never received low tidal volume ventilation. Compared with these nonadherent patients, the estimated absolute risk reduction in 2 year mortality for a prototypical patient with 50% adherence to lung protective ventilation was 4.0% (0.8% to 7.2%; $P = .012$) and with 100% adherence was 7.8% (1.6% to 14.0%; $P = .011$).

In conclusion there are no published data to support the superiority of VCV over PCV or vice versa. Noncompliance with tidal volume standards is alarmingly common and arguably more likely with PCV.

HIGH FREQUENCY VENTILATION

High frequency ventilation is defined as mechanical ventilation with higher than normal breathing frequencies: in practice, between 100 and 600 breaths per minute. There are two types of high frequency ventilators used in clinical practice: jet ventilators, used in airway surgery, and oscillators, used in ICUs.

There has been considerable interest in the past 15 years in the use of high frequency oscillation ventilation (HFOV) in the management of ARDS, as part of the open lung approach. HFOV is unique in mechanical ventilation in that expiration and inspiration are active, as an oscillating diaphragm produces a sinusoidal airflow from a continuous pressurized circuit. Tidal volumes generated with HFOV are typically 1 to 2 mL/kg and are delivered at rates of 3 to 15 Hz (180 to 900 breaths per minute).[37] Theoretically, HFOV is ideal for lung protection as incremental alveolar stretch during inspiration is minimal, and clinicians can set the mean airway pressure on HFOV significantly higher than they are able to set PEEP on conventional ventilation. Hypothetically, this can minimize cyclical collapse (atelectrauma), while simultaneously avoiding very high inspiratory pressures (barotrauma) and lung stretch (volutrauma). HFOV represents full vital capacity mechanical ventilation—on the expiratory limb of the volume-pressure curve. Once HFOV is commenced, ventilation-perfusion mismatch and shunt typically improve. One would expect that these apparent advantages would facilitate ventilation within the "safe window" of lung protection.

On the basis of impressive anecdotal reports and positive outcomes in neonates, HFOV became widely used in the 2000s, when it was used principally as rescue therapy in severe ARDS. Two small RCTs appeared to demonstrate the safety of HFOV but were underpowered to detect outcome differences.[25,38]

Two major multicenter trials investigating the role of HFOV in moderate to severe ARDS have now been published. The OSCILLATE trial, an international study led by members of the Canadian Critical Care Trials Group,[39] studied the use of HFOV in early, moderate to severe ARDS Pao_2/Fio_2 ratio ≤200 mm Hg) compared with conventional, protective ventilation management. Patients were randomized to HFOV or pressure-controlled ventilation (at 6 mL/kg, although volume control and pressure support could also be used). The HFOV patients received a recruitment maneuver and then underwent HFOV at a mean airway pressure of 30 cm H_2O, which was adjusted to keep the Pao_2 (partial pressure of arterial oxygen) between 55 and 80 mm Hg. The study was terminated early, following interim analysis. Of the originally planned 1200 patient cohort, 548 patients were recruited. In-hospital mortality was 47% in the HFOV group versus 35% in the conventional ventilation (CV)—an absolute risk increase of 12% (number needed to injure 8, $P = .005$). The 28 day mortality rate was 40% versus 29% (HFOV vs. CV) (RR, 1.41 [1.12 to 1.79]; $P = .004$). Patients who received HFOV were more likely treated with neuromuscular blockade and vasopressors and received higher doses of sedatives compared with controls. Of note, 12% of patients in the CV group were treated with HFOV.

The OSCAR study (n = 798) was conducted simultaneously in the United Kingdom,[36] and involved a similar population of patients. Patients receiving HFOV in this study were started at a mean airway pressure 5 cm H_2O above their baseline. Patients in the CV group were administered PCV at targeted tidal volumes of <6 mL/kg. The investigators reported a 30 day mortality rate of 41.7% in the HFOV group and 41.1% in the conventional ventilation group ($P = .85$ by the chi-square test). Mortality increased to 48.4% (HFOV) and 48.4% (CV) (not significant) at first hospital discharge. There did not appear to be any differences between the groups in terms of vasopressor support or fluid administration. Although equipoise may be apparent from these data, it is unclear whether the "conventional" group truly had a lung protective ventilator strategy (6 mL/kg, P_{plat}<30 cm H_2O) because baseline tidal volumes were >8 mL/kg in both groups and the plateau pressure in the CV group was the same on days 1 to 3. The PROSEVA trial,[40] published subsequently, looked at conventional low stretch ventilation with or without prone positioning. The 28 day mortality was 16.0% in the prone group and 32.8% in the conventional group ($P < .001$). The severity of illness and oxygenation index was comparable to the control group in the OSCAR trial, with substantially better outcomes.

It is unclear why the HFOV trials failed. The relatively high mean airway pressures may have been associated with increased regional overdistension and VILI. Alternatively, increased intrathoracic pressures may have resulted in hypotension, right ventricular dysfunction, fluid overload, hypoperfusion, and multiple organ dysfunction syndrome (MODS).

In the intermediate term, we cannot recommend the use of HFOV in early ARDS. Alternative strategies such as neuromuscular blockade[41] and prone positioning[40] should be used first. HFOV may have a role as a rescue therapy or as a bridge to extracorporeal membrane oxygenation (ECMO), but this is based on anecdote (improved oxygenation), rather than evidence.

In conclusion, on the basis of current evidence, HFOV should not be used as a primary mechanical ventilation mode in ARDS, and its use as rescue therapy should be reserved until after proven strategies have been exhausted.

PRONE POSITIONING

Patient positioning, in addition to careful mechanical ventilation, results in better outcomes in patients with severe ARDS. It has been observed that in a significant proportion of patients with ARDS, ventilating in the prone position can induce transient or sustained improvement in oxygenation by 20% to 30%. Prone positioning is attractive because it requires no special equipment—only a coordinated ICU team. Initial multicentered trials involving more than a thousand patients with ARDS tested the hypothesis that prone positioning for 6[10] or 8 hours[9] per day for 10 days would enhance survival. Both trials demonstrated that prone positioning significantly improved oxygen tension each day, but there was no difference in mortality at ICU days 10 and 28, or after 6 months. A 2006 meta-analysis suggested a survival benefit for prone positioning in patients with more severe lung injury.[42] This prompted the PROSEVA investigators,[40] in France, to undertake a multicenter trial of prone positioning for 16 hours per day in severely hypoxemic patients (PF ratio, 100 mm Hg±30). Patients received VCV with constant inspiratory flow, with tidal volume targeted at 6 mL per kilogram of predicted body weight and the PEEP level selected from a PEEP-Fio_2 table. Members of the intervention group were turned prone, if tolerated, for 16 hours per day; on average

4 times in total. There was a substantial 28 day mortality benefit (16% vs. 33%; ARR, 17%; NNT, 6; $P < .001$) for patients undergoing this intervention. These data provide the lowest reported mortality rate at 28 days in ARDS. Patients in the prone group were less likely to receive rescue therapy with inhaled nitric oxide, required less oxygen and PEEP, and had lower airway pressures than patients kept supine. Proned patients were more likely to be successfully extubated and had significantly fewer cardiac arrests, overall. These benefits likely resulted from reduced incidence of VILI.

In conclusion, prone positioning should be considered a "standard of care" in patients with severe (PF ratio of <150 mm Hg) ARDS. Currently no data exist to support prone positioning in patients with mild to moderate hypoxemia.

NEUROMUSCULAR BLOCKADE

Spontaneous ventilation in the early acute phase of ARDS may improve overall oxygenation but results in greater transpulmonary pressure and, potentially, higher end-inspiratory lung volumes despite apparently "safe" levels of plateau pressure. Deep sedation and neuromuscular blockade, early in ARDS, ensure tighter control of tidal ventilation and airway pressure. Papazian and colleagues,[42] demonstrated that early, short-term use of neuromuscular blockade in severe ARDS (PF ratio, <150 mm Hg) reduced adjusted 90-day mortality (hazard ratio for death at 90 days was 0.68; CI, 0.48 to 0.98; $P = .04$) and mechanical ventilation days, without an associated increase in ICU-acquired weakness.[43] These data were confirmed by a subsequent systematic review.[58] In conclusion, in addition to a low stretch mechanical ventilation strategy, early and limited duration use of neuromuscular blockade may improve outcomes in ARDS.

AIRWAY PRESSURE RELEASE VENTILATION IN ARDS

Airway pressure release ventilation (APRV) is a form of extreme inverse ratio ventilation that inverts the respiratory cycle such that the baseline airway pressure (high CPAP) is set at a high level: typically 25 to 40 cm H_2O. A very short expiratory time (usually <0.8 seconds) is used to "release" pressure, tidally ventilate, and expel carbon dioxide. On modern mechanical ventilators, an active expiratory "flutter" valve is used to facilitate spontaneous ventilation, even at high lung volumes. Used in this manner, APRV is analogous to CPAP, albeit at a high pressure level, with occasional (6 to 8 per minute) pressure releases. APRV is widely used as a rescue therapy in ARDS,[30,46] although its use is not supported by randomized controlled trials.

Mandatory breaths during mechanical ventilation preferentially ventilate the anterior apical segments of the lung, and this may lead to progressive derecruitment of the posterior dorsal segments. Spontaneous breathing during APRV redistributes ventilation and aeration to dependent, usually well-perfused, juxtadiaphragmatic lung regions, resulting in improved arterial oxygenation.[47]

Putensen and colleagues[48] randomized 24 patients to receive APRV and PSV with equal airway pressure limits (Paw) (n=12) or minute ventilation (VE) (n=12). In both groups spontaneous breathing during APRV was associated with increases ($P < .05$) in right ventricular end-diastolic volume, stroke volume, CI, PaO_2, oxygen delivery (DO_2), and mixed venous oxygen tension (PvO_2) and with reductions ($P < .05$) in pulmonary vascular resistance and oxygen extraction. Subsequently, Putensen and colleagues[49] studied 30 trauma patients who were randomized either to breathe spontaneously with APRV (APRV group) (n=15) or to receive PCV for 72hours followed by weaning with APRV (PCV group) (n=15). Absence of spontaneous breathing (PCV group) was induced with sufentanil and midazolam (Ramsay sedation score [RSS] of 5) and neuromuscular blockade. Primary use of APRV was associated with increased ($P < .05$) respiratory system compliance, arterial oxygen tension (PaO_2), CI, and DO_2, and with reductions ($P < .05$) in right to left shunt venous admixture (QVA/QT), and oxygen extraction. Primary use of APRV was also associated with a shorter duration of ventilatory support, reduced sedation, and length of ICU stay.

Is APRV the optimal mode of mechanical ventilation in ARDS? It is important to stress that APRV has not been subjected to large scale randomized controlled investigation. Most of the clinical and experimental data have come from a single group in Germany. The scientific rationale for APRV is similar to that of HFOV, enthusiasm for which has cooled significantly since the OSCILLATE (Oscillation for ARDS Treated Early) trial.[49] Similar to HFOV, oxygenation improves, sometimes spectacularly, with APRV, but no data exist that demonstrate a mortality benefit. End-inspiratory lung volumes, when augmented with spontaneous breaths, cannot be measured or estimated. Release volumes frequently exceed 6 mL/kg and, if expiratory times are too long, atelectrauma may be an issue. Many of the potential benefits of APRV with spontaneous ventilation can be achieved with prone positioning, at lower mean airway pressures, with compelling outcome data.[40] Moreover, spontaneous breathing, in early ARDS, is not currently recommended, on the basis of the data from the ACURYSYS study.[41] It is unclear whether any real benefit exists if a patient ventilated with APRV is given neuromuscular blockade. Sedation regimens have improved significantly since the late 1990s/early 2000s, when these studies were performed.

In conclusion, we would recommend against using APRV as primary mechanical ventilation strategy in ARDS until outcomes data become available. Like HFOV, APRV continues to have a role as rescue therapy (after prone positioning) or as a bridge to ECMO.

SUMMARY

Ventilatory strategies that minimize damage to the lung are essential for reducing the morbidity and mortality from acute respiratory distress syndrome. There is strong evidence that the manner in which ARDS patients undergo ventilation has a large impact on their mortality. Limiting tidal volumes and inspiratory pressures are fundamental tenets of lung protection, along with at least low-moderate levels of PEEP. Attempts to open the lung with higher levels of PEEP with or without recruitment maneuvers may be beneficial in patients with moderate-severe ARDS. Neuromuscular blockade, early in ARDS, and prone positioning for severe hypoxemia appear to improve outcomes. There is likely no difference in outcome between VCV and PCV, but alternative modes, such as HFOV and APRV, should be used with caution, and only as rescue therapy.

AUTHORS' RECOMMENDATIONS

- Ventilator-associated lung injury is an important contributor to mortality in patients with ARDS.
- The current standard of mechanical ventilation care for most patients with ARDS involves setting tidal volumes at < 6 mL/kg and plateau pressure below 30 cm H_2O.
- PEEP is an essential component of mechanical ventilation strategy in ARDS. There is no widely accepted method of achieving optimal PEEP. There is no clear evidence that high versus low PEEP improves outcomes in ARDS.
- The routine use of RMs is not supported by clinical evidence. RMs should only be used in situations of potentially catastrophic hypoxemia.
- There are no published data to support the superiority of VCV over PCV or vice versa. Noncompliance with tidal volume standards is alarmingly common.
- HFOV should not be used as a primary mechanical ventilation mode in ARDS, and its use as rescue therapy should be reserved until after proven strategies have been exhausted.
- Prone positioning should be considered a standard of care in patients with severe (PF ratio of <150 mm Hg) ARDS. Currently no data exist to support prone positioning in patients with mild to moderate hypoxemia.
- Early and limited duration use of neuromuscular blockade may improve outcomes in ARDS.
- APRV is not currently supported by outcomes data in ARDS, and its use should be limited to rescue therapy.

REFERENCES

1. Ashbaugh DG, Bigelow DB, Petty TL, Levine BE. Acute respiratory distress in adults. *The Lancet.* 1967;2:319–323.
2. Rubenfeld GD, et al. Incidence and outcomes of acute lung injury. *N Engl J Med.* 2005;353:1685–1693.
3. Herridge MS, et al. One-year outcomes in survivors of the acute respiratory distress syndrome. *N Engl J Med.* 2003;348:683–693.
4. Cheung AM, et al. Two-year outcomes, health care use, and costs of survivors of acute respiratory distress syndrome. *Am J Respir Crit Care Med.* 2006;174:538–544.
5. Rouby JJ, et al. Histologic aspects of pulmonary barotrauma in critically ill patients with acute respiratory failure. *Intensive Care Med.* 1993;19:383–389.
6. Webb HH, Tierney DF. Experimental pulmonary edema due to intermittent positive pressure ventilation with high inflation pressures. Protection by positive end-expiratory pressure. *Am Rev Respir Dis.* 1974;110:556–565.
7. Gattinoni L, Caironi P, Pelosi P, Goodman LR. What has computed tomography taught us about the acute respiratory distress syndrome? *Am J Respir Crit Care Med.* 2001;164:1701–1711.
8. Gattinoni L, Pesenti A. The concept of "baby lung. *Intensive Care Med.* 2005;31:776–784.
9. Brochard L, et al. Tidal volume reduction for prevention of ventilator-induced lung injury in acute respiratory distress syndrome. The Multicenter Trail Group on Tidal Volume reduction in ARDS. *Am J Respir Crit Care Med.* 1998;158:1831–1838.
10. Stewart TE, et al. Evaluation of a ventilation strategy to prevent barotrauma in patients at high risk for acute respiratory distress syndrome. Pressure- and Volume-Limited Ventilation Strategy Group. *N Engl J Med.* 1998;338:355–361.
11. Brower RG, et al. Prospective, randomized, controlled clinical trial comparing traditional versus reduced tidal volume ventilation in acute respiratory distress syndrome patients. *Crit Care Med.* 1999;27:1492–1498.
12. Amato MB, et al. Effect of a protective-ventilation strategy on mortality in the acute respiratory distress syndrome. *N Engl J Med.* 1998;338:347–354.
13. Ventilation with lower tidal volumes as compared with traditional tidal volumes for acute lung injury and the acute respiratory distress syndrome. The Acute Respiratory Distress Syndrome Network. *N Engl J Med.* 2000;342:1301–1308.
14. Ferguson ND, et al. Airway pressures, tidal volumes, and mortality in patients with acute respiratory distress syndrome. *Crit Care Med.* 2005;33:21–30.
15. Villar J, Kacmarek RM, Pérez-Méndez L, Aguirre-Jaime A. A high positive end-expiratory pressure, low tidal volume ventilatory strategy improves outcome in persistent acute respiratory distress syndrome: a randomized, controlled trial. *Crit Care Med.* 2006;34:1311–1318.
16. Brower RG, et al. Higher versus lower positive end-expiratory pressures in patients with the acute respiratory distress syndrome. *N Engl J Med.* 2004;351:327–336.
17. Meade MO, et al. Ventilation strategy using low tidal volumes, recruitment maneuvers, and high positive end-expiratory pressure for acute lung injury and acute respiratory distress syndrome: a randomized controlled trial. *JAMA.* 2008;299:637–645.
18. Mercat A, et al. Positive end-expiratory pressure setting in adults with acute lung injury and acute respiratory distress syndrome: a randomized controlled trial. *JAMA.* 2008;299:646–655.
19. Briel M, et al. Higher vs lower positive end-expiratory pressure in patients with acute lung injury and acute respiratory distress syndrome: systematic review and meta-analysis. *JAMA.* 2010;303:865–873.
19a. Santa Cruz R, et al. High versus low positive end-expiratory pressure (PEEP) levels for mechanically ventilated adult patients with acute lung injury and acute respiratory distress syndrome. *Cochrane Database Syst Rev.* 2013 Jun 6;6: CD009098.
20. Brower RG, et al. Effects of recruitment maneuvers in patients with acute lung injury and acute respiratory distress syndrome ventilated with high positive end-expiratory pressure. *Crit Care Med.* 2003;31:2592–2597.
21. Foti G, et al. Effects of periodic lung recruitment maneuvers on gas exchange and respiratory mechanics in mechanically ventilated acute respiratory distress syndrome (ARDS) patients. *Intensive Care Med.* 2000;26:501–507.
22. Dreyfuss D, Soler P, Basset G, Saumon G. High inflation pressure pulmonary edema. Respective effects of high airway pressure, high tidal volume, and positive end-expiratory pressure. *Am Rev Respir Dis.* 1988;137:1159–1164.
23. Fan E, et al. Complications from recruitment maneuvers in patients with acute lung injury: secondary analysis from the lung open ventilation study. *Respir Care.* 2012;57:1842–1849.
24. Fan E, et al. Recruitment maneuvers for acute lung injury: a systematic review. *Am J Respir Crit Care Med.* 2008;178:1156–1163.
25. Suzumura EA, et al. Effects of alveolar recruitment maneuvers on clinical outcomes in patients with acute respiratory distress syndrome: a systematic review and meta-analysis. *Intensive Care Med.* 2014;40:1227–1240.
26. Hodgson C, et al. Recruitment maneuvers for adults with acute lung injury receiving mechanical ventilation. *Cochrane Database Syst Rev.* 2009:CD006667. http://dx.doi.org/10.1002/14651858. CD006667.pub2.
27. Hodgson CL, et al. A randomised controlled trial of an open lung strategy with staircase recruitment, titrated PEEP and targeted low airway pressures in patients with acute respiratory distress syndrome. *Crit Care.* 2011;15:R133.
28. ART Investigators. Rationale, study design, and analysis plan of the Alveolar Recruitment for ARDS Trial (ART): study protocol for a randomized controlled trial. *Trials.* 2012;13:153.
29. Claesson J, et al. *Acta Anaesthetesiol Scand.* March 2015;59(3): 286–297.

30. Kredel M, et al. Therapy of acute respiratory distress syndrome : Survey of German ARDS centers and scientific evidence. *Anaesthesist*. April 2015;64(4):277–285.
31. Sharma NS et al. Use of ECMO in the Management of Severe Acute Respiratory Distress Syndrome: A Survey of Academic Medical Centers in the United States. *ASAIO J*. 2015;61:556–563.
32. Amato MBP, et al. Driving Pressure and Survival in the Acute Respiratory Distress Syndrome. *N Engl J Med*. 2015;372:747–755.
33. Chacko B, et al. Pressure-controlled versus volume-controlled ventilation for acute respiratory failure due to acute lung injury (ALI) or acute respiratory distress syndrome (ARDS). *Cochrane Database Syst Rev*. January 14, 2015;1:CD008807. http://dx.doi.org/10.1002/14651858.CD008807.pub2.
34. McAuley DF, et al. Simvastatin in the Acute Respiratory Distress Syndrome. Harp-2. *N Engl J Med*. 2014;371:1695–1703.
35. Needham DM, et al. Lung protective mechanical ventilation and two year survival in patients with acute lung injury: prospective cohort study. *BMJ*. 2012;344:e2124.
36. Young D, et al. High-Frequency Oscillation for Acute Respiratory Distress Syndrome. *N Engl J Med*. 2013;368:806–813.
37. Hickling KG, Henderson SJ, Jackson R. Low mortality associated with low volume pressure limited ventilation with permissive hypercapnia in severe adult respiratory distress syndrome. *Intensive Care Med*. 1990;16:372–377.
38. Tremblay L, Valenza F, Ribeiro SP, Li J, Slutsky AS. Injurious ventilatory strategies increase cytokines and c-fos m-RNA expression in an isolated rat lung model. *J Clin Invest*. 1997;99:944–952.
39. Ferguson ND, et al. High-frequency oscillation in early acute respiratory distress syndrome. *N Engl J Med*. 2013;368:795–805.
40. Guérin C, et al. Prone positioning in severe acute respiratory distress syndrome. *N Engl J Med*. June 6, 2013;368(23):2159–2168.
41. Sud S, et al. Prone ventilation reduces mortality in patients with acute respiratory failure and severe hypoxemia: systematic review and meta-analysis. *Intensive Care Med*. 2010;36:585–599.
42. Papazian L, et al. Neuromuscular blockers in early acute respiratory distress syndrome. *N Engl J Med*. 2010;363:1107–1116.
43. Ware LB, Matthay MA. The acute respiratory distress syndrome. *N Engl J Med*. 2000;342:1334–1349.
44. Hudson LD, Milberg JA, Anardi D, Maunder RJ. Clinical risks for development of the acute respiratory distress syndrome. *Am J Respir Crit Care Med*. 1995;151:293–301.
45. Alhazzani W, et al. Neuromuscular blocking agents in acute respiratory distress syndrome: a systematic review and meta-analysis of randomized controlled trials. *Crit Care*. 2013;17:R43.
46. González M, et al. Airway pressure release ventilation versus assist-control ventilation: a comparative propensity score and international cohort study. *Intensive Care Med*. May 2010;36(5):817–827.
47. Wrigge H, Zinserling J, Neumann P, et al. Spontaneous breathing improves lung aeration in oleic acid-induced lung injury. *Anesthesiology*. 2003;99:376–384.
48. Putensen C, Mutz NJ, Putensen-Himmer G, Zinserling J. Spontaneous breathing during ventilatory support improves ventilation-perfusion distributions in patients with acute respiratory distress syndrome. *Am J Respir Crit Care Med*. April 1999;159(4 Pt 1): 1241–1248.
49. Putensen C, Zech S, Wrigge H, et al. Long-term effects of spontaneous breathing during ventilatory support in patients with acute lung injury. *Am J Respir Crit Care Med*. 2001;164:43–49.

31 Is Permissive Hypercapnia Useful in ARDS?

Maya Contreras, Claire Masterson, John G. Laffey

Traditional approaches to the carbon dioxide (CO_2) management of adults with acute respiratory failure have focused on the potential for hypercapnia to exert deleterious effects. Support for this paradigm is derived from the association between hypercapnia and adverse outcome in diverse clinical contexts, including cardiac arrest, sepsis, and neonatal asphyxia. However, this approach has been increasingly questioned, particularly in the setting of acute severe respiratory failure. Accumulating evidence from experimental[1,2] and clinical[3-6] studies clearly demonstrates that high-stretch mechanical ventilation can directly injure the lungs, a phenomenon termed *ventilator-induced lung injury.* Mechanical ventilation strategies that reduce the intensity of mechanical ventilation, resulting in a respiratory acidosis termed *permissive hypercapnia* (PHC), improve outcome.[3,4] Consequently, PHC has been progressively accepted in critical care for patients requiring mechanical ventilation. Conventionally, the protective effect of ventilatory strategies incorporating PHC is considered to be due solely to reduction in lung stretch, with hypercapnia "permitted" to achieve this goal. However, CO_2 is a potent biologic agent with the potential to exert beneficial and harmful effects. Furthermore, it is possible to minimize the potential for hypercapnia in the context of low-stretch ventilatory strategies by manipulating the respiratory frequency or by incorporating extracorporeal CO_2 removal (ECCO$_2$R) technologies.[7,8] Therefore it is important to fully understand the biologic effects of hypercapnia in the critically ill.[9] To address these issues, we examine the physiologic effects of hypercapnia, insights that have emerged from studies of hypercapnic acidosis (HCA) in preclinical models, and data from clinical studies.

PHYSIOLOGY AND MOLECULAR BIOLOGY OF HYPERCAPNIA

Respiratory System

HCA improves oxygenation by reducing ventilation-perfusion ($\dot{V}/\dot{Q}$) heterogeneity.[10-12] HCA increases parenchymal lung compliance by enhancing alveolar surfactant secretion and function[13] and by inhibiting actin-myosin interactions.[14] Although, HCA can increase pulmonary vascular resistance and worsen pulmonary hypertension (PH), recent laboratory data suggest that moderate hypercapnia attenuates structural and functional changes in the pulmonary vasculature and reverses impaired right ventricular function in preclinical models.[15-19] In acute respiratory distress syndrome (ARDS), PHC appears to increase shunt fraction because of a reduction in tidal volume (V_t) and airway closure rather than to hypercapnia per se.[20] Hypercapnia directly dilates small airways but also stimulates vagal-mediated large airway constriction with an overall minor net effect on airway resistance.[21,22] The impact of HCA on diaphragmatic function is controversial. HCA impairs diaphragmatic contractility and increases diaphragmatic fatigue in spontaneously breathing subjects.[23,24] In contrast, it restores diaphragmatic dysfunction induced by prolonged mechanical ventilation in experimental models when minute ventilation is controlled.[25] HCA also prevents myosin loss and inflammation in diaphragmatic tissue after prolonged ventilation.[26] The clinical impact of hypercapnia on diaphragmatic function, especially with regard to weaning from mechanical ventilation, has yet to be elucidated.

Cardiovascular System

The direct depressive effects of HCA on the cardiovascular system are counterbalanced by its stimulatory effects on the sympathetic nervous system. HCA directly reduces the contractility of cardiac[27] and vascular smooth muscle.[21] However, hypercapnia-mediated sympathoadrenal effects, including increased preload and heart rate, increased myocardial contractility, and decreased afterload, lead to a net increase in cardiac output.[21,28] Hypercapnia also results in a net increase in the partial pressure of oxygen in arterial blood (Pao$_2$) and increases global O_2 delivery by elevating cardiac output. Hypercapnia and acidosis shift the hemoglobin-O_2 dissociation curve rightward, reducing the O_2 affinity of hemoglobin, and may cause an elevation in hematocrit level,[29] further increasing tissue O_2 delivery. The concurrent reduced cellular respiration and O_2 consumption observed during acidosis may further improve O_2 supply-demand balance, particularly in the setting of compromised supply.[30]

Tissue Oxygenation

CO_2 increases the cardiac index by 10% to 15% by each 10 mm Hg of partial pressure of oxygen in arterial blood (Pao$_2$) increase[31,32] and consequently improves subcutaneous tissue O_2 tension and muscle tissue O_2 saturation.[31-35] In contrast, even a short period of hypocapnic alkalosis significantly reduces cardiac output, portal blood flow, gut perfusion, and O_2 delivery.[32,36] Although a small randomized study (n = 30), suggested that mild intraoperative hypercapnia improves colon tissue oxygenation in nonselected[34] and morbidly obese surgical patients,[35] this effect did not reduce surgical site infection in a large recent multicenter randomized controlled trial (RCT) (n = 1206) of patients undergoing colon surgery.[37]

Central Nervous System

Hypercapnia is a potent ventilatory stimulant. HCA improves cerebral tissue oxygenation by augmenting Pao_2 and cerebral blood flow (CBF).[38] HCA dilates precapillary cerebral arterioles, a function attributed to acidosis rather than hypercapnia per se.[39] Indeed, cerebral vascular reactivity to CO_2 measured by transcranial Doppler ultrasound may be used as a risk predictor for ischemic stroke.[40] HCA-mediated increases in CBF are a clear concern in the setting of reduced intracranial compliance in which increased global CBF may critically elevate intracranial pressure. Therefore traditional management of traumatic brain injury recommended sustained hypocapnia to reduce cerebral blood volume.[41] However, this technique has fallen out of favor as a result of concerns over hypocapnia-induced hypoperfusion, resulting in cerebral tissue ischemia, increased risk of vasospasm, neuronal excitability, and seizures.[42]

INTRACELLULAR MECHANISMS OF ACTION OF CARBON DIOXIDE

The molecular effects of hypercapnia—both beneficial and harmful—are increasingly well understood. Hypercapnia inhibits nuclear factor-κB (NF-κB), a key transcriptional protein regulating gene transcription in lung injury, inflammation, and repair via mechanisms that include reduced degradation of its cytosolic inhibitor, IκBα.[43] This mechanism protects the lung in the setting of ventilator-induced and ischemia-reperfusion–induced injury,[44,45] but it also delays pulmonary epithelial wound repair after injury.[46] Hypercapnia-mediated NF-κB inhibition may contribute to its immunosuppressive effects,[47,48] by decreasing NF-κB–dependent antimicrobial peptide gene expression in *Drosophila*,[49] and it decreases macrophage phagocytic activity and cytokine production.[50] These effects may reduce injury in early pulmonary[51-53] and systemic[54,55] sepsis but worsen injury in prolonged untreated pneumonia[47,48] in preclinical models.

Alveolar fluid clearance is an important step for the resolution of ARDS.[56] Recent data indicate that CO_2 may facilitate Na^+/K^+-ATPase (sodium-potassium adenosine triphosphatase) pump endocytosis—a key ion pump responsible for Na^+ and fluid shift across alveolar epithelial cells—and delays fluid absorption by activation of protein kinases C and A and extracellular signal-regulated kinase (ERK)–mediated mitogen-activated protein (MAP)–kinase pathways.[57-59]

Mechanical stretch has been shown to activate "shedding" of endogenous ligands, such as tumor necrosis factor receptor (TNFR), by metalloproteases (ADAM-17)[60] that upregulate the epidermal growth factor receptor (EGFR) pathway[61] and drive the inflammatory response. HCA inhibits shedding in stretch-induced lung injury, resulting in reduced activation of EGFR and P44/42 MAP-kinase pathways[62] (Fig. 31-1).

ROLE OF PERMISSIVE HYPERCAPNIA IN ADULT CRITICAL CARE

Acute Respiratory Distress Syndrome

The only therapeutic intervention to convincingly demonstrate a significant reduction in mortality in patients with ARDS and acute lung injury is lung-protective mechanical ventilation. The potential for protective lung ventilation strategies incorporating PHC to improve survival in patients with ARDS was suggested initially by Hickling and colleagues.[5,6] Of the subsequent five prospective randomized controlled trials of protective ventilatory strategies, two demonstrated an impact of ventilator strategy on mortality,[3,4] although three did not.[63-65] Although to some extent PHC developed in all of the trials, there was much variability (Table 31-1). Therefore, although it is clear that ventilation strategy can definitely affect mortality—in the positive trials—there is no discernible relationship between levels of CO_2 and survival among these data.

The database of the largest of these studies (ARMA)[3] has been subsequently analyzed to determine whether, in addition to the effect of V_t, there might also be an independent effect of HCA.[66] Mortality was examined as a function of PHC on the day of enrollment using multivariate analysis and controlling for other comorbidities and severity of lung injury. It was found that PHC reduced 28-day mortality in patients randomized to the higher V_t but not in those receiving lower V_t.[66] A recent pilot study including 20 ARDS patients compared the effectiveness of a new open lung ventilation strategy—a combination of PHC, staircase recruitment maneuvers, positive end-expiratory pressure (PEEP) titration, and targeted low plateau pressure—with lung-protective ventilation applied in the ARMA trial.[67] During the 7-day observation period of lung compliance, the Pao_2/Fio_2 (fraction of inspired oxygen) ratio was significantly better with the new open lung strategy. Of note, both ventilation strategies resulted in similar arterial CO_2 and pH values, suggesting that the observed benefits were more likely related to better lung recruitment than to PHC per se. Overall, although these clinical studies suggest that PHC may be beneficial in ARDS, they do not confirm it. Further appropriately designed randomized clinical studies are needed to elucidate the direct effect of PHC on acute lung injury.

Acute Severe Asthma

Controlled hypoventilation with PHC was first described in severe asthma by Darioli and Perret in 1984,[68] predating its described use in ARDS. PHC facilitates a reduction of dynamic hyperinflation during mechanical ventilation in acute severe asthma by increasing the expiratory time, reducing inspiratory flow rates and V_t.[69] Multiple reports exist of the successful use of PHC in severe asthma,[70] and modest levels of PHC (mean highest levels 62 mm Hg) are routinely used for patients in Europe[71] and North America[72] with acute severe asthma that requires assisted ventilation.

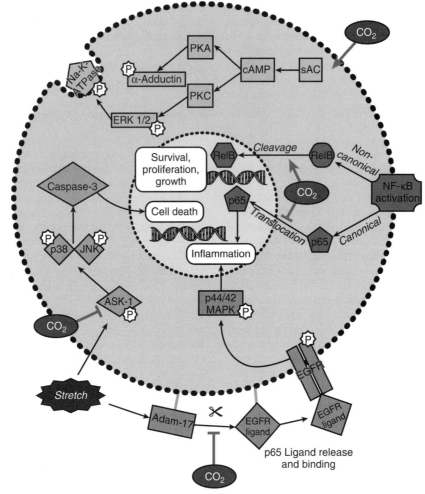

Figure 31-1. Potential molecular mechanisms of hypercapnia. Hypercapnia or acidosis inhibits nuclear factor-κB (*NF-κB*) signal transduction pathways at multiple levels. Hypercapnia prevents p65 translocation to the nucleus (canonical pathway) and reduces inflammatory gene expressions, whereas inhibition of RelB activation (noncanonical pathway) influences gene expressions responsible for survival, proliferation, and cell growth. Carbon dioxide (CO_2) activates soluble adenylate cyclase (*sAC*) and increases intracellular cyclic adenosine monophosphate (*cAMP*) levels, which in turn activate protein kinases (*PKA* and *PKC*). Phosphorylation of α-adductin and extracellular signal-regulated kinase (*ERK 1/2*) by PKA/C initiates the endocytosis of sodium-potassium adenosine triphosphatase (Na$^+$/K$^+$-ATPase), leading to reduced alveolar fluid transport. Mechanical stretch-induced inflammatory response and apoptosis are also inhibited by hypercapnia. Hypercapnia prevents shedding of TNFR by inhibiting metalloproteases (*ADAM-17*). This, in turn, leads to reduced activation of p44/42 mitogen-activated protein —kinase (*MAPK*) pathway–dependent inflammatory gene expression. Hypercapnia reduces cell death by inhibiting apoptosis signal-regulating kinase 1 (*ASK-1*) and intracellular caspase-3 activity. *EGFR*, epidermal growth factor receptor

Table 31-1 Ventilatory Strategies and Management of CO$_2$ in Clinical Trials

Trial	Mortality Benefit	Control Paco$_2$ (mm Hg, mean ± SD)	"Protective" Paco$_2$ (mm Hg, mean ± SD)	Buffering Permitted
ARDSnet Trial[3]	Yes	35.8 ± 8.0	40.0 ± 10.0	Yes
Amato et al.[4]	Yes	36.0 ± 1.5	58.0 ± 3.0	No
Stewart et al.[65]	No	46.0 ± 10.0	54.5 ± 15.0	No
Brochard et al.[63]	No	41.0 ± 7.5	59.5 ± 19.0	No
Brower et al.[64]	No	40.1 ± 1.6	50.3 ± 3.5	Yes

CO_2, carbon dioxide; Paco$_2$, partial pressure of carbon dioxide in arterial blood.

Chronic Obstructive Pulmonary Disease

Acute exacerbations of chronic obstructive pulmonary disease (COPD) result in diffuse airway narrowing, which increases airway resistance and respiratory workload, causing muscle fatigue and respiratory failure. Although noninvasive ventilation is the first-line ventilation strategy,[73] extreme respiratory muscle fatigue may necessitate invasive ventilation. The rationale for the use of PHC in COPD is similar to that for acute severe asthma (i.e., it can reduce dynamic hyperinflation).

ROLE OF PERMISSIVE HYPERCAPNIA IN PEDIATRIC CRITICAL CARE

Neonatal Respiratory Distress Syndrome

Acute respiratory failure in the preterm newborn is most commonly associated with sepsis and meconium aspiration. Ventilation strategies involving PHC are well tolerated and may lower the risk of chronic lung disease (CLD) in preterm infants.[74] In contrast, hypocapnia has been shown to be a strong prognostic factor for CLD in neonates.[75] Mariani et al.[76] demonstrated that PHC reduces the duration of ventilation support and speeds weaning from ventilation in preterm infants. A multicenter factorial trial of PHC and dexamethasone was stopped early because of unanticipated nonrespiratory adverse events related to dexamethasone therapy.[77] In the trial, there was a trend toward a lower incidence of death and CLD in the PHC group, and only 1% of the PHC group patients required mechanical ventilation at 36 weeks' gestational age compared with 16% in the normocapnia group.[77] A Danish study demonstrated that a ventilatory strategy incorporating PHC, nasal continuous positive airway pressure, and surfactant therapy reduced the incidence of CLD.[78] Of concern is the potential of severe hypercapnia to cause intracranial hemorrhage in premature infants. An early meta-analysis of PHC in newborn infants suggested that PHC may decrease the incidence of intracranial hemorrhage.[79] However, more severe hypercapnia (55 to 65 mm Hg) can worsen neurologic outcomes and increase the incidence of combined mental impairment and death compared with normocapnia.[80] Further research is needed to determine safe levels of hypercapnia to harness the beneficial and reduce the potentially harmful effects of PHC in preterm infants.

Congenital Diaphragmatic Hernia

Congenital diaphragmatic hernia (CDH) occurs in approximately 1 in every 3000 to 4000 births. Traditional approaches to CDH, which advocated aggressive control of PH with hyperventilation and alkalinization, have been largely abandoned because of concerns regarding increased mortality secondary to barotrauma.[81] PHC (60 to 80 mm Hg) ventilation strategies can reduce barotrauma to the hypoplastic lung,[82] and, in combination with delayed surgery, it increases survival and decreases the need for extracorporeal membrane oxygenation (ECMO) lower airway pressure ventilation.[83-87] Consequently, PHC strategies remain the standard of care for pediatric patients with CDH.

Persistent Pulmonary Hypertension of the Newborn

Persistent pulmonary hypertension (PPH) of the newborn is a clinical syndrome of multifactorial etiology characterized by hypoxemia secondary to elevated pulmonary vascular resistance and right-to-left shunting of blood across the foramen ovale and/or ductus arteriosus. Traditional management strategies, which emphasized the use of hyperventilation to decrease pulmonary arterial pressure, have been superseded by concerns regarding adverse neurologic outcomes with hypocapnia.[88-90] The safety of strategies limiting ventilator intensity, with resultant PHC, is supported by a number of relatively small clinical studies.[81,91,92] In one study of 40 infants, less aggressive ventilation increased the survival of the sickest infants with PPH from 17% to 90%.[91] Marron et al.[92] reported 100% survival, better neurologic outcome with reduced sensorineural deafness, and less CLD in a case series of 34 infants with severe PPH and severe respiratory failure at birth managed with PHC.

Congenital Heart Disease

Manipulation of arterial CO_2 tension has traditionally played an integral role in the management of patients with complex congenital heart defects. Impaired neurodevelopmental outcome remains the major cause of morbidity in survivors after heart surgery. In this regard, the potential of hypercapnia to improve brain and other systemic organ oxygenation is increasingly recognized. Licht et al.[93] have demonstrated that inspired CO_2 reverses the periventricular leukomalacia caused by low CBF in neonates with severe CHD. Hypercapnia increased cerebral oxygenation and mean arterial pressure in patients with hypoplastic left heart syndrome[94] and after cavopulmonary connection.[95] Hypoventilation improved systemic oxygenation after bidirectional superior cavopulmonary shunt, potentially via a hypercarbia-induced decrease in cerebral vascular resistance, thus increasing cerebral, superior vena caval, and pulmonary blood flow.[96] Finally, inspired CO_2 improved CBF and systemic oxygenation after cavopulmonary shunt.[97] Taken together, these studies raise the potential that inhaled CO_2 might have a future therapeutic role in this context.

CONTROVERSIES AND AREAS OF UNCERTAINTY

Permissive Hypercapnia and Intracranial Pressure Regulation

A key concern is the potential for hypercapnia to increase CBF and critically elevate intracranial pressure. Intracranial hypertension constitutes a relative rather than an absolute contraindication to PHC. Consideration should be given to the insertion of an intracranial pressure monitor or a jugular venous oximetry catheter because these can facilitate the gradual titration—or clearly avoidance—of PHC in a patient with a brain injury.

Permissive Hypercapnia and Pulmonary Vascular Resistance

Clinical conditions predisposing to PH are a relative rather than absolute contraindication to PHC. Where concerns exist regarding PH, a useful approach is to measure pulmonary pressures and accordingly titrate the degree of hypercapnia. In this context, monitoring with transthoracic echocardiography or placement of a pulmonary artery catheter may be indicated.

Permissive Hypercapnia and the Role of Buffering

Buffering of the acidosis induced by hypercapnia remains a common, albeit controversial, clinical practice. There is some evidence that the protective effects of HCA in ARDS are a function of the acidosis rather than elevated CO_2.[98,99] Buffering may simply ablate any protective effects of acidosis while not addressing the primary problem. Specific concerns exist regarding sodium bicarbonate ($NaHCO_3$), the buffer used most frequently in the clinical setting. Although the physiochemical effect of $NaHCO_3$ is to increase the strong ion difference, the net effect is the generation of CO_2. Hence, $NaHCO_3$ is an inappropriate therapy in patients with HCA. Tromethamine may be a better choice of buffer if available in situations in which buffering of HCA is considered.[100]

Extracorporeal Carbon Dioxide Removal

Recent advancements in technology have provided more widespread use of new-generation ECMO and selective $ECCO_2R$ devices in severe respiratory failure.[101] The rationale for integrating $ECCO_2R$ into the management of severe ARDS is to allow more protective ventilation (i.e., providing very low V_t with conventional mechanical ventilation while avoiding extreme levels of respiratory acidosis). A recent study suggested that at least one third of ARDS patients ventilated with lung-protective ventilation still have significant lung hyperinflation.[102] Terragni et al.[8] subsequently demonstrated in a small cohort of ARDS patients (n = 10) that application of $ECCO_2R$ can further reduce lung injury by allowing very low V_t ventilation (3.5 to 5 mL/kg). Most recently, Bein et al.[7] showed that combining $ECCO_2R$ with a very low V_t ventilation strategy in patients with established ARDS was safe. Importantly, a subset of patients with more severe hypoxemia had significantly more ventilator-free days when a combination of $ECCO_2R$ and very low V_t was used (40.9 vs. 28 days).

PERMISSIVE HYPERCAPNIA AT THE BEDSIDE: PRACTICAL ISSUES

Application of hypercapnia in the critically ill patient with severe respiratory failure requires several practical considerations. First, there is considerable evidence that patients generally tolerate HCA to pH values of 7.2 and even lower very well. The reported levels of $Paco_2$ and pH in the study of Hickling et al.[6] reflect reasonable initial goals ($Paco_2$: 67 mm Hg; mean pH, 7.2). However, a more useful approach is to individualize $Paco_2$ and pH goals in each patient, with great care required in settings where hypercapnia may have deleterious effects, such as the setting of combined lung and head injury.

Second, rapid induction of HCA in ARDS patients can have profound adverse hemodynamic effects. Therefore, when PHC is instituted, the degree of hypercapnia should be gradually titrated upward over a period of at least several hours until the ventilatory goals to minimize the potential for ventilator-induced lung injury have been achieved.

Third, in regard to altering the ventilatory strategy to produce PHC, the first priority in ARDS patients is to reduce V_t to reduce plateau pressures below 30 cm H_2O where possible. Tidal volumes should be reduced to 6 mL/kg ideal body weight (BW) and may need to be decreased further if plateau pressures remain unacceptably high.[3] It is important to remember that 30% of patients ventilated with the ARDSnet strategy still have significant hyperinflation; these patients may benefit from very low V_t ventilation (3 mL/kg ideal BW).[102] For the prevention of excessive hypercapnia and acidosis in these situations, or where there are specific concerns regarding hypercapnia, application of selective CO_2 removal by $ECCO_2R$ is an increasingly feasible option.[7]

Fourth, the effect of the disease process on the optimal ventilatory strategy must be considered. The management of ventilatory rate will differ in patients with ARDS compared with acute bronchial asthma or COPD. ARDS is characterized by a predominance of alveoli with short time constants due to low compliance with normal airway resistance. Therefore, it is possible to ventilate at relatively high ventilatory rates and to prolong inspiration to maintain oxygenation. Conversely, asthma or COPD is characterized by a predominance of alveoli with long time constants because of normal or elevated compliance with high airway resistance. In these patients, greater time is required for alveolar emptying in expiration to reduce the risk of auto-PEEP and dynamic hyperinflation. This is achieved by using lower respiratory rates and by prolonging expiration to allow complete alveolar emptying.

AUTHORS' RECOMMENDATIONS

- PHC is a common consequence of lung-protective ventilation that has been associated with improved outcome in ARDS patients.
- Evidence also supports the use of PHC strategies in acute severe asthma, COPD, and in pediatric intensive care.
- Hypercapnia is a potent biologic agent, and there is substantial evidence from laboratory studies that hypercapnia attenuates lung and systemic organ injury. However, recent experimental data suggest that hypercapnia may be harmful by delaying wound repair and suppressing innate immune responses to bacterial infection.
- The potential for hypercapnia to exert deleterious physiologic effects in cases of raised intracranial pressure or PH should be considered.
- There is no clinical evidence to support the clinical practice of buffering HCA with bicarbonate.
- A clearer understanding of the effects and mechanisms of action of hypercapnia is central to determining its safety and therapeutic utility.
- The potential for extracorporeal CO_2 removal technologies to facilitate even greater reductions in tidal and minute ventilation is clear, but this awaits definitive studies.

REFERENCES

1. Dreyfuss D, Saumon G. Ventilator-induced lung injury: lessons from experimental studies. *Am J Respir Crit Care Med.* 1998;157(1):294–323.
2. Pinhu L, Whitehead T, Evans T, Griffiths M. Ventilator-associated lung injury. *Lancet.* 2003;361(9354):332–340.
3. Ventilation with lower tidal volumes as compared with traditional tidal volumes for acute lung injury and the acute respiratory distress syndrome. The Acute Respiratory Distress Syndrome Network. *N Engl J Med.* 2000;342(18):1301–1308.
4. Amato MBP, Barbas CS, Medeiros DM, et al. Effect of protective-ventilation strategy on mortality in the acute respiratory distress syndrome. *N Engl J Med.* 1998;338(6):347–354.
5. Hickling KG, Henderson SJ, Jackson R. Low mortality associated with low volume pressure limited ventilation with permissive hypercapnia in severe adult respiratory distress syndrome. *Intensive Care Med.* 1990;16(6):372–377.
6. Hickling KG, Walsh J, Henderson S, Jackson R. Low mortality rate in adult respiratory distress syndrome using low-volume, pressure-limited ventilation with permissive hypercapnia: a prospective study. *Crit Care Med.* 1994;22(10):1568–1578.
7. Bein T, Weber-Carstens S, Goldmann A, et al. Lower tidal volume strategy (approximately 3 ml/kg) combined with extracorporeal CO2 removal versus 'conventional' protective ventilation (6 ml/kg) in severe ARDS: the prospective randomized Xtravent-study. *Intensive Care Med.* 2013;39(5):847–856. {Helenius, 2009 #1211}.
8. Terragni PP, Del Sorbo L, Mascia L, et al. Tidal volume lower than 6 ml/kg enhances lung protection: role of extracorporeal carbon dioxide removal. *Anesthesiology.* 2009;111(4):826–835.
9. Ferring M, Vincent JL. Is outcome from ARDS related to the severity of respiratory failure? *Eur Respir J.* 1997;10(6):1297–1300.
10. Brogan TV, Hedges RG, McKinney S, Robertson HT, Hlastala MP, Swenson ER. Pulmonary NO synthase inhibition and inspired CO$_2$: effects on V′/Q′ and pulmonary blood flow distribution. *Eur Respir J.* 2000;16(2):288–295.
11. Brogan TV, Robertson HT, Lamm WJ, Souders JE, Swenson ER. Carbon dioxide added late in inspiration reduces ventilation-perfusion heterogeneity without causing respiratory acidosis. *J Appl Physiol.* 2004;96(5):1894–1898.
12. Swenson ER, Robertson HT, Hlastala MP. Effects of inspired carbon dioxide on ventilation-perfusion matching in normoxia, hypoxia, and hyperoxia. *Am J Respis Crit Care Med.* 1994;149(6):1563–1569.
13. Wildeboer-Venema F. The influences of temperature and humidity upon the isolated surfactant film of the dog. *Respir Physiol.* 1980;39(1):63–71.
14. Emery MJ, Eveland RL, Min JH, Hildebrandt J, Swenson ER. CO$_2$ relaxation of the rat lung parenchymal strip. *Respir Physiol Neurobiol.* 2013;186(1):33–39.
15. Ketabchi F, Ghofrani HA, Schermuly RT, et al. Effects of hypercapnia and NO synthase inhibition in sustained hypoxic pulmonary vasoconstriction. *Respir Res.* 2012;13(7).
16. Masood A, Yi M, Lau M, et al. Therapeutic effects of hypercapnia on chronic lung injury and vascular remodeling in neonatal rats. *Am J Physiol Lung Cell Mol Physiol.* 2009;297(5):L920–L930.
17. Ooi H, Cadogan E, Sweeney M, Howell K, O'Regan RG, McLoughlin P. Chronic hypercapnia inhibits hypoxic pulmonary vascular remodeling. *Am J Physiol Heart Circ Physiol.* 2000;278(2):H331–H338.
18. Peng G, Ivanovska J, Kantores C, et al. Sustained therapeutic hypercapnia attenuates pulmonary arterial Rho-kinase activity and ameliorates chronic hypoxic pulmonary hypertension in juvenile rats. *Am J Physiol Heart Circ Physiol.* 2012;302(12):H2599–H2611.
19. Sewing AC, Kantores C, Ivanovska J, et al. Therapeutic hypercapnia prevents bleomycin-induced pulmonary hypertension in neonatal rats by limiting macrophage-derived tumor necrosis factor-alpha. *Am J Physiol Lung Cell Mol Physiol.* 2012;303(1):L75–L87.
20. Feihl F, Eckert P, Brimiouelle S, et al. Permissive hypercapnia impairs pulmonary gas exchange in the acute respiratory distress syndrome. *Am J Respis Crit Care Med.* 2000;162:209–215.
21. Kregenow DA, Swenson ER. The lung and carbon dioxide: implications for permissive and therapeutic hypercapnia. *Eur Respir J.* 2002;20(1):6–11.
22. Lele EE, Hantos Z, Bitay M, et al. Bronchoconstriction during alveolar hypocapnia and systemic hypercapnia in dogs with a cardiopulmonary bypass. *Respir Physiol Neurobiol.* 2011;175(1):140–145.
23. Jonville S, Delpech N, Denjean A. Contribution of respiratory acidosis to diaphragmatic fatigue at exercise. *Eur Respir J.* 2002;19(6):1079–1086.
24. Juan G, Calverley P, Talamo C, Schnader J, Roussos C. Effect of carbon dioxide on diaphragmatic function in human beings. *N Engl J Med.* 1984;310(14):874–879.
25. Jung B, Sebbane M, Goff CL, et al. Moderate and prolonged hypercapnic acidosis may protect against ventilator-induced diaphragmatic dysfunction in healthy piglet: an in vivo study. *Crit Care.* 2013;17(1):R15.
26. Schellekens WJ, van Hees HW, Kox M, et al. Hypercapnia attenuates ventilator-induced diaphragm atrophy and modulates dysfunction. *Crit Care.* 2014;18(1):R28.
27. Tang WC, Weil MH, Gazmuri RJ, Bisera J, Rackow EC. Reversible impairment of myocardial contractility due to hypercarbic acidosis in the isolated perfused rat heart. *Crit Care Med.* 1991;19(2):218–224.
28. Cullen DJ, Eger 2nd EI. Cardiovascular effects of carbon dioxide in man. *Anesthesiology.* 1974;41(4):345–349.
29. Torbati D, Mangino MJ, Garcia E, Estrada M, Totapally BR, Wolfsdorf J. Acute hypercapnia increases the oxygen-carrying capacity of the blood in ventilated dogs. *Crit Care Med.* 1998;26(11):1863–1867.
30. Hood VL, Tannen RL. Protection of acid-base balance by pH regulation of acid production. *N Engl J Med.* 1998;339(12):819–826.
31. Akca O, Doufas AG, Morioka N, Iscoe S, Fisher J, Sessler DI. Hypercapnia improves tissue oxygenation. *Anesthesiology.* 2002;97(4):801–806.
32. Mas A, Saura P, Joseph D, et al. Effect of acute moderate changes in PaCO$_2$ on global hemodynamics and gastric perfusion. *Crit Care Med.* 2000;28(2):360–365.
33. Akca O, Sessler DI, Delong D, Keijner R, Ganzel B, Doufas AG. Tissue oxygenation response to mild hypercapnia during cardiopulmonary bypass with constant pump output. *Br J Anaesth.* 2006;96(6):708–714.
34. Fleischmann E, Herbst F, Kugener A, et al. Mild hypercapnia increases subcutaneous and colonic oxygen tension in patients given 80% inspired oxygen during abdominal surgery. *Anesthesiology.* 2006;104(5):944–949.
35. Hager H, Reddy D, Mandadi G, et al. Hypercapnia improves tissue oxygenation in morbidly obese surgical patients. *Anesth Analg.* 2006;103(3):677–681.
36. Guzman JA, Kruse JA. Splanchnic hemodynamics and gut mucosal-arterial PCO(2) gradient during systemic hypocapnia. *J Appl Physiol (1985).* 1999;87(3):1102–1106.
37. Akca O, Kurz A, Fleischmann E, et al. Hypercapnia and surgical site infection: a randomized trial. *Br J Anaesth.* 2013;111(5):759–767.
38. Hare GM, Kavanagh BP, Mazer CD, et al. Hypercapnia increases cerebral tissue oxygen tension in anesthetized rats. *Can J Anaesth.* 2003;50(10):1061–1068.
39. Nakahata K, Kinoshita H, Hirano Y, Kimoto Y, Iranami H, Hatano Y. Mild hypercapnia induces vasodilation via adenosine triphosphate-sensitive K+ channels in parenchymal microvessels of the rat cerebral cortex. *Anesthesiology.* 2003;99(6):1333–1339.
40. Reinhard M, Schwarzer G, Briel M, et al. Cerebrovascular reactivity predicts stroke in high-grade carotid artery disease. *Neurology.* 2014;83:1424–1431.
41. Raichle ME, Posner JB, Plum F. Cerebral blood flow during and after hyperventilation. *Arch Neurol.* 1970;23(5):394–403.
42. Curley G, Kavanagh BP, Laffey JG. Hypocapnia and the injured brain: more harm than benefit. *Crit Care Med.* 2010;38(5):1348–1359.
43. Takeshita K, Suzuki Y, Nishio K, et al. Hypercapnic Acidosis Attenuates Endotoxin-induced Nuclear Factor-kB Activation. *Am J Respir Cell Mol Biol.* 2003;29(1):124–132.
44. Contreras M, Ansari B, Curley G, et al. Hypercapnic acidosis attenuates ventilation-induced lung injury by a nuclear factor-kappaB-dependent mechanism. *Crit Care Med.* 2012;40(9):2622–2630.
45. Wu SY, Li MH, Ko FC, Wu GC, Huang KL, Chu SJ. Protective effect of hypercapnic acidosis in ischemia-reperfusion lung injury is attributable to upregulation of heme oxygenase-1. *PLoS One.* 2013;8(9):e74742.

46. O'Toole D, Hassett P, Contreras M, et al. Hypercapnic acidosis attenuates pulmonary epithelial wound repair by an NF-kappaB dependent mechanism. *Thorax.* 2009;64(11):976–982.

47. O'Croinin DF, Nichol AD, Hopkins N, et al. Sustained hypercapnic acidosis during pulmonary infection increases bacterial load and worsens lung injury*. *Crit Care Med.* 2008;36(7):2128–2135.

48. Cummins EP, Oliver KM, Lenihan CR, et al. NF-kappaB links CO_2 sensing to innate immunity and inflammation in mammalian cells. *J Immunol.* 2010;185(7):4439–4445.

49. Helenius IT, Krupinski T, Turnbull DW, et al. Elevated CO_2 suppresses specific Drosophila innate immune responses and resistance to bacterial infection. *Proc Natl Acad Sci USA.* 2009;106(44):18710–18715.

50. Wang N, Gates KL, Trejo H, et al. Elevated CO_2 selectively inhibits interleukin-6 and tumor necrosis factor expression and decreases phagocytosis in the macrophage. *FASEB J.* 2010;24(7): 2178–2190.

51. Ni Chonghaile M, Higgins BD, Costello J, Laffey JG. Hypercapnic acidosis attenuates severe acute bacterial pneumonia induced lung injury by a neutrophil independent mechanism. *Crit Care Med.* 2008;36(12):3135–3144.

52. Ni Chonghaile M, Higgins BD, Costello J, Laffey JG. Hypercapnic acidosis attenuates lung injury induced by established bacterial pneumonia. *Anesthesiology.* 2008;109(5):837–848.

53. O'Croinin DF, Hopkins NO, Moore MM, Boylan JF, McLoughlin P, Laffey JG. Hypercapnic acidosis does not modulate the severity of bacterial pneumonia-induced lung injury. *Crit Care Med.* 2005;33(11):2606–2612.

54. Costello J, Higgins B, Contreras M, et al. Hypercapnic acidosis attenuates shock and lung injury in early and prolonged systemic sepsis. *Crit Care Med.* 2009;37(8):2412–2420.

55. Higgins BD, Costello J, Contreras M, Hassett P, OT D, Laffey JG. Differential effects of buffered hypercapnia versus hypercapnic acidosis on shock and lung injury induced by systemic sepsis. *Anesthesiology.* 2009;111(6):1317–1326.

56. Ware LB, Matthay MA. Alveolar fluid clearance is impaired in the majority of patients with acute lung injury and the acute respiratory distress syndrome. *Am J Respir Crit Care Med.* 2001;163(6):1376–1383.

57. Lecuona E, Sun H, Chen J, Trejo HE, Baker MA, Sznajder JI. Protein kinase A-Ialpha regulates Na,K-ATPase endocytosis in alveolar epithelial cells exposed to high CO(2) concentrations. *Am J Respir Cell Mol Biol.* 2013;48(5):626–634.

58. Vadasz I, Dada LA, Briva A, et al. Evolutionary conserved role of c-Jun-N-terminal kinase in CO(2)-induced epithelial dysfunction. *PLoS One.* 7(10):e46696.

59. Welch LC, Lecuona E, Briva A, Trejo HE, Dada LA, Sznajder JI. Extracellular signal-regulated kinase (ERK) participates in the hypercapnia-induced Na,K-ATPase downregulation. *FEBS Lett.* 2010;584(18):3985–3989.

60. Shiomi T, Tschumperlin DJ, Park JA, et al. TNF-alpha-converting enzyme/a disintegrin and metalloprotease-17 mediates mechanotransduction in murine tracheal epithelial cells. *Am J Respir Cell Mol Biol.* 45(2):376–385.

61. Correa-Meyer E, Pesce L, Guerrero C, Sznajder JI. Cyclic stretch activates ERK1/2 via G proteins and EGFR in alveolar epithelial cells. *Am J Physiol Lung Cell Mol Physiol.* 2002;282(5):L883–L891.

62. Otulakowski G, Engelberts D, Gusarova GA, Bhattacharya J, Post M, Kavanagh BP. Hypercapnia attenuates ventilator-induced lung injury via a disintegrin and metalloprotease-17. *J Physiol.* 2014;592:4507–4521.

63. Brochard L, Roudot-Thoraval F, Roupie E, et al. Tidal volume reduction for prevention of ventilator-induced lung injury in acute respiratory distress syndrome. *Am J Respis Crit Care Med.* 1998;158:1831–1838.

64. Brower RG, Shanholtz CB, Fessler HE, et al. Prospective, randomized, controlled clinical trial comparing traditional versus reduced tidal volume ventilation in acute respiratory distress syndrome patients. *Crit Care Med.* 1999;27(8):1492–1498.

65. Stewart TE, Meade MO, Cook DJ, et al. Evaluation of a ventilation strategy to prevent barotrauma in patients at high risk for acute respiratory distress syndrome. *N Engl J Med.* 1998;338(6): 355–361.

66. Kregenow DA, Rubenfeld G, Hudson L, Swenson ER. Permissive hypercapnia reduces mortality with 12 ml/kg tidal volumes in acute lung injury. *Am J Resp Crit Care Med.* 2003;167:A616.

67. Hodgson CL, Tuxen DV, Davies AR, et al. A randomised controlled trial of an open lung strategy with staircase recruitment, titrated PEEP and targeted low airway pressures in patients with acute respiratory distress syndrome. *Crit Care.* 2011;15(3):R133.

68. Darioli R, Perret C. Mechanical controlled hypoventilation in status asthmaticus. *Am Rev Respir Dis.* 1984;129(3):385–387.

69. Tuxen DV, Williams TJ, Scheinkestel CD, Czarny D, Bowes G. Use of a measurement of pulmonary hyperinflation to control the level of mechanical ventilation in patients with acute severe asthma. *Am Rev Respir Dis.* 1992;146(5 Pt 1):1136–1142.

70. Mutlu GM, Factor P, Schwartz DE, Sznajder JI. Severe status asthmaticus: management with permissive hypercapnia and inhalation anesthesia. *Crit Care Med.* 2002;30(2):477–480.

71. Gupta D, Keogh B, Chung KF, et al. Characteristics and outcome for admissions to adult, general critical care units with acute severe asthma: a secondary analysis of the ICNARC Case Mix Programme Database. *Crit Care.* 2004;8(2):R112–R121.

72. Peters JI, Stupka JE, Singh H, et al. Status asthmaticus in the medical intensive care unit: a 30-year experience. *Respir Med.* 2012;106(3):344–348.

73. Lightowler JV, Wedzicha JA, Elliott MW, Ram FS. Non-invasive positive pressure ventilation to treat respiratory failure resulting from exacerbations of chronic obstructive pulmonary disease: cochrane systematic review and meta-analysis. *BMJ.* 2003;326(7382):185.

74. Avery ME, Tooley WH, Keller JB, et al. Is chronic lung disease in low birth weight infants preventable? A survey of eight centers. *Pediatrics.* 1987;79(1):26–30.

75. Kraybill EN, Runyan DK, Bose CL, Khan JH. Risk factors for chronic lung disease in infants with birth weights of 751 to 1000 grams. *J Pediatr.* 1989;115(1):115–120.

76. Mariani G, Cifuentes J, Carlo WA. Randomized trial of permissive hypercapnia in preterm infants. *Pediatrics.* 1999;104(5 Pt 1):1082–1088.

77. Carlo WA, Stark AR, Wright LL, et al. Minimal ventilation to prevent bronchopulmonary dysplasia in extremely-low-birth-weight infants. *J Pediatr.* 2002;141(3):370–374.

78. Kamper J, Feilberg Jorgensen N, Jonsbo F, Pedersen-Bjergaard L, Pryds O. The Danish national study in infants with extremely low gestational age and birthweight (the ETFOL study): respiratory morbidity and outcome. *Acta Paediatr.* 2004;93(2):225–232.

79. Woodgate PG, Davies MW. Permissive hypercapnia for the prevention of morbidity and mortality in mechanically ventilated newborn infants. *Cochrane Database Syst Rev.* 2001;2:CD002061.

80. Thome UH, Carroll W, Wu TJ, et al. Outcome of extremely preterm infants randomized at birth to different $PaCO_2$ targets during the first seven days of life. *Biol Neonate.* 2006;90(4): 218–225.

81. Wung JT, James LS, Kilchevsky E, James E. Management of infants with severe respiratory failure and persistence of the fetal circulation, without hyperventilation. *Pediatrics.* 1985;76(4): 488–494.

82. Bohn D. Congenital diaphragmatic hernia. *Am J Respir Crit Care Med.* 2002;166(7):911–915.

83. Kays DW, Langham Jr MR, Ledbetter DJ, Talbert JL. Detrimental effects of standard medical therapy in congenital diaphragmatic hernia. *Ann Surg.* 1999;230(3):340–348. discussion 348–351.

84. Wilson JM, Lund DP, Lillehei CW, Vacanti JP. Congenital diaphragmatic hernia–a tale of two cities: the Boston experience. *J Pediatr Surg.* 1997;32(3):401–405.

85. Bagolan P, Casaccia G, Crescenzi F, Nahom A, Trucchi A, Giorlandino C. Impact of a current treatment protocol on outcome of high-risk congenital diaphragmatic hernia. *J Pediatr Surg.* 2004;39(3):313–318. discussion 313–318.

86. Boloker J, Bateman DA, Wung JT, Stolar CJ. Congenital diaphragmatic hernia in 120 infants treated consecutively with permissive hypercapnea/spontaneous respiration/elective repair. *J Pediatr Surg.* 2002;37(3):357–366.

87. Guidry CA, Hranjec T, Rodgers BM, Kane B, McGahren ED. Permissive hypercapnia in the management of congenital diaphragmatic hernia: our institutional experience. *J Am Coll Surg,* 214(4):640–645, 647.e641; discussion 646–647.

88. Ferrara B, Johnson DE, Chang PN, Thompson TR. Efficacy and neurologic outcome of profound hypocapneic alkalosis for the treatment of persistent pulmonary hypertension in infancy. *J Pediatr.* 1984;105(3):457–461.

89. Hendricks-Munoz KD, Walton JP. Hearing loss in infants with persistent fetal circulation. *Pediatrics.* 1988;81(5):650–656.
90. Leavitt AM, Watchko JF, Bennett FC, Folsom RC. Neurodevelopmental outcome following persistent pulmonary hypertension of the neonate. *J Perinatol.* 1987;7(4):288–291.
91. Dworetz AR, Moya FR, Sabo B, Gladstone I, Gross I. Survival of infants with persistent pulmonary hypertension without extracorporeal membrane oxygenation. *Pediatrics.* 1989;84(1):1–6.
92. Marron MJ, Crisafi MA, Driscoll Jr JM, et al. Hearing and neurodevelopmental outcome in survivors of persistent pulmonary hypertension of the newborn. *Pediatrics.* 1992;90(3):392–396.
93. Licht DJ, Wang J, Silvestre DW, et al. Preoperative cerebral blood flow is diminished in neonates with severe congenital heart defects. *J Thorac Cardiovasc Surg.* 2004;128(6):841–849.
94. Tabbutt S, Ramamoorthy C, Montenegro LM, et al. Impact of inspired gas mixtures on preoperative infants with hypoplastic left heart syndrome during controlled ventilation. *Circulation.* 2001;104(12 suppl 1):I159–I164.
95. Ramamoorthy C, Tabbutt S, Kurth CD, et al. Effects of inspired hypoxic and hypercapnic gas mixtures on cerebral oxygen saturation in neonates with univentricular heart defects. *Anesthesiology.* 2002;96(2):283–288.
96. Bradley SM, Simsic JM, Mulvihill DM. Hypoventilation improves oxygenation after bidirectional superior cavopulmonary connection. *J Thorac Cardiovasc Surg.* 2003;126(4):1033–1039.
97. Hoskote A, Li J, Hickey C, et al. The effects of carbon dioxide on oxygenation and systemic, cerebral, and pulmonary vascular hemodynamics after the bidirectional superior cavopulmonary anastomosis. *J Am Coll Cardiol.* 2004;44(7):1501–1509.
98. Laffey JG, Engelberts D, Kavanagh BP. Buffering hypercapnic acidosis worsens acute lung injury. *Am J Respir Crit Care Med.* 2000;161(1):141–146.
99. Nichol AD, O'Cronin DF, Howell K, et al. Infection-induced lung injury is worsened after renal buffering of hypercapnic acidosis. *Crit Care Med.* 2009;37(11):2953–2961.
100. Weber T, Tschernich H, Sitzwohl C, et al. Tromethamine buffer modifies the depressant effect of permissive hypercapnia on myocardial contractility in patients with acute respiratory distress syndrome. *Am J Respir Crit Care Med.* 2000;162(4 Pt 1):1361–1365.
101. MacLaren G, Combes A, Bartlett RH. Contemporary extracorporeal membrane oxygenation for adult respiratory failure: life support in the new era. *Intensive Care Med.* 38(2):210–220.
102. Terragni PP, Rosboch G, Tealdi A, et al. Tidal hyperinflation during low tidal volume ventilation in acute respiratory distress syndrome. *Am J Respir Crit Care Med.* 2007;175(2):160–166.

32 Do Patient Positioning in General and Prone Positioning in Particular Make a Difference in ARDS?

Alain F. Broccard, Maneesh Bhargava

Changes in posture and position invariably accompany activity in healthy adults, with likely salutary effects on physiology. Similar changes in position during illness have important effects on cardiovascular and pulmonary physiology because of interactions between gravitational forces and chest mechanics. Such changes can improve oxygenation in patients with hypoxemic respiratory failure and may reduce the risk of ventilator-associated pneumonia. We review the salient effects of positioning on respiratory physiology and outline the clinical evidence supporting active positioning as a therapeutic or supportive intervention.

EFFECTS OF POSITION ON NORMAL RESPIRATORY PHYSIOLOGY

Airspace Mechanics

Gravity interacts with thoracic structures and transdiaphragmatic forces to modulate regional lung volume, distribution of ventilation, and ventilation-perfusion matching.[1,2] The local transpulmonary pressure gradient (alveolar pressure–pleural pressure), in concert with the corresponding regional lung compliance, is the major determinant of regional lung volume. Under "relaxed" conditions, the total aerated lung volume is denoted as functional residual capacity (FRC). During active inspiration, the transpulmonary pressure gradient determines the regional distribution of inspiratory flow, an important component of ventilation-perfusion matching and the distribution of peak alveolar strain during positive pressure ventilation. Conversely, at end expiration (or during the expiratory phase in the context of pulmonary disease), an unfavorable transpulmonary pressure gradient arising from abnormal pleural or diaphragmatic mechanics can promote airspace collapse, compromising oxygenation by increasing shunt fraction. Regardless of the position, regional pleural pressure tends to be less negative; therefore alveolar dimensions are smaller in the dependent than in the nondependent lung regions because of the effects of gravity on the adjacent abdominal structure and the heart on the most dependent pleural space.

Positional changes affect the gradients of regional pleural pressure and thus regional lung volume. For example, the heart rests on the lungs in the supine position and primarily on the sternum in the prone position.[3] This partially explains the observation that gravitational pleural pressure gradients are consistently less in the prone than the supine position.[4] In addition, the prone position reduces the pressure the abdominal contents exert on the diaphragm, a pressure that is transmitted to the pleural space. Consequently, when in the supine position, the dorsal lung regions are surrounded by a less negative pleural pressure (and a smaller transpulmonary pressure gradient). The prone position results in a more negative pleural pressure adjacent to the dorsal lung zones. The increased ventral pleural pressure in the prone position has less effect on FRC because there is less lung at risk of compression by the heart. The improved aeration of the dorsal lung regions, combined with the smaller effect of cardiac weight on the ventral lung regions, tends to increase FRC. The effect of position on FRC is significant. In healthy subjects, FRC is reduced by approximately 30% on transition from the sitting to the supine, horizontal posture.[5] Anesthesia or neuromuscular blocking agents tend to enhance this effect, presumably by reducing the tone of the diaphragm. When compared with the horizontal supine position, total FRC is approximately 20% greater in the lateral decubitus and prone positions.[5,6] Not surprisingly, abdominal distension and obesity reduce FRC further, and prone positioning may help offset the consequences of reclining on lung mechanics and gas exchange.[7,8]

In healthy, spontaneously breathing adults, ventilation distributes preferentially to the dependent lung regions in the upright, supine, prone, and lateral decubitus position. This effect is partially attributable to the phasic swings in pleural pressure that attend respiratory muscle activity.[2] In contrast, elimination of the normal phasic changes in pleural pressure that accompany the pharmacologic paralysis and mechanical ventilation of healthy patients[9,10] or the altered parenchymal characteristics in the setting of lung injury[11,12] can markedly attenuate or even reverse the predominantly dependent distribution of ventilation. The changes in the distribution of ventilation during the positive pressure mechanical ventilation of nonparalyzed, partially assisted patients are complex. They vary with the specifics of the applied ventilatory support and regional lung mechanics. For instance, positive end-expiratory pressure (PEEP) can help redistribute ventilation in the dependent regions in patients with acute respiratory distress syndrome (ARDS) but only if those regions are recruitable and the level of PEEP used is sufficient to maintain alveolar patency. Active diaphragmatic contraction, through its effects on pleural pressure, can increase transpulmonary pressure and help preserve alveolar patency.

Distribution of Blood Flow and Ventilation-Perfusion Ratio

Until recently, gravity was thought to be the main determinant of blood flow distribution within the lungs. It has now been shown that perfusion tends to distribute preferentially to the dorsal regions in the supine and prone positions. This distribution cannot be explained by gravity alone.[13,14] Regional differences in vascular development and geometry[15] and/or vasoregulation by nitric oxide[16] appear to contribute to regional distribution of perfusion within the lungs.

The modulation of airspace events combined with the less marked effect of gravity on distribution of pulmonary blood flow render the overall ventilation-perfusion ratio ($\dot{V}/\dot{Q}$) sensitive to position.[17] Overall, the ventilation perfusion relationship is less favorable in the supine than in the upright and prone positions. The effects of recumbency on oxygenation are complex and depend on the interrelationship of closing volume, FRC, and tidal volume.[18] Interindividual variations in the relations between these variables contribute to the variable effects of reclining on the partial pressure of oxygen in arterial blood (Pao_2) between subjects.

POSITIONING IN CRITICALLY ILL PATIENTS WITH RESPIRATORY FAILURE: GENERAL OVERVIEW

Judicious positioning of critically ill patients might reduce atelectasis, improve gas exchange, and decrease the threat of ventilator-associated pneumonia. The lateral and prone positions have the potential to improve gas exchange in selected patients with respiratory failure. "Head-up" positioning (tilting the patient upright) to alleviate diaphragmatic compression by the abdominal contents has been demonstrated to have some benefits. We briefly review the mechanisms that account for these observations and the outcome studies, when available, with an emphasis on the prone position—the best-studied position in the intensive care unit (ICU).

Respiratory Effects of Frequent Posture Changes

In anesthetized dogs, immobility is associated with a deterioration of gas exchange that can be prevented by turning every half hour.[19] Frequent changes in position are likely to be similarly important in maintaining normal respiratory function in humans. The effect of frequent positional changes has been tested in the clinical arena with continuous oscillating beds with promising results. Such "kinetic therapy" appears to be well tolerated hemodynamically and has been reported to improve oxygenation,[20] decrease the risk of atelectasis and pulmonary infections,[21,22] and reduce the duration of intubation and resource utilization in trauma patients.[19,23] Kinetic therapy also has been used to treat established atelectasis.[24] A reduction in the incidence of pneumonia and improved oxygenation was observed in medical ICU patients.[25,26] It has been suggested that this modality may improve outcome in the sickest patients ($P = 0.056$ for subgroup with APACHE [Acute Physiology and Chronic Health Evaluation] II score >20),[27] but more studies are needed to conclude that it does. Most available studies are relatively small sized and have limitations, and the results are not always consistent. For example, the use of a kinetic therapy bed has been associated with more frequent infectious complications, respiratory failure, and more ventilator support days in patients with thoracolumbar spinal column injuries.[28] In summary, the efficacy of position changes in protecting pulmonary function[29] or improving outcome remains uncertain.

Lateral Position

Because perfusion and ventilation distribute preferentially to the dependent lung during active breathing, $\dot{V}/\dot{Q}$ mismatching and intrapulmonary shunting can be significantly reduced by lateral positioning of patients with unilateral or asymmetrical lung disease with the good lung down (GLD).[30-32] This therapeutic adjunct may significantly improve Pao_2 and even preclude the need for intubation and mechanical ventilation.[30] Arterial and mixed venous oxygen content usually increase, without significant hemodynamic changes, in the GLD position.[33] On occasion, critically ill patients fail to improve with GLD (paradoxically); improve with the bad lung down; or develop arrhythmias, hypotension, or a marked reduction in mixed venous saturation of O_2 (SvO_2),[34] necessitating prompt return to the supine position. The slight and usually transient decrements in SvO_2 reported after postural changes in critically ill patients do not explain the occasional persistent failure of blood gases to improve in the lateral position with GLD. Atelectasis due to unusual pressure distributions generated by the abdominal contents or increased pressure transmission to the thorax is more likely responsible. In such circumstances, PEEP may prove beneficial. Fortunately, in patients with predominant unilateral alveolar consolidation or flooding, PEEP is less likely to detrimentally affect the distribution of perfusion in the lateral than when the patient is in the supine position. When the patient is supine, an inappropriately high level of PEEP may redistribute blood flow to the diseased lung by promoting zone 1 conditions in the spared lung.[35] However, in unilateral pneumonia, PEEP may help limit contamination of the good lung by the diseased lung[36] and may theoretically be more effective when used in combination with the lateral position.

The practice of positioning of patients with the GLD has notable exceptions. Children, some patients with chronic airflow obstruction,[37] and anesthetized-paralyzed patients share a tendency to have higher ventilation to the nondependent lung. In the presence of a moderate unilateral pleural effusion, $\dot{V}/\dot{Q}$ matching during spontaneous breathing appears to be similar in the lateral position with the affected side up or down,[31] suggesting that moderate pleural effusions have little effect on gas exchange. Studies of regional lung function in seated patients with unilateral pleural effusions demonstrate that although the overall lung volume on the side of effusion is reduced, the residual volume/total lung capacity (RV/TLC) and FRC/TLC ratios on both sides are very similar.[38] This may explain the poor correlations among posture, pleural effusion size, and gas exchange in patients with unilateral pleural effusion without marked underlying infiltrates or hypoxemia. Patients with whole lung collapse secondary to unilateral central airway obstruction may not improve or may even deteriorate when positioned with the spared lung down.[39] Patients with unilateral massive pulmonary embolism requiring mechanical ventilation have been reported to have better gas exchange with the diseased lung down.[40] Finally, lateral positioning with the GLD is contraindicated in hemoptysis and lung abscess because of the risk of spillage into the unaffected lung.

Elevation of the Head of the Bed

Elevating the head of the bed can improve oxygenation in ARDS, probably by promoting lung recruitment at the bases.[41] In 16 patients with ARDS, vertical positioning (trunk elevated at 45 degrees and legs down at 45 degrees) significantly increased Pao_2 from 94 ± 33 to 142 ± 49 mm Hg, with an increase higher than 40% in 11 patients. The semirecumbent position may also help reduce gastric content aspiration.[42] Conversely, head position less than 30 degrees in the first 24 hours after intubation was found to be an independent risk factor for development of ventilator-associated pneumonia.[43] In a subsequent randomized prospective trial, the semirecumbent position was reported to significantly reduce the rate of ventilator-associated pneumonia (odds ratio [OR] 6.8 for the supine body position).[44] On the basis of this evidence, head-of-the-bed elevation has been endorsed by medical societies such as the Society of Critical Care Medicine. However, this approach has not been universally endorsed because of persistent questions about efficacy.[45,46] Many queries remain unanswered, such as how many hours per day the head of the bed must be elevated and what the optimal angle of elevation is for the head of the bed. Nonetheless, given that head-of-the-bed elevation is cheap, benign, and potentially helpful, it seems a reasonable intervention even in the absence of definitive data.

PRONE POSITION IN ARDS

Physiology and Physiopathology of Prone Positioning

In 1976, Piehl and Brown[47] first described improved oxygenation in patients with acute hypoxemic respiratory failure who were ventilated in the prone position. This has been confirmed in subsequent studies; overall, oxygenation improves in approximately two thirds of patients when placed in the prone position.[48] The mechanisms underlying this improvement have been most extensively studied in large animal models. Complex interactions between regional aeration and the modulation of perfusion during positive pressure ventilation determine the effects of prone positioning on gas exchange. These mechanisms have been reviewed by Guerin and colleagues.[49]

The improved oxygenation associated with prone positioning appears to be primarily related to regional differences in FRC alongside relatively unchanged distribution of dorsal-ventral perfusion. The largest proportion of pulmonary blood flow is directed to the dorsal lung regions in the supine and prone positions.[14] The predominance of dorsal perfusion is preserved when the animal is turned prone.[50] In a canine model of lung injury induced by oleic acid, the prone position was found to improve gas exchange by reducing shunt.[51] In the setting of lung injury, both animals and patients with ARDS tend to have less aerated lung in the dependent regions because of the effects of gravity on the edematous lungs. The time constant of the dependent collapsed/flooded lung units is such that tidal ventilation distributes preferentially to the "open" nondependent lung units,[11] namely, to ventral regions when supine and to dorsal regions when prone. Accordingly, the increase in FRC seen when an injured animal or patient is turned prone (because of changes in transpulmonary pressure favoring "opening" of the now nondependent dorsal regions, vide supra) is accompanied by an increase in perfusion to aerated lung units, with an accompanying decrease in shunt fraction.

In addition, positive pressure ventilation tends to create West zone 1 or 2 conditions and can redistribute blood flow from the nondependent region to the dependent regions. Positive airway pressure decreases the vertical perfusion gradient when in the prone position whereas it increases the vertical perfusion gradient in the supine position.[52] Positive pressure ventilation of regionally heterogeneous ARDS lungs creates opposing gradients of ventilation and perfusion along the vertical axis, promoting ventilation-perfusion mismatch and shunting. This effect of positive pressure is more marked in the supine position than in the prone position. Indeed, regional ventilation (V_r) and regional perfusion (Q_r) assessed by single-photon emission computed tomography showed that the prone position improved dorsal V_r to a greater extent than ventral V_r, whereas Q_r remained essentially unchanged.[53] In other words, recruitment of dorsal lung units associated with preserved dorsal perfusion largely explains why prone positioning improves gas exchange in experimental models and why an overall increase in FRC is not required for prone positioning to improve $\dot{V}/\dot{Q}$ matching (vide infra).[54]

However, additional factors may contribute to the improved gas exchange afforded by prone positioning. The pleural pressure gradient is smaller along the vertical axis[4] and pleural pressure is more negative in the dependent regions in the prone than in the supine position.[55] This favors lung recruitment and accounts for the increase in FRC sometimes observed after turning to the prone position.[56] The effect of prone positioning on gas exchange during positive pressure ventilation of pharmacologically paralyzed subjects appears to be further modulated by changes in thoracicoabdominal compliance that accompany the prone position. Pelosi et al.[56] found that the improvement in oxygenation attending prone positioning correlated with a high supine thoracicoabdominal compliance. A very compliant anterior chest tends to redistribute the tidal volume toward the nondependent, less well perfused lung regions, promoting $\dot{V}/\dot{Q}$ mismatching in the supine position. Constraint of the flexible ventral chest wall by contact with the bed during prone positioning "stiffens" the anterior chest wall. Such stiffening redirects tidal ventilation toward the better perfused dorsal regions, improving $\dot{V}/\dot{Q}$ matching.[57] These data do not suggest that minimizing abdominal contact, as proposed by some, is a prerequisite for improved gas exchange. Finally, the properties of the lung (e.g., cause of ARDS or phase of the disease [edema vs. fibrosis]) tend to alter the response to prone positioning.[58] In general, patients in the early edematous phase of ARDS are more likely to experience improved gas exchange when turned prone than patients who have pulmonary fibrosis.

Which of these mechanisms prevails in individual patients and best accounts for the improved Pao_2/fraction of inspired oxygen (Fio_2) ratio associated with prone positioning is not always clear, but it is potentially important. It has been suggested that a reduction in the partial pressure of carbon dioxide in arterial blood ($Paco_2$) after prone positioning may indicate the presence of recruitment and improved outcome.[59] Better recruitment distributes a given tidal volume to a larger number of alveoli, thereby reducing alveolar strain and the risk of epithelial and endothelial injury. Mentzelopoulos et al.[60] measured tidal transpulmonary pressures as a function of end expiratory lung volume as a marker for lung mechanical stress and found this to be reduced during prone positioning. More uniform distribution of blood flow may also be important given the potential importance of ventilation and perfusion interaction in the pathogenesis of ventilator-induced lung injury (VILI).[61] Regardless of the mechanisms, prone positioning has been found to attenuate VILI in large animals with normal[62] or injured lungs.[63] Overall, the protective effect of prone positioning is consistent with the post hoc findings of Gattinoni and colleagues,[48] who reported reduced mortality in a subset of patients who received excessive tidal volume (large tidal volume relative to the size of lung) either because of the large tidal volume used (largest tidal volume subgroup) or the small size of the lungs (severest form of ARDS subgroup).

Prone Position and Outcome

Prone ventilation improves oxygenation in most patients and mortality in those with severe ARDS. Multiple randomized trials[48,64-70] addressing the effect of prone positioning on outcomes have been published. Patient characteristics and the main results of these trials are summarized in Table 32-1. Several initial studies demonstrated either no difference[64-66] or only a trend toward improved mortality in subsets of patients with ARDS.[48,67] Taken together, the data suggested that the prone position may improve outcome in subgroups of patients with severe ARDS,[48] and multivariate analysis of data from the study by Mancebo and colleagues[67] showed that randomization to the supine position was an independent risk factor for mortality. This hypothesis has been confirmed by the landmark study by Guerin and colleagues.[69] In this study, a standardized protocol for prolonged daily prone ventilation, neuromuscular blockade, and lung-protective ventilation was instituted by trained medical staff within 36 hours for severe ARDS. This study demonstrated a dramatic improvement in 28-day (16% vs 32.8%, OR, 0.39; confidence interval [CI], 0.25 to 0.63) and 90-day (23.6 vs. 41%, OR, 0.44; CI, 0.29 to 0.70) mortality with prone ventilation.[69]

In addition to improving gas exchange and reducing mortality, the prone position has also been shown to have the potential to have favorable hemodynamic effects. In a study of 18 patients with ARDS, the prone position was associated with reduced right ventricular afterload and pulmonary vascular resistance; interestingly, only patients with preload reserve increased their cardiac index.[71]

Although early studies reported a high rate of complications, it now appears that, when carefully done by trained personnel, the prone position may not increase the rate of major complications.[72-75] Many complications, such as pressure ulcers, which have been reported to be significantly more common in two meta-analyses,[74,75] are preventable. Indeed, in the latest multicenter randomized trial by Guerin et al.,[69] the rate of complications was not higher in the prone group, which suggests that excess complications reflect inexperience with the technique.

Several meta-analyses[72-76] have been published, including one subsequent to the study by Guerin et al.[69] The prone position clearly improves gas exchange[72-76] and mortality.[72-75] In addition, all-cause mortality was improved when the daily duration of prone ventilation was prolonged (>16 hours per day; relative risk [RR], 0.77; CI, 0.64 to 0.92)[76] in cases with moderate and severe hypoxemia (RR, 0.76; CI, 0.61 to 0.94).

Overall, current randomized trials are difficult to compare (e.g., patients enrolled had different cause for ARDS and severity, and they were at different stages in the course of ARDS), and prone positioning lacks standardization in regard to its duration and to ventilatory strategy.[72] Pooled together, the data suggest that the prone position is not needed in all and is unlikely to benefit mild ARDS. Although the prone position significantly improved the Pao_2/Fio_2 ratio and reduced the mortality in patients with severe ARDS, the observed improvement in gas exchange was not found to be a predictor of improved survival. This suggests that prone ventilation improves survival by decreasing VILI[77] and that protecting the lungs may be more important than achieving the best possible blood gas, a lesson learned in patients with status asthmaticus decades ago with permissive hypercapnia.

The evidence has clearly evolved to strongly support the use of prone ventilation in severe ARDS. The prone position is best implemented by trained personnel as a carefully planned lung-protective strategy for ARDS. Such a protocol should include specific directions regarding indications and contraindications to initiating the prone position as well as the duration (dose) and rationale for discontinuation based on the risk for VILI as opposed to gas exchange alone. Close attention to preventable complications during turning and throughout the duration of prone ventilation is essential. The optimal duration of prone ventilation remains unknown, but a minimum of 16 hours per day appears reasonable given that such duration has been associated with improved outcome. Careful considerations also need to be given to other lung-protective measures. It remains unknown if combining the prone position with another modality such as the upright position may convey additional benefits as suggested in a small study.[78] Finally, proning should be considered early on in patients with severe ARDS. Although the prone position is unlikely to be helpful in patients with mild ARDS, further studies are needed to determine which patients with moderate ARDS, if any, might benefit from this approach.

Table 32-1 Summary of Randomized Controlled Trials

Study	Type of Respiratory Failure	Number of Subjects (Supine/Prone)	Study Design	Duration of Daily Prone Positioning	OUTCOME		COMPLICATIONS		
					Mortality	Results Supine/Prone n/n (%)	VAP (%)	Major Respiratory Complication (Extubation and ET Obstruction) (%)	Pressure Sores (%)
Gattinoni, 2001	ALI and ARDS	152/152	MRC	7.0±1.8 hr for 10 days	10-day	73/152 (48) vs. 77/152 (51)	NA	10 vs. 8	36 vs. 28
Guerin, 2004	Acute hypoxemic respiratory failure	378/413	MRC	8 hours per day for 4.0 days (range, 2.0-6.0)	28-day	119/378 (32) vs. 134/413 (32)	24 vs. 21	16 vs. 20	50 vs. 42
Voggenreiter, 2005	ALI and ARDS (trauma)	19/21	SR	11±5 hours	ICU	3/19(16) vs. 1/21 (5)	89 vs. 62	5 vs. 5	91 vs. 63
Curley, 2005	ALI (pediatric study)	51/51	SR	18±4 hours	28-day	4/50 (8) vs. 4/51 (7.8)	NA	10 vs. 12	16 vs. 20
Mancebo, 2006	ARDS	60/76	MR	17 hours for 10.1 days	ICU	35/60 (58) vs. 33/76 (43)	15 vs. 18	2 vs. 8	3 vs. NA
Fernandez, 2008	ARDS	19/21	MRC	Up to 20 hours per day	60-day	10/19 (53) vs. 8/21 (38)	5 vs.14	10 vs. 5	Very common (prone)
Taccone, 2009	Moderate and severe ARDS	174/168	MR	At least 20 hours per day	28-day	57174 (32.8) vs. 52/168 (31)	NA	61.3 vs. 38.5	NA
Guerin, 2013	Severe ARDS (PF ratio <150)	220/237	MR	16 hours per day	28-day	75/229 (32.8) vs. 38/237 (16)	NA	20.7 vs. 15.3	NA

ALI, acute lung injury; ARDS, acute respiratory distress syndrome; C, crossover allowed; ET, endotracheal tube; ICU, intensive care unit; M, metacentric; NA, not applicable; PF, Pao_2/Fio_2; R, randomized; S, single center; VAP, ventilator-associated pneumonia.

AUTHORS' RECOMMENDATIONS

- Overall, in the last few decades, significant progress in our understanding of the physiologic effects of positioning on the respiratory system has been made. Judicious use of positioning can improve gas exchange in ventilated critically ill patients. Whether positioning improves outcome in most patients with acute respiratory failure remains unproven and is very unlikely.
- Limited clinical data suggest that the semirecumbent position helps to reduce the risk of ventilator-associated pneumonia in intubated and mechanically ventilated ICU patients. Although many questions remain and more evidence is needed, this practice has been widely adopted. However, more studies are needed.
- Prone positioning significantly improves gas exchange, defined by improved Pao_2/Fio_2.
- There are compelling data to conclude that the mortality of patients with severe ARDS is reduced with the judicious use of prone positioning as part of a multimodal protocol that includes lung-protective ventilator strategy.
- Prone positioning should be used for 16 hours or more per day.
- For this approach to be kept safe and effective, training of bedside staff and close attention to preventable complications are needed.

REFERENCES

1. Milic-Emili J, Henderson JA, Dolovich MB, Trop D, Kaneko K. Regional distribution of inspired gas in the lung. *J Appl Physiol.* 1966;21:749–759.
2. Kaneko K, Milic-Emili J, Dolovich MB, Dawson A, Bates DV. Regional distribution of ventilation and perfusion as a function of body position. *J Appl Physiol.* 1966;21:767–777.
3. Albert RK, Hubmayr RD. The prone position eliminates compression of the lungs by the heart. *Am J Respir Crit Care Med.* 2000;161:1660–1665.
4. Mutoh T, Guest RJ, Lamm WJ, Albert RK. Prone position alters the effect of volume overload on regional pleural pressures and improves hypoxemia in pigs in vivo. *Am Rev Respir Dis.* 1992;146:300–306.
5. Marini JJ, Tyler ML, Hudson LD, Davis BS, Huseby JS. Influence of head-dependent positions on lung volume and oxygen saturation in chronic air-flow obstruction. *Am Rev Respir Dis.* 1984;129:101–105.
6. Lumb AB, Nunn JF. Respiratory function and ribcage contribution to ventilation in body positions commonly used during anesthesia. *Anesth Analg.* 1991;73:422–426.
7. Mure M, Glenny RW, Domino KB, Hlastala MP. Pulmonary gas exchange improves in the prone position with abdominal distension. *Am J Respir Crit Care Med.* 1998;157:1785–1790.
8. Pelosi P, Croci M, Calappi E, et al. Prone positioning improves pulmonary function in obese patients during general anesthesia. *Anesth Analg.* 1996;83:578–583.
9. Bindslev L, Santesson J, Hedenstierna G. Distribution of inspired gas to each lung in anesthetized human subjects. *Acta Anaesthesiol Scand.* 1981;25:297–302.
10. Rehder K, Knopp TJ, Sessler AD, Didier EP. Ventilation-perfusion relationship in young healthy awake and anesthetized-paralyzed man. *J Appl Physiol.* 1979;47:745–753.
11. Martynowicz MA, Minor TA, Walters BJ, Hubmayr RD. Regional expansion of oleic acid-injured lungs. *Am J Respir Crit Care Med.* 1999;160:250–258.
12. Pelosi P, Crotti S, Brazzi L, Gattinoni L. Computed tomography in adult respiratory distress syndrome: what has it taught us? *Euro Respir J.* 1996;9:1055–1062.
13. Glenny RW. Blood flow distribution in the lung. *Chest.* 1998;114:8S–16S.
14. Glenny RW, Lamm WJ, Albert RK, Robertson HT. Gravity is a minor determinant of pulmonary blood flow distribution. *J Appl Physiol.* 1985;1991(71):620–629.
15. Glenny RW, Bernard SL, Luchtel DL, Neradilek B, Polissar NL. The spatial-temporal redistribution of pulmonary blood flow with postnatal growth. *J Appl Physiol.* 1985;2007(102):1281–1288.
16. Rimeika D, Nyren S, Wiklund NP. Regulation of regional lung perfusion by nitric oxide. *Am J Respir Crit Care Med.* 2004;170:450–455.
17. Amis TC, Jones HA, Hughes JM. Effect of posture on inter-regional distribution of pulmonary perfusion and VA/Q ratios in man. *Respir Physiol.* 1984;56:169–182.
18. Craig DB, Wahba WM, Don HF, Couture JG, Becklake MR. "Closing volume" and its relationship to gas exchange in seated and supine positions. *J Appl Physiol.* 1971;31:717–721.
19. Ray 3rd JF, Yost L, Moallem S, et al. Immobility, hypoxemia, and pulmonary arteriovenous shunting. *Arch Surg.* 1974;109:537–541.
20. Stiletto R, Gotzen L, Goubeaud S. Kinetic therapy for therapy and prevention of post-traumatic lung failure. Results of a prospective study of 111 polytrauma patients. *Der Unfallchirurg.* 2000;103:1057–1064.
21. Fink MP, Helsmoortel CM, Stein KL, Lee PC, Cohn SM. The efficacy of an oscillating bed in the prevention of lower respiratory tract infection in critically ill victims of blunt trauma. A prospective study. *Chest.* 1990;97:132–137.
22. Gentilello L, Thompson DA, Tonnesen AS, et al. Effect of a rotating bed on the incidence of pulmonary complications in critically ill patients. *Crit Care Med.* 1988;16:783–786.
23. Nelson LD, Choi SC. Kinetic therapy in critically ill trauma patients. *Clin Intensive Care.* 1992;3:248–252.
24. Raoof S, Chowdhrey N, Raoof S, et al. Effect of combined kinetic therapy and percussion therapy on the resolution of atelectasis in critically ill patients. *Chest.* 1999;115:1658–1666.
25. deBoisblanc BP, Castro M, Everret B, Grender J, Walker CD, Summer WR. Effect of air-supported, continuous, postural oscillation on the risk of early ICU pneumonia in nontraumatic critical illness. *Chest.* 1993;103:1543–1547.
26. Wang JY, Chuang PY, Lin CJ, Yu CJ, Yang PC. Continuous lateral rotational therapy in the medical intensive care unit. *J Formos Med Assoc.* 2003;102:788–792.
27. Traver GA, Tyler ML, Hudson LD, Sherrill DL, Quan SF. Continuous oscillation: outcome in critically ill patients. *J Crit Care.* 1995;10:97–103.
28. Chipman JG, Taylor JH, Thorson M, Skarda DE, Beilman GJ. Kinetic therapy beds are associated with more complications in patients with thoracolumbar spinal column injuries. *Surgical Infect.* 2006;7:513–518.
29. Dolovich M, Rushbrook J, Churchill E, Mazza M, Powles AC. Effect of continuous lateral rotational therapy on lung mucus transport in mechanically ventilated patients. *J Crit Care.* 1998;13:119–125.
30. Dhainaut JF, Bons J, Bricard C, Monsallier JF. Improved oxygenation in patients with extensive unilateral pneumonia using the lateral decubitus position. *Thorax.* 1980;35:792–793.
31. Gillespie DJ, Rehder K. Body position and ventilation-perfusion relationships in unilateral pulmonary disease. *Chest.* 1987;91:75–79.
32. Seaton D, Lapp NL, Morgan WK. Effect of body position on gas exchange after thoracotomy. *Thorax.* 1979;34:518–522.
33. Dreyfuss D, Djedaini K, Lanore JJ, Mier L, Froidevaux R, Coste F. A comparative study of the effects of almitrine bismesylate and lateral position during unilateral bacterial pneumonia with severe hypoxemia. *Am Rev Respir Dis.* 1992;146:295–299.
34. Winslow EH, Clark AP, White KM, Tyler DO. Effects of a lateral turn on mixed venous oxygen saturation and heart rate in critically ill adults. *Heart Lung.* 1990;19:557–561.
35. Hasan FM, Weiss WB, Braman SS, Hoppin Jr FG. Influence of lung injury on pulmonary wedge-left atrial pressure correlation during positive end-expiratory pressure ventilation. *Am Rev Respir Dis.* 1985;131:246–250.
36. Schortgen F, Bouadma L, Joly-Guillou ML, Ricard JD, Dreyfuss D, Saumon G. Infectious and inflammatory dissemination are affected by ventilation strategy in rats with unilateral pneumonia. *Intensive Care Med.* 2004;30:693–701.
37. Shim C, Chun KJ, Williams Jr MH, Blaufox MD. Positional effects on distribution of ventilation in chronic obstructive pulmonary disease. *Ann Intern Med.* 1986;105:346–350.
38. Anthonisen NR, Martin RR. Regional lung function in pleural effusion. *Am Rev Respir Dis.* 1977;116:201–207.

39. Chang SC, Chang HI, Shiao GM, Perng RP. Effect of body position on gas exchange in patients with unilateral central airway lesions. Down with the good lung? *Chest.* 1993;103:787–791.

40. Badr MS, Grossman JE. Positional changes in gas exchange after unilateral pulmonary embolism. *Chest.* 1990;98:1514–1516.

41. Richard JC, Maggiore SM, Mancebo J, Lemaire F, Jonson B, Brochard L. Effects of vertical positioning on gas exchange and lung volumes in acute respiratory distress syndrome. *Intensive Care Med.* 2006;32:1623–1626.

42. Torres A, El-Ebiary M, Soler N, Monton C, Fabregas N, Hernandez C. Stomach as a source of colonization of the respiratory tract during mechanical ventilation: association with ventilator-associated pneumonia. *Euro Respir J.* 1996;9:1729–1735.

43. Kollef MH. Ventilator-associated pneumonia. A multivariate analysis. *JAMA.* 1993;270:1965–1970.

44. Drakulovic MB, Torres A, Bauer TT, Nicolas JM, Nogue S, Ferrer M. Supine body position as a risk factor for nosocomial pneumonia in mechanically ventilated patients: a randomised trial. *Lancet.* 1999;354:1851–1858.

45. Heyland DK, Cook DJ, Dodek PM. Prevention of ventilator-associated pneumonia: current practice in Canadian intensive care units. *J Crit Care.* 2002;17:161–167.

46. van Nieuwenhoven CA, Vandenbroucke-Grauls C, van Tiel FH, et al. Feasibility and effects of the semirecumbent position to prevent ventilator-associated pneumonia: a randomized study. *Crit Care Med.* 2006;34:396–402.

47. Piehl MA, Brown RS. Use of extreme position changes in acute respiratory failure. *Crit Care Med.* 1976;4:13–14.

48. Gattinoni L, Tognoni G, Pesenti A, et al. Effect of prone positioning on the survival of patients with acute respiratory failure. *New Engl J Med.* 2001;345:568–573.

49. Guerin C, Baboi L, Richard JC. Mechanisms of the effects of prone positioning in acute respiratory distress syndrome. *Intensive Care Med.* 2014;40:1634–1642.

50. Wiener CM, Kirk W, Albert RK. Prone position reverses gravitational distribution of perfusion in dog lungs with oleic acid-induced injury. *J Appl Physiol.* 1985;1990(68):1386–1392.

51. Albert RK, Leasa D, Sanderson M, Robertson HT, Hlastala MP. The prone position improves arterial oxygenation and reduces shunt in oleic-acid-induced acute lung injury. *Am Rev Respir Dis.* 1987;135:628–633.

52. Nyren S, Mure M, Jacobsson H, Larsson SA, Lindahl SG. Pulmonary perfusion is more uniform in the prone than in the supine position: scintigraphy in healthy humans. *J Appl Physiol.* (1985) 1999;86:1135–1141.

53. Lamm WJ, Graham MM, Albert RK. Mechanism by which the prone position improves oxygenation in acute lung injury. *Am J Respir Crit Care Med.* 1994;150:184–193.

54. Pappert D, Rossaint R, Slama K, Gruning T, Falke KJ. Influence of positioning on ventilation-perfusion relationships in severe adult respiratory distress syndrome. *Chest.* 1994;106:1511–1516.

55. Mutoh T, Lamm WJ, Embree LJ, Hildebrandt J, Albert RK. Volume infusion produces abdominal distension, lung compression, and chest wall stiffening in pigs. *J Appl Physiol.* (1985) 1992;72:575–582.

56. Pelosi P, Croci M, Calappi E, et al. The prone positioning during general anesthesia minimally affects respiratory mechanics while improving functional residual capacity and increasing oxygen tension. *Anesth Analg.* 1995;80:955–960.

57. Pelosi P, Tubiolo D, Mascheroni D, et al. Effects of the prone position on respiratory mechanics and gas exchange during acute lung injury. *Am J Respir Crit Care Med.* 1998;157:387–393.

58. Nakos G, Tsangaris I, Kostanti E, et al. Effect of the prone position on patients with hydrostatic pulmonary edema compared with patients with acute respiratory distress syndrome and pulmonary fibrosis. *Am J Respir Crit Care Med.* 2000;161:360–368.

59. Gattinoni L, Vagginelli F, Carlesso E, Prone-Supine Study G, et al. Decrease in PaCO2 with prone position is predictive of improved outcome in acute respiratory distress syndrome. *Crit Care Med.* 2003;31:2727–2733.

60. Mentzelopoulos SD, Roussos C, Zakynthinos SG. Prone position reduces lung stress and strain in severe acute respiratory distress syndrome. *Euro Respir J.* 2005;25:534–544.

61. Broccard AF, Vannay C, Feihl F, Schaller MD. Impact of low pulmonary vascular pressure on ventilator-induced lung injury. *Crit Care Med.* 2002;30:2183–2190.

62. Broccard AF, Shapiro RS, Schmitz LL, Ravenscraft SA, Marini JJ. Influence of prone position on the extent and distribution of lung injury in a high tidal volume oleic acid model of acute respiratory distress syndrome. *Crit Care Med.* 1997;25:16–27.

63. Broccard A, Shapiro RS, Schmitz LL, Adams AB, Nahum A, Marini JJ. Prone positioning attenuates and redistributes ventilator-induced lung injury in dogs. *Crit Care Med.* 2000;28:295–303.

64. Curley MA, Hibberd PL, Fineman LD, et al. Effect of prone positioning on clinical outcomes in children with acute lung injury: a randomized controlled trial. *JAMA.* 2005;294:229–237.

65. Fernandez R, Trenchs X, Klamburg J, et al. Prone positioning in acute respiratory distress syndrome: a multicenter randomized clinical trial. *Intensive Care Med.* 2008;34:1487–1491.

66. Guerin C, Gaillard S, Lemasson S, et al. Effects of systematic prone positioning in hypoxemic acute respiratory failure: a randomized controlled trial. *JAMA.* 2004;292:2379–2387.

67. Mancebo J, Fernandez R, Blanch L, et al. A multicenter trial of prolonged prone ventilation in severe acute respiratory distress syndrome. *Am J Respir Crit Care Med.* 2006;173:1233–1239.

68. Voggenreiter G, Aufmkolk M, Stiletto RJ, et al. Prone positioning improves oxygenation in post-traumatic lung injury–a prospective randomized trial. *J Trauma.* 2005;59:333–341. discussion 341–333.

69. Guerin C, Reignier J, Richard JC, et al. Prone positioning in severe acute respiratory distress syndrome. *N Engl J Med.* 2013;368:2159–2168.

70. Taccone P, Pesenti A, Latini R, et al. Prone positioning in patients with moderate and severe acute respiratory distress syndrome: a randomized controlled trial. *JAMA.* 2009;302:1977–1984.

71. Jozwiak M, Teboul JL, Anguel N, et al. Beneficial hemodynamic effects of prone positioning in patients with acute respiratory distress syndrome. *Am J Respir Crit Care Med.* 2013;188:1428–1433.

72. Abroug F, Ouanes-Besbes L, Elatrous S, Brochard L. The effect of prone positioning in acute respiratory distress syndrome or acute lung injury: a meta-analysis. Areas of uncertainty and recommendations for research. *Intensive Care Med.* 2008;34:1002–1011.

73. Alsaghir AH, Martin CM. Effect of prone positioning in patients with acute respiratory distress syndrome: a meta-analysis. *Crital Care Med.* 2008;36:603–609.

74. Sud S, Sud M, Friedrich JO, Adhikari NK. Effect of mechanical ventilation in the prone position on clinical outcomes in patients with acute hypoxemic respiratory failure: a systematic review and meta-analysis. *CMAJ.* 2008;178:1153–1161.

75. Tiruvoipati R, Bangash M, Manktelow B, Peek GJ. Efficacy of prone ventilation in adult patients with acute respiratory failure: a meta-analysis. *J Crit Care.* 2008;23:101–110.

76. Sud S, Friedrich JO, Adhikari NK, et al. Effect of prone positioning during mechanical ventilation on mortality among patients with acute respiratory distress syndrome: a systematic review and meta-analysis. *CMAJ.* 2014;186:E381–E390.

77. Albert RK, Keniston A, Baboi L, Ayzac L, Guerin C, Proseva I. Prone position-induced improvement in gas exchange does not predict improved survival in the acute respiratory distress syndrome. *Am J Respir Crit Care Med.* 2014;189:494–496.

78. Robak O, Schellongowski P, Bojic A, Laczika K, Locker GJ, Staudinger T. Short-term effects of combining upright and prone positions in patients with ARDS: a prospective randomized study. *Crit Care.* 2011;15:R230.

33 Is Pulmonary Hypertension Important in ARDS? Should We Treat It?

Criona M. Walshe, Leo G. Kevin

In this chapter, we systematically examine the evidence linking acute respiratory distress syndrome (ARDS) with pulmonary hypertension, the implications of pulmonary hypertension and consequent right ventricular failure for patient outcomes, and the data related to pulmonary vasodilator therapies in this patient group.

PULMONARY HYPERTENSION IN ARDS

Pulmonary hypertension in ARDS was described in the late 1970s and was soon accepted as a key cause of death.[1] A consistent observation in reports at the time was that nonsurvivors of ARDS demonstrated pulmonary artery pressures that continued to increase throughout the early phase of the illness. Later, systematic studies, such as the European Collaborative ARDS study,[2] confirmed the prognostic significance of pulmonary artery pressures for these patients. In that report, a logistic regression analysis that included multiple hemodynamic measures and other factors identified day 2 systolic pulmonary artery pressure (24.1 ± 6.7 mm Hg for eventual survivors compared with 28.4 ± 8.5 mm Hg for eventual nonsurvivors) as a potent independent predictor of mortality. More recently, a secondary analysis[3] of results from the Fluid and Catheter Treatment Trial[4] found that pulmonary vascular resistance was elevated early in the course of ARDS and was statistically higher in patients who died. In multivariate prediction models, pulmonary vascular resistance was a strong independent risk factor for 60-day mortality.

How common is pulmonary hypertension in ARDS? There are surprisingly few data to accurately answer this question. Zapol and Snider[5] found that all of the 30 ARDS patients in their series had elevated pulmonary artery pressures, even after correction of hypoxemia. Clinical trials in ARDS have consistently reported baseline mean pulmonary pressures of 29 to 30 mm Hg.[6,7] More recently, with a cutoff mean pulmonary artery pressure of 25 mm Hg, 92.2% of ARDS patients had pulmonary hypertension, although this was severe (defined by a mean pulmonary artery pressure of >45 mm Hg) in only 7.4%.[6]

A combination of factors may contribute to the development of pulmonary hypertension in patients with ARDS. Correlations between lung edema and pulmonary artery pressures have been demonstrated.[7] Intravascular thrombosis causing microvascular occlusion was an important factor in pulmonary vascular resistance in a pig model,[8] and postmortem studies have demonstrated widespread pulmonary thromboembolism in 95% of cases of ARDS.[9] Although marked hypoxic pulmonary vasoconstriction has been demonstrated in nonventilated areas of the lung in patients with ARDS,[10] the effect of this phenomenon on overall pulmonary hemodynamic measures is uncertain. For example, Sibbald and colleagues[1] reported that the severity of pulmonary hypertension occurring in ARDS correlated poorly with the degree of hypoxia. Hypoxic pulmonary vasoconstriction may be a weak contributor because it is partially or wholly inhibited by factors such as locally released nitric oxide (NO) or prostaglandin. Furthermore, pulmonary hypertension in ARDS may persist, even after the resolution of hypoxemia. One possible explanation is that pulmonary vascular smooth muscle cells proliferate over time. This results in a diminution in wall compliance.

Inflammatory mediators released in sepsis may increase vascular tone in the pulmonary circulation while decreasing it in the systemic circulation. Cytokines such as tumor necrosis factor-α have been implicated, but their exact role is unclear. Endothelin-1 (ET-1) is a potent pulmonary vasoconstrictor and activator of vascular smooth muscle proliferation. ET-1 expression is upregulated in patients with ARDS, although there is currently no evidence directly implicating ET-1 in ARDS-related pulmonary hypertension.

PULMONARY HYPERTENSION, RIGHT HEART FAILURE, AND DEATH

The thin-walled right ventricle is accustomed to pumping into a low-pressure circuit; therefore it responds poorly to increases in afterload. In the critically ill patient, multiple factors, such as fluid overload, negative inotropy associated with sepsis, and elevated mean airway pressures, may impair right ventricular function. This is supported by data indicating that right ventricular failure both predicts and appears to cause the death of 30% of patients with ARDS.[6,11] In an echocardiography-based study that evaluated the right side of the heart in 23 patients with ARDS,[12]

9 patients were found to have normal right ventricular function, whereas 9 other patients had a slightly enlarged right ventricle with normal systolic function. The remaining five patients had a severely enlarged right ventricle with contractile dysfunction and reductions in left ventricular size. These findings suggest detrimental ventricular interdependence. Of note, all of the patients in that study had normal left ventricular systolic function by two-dimensional echocardiography. Severe right ventricular failure was strongly associated with death.

Vieillard-Baron and associates[13] used echocardiography to evaluate the right side of the heart in ARDS. Right ventricular dysfunction was present in 19 (25%) of 75 patients on day 2. Many of these patients also had evidence of left ventricular diastolic dysfunction. Although mortality was the same as that for patients without right ventricular dysfunction, duration of respiratory support was longer. Of particular interest in this study, elevated partial pressure of carbon dioxide in arterial blood ($Paco_2$) was identified as the sole independent predictor of acute right ventricular failure. This may reflect increased dead space, associated with high levels of positive end-expiratory pressure (PEEP) and worse outcomes with ARDS. For example, Poelaert and coworkers[14] found incremental PEEP-induced cyclic augmentation of right ventricular outflow impedance. Jardin and Vieillard-Baron[15] illustrated that higher plateau pressures were associated with marked increases in acute right heart failure and death. These authors recently proposed the concept of a "right ventricular protective approach" to mechanical ventilation for the patient with ARDS.[16]

PULMONARY VASODILATOR THERAPIES IN ARDS

Inhaled Nitric Oxide

NO is a free radical gas that was identified in 1987 as the elusive endothelium-derived relaxing factor.[17] After native generation in the endothelium, NO enters local vascular smooth cells where it activates soluble guanylate cyclase. This enzyme stimulates the conversion of guanosine 5′-triphosphate to cyclic guanosine monophosphate (cGMP), which causes hyperpolarization and attenuates calcium entry to the muscle cytoplasm. The net result is vasodilation. Deficiencies in NO production[18] and attenuated responsiveness to NO[19] in the pulmonary circulation have been identified and are now accepted as important factors in the pathogenesis of primary and secondary pulmonary hypertension.

Within a year of the discovery of NO, inhaled NO was confirmed as an effective pulmonary vasodilator in patients with primary pulmonary hypertension.[20] Shortly thereafter, several small case series describing the use of NO therapy for patients with ARDS and pulmonary hypertension appeared in the literature.[21-23] Studies reported not only decreases in pulmonary vascular resistance and pulmonary artery pressures but also significant improvements in oxygenation. For example, in 1993, Rossaint and colleagues[23] gave 18 ppm inhaled NO to 10 patients with ARDS. Pulmonary artery pressures decreased by an average of 6 mm Hg, and pulmonary vascular resistance decreased by an average of 71 dyn sec cm^{-5} from baseline. There were no significant changes in systemic blood pressure or cardiac output. However, most compelling to clinicians at the time was an average increase in the partial pressure of oxygen in arterial blood (Pao_2)/fraction of inspired oxygen (Fio_2) of 51 mm Hg. Inhaled NO was rapidly adopted for the treatment of severe ARDS. Indeed, a survey of intensive care physicians' practices across Europe showed that, by 1998, 98.5% of respondents considered ARDS an indication for inhaled NO. Moreover, 71% considered that Pao_2/Fio_2 ratios were sufficient criteria for initiating treatment.[24]

In these early studies, three observations were made that would later become contentious. The first of these was that the response to NO, whether based on decreased pulmonary artery pressures or on improved oxygenation, was largely predictable and almost universal. It was later established that, at most, 40% to 60% of ARDS patients responded to inhaled NO with an improvement in one or both of these parameters.[25] Prediction of likely responders was difficult.[26] The second observation was that the response to inhaled NO was sustained over a prolonged period of treatment. In contrast, later data demonstrated the development of tachyphylaxis within 2 to 3 days.[25] The final observation was that although daily interruptions of inhaled NO were noted to cause increases in pulmonary artery pressures,[23] these changes were not thought to be particularly problematic. Rebound pulmonary hypertension after withdrawal was later appreciated as a phenomenon of real consequence, albeit one that could be overcome.

Early enthusiasm for inhaled NO was curtailed by negative Phase II[27,28] and Phase III[25,29] trials showing that NO did not improve overall survival in ARDS. This was supported by meta-analyses of trials of NO therapy in ARDS.[30,31] In addition, NO may have an adverse effect on renal function[31,32] In the United States, concerns about clinical efficacy of NO have been reinforced by the high costs associated with the delivery system. The results of a Canadian survey were likely representative of worldwide practice: By 2004, less than 40% of critical care physicians were using NO as therapy in ARDS and then only selectively.[32]

Prostaglandins

Prostaglandins are vasodilators that act through intracellular adenylate cyclase, leading to a decrease in intracellular calcium. Various prostaglandins and their analogs have been shown to improve exercise capacity and quality of life in chronic pulmonary hypertension[33] but with little effect on mortality.

During the late 1980s, several reports described the use of intravenous prostaglandin E_1 (PGE_1) for ARDS. PGE_1 appeared to exert its effects but as an anti-inflammatory and as a pulmonary vasodilator. The finding that pulmonary artery pressures were indeed decreased—by approximately 15% when given in the typical dose range[34]—prompted two randomized controlled trials. The first, and the smaller of the two, was limited to ARDS in surgical patients and suggested a survival advantage.[35] The subsequent, larger, and more inclusive trial failed to confirm this. Indeed, the authors reported systemic hypotension and increases in intrapulmonary shunting.[36] As these results were emerging, reported successes with inhaled NO fueled attempts to find an inhaled prostaglandin. Iloprost, a synthetic analog of prostacyclin, emerged as a drug stable in aerosolization and suitable for inhalation. In 1993, Walmrath and coworkers[37] first reported the use of aerosolized iloprost in three patients with ARDS. Pulmonary vascular resistance and intrapulmonary shunt decreased and oxygenation improved, all by 30% to 40%. These findings were confirmed 3 years later by 2 reports, both involving rather few patients.[38] In a more recent report, 10 mg nebulized iloprost was administered to a series of 20 ARDS patients with pulmonary hypertension identified by echocardiography. Pao_2 increased by a mean of 18 mm Hg without demonstrable adverse effects.[39]

Iloprost compares well with inhaled NO for the treatment of pulmonary hypertension in ARDS. Prostacyclin and its analogs have a longer half-life (2 to 3 minutes) compared with NO (seconds). Although this could increase the risk for systemic vasodilation and hypotension, in practice this does not appear to be a significant problem.[40,41] Indeed, 50 ng/kg/min, the upper end of the dose range for iloprost, caused no systemic hemodynamic effects in children with acute lung injury.[40] Prostacyclin is also a potent inhibitor of platelet aggregation. In the absence of increased bleeding, this may be of benefit.

Nonetheless, comparisons of iloprost and NO are complicated by the limited published data. There are several small studies. Van Heerden and colleagues[38] showed drug equivalency for iloprost at 50 ng/kg/min and NO at 10 ppm in five hypoxemic ARDS patients. Zwissler and associates[42] compared 1, 10, and 25 ng/kg/min iloprost with NO at 1, 4, and 8 ppm, respectively, and found that both drugs produced roughly comparable effects. This also established limited dose-response curves for ARDS patients. Likewise, in 16 ARDS patients, Walmrath and coworkers[43] found that iloprost (average dose 7.5±2.5 ng/kg/min) and inhaled NO (average dose 18 ppm) were equally effective. Finally, similar comparative studies in primary pulmonary hypertension point to roughly comparable clinical effects of the two agents.[44]

NO is degraded to nitrogen dioxide, a potential toxin. NO also requires an expensive delivery and monitoring system. Iloprost does not have this problem because it can be delivered by simple nebulizer systems. However, as with inhaled NO, rebound hypertension on drug withdrawal has been reported.[45] What remains to be conclusively demonstrated is whether prostaglandins may succeed in NO-unresponsive patients and vice versa. Because NO and prostaglandins exert their effects by entirely different mechanisms, the hypothesis is an attractive one, but which patients will respond to either remains difficult to predict. Data from Domenighetti and colleagues[46] suggest that patients with ARDS of pulmonary origin are less likely to respond than those with ARDS of extrapulmonary origin, but a direct comparison with NO was not performed. Of note, Brett and associates[26] found no predictors of response to inhaled NO. Finally, as with NO, there are no data suggesting that inhaled prostacyclin alters outcome in ARDS.

Phosphodiesterase Inhibitors

Enoximone, amrinone, and milrinone are inhibitors of phosphodiesterase type 3 PDE-3, the enzyme that catalyzes the breakdown of cyclic adenosine monophosphate in myocardium and vascular smooth muscle. Inhibition of this enzyme increases myocardial contractility and causes widespread vasodilation. Although long-term survival rates are not improved for patients with chronic cardiac failure taking oral milrinone, this class of drugs is widely used in the setting of acute cardiac failure in cardiac surgical patients.[47,48] Decreases in output impedance should particularly favor the failing right ventricle. In a retrospective comparison of milrinone and dobutamine in 329 patients with acutely decompensated cardiac failure, milrinone produced greater decreases in pulmonary vascular resistance with greater improvements in cardiac output.[49] Likewise, in patients with severe pulmonary hypertension undergoing transplantation, milrinone[50] or enoximone[51] potently decreased pulmonary vascular resistance and increased cardiac index.

Sildenafil is an orally administered, highly selective inhibitor of PDE-5. This subtype of PDE is present in abundance in the smooth muscle cells of the pulmonary vasculature. Inhibition of PDE-5 prevents the breakdown of cGMP, thereby augmenting the vasodilating effects of native and inhaled NO.

There are some reports of sildenafil treatment for patients with new-onset, life-threatening pulmonary hypertension related to acute lung injury or ARDS. Giacomini and associates[52] gave enteral vardenafil, a sildenafil analog, to a single patient with ARDS and pulmonary hypertension in whom weaning of inhaled NO had proved impossible. Vardenafil permitted withdrawal of the inhaled NO and was itself eventually tapered. However, a recent open-label study evaluated the effect of a single 50-mg dose of sildenafil in 10 patients with ARDS and pulmonary hypertension.[53] Although pulmonary artery pressures decreased significantly, from means of 25 to 22 mm Hg, systemic arterial blood pressures also decreased, whereas shunt fraction increased. In the absence of further evidence, sildenafil remains an unproven therapy for pulmonary hypertension in ARDS.

Levosimendan

Levosimendan is an inodilator. The inotropic effect occurs through sensitization of troponin C in the myocardium. Contractility is improved, but this uniquely occurs without a concomitant increase in intracellular calcium or in energy consumption. Vasodilation occurs through activation of potassium–adenosine triphosphate channels in the vasculature. Activation of these channels may also account for the cardioprotective effect reported in laboratory[54] and clinical studies.[55] An immunomodulatory effect is also described, although the mechanism is unknown.

The LIDO (Levosimendan Infusion versus Dobutamine) study was a double-blind randomized controlled trial that compared levosimendan with dobutamine in cardiogenic shock.[56] Not only were predetermined hemodynamic goals achieved more successfully with levosimendan, but there was also a significant survival benefit. The extreme sensitivity of the right ventricle to modest changes in afterload suggests a particular potential for levosimendan in the treatment of right ventricular failure complicating pulmonary hypertension.

There are several clinical studies describing the use of levosimendan specifically for pulmonary hypertension and right ventricular failure. In a small placebo-controlled trial, Ukkonen and associates[57] reported marked decreases in pulmonary vascular resistance along with improvements in right ventricular mechanical efficiency and cardiac output in patients with severe right heart failure. Morelli and colleagues[58] performed a randomized placebo-controlled trial in 35 patients with ARDS. Levosimendan decreased mean pulmonary artery pressures from 29 ± 3 to 25 ± 3 mm Hg while increasing the right ventricular ejection fraction from 45 ± 10 to $59 \pm 10\%$. Cardiac index and mixed venous oxygen saturations also significantly increased.

AUTHORS' RECOMMENDATIONS

- Pulmonary hypertension is frequently unrecognized in ARDS.
- Pulmonary hypertension undoubtedly contributes to poor outcomes in some patients.
- Optimal treatment is unclear. Large randomized controlled trials failed to show survival benefits of pulmonary vasodilators. However, these trials enrolled all ARDS patients, with or without pulmonary hypertension, and primarily targeted oxygenation indices.
- Although unproven, recognition and treatment of pulmonary hypertension in selected patients with ARDS may improve survival.
- A modern approach emphasizes attention to the effects of ventilatory parameters on right ventricular function.

REFERENCES

1. Sibbald W, Paterson NA, Holliday RL, Anderson RA, Lobb TR, Duff JH. Pulmonary hypertension in sepsis: measurement by the pulmonary arterial diastolic-pulmonary wedge pressure gradient and the influence of passive and active factors. *Chest.* 1978;73:583–591.
2. Squara P, Dhainaut JF, Artigas A, Carlet J. Hemodynamic profile in severe ARDS: results of the European Collaborative ARDS Study. *Intensive Care Med.* 1998;24:1018–1028.
3. Bull TM, Clark B, McFann K, Moss M. National Institutes of Health/National Heart, Lung, and Blood Institute ARDS Network: pulmonary vascular dysfunction is associated with poor outcomes in patients with acute lung injury. *Am J Respir Crit Care Med.* 2010;182:1123–1128.
4. Wiedemann HP, Wheeler AP, Bernard GR, et al. Comparison of two fluid-management strategies in acute lung injury. National Heart, Lung, and Blood Institute Acute Respiratory Distress Syndrome (ARDS) Clinical Trials Network. *N Engl J Med.* 2006;354:2564–2575.
5. Zapol W, Snider M. Pulmonary hypertension in severe acute respiratory failure. *N Engl J Med.* 1977;296:476–480.
6. Beiderlinden M, Kuehl H, Boes T, Peters J. Prevalence of pulmonary hypertension associated with severe acute respiratory distress syndrome: predictive value of computed tomography. *Intensive Care Med.* 2006;32:852–857.
7. Prewitt R, McCarthy J, Wood LD. Treatment of acute low pressure pulmonary edema in dogs: relative effects of hydrostatic and oncotic pressure, nitroprusside, and positive end-expiratory pressure. *J Clin Invest.* 1981;67:409–418.
8. Hardaway R, Williams CH, Marvasti M, et al. Prevention of adult respiratory distress syndrome with plasminogen activator in pigs. *Crit Care Med.* 1990;18:1413–1418.
9. Tomashefski JJ, Davies P, Boggis C, Greene R, Zapol WM, Reid LM. The pulmonary vascular lesions of the adult respiratory distress syndrome. *Am J Pathol.* 1983;112:112–126.
10. Benzing A, Mols G, Brieschal T, Geiger K. Hypoxic pulmonary vasoconstriction in nonventilated lung areas contributes to differences in hemodynamic and gas exchange responses to inhalation of nitric oxide. *Anesthesiology.* 1997;86:1254–1261.
11. Monchi M, Bellenfant F, Cariou A, et al. Early predictive factors of survival in the acute respiratory distress syndrome. *Am J Respir Crit Care Med.* 1998;158:1076–1081.
12. Jardin F, Gueret P, Dubourg O, Farcot JC, Margairaz A, Bourdarias JP. Two-dimensional echocardiographic evaluation of right ventricular size and contractility in acute respiratory failure. *Crit Care Med.* 1985:13.
13. Vieillard-Baron A, Schmitt JM, Augarde R, et al. Acute cor pulmonale in acute respiratory distress syndrome submitted to protective ventilation Incidence, clinical implications, and prognosis. *Crit Care Med.* 2001;29:1551–1555.
14. Poelaert JV, Everaert JA, DeDeyne CS, Decruyenaere J, Colardyn FA. Doppler evaluation of right ventricular outflow impedance during positive-pressure ventilation. *J Cardiothorac Vasc Anesth.* 1994;8:392–397.
15. Jardin F, Vieillard-Baron A. Is there a safe plateau pressure in ARDS? The right heart only knows. *Intensive Care Med.* 2007;33:444–447.
16. Repessé X, Charron C, Vieillard-Baron A. Right ventricular failure in acute lung injury and acute respiratory distress syndrome. *Minerva Anestesiol.* 2012;78:941–948.
17. Ignarro L, Buga GM, Wood KS, Byrns RE, Chaudhuri G. Endothelium-derived relaxing factor produced and released from artery and vein is nitric oxide. *Proc Natl Acad Sci USA.* 1987;84:9265–9269.
18. Kaneko F, Arroliga AC, Dweik RA, et al. Biochemical reaction products of nitric oxide as quantitative markers of primary pulmonary hypertension. *Am J Respir Crit Care Med.* 1998;158:917–923.
19. Carville C, Raffestin B, Eddahibi S, Blouquit Y, Adnot S. Loss of endothelium-dependent relaxation in proximal pulmonary arteries from rats exposed to chronic hypoxia: effects of in vivo and in vitro supplementation with L-arginine. *J Cardiovasc Pharmacol.* 1993;22:889–896.
20. Higenbottam T, Pepke-Zaba J, Scott J, Woolman P, Coutts C, Wallwork J. Inhaled endothelial derived-relaxing factor (EDRF) in primary pulmonary hypertension (PPH). *Am Rev Respir Dis.* (suppl). 1988: A107.
21. Young JD, Brampton WJ, Knighton JD, Finfer SR. Inhaled nitric oxide in acute respiratory failure in adults. *Br J Anaesth.* 1994;73:499–502.
22. Gerlach H, Pappert D, Lewandowski K, Rossaint R, Falke KJ. Long-term inhalation with evaluated low doses of nitric oxide for selective improvement of oxygenation in patients with adult respiratory distress syndrome. *Intensive Care Med.* 1993;19:443–449.
23. Rossaint RFK, Lopez F, Slama K, Pison U, Zapol WM. Inhaled nitric oxide for the adult respiratory distress syndrome. *N Engl J Med.* 1993;328:399–405.
24. Beloucif S, Payen D. European survey of the use of inhaled nitric oxide in the ICU. Working Group on Inhaled NO in the ICU of the European Society of Intensive Care Medicine. *Intensive Care Med.* 1998;24:864–877.
25. Taylor R, Zimmerman JL, Dellinger RP, et al. Low-dose inhaled nitric oxide in patients with acute lung injury: a randomized controlled trial. *JAMA.* 2004;291:1603–1609.
26. Brett S, Hansell DM, Evans TW. Clinical correlates in acute lung injury: response to inhaled nitric oxide. *Chest.* 1998;114:1397–1404.
27. Payen D, Vallet B, Groupe d'Etude sur le NO inhale au cours de l'ARDS (GENOA). Results of the French prospective multicentric randomized doubleblind placebo-controlled trial on inhaled nitric oxide (NO) in ARDS [abstract 645]. *Intensive Care Med.* 1999;25:S166.
28. Dellinger R, Zimmerman JL, Taylor RW, et al. Effects of inhaled nitric oxide in patients with acute respiratory distress syndrome: results of a randomized phase II trial. *Crit Care Med.* 1998;26:15–23.
29. Lundin S, Mang H, Smithies M, Stenqvist O, Frostell C. Inhalation of nitric oxide in acute lung injury: results of a European multicentre study. The European Study Group of Inhaled Nitric Oxide. *Intensive Care Med.* 1999;25:911–919.
30. Sokol J, Jacobs SE, Bohn D. Inhaled nitric oxide for acute hypoxic respiratory failure in children and adults: a meta-analysis. *Anesth Analg.* 2003;97:989–998.
31. Adhikari NK, Burns KE, Friedrich JO, Granton JT, Cook DJ, Meade MO. Effect of nitric oxide on oxygenation and mortality in acute lung injury: systematic review and meta-analysis. *BMJ.* 2007;334:779.

32. Meade M, Jacka MJ, Cook DJ, Dodek P, Griffith L, Guyatt GH. Canadian Critical Care Trials Group: Survey of interventions for the prevention and treatment of acute respiratory distress syndrome. *Crit Care Med.* 2004;32:946–954.

33. Olschewski H, Simonneau G, Galie N, et al. Aerosolized Iloprost Randomized Study Group: Inhaled iloprost for severe pulmonary hypertension. *N Engl J Med.* 2002;347:322–329.

34. Mélot C, Lejeune P, Leeman M, Moraine JJ, Naeije R. Prostaglandin E1 in the adult respiratory distress syndrome. Benefit for pulmonary hypertension and cost for pulmonary gas exchange. *Am Rev Respir Dis.* 1989;139:106–110.

35. Holcroft J, Vassar MJ, Weber CJ. Prostaglandin E1 and survival in patients with the adult respiratory distress syndrome. A prospective trial. *Ann Surg.* 1986;203:371–378.

36. Bone R, Slotman G, Maunder R, et al. Randomized double-blind, multicenter study of prostaglandin E1 in patients with the adult respiratory distress syndrome. Prostaglandin E1 Study Group. *Chest.* 1989;96:114–119.

37. Walmrath DST, Pilch J, Grimminger F, Seeger W. Aerosolised prostacyclin in adult respiratory distress syndrome. *Lancet.* 1993;342:961–962.

38. Van Heerden P, Blythe D, Webb SA. Inhaled aerosolized prostacyclin and nitric oxide as selective pulmonary vasodilators in ARDS–a pilot study. *Anaesth Intensive Care.* 1996;24:564–568.

39. Sawheny E, Ellis AL, Kinasewitz GT. Iloprost improves gas exchange in patients with pulmonary hypertension and ARDS. *Chest.* 2013;144:55–62.

40. Dahlem P, van Aalderen WM, de Neef M, Dijkgraaf MG, Bos AP. Randomized controlled trial of aerosolized prostacyclin therapy in children with acute lung injury. *Crit Care Med.* 2004;32:1055–1060.

41. Pappert DB, Gerlach H, Lewandowski K, Radermacher P, Rossaint R. Aerosolized prostacyclin versus inhaled nitric oxide in children with severe acute respiratory distress syndrome. *Anesthesiology.* 1995;82:1507–1511.

42. Zwissler B, Kemming G, Habler O, et al. Inhaled prostacyclin (PGI2) versus inhaled nitric oxide in adult respiratory distress syndrome. *Am J Respir Crit Care Med.* 1996;154:1671–1677.

43. Walmrath D, Schneider T, Schermuly R, Olschewski H, Grimminger F, Seeger W. Direct comparison of inhaled nitric oxide and aerosolized prostacyclin in acute respiratory distress syndrome. *Am J Respir Crit Care Med.* 1996;153:991–996.

44. Hoeper M, Olschewski H, Ghofrani HA, et al. A comparison of the acute hemodynamic effects of inhaled nitric oxide and aerosolized iloprost in primary pulmonary hypertension. German PPH Study Group. *J Am Coll Cardiol.* 2000;35:176–182.

45. Augoustides J, Culp K, Smith S. Rebound pulmonary hypertension and cardiogenic shock after withdrawal of inhaled prostacyclin. *Anesthesiology.* 2004;100:1023–1025.

46. Domenighetti G, Stricker H, Waldispuehl B. Nebulized prostacyclin (PGI2) in acute respiratory distress syndrome: impact of primary (pulmonary injury) and secondary (extrapulmonary injury) disease on gas exchange response. *Crit Care Med.* 2001;29:57–62.

47. Kastrup M, Markewitz A, Spies C, et al. Current practice of hemodynamic monitoring and vasopressor and inotropic therapy in post-operative cardiac surgery patients in Germany: results from a postal survery. *Acta Anaesthesiol Scand.* 2007;51:347–358.

48. Kwak Y, Oh YJ, Kim SH, Shin HK, Kim JY, Hong YW. Efficacy of pre-emptive milrinone in off-pump coronary artery bypass surgery: comparison between patients with a low and normal pregraft cardiac index. *Eur J Cardiothorac Surg.* 2004;26:687–693.

49. Yamani MH, Haji SA, Starling RC, et al. Comparison of dobutamine-based and milrinone-based therapy for advanced decompensated congestive heart failure: Hemodynamic efficacy, clinical outcome, and economic impact. *Am Heart J.* 2001;142:998–1002.

50. Pamboukian SV, Carere RG, Webb JG, et al. The use of milrinone in pre-transplant assessment of patients with congestive heart failure and pulmonary hypertension. *J Heart Lung Transplant.* 1999;18:367–371.

51. Schulz O, Mitrovic V, Schonburg M, Thormann J. High-dose enoximone to evaluate reversibility of pulmonary hypertension: is there a diagnostic value of neurohormonal measurements? *Am Heart J.* 1999;137:887–894.

52. Giacomini M, Borotto E, Bosotti L, et al. Vardenafil and weaning from inhaled nitric oxide: effect on pulmonary hypertension in ARDS. *Anaesth Intensive Care.* 2007;35:91–93.

53. Cornet AD, Hofstra JJ, Swart EL, Girbes AR, Juffermans NP. Sildenafil attenuates pulmonary arterial pressure but does not improve oxygenation during ARDS. *Intensive Care Med.* 2010;36:758–764.

54. Yapici D, Altunkan Z, Ozeran M, et al. Effects of levosimendan on myocardial ischaemia-reperfusion injury. *Eur J Anaesthesiol.* 2008;25:8–14.

55. Tritapepe L, DeSantis V, Vitale D, et al. Levosimendan pre-treatment improves outcomes in patients undergoing coronary surgery. *Br J Anaesth.* 2009;102:198–204.

56. Follath F, Cleland JGF, Just H, et al. Efficacy and safety of intravenous levosimendan compared with dobutamine in severe low-output heart failure (the LIDO study): a randomised double-blind trial. *Lancet.* 2002;360:196–202.

57. Ukkonen H, Saraste M, Akkila J, et al. Myocardial efficiency during levosimendan infusion in congestive heart failure. *Clin Pharmacol Ther.* 2000;68:522–531.

58. Morelli A, Teboul JL, Maggiore SM, et al. Effects of levosimendan on right ventricular afterload in patients with acute respiratory distress syndrome: a pilot study. *Crit Care Med.* 2006;34:2287–2293.

34 Inhaled Vasodilators in ARDS: Do They Make a Difference?

Francois Lamontagne, Maureen O. Meade

Inhaled vasodilators have a compelling physiologic rationale in the management of critically ill patients with acute respiratory distress syndrome (ARDS). A 20-year accumulation of rigorous research has helped to clarify their role in this setting, which is significantly more limited than original reports suggested.

PHYSIOLOGIC RATIONALE

Lung imaging studies in patients with ARDS show that alveoli that are poorly aerated because of exudative edema, hyaline membranes, and microatelectasis are not homogeneously distributed throughout the lung parenchyma. Instead, certain zones are relatively preserved and remain compliant, allowing them to receive disproportionately large fractions of the minute ventilation.[1,2] The more diseased lung regions, located predominantly in the dependent areas of the lungs, may be poorly ventilated and yet receive much of the right ventricular cardiac output, resulting in a significant ventilation-perfusion mismatch.

Heart-lung interactions are also part of the pathology of ARDS. Laboratory research has shown that hypoxia-induced vasoconstriction leads to pulmonary hypertension.[3,4] This is compounded by the dysregulation of constricting and dilating mediators, which contribute to a pathologic increase in the pulmonary vascular resistance.[5] In severe ARDS, these effects may lead to right ventricular failure, a plausible independent predictor for death.[6]

Theoretically, selective vasodilatation of vessels perfusing aerated lung tissue would redistribute blood from poorly ventilated regions, reducing the shunt fraction and at the same time correcting pulmonary hypertension. Improved oxygenation would reduce the mortality risk that is directly attributable to respiratory and right ventricular failure, whereas quicker resolution of ARDS would reduce the complications and morbidities associated with prolonged mechanical ventilation.[7] Unfortunately, these are not the effects that investigators have observed in randomized clinical trials.

The following discussion focuses mainly on inhaled nitric oxide (NO), which is by far the most extensively studied inhaled vasodilator in the context of ARDS. Fewer data are available for nebulized prostaglandins, specifically prostaglandin I_2 (PGI$_2$; prostacyclin), prostaglandin

E_1 (PGE$_1$; alprostadil), and prostaglandin E_2 (PGE$_2$; dinoprostone).

NITRIC OXIDE

In 1993, Rossaint et al.[8] demonstrated in a prospective cohort of 10 patients that inhaled NO, as opposed to intravenous prostacyclin, improved oxygenation in adult patients with ARDS. This report supported the potential benefit of selective pulmonary vasodilatation. Other preclinical and clinical observational studies confirmed the effects of inhaled NO on arterial oxygenation.[9-11] Added to further laboratory investigations finding additional benefits of NO on platelet and leukocyte function,[12] these results inspired the conduct of several randomized clinical trials.

Two systematic reviews have evaluated inhaled NO in ARDS.[13,14] Among the included randomized trials, the study populations varied to some extent. Most included adults with moderate to severe ARDS; however, some included children,[15-17] those with less severe ARDS,[18,19] or patients with a demonstrated favorable physiologic response to inhaled NO.[20] Protocols for the dose and duration of therapy also varied from 1 to 80 ppm and less than 1 day to 28 days, respectively. One trial was a "dose-finding" study.[20] Lastly, efforts to minimize bias ranged across the studies: 10 had concealed allocation,[15,16,18-25] 5 studies blinded caregivers,[16,19,21,24,25] and 6 reported on the use of alternative experimental therapies for ARDS.[18,19,21-23,26]

Despite the nuances of study populations, therapeutic protocols, and methodological rigor, the results related to mortality were strikingly consistent. The relative similarity of patients, methods, and results supports the decision to statistically aggregate results for this outcome. With or without statistical pooling, a visual review of the meta-analytical results provides a strong impression (Figure 34-1). The aggregate results further suggest that inhaled NO does not improve survival despite a demonstration of improved oxygenation. In fact, trends were more in keeping with increased mortality (relative risk 1.06; 95% confidence interval [CI], 0.93 to 1.22).[14] Likewise, the pooled results suggest that inhaled NO is not beneficial in terms of duration of mechanical ventilation (mean difference 1.02 days; 95% CI, −2.08 to 4.12) or ventilator-free-days (mean difference −0.57; 95% CI, −1.82 to 0.69).[14]

Analysis I.I
Comparison I Mortality: iNO versus control group, outcome I Longest follow-up mortality
(complete case analysis): iNO versus control

Review: Inhaled nitric oxide for acute respiratory distress syndrome (ARDS) and acute lung injury in children and adults

Comparison: I Mortality: iNO versus control group

Outcome: I Longest follow up mortality (complete case analysis): iNO versus control

Study or subgroup	iNO n/N	Control n/N	Risk ratio M-H, Fixed, 95% CI	Weight	Risk ratio M-H, Fixed, 95% CI
Cuthbertson 2000	8/15	7/15		3.0%	1.14 [0.56, 2.35]
Day 1997	1/12	2/12		0.9%	0.50 [0.05, 4.81]
Dellinger 1998	35/120	17/57		9.8%	0.98 [0.60, 1.59]
Dobyns 1999	22/53	24/55		10.1%	0.95 [0.61, 1.47]
Gerbach 2003	3/20	4/20		1.7%	0.75 [0.19, 2.93]
Ibrahim 2007	9/15	8/15		3.4%	1.13 [0.60, 2.11]
Lundin 1999	48/93	38/87		16.8%	1.18 [0.87, 1.61]
Mehta 2001	4/8	3/6		1.5%	1.00 [0.35, 2.88]
Michael 1998	11/20	9/20		3.8%	1.22 [0.65, 2.29]
Park 2003	8/17	2/6		1.3%	1.41 [0.41, 4.87]
Payen 1999	53/98	53/105		21.9%	1.07 [0.82, 1.39]
Schwebel 1997	0/9	0/10			Not estimable
Taylor 2004	54/165	53/167		22.5%	1.03 [0.75, 1.41]
Troncy 1998	9/15	8/15		3.4%	1.13 [0.60, 2.11]
Total (95% CI)	**660**	**590**		**100.0%**	**1.06 [0.93, 1.22]**

Total events: 265 (iNO), 228 (Control)
Heterogencity: Chi^2 = 203, df = 12 (P = 1.00); I^3 = 0.0%
Test for overall effect: Z = 0.90 (P = .37)
Test for subgroup differences: Not applicable

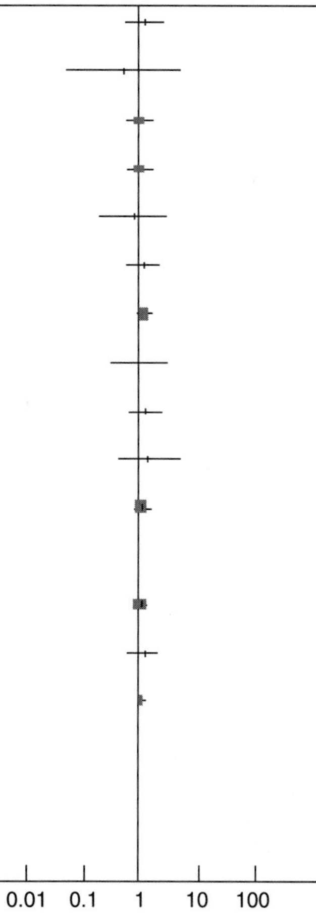

0.01   0.1   1   10   100
Favors experimental   Favors control

Figure 34-1. Inhaled nitric oxide (*iNO*) for acute respiratory distress syndrome (*ARDS*) and acute lung injury in children and adults. (Review) *(Copyright 2013 The Cochrane Collaboration. Published by John Wiley & Sons, Ltd.)*

Both systematic reviews suggest a statistically significant increase in the risk of renal dysfunction with inhaled NO therapy in the four studies that evaluated this outcome (relative risk 1.59; 95% CI, 1.17 to 2.16).[14] One unblinded and three blinded trials observed this effect.[19-21,24]

The generalizability of these results to clinical practice is high. The studies included patients across the spectrum of ARDS who clinicians commonly considered (before the publication of these studies) for inhaled NO therapy. Moreover, the treatment effects were strikingly similar across studies, notwithstanding the variations in populations, drug administration protocols, and methodological quality.

In parallel with these systematic reviews, data on the long-term quality of life outcomes and costs of inhaled NO have emerged.[27] Using the dataset of a previously published trial of inhaled NO in ARDS,[19] Angus et al.[27] performed a cost-effectiveness analysis suggesting that inhaled NO did not modify long-term outcomes or posthospital discharge costs. In a separate retrospective analysis of the same dataset, Dellinger et al.[28] reported on the long-term pulmonary function of ARDS survivors who had participated in the trial. At 6 months, the 51 survivors treated with inhaled NO (compared with 41 who were not) had a greater mean (standard deviation [SD]) (1) total lung capacity (TLC; 5.54 [1.42] vs. 4.81 [1.0], *P* = 0.026), (2) percentage of predicted forced expiratory volume in 1 second (FEV_1; 80.2 [21.2] vs. 69.5 [29.0], $P = 0.042$), (3) percentage of predicted forced vital capacity (FVC; 83.8 [19.4] vs. 69.8 [27.4], $P = 0.02$), (4) percentage of predicted FEV_1/FVC (96.1 [13.8] vs. 87.9 [19.8], $P = 0.03$), and (5) percentage of predicted TLC (93.3 [18.2] vs. 76.1 [21.8], $P < 0.001$). Most recently, Medjo and colleagues[29] reported on a prospective observational study of inhaled NO in 16 children with ARDS who were compared with historic controls.[29] Although oxygenation improved for up to 4 hours with inhaled NO, values had returned to baseline 24 hours after the onset of therapy and survival was not improved.

In summary, current clinical trials do not support a role for inhaled NO in the routine management of patients with acute lung injury and ARDS. In fact, meta-analyses suggest this approach to patient care is more likely to cause harm.[13,14]

PROSTAGLANDINS

Bearing the same physiologic rationale as inhaled NO in ARDS, three vasodilating prostaglandin molecules are a focus of interest in ARDS research: prostaglandin I_2 (PGI_2), alprostadil (PGE_1), and dinoprostone (PGE_2). In addition, PGI_2 blocks platelet aggregation and neutrophil migration, and PGE_2 has anti-inflammatory properties. For these reasons, many investigators have hypothesized that nebulized prostaglandins would serve as selective vasodilators; therefore, they would be useful adjuncts in the context of ARDS.

The body of literature evaluating a role for inhaled prostaglandins in the management of patients with ARDS is limited. Dahlem et al.[30] reported that among 14 children with ARDS randomized to nebulized prostacyclin or placebo, oxygenation did improve with prostacyclin (median change in oxygen index −2.5, interquartile range −5.8 to −0.2), but mortality was unchanged. Other uncontrolled trials led to similar results. In a dose-finding study, Van Heerden et al.[31] treated nine adult patients who had ARDS with inhaled prostacyclin. The partial pressure of oxygen in arterial blood (PaO_2)/fraction of inspired oxygen (FIO_2) increased, but prostacyclin had no effect on hemodynamic variables or on platelet function. Sawheny et al.[32] treated 20 patients with ARDS and elevated pulmonary arterial pressures with PGI_2. The mean PaO_2/FIO_2 ratio increased from 177 (SD 60) to 213 (SD 67), but the partial pressure of carbon dioxide in arterial blod ($PaCO_2$), peak and plateau airway pressures, systemic blood pressure, and heart rate did not significantly change. Using a different prostaglandin, Meyer et al.[33] treated 15 adult patients with acute lung injury with inhaled PGE_2. The mean PaO_2/FIO_2 ratio increased from 105 (standard error [SE] 9) to 160 (SE 17) ($P < 0.05$) after 4 hours and to 189 (SE 25) ($P < 0.05$) after 24 hours.

In contrast, Camamo et al.[34] reviewed the charts of 27 patients treated with PGI_2 or PGE_1 (alprostadil) for a primary or secondary diagnosis of ARDS and found no statistically significant improvement in oxygenation. Likewise, in a prospective uncontrolled trial of nebulized PGI_2 to 15 consecutive patients with ARDS and severe hypoxemia, Domenighetti et al.[35] found no improvement in oxygenation.

COMPARISONS OF INHALED NITRIC OXIDE AND PROSTAGLANDIN

Comparisons between nebulized PGI_2 and inhaled NO suggest that these agents have similar effects. Walmrath et al. individually titrated doses of both agents sequentially. The effects on pulmonary arterial pressure and distribution of blood flow were nearly identical.[36,37] Torbic et al.[38] compared the effects and costs of inhaled NO and PGI_2 in 105 patients. There was no difference in the change in PaO_2/FIO_2, duration of mechanical ventilation, and intensive care unit and hospital lengths of stay. The authors did observe that inhaled NO was 4.5 to 17 times more expensive than nebulized PGI_2.

RECONCILING THE RATIONALE WITH CLINICAL RESEARCH FINDINGS

This discordance between physiologic outcomes and mortality is not without precedent in critical care. In a landmark study of low tidal volume ventilation conducted by the ARDS Network, patients who underwent ventilation with low tidal volumes had lower O_2 levels but an increased survival when compared with those patients receiving traditionally larger tidal volumes.[39] A disconnect between effects of inhaled NO on physiologic outcomes and survival fits with the understanding that ARDS patients seldom die of respiratory failure.[40] However, for the minority of patients with profound and refractory hypoxemia threatening immediate survival, the question remains unanswered. There are insufficient research data in this specific at-risk subgroup to conclude that inhaled NO is on balance more likely to benefit or to harm.

There are several plausible explanations for the lack of benefit of inhaled NO as well as, prostaglandins in most patients with ARDS. It is conceivable that the purported physiologic benefits are offset by relatively hidden deleterious effects on other organ systems. Contrary to common belief, recent experiments have shown that inhaled NO does not act strictly within the pulmonary vasculature; rather, it reacts with various molecules to produce nitrosothiol compounds that share many properties of NO donors but have longer half-lives.[41-44] In keeping with the unexpected association between inhaled NO administration and renal dysfunction, this evidence suggests that the pharmacodynamic effects of inhaled NO are likely more complex than originally understood. The data on inhaled prostaglandins are less clear, but the same principles may apply.

CONCLUSION

The use of inhaled vasodilators appeals to our current understanding of ARDS physiopathology. Caregivers expect that by limiting ventilation-perfusion mismatch, these medications will improve survival. There are also hypotheses related to pleiotropic effects on leukocyte migration, platelet adhesion, and overall inflammation. Therefore inhaled vasodilator therapies have been subjected to wide and rapid dissemination.[45] However, a careful examination of randomized trials reveals disappointing results. In the case of NO, in which the overall trend is indicative of harm, there are now sufficient data—in quantity and quality—to suggest that inhaled NO should not be used in the routine management of patients with ARDS. Whether this therapy can make a difference in the setting of severe, life-threatening refractory hypoxemia is uncertain, but any potential benefit should be weighed against the risk for extrapulmonary side effects (e.g., kidney injury) and its high cost. Fewer data are available to address the potential role for nebulized prostaglandin therapy.

AUTHORS' RECOMMENDATIONS

- Inhaled NO frequently improves oxygenation.
- Inhaled NO likely causes more harm than good in routine care.
- The role of inhaled NO as a rescue therapy is unclear.
- No evidence suggests that prostaglandins are superior or inferior to inhaled NO.

REFERENCES

1. Gattinoni L, Pesenti A, Bombino M, et al. Relationships between lung computed tomographic density, gas exchange, and PEEP in acute respiratory failure. *Anesthesiology.* 1988;69(6):824–832. PubMed PMID: 3057937.
2. Maunder RJ, Shuman WP, McHugh JW, Marglin SI, Butler J. Preservation of normal lung regions in the adult respiratory distress syndrome. Analysis by computed tomography. *JAMA.* 1986;255(18):2463–2465. PubMed PMID: 3701964.
3. Tomashefski Jr JF, Davies P, Boggis C, Greene R, Zapol WM, Reid LM. The pulmonary vascular lesions of the adult respiratory distress syndrome. *Am J Pathol.* 1983;112(1):112–126. PubMed PMID: 6859225.
4. Zapol WM, Snider MT. Pulmonary hypertension in severe acute respiratory failure. *N Engl J Med.* 1977;296(9):476–480. PubMed PMID: 834225.
5. Moloney ED, Evans TW. Pathophysiology and pharmacological treatment of pulmonary hypertension in acute respiratory distress syndrome. *Eur Respir J.* 2003;21(4):720–727. PubMed PMID: 12762363.
6. Boissier F, Katsahian S, Razazi K, et al. Prevalence and prognosis of cor pulmonale during protective ventilation for acute respiratory distress syndrome. *Intensive Care Med.* 2013;39(10):1725–1733. http://dx.doi.org/10.1007/s00134-013-2941-9. Epub 2013/05/16. PubMed PMID: 23673401.
7. Siobal MS, Hess DR. Are inhaled vasodilators useful in acute lung injury and acute respiratory distress syndrome? *Respir Care.* 2010;55(2):144–157. discussion 57-61. Epub 2010/01/29. PubMed PMID: 20105341.
8. Rossaint R, Falke KJ, Lopez F, Slama K, Pison U, Zapol WM. Inhaled nitric oxide for the adult respiratory distress syndrome. *N Engl J Med.* 1993;328(6):399–405. PubMed PMID: 8357359.
9. Bigatello LM, Hurford WE, Kacmarek RM, Roberts Jr JD, Zapol WM. Prolonged inhalation of low concentrations of nitric oxide in patients with severe adult respiratory distress syndrome. Effects on pulmonary hemodynamics and oxygenation. *Anesthesiology.* 1994;80(4):761–770. PubMed PMID: 8024129.
10. Rossaint R, Gerlach H, Schmidt-Ruhnke H, et al. Efficacy of inhaled nitric oxide in patients with severe ARDS. *Chest.* 1995;107(4):1107–1115. PubMed PMID: 7705124.
11. Puybasset L, Stewart T, Rouby JJ, et al. Inhaled nitric oxide reverses the increase in pulmonary vascular resistance induced by permissive hypercapnia in patients with acute respiratory distress syndrome. *Anesthesiology.* 1994;80(6):1254–1267. PubMed PMID: 8010472.
12. Bigatello LM, Hurford WE, Hess D. Use of inhaled nitric oxide for ARDS. *Respir Care Clin North Am.* 1997;3(3):437–458. PubMed PMID: 9390919.
13. Adhikari NK, Burns KE, Friedrich JO, Granton JT, Cook DJ, Meade MO. Effect of nitric oxide on oxygenation and mortality in acute lung injury: systematic review and meta-analysis. *BMJ.* 2007;334(7597):779. http://dx.doi.org/10.1136/bmj.39139.716794.55. Epub 2007/03/27. PubMed PMID: 17383982; PubMed Central PMCID: PMC1852043.
14. Afshari A, Brok J, Moller AM, Wetterslev J. Inhaled nitric oxide for acute respiratory distress syndrome (ARDS) and acute lung injury in children and adults. *Cochrane Database Syst Rev.* 2010;7. http://dx.doi.org/10.1002/14651858.CD002787. CD002787. Epub 2010/07/09. pub2. PubMed PMID: 20614430.
15. Day RW, Allen EM, Witte MK. A randomized, controlled study of the 1-hour and 24-hour effects of inhaled nitric oxide therapy in children with acute hypoxemic respiratory failure. *Chest.* 1997;112(5):1324–1331. PubMed PMID: 9367476.
16. Dobyns EL, Cornfield DN, Anas NG, et al. Multicenter randomized controlled trial of the effects of inhaled nitric oxide therapy on gas exchange in children with acute hypoxemic respiratory failure. *J Pediatr.* 1999;134(4):406–412. PubMed PMID: 10190913.
17. Ibrahim T, El-Mohamady H. Inhaled nitric oxide and prone position: how far they can improve oxygenation in pediatric patients with acute respiratory distress syndrome? *J Med Sci.* 2007;7:390–395.
18. Troncy E, Collet JP, Shapiro S, et al. Inhaled nitric oxide in acute respiratory distress syndrome: a pilot randomized controlled study. *Am J Respir Crit Care Med.* 1998;157(5 Pt 1):1483–1488. PubMed PMID: 9603127.
19. Taylor RW, Zimmerman JL, Dellinger RP, et al. Low-dose inhaled nitric oxide in patients with acute lung injury: a randomized controlled trial. *JAMA.* 2004;291(13):1603–1609. http://dx.doi.org/10.1001/jama.291.13.1603. Epub 2004/04/08. PubMed PMID: 15069048.
20. Lundin S, Mang H, Smithies M, Stenqvist O, Frostell C. Inhalation of nitric oxide in acute lung injury: results of a European multicentre study. The European Study Group of Inhaled Nitric Oxide. *Intensive Care Med.* 1999;25(9):911–919. PubMed PMID: 10501745.
21. Dellinger RP, Zimmerman JL, Taylor RW, et al. Effects of inhaled nitric oxide in patients with acute respiratory distress syndrome: results of a randomized phase II trial. Inhaled Nitric Oxide in ARDS Study Group. *Crit Care Med.* 1998;26(1):15–23. PubMed PMID: 9428538.
22. Gerlach H, Keh D, Semmerow A, et al. Dose-response characteristics during long-term inhalation of nitric oxide in patients with severe acute respiratory distress syndrome: a prospective, randomized, controlled study. *Am J Respir Crit Care Med.* 2003;167(7):1008–1015. PubMed PMID: 12663340.
23. Park KJ, Lee YJ, Oh YJ, Lee KS, Sheen SS, Hwang SC. Combined effects of inhaled nitric oxide and a recruitment maneuver in patients with acute respiratory distress syndrome. *Yonsei Med J.* 2003;44(2):219–226. PubMed PMID: 12728461.
24. Payen D, Vallet B, Groupe d'étude du NO dans l'ARDS. Results of the French prospective multicentric randomized double-blind placebo-controlled trial on inhaled nitric oxide (NO) in ARDS [abstract]. *Intensive Care Med.* 1999;25(suppl. 1):S166.
25. Schwebel C, Beuret P, Perdrix JP, Jospe R, Duperret S, Fogliani J. Early inhaled nitric oxide inhalation in acute lung injury: results of a double-blind randomized study [abstract]. *Intensive Care Med.* 1997;23(suppl. 1):S2.
26. Mehta S, Simms HH, Levy MM, Hill NS, Schwartz W, Nelson D. Inhaled nitric oxide improves oxygenation acutely but not chronically in acute respiratory syndromes: a randomized controlled trial. *J Appl Res.* 2001;1:73–84.
27. Angus DC, Clermont G, Linde-Zwirble WT, et al. Healthcare costs and long-term outcomes after acute respiratory distress syndrome: a phase III trial of inhaled nitric oxide. *Crit Care Med.* 2006;34(12):2883–2890.
28. Dellinger RP, Trzeciak SW, Criner GJ, et al. Association between inhaled nitric oxide treatment and long-term pulmonary function in survivors of acute respiratory distress syndrome. *Crit Care.* 2012;16(2):R36. http://dx.doi.org/10.1186/cc11215. Epub 2012/03/06. PubMed PMID: 22386043; PubMed Central PMCID: PMC3681348.
29. Medjo B, Atanaskovic-Markovic M, Nikolic D, Cuturilo G, Djukic S. Inhaled nitric oxide therapy for acute respiratory distress syndrome in children. *Indian Pediatr.* 2012;49(7):573–576. Epub 2012/08/14. PubMed PMID: 22885439.
30. Dahlem P, van Aalderen WM, de Neef M, Dijkgraaf MG, Bos AP. Randomized controlled trial of aerosolized prostacyclin therapy in children with acute lung injury. *Crit Care Med.* 2004;32(4):1055–1060. PubMed PMID: 15071401.

31. van Heerden PV, Barden A, Michalopoulos N, Bulsara MK, Roberts BL. Dose-response to inhaled aerosolized prostacyclin for hypoxemia due to ARDS. *Chest.* 2000;117(3):819–827. PubMed PMID: 10713012.

32. Sawheny E, Ellis AL, Kinasewitz GT. Iloprost improves gas exchange in patients with pulmonary hypertension and ARDS. *Chest.* 2013;144(1):55–62. http://dx.doi.org/10.1378/chest.12-2296. Epub 2013/02/02. PubMed PMID: 23370599.

33. Meyer J, Theilmeier G, Van Aken H, et al. Inhaled prostaglandin E1 for treatment of acute lung injury in severe multiple organ failure. *Anesth Analg.* 1998;86(4):753–758. PubMed PMID: 9539597.

34. Camamo JM, McCoy RH, Erstad BL. Retrospective evaluation of inhaled prostaglandins in patients with acute respiratory distress syndrome. *Pharmacotherapy.* 2005;25(2):184–190. PubMed PMID: 15767234.

35. Domenighetti G, Stricker H, Waldispuehl B. Nebulized prostacyclin (PGI2) in acute respiratory distress syndrome: impact of primary (pulmonary injury) and secondary (extrapulmonary injury) disease on gas exchange response. *Crit Care Med.* 2001;29(1):57–62. PubMed PMID: 11176161.

36. Eichelbronner O, Reinelt H, Wiedeck H, et al. Aerosolized prostacyclin and inhaled nitric oxide in septic shock–different effects on splanchnic oxygenation?. *Intensive Care Med.* 1996;22(9):880–887. PubMed PMID: 8905421.

37. Walmrath D, Schneider T, Schermuly R, Olschewski H, Grimminger F, Seeger W. Direct comparison of inhaled nitric oxide and aerosolized prostacyclin in acute respiratory distress syndrome. *Am J Respir Crit Care Med.* 1996;153(3):991–996. PubMed PMID: 8630585.

38. Torbic H, Szumita PM, Anger KE, Nuccio P, LaGambina S, Weinhouse G. Inhaled epoprostenol vs inhaled nitric oxide for refractory hypoxemia in critically ill patients. *J Crit Care.* 2013;28(5):844–848. http://dx.doi.org/10.1016/j.jcrc.2013.03.006. Epub 2013/05/21. PubMed PMID: 23683572.

39. Ventilation with lower tidal volumes as compared with traditional tidal volumes for acute lung injury and the acute respiratory distress syndrome. The Acute Respiratory Distress Syndrome Network. *N Engl J Med.* 2000;342(18):1301–1308. PubMed PMID: 10793162.

40. Montgomery AB, Stager MA, Carrico CJ, Hudson LD. Causes of mortality in patients with the adult respiratory distress syndrome. *Am Rev Respir Dis.* 1985;132(3):485–489. PubMed PMID: 4037521.

41. Fox-Robichaud A, Payne D, Hasan SU, et al. Inhaled NO as a viable antiadhesive therapy for ischemia/reperfusion injury of distal microvascular beds. *J Clin Invest.* 1998;101(11):2497–2505. PubMed PMID: 9616221.

42. Keaney Jr JF, Simon DI, Stamler JS, et al. NO forms an adduct with serum albumin that has endothelium-derived relaxing factor-like properties. *J Clin Invest.* 1993;91(4):1582–1589. PubMed PMID: 8473501.

43. Kubes P, Payne D, Grisham MB, Jourd-Heuil D, Fox-Robichaud A. Inhaled NO impacts vascular but not extravascular compartments in postischemic peripheral organs. *Am J Physiol.* 1999;277(2 Pt 2):H676–H682. PubMed PMID: 10444494.

44. Jia L, Bonaventura C, Bonaventura J, Stamler JS. S-nitrosohaemoglobin: a dynamic activity of blood involved in vascular control. *Nature.* 1996;380(6571):221–226. PubMed PMID: 8637569.

45. Beloucif S, Payen DA. European survey of the use of inhaled nitric oxide in the ICU. Working Group on Inhaled NO in the ICU of the European Society of Intensive Care Medicine. *Intensive Care Med.* 1998;24(8):864–877. PubMed PMID: 9757934.

35 Do Nonventilatory Strategies for Acute Respiratory Distress Syndrome Work?

Rob Mac Sweeney, Danny McAuley

The inflammatory injury suffered by the alveolar epithelium–endothelium complex provides multiple potential therapeutic targets. The inflammatory process could be inhibited at any stage from the genome to inflammatory signaling to leukocyte activation. Likewise, the various pathophysiologic consequences of alveolar injury could be amenable to pharmacologic intervention. The injurious process affects local alveolar ventilation, gaseous diffusion, and perfusion, leading to reduced compliance, ventilation-perfusion mismatch, and respiratory failure. This chapter reviews the evidence for past, present, and potential future pharmacologic therapies for acute respiratory distress syndrome (ARDS). Therapies can be classified as those that aim to improve the pathophysiologic consequences of ARDS or those that are anti-inflammatory, although a large degree of overlap exists.

THERAPIES TO TREAT THE PATHOPHYSIOLOGIC CONSEQUENCES OF ARDS

Surfactant Deficiency

Surfactant is an endogenous mixture of phospholipids and proteins A-D produced by type 2 alveolar cells. It reduces alveolar surface tension, preventing alveolar collapse, and has anti-inflammatory and antimicrobial properties. Exogenous surfactant administration has been successfully used in neonatal respiratory distress syndrome, a condition of reduced surfactant production. Early trials in ARDS demonstrated physiologic improvements[1-7]; however, later phase III trials failed to show an improvement in mortality.[8-12] A meta-analysis of surfactant trials in ARDS reported an increase in oxygenation, without an improvement in duration of ventilation or mortality, at a cost of more frequent complications.[13]

Various reasons have been proposed for these results. Although the neonatal syndrome is due to reduced production, the situation is more complex in ARDS. Surfactant is affected by increased removal, altered composition, reduced efficacy, and reduced production.

Potential limitations of these phase III studies include the use of suboptimal surfactant formulation, dose and duration of therapy, inadequate alveolar delivery, and late initiation of therapy. Pending new research, surfactant therapy is not recommended.

Limitation of Generation of Alveolar Edema

Although an increasing appreciation of the endothelial glycocalyx has modified our understanding of microvascular fluid fluxes, alveolar flooding had previously been thought to be primarily dependent on three factors: capillary hydrostatic pressure, oncotic pressure, and alveolar capillary permeability. Capillary permeability is increased in ARDS. Reducing hydrostatic pressure, increasing oncotic pressure, or both have been tested to ameliorate the development of pulmonary edema.

Reducing capillary hydrostatic pressure targeted to pulmonary artery occlusion pressure (PAOP)[14] and central venous pressure[15] may be associated with improved outcome in ARDS, although fluid management guided by a pulmonary artery catheter compared with a central venous catheter offers no advantage in ARDS.[16] A positive fluid balance[17-20] and increased extravascular lung water (EVLW)[21] are associated with poor outcomes in ARDS. Guiding fluid therapy with EVLW measurement rather than with PAOP may be better.[22]

Hydrostatic pressure may be reduced by restricting fluid intake, increasing fluid output with either diuretics or renal replacement therapy (RRT), or decreasing vasomotor tone with vasodilators. The phase III FACTT (Fluid and Catheters Treatment Trial) study demonstrated improvements in secondary outcomes such as duration of ventilation and intensive care unit (ICU) stay with a restrictive fluid strategy. Fluid balance was dictated by a protocol of diuretic administration based on filling pressures.[15] Total 7-day fluid balance was approximately 0 mL compared with approximately 7000 mL in the liberal fluid strategy. Although there was no difference in mortality, importantly, there was no increase in renal failure or organ hypoperfusion with fluid restriction.

Animal models have demonstrated reduced pulmonary edema through reductions in pulmonary vascular pressures and permeability with RRT. Two small observational studies in humans have provided mixed results. Ten children with ARDS after bone marrow transplantation or chemotherapy who were treated with RRT had an 80% survival rate in contrast to a historic survival of 15%.[23] Thirty-seven adults with renal failure and acute lung injury (ALI)/ARDS who were treated with RRT and a zero fluid balance had no pulmonary improvements within the first 24 hours of treatment.[24] The role of RRT in the management of ARDS remains uncertain.

The choice of fluid for resuscitation in ARDS has been indirectly informed by recent large, multicenter randomized controlled trials on fluid therapy in the critically ill. The traditional Starling forces–based understanding of capillary fluid flux has been challenged,[25] questioning an edema-sparing effect from colloid fluids. With clear signals of harm from hydroxyethyl starches,[26,27] a lack of safety data for gelatins,[28] and an absence of benefit from albumin over crystalloids,[29,30] balanced crystalloid solutions[31] are arguably the fluid of choice for all nonexsanguinating patients.

Hypoproteinemia is associated with the development of lung injury and is a marker of weight gain and death. Two small studies have investigated the use of furosemide with albumin infusions in patients with hypoproteinemia who have ALI. Both showed increases in total serum protein and more negative fluid balances with furosemide and albumin administration. This was associated with increased oxygenation but without improving mortality.[32,33]

Albumin also exerts antioxidant effects via its thiol group. Nonsurvivors of ALI/ARDS have reduced thiol values.[34] The infusion of albumin is associated with increased plasma thiol levels in sepsis[35] and ARDS[36] and decreased markers of oxidant injury. In the recently published ALBIOS (Albumin Italian Outcome Sepsis) study,[30] comparing albumin with crystalloid administration in sepsis, there was no difference in the respiratory SOFA (Sequential Organ Failure Assessment) score between groups.

Lung injury is often heralded by an increase in pulmonary vascular resistance, with an imbalance between pulmonary vasoconstrictors and vasodilators seen in animal endotoxin shock models. Intravenous adenosine reduces EVLW, whereas intravenous nitroprusside and nitroglycerin also reduce pulmonary edema generation but at the expense of increasing ventilation-perfusion mismatch. To date, there is no clear evidence to support the role of vasodilator treatment in ARDS.

MAXIMIZING ALVEOLAR FLUID CLEARANCE

Alveolar fluid clearance (AFC) is impaired in more than 50% of those with ARDS, with this group having higher mortality rates.[37] Beta agonists upregulate AFC by increasing sodium ion transport from the alveolar space. A clinical trial of intravenous salbutamol in ARDS demonstrated reduced EVLW and a trend toward increased survival.[38] A retrospective study of salbutamol exposure in ARDS suggested an association between higher exposure and improved outcome.[39] Beta-2 agonists may cause several other beneficial effects in ARDS, including increased surfactant secretion, decreased lung endothelial permeability, decreased airway resistance, and decreased airway pressures. Unfortunately, despite a wealth of lower level evidence, two large beta-2 agonist multicenter studies in the United States (ALTA [Albuterol to Treat Acute Lung Injury] study,[40] investigating aerosolized albuterol in ARDS) and the United Kingdom (BALTI-2 [Beta Agonist Lung Injury Trial-2] study,[41] investigating intravenous salbutamol in ARDS) were stopped early for futility and harm, respectively.

Another future potential treatment is gene therapy to increase the expression of the ion channels and pumps needed for AFC. An animal study investigating overexpression of the beta-1 subunit of the sodium-potassium adenosine triphosphatase (Na^+,K^+-ATPase) pump demonstrated increased rates of AFC and improved survival.[42] If the alveolar epithelium is severely injured, then cellular regeneration may be required before a functioning epithelial layer can be manipulated.

Epithelial and Endothelial Repair

Stem cells have the capacity for limitless self-renewal and differentiation. Embryonic stem cells are pluripotent and have the ability to differentiate into any cell type in the body. Adult stem cells are multipotent and have the ability to differentiate into several cell types, including cell types of other organ systems.

Stem cells provide three therapeutic opportunities.[43] First, endogenous stem cells may be stimulated via exogenously administered growth factors. Keratinocyte growth factor (KGF), hepatocyte growth factor, and transforming growth factor-α (TGF-α) have all been shown to reduce the effects of ALI in animal models. Epidermal growth factor, TGF-α, and KGF can all upregulate AFC. KGF has other potentially useful effects, including cytoprotection, augmented surfactant secretion, and an antioxidant effect. A randomized, controlled phase II study of intravenous KGF (palifermin) in ARDS (KARE study) has recently completed with publication imminent.[44] Vascular endothelial growth factor (VEGF) promotes angiogenesis and regulates vascular permeability. Genetic polymorphisms of the VEGF gene are associated with lower levels of VEGF and increased mortality in ARDS.[45] Although VEGF increases alveolar permeability in ARDS,[46] its administration enhances alveolar repair in vitro and in animal models. The role of VEGF in ARDS is currently being studied (NCT00319631).

Second, administration of exogenous stem cells, either embryonic or adult, can provide repair to an injured alveolus. Animal studies have been promising. In a lipopolysaccharide (LPS)–induced ARDS model, bone marrow progenitor cells localized to the site of injury and differentiated into endothelial and epithelial cells. Autologous transplantation of endothelial progenitor cells preserves endothelial function and maintains the integrity of the pulmonary alveolar-capillary barrier, whereas administration of mesenchymal stem cells reduces the severity of ARDS in mice.[47] Patients with pneumonia[48] and

ARDS[49] have higher levels of endothelial progenitor cells, and this higher level correlates with improved outcome. Mesenchymal stem cells were originally thought to act as a source of regenerative cells by differentiating into, and locally replacing, lethally injured cells. However, their primary mechanism of action may be through the secretion of growth factors, cytokines, and other signaling molecules causing trophic modulation of inflammation, cell death, fibrosis, and tissue repair.[50]

The third role of stem cells is their ability to deliver gene therapy to the injured lung. Endothelial progenitor cells have been used to deliver vasodilatory genes to the pulmonary vasculature with resultant decreases in pulmonary artery pressures in experimental pulmonary hypertension. In one study, nontransfected mesenchymal stem cells reduced the severity of ARDS in a mouse LPS model, whereas administration of mesenchymal stem cells transfected with the human angiopoietin-1 gene only demonstrated a small additional improvement.[47] Human studies are awaited.

Vasodilators

Nitric oxide (NO) is an endogenous vasodilator produced by the endothelium. When administered by inhalation, it vasodilates the circulation of ventilated alveoli, thus potentially reducing shunt and pulmonary hypertension. Early studies demonstrated physiologic improvements with NO in ARDS[51-55]; however, mortality remained unchanged. Two meta-analyses showed no mortality benefit[56,57] and reported possible harm due to methemoglobinemia, toxic nitrogen compounds, increased pulmonary edema, rebound pulmonary hypertension, and renal failure. Because NO is expensive, possibly harmful, and without a mortality benefit, its routine use is not recommended. It may have a place as salvage therapy for severe hypoxemia given its ability to increase oxygenation,[58] although a recent meta-analysis failed to show a benefit in the most hypoxic patient group.[59]

Prostacylins are derivatives of arachidonic acid and have potentially beneficial effects, including vasodilation, inhibition of platelet aggregation, reduction of neutrophil adhesion, and inhibition of macrophage and neutrophil activation. Inhaled prostaglandin I_2 (PGI$_2$, or prostacyclin) has been compared with inhaled NO in ARDS.[60-62] PGI$_2$ has similar efficacy, and some advantages including minimal systemic effects, absence of platelet dysfunction, easy administration, harmless metabolites, and no requirement for monitoring. A small study published in 2013 showed nebulized PGI$_2$ (iloprost) selectively decreases pulmonary hypertension and improves myocardial diastolic dysfunction but without a significant effect on oxygenation in ARDS.[63]

Intravenous prostacyclin in the form of prostaglandin E_1 (PGE$_1$) has also been investigated in ARDS. Although vasodilatory effects can cause hypotension and increase pulmonary shunting, prostacyclin is anti-inflammatory and can increase both cardiac output and oxygen delivery and improve oxygen extraction during reduced oxygen delivery. Early studies[64-66] in ARDS showed no significant benefit, although the dose delivered was questioned.[67] PGE$_1$ was reformulated as liposomal PGE$_1$ to increase pulmonary

drug delivery and minimize side effects. Again, despite a promising preclinical study,[68] results of subsequent studies were negative.[69,70]

Endothelin-1 is a potent vasoconstrictor that has been implicated in the pathophysiology of lung injury. Tezosentan, an endothelin receptor antagonist, has been investigated in animal models of lung injury with mixed results thus far.

Vasoconstrictors

Almitrine is a pulmonary vasoconstrictor that may increase hypoxic pulmonary vasoconstriction and reduce shunt. In a small ARDS study, oxygenation was improved with minimal increase in pulmonary vascular pressures.[71] The combination of intravenous almitrine to decrease blood flow to hypoxic lung units and inhaled NO to increase blood flow to ventilated lung units has been investigated in experimental lung injury and a small clinical study.[72] Both found the combination superior to either therapy alone at increasing the partial pressure of oxygen in arterial blood (Pao$_2$) with minimal increase in pulmonary artery pressure. Further research is required.

Coagulation

An imbalance between fibrinogenesis and fibrinolysis in ARDS results in widespread fibrin deposition in the alveolar airspace, interstitium, and blood vessels. Pulmonary intravascular thrombosis and vasoconstriction can lead to the development of increased pulmonary vascular dead space, an independent predictor of mortality in ARDS. Several anticoagulants have been proposed as potential therapies in ARDS and have undergone investigation in animal models. Tissue factor pathway inhibitor (TFPI), factor VIIai, heparin, antithrombin III, activated protein C (APC), and thrombomodulin have all been shown to have beneficial effects at this level of investigation.[73]

Protein C levels are lower in patients with ARDS than in normal controls, and the level of protein C correlates with clinical outcome.[74] However, a small randomized controlled trial of APC in ARDS did not reduce either duration of ventilation or mortality, although pulmonary vascular dead space was decreased.[75] A further small study investigating APC in inflammatory and infectious ARDS also failed to demonstrate benefit.[76] After the disappointing results of the PROWESS-SHOCK (Prospective Recombinant Human Activated Protein C Worldwide Evaluation in Severe Sepsis and Septic Shock) study,[77] recombinant APC (Xigris) has been withdrawn from the market. A phase II trial of recombinant TFPI demonstrated improvements in lung dysfunction score and survival.[78]

The pathophysiologic role played by platelets, as both proinflammatory and prothrombotic effectors, could potentially allow for a therapeutic effect for antiplatelet agents. Aspirin is currently being examined in a human preclinical ARDS model (NCT01659307) and an ARDS prevention clinical study (NCT01504867). Therapeutic modulation of the hemostatic system is not currently recommended in ARDS.

Neuromuscular Blockade

Ventilator-induced lung injury can be a significant problem for patients with ARDS, with levels of mechanical ventilation required for maintenance of adequate gas exchange producing volutrauma, barotrauma, and biotrauma. Inhibition of skeletal muscle activity attenuates numerous pathophysiologic mechanisms, such as elevated airway pressures, regional hyperventilation, reduced compliance, and patient-ventilator dyssynchrony. Two small randomized controlled trials demonstrated improved oxygenation[79] and decreased pulmonary inflammation,[80] leading to a large multicenter randomized controlled trial in 340 patients with severe ARDS investigating early paralysis for 48 hours with cisatracurium. Neuromuscular blockade was associated with improved adjusted 90-day mortality, with no difference in rates of ICU-acquired weakness.[81]

ANTI-INFLAMMATORY THERAPY

Glucocorticoids

Steroids possess a myriad of anti-inflammatory properties, stretching from the genome to the macrophage. In the 1980s, several trials unsuccessfully examined the role of short-course, high-dose methylprednisolone in preventing the development of ARDS in high-risk patients.[82-85] A trial of high-dose steroids early in the course of ARDS had negative results,[86] but a recent study in 91 patients with prolonged low-dose methylprednisolone showed reduced inflammation and organ dysfunction, plus reduced duration of mechanical ventilation and ICU stay.[87]

Excessive alveolar fibrosis is a feature of established ARDS, and the antifibrotic properties of steroids have been investigated in this setting. Observational studies[88-90] showed promising results and were followed by a small randomized controlled trial that suggested a beneficial effect on outcome.[91] However, the ARDSnet Late Steroid Rescue Study demonstrated no overall effect on mortality, with increased mortality when steroids were commenced 7 days after the onset of ARDS.[92] A meta-analysis[93] and systematic review[94] concluded that steroids have no role in preventing ARDS but that they may have a role in treating ARDS. Further studies are required to definitively answer this question.

Proinflammatory Mediator Inhibition

Eicosanoids are derivatives of arachidonic acid and act as proinflammatory mediators. They are produced via the activity of either 5-lipoxygenase to produce the leukotrienes or cyclooxygenase to produce prostanoids.

Ketoconazole is an imidazole antifungal agent with anti-inflammatory properties, specifically an ability to block leukotriene and thromboxane A_2 synthesis, and an antimacrophage effect by which proinflammatory cytokine secretion is reduced. Small studies reported positive results for the prevention of ARDS in high-risk patients.[95-97] A large subsequent study by the ARDSnet group of ketoconazole in 234 patients with ARDS demonstrated no beneficial effects.[98]

Ibuprofen is a nonsteroidal anti-inflammatory agent that inhibits cyclooxygenase. In a large sepsis study of 448 patients, ibuprofen diminished prostanoid production and was associated with a trend toward decreased duration of pulmonary dysfunction and ARDS, but this did not reach statistical significance.[99] Modulation of other inflammatory mediators has also been investigated, but to date no treatment has been shown to effectively reduce mortality.

Complement can contribute to ARDS by the generation of C3a and C5a, which attract neutrophils to the lungs and activate them. Complement can also cause cellular injury through the production of the membrane attack complex, C5b-9. Complement receptor 1 is a cell surface receptor on erythrocytes and leukocytes that can inhibit classic and alternative complement pathways. Animal studies have provided a basis for further investigation, and a human phase I study in 24 patients with ARDS has demonstrated the safety of recombinant soluble cytokine receptor 1 and its ability to inhibit the complement cascade.[100] Further studies are awaited.

Interferon β-1a may reduce lung endothelial barrier dysfunction and minimize lung edema through the generation of adenosine, which reduces vascular permeability. An open-label phase II study investigating this intervention reported increased lung CD73 expression, which produces adenosine, and lessened mortality in ARDS.[101] Anti-inflammatory therapy for ARDS is not recommended pending further research.

Immunonutrition

Nutrition has been suggested to play various roles in the management of ARDS. The use of a feed high in fat and low in carbohydrate can reduce carbon dioxide (CO_2) production and thus ventilatory requirements.[102] Enteral nutrition can stimulate gut and lung immunoglobulin A defense mechanisms.[103] The omega-3 polyunsaturated fatty acids found in fish oil, eicosapentaenoic acid, γ-linolenic acid, and docosahexaenoic acid can reduce the production of arachidonic acid from membrane phospholipids, with potential effects on inflammation. On the basis of these findings, several recent studies in ARDS and general ICU populations have investigated various elements of nutrition such as intensity, feeding route, and formulation, including pharmaconutrition. The EDEN (Early vs. Delayed Enteral Feeding) study compared early enteral trophic feeding with full enteral feeding in 1000 patients with ARDS and found that trophic feeding was associated with reduced gastrointestinal intolerance but no improvement in ventilator-free days, infections, or 60-day mortality.[104] The very recently completed CALORIES trial demonstrated no difference in duration of advanced respiratory support in 2388 critically ill patients randomized to either early enteral or parenteral nutrition.[105] Three major pharmaconutrition studies (OMEGA[106] in an ARDS population, as well as REDOX[107] [Reducing Deaths due to Oxidative Stress] and METAPLUS[108] in non-ARDS, mechanically ventilated populations) all reported harm from a range of interventions.

Despite various purported physiologic advantages, including reductions in pulmonary neutrophil infiltration, microvascular permeability, and pulmonary vascular resistance, numerous clinical studies of omega-3 fatty acids in

ARDS have failed to clearly show benefit from this intervention, a finding confirmed in separate meta-analyses of enteral[109] and parenteral[110] administration studies.

Antiadhesion Molecule Therapy

The adhesion of immune cells to the endothelium to facilitate diapedesis is a vital step in the accumulation of neutrophils in the alveolus. The blockage of adhesion molecules is a potential therapeutic target in ARDS. Blockage of CD18, a neutrophil adhesion molecule, has been shown to attenuate the development of experimental lung injury. To date, there are no human studies.

Effector Cell Inhibition

Pentoxifylline is a phosphodiesterase inhibitor with anti-inflammatory effects, acting against neutrophils and macrophages. A small phase I study of pentoxifylline in six ARDS patients did not show any advantage in either gas exchange or hemodynamic parameters.[111]

Lisofylline is a pentoxifylline derivative with slightly differing anti-inflammatory mechanisms. Although it also inhibits neutrophil accumulation and downregulates pro-inflammatory cytokines, it additionally has an effect on reducing levels of oxidized free fatty acids. Animal studies of lisofylline in the treatment of ARDS were promising, but again a large multicenter study by the ARDSnet group in 235 patients with ARDS had negative results.[112]

Granulocyte-macrophage colony stimulating factor (GM-CSF) is involved in the development and homeostasis of alveolar macrophages. It also plays a role in the prevention of alveolar epithelial apoptosis. A small study of 10 patients with ALI demonstrated an improvement in oxygenation with GM-CSF over a 5-day period.[113] A further study of GM-CSF in 130 patients with ARDS failed to demonstrate benefit, although it was underpowered, with nonsignificant signals of benefit evident.[114]

Activated neutrophils release neutrophil elastase, which plays a key role in alveolar injury leading to increased vascular permeability and alveolar flooding. EPI-hNE-4 is a neutrophil elastase inhibitor that improved pulmonary compliance without affecting immune function during *Pseudomonas aeruginosa*–induced pneumonia in rats. A phase III multicenter trial of depelestat (EPI-hNE-4) in ARDS has completed and is awaiting publication (NCT 00455767). Sivelestat is a reversible, competitive inhibitor of neutrophil elastase. After promising animal studies, sivelestat underwent a phase III study in which it improved pulmonary function and reduced duration of ICU stay, with trends toward a reduction in duration of mechanical ventilation and mortality.[115] However, the international STRIVE (Sivelestat Trial in ALI Patients Requiring Mechanical Ventilation) study in 492 ALI patients was prematurely stopped after an increase in 180-day all-cause mortality was noted.[116] No pulmonary improvements occurred, and 28-day mortality was not reduced.

Antioxidant Therapy

Activated neutrophils and macrophages partly exert their injurious effects through the generation of reactive oxygen species. Pulmonary glutathione, an antioxidant, is reduced in ARDS. *N*-acetylcysteine and procysteine are precursors for glutathione, and their administration can replete pulmonary glutathione levels in ARDS. Small studies of *N*-acetylcysteine in ARDS reported mixed results,[117-120] whereas a study of procysteine in ARDS was halted in 1998 because of increased mortality (unpublished data). *N*-acetylcysteine can also downregulate nuclear factor-κB with resultant reduction in neutrophil chemoattractant mRNA and alveolitis in a rat model of lung injury.

In a study of critically ill surgical patients, vitamin C and E administration reduced the duration of mechanical ventilation and ICU stay without decreasing the incidence of ARDS.[121] The more recent REDOX study reported no efficacy from antioxidant administration in a general ICU population,[107] whereas a high-protein enteral diet enriched with pharmaconutrients including antioxidants also failed to demonstrate efficacy.

Statins

Statins were introduced into clinical practice as cholesterol-lowering agents through the inhibition of 3-hydroxy-3-methylglutaryl-coenzyme A (HMG CoA) reductase and have since been shown to possess pleotropic actions both dependent and independent of HMG CoA reductase inhibition. Statins exert beneficial effects on inflammation and coagulation as well as epithelial, endothelial, and immune cell function.[122] Several retrospective studies have demonstrated that prior statin therapy is associated with improved survival in sepsis, including pneumonia.[123-127] In a healthy-volunteer, inhaled LPS-induced model of lung injury, pretreatment with a statin reduced pulmonary markers of inflammation[128] Despite this promising background, two large, multicenter randomized controlled trials published in 2014 did not demonstrate any advantage to statin therapy in ARDS. The American SAILS (Statins for Acutely Injured Lungs from Sepsis) study,[129] investigating rosuvastatin, reported no mortality benefit and possible renal harm, whereas the Irish Critical Care Trials Group HARP-2 (Hydroxymethyl-glutaryl-CoA reductase inhibition with simvastatin in Acute lung injury to Reduce Pulmonary dysfunction) study,[130] examining simvastatin, showed no statistically significant improvement in ventilator-free days, although it was potentially underpowered to detect a small difference in mortality.

Angiotensin-Converting Enzyme Inhibitors

The severe acute respiratory syndrome epidemic led to the discovery of a novel coronavirus, the receptor for which is a variant of the angiotensin-converting enzyme (ACE), implicating the renin-angiotensin system (RAS) in ARDS. ACE converts angiotensin I into angiotensin II, and angiotensin II, acting through the angiotensin-1 receptor (AT1R), mediates vasoconstriction, alveolar permeability, and lung injury. ACE2 degrades angiotensin II; therefore excessive ACE activity or ACE2 deletion is associated with worse lung injury.

Genetic observational studies in humans have supported the concept that the RAS is important in the development and outcome of ARDS. The ACE DD genotype is associated with increased ACE activity and worse outcome in ARDS.[131-133] A retrospective study has shown that prior treatment with an ACE inhibitor was associated with decreased mortality in

Table 35-1 Summary of Nonventilatory Strategies for ALI/ARDS

Recommended	Not Recommended as Routine Therapy	Investigational
Restrictive fluid strategy	Intravenous vasodilators	Guided fluid strategy
Diuretics	Pulmonary artery catheter guided management	Lung ultrasound
Neutral to negative fluid balance	—	EVLW
Neuromuscular blockade in severe ARDS	—	RRT
—	—	Albumin
—	—	Beta-2 agonists
—	Inhaled NO	Inhaled prostacyclin
—	APC	Almitrine
—	Antithrombin III	TFPI
—	—	Factor VIIai
—	—	Heparin
—	—	Thrombomodulin
—	—	Aspirin
—	Steroids (for established ARDS)	Steroids (for early ARDS)
—	Ketoconazole	Complement antagonism
—	Ibuprofen	Anti-CD14 antibody
—	N-Acetylcysteine	Anti-CD18 antibody
—	Procysteine	Pentoxifylline
—	Lisofylline	GM-CSF
—	Silvelestat	Depelestat
—	Statins	Vitamins C and E
—	Omega-3 fatty acids	RAS modulation
—	Glutamine	Induced hypothermia
—	Artificial colloid solutions	—
—	—	—

Therapies with mixed results in clinical studies (e.g., steroids) require further evaluation before a specific recommendation can be made.
ALI, acute lung injury; *APC*, activated protein C; *ARDS*, acute respiratory distress syndrome; *EVLW*, extravascular lung water; *GM-CSF*, granulocyte-macrophage colony stimulating factor; *NO*, nitric oxide; *RRT*, renal replacement therapy; *TFPI*, tissue factor pathway inhibitor.

patients requiring hospitalization for community-acquired pneumonia.[127] Therapeutic modulation of the RAS with recombinant ACE2, ACE inhibition, and AT1R blockade with losartan attenuate pulmonary inflammation in rodent models of LPS-induced ARDS and ventilator-induced lung injury. Human studies are awaited.

Induced Hypothermia

Hypothermia decreases metabolism by 25% at 33° C, reducing oxygen consumption and CO_2 production and thus ventilatory demand. It also decreases proinflammatory gene transcription and exerts an anti-inflammatory effect. In animal models, induced hypothermia reduces the expression of intracellular adhesion molecule-1, interleukin-1β levels, the pulmonary accumulation of neutrophils, and histologic lung damage. Several case reports have documented the successful use of hypothermia (33 to 34° C) for severe ARDS.[134-136] To date, there has been only one small study of 19 patients with sepsis-associated severe ARDS treated with induced hypothermia.[137] Mortality was reduced by 33% at a mean temperature of 33.7° C. The reduction in body temperature was associated with a reduction in alveolar-arterial oxygen gradient, heart rate, and cardiac index and an increase in oxygen extraction, although oxygen consumption interestingly remained unchanged. Further research is required.

REASONS WHY PHARMACOLOGIC THERAPY IS INEFFECTIVE IN ALI/ARDS

Despite repeated promising preclinical and clinical phase I and II studies of therapies for ARDS, no nonventilatory strategy has yet convincingly been shown to improve outcome, with the possible exception of early neuromuscular blockade. There are many reasons for the scientific failure of translation from bench to bedside. These include limitations of animal models, poorly understood human factors, study methodological flaws, and the use of oxygenation as an outcome measure in a condition in which only a small minority die from refractory hypoxemia.[138,139] The use of pharmacologic agents as adjuncts to increase oxygenation allowing the limitation of injurious ventilation may be associated with improved outcomes, but this remains to be tested (Table 35-1).

AUTHORS' RECOMMENDATIONS

- Despite promising scientific advances, nonventilatory strategies for ARDS remain elusive.
- The best evidence we have is for minimizing pulmonary edema through fluid restriction when appropriate, and early use of neuromuscular blockade to minimize ventilator-induced lung injury.
- Other therapies may occasionally be justified as salvage therapy in severe ARDS, but with the knowledge that their risk/benefit ratio remains unclear.

REFERENCES

1. Reines HD, Silverman H, Hurst J, et al. Effects of two concentrations of nebulized surfactant (Exosurf) in sepsis-induced adult respiratory distress syndrome (ARDS). *Crit Care Med.* 1992;20:S61.
2. Spragg RG, Gilliard N, Richman P, et al. Acute effects of a single dose of porcine surfactant on patients with the adult respiratory distress syndrome. *Chest.* 1994;105(1):195–202.
3. Weg JG, Balk RA, Tharratt RS, et al. Safety and potential efficacy of an aerosolized surfactant in human sepsis-induced adult respiratory distress syndrome. *JAMA.* 1994;272(18):1433–1438.
4. Walmrath D, Günther A, Ghofrani HA, et al. Bronchoscopic surfactant administration in patients with severe adult respiratory distress syndrome and sepsis. *Am J Respir Crit Care Med.* 1996;154(1):57–62.
5. Wiswell TE, Smith RM, Katz LB, et al. Bronchopulmonary segmental lavage with Surfaxin (KL4-surfactant) for acute respiratory distress syndrome. *Am J Respir Crit Care Med.* 1999;160(4):1188–1195.
6. Gregory TJ, Steinberg KP, Spragg R, et al. Bovine surfactant therapy for patients with acute respiratory distress syndrome. *Am J Respir Crit Care Med.* 1997;155(4):1309–1315.
7. Walmrath D, Grimminger F, Pappert D, et al. Bronchoscopic administration of bovine natural surfactant in ARDS and septic shock: impact on gas exchange and haemodynamics. *Eur Respir J.* 2002;19(5):805–810.
8. Anzueto A, Baughman RP, Guntupalli KK, et al. Aerosolized surfactant in adults with sepsis-induced acute respiratory distress syndrome. *N Engl J Med.* 1996;334(22):1417–1422.
9. Spragg RG, Lewis JF, Wurst W, et al. Treatment of acute respiratory distress syndrome with recombinant surfactant protein C surfactant. *Am J Respir Crit Care Med.* 2003;167(11):1562–1566.
10. Willson DF, Thomas NJ, Tamburro R, et al. Pediatric calfactant in acute respiratory distress syndrome trial. *Pediatr Crit Care Med.* 2013;14(7):657–665.
11. Kesecioglu J, Beale R, Stewart TE, et al. Exogenous natural surfactant for treatment of acute lung injury and the acute respiratory distress syndrome. *Am J Respir Crit Care Med.* 2009;180(10):989–994.
12. Spragg RG, Taut FJH, Lewis JF, et al. Recombinant surfactant protein C–based surfactant for patients with severe direct lung injury. *Am J Respir Crit Care Med.* 2011;183(8):1055–1061.
13. Meng H, Sun Y, Lu J, et al. Exogenous surfactant may improve oxygenation but not mortality in adult patients with acute lung injury/acute respiratory distress syndrome: a meta-analysis of 9 clinical trials. *J Cardiothorac Vasc Anesth.* 2012;26(5):849–856.
14. Humphrey H, Hall J, Sznajder I, Silverstein M, Wood L. Improved survival in ARDS patients associated with a reduction in pulmonary capillary wedge pressure. *Chest.* 1990;97(5):1176–1180.
15. Wiedemann HP, Wheeler AP, Bernard GR, et al. National Heart, Lung, and Blood Institute Acute Respiratory Distress Syndrome (ARDS) Clinical Trials Network, Comparison of two fluid-management strategies in acute lung injury. *N Engl J Med.* 2006;354(24):2564–2575.
16. Wheeler AP, Bernard GR, Thompson BT, et al. Pulmonary-artery versus central venous catheter to guide treatment of acute lung injury. *N Engl J Med.* 2006;354(21):2213–2224.
17. Rosenberg AL, Dechert RE, Park PK, Bartlett RH. Review of a large clinical series: association of cumulative fluid balance on outcome in acute lung injury: a retrospective review of the ARDSnet tidal volume study cohort. *J Intensive Care Med.* 2009;24(1):35–46.
18. Schuller D, Mitchell JP, Calandrino FS, Schuster DP. Fluid balance during pulmonary edema. Is fluid gain a marker or a cause of poor outcome? *Chest.* 1991;100(4):1068–1075.
19. Sakr Y, Vincent J-L, Reinhart K, et al. High tidal volume and positive fluid balance are associated with worse outcome in acute lung injury. *Chest.* 2005;128(5):3098–3108.
20. Simmons RS, Berdine GG, Seidenfeld JJ, et al. Fluid balance and the adult respiratory distress syndrome. *Am Rev Respir Dis.* 1987;135(4):924–929.
21. Davey-Quinn A, Gedney JA, Whiteley SM, Bellamy MC. Extravascular lung water and acute respiratory distress syndrome–oxygenation and outcome. *Anaesth Intensive Care.* 1999;27(4):357–362.
22. Mitchell JP, Schuller D, Calandrino FS, Schuster DP. Improved outcome based on fluid management in critically Ill patients requiring pulmonary artery catheterization. *Am Rev Respir Dis.* 1992;145(5):990–998.
23. DiCarlo JV, Alexander SR, Agarwal R, Schiffman JD. Continuous veno-venous hemofiltration may improve survival from acute respiratory distress syndrome after bone marrow transplantation or chemotherapy. *J Pediatr Hematol Oncol.* 2003;25(10):801–805.
24. Hoste EA, Vanholder RC, Lameire NH, et al. No early respiratory benefit with CVVHDF in patients with acute renal failure and acute lung injury. *Nephrol Dial Transplant.* 2002;17(12):2153–2158.
25. Levick JR, Michel CC. Microvascular fluid exchange and the revised Starling principle. *Cardiovasc Res.* 2010;87(2):198–210.
26. Myburgh JA, Finfer S, Bellomo R, et al. Hydroxyethyl starch or saline for fluid resuscitation in intensive care. *N Engl J Med.* 2012;367(20):1901–1911.
27. Perner A, Haase N, Guttormsen AB, et al. Hydroxyethyl starch 130/0.42 versus Ringer's acetate in severe sepsis. *N Engl J Med.* 2012;367(2):124–134.
28. Thomas-Rueddel DO, Vlasakov V, Reinhart K, et al. Safety of gelatin for volume resuscitation—a systematic review and meta-analysis. *Intensive Care Med.* 2012;38(7):1134–1142.
29. Finfer S, Bellomo R, Boyce N, et al. A comparison of albumin and saline for fluid resuscitation in the intensive care unit. *N Engl J Med.* 2004;350(22):2247–2256.
30. Caironi P, Tognoni G, Masson S, et al. Albumin replacement in patients with severe sepsis or septic shock. *N Engl J Med.* 2014;370(15):1412–1421.
31. Yunos NM, Bellomo R, Hegarty C, et al. Association between a chloride-liberal vs chloride-restrictive intravenous fluid administration strategy and kidney injury in critically ill adults. *JAMA.* 2012;308(15):1566–1572.
32. Martin GS, Mangialardi RJ, Wheeler AP, Dupont WD, Morris JA, Bernard GR. Albumin and furosemide therapy in hypoproteinemic patients with acute lung injury. *Crit Care Med.* 2002;30(10):2175–2182.
33. Martin GS, Moss M, Wheeler AP, Mealer M, Morris JA, Bernard GR. A randomized, controlled trial of furosemide with or without albumin in hypoproteinemic patients with acute lung injury. *Crit Care Med.* 2005;33(8):1681–1687.

34. Quinlan GJ, Evans TW, Gutteridge JM. Oxidative damage to plasma proteins in adult respiratory distress syndrome. *Free Radic Res*. 1994;20(5):289–298.

35. Quinlan GJ, Mumby S, Martin GS, Bernard GR, Gutteridge JM, Evans TW. Albumin influences total plasma antioxidant capacity favorably in patients with acute lung injury. *Crit Care Med*. 2004;32(3):755–759.

36. Quinlan GJ, Margarson MP, Mumby S, Evans TW, Gutteridge JM. Administration of albumin to patients with sepsis syndrome: a possible beneficial role in plasma thiol repletion. *Clin Sci*. 1998;95:459–465.

37. Ware LB, Matthay MA. Alveolar fluid clearance is impaired in the majority of patients with acute lung injury and the acute respiratory distress syndrome. *Am J Respir Crit Care Med*. 2001;163(6):1376–1383.

38. Perkins GD, McAuley DF, Richter A, Thickett DR, Gao F. Bench-to-bedside review: β2-agonists and the acute respiratory distress syndrome. *Crit Care*. 2003;8(1):25.

39. Manocha S, Gordon AC, Salehifar E, Groshaus H, Walley KR, Russell JA. Inhaled beta-2 agonist salbutamol and acute lung injury: an association with improvement in acute lung injury. *Crit Care*. 2006;10(1):R12.

40. Matthay MA, Brower RG, Carson S, et al. Randomized, placebo-controlled clinical trial of an aerosolized β-agonist for treatment of acute lung injury. National Heart, Lung, and Blood Institute Acute Respiratory Distress Syndrome (ARDS) Clinical Trials Network. *Am J Respir Crit Care Med*. 2011;184:561–568.

41. Smith FG, Perkins GD, Gates S, et al. Effect of intravenous β-2 agonist treatment on clinical outcomes in acute respiratory distress syndrome (BALTI-2): a multicentre, randomised controlled trial. *Lancet*. 2012;379(9812):229–235.

42. Factor P, Dumasius V, Saldias F, Brown LAS, Sznajder JI. Adenovirus-mediated transfer of an Na$^+$/K$^+$-ATPase β1 subunit gene improves alveolar fluid clearance and survival in hyperoxic rats. *Hum Gene Ther*. 2000;11(16):2231–2242.

43. Yen CC, Yang SH, Lin CY, Chen CM. Stem cells in the lung parenchyma and prospects for lung injury therapy. *Eur J Clin Invest*. 2006;36(5):310–319.

44. Cross L, O'Kane C, McDowell C, Elborn J, Matthay M, McAuley D. Keratinocyte growth factor in acute lung injury to reduce pulmonary dysfunction – a randomised placebo-controlled trial (KARE): study protocol. *Trials*. 2013;14(1):51.

45. Zhai R, Gong MN, Zhou W, et al. Genotypes and haplotypes of the VEGF gene are associated with higher mortality and lower VEGF plasma levels in patients with ARDS. *Thorax*. 2007;62(8):718–722.

46. Thickett DR, Armstrong L, Christie SJ, Millar AB. Vascular endothelial growth factor may contribute to increased vascular permeability in acute respiratory distress syndrome. *Am J Respir Crit Care Med*. 2001;164(9):1601–1605.

47. Mei SH, McCarter SD, Deng Y, Parker CH, Liles WC, Stewart DJ. Prevention of LPS-induced acute lung injury in mice by mesenchymal stem cells overexpressing angiopoietin 1. *PLoS Med*. 2007;4(9):e269.

48. Yamada M, Kubo H, Ishizawa K, Kobayashi S, Shinkawa M, Sasaki H. Increased circulating endothelial progenitor cells in patients with bacterial pneumonia: evidence that bone marrow derived cells contribute to lung repair. *Thorax*. 2005;60(5):410–413.

49. Burnham EL, Taylor WR, Quyyumi AA, Rojas M, Brigham KL, Moss M. Increased circulating endothelial progenitor cells are associated with survival in acute lung injury. *Am J Respir Crit Care Med*. 2005;172(7):854–860.

50. Van Poll D, Parekkadan B, Rinkes IB, Tilles AW, Yarmush ML. Mesenchymal stem cell therapy for protection and repair of injured vital organs. *Cell Mol Bioeng*. 2008;1(1):42–50.

51. Dellinger RP, Zimmerman JL, Taylor RW, et al. Effects of inhaled nitric oxide in patients with acute respiratory distress syndrome: results of a randomized phase II trial. *Crit Care Med*. 1998;26(1):15–23.

52. Michael JR, Barton RG, Saffle JR, et al. Inhaled nitric oxide versus conventional therapy: effect on oxygenation in ARDS. *Am J Respir Crit Care Med*. 1998;157(5):1372–1380.

53. Troncy E, Collet J-P, Shapiro S, et al. Inhaled nitric oxide in acute respiratory distress syndrome: a pilot randomized controlled study. *Am J Respir Crit Care Med*. 1998;157(5):1483–1488.

54. Dobyns EL, Cornfield DN, Anas NG, et al. Multicenter randomized controlled trial of the effects of inhaled nitric oxide therapy on gas exchange in children with acute hypoxemic respiratory failure. *J Pediatr*. 1999;134(4):406–412.

55. Lundin S, Mang H, Smithies M, Stenqvist O, Frostell C. Inhalation of nitric oxide in acute lung injury: results of a European multicentre study. *Intensive Care Med*. 1999;25(9):911–919.

56. Sokol J, Jacobs SE, Bohn D. Inhaled nitric oxide for acute hypoxic respiratory failure in children and adults: a meta-analysis. *Anesth Analg*. 2003;97(4):989–998.

57. Adhikari N, Granton JT. Inhaled nitric oxide for acute lung injury: no place for NO? *JAMA*. 2004;291(13):1629–1631.

58. Ferguson ND. Inhaled nitric oxide for acute respiratory distress syndrome. *BMJ*. 2007;334(7597):757–758.

59. Adhikari NKJ, Dellinger RP, Lundin S, et al. Inhaled nitric oxide does not reduce mortality in patients with acute respiratory distress syndrome regardless of severity: systematic review and meta-analysis. *Crit Care Med*. 2014;42(2):404–412.

60. Zwissler B, Kemming G, Habler O, et al. Inhaled prostacyclin (PGI2) versus inhaled nitric oxide in adult respiratory distress syndrome. *Am J Respir Crit Care Med*. 1996;154(6):1671–1677.

61. Walmrath D, Schneider T, Schermuly R, Olschewski H, Grimminger F, Seeger W. Direct comparison of inhaled nitric oxide and aerosolized prostacyclin in acute respiratory distress syndrome. *Am J Respir Crit Care Med*. 1996;153(3):991–996.

62. Van Heerden PV, Blythe D, Webb SA. Inhaled aerosolized prostacyclin and nitric oxide as selective pulmonary vasodilators in ARDS—a pilot study. *Anaesth Intensive Care*. 1996;24(5):564–568.

63. Siddiqui S, Salahuddin N, Zubair S, Yousef M, Azam I, Gilani A. Use of inhaled PGE1 to improve diastolic dysfunction, LVEDP, pulmonary hypertension and hypoxia in ARDS—a randomised clinical trial. *Open J Anesthesiol*. 2013;3(2):109–115.

64. Holcroft JW, Vassar MJ, Weber CJ. Prostaglandin E1 and survival in patients with the adult respiratory distress syndrome. A prospective trial. *Ann Surg*. 1986;203(4):371.

65. Bone RC, Slotman G, Maunder R, et al. Randomized double-blind, multicenter study of prostaglandin E1 in patients with the adult respiratory distress syndrome. Prostaglandin E1 Study Group. *Chest*. 1989;96(1):114–119.

66. Slotman GJ, Kerstein MD, Bone RC, et al. The effects of prostaglandin E1 on non-pulmonary organ function during clinical acute respiratory failure. *J Trauma*. 1992;32(4):480–489.

67. Rossignon M-D, Khayat D, Royer C, Rouby J-J, Jacquillat C, Viars P. Functional and metabolic activity of polymorphonuclear leukocytes from patients with adult respiratory distress syndrome: results of a randomized double-blind placebo-controlled study on the activity of prostaglandin E1. *Anesthesiology*. 1990;72(2):276–281.

68. Leff JA, Baer JW, Kirkman JM, et al. Liposome-entrapped PGE1 posttreatment decreases IL-1 alpha-induced neutrophil accumulation and lung leak in rats. *J Appl Physiol*. 1994;76(1):151–157.

69. Abraham E, Baughman R, Fletcher E, et al. Liposomal prostaglandin E1 (TLC C-53) in acute respiratory distress syndrome: a controlled, randomized, double-blind, multicenter clinical trial. *Crit Care Med*. 1999;27(8):1478–1485.

70. Vincent J-L, Brase R, Santman F, et al. A multi-centre, double-blind, placebo-controlled study of liposomal prostaglandin E1 (TLC C-53) in patients with acute respiratory distress syndrome. *Intensive Care Med*. 2001;27(10):1578–1583.

71. Reyes A, Roca J, Rodriguez-Roisin R, Torres A, Ussetti P, Wagner PD. Effect of almitrine on ventilation-perfusion distribution in adult respiratory distress syndrome. *Am Rev Respir Dis*. 1988;137(5):1062–1067.

72. Gallart L, Lu QIN, Puybasset L, Umamaheswara Rao GS, Coriat P, Rouby J-J. Intravenous almitrine combined with inhaled nitric oxide for acute respiratory distress syndrome. *Am J Respir Crit Care Med*. 1998;158(6):1770–1777.

73. Laterre P-F, Wittebole X, Dhainaut J-F. Anticoagulant therapy in acute lung injury. *Crit Care Med*. 2003;31(4):S329–S336.

74. Ware LB, Fang X, Matthay MA. Protein C and thrombomodulin in human acute lung injury. *Am J Physiol-Lung Cell Mol Physiol*. 2003;285(3):L514–L521.

75. Liu KD, Levitt J, Zhuo H, et al. Randomized clinical trial of activated protein C for the treatment of acute lung injury. *Am J Respir Crit Care Med*. 2008;178(6):618–623.

76. Cornet AD, Groeneveld AJ, Hofstra JJ, et al. Recombinant human activated protein C in the treatment of acute respiratory distress syndrome: a randomized clinical trial. *PloS One.* 2014;9(3):e90983.

77. Ranieri VM, Thompson BT, Barie PS, et al. Drotrecogin alfa (activated) in adults with septic shock. *N Engl J Med.* 2012;366(22):2055–2064.

78. Abraham E, Reinhart K, Svoboda P, et al. Assessment of the safety of recombinant tissue factor pathway inhibitor in patients with severe sepsis: a multicenter, randomized, placebo-controlled, single-blind, dose escalation study. *Crit Care Med.* 2001;29(11):2081–2089.

79. Gainnier M, Roch A, Forel J-M, et al. Effect of neuromuscular blocking agents on gas exchange in patients presenting with acute respiratory distress syndrome. *Crit Care Med.* 2004;32(1):113–119.

80. Forel J-M, Roch A, Marin V, et al. Neuromuscular blocking agents decrease inflammatory response in patients presenting with acute respiratory distress syndrome. *Crit Care Med.* 2006;34(11):2749–2757.

81. Papazian L, Forel J-M, Gacouin A, et al. Neuromuscular blockers in early acute respiratory distress syndrome. *N Engl J Med.* 2010;363(12):1107–1116.

82. Weigelt JA, Norcross JF, Borman KR, Snyder WH. Early steroid therapy for respiratory failure. *Arch Surg.* 1985;120(5):536–540.

83. Sprung CL, Caralis PV, Marcial EH, et al. The effects of high-dose corticosteroids in patients with septic shock: a prospective, controlled study. *N Engl J Med.* 1984;311(18):1137–1143.

84. Bone RC, Fisher CJ, Clemmer TP, Slotman GJ, Metz CA. Early methylprednisolone treatment for septic syndrome and the adult respiratory distress syndrome. *Chest.* 1987;92(6):1032–1036.

85. Luce JM, Montgomery AB, Marks JD, Turner J, Metz CA, Murray JF. Ineffectiveness of high-dose methylprednisolone in preventing parenchymal lung injury and improving mortality in patients with septic shock. *Am Rev Respir Dis.* 1988;138(1):62–68.

86. Bernard GR, Luce JM, Sprung CL, et al. High-dose corticosteroids in patients with the adult respiratory distress syndrome. *N Engl J Med.* 1987;317(25):1565–1570.

87. Meduri GU, Golden E, Freire AX, et al. Methylprednisolone infusion in early severe ARDS results of a randomized controlled trial. *Chest.* 2007;131(4):954–963.

88. Hooper RG, Kearl RA. Established ARDS treated with a sustained course of adrenocortical steroids. *Chest.* 1990;97(1):138–143.

89. Meduri GU, Belenchia JM, Estes RJ, Wunderink RG, El Torky M, Leeper KV. Fibroproliferative phase of ARDS. Clinical findings and effects of corticosteroids. *Chest.* 1991;100(4):943–952.

90. Meduri GU, Chinn AJ, Leeper KV, et al. Corticosteroid rescue treatment of progressive fibroproliferation in late ARDS. Patterns of response and predictors of outcome. *Chest.* 1994;105(5):1516–1527.

91. Meduri GU, Headley AS, Golden E, et al. Effect of prolonged methylprednisolone therapy in unresolving acute respiratory distress syndrome: a randomized controlled trial. *JAMA.* 1998;280(2):159–165.

92. Steinberg KP, Hudson LD, Goodman R, et al. National Heart, Lung, and Blood Institute Acute Respiratory Distress Syndrome (ARDS) Clinical Trials Network. Efficacy and safety of corticosteroids for persistent acute respiratory distress syndrome. *N Engl J Med.* 2006;354(16):1671–1684.

93. Peter JV, John P, Graham PL, Moran JL, George IA, Bersten A. Corticosteroids in the prevention and treatment of acute respiratory distress syndrome (ARDS) in adults: meta-analysis. *BMJ.* 2008;336(7651):1006–1009.

94. Deal EN, Hollands JM, Schramm GE, Micek ST. Role of corticosteroids in the management of acute respiratory distress syndrome. *Clin Ther.* 2008;30(5):787–799.

95. Slotman GJ, Burchard KW, D'arezzo A, Gann DS. Ketoconazole prevents acute respiratory failure in critically ill surgical patients. *J Trauma Acute Care Surg.* 1988;28(5):648–654.

96. Yu M, Tomasa G. A double-blind, prospective, randomized trial of ketoconazole, a thromboxane synthetase inhibitor, in the prophylaxis of the adult respiratory distress syndrome. *Crit Care Med.* 1993;21(11):1635–1641.

97. Sinuff T, Cook DJ, Peterson JC, Fuller HD. Development, implementation, and evaluation of a ketoconazole practice guideline for ARDS prophylaxis. *J Crit Care.* 1999;14(1):1–6.

98. Network A. Ketoconazole for early treatment of acute lung injury and acute respiratory distress syndrome: a randomized controlled trial. The ARDS Network. *JAMA.* 2000;283(15):1995–2002.

99. Bernard GR, Wheeler AP, Russell JA, et al. The effects of ibuprofen on the physiology and survival of patients with sepsis. *N Engl J Med.* 1997;336(13):912–918.

100. Zimmerman JL, Dellinger RP, Straube RC, Levin JL. Phase I trial of the recombinant soluble complement receptor 1 in acute lung injury and acute respiratory distress syndrome. *Crit Care Med.* 2000;28(9):3149–3154.

101. Bellingan G, Maksimow M, Howell DC, et al. The effect of intravenous interferon-beta-1a (FP-1201) on lung CD73 expression and on acute respiratory distress syndrome mortality: an open-label study. *Lancet Respir Med.* 2014;2(2):98–107.

102. Al-Saady NM, Blackmore CM, Bennett ED. High fat, low carbohydrate, enteral feeding lowers PaCO$_2$ and reduces the period of ventilation in artificially ventilated patients. *Intensive Care Med.* 1989;15(5):290–295.

103. King BK, Kudsk KA, Li J, Wu Y, Renegar KB. Route and type of nutrition influence mucosal immunity to bacterial pneumonia. *Ann Surg.* 1999;229(2):272.

104. Heart TN. Initial trophic vs full enteral feeding in patients with acute lung injury: the EDEN randomized trial. *JAMA.* 2012;307(8):795.

105. Harvey SE, Parrott F, Harrison DA, et al. Trial of the route of early nutritional support in critically ill adults. *N Engl J Med.* 2014;371(18):1673–1684.

106. Rice TW, Wheeler AP, Thompson BT, et al. Enteral omega-3 fatty acid, γ-linolenic acid, and antioxidant supplementation in acute lung injury. *JAMA.* 2011;306(14):1574.

107. Heyland D, Muscedere J, Wischmeyer PE, et al. A randomized trial of glutamine and antioxidants in critically ill patients. *N Engl J Med.* 2013;368(16):1489–1497.

108. Van Zanten AR, Sztark F, Kaisers UX, et al. High-protein enteral nutrition enriched with immune-modulating nutrients vs standard high-protein enteral nutrition and nosocomial infections in the ICU: a randomized clinical trial. *JAMA.* 2014;312(5):514–524.

109. Zhu D, Zhang Y, Li S, Gan L, Feng H, Nie W. Enteral omega-3 fatty acid supplementation in adult patients with acute respiratory distress syndrome: a systematic review of randomized controlled trials with meta-analysis and trial sequential analysis. *Intensive Care Med.* 2014;40(4):504–512.

110. Palmer AJ, Ho CKM, Ajibola O, Avenell A. The role of ω-3 fatty acid supplemented parenteral nutrition in critical illness in adults: a systematic review and meta-analysis. *Crit Care Med.* 2013;41(1):307–316.

111. Montravers P, Fagon JY, Gilbert C, Blanchet F, Novara A, Chastre J. Pilot study of cardiopulmonary risk from pentoxifylline in adult respiratory distress syndrome. *Chest.* 1993;103(4):1017–1022.

112. Network ACT. Randomized, placebo-controlled trial of lisofylline for early treatment of acute lung injury and acute respiratory distress syndrome. *Crit Care Med.* 2002;30(1):1–6.

113. Presneill JJ, Harris T, Stewart AG, Cade JF, Wilson JW. A randomized phase II trial of granulocyte-macrophage colony-stimulating factor therapy in severe sepsis with respiratory dysfunction. *Am J Respir Crit Care Med.* 2002;166(2):138–143.

114. Paine RI, Standiford TJ, Dechert RE, et al. A randomized trial of recombinant human granulocyte-macrophage colony stimulating factor for patients with acute lung injury. *Crit Care Med.* 2012;40(1):90–97.

115. Tamakuma S, Shiba T, Hirasawa H, Ogawa M, Nakajima M. A phase III clinical study of neutrophil elastase inhibitor ONO-5046 Na in SIRS patients. *J Clin Ther Med Jpn.* 1998;14:289–318.

116. Zeiher BG, Artigas A, Vincent J-L, et al. Neutrophil elastase inhibition in acute lung injury: results of the STRIVE study. *Crit Care Med.* 2004;32(8):1695–1702.

117. Ortolani O, Conti A, De Gaudio AR, Masoni M, Novelli G. Protective effects of N-acetylcysteine and rutin on the lipid peroxidation of the lung epithelium during the adult respiratory distress syndrome. *Shock.* 2000;13(1):14–18.

118. Jepsen S, Herlevsen P, Knudsen P, Bud MI, Klausen N-O. Antioxidant treatment with N-acetylcysteine during adult respiratory distress syndrome: a prospective, randomized, placebo-controlled study. *Crit Care Med.* 1992;20(7):918–923.

119. Suter PM, Domenighetti G, Schaller M-D, Ritz R, Perret C. N-acetylcysteine enhances recovery from acute lung injury in man. A randomized, double-blind, placebo-controlled clinical study. *Chest.* 1994;105(1):190–194.

120. Bernard GR, Wheeler AP, Arons MM, et al. A trial of antioxidants N-acetylcysteine and procysteine in ARDS. *Chest*. 1997;112(1):164–172.

121. Nathens AB, Neff MJ, Jurkovich GJ, et al. Randomized, prospective trial of antioxidant supplementation in critically ill surgical patients. *Ann Surg*. 2002;236(6):814.

122. Craig T, O'Kane C, McAuley D. Potential mechanisms by which statins modulate the development of acute lung injury. In: *Intensive Care Medicine*. Springer; 2007:276–288.

123. Almog Y, Shefer A, Novack V, et al. Prior statin therapy is associated with a decreased rate of severe sepsis. *Circulation*. 2004;110(7):880–885.

124. Liappis AP, Kan VL, Rochester CG, Simon GL. The effect of statins on mortality in patients with bacteremia. *Clin Infect Dis*. 2001;33(8):1352–1357.

125. Kruger P, Fitzsimmons K, Cook D, Jones M, Nimmo G. Statin therapy is associated with fewer deaths in patients with bacteraemia. *Intensive Care Med*. 2006;32(1):75–79.

126. Hackam DG, Mamdani M, Li P, Redelmeier DA. Statins and sepsis in patients with cardiovascular disease: a population-based cohort analysis. *Lancet*. 2006;367(9508):413–418.

127. Mortensen EM, Pugh MJ, Copeland LA, et al. Impact of statins and angiotensin-converting enzyme inhibitors on mortality of subjects hospitalised with pneumonia. *Eur Respir J*. 2008;31(3):611–617.

128. Shyamsundar M, McKeown STW, O'Kane CM, et al. Simvastatin decreases lipopolysaccharide-induced pulmonary inflammation in healthy volunteers. *Am J Respir Crit Care Med*. 2009;179(12):1107–1114.

129. Rosuvastatin for sepsis-associated acute respiratory distress syndrome. *N Engl J Med*. 2014;370(23):2191–2200.

130. McAuley DF, Laffey JG, O'Kane CM, et al. Simvastatin in the acute respiratory distress syndrome. *N Engl J Med*. 2014. Epub September 30, 2014.

131. Marshall RP, Webb S, Bellingan GJ, et al. Angiotensin converting enzyme insertion/deletion polymorphism is associated with susceptibility and outcome in acute respiratory distress syndrome. *Am J Respir Crit Care Med*. 2002;166(5):646–650.

132. Jerng J-S, Yu C-J, Wang H-C, Chen K-Y, Cheng S-L, Yang P-C. Polymorphism of the angiotensin-converting enzyme gene affects the outcome of acute respiratory distress syndrome. *Crit Care Med*. 2006;34(4):1001–1006.

133. Orfanos SE, Armaganidis A, Glynos C, et al. Pulmonary capillary endothelium-bound angiotensin-converting enzyme activity in acute lung injury. *Circulation*. 2000;102(16):2011–2018.

134. Gilston A. A hypothermic regime for acute respiratory failure. *Intensive Care Med*. 1983;9(1):37–39.

135. Hurst JM, DeHaven CB, Branson R, Solomkin RJS. Combined use of high-frequency jet ventilation and induced hypothermia in the treatment of refractory respiratory failure. *Crit Care Med*. 1985;13(9):771–772.

136. Wetterberg T, Steen S. Combined use of hypothermia and buffering in the treatment of critical respiratory failure. *Acta Anaesthesiol Scand*. 1992;36(5):490–492.

137. Villar J, Slutsky AS. Effects of induced hypothermia in patients with septic adult respiratory distress syndrome. *Resuscitation*. 1993;26(2):183–192.

138. Montgomery AB, Stager MA, Carrico CJ, Hudson LD. Causes of mortality in patients with the adult respiratory distress syndrome. *Am Rev Respir Dis*. 1985;132(3):485–489.

139. Stapleton RD, Wang BM, Hudson LD, Rubenfeld GD, Caldwell ES, Steinberg KP. Causes and timing of death in patients with ARDS. *Chest J*. 2005;128(2):525–532.

36 Are Anti-inflammatory Therapies in ARDS Effective?

Tom Doris, B. Messer, S.V. Baudouin

The acute respiratory distress syndrome (ARDS) is a syndrome of acute lung injury (ALI) caused by direct or indirect damage to the lung parenchyma. It is characterized clinically by acute onset of hypoxemic respiratory failure that cannot be explained by heart failure or volume overload and by bilateral infiltrative changes on chest radiographs not explained by other pulmonary disease. Pathologically, the findings include diffuse alveolar damage, with neutrophil and macrophage infiltration and protein-rich edema fluid in the alveolar spaces. This is associated with both capillary injury and disruption of the alveolar epithelium.

ARDS is an inflammatory condition. Lung biopsy demonstrates an intense cellular infiltrate in the airspaces, consisting of granulocytes and mononuclear cells. Bronchoalveolar lavage (BAL) confirms the inflammatory nature of the lung injury with the presence of neutrophils, monocytes, and several pro- and anti-inflammatory mediators detected in lavage fluid. In addition, reactive oxygen species, their by-products, and changes in oxidant/antioxidant balance have also been frequently reported. Similar pro- and anti-inflammatory changes can also be found systemically in patients with ARDS and mirror those found in the lung. In parallel with these inflammatory changes, a potentially fibrotic healing process is also initiated at an early stage of lung injury. Ultimately, ARDS may completely resolve with little evidence of permanent lung damage or evolve into a stage of irreversible lung fibrosis. The factors that govern these transitions are poorly understood.[1]

The basic science of ARDS therefore suggests that anti-inflammatory agents should be effective in preventing the initiation and progression of lung injury. In this chapter, we review the evidence for the use of anti-inflammatory therapies in ARDS. We particularly concentrate on the role of corticosteroids in the treatment of ARDS because these have been widely studied and have generated much debate. We limit the review to anti-inflammatory therapies and exclude other pharmacologic strategies, such as the use of anticoagulants in ARDS and the use of physiologic antagonists of other parts of the pathologic process such as nitric oxide and surfactant administration. However, it should be acknowledged that these agents have multiple actions, which, in many cases, include significant effects on the inflammatory process.

STEROIDS

Steroids in Early ARDS

The long-established anti-inflammatory actions of corticosteroids have made these drugs the most well studied of potential therapies for ARDS. Initial studies examined the use of high dose methylprednisolone in early ARDS. In 1987, Bernard and colleagues[2] published a placebo-controlled trial of four doses of 30 mg/kg of methylprednisolone (Table 36-1). Ninety-nine patients were randomized within 3 days of having ARDS. At 45 days, there were no differences in mortality, pulmonary compliance, or severity of ARDS as determined by arterial blood gas analysis or chest X-ray appearance. Similar results had been observed with high-dose steroids in patients with septic shock who commonly have ARDS.[3]

Further trials of corticosteroids in ARDS followed this initial study. These trials have used lower steroid doses than the original study, but these remain significantly greater than normal physiologic levels, even under stress. In 2006, a retrospective subgroup analysis of patients with ARDS in a study of corticosteroids in sepsis found that in early ARDS patients there was a reduction in mortality in those patients treated with 7 days of low-dose corticosteroids and mineralosteroids.[4] This effect was only seen in the patients who did not show a response to a short Synacthen (ACTH) test.[5]

In 2007, Meduri and colleagues[6] reexamined the use of corticosteroids in early ARDS with patients recruited within 72 hours of onset of ARDS. Ninety-one patients were randomized with a ratio of two patients in the treatment group for each one in the placebo group. The dose of methylprednisolone was 1 mg/kg/day for 2 weeks, which was tapered over a further 2 weeks. Compared with placebo, there was a significant improvement in intensive care unit (ICU) survival and a trend toward an increased hospital survival in the steroid group. At day 7, there were also improvements in length of ICU stay, ventilator-free days, Pao_2/Fio_2 (partial pressure of oxygen in arterial blood/fraction of inspired oxygen) ratio, lung injury score, and multiorgan dysfunction score in the treatment arm of the study compared with placebo.

Table 36-1 Summary of Major Clinical Trials of Steroid Therapy in ARDS

Trial	Design	Number of Patients	Timing of Steroids	Duration of Therapy (days)	Dose of Steroids	Taper (Yes/No)	Results
Bernard 1987[2]	Randomized, placebo controlled	99	Early (3 days)	1	120 mg/kg/day methylprednisolone	No	No mortality difference
Meduri 1991[7]	Case series	9	Medium (more than 3 days)	Variable	2 to 3 mg/kg/day methylprednisolone	Yes	Improved indices of lung function
Meduri 1994[8]	Case series	25	Late	Until extubation	2 to 3 mg/kg/day methylprednisolone	Yes	Improved indices of lung function
Meduri 1998[9]	Randomized, placebo controlled with crossover	24	Late	14	2 mg/kg/day methylprednisolone	Yes	Improved ICU and hospital mortality
Annane 2006[5]	Post hoc analysis of randomized, placebo controlled	177	Early	7	200 mg/day hydrocortisone 50 µg/day fludrocortisone	No	Improved mortality in nonresponders to short Synacthen test
ARDSnet 2006[10]	Randomized, placebo controlled	180	Late	14	2 mg/kg/day methylprednisolone	Yes	No mortality difference
Meduri 2007[6]	Randomized, placebo controlled	91	Early (within 72 hours)	14	1 mg/kg/day methylprednisolone	Yes	Improved ICU survival

ARDS, acute respiratory stress disorder; *ICU*, intensive care unit.

At longer term follow-up (up to 12 months), there was no significant mortality benefit but a trend to improved survival in the steroid-treated patients. The significantly higher baseline incidence of shock in the placebo group may have contributed to this trend. There were significantly fewer infectious complications in the methylprednisolone group but a nonsignificant trend toward more ventilator-associated pneumonia in this group.

Steroids in Late ARDS

The lack of efficacy of steroid therapy in preventing the development of ARDS prompted researchers to investigate their potential in the later, so-called fibroproliferative stage of lung injury. Steroid therapy has an established, if somewhat controversial, role in the treatment of other causes of pulmonary fibrosis. Meduri and colleagues[7] reported a case series of nine patients with ARDS and fibrotic changes on open lung biopsy. The use of 2 to 3 mg/kg/day of methylprednisolone resulted in improvement in lung injury scores, chest X-ray appearance, and oxygenation in all patients. A reduction in neutrophil levels in BAL specimens was also noted. A larger case series of 25 patients was published by the same author in 1994 using similar doses of methylprednisolone followed by a tapering dose over 6 weeks, resulting in marked improvement in most indices of lung function.[8]

In a further randomized placebo-controlled trial of 24 patients (with 2:1 randomization to the methylprednisolone group), low-dose methylprednisolone, of at least a 7-day duration, improved hospital mortality and indices

of lung function.[9] Mortality in the control group was due to unresolved ARDS, with four of five deaths associated with hypercapnic respiratory failure. There was, however, a nonsignificant trend toward increased ventilator-associated pneumonia in the treatment group.

These small studies and case series prompted a larger trial into the use of steroids in late, nonresolving ARDS that was conducted by the ARDS Clinical Trials Network and published in 2006.[10] This was a 25 center trial of methylprednisolone in patients recruited 7 to 28 days after the diagnosis of ARDS. ARDS was due to direct causes of lung injury in 55% of patients. Patients were followed up until death, discharge, or 180 days. Of 4123 patients screened for the trial, only 180 patients were randomized to receive 2 mg/kg/day methylprednisolone or placebo. Major causes of exclusion were due to previous steroids or immunosuppression (22%), chronic lung disease (15%), and physician refusal (8%). The steroids were tapered over a 3 week period unless the patient remained ventilated at 21 days when the steroids were tapered over 4 days.

At 60 days, mortality was 28.6% in the placebo group and 29.2% in the treatment group (nonsignificant difference). Patients who had had ARDS for more than 13 days and received steroids had a statistically significant increased 60-day mortality compared with the placebo group. Patients with a raised procollagen type III in BAL specimens (a biologic marker of collagen synthesis and thus pulmonary fibrosis) showed an improvement in mortality in the treatment group.

A number of secondary endpoints were significantly better in the treatment group. These included ventilator-free days during the first 28 days as well as at 180 days. Patients in the treatment group were able to breathe without assistance earlier than patients given placebo. Compared with the placebo group, the methylprednisolone group had significantly fewer days in the ICU during the first 28 days. Indices of oxygenation and respiratory mechanics were improved in the patients receiving steroids. However, more patients in the treatment group required resumption of ventilatory support, and these patients were more likely to be shocked. There was no increase in infectious complications in the steroid group; in fact, there were fewer cases of pneumonia and fewer incidences of septic shock.

The main conclusions drawn from this trial were that administration of methylprednisolone in late ARDS did not result in any survival improvement, and when patients were treated with steroids at later than 13 days into their illness, there was an increase in mortality. It should, however, be noted that there was a high exclusion rate for patients, raising the question of the wider applicability of these data to clinical practice. Second, the rapid tapering of steroids after extubation may have been a factor in causing the higher levels of reintubation in the steroid group.

STEROID TRIALS APPRAISAL

The use of steroids in ARDS still remains controversial with some polarization of views occurring.[11,12] One evidence-based approach is to use the techniques of systematic review and meta-analysis to reach a robust recommendation. There have been a number of such reviews published. One such study, which included published studies to December 2013, identified five cohort and four randomized controlled trial (RCTs).[13] Meta-analysis of RCT and cohort studies both reported "trends" to improved outcome with steroids but confidence intervals both crossed the no effect line. No excess adverse events were found. Marked heterogeneity was noted in the studies reviewed. A further systematic review and meta-analysis reached similar conclusions on the basis of pooled data from eight RCTs and 10 cohort studies.[14] Again, there was no significant benefit of steroids and possible worse outcome in influenza-related ARDS.

A key to understanding these differences is a critical examination of several aspects of the trial designs. The studies show marked heterogeneity including in the timing of the administration of steroids, the length of the course of steroids, the dose of steroids, the patients to whom steroids are administered, and the cause of ARDS. A discussion of these topics follows.

Timing of Doses

Experimental studies of anti-inflammatory agents in lung injury emphasize that the timing of the intervention is important. Anti-inflammatories are often effective if given before or during the initiation of the injury-inducing agent. Given at a later period, they are commonly ineffective. These studies suggest that earlier intervention is more likely to prevent the progression of ALI. Evidence that lung fibrosis begins at a very early stage of ALI would also support the earliest possible use of anti-inflammatories.

Clinical data in ARDS also support this. Inflammatory cytokines are present in the plasma and in the BAL specimens of patients with ARDS from the outset of their illness,[15] and their presence may predate the clinical manifestation of ALI. For example, Park and coworkers[16] found that in patients at risk of ARDS (patients with sepsis or trauma), levels of tumor necrosis factor α (TNF-α) and interleukin 1 (IL-1) β were elevated in BAL specimens before the onset of clinical lung injury.

The timing of steroid dose differed significantly in two major studies.[6,10] The ARDS net study recruited patients at least 7 days into the course of their disease, whereas Meduri's group recruited patients within 3 days of diagnosis. One interpretation of these trials is that steroids may only be effective if given early in lung injury, before the inflammatory process has caused irreversible damage to the alveoli.

Duration of Treatment

Proinflammatory and anti-inflammatory cytokines are present at raised levels in BAL specimens until at least 21 days into the course of ARDS.[16] If the rationale for treatment is to reduce inflammation in the lungs, then a prolonged course is more likely to be of benefit. However, steroid-related side effects will increase with duration of therapy and could negate any potential benefits.

Steroid Dose

Very little is known about steroid dose/response relationships in the critically ill. Metabolism and tissue distribution of steroids will change in this population. In addition, the principal target of anti-inflammatories remains uncertain with both local (lung) and systemic actions of possible importance. Furthermore, the inflammatory response is extremely complex and multifaceted. Overlapping and redundant pathways are common, and it may be naive to presume that a "one-dose-fits-all strategy" of anti-inflammatory treatment will be successful.

Physiologic Response

In the retrospective analysis of ARDS patients from the sepsis trial conducted by Annane in 2002,[4] there was a difference in outcome from steroid treatment in subgroups depending on their response to a corticotrophin test.[5] Furthermore, the ARDSnet study found different results depending on whether patients had greater than or less than median levels of procollagen type III in BAL specimens.[10] Selection of patients dependent on inflammatory cytokine levels or other biomarkers of inflammation may in the future help predict response to steroids in ARDS.

Direct and Indirect Lung Injury

ARDS is a heterogeneous syndrome with outcome determined by multiple factors including the nature of the initial insult. The mortality of patients with direct lung injury (e.g., pneumonia) may be greater than those with indirect injury (e.g., sepsis). This suggests that different inflammatory pathways may be involved in the pathogenesis of lung injury. The trials differ, to some extent, in recruitment in terms of the cause of lung injury. There is a slightly higher proportion of direct lung injury in one positive study of steroids in ARDS.[6] It may be that the two causes of lung injury behave differently in their response to steroids and other treatments. For example, there are data to suggest that different patterns of lung injury respond differently to lung recruitment strategies.[17]

OTHER ANTI-INFLAMMATORY AGENTS

Statins

The mechanism of action of statins is the inhibition of hydroxyl methylglutaryl coenzyme A reductase. They have been shown in animal models to modify the inflammatory processes involved in ARDS. The HARP-2 trial was a multicenter RCT of simvastatin (80 mg once daily) versus placebo within 48 hours of a diagnosis of ALI or ARDS.[18] The study recruited 540 patients, with 259 patients assigned to simvastatin and 281 to placebo. There was no significant difference between the study groups in the mean (±SD) number of ventilator-free days (12.6 ± 9.9 with simvastatin and 11.5 ± 10.4 with placebo, $P = .21$) or days free of nonpulmonary organ failure (19.4 ± 11.1 and 17.8 ± 11.7, respectively; $P = .11$) or in mortality at 28 days (22.0% and 26.8%, respectively; $P = .23$). There was no significant difference between the two groups in the incidence of serious adverse events related to the study drug.

A similar study comparing rosuvastatin with placebo in sepsis-associated ARDS was conducted with the primary outcome of hospital mortality or mortality within 60 days if the patient remained in a health-care facility.[19] Patients were randomized to receive rosuvastatin 20 mg per day (following a 40-mg loading dose) or placebo. The trial was terminated after recruitment of 745 patients because of futility. It showed no improvement in mortality or ventilator-free days, but the patients in the rosuvastatin group did show a trend toward fewer days free of renal and hepatic failure. The lack of improvement in outcomes was also seen in the post hoc subgroup of patients who were already receiving a statin before enrollment in the study. The study conclusion was that the data do not support the initiation or continuation of statin therapy in patients with sepsis-associated ARDS.

Prostaglandin E$_1$

Prostaglandin E$_1$ (PGE$_1$) has been found in experimental trials to modulate neutrophil function.[20,21] The neutrophil has previously been implicated in the pathogenesis of ARDS, and modulation of neutrophil function is an attractive therapeutic strategy. In 1989, a multicenter trial of PGE$_1$ versus placebo in ARDS following trauma was carried out. At 6 months there was no significant difference in survival between the two groups, though the patients in the PGE$_1$ group were older, had a greater incidence of sepsis, and had more severe derangements of oxygenation than the placebo group.[20]

In 1999, a randomized double-blind trial was conducted of liposomal PGE$_1$ versus placebo in ARDS of less than 24 hours' duration. No difference in mortality was seen at 28 days.[22] No difference in time to cessation of respiratory support and no difference in pulmonary compliance were seen between the groups. The treatment group attained a Pao$_2$/Fio$_2$ ratio of greater than 300 in significantly fewer days than the placebo group. This study was well powered, achieving its target of 350 patients randomized (348 analyzed), which gave an 80% power to detect a 26% difference in time to discontinuation of mechanical ventilation for 24 hours. It was not powered to detect a mortality difference.

Ketoconazole

Ketoconazole has anti-inflammatory actions including inhibition of thromboxane synthase and lipoxygenase and decreases procoagulant activity.[23] In 2000, the ARDSnet group recruited 234 patients with ARDS into an RCT, in a 2×2 trial design, that also examined the effect of low tidal volumes in ALI.[24] Patients were recruited early (within 36 hours) in the course of ALI. Treatment, which was double-blinded, was randomized to 400 mg orally of ketoconazole or placebo. Treatment was for 21 days or until the patient was no longer ventilator dependent. In-hospital mortality, ventilator-free days, and indices of lung injury were not significantly different between the two groups. In terms of adverse effects, there was a nonsignificant trend toward an increase in cardiovascular complications in the treatment group.

Antioxidants

The proposed role of oxygen free radical species in the pathogenesis of ARDS[25] prompted interest in the use of N-acetylcysteine (NAC) and procysteine in the treatment of ARDS to increase intracellular glutathione and reduce the load of free radicals. A placebo-controlled trial of NAC that recruited 66 patients was conducted in 1992, and no 60-day mortality benefit of NAC was found.[26] Similarly, in 1997, NAC was trialled against procysteine and placebo without an improvement in mortality, though there was a trend toward less organ failure, sepsis, ventilator dependency, and ICU stay in the treatment groups.[27]

Lisofylline

Circulating free fatty acids (FFA) have been shown to cause lung damage and may predict the development of ARDS.[28] Lisofylline reduces levels of FFA and also decreases levels of some inflammatory cytokines.[28] A placebo-controlled trial of 235 patients was carried out in 2002 by the ARDSnet group that failed to show any benefit in mortality, organ failure, ventilator-free days, or infections in the lisofylline group.[29] Interestingly, there was no change in FFA levels in the trial, suggesting that the dose of lisofylline used may have been too low. However, the authors stated that higher doses of the study drug could be associated with gastrointestinal and cardiovascular toxicity.

Macrolides

Macrolide antibiotics are thought to have anti-inflammatory actions on the lung because of inhibition of chemokine production. A secondary analysis of the ARDSnet LARMA (Lisofylline and Respiratory Management of Acute Lung Injury) trial database looked at those that had received a macrolide antibiotic within the first 24 hours of trial enrollment.[30] There was a significant mortality reduction in the macrolide group only after adjusting for covariates. The macrolide recipients also had a shorter time to successful discontinuation of mechanical ventilation. Those receiving fluoroquinolones did not have such differences, suggesting that it is not simply the antimicrobial action of macrolides that results in this potential benefit.

Activated Protein C

As well as its anticoagulant effect, activated protein C (APC) also has anti-inflammatory properties, and its effect in sepsis has been extensively studied.[31-33] It has not been trialled specifically in ARDS, nor were ARDS patients subjected to any detailed subgroup analysis in any of the trials of APC. In PROWESS, the absolute risk reduction of death in APC-treated patients who were ventilated was greater than that seen in all patients (7.4% reduction vs. 6.1% reduction overall).[31] However, the subsequent PROWESS-SHOCK[32] trial showed that there were no benefits to the use of activated protein C, and the product was voluntarily withdrawn by the manufacturer.

Neutrophil Elastase Inhibitors

Neutrophil elastase is an important mediator in ALI. Sivelestat is a small molecular weight inhibitor of neutrophil elastase. The STRIVE study[34] compared the use of sivelestat to placebo for use in patients within 48 hours of diagnosis of ALI. The study was terminated early due to an increased longer term mortality in the treatment group. There was no difference in mortality between the groups before day 28.

Beta-2 Adrenoreceptor Agonists

Preclinical studies had suggested that beta-2 agonists may decrease the degree of pulmonary edema seen in ALI, possibly because of the drug's action on cyclic adenosine monophosphate (AMP). Several studies had aimed to show an outcome benefit associated with their use in ARDS. A multicenter RCT comparing nebulized albuterol and saline for used in patients with ARDS did not show any improvement in hospital mortality or in ventilator-free days in the albuterol group.[35] The BALTI (Beta-Agonist Lung Injury Trial) was a single-center study comparing intravenous salbutamol to placebo for use in early ARDS.[36] The treatment group had significantly lower lung water, a lower plateau airway pressure at day 7, and a nonsignificant trend toward lower Murray scores, but also had a higher incidence of supraventricular tachycardias. Following these initially promising findings, a multicenter trial was conducted. BALTI-2 investigated the effect of intravenous salbutamol on 28-day mortality in early ARDS.[37] The trial was terminated after the recruitment of 326 patients due to a 10.9% absolute mortality increase at day 28 in the treatment group on interim analysis. Significantly increased adverse effects of salbutamol treatment were tachycardia, dysrhythmia, and lactic acidosis.

BALTI-Prevention also suggested that the use of inhaled salmeterol in patients undergoing esophagectomy did not reduce the risk of the development of early ALI postoperatively.[38] It did suggest that there was a lower rate of adverse effects in the treatment group, largely due to a reduction in postoperative pneumonias.

In summary, beta-2 agonists have not been shown to be helpful in the treatment or prevention of ARDS. Table 36-2 is a summary of the major trials of nonsteroid anti-inflammatories.

DISCUSSION

Despite significant experimental evidence that anti-inflammatories are effective in ALI, no clinical trial has produced unequivocal evidence for a therapeutic effect in man. There are several possible explanations for these disappointing results:

1. The hypothesis is wrong. Inflammation is not causal in lung injury, but just an "innocent bystander." An extreme view would emphasize the role of inflammation in lung repair and regeneration and suggest that anti-inflammatories could be harmful in ALI.
2. Inflammation is too complex a process to be manipulated successfully by single agents. In this view, there is no final common pathway that can be simply targeted by a single agent.
3. ARDS is a syndrome not a disease. Clinical definitions of ARDS are useful for trial recruitment but may not define a specific disease entity. The comparison with acute myocardial infarction is useful. Here, a uniform pathophysiologic process (thrombotic artery occlusion) is easily identified by a simple, reliable test (electrocardiogram [ECG]).
4. Interventions are given at an irreversible stage of illness. Inflammation occurs at an early preclinical stage of the disease. Even "early" ARDS trials start treatment at a relatively late stage of disease evolution. In this scenario, better markers of early, subclinical lung injury are needed to guide therapy.
5. Side effects of anti-inflammatories outweigh benefits. Most anti-inflammatory agents have immunosuppressive effects. It is possible that any potential benefits, in terms of reducing the severity of lung injury, are offset by infection and other side effects. Although most studies have not reported excessive infections in the treatment group, more subtle complications cannot be fully excluded.
6. The extent of lung injury is not the main determinant of outcome in ARDS. Multiorgan failure is common in ARDS, and outcome is heavily determined by the involvement of other organs. In this situation, a reduction in lung injury may have only minimal effects on survival.

The inflammatory response appears to be an attractive target in the treatment of ALI. However, the translation of approaches developed in basic science laboratories into better clinical outcomes remains elusive. The possibility that anti-inflammatory strategies in ARDS are ineffective needs to be seriously considered by the research community.

Table 36-2 Summary of Major Trials of Nonsteroid Anti-inflammatory in ARDS

Trial	Design	Number of Patients	Treatment	Early/Late ARDS	Results
Bone 1989[39]	Randomized, placebo controlled	100	Prostaglandin E$_1$	Early	No mortality difference
Abraham 1999[22]	Randomized, placebo controlled	348	Prostaglandin E$_1$	Early	No mortality difference
ARDSnet 2000[24]	Randomized, placebo controlled	234	Ketoconazole	Early	No mortality difference
Jepsen 1992[26]	Randomized, placebo controlled	66	N-Acetylcysteine	Early	No mortality difference
Bernard 1997[27]	Randomized, placebo controlled	46	N-Acetylcysteine Procysteine	Early	No mortality difference
Perkins 2006[36]	Randomized, placebo controlled	235	Lisofylline	Early	No mortality difference
MacAuley 2014[18]	Randomized, placebo controlled	540	Simvastatin	Early	No mortality difference
Walkley 2012[30]	Secondary analysis LARMA	235	Macrolide	Early	Mortality improvement only after adjusting for covariates
Zeiher 2004[34]	Randomized, placebo controlled	487	Sivelestat	Early	Increased mortality in treatment group
Truwit 2014[19]	Randomized, placebo controlled	745	Rosuvastatin	Early	No mortality benefit; trend toward more renal and hepatic failure
Matthay 2011[35]	Randomized, placebo controlled	282	Nebulized albuterol	Early	No mortality difference
Perkins 2006[36]	Randomized, placebo controlled	40	Intravenous salbutamol	Early	Lower plateau pressure
Smith 2012[37]	Randomized, placebo controlled	326	Intravenous salbutamol	Early	Increased mortality in treatment group
Perkins 2014[38]	Randomized, placebo controlled	179	Inhaled salmeterol	Early	No mortality difference

ARDS, acute respiratory distress syndrome.

AUTHORS' RECOMMENDATIONS

- ARDS involves an inflammatory process. Modification of the inflammatory process could, theoretically, ameliorate the damage resulting from ARDS. This makes it an attractive target for pharmacotherapy.
- There are no anti-inflammatory agents that have strong evidence to support their use in ARDS.
- The research community needs to further reflect on the lack of success of anti-inflammatory strategies in ARDS. If further studies are performed, they should only recruit specific subgroups of patients with ARDS where there is direct biological evidence of lung inflammation at an early stage of disease.

REFERENCES

1. Ware LB, Matthay MA. The acute respiratory distress syndrome. *N Engl J Med.* 2000;342:1334–1349.
2. Bernard GR, Luce JM, Sprung CL, et al. High-dose corticosteroids in patients with the adult respiratory distress syndrome. *N Engl J Med.* 1987;317:1565–1570.
3. Sprung CL, Caralis PV, Marcial EH, et al. The effects of high-dose corticosteroids in patients with septic shock. A prospective, controlled study. *N Engl J Med.* 1984;311:1137–1143.
4. Annane D, Sebille V, Charpentier C, et al. Effect of treatment with low doses of hydrocortisone and fludrocortisone on mortality in patients with septic shock. *JAMA.* 2002;288:862–871.
5. Annane D, Sebille V, Bellissant E. Effect of low doses of corticosteroids in septic shock patients with or without early acute respiratory distress syndrome. *Crit Care Med.* 2006;34:22–30.
6. Meduri GU, Golden E, Freire AX, et al. Methylprednisolone infusion in early severe ARDS: results of a randomized controlled trial. *Chest.* 2007;131:954–963.
7. Meduri GU, Belenchia JM, Estes RJ, Wunderink RG, el Torky M, Leeper Jr KV. Fibroproliferative phase of ARDS. Clinical findings and effects of corticosteroids. *Chest.* 1991;100:943–952.
8. Meduri GU, Chinn AJ, Leeper KV, et al. Corticosteroid rescue treatment of progressive fibroproliferation in late ARDS. Patterns of response and predictors of outcome. *Chest.* 1994;105:1516–1527.
9. Meduri GU, Headley AS, Golden E, et al. Effect of prolonged methylprednisolone therapy in unresolving acute respiratory distress syndrome: a randomized controlled trial. *JAMA.* 1998;280:159–165.
10. Steinberg KP, Hudson LD, Goodman RB, et al. Efficacy and safety of corticosteroids for persistent acute respiratory distress syndrome. *N Engl J Med.* 2006;354:1671–1684.

11. Meduri GU, Marik PE, Chrousos GP, et al. Steroid treatment in ARDS: a critical appraisal of the ARDS network trial and the recent literature (Structured abstract). *Intensive Care Med.* 2008:61–69.

12. Suter PM. Lung Inflammation in ARDS–friend or foe? *N Engl J Med.* 2006;354:1739–1742.

13. Tang BM, Craig JC, Eslick GD, Seppelt I, McLean AS. Use of corticosteroids in acute lung injury and acute respiratory distress syndrome: a systematic review and meta-analysis (Structured abstract). *Crit Care Med.* 2009:1594–1603.

14. Ruan SY, Lin HH, Huang CT, Kuo PH, Wu HD, Yu CJ. Exploring the heterogeneity of effects of corticosteroids on acute respiratory distress syndrome: a systematic review and meta-analysis (Provisional abstract). *Crit Care.* 2014:R63.

15. Headley AS, Tolley E, Meduri GU. Infections and the inflammatory response in acute respiratory distress syndrome. *Chest.* 1997;111:1306–1321.

16. Park WY, Goodman RB, Steinberg KP, et al. Cytokine balance in the lungs of patients with acute respiratory distress syndrome. *Am J Respir Crit Care Med.* 2001;164:1896–1903.

17. Gattinoni L, Caironi P, Cressoni M, et al. Lung recruitment in patients with the acute respiratory distress syndrome. *N Engl J Med.* 2006;354:1775–1786.

18. McAuley DF, Laffey JG, et al. HARP-2 Investigators; Irish Critical Care Trials Group. Simvastatin in the acute respiratory distress syndrome. *N Engl J Med.* October 30, 2014;371(18):1695–1703.

19. National Heart L, Blood Institute ACTN, Truwit JD, et al. Rosuvastatin for sepsis-associated acute respiratory distress syndrome. *N Engl J Med.* 2014;370:2191–2200.

20. Eierman DF, Yagami M, Erme SM, et al. Endogenously opsonized particles divert prostanoid action from lethal to protective in models of experimental endotoxemia. *Proc Natl Acad Sci USA.* 1995;92:2815–2819.

21. Rossetti RG, Brathwaite K, Zurier RB. Suppression of acute inflammation with liposome associated prostaglandin E1. *Prostaglandins.* 1994;48:187–195.

22. Abraham E, Baughman R, Fletcher E, et al. Liposomal prostaglandin E1 (TLC C-53) in acute respiratory distress syndrome: a controlled, randomized, double-blind, multicenter clinical trial. TLC C-53 ARDS Study Group. *Crit Care Med.* 1999;27:1478–1485.

23. Williams JG, Maier RV. Ketoconazole inhibits alveolar macrophage production of inflammatory mediators involved in acute lung injury (adult respiratory distress syndrome). *Surgery.* 1992;112:270–277.

24. Ketoconazole for early treatment of acute lung injury and acute respiratory distress syndrome: a randomized controlled trial. The ARDS Network. *JAMA.* 2000;283:1995–2002.

25. Brigham KL. Role of free radicals in lung injury. *Chest.* 1986;89:859–863.

26. Jepsen S, Herlevsen P, Knudsen P, Bud MI, Klausen NO. Antioxidant treatment with N-acetylcysteine during adult respiratory distress syndrome: a prospective, randomized, placebo-controlled study. *Crit Care Med.* 1992;20:918–923.

27. Bernard GR, Wheeler AP, Arons MM, et al. A trial of antioxidants N-acetylcysteine and procysteine in ARDS. The Antioxidant in ARDS Study Group. *Chest.* 1997;112:164–172.

28. Bursten SL, Federighi D, Wald J, Meengs B, Spickler W, Nudelman E. Lisofylline causes rapid and prolonged suppression of serum levels of free fatty acids. *J Pharmacol Experiment Therapeut.* 1998;284:337–345.

29. Randomized, placebo-controlled trial of lisofylline for early treatment of acute lung injury and acute respiratory distress syndrome. *Crit Care Med.* 2002;30:1–6.

30. Walkey AJ, Wiener RS. Macrolide antibiotics and survival in patients with acute lung injury. *Chest.* 2012;141:1153–1159.

31. Bernard GR, Vincent JL, Laterre PF, et al. Efficacy and safety of recombinant human activated protein C for severe sepsis. *N Engl J Med.* 2001;344:699–709.

32. Ranieri VM, Thompson BT, Barie PS, et al. Drotrecogin alfa (activated) in adults with septic shock. *N Engl J Med.* 2012;366:2055–2064.

33. Bernard GR, Margolis BD, Shanies HM, et al. Extended evaluation of recombinant human activated protein C United States Trial (ENHANCE US): a single-arm, phase 3B, multicenter study of drotrecogin alfa (activated) in severe sepsis. *Chest.* 2004;125:2206–2216.

34. Zeiher BG, Artigas A, Vincent JL, et al. Neutrophil elastase inhibition in acute lung injury: results of the STRIVE study. *Crit Care Med.* 2004;32:1695–1702.

35. National Heart L, Blood Institute Acute Respiratory Distress Syndrome Clinical Trials N, Matthay MA, et al. Randomized, placebo-controlled clinical trial of an aerosolized beta(2)-agonist for treatment of acute lung injury. *Am J Respir Crit Care Med.* 2011;184:561–568.

36. Perkins GD, McAuley DF, Thickett DR, Gao F. The beta-agonist lung injury trial (BALTI): a randomized placebo-controlled clinical trial. *Am J Respir Crit Care Med.* 2006;173:281–287.

37. Gao Smith F, Perkins GD, Gates S, et al. Effect of intravenous beta-2 agonist treatment on clinical outcomes in acute respiratory distress syndrome (BALTI-2): a multicentre, randomised controlled trial. *Lancet.* 2012;379:229–235.

38. Perkins GD, Gates S, Park D, et al. The beta agonist lung injury trial prevention. A randomized controlled trial. *Am J Respir Crit Care Med.* 2014;189:674–683.

39. Bone RC, Slotman G, Maunder R, et al. Randomized double-blind, multicenter study of prostaglandin E1 in patients with the adult respiratory distress syndrome. Prostaglandin E1 Study Group. *Chest.* 1989;96:114–119.

SECTION VII

SEPSIS

37 What Is Sepsis? What Is Septic Shock? What Are MODS and Persistent Critical Illness?

Clifford S. Deutschman

"I can't define pornography, but I know it when I see it."
Potter Stewart, Associate Justice of the U.S. Supreme Court
Jacobellis vs. Ohio, 1964

Sepsis is part of every critical care practice. Care for septic patients is provided by internists, anesthesiologists, surgeons, pediatricians, neurologists, neurosurgeons, emergency physicians, nurses, respiratory therapists, and pharmacists. The disorder effects patients of all ages—babies, children, adolescents, young adults, older adults, and geriatric patients. It presents in every type of intensive care unit (ICU)—medical ICUs (MICUs), surgical ICUs (SICUs), pediatric ICUs (PICUs), trauma ICUs, coronary care and cardiac surgical ICUs, mixed (Med/Surg) ICUs, and neonatal ICUs (NICUs). Caring for septic patients is expensive. In 2011, managing septic patients in hospitals in the United States cost more than $20 billion, 5.2% of total hospital costs.[1] Sepsis is common, but it is difficult to determine just how common. Four large U.S. population studies reported that the incidence of sepsis rose an average of 13% per year between 2004 and 2009.[2] Iwashyna et al. determined that, over a 12-year period beginning in 1996, the incidence of sepsis increased threefold among patients receiving Medicare; by 2008, there were nearly 1,000,000 new cases each year in the United States[2] and untold numbers worldwide.[3] However, Gaieski et al. reported that, depending on the method of database abstraction used, the incidence of sepsis varied 3.5-fold, from 300 to 1031/100,000 population, and in-hospital mortality varied twofold, from 14.7% to 29.9%.[4] Nonetheless, even conservative estimates indicate that sepsis is a major cause of mortality and morbidity worldwide.[5,6] In the United States, the annual number of sepsis-associated deaths likely rivals that for coronary heart disease (375,000)[7] and may exceed the mortality attributable to the four deadliest forms of cancer combined.[8] It is also now recognized that sepsis survivors are plagued by functional, cognitive, and emotional disabilities[9-11] that constitute an additional burden on the health care system.[12] In short, "sepsis" identifies a syndrome that constitutes an increasingly important public health concern.

If asked to define sepsis, however, most ICU providers would struggle. They would likely invoke some combination of infection and inflammatory markers—temperature, heart rate, respiratory rate, and white blood cell count—the so-called SIRS (systemic inflammatory response syndrome)

criteria. Most would also acknowledge that this definition, first articulated in a 1992 paper,[13] identifies a large number of patients who are not septic. A more detailed discussion is clearly in order.

The term *sepsis* is generically used to describe a set of clinical, pathologic, and biochemical changes that may accompany infection. The root of the word is derived from the ancient Greek for "to decay" or "to putrefy." Over the years, sepsis has been used to describe a wide and often bewildering array of medical conditions. Consensus conferences convened in 1991[13] and 2001[14] to provide structure and clarity focused on the then-accepted view that sepsis represented a generalized inflammatory host response to infection. The emphasis of the initial consensus conference[13] on deriving a clinically useful construct resulted in the creation of SIRS. Sepsis was defined as "the systemic response to infection," that is, SIRS in a patient with suspected, presumed, or identified infection. Sepsis could progress until patients had organ dysfunction or "organ failure." When organ dysfunction was present, the syndrome was termed *severe sepsis*. Severe sepsis could continue to progress across a continuum to septic shock, defined as "sepsis-induced hypotension persisting despite adequate fluid resuscitation." Finally, patients with sepsis could progress to develop a disorder where most organ systems function abnormally, the multiple organ dysfunction syndrome (MODS). Issues with these definitions, in particular with the nonspecific nature of SIRS, arose almost immediately. Indeed, soon after their publication, the primary architect of the 1991 definitions, Roger Bone, proposed the existence of a compensatory anti-inflammatory response syndrome (CARS),[15] while others noted that changes in organ function corrected with survival, a finding not thought to be consistent with organ failure. Ongoing concerns ultimately led to the 2001 consensus conference. The participants noted that SIRS was present in the great majority of critically ill patients—indeed, 93% fulfill criteria on admission as part of the host response to any critical illness.[16] The identified limitations in SIRS were addressed by expanding the list of defining criteria used. The determinants of severe sepsis were left unchanged, whereas criteria to characterize the "state of acute circulatory failure" of septic shock were expanded incrementally. Despite a number of developments suggesting that reassessment was needed, no formal attempt to revisit the definitions was subsequently undertaken. In effect, the definitions of sepsis, septic shock, and organ dysfunction remained largely unchanged for two decades.

Because of these inherent concerns, a Task Force of intensivists, infectious disease experts, and pulmonologists was convened in January 2014. The group was provided unrestricted support by the Society of Critical Care Medicine (SCCM) and the European Society of Intensive Care Medicine (ESICM), and was charged to reexamine and, as deemed appropriate, revise existing definitions of sepsis, severe sepsis, septic shock, and organ dysfunction. Proposed changes were to reflect a deeper understanding of the pathophysiology of sepsis and the availability of large electronic health records, clinical databases, and patient registries. Endorsement of the document from major international societies focused on intensive care and other relevant disciplines was then obtained, and the document was published in 2016.[17]

WHY IS REASSESSING THE DEFINITIONS OF SEPSIS AND SEPSIS-RELATED CONDITIONS SO ESSENTIAL—AND SO DIFFICULT?

Variability in Terminology

Sepsis. A patient is currently defined as having sepsis if she or he has presumed or demonstrated infection in the presence of two or more SIRS criteria. This approach is problematic. SIRS reflects inflammation, a normal response to "danger," and thus is neither pathologic nor necessarily infection driven. Further, the current reliance on SIRS has led to inconsistencies in hospital reporting and in accruing epidemiologic data. As noted, Giaeiski et al. found a 3.5-fold variation in the incidence of sepsis and a twofold variation in hospital mortality when different abstraction methods were applied to the same patient population.[4] In addition, a recent study showed that a significant number of patients admitted to critical care units with infection and organ failure did not meet SIRS criteria.[18] Thus, current definitions impede diagnosis, assessment of outcome, and the gathering of epidemiologic data.

Organ Dysfunction. Although identifying sepsis-induced organ-specific abnormalities as "failure" has become infrequent, several issues arise when considering organ dysfunction. Perhaps most important is a lack of reliable criteria to identify "dysfunction" that is evident when one examines the selected clinical findings, laboratory data, or therapeutic interventions in current use. Many abnormalities are nonspecific, and basing assessment of severity on intervention is subject to a host of concerns, especially when therapeutic approaches are changing and their application is not subject to uniform guidelines. It has also become common practice to combine organ-based abnormalities into scoring systems. Perhaps the most frequently used system is the Sequential Organ Failure Assessment Score (SOFA), which was originally called the Sepsis-related Organ Failure Assessment Score.[19] SOFA, however, illustrates many of the concerns with current approaches to organ dysfunction.

For example, an elevation in serum bilirubin levels, which in SOFA is used to demonstrate hepatic dysfunction, can arise from hemolysis. Coagulation abnormalities are noted by a decrease in platelet counts, which is just as likely to reflect an effect on bone marrow, especially when noted in conjunction with anemia or neutropenia. The progression of cardiovascular dysfunction is based on escalating doses of vasopressors, which may be managed in different ways according to local custom. Indeed, the reliance of the SOFA cardiovascular score is based on the dose of dopamine, a drug that is no longer routinely administered. Finally, most indices, and SOFA in particular, were not derived based on data but rather reflected consensus, especially with regard to variable selection and cutoff values. That said, a higher SOFA score does seem to indicate an increasing probability of mortality.[20]

Septic Shock. Problems with the existing definitions are particularly evident when septic shock is examined. As part of the Task Force effort, Shankar-Hari et al.[21] undertook a systemic review of the literature. The results indicate that septic shock is defined by the presence of infection (presumed or confirmed) in conjunction with combinations of terms that are themselves defined with distressing variability, namely:

- Hypotension (SBP [systolic blood pressure] <90 mm Hg *or* MAP [mean arterial pressure] <60 or <70 mm Hg *or* fall in SAP pressure >40 mm Hg from baseline or >2 standard deviations from the norm for age despite "adequate fluid resuscitation")
- The presence of abnormal biochemical variables (e.g., lactate >2 or >4 mmol/L or base deficit >5 mmol/L)
- The use of inotropes or vasopressors (not necessarily above a prespecified dose)
- New onset organ dysfunction (defined variably with various scoring systems such as APACHE [Acute Physiology and Chronic Health Evaluation] II, APACHE III, or the cardiovascular component of the SOFA score)

Further complicating matters are the following:

- Variable endpoints of adequacy of fluid resuscitation (rarely defined or reported)
- Variable durations of hypotension or vasopressor therapy
- Failure to account for the underlying blood pressure of the patient or other comorbidities
- Failure to account for the hypotensive effect of cointerventions such as vasodilating and/or cardiodepressant sedative agents.

In effect, issues with terminology are even more problematic for septic shock than for sepsis.

Improved Understanding of Sepsis Pathobiology

There are inherent challenges in defining sepsis. First and foremost, the term *sepsis* describes a complex and poorly understood process. There are no simple or unambiguous clinical criteria or biological characteristics that differentiate patients who are "septic" from those who are not. That is, clinical features or current animal models poorly delineate the complexity, variability, and time dependence of the sepsis phenotype.[22]

The original conceptualization of sepsis as infection with SIRS focused solely on immune excess. Recent advances have demonstrated that sepsis involves early activation of both proinflammatory and anti-inflammatory responses,[23] of nonimmunologic pathways such as cardiovascular, neuronal, autonomic, hormonal, bioenergetic, metabolic, and coagulation,[22-25] all of which carry prognostic significance. Modulation of septic response involves not only the immune system but also the endocrine and central nervous systems.[26,27] Organ dysfunction, even when severe, is not necessarily associated with significant cell damage,[28] whereas a sepsislike biological response may be triggered by noninfectious host factors (damage-associated molecular patterns).[29] In short, criteria currently in use are no longer consistent with what we understand about the pathobiologic of sepsis.

A Need for Sepsis Definitions for the Lay Public and for Health-care Practitioners

Despite its prevalence, associated morbidity, contribution to the rising cost of health care, worldwide importance,[5,6] and recent high-profile cases,[30] public awareness of sepsis is poor,[31] and limited resources are directed toward sepsis-associated research.[32] Furthermore, recognition of clinical sepsis is difficult for trained medical personnel and can be entirely obscure to the populace at large. There is thus a glaring need for a description of sepsis that can be appreciated by the nonmedical public.

In addition, the diagnosis of sepsis is problematic even for experienced practitioners. A recent high-profile death of a 12-year-old boy (Rory Staunton) from sepsis[30] at least in part reflects this difficulty—sepsis is a condition that can confound the most experienced practitioners, especially at times of the year when other conditions that present with similar protean signs and symptoms are common (e.g., during flu season). Thus, health-care practitioners would benefit greatly from a simple, validated set of bedside criteria that directs them to consider sepsis when presented with infected patients.

Availability of Patient Data

Although there have been a number of important clinical trials regarding therapy for sepsis, a great deal of the material on which the definitions of sepsis are based reflects findings from small studies or expert opinion. By their nature, it is difficult to validate such studies. However, there are now in existence a number of large electronic health record (EHR) databases and patient registries that either relate directly to sepsis itself (e.g., the Surviving Sepsis Campaign [SSC] database[33]) or contain general information that could be leveraged to study patients with sepsis. These datasets enable the derivation and validation of variables that better capture the incidence, severity, and trajectory of sepsis.

Nature of the Problem: What Is a "Definition"?

Per the Merriam-Webster dictionary, a definition is "a statement expressing the essential nature of something." In effect, a definition is the "gold standard" to be compared with any other descriptions or collection of signs and symptoms used to identify something. There is no such gold standard for sepsis. In contrast to "cancer," there is no tissue specimen that, if examined under a microscope or in some other manner, can be unambiguously identified as sepsis. Unlike cystic fibrosis, there is no specific, characteristic genetic abnormality. Sepsis even differs from infection, where a culture can identify the offending microorganism. Thus, by its very nature, any current definition of sepsis cannot be validated in the clinical realm. The best that can be hoped for is to delineate characteristics or criteria to identify patients with some proxy for sepsis, and who are thus highly likely to have sepsis.

UPDATED DEFINITIONS OF SEPSIS, SEPTIC SHOCK, AND ORGAN DYSFUNCTION IN ADULTS: FINDINGS OF THE SCCM/ESICM SEPSIS DEFINITIONS TASK FORCE

Sepsis: A Life-Threatening Organ Dysfunction Due to a Dysregulated Host Response to Infection.

On the basis of improving the understanding of the pathobiology of sepsis, the Task Force shifted the focus from infection and inflammation to aberrant or dysregulated host responses. It was recognized that inflammation, as identified by the SIRS criteria, is an adaptive response not only to infection but also to a myriad of other threats to the viability of the organism. In contrast, sepsis reflects a more complex and threatening state; in effect, sepsis is "maladaptive inflammation." The biological underpinnings of this difference are unknown but represent an active area of investigation. The septic response may be influenced by the nature of the pathogen and the genetics and age of the host as well as preexisting acute and chronic conditions and comorbidities. Interventions such as administration of medications and procedures can alter the clinical presentation. Finally, the septic response follows a time course that can, in some instances, be predicted and modified. The clinical course can thus also reflect the trajectory of the response.

Importantly, the old term *severe sepsis* has been replaced by *sepsis* in the new definitions and should no longer be used.

Sepsis is the primary cause of death from infection and is especially deadly if not recognized and treated promptly. Data from the SSC database indicate that mortality from sepsis increases for each 30-minute delay in the initiation of broad-spectrum antibiotics.[34] Although three recent studies that focused on patients with septic shock failed to confirm the value of a fluid replacement strategy called *early goal-directed therapy*, [35-37] this outcome should probably be applied only when the complete management protocol is used. The treatment of the control groups reflected administration of a substantial amount of fluid. Thus, as with antibiotics, timely fluid resuscitation is essential.

A patient who receives a diagnosis of sepsis in general warrants an escalating level of monitoring and intervention, including referral/admission to critical care/high dependency facilities. Importantly, there may be occult, early organ dysfunction in any patient presenting with infection. Therefore, assessment of organ function should be considered in patients with suspected infection because the presence of dysfunction would fulfill the criteria for sepsis. Conversely, unrecognized infection may underlie new-onset organ dysfunction, and therefore unexplained organ dysfunction might prompt a search for infection.

qSOFA: Clinical Criteria to Aid in the Identification of Patients Likely to Have Sepsis

The revised definition of sepsis detailed above may indeed encompass the "essential nature" of sepsis, but its utility in the clinical arena is limited. It is impossible to apply the definition because a "dysregulated host response" cannot be identified clinically—at this time. However, it is essential that clinicians be able to identify sepsis from among all infected patients as early as possible.[34] To circumvent this problem, the Task Force members first identified 21 variables that had been associated with sepsis in prior studies. They further reasoned that patients with sepsis could, after the fact, be distinguished from patients who merely had infection by a number of adverse outcomes: hospital mortality, mortality, ICU stay of 3 days or longer, or an administrative discharge code explicit for severe sepsis. Seymour et al.[38] queried a large EHR, identified all patients with suspected infection (i.e., patients who, on hospital admission, were cultured and received broad-spectrum antibiotics), and used these proxy outcomes to identify those most likely to have sepsis. They applied receiver-operator curve analysis to combinations of the 21 variables and determined what combinations best indicated risk of death or an ICU stay of longer than 3 days. The performance of these combinations was compared with background risk, reflecting age, gender, and comorbidities, and with a number of other constructs such as SIRS or the SOFA score. High performing combinations were then tested in several other datasets, including one compiled in Germany. A combination of three simple bedside measures—systolic blood pressure (SBP) of 100 mm Hg or less, respiratory rate of 22 or more breaths/min, and Glasgow Coma Score (GCS) of 13 or less—robustly identified patients with suspected infection who were most likely to die or to require an ICU stay of more than 3 days. Additional applications of multiple sensitivity analyses indicated that a GCS less than15—that is, any alteration in mental status—provided equivalent discrimination.

This combination—otherwise unexplained altered mentation, SBP of 100 mm Hg or less, and respiratory rate of 22 or fewer breaths/min—was designated as qSOFA (for quick SOFA). qSOFA was equivalent to the full SOFA score, which requires additional measurements and laboratory data, and outperformed SIRS. qSOFA is particularly accurate when applied to patients in the emergency department or the wards; it was less robust and was surpassed by the full SOFA when used in the ICU itself, in part because of the use of interventions such as vasopressors, sedation, and mechanical ventilation that alter SBP, GCS, and respiratory rate. Interestingly, adding lactate concentration (or substituting it for one of the other elements) did not improve the performance of qSOFA.

Thus qSOFA, which consists of three simple measures easily obtained at the bedside, can be used to identify infected patients who are at risk of significant clinical deterioration and thus are highly likely to be septic. The qSOFA

model offers considerable advantages over the full SOFA score; it consists of fewer variables and does not require laboratory results. qSOFA is *not*, however, a stand-alone definition of sepsis or of organ dysfunction. The measure is probably best used to alert practitioners about the potential for organ dysfunction or a source of infection, to identify the need for appropriate therapy, and to consider that a higher level of care might be appropriate.

Organ Dysfunction (and MODS) Can, for the Moment, Be Approximated with the SOFA Score

The emphasis on organ dysfunction is the most important conceptual change in the new definition of sepsis. This change reflects the Task Force view that underlying cellular defects are the source of the physiologic and biochemical abnormalities that develop within specific organ systems. At present, definitions of dysfunction in individual organ systems are lacking, and clinical criteria to identify patients with organ dysfunction are problematic and badly need updating. In contrast to sepsis, there are aspects of organ dysfunction that are directly demonstrable. In particular, lung dysfunction, in the form of acute respiratory distress syndrome (ARDS), produces a characteristic pathologic picture: neutrophil infiltration, macrophage activation, apoptosis and necrosis of type I pulmonary epithelial cells with patchy denuding of the underlying basement membrane, overexuberant proliferation of type II cells to cover the defect, and the accumulation of cellular debris into a "hyaline membrane." However, ARDS develops in settings other than sepsis, and there are truly no other organ-specific lesions in sepsis. Indeed, recovery from sepsis is often associated with a pathologic and pathophysiologic picture that appears, for all intents and purposes, normal.

It is tempting to apply the tools developed in identifying clinical criteria most likely to identify patients with sepsis to each individual organ system. Use of that approach is hampered by uncertainty about putative "biomarkers" and a lack of robust validation data. Simply put, there are no viable proxies for dysfunction in organs such as the heart, liver, kidney, and gut. Currently used biomarkers are important components of SOFA, but they suffer from lack of specificity (e.g., platelet count = coagulation dysfunction), lack of sensitivity (elevations in bilirubin = liver dysfunction), reliance on support modalities whose use differs from practitioner to practitioner (Pao_2/Fio_2 [partial pressure of oxygen in arterial blood/fraction of inspired oxygen] ratio = lung injury) or on therapeutic interventions that are rarely used at all (dopamine infusion at a rate <5 μg/kg/min = cardiovascular dysfunction), or use of biochemical abnormalities that change only when function is severely disturbed (creatinine elevation = renal dysfunction). Potentially more useful alternatives, for example, neutrophil gelatinase-associated lipocalin, have not been incorporated into routine practice. Finally, most large EHRs and clinical registries lack the specific data that would be needed to validate improved definitions for dysfunction in individual organ systems.

Therefore the Task Force recommended that a change in baseline of the total SOFA score of 2 points or more be taken as the clinical criterion needed to identify a high likelihood[19,20] of "life-threatening organ dysfunction." This decision was not entirely without controversy. A number of Task Force members, including me, thought that a SOFA score of 2 or less for an individual organ system could be used as a surrogate for dysfunction within that system alone but were uncomfortable with the decision that a composite score of 2 or more was indicative of some sort of "global" organ dysfunction. Nevertheless, SOFA's strengths offset the previously noted issues, as well as concerns that optimal variable selection, cutoff values, and weighting have not been formally validated.

In the aggregate, dysfunction in more than one organ system constitutes MODS. The term was first coined in the 1991 consensus definitions, replacing a number of terms: sequential organ failure, multiple organ failure, multiple systems organ failure, and others.[13] The term *failure* was abandoned because it connoted a dichotomous event, either present or absent, as opposed to a continuum of abnormalities, but the authors explicitly declined to enumerate characteristics that could be used to identify dysfunction in individual organ systems. The participants in the 2001 consensus conference provided a short list of "organ dysfunction variables" that could be nominally applied to individual organ systems (e.g., hypoxemia, oliguria, hyperbilirubinemia). In reality, these variables were derived from either the SOFA[14] or the multiple organ dysfunction score (a different but related MODS).[39] Since that time, SOFA has become the more commonly used approach, and its constituent abnormalities have been used both to define dysfunction in individual organ systems and to provide an index of global organ dysfunction. As previously discussed, SOFA has a number of drawbacks and deficiencies, and although it remains the best available method for identifying individual and global organ dysfunction, it is far from sufficient. Addressing these issues and developing and validating a more robust set of definitions and clinical criteria for organ dysfunction should be undertaken in the very near future.

Definition of Septic Shock

Septic shock **is defined as a subset of sepsis where underlying circulatory and cellular abnormalities are profound enough to substantially increase mortality.**

The definition of septic shock contained in the 2001 consensus statement described septic shock as "a state of acute circulatory failure."[14] However, insight into the pathobiology of sepsis suggests that limiting the concept of "shock" to circulatory abnormalities is problematic. This topic was discussed in depth during the Task Force deliberations. A number of members, including me, favored a view that emphasized cellular dysfunction alone, reasoning that cardiovascular dysfunction is simply cell dysfunction where the cells in question are part of the circulatory system. Thus, hypotension, rather than specifically characterizing cardiovascular dysfunction, reflects how a global cellular defect specifically alters vascular smooth muscle, endothelial cells, and cardiomyocytes. This conceptualization reflects trends in cellular biology (e.g., heat shock) and is consistent with the recognition that shock in some clinical situations does not involve the circulation (e.g., insulin shock) Similarly,

a sepsis-induced rise in blood lactate level reflects dysfunction in a number of different types of cells: limited oxygen uptake by pulmonary endothelial cells, altered oxygen-carrying capacity in red blood cells, impaired aerobic respiration and accelerated aerobic glycolysis in virtually all cells, reduced lactate biotransformation in the liver, altered renal clearance for substrate, etc.[40] That said, an elevation in serum lactate is a marker of illness severity that parallels mortality.[41]

Clinical Criteria to Aid in the Identification of Patients with Septic Shock

As with sepsis, the revised definition of septic shock may have limited practical utility because it invokes abnormalities that cannot be measured clinically, in particular the concept of cellular dysfunction. Therefore, as noted previously, Shankar-Hari et al. used a slightly different approach to develop clinically useful criteria to identify the septic patients most likely to have septic shock.[21] Some elements of the systematic review of current use of the term *septic shock* were detailed earlier in this chapter. In addition, this review highlighted the overwhelming need for a revised definition. The variable meaning attached to terminology identifying patients with septic shock is reflected in large disparities in reported outcomes. To illustrate, the 2012 mortality rate for septic shock patients admitted to intensive care units in Australia and New Zealand (171 ICUs; n=6757) was 22%.[18] Similar data from Italy (190 ICUs; n=3596) and Germany revealed a fatal outcome in 57.4% and 60.5%, respectively.[42]

The systematic review was followed by use of a modified Delphi process among Task Force members. It was agreed that, as reflected in the revised definition, mortality from septic shock should be substantially higher than from sepsis and that the ability of clinical findings such as "hypotension," "need for vasopressor therapy," "raised lactate," and "adequate fluid resuscitation" to identify septic patients with a particularly high risk of death should be tested. Furthermore, there was consensus to use a MAP of less than 65 mm Hg but that the volume of resuscitative fluid or dose of vasopressor would not be specified. Quantification was thought to be highly user dependent, relying on variable application of different monitors, inconsistent hemodynamic targets, and unspecified approaches to other support measures (e.g., sedation volume status assessment, PEEP [positive end-expiratory pressure] level). It was also agreed that, in the databases examined, an attempt be made to identify an optimal threshold to identify an elevation in serum lactate levels.

Interrogation of the SSC international multicenter database, where all 28,150 patients had infection, two or more SIRS criteria, and at least one dysfunctional organ system, identified about 19,000 patients with some combination of hypotension (MAP <65 mm Hg, the only available cutoff), ongoing vasopressor therapy, and/or hyperlactatemia (>2 mmol/L) after volume resuscitation. Analysis revealed that mortality in patients who had both fluid-resistant hypotension (i.e., who required vasopressors to maintain a MAP >65 mm Hg) *and* elevated lactate levels was 42.3%, significantly higher than in patients who had either isolated hyperlactatemia or fluid-resistant hypotension requiring vasopressors without an elevated serum lactate level. This difference (fluid-resistant hypotension requiring vasopressors *and* hyperlactatemia vs. either alone) also identified patients with a higher mortality when we isolated data from the EHRs from two health systems perused to identify patients carrying a diagnosis of sepsis (University of Pittsburgh Medical Center, 54% vs. 20%; Kaiser Permanente Northern California, 34% vs. 8%).

Many members of the Task Force opined that either hypotension or hyperlactatemia should be used to identify patients with septic shock (hyperlactatemia alone was said to identify "cryptic" shock). However, application of the one easily measured element in the new definition—substantially increased mortality—did not support these positions. The Task Force recognized that blood lactate is commonly, but not universally, available. Nonetheless, the decision to limit the clinical criteria to the combination was preferred by only a small majority of Task Force members, and the issue should be readdressed in the future.

Persistent Critical Illness

The final syndrome that requires description is the most recently identified and the most poorly described. It has been noted that sepsis is the most common cause of death from infection. However, the most common cause of death in critically ill patients is not sepsis, or septic shock, or respiratory failure, or any of a number of other specific maladies. Critically ill patients may die with ARDS, or infection, or sepsis, but they do not appear to die from them. Rather, in the most common scenario, a patient is admitted to the ICU with sepsis, or, perhaps, with something else (e.g., polytrauma, respiratory failure, GI bleeding), and support is initiated. The patient undergoes intubation and mechanical ventilation and is perhaps supported with vasopressors and almost certainly intravenous (IV) fluids. Sedation is provided at variable doses (certainly far less than was used when previous consensus conferences compiled their definitions). Nutrition is delivered by feeding tube or intravenously. A number of different infections are suspected, and confirmation is sought. In the meantime, different antibiotics are started and discontinued. Renal function may decline, and dialysis for acidosis, fluid overload, electrolyte abnormalities, or "uremia" may be initiated. Problems and complications related to preexisting conditions and comorbidities arise and are managed. And so it goes: the patient settles into a remarkably stable yet remarkably abnormal state in which she or he may remain for weeks, not getting worse but certainly not getting better. The patients can remain in this condition for weeks, even months. Ultimately, the patient recovers sufficiently to be transferred to a skilled nursing facility or a chronic respiratory unit, where ventilators can be managed or someone in the patient's family decides that it is time to stop, and life-supporting interventions such as mechanical ventilation and dialysis are stopped. Thus, the most common cause of death in ICUs is discontinuation of exogenous support. The syndrome afflicting these patients is *persistent critical illness*.

Persistent critical illness is poorly defined. Data on incidence, outcomes, and consequences have yet to be collected. Just as improved treatment in previous eras, when patients with once fatal conditions could be kept alive, led to the emergence of new disorders (e.g., fluid resuscitation, acute renal failure, mechanical ventilation, ARDS, cardiopulmonary resuscitation [CPR], myocardial "stunning" and anoxic brain injury, massive resuscitation, and coagulopathy), our ability to acutely manage sepsis, septic shock, and other related disorders has given rise to persistent critical illness. The pathogenesis and pathophysiology are poorly understood and meaningful therapy is unknown, but understanding and treating this condition represent the next challenge in intensive care medicine.

AUTHOR'S RECOMMENDATIONS

- Current definitions of sepsis, septic shock, and organ dysfunction suffer from inconsistencies and a lack of precision, reliance on outdated models of the disorders, limited use of data-driven approaches, and the inability to test validity because of the lack of a "gold standard."
- **Sepsis is defined as life-threatening organ dysfunction due to a dysregulated host response to infection.**
- The term *sepsis* replaces the older term *severe sepsis*, which should no longer be used.
- A prolonged ICU course or death during the acute hospitalization can serve as a proxy for sepsis in patients with suspected, presumed, or documented infection.
- Patients with suspected infection who are likely to have a prolonged ICU course or to die during the acute hospitalization can be clinically identified in the emergency department or on the wards with qSOFA, a combination of three abnormalities—hypotension, increased respiratory rate, and altered mental status—that can be measured at the bedside. Similar patients in the ICU are more reliably identified with the full SOFA score.
- **Septic shock is defined as a subset of sepsis where underlying circulatory and cellular abnormalities are profound enough to substantially increase mortality.**
- Patients with sepsis who are most likely to have septic shock can be identified by a combination of hypotention/a requirement for vasopressors to maintain MAP above 65 mm Hg and an elevated serum lactate level.
- In the absence of fully validated choices, organ dysfunction can be identified with criteria detailed in the SOFA score. Nevertheless, it is imperative that a data-driven, validated alternative be developed in the near future.
- Patients who become septic may evolve to a state where they require prolonged intensive care support. This newly described condition is called persistent critical illness.

REFERENCES

1. Torio CM, Andrews RM. Healthcare Cost and Utilization Project (HCUP) Statistical Briefs. National Inpatient Hospital Costs: The Most Expensive Conditions by Payer, 2011. Statistical Brief #160. http://www.ncbi.nlm.nih.gov/books/NBK169005/; August 2013 (last accessed 31.03.15).
2. Iwashyna TJ, Cooke CR, Wunsch H, Kahn JM. Population burden of long-term survivorship after severe sepsis in older Americans. *J Am Geriatr Soc.* 2012;60:1070–1077.
3. Fleischmann C, Scherag A, Adhikari NK, et al. International Forum of Acute Care Trialists: Assessment of Global Incidence and Mortality of Hospital-treated Sepsis—Current Estimates and Limitations. *Am J Respir Crit Care Med.* 2015 Sep 28. [Epub ahead of print].
4. Gaieski DF, Edwards JM, Kallan MJ, Carr BG. Benchmarking the incidence and mortality of severe sepsis in the United States. *Crit Care Med.* 2013;41:1167–1174.

5. Adhikari NKJ, Fowler RA, Bhagwanjee S, Rubenfeld GD. Critical care and the global burden of critical illness in adults. *Lancet*. 2010;376:1339–1346.

6. Vincent J-L, Marshall JC, Namendys-Silva SA, et al. Assessment of the worldwide burden of critical illness: the intensive care over nations (ICON) audit. *Lancet Respir Med*. 2014;2:380–386.

7. Mozaffarien D, Benjamin EJ, Go AS, et al. Heart disease and stroke statistics–2015 update. A report from the American Heart Association. *Circulation*. 2015;131:e29–e322.

8. American Cancer Society. *Cancer Facts & Figures 2015*. Atlanta: American Cancer Society; 2015.

9. Odden AJ, Rohde JM, Bonham C, et al. Functional outcomes of general medical patients with severe sepsis. *BMC Infect Dis*. December 12, 2013;13:588.

10. Iwashyna TJ, Ely EW, Smith DM, Langa KM. Long-term cognitive impairment and functional disability among survivors of severe sepsis. *JAMA*. 2010;304:1787–1794.

11. Rosendahl J, Brunkhorst FM, Jaenichen D, Strauss B. Physical and mental health in patients and spouses after intensive care of severe sepsis: a dyadic perspective on long-term sequelae testing the Actor-Partner Interdependence Model. *Crit Care Med*. 2013;41:69–75.

12. Prescott HC, Langa KM, Liu V, Escobar GJ, Iwashyna TJ. Increased 1-year healthcare use in survivors of severe sepsis. *Am J Respir Crit Care Med*. July 1, 2014;190(1):62–69.

13. Bone RC, Balk RA, Cerra FB, et al. American College of Chest Physicians/Society of Critical Care Medicine Consensus Conference: definitions for sepsis and organ failure and guidelines for the use of innovative therapies in sepsis. *Crit Care Med*. 1992;20:864–874.

14. Levy MM, Fink MP, Marshall JC, et al. SCCM/ESICM/ACCP/ATS/SIS International Sepsis Definitions Conference. *Intensive Care Med*. 2003;29(4):530–538. and Crit Care Med. 2003;31:1250–1256.

15. Bone RC. Immunologic dissonance: a continuing evolution in our understanding of the systemic inflammatory response syndrome (SIRS) and the multiple organ dysfunction syndrome (MODS). *Ann Intern Med*. 1996;125:680–687.

16. Sprung CL, Sakr Y, Vincent JL, et al. An evaluation of systemic inflammatory response syndrome signs in the Sepsis Occurrence In Acutely Ill Patients (SOAP) study. *Intensive Care Med*. 2006;32:421–427.

17. Singer M, Deutschman CS, et al. *Sepsis 3.0–New International Definitions of Sepsis and Septic Shock*; 2015. to be submitted.

18. Kaukonen K-M, Bailey M, Pilcher D, Cooper DJ, Bellomo R. Systemic inflammatory response syndrome criteria in defining severe sepsis. *N Engl J Med*. 2015;372(17):1629–1638.

19. Vincent JL, Moreno R, Takala J, et al. The SOFA (Sepsis-related Organ Failure Assessment) score to describe organ dysfunction/failure. On behalf of the Working Group on Sepsis-Related Problems of the European Society of Intensive Care Medicine. *Intensive Care Med*. 1996;22:707–710.

20. Vincent JL, de Mendonça A, Cantraine F, Moreno R, Takala J, Suter PM. Use of the SOFA score to assess the incidence of organ dysfunction/failure in intensive care units: results of a multicenter, prospective study. Working group on "sepsis-related problems" of the European Society of Intensive Care Medicine. *Crit Care Med*. 1998;26:1793–1800.

21. Shankar-Hari M, Deutschman CS, Singer M. Do we need a new definition of sepsis? *Intensive Care Med*. 2015;41:909–911.

22. Angus DC, Van der Poll T. Severe sepsis and septic shock. *N Engl J Med*. 2013;369:840–851.

23. Hotchkiss RS, Monneret G, Payen D. Sepsis-induced immunosuppression: from cellular dysfunctions to immunotherapy. *Nat Rev Immunol*. 2013;13:862–874.

24. Deutschman CS, Tracey KJ. Sepsis: current dogma and new perspectives. *Immunity*. 2014;40:463–475.

25. Singer M, De Santis V, Vitale D, Jeffcoate W. Multi-organ failure is an adaptive, endocrine-mediated, metabolic response to overwhelming systemic inflammation. *Lancet*. 2004;364:545–548.

26. Pavlov VA, Tracey KJ. The vagus nerve and the inflammatory reflex–linking immunity and metabolism. *Nat Rev Endocrinol*. 2012;8:743–754.

27. Deutschman CS, Raj NR, McGuire EO, Kelz MB. Orexinergic activity modulates altered vital signs and pituitary hormone secretion in experimental sepsis. *Crit Care Med*. 2013;41:e368–e375.

28. Hotchkiss RS, Swanson PE, Freeman BD, Tinsley KW, Cobb JP, Matuschak GM. Apoptotic cell death in patients with sepsis, shock, and multiple organ dysfunction. *Crit Care Med*. 1999;27:1230–1251.

29. Wiersinga WJ, Leopold SJ, Cranendonk DR, van der Poll T. Host innate immune responses to sepsis. *Virulence*. 2014;5:36–44.

30. Staunton R, Dwyer J. An infection, unnoticed, turns unstoppable. *New York Times*. July 11, 2012.

31. Rubulotta FM, Ramsey G, Parker MM, et al. An international survey: public awareness and perception of sepsis. *Crit Care Med*. 2009;37:167–170.

32. Coopersmith CM, Wunsch H, Fink MP, et al. A comparison of critical care research funding and the financial burden of critical illness in the United States. *Crit Care Med*. 2012;40(4):1072–1079.

33. Levy MM, Rhodes A, Phillips GS, et al. Surviving Sepsis Campaign: association between performance metrics and outcomes in a 7.5-year study. *Crit Care Med*. 2015;43:3–12.

34. Ferrer R, Martin-Loeches I, Phillips G, et al. Empiric antibiotic treatment reduces mortality in severe sepsis and septic shock from the first hour: results from a guideline-based performance improvement program. *Crit Care Med*. 2014;42:1749–1755.

35. ProCESS Investigators, Yealy DM, Kellum JA, Huang DT, et al. A randomized trial of protocol-based care for early septic shock. *N Engl J Med*. 2014;370:1683–1693.

36. Mouncey PR, Osborn TM, Power GS, et al. ProMISe Trial Investigators. Trial of early, goal-directed resuscitation for septic shock. *N Engl J Med*. 2015;372:1301–1311.

37. ARISE Investigators; ANZICS Clinical Trials Group, Peake SL, Delaney A, Bailey M, et al. Goal-directed resuscitation for patients with early septic shock. *N Engl J Med*. 2014;371:1496–1506.

38. Seymour CW, Rosengart MR. Septic Shock: Advances in Diagnosis and Treatment. *JAMA*. 2015;314:708–717.

39. Marshall JC, Cook DJ, Christou NV, et al. Multiple organ dysfunction score: a reliable descriptor of a complex clinical outcome. *Crit Care Med*. 1995;23:1638–1652.

40. Kraut JA, Midias NE. Lactic acidosis. *N Engl J Med*. 2014;371:2309–2319.

41. Casserly B, Phillips GS, Schorr C, et al. Lactate measurement in sepsis-induced tissue hypoperfusion: results from the Surviving Sepsis Campaign database. *Crit Care Med*. 2015;43:567–573.

42. Shankar-Hari M, Deutschman CS, Singer M. Do we need a new definition of sepsis? *Intensive Care Med*. 2015;41:909–911.

38 Is There Immune Suppression in the Critically Ill Patient?

Isaiah R. Turnbull, Richard S. Hotchkiss

In his seminal 1876 work defining germ theory, Dr. Robert Koch described experiments in which he established the causative role of infecting microorganisms in septic shock.[1] Infection was accepted as the cause of sepsis until 1957, when bacterial endotoxin was discovered and demonstrated to recapitulate the pathophysiology of septic shock in the absence of a live replicating bacterial infection.[2] The link between septic shock and the immune system was established 30 years later when Cerami and colleagues demonstrated that endotoxin activated macrophages to release the inflammatory cytokine tumor necrosis factor α (TNF-α), later found to be a primary endogenous mediator of endotoxic shock.[3] Subsequent studies established elevated levels of inflammatory cytokines in the blood of patients with sepsis. The prevailing theory regarding the pathogenesis of sepsis at that time was that bacterial infection induced an inflammatory cytokine storm that caused septic shock.[4] Subsequently, sepsis researchers sought to treat sepsis by attenuating the inflammatory response. Unfortunately, in numerous clinical trials, anti-inflammatory strategies have failed to improve sepsis survival, and in some cases treatment with anti-inflammatory agents increased sepsis mortality.[5-10]

The failure of anti-inflammatory strategies alone to improve sepsis survival led to a reevaluation of the role of the immune system in the pathogenesis of sepsis.[11] Mounting evidence suggests that suppression is the primary immune derangement in the septic patient and that the pathophysiology of sepsis results as much or more from an immunocompromised state than from a systemic inflammatory response.[12,13]

A wealth of evidence supports a role for immune dysfunction in sepsis, with data demonstrating exaggerated and suppressed immune responses. The state of the immune system in sepsis, though, remains incompletely understood. This chapter reviews the available basic and clinical evidence indicating that immunosuppression is the overriding immunologic derangement septic patients. We also highlight potential methods to monitor the immune status of a critically ill patient. We review potential therapies aimed at stimulating the immune system of the septic patient.

IMMUNE SYSTEM IN SEPSIS: SYSTEMIC INFLAMMATORY RESPONSE SYNDROME TO COMPENSATORY ANTI-INFLAMMATORY RESPONSE SYNDROME

The host response to infection is complex and varies depending on the type of infection, bacterial load, and host genetic factors.[11] Cells of the innate immune system, including granulocytes, macrophages, dendritic cells, and innate lymphoid cells such as natural killer cells express germ-line-encoded receptors that recognize pathogen-associated molecular patterns and host-derived molecules associated with tissue damage (damage-associated molecular patterns).[14] These innate immune cells are tasked with the early recognition of microbial infection and the tissue damage associated with infection or injury.[14] Activation of the innate immune system causes release of a diverse range of inflammatory mediators including those canonically associated with sepsis: TNF-α and interleukin 6 (IL-6).[15] The proximal signaling mechanisms of the innate immune system form a positive feedback loop that serves to amplify the response to minor injuries and infections to facilitate early clearance of infecting organisms and damaged tissue. This innate inflammatory response activates the adaptive immune system, inducing proliferation of antigen-specific T cells and B cells that acutely combat infection and provide long-term memory cells, improving future immunity.[15] Under normal physiologic conditions, progression of the immune response leads to activation of negative feedback pathways that downregulate inflammation. Innate immune cells switch from production of inflammatory cytokines to production of anti-inflammatory cytokines such as IL-10 and transforming growth factor β (TGF-β).[16] Innate immune cells, including antigen-presenting cells, undergo programmed cell death through apoptosis, which removes the stimulation to the adaptive immune cells.[17] Without activation, T and B cells become less responsive. A subset of these cells transition to a memory phenotype, and effector B and T cells, no longer required to fight infection, undergo apoptosis.

With the discovery that TNF-α can induce a syndrome similar to endotoxic shock, a theory of sepsis as an overexuberant inflammatory reaction developed.[4] It was hypothesized that in response to severe infections or significant tissue damage, the positive feedback loops of the innate immune response drove activation of the inflammatory response beyond the local environment. This change led to a pathologic organism-wide activation of innate immunity, termed the systemic inflammatory response syndrome (SIRS).[18] Inflammatory cytokines that normally function in the local environment were systemically disseminated, causing fever, leukocytosis, and tachycardia while contributing to capillary leak, vasogenic shock, and remote organ damage.[4] To explain the persistence of SIRS in sepsis, Bone hypothesized that, under normal conditions, inflammation was followed by immune downregulation that limited the inflammatory response. Just as SIRS represented exaggeration of normal, adaptive, proinflammatory pathways, a new syndrome, the compensatory anti-inflammatory response syndrome (CARS), reflected a pathologic downregulation of immune function.[19]

Since the development of the SIRS-CARS model, ongoing research has clarified the relationship among the severe infections that cause sepsis, the state of the immune system, and the clinical course of septic patients. Clinically, septic patients exhibit clear evidence of immune dysfunction. The signs include a loss of delayed hypersensitivity, an

inability to clear microorganisms, and a predisposition to secondary infections.[20-22] Postmortem studies demonstrate that 80% of patients who die with sepsis have a persistent focus of infection.[23] With ongoing sepsis, infectious burden increases, with increased frequency of positive blood cultures and increased infections with opportunistic organisms.[24] Septic patients also demonstrate viral DNAemia; viral DNA from latent herpes family viruses (presumably reactivated during sepsis-induced immunosuppression) are recovered in the blood of 42% of sepsis patients, as compared with 5% of critically ill nonseptic controls.[25] The immune state of the septic patient is characterized by impairment of neutrophil functions, increased lymphocyte and dendritic cell apoptosis, a shift from a T_H1 (T helper cell type 1) to a T_H2 (T helper cell type 2) cytokine profile, an increase in the proportion of T regulatory cells, a release of anti-inflammatory mediators, lymphocyte anergy, and monocyte deactivation (Table 38-1).[12,13] Most deaths in sepsis occur late in the course of the syndrome, well after resuscitation. Those patients who survive show evidence of immune function recovery.[20]

MECHANISMS OF IMMUNE DYSFUNCTION

In animal and human studies, sepsis induces apoptosis in lymphocytes and gastrointestinal epithelial cells (Fig. 38-1).[26-28] Examination of the spleen of patients who died from sepsis reveals a profound depletion of B cells, CD4 T cells, and follicular dendritic cells from the innate and adaptive immune systems that is not observed in the spleen of patients who died after trauma.[28] Septic patients also have absolute lymphocyte counts well below normal. This lymphopenia is associated with poor outcome and the degree of lymphocyte apoptosis correlates with the severity of sepsis.[29] Loss of these cells impairs antibody production, macrophage activation, and antigen presentation. Apoptosis also impairs innate immunity by disrupting the crosstalk between the innate and adaptive

Table 38-1 **Mechanisms of Immunosuppression in Sepsis**
Lymphocyte (CD4 T cells, B cells) and dendritic cell apoptosis
Switch to T_H2, or immunosuppressive, cytokine profile and release of anti-inflammatory mediators
Lymphocyte anergy increased proportion of regulatory T cells
Monocyte deactivation evidenced by decreased expression of mHLA-DR Impairment of neutrophil functions
Expansion of immature myeloid suppressor cell populations

mHLA-DR, monocyte human leukocyte antigen type DR.

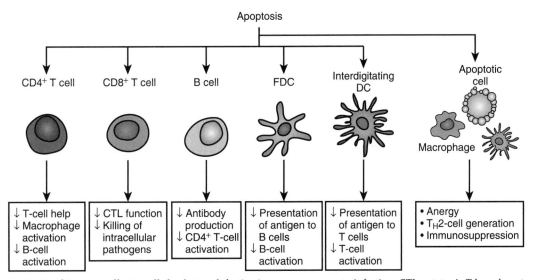

Apoptosis

CD4⁺ T cell	CD8⁺ T cell	B cell	FDC	Interdigitating DC	Apoptotic cell

Macrophage

| ↓ T-cell help
↓ Macrophage activation
↓ B-cell activation | ↓ CTL function
↓ Killing of intracellular pathogens | ↓ Antibody production
↓ CD4⁺ T-cell activation | ↓ Presentation of antigen to B cells
↓ B-cell activation | ↓ Presentation of antigen to T cells
↓ T-cell activation | • Anergy
• T_H2-cell generation
• Immunosuppression |

Figure 38-1. Apoptosis of immune effector cells leads to a defective immune response to infection. *CTL,* cytotoxic T lymphocyte; *DC,* dendritic cell; *FDC,* follicular dendritic cell. *(From Hotchkiss RS, Nicholson DW. Apoptosis and caspases regulate death and inflammation in sepsis.* Nat Rev Immunol. *2006; 6:813-822.)*

immune systems. As a result, sepsis is associated with T cell anergy.[30] Macrophages and dendritic cells that take up and eliminate apoptotic cells release anti-inflammatory cytokines such as IL-10 and TGF-β while suppressing proinflammatory cytokines.[31] T cells that come into contact with these macrophages and dendritic cells become anergic or undergo apoptosis. T cells of patients with peritonitis also have decreased T_H1 function even in the absence of T_H2 cytokines. These T cells fail to proliferate. These T cell findings positively correlate with mortality.[32] Studies in a clinically relevant mouse model of sepsis confirm the significance of lymphocyte apoptosis to sepsis pathophysiology.[33] Mice were injected with either apoptotic or necrotic cells before induction of sepsis and survival was recorded. Mice adopting transferred apoptotic cells had greater mortality compared with mice that received necrotic cells. Significantly, mice that received apoptotic as opposed to necrotic cells also exhibited T_H2 cytokine profiles and decreased interferon γ (IFN-γ) production by spleen cells. In several animal studies, apoptosis was reversed.[34-36] In such investigations, mice that overexpressed BCL-2, an antiapoptotic protein, in lymphocytes had lower mortality rates in pneumonia and cecal ligation and puncture models of sepsis.[36,37] Similar data were reported in mice that overexpressed BCL-2 (B cell lymphoma 2) in gut epithelia.[28,35] The cellular mechanisms of apoptosis in sepsis are incompletely understood, but there is evidence that the extrinsic death receptor and the intrinsic, or mitochondrial, pathways are being activated.[38] Death receptors activated by circulating TNF and CD95 (FasL) activate caspase-8, which then sets off an apoptotic cascade.[30] The mitochondrial pathway can be stimulated by several different agents. These include reactive oxygen species, radiation, chemotherapeutic agents, cytochrome *c*, and cytokine withdrawal. It appears that there is significant crosstalk between the two pathways and that sepsis acts through multiple mechanisms to induce cell apoptosis.

Although controversial, some investigators have reported that T regulatory (CD4+ and CD25+) cells play an important role in the immunosuppression that occurs during sepsis. T regulatory cells modulate the immune response to pathogens by acting on other T cells and antigen-presenting cells.[39] T regulatory cells release cytokines such as IL-10, TGF-β, and IL-4 and thereby mediate responses in CD4 and CD8 T cells. One study revealed that the proportion of T regulatory cells was increased in the blood of septic patients immediately after diagnosis and persisted only in nonsurvivors.[40] This increase in T regulatory cells also has been shown in clinically relevant animal models of sepsis.[41-44] T regulatory cells may be important in the switch from a hyperinflammatory state to immune dysfunction in sepsis. A study demonstrated improved survival in septic mice given an antibody to the glucocorticoid-induced TNF receptor that is highly expressed on T regulatory cells.[44] This antibody restored CD4+ T cell proliferation and increased T_H1 and T_H2 cytokines. This approach reversed the adaptive immune dysfunction seen in sepsis. T regulatory cells may prove to play a crucial role in the development and treatment of immune dysfunction in severe sepsis. Our group performed functional studies on leukocytes isolated from immediate postmortem autopsies

of critically ill patients.[45] As compared with noncritically ill control patients, splenocytes from septic patients were profoundly anergic. When stimulated ex vivo, cytokine elaborated by cells from septic patients was generally less than 10% of that produced by cells isolated from noncritically ill controls. These differences included proinflammatory and anti-inflammatory cytokines, demonstrating that these lymphocytes are globally suppressed and not simply skewed to a pro- or anti-inflammatory phenotype. This phenotype has been hypothesized to result from either T cell exhaustion or from a global slow-down in cellular function and is termed *hibernation.* Phenotypic evaluation of cells from septic patients found increased expression of the inhibitory receptor programmed cell death protein-1 (PD-1), suggesting that sepsis results in a lymphocyte cohort that suppresses cellular activation. Administration of antibodies designed to block PD-1 activity restored adaptive immune function, suggesting that PD-1 inhibited lymphocyte activation. These data are consistent with a T cell "exhaustion" phenotype and provide a possible means to reverse T cell dysfunction in patients using anti–PD-1 antibodies.

In addition to the demonstrated effects of sepsis on splenocytes, recent studies have found expansion of immature myeloid suppressor cells (Gr-1+, CD11b+ cells) in the spleen, lymph nodes, and bone marrow in prolonged sepsis. Studies of lung tissue from septic patients demonstrated increased numbers of myeloid-derived suppressor cells (MDSCs) in the lung as compared with healthy controls. Depletion of these cells in septic mice challenged with T-cell-dependent antigens blocked a T_H2 response. This evidence suggests a role for immature myeloid suppressor cells in sepsis-induced immune suppression.[46]

Monocytes from septic patients also are dramatically affected. In patients with postoperative sepsis, there is an immediate suppression of proinflammatory and anti-inflammatory cytokines after lipopolysaccharide stimulation.[47] Survival among these patients correlated with a recovery of the proinflammatory, but not the anti-inflammatory, response. Monocytes from septic patients have decreased cell surface markers, notably monocyte human leukocyte antigen type DR (mHLA-DR).[48] These monocytes produce only small amounts of TNF-α and IL-1 in response to bacterial challenges.[49] T cells from septic patients also have decreased human leukocyte antigen type DR (HLA-DR) expression, and ex vivo studies demonstrate that these cells are defective for antigen presentation.[49] Numerous characteristics of immune suppression in sepsis have been identified. Nonetheless, researchers have yet to find diagnostic tests that can inform clinicians about the state of the immune system in septic patients. There are no discrete clinical signs or symptoms of immune dysfunction, and there is no gold standard available that can identify a patient in a state of immune suppression.[12]

Identifying Immune Dysfunction in the Septic Patient

The host immune response to sepsis is complex and involves many circulating mediators and cells. Various cytokines and their correlation with mortality have been studied. Baseline circulating IL-6 and soluble TNF receptor have been shown to correlate with disease severity and 28-day all-cause mortality,[50] and they may help in determining when an anti-inflammatory therapy may be of benefit. Levels of anti-inflammatory cytokines such as IL-10 may be more helpful in determining whether a patient is immunosuppressed (Table 38-2). Elevated and sustained levels of IL-10[51,52] and high IL-10/TNF-α ratios were predictive of poor outcome.[53] IL-10 correlated with the decreased expression of mHLA-DR in septic patients (another marker of sepsis-induced immunosuppression; see following paragraph) and may have mediated this finding.[54] IL-10 may prove to be a useful marker of immune dysfunction, but it needs to be evaluated in larger clinical trials. For both pro- and anti-inflammatory cytokines, changes in circulating mediator levels may not correlate with biological activity. Sepsis is associated with changes in cytokine receptor levels[45] and alterations in intracellular signaling pathways[55] that make the biological consequence of circulating cytokine levels difficult to interpret.

Another possibility for evaluating the robustness of the immune response is quantitation of the mHLA-DR cell surface expression in the septic patient. mHLA-DR expression was reduced in patients who develop nosocomial infections after trauma, surgery, and pancreatitis.[56] Patients who recovered from these complications also recovered mHLA-DR expression.[56] This finding became apparent only 48 hours after the onset of sepsis.[57] Therefore sequentially measuring mHLA-DR expression in critically ill patients with concern for sepsis over time may help to identify patients in the early phases of sepsis, but monitoring mHLA-DR is difficult because there is no reliable, standardized testing system at this time.

Procalcitonin has been widely investigated as a serum marker to differentiate SIRS from sepsis. Several small trials indicate that procalcitonin predicts mortality in critically ill patients.[58-60] A recent meta-analysis reviewed the available clinical data and concluded that procalcitonin cannot be used to distinguish sepsis from SIRS and that more studies are needed.[58]

Some investigators have advocated a genomic approach to monitoring immune function. Preliminary studies involving small cohorts of patients indicate that 95% of patients with the same outcome show similar change in the messenger RNA expression of 10 specific genes.[61] Gene chip analysis allows for the comparison of thousands of genes and may eventually reveal sepsis-associated differences in gene expression related to immune dysfunction. This direction may be limited by genetic variability and heterogeneity. This technology is still under development, but it may prove useful in the future.

POTENTIAL THERAPIES AIMED AT SEPSIS-INDUCED IMMUNOSUPPRESSION

Anti-inflammatory therapies, including TNF-α antagonists, IL-1 receptor antagonists, antiendotoxin antibodies, and corticosteroids, have not been shown to decrease overall mortality in patients with sepsis. It is possible that new approaches aimed at stimulating the immune system may succeed where interventions based on inhibiting the immune response have failed. In septic patients demonstrated to be immunocompromised based on decreased expression of HLA-DR, treatment with granulocyte macrophage colony-stimulating factor (GM-CSF) was associated with a decrease in the number of ICU days and decreased APACHE (Acute Physiology and Chronic Health Evaluation) II score.[62] On the basis of these encouraging results, a large multicenter trial of GM-CSF is beginning in 2015, assessing restoration of immune function and improvement in clinical outcomes from sepsis (Does GM-CSF Restore Neutrophil Phagocytosis in Critical Illness In: ClinicalTrials.gov [Internet]. Bethesda [MD]: National Library of Medicine [US]. 2000- [cited 2015 Jan 6]. Available from: http://clinicaltrials.gov/show/NCT01653665 NLM Identifier: NCT01653665). Treatment with IFN-γ improved mHLA-DR expression and mortality in a small group of septic patients, but this has not been studied in a large clinical trial.[63] A case report suggests that IFN-γ can be effective in treating staphylococcal sepsis.[64] The potential for IFN-γ treatment to improve outcomes from sepsis is currently being evaluated in a large RCT.[65]

Blockade of the interaction between the inhibitory receptor PD-1 and its cognate receptor PD-L1 is also being evaluated as a potential therapeutic avenue in sepsis.[13] PD-1 is an inhibitory costimulatory molecule expressed by T cells. PD-1 is expressed after persistent antigenic stimulation of a T cell and ligation of PD-1 by its cognate ligand results in T cell anergy with abrogation of proliferation and cytokine secretion.[13] An increased proportion of splenocytes from septic patients express PD-1, and its ligand PD-L1 is upregulated on antigen-presenting cells and macrophages isolated from septic patients.[45] Blockade of PD-1/PD-L1 interactions has been demonstrated by several groups to improve survival in animal models of sepsis.[66-68] Antibodies blocking the PD-1/PD-L1 interaction have been used successfully as an immunostimulant in cancer patients.[69] Clinical studies to evaluate the efficacy of PD-1 modulation in sepsis are under development.

Researchers are also initiating clinical trials of the cytokine IL-7 as an immunomodulator in sepsis. IL-7 acts broadly on cells of the adaptive immune system, driving proliferation and survival of T cells, B cells, and innate lymphoid cells, including natural killer cells. IL-7 has been demonstrated to increase lymphocyte counts in cancer patients and in HIV-positive patients with persistently low CD4+ T cell counts. Therapeutic exogenous IL-7 leads to a predominate increase in CD4+ and CD8+ T cells with no significant increase in B cell numbers.[70] Ex vivo studies have demonstrated that IL-7 can reverse sepsis-induced lymphocyte hyporesponsiveness. Ex vivo treatment of lymphocytes isolated from septic patients with IL-7 increased levels of the anti-apoptotic molecule BCL-2 to that seen in healthy controls.[71] Ex vivo treatment with IL-7 also improved sepsis-induced deficits in lymphocyte

Table 38-2 **Possible Diagnostic Markers of Sepsis-Induced Immunosuppression**
Increased initial and sustained IL-10 levels
High IL-10/TNF-α ratios
Decreased mHLA-DR expression

IL-10, interleukin-10; *mHLA-DR,* monocyte human leukocyte antigen type DR; *TNF-α,* tumor necrosis factor α.

IFN-γ production.[71] IL-7 treatment has been demonstrated to improve sepsis survival and improve lymphocyte function in a clinically relevant animal model of sepsis.[72]

IL-7 therapy has been efficacious in the treatment of chronic viral infections, including hepatitis, HIV, and JC virus–induced progressive multifocal encephalopathy.[73] IL-7 is also being evaluated as a treatment for chemotherapy-induced lymphopenia and as a treatment of aging-induced immunosenescence.[73] These early studies have suggested that IL-7 is safe and effective in reversing a wide range of immunosuppressive conditions. Taken together, these data make IL-7 a promising candidate for the treatment of sepsis-induced immunosuppression.

CONCLUSION

Previous theories regarding the pathophysiology of sepsis failed to appropriately characterize sepsis-associated immune dysfunction. Most deaths in sepsis occur after the initial hyperdynamic, proinflammatory phase when patients are unable to clear either primary infection or develop secondary, nosocomial infections. This period of immunosuppression is an important cause of mortality, and patients who recover immune function tend to resolve their infections and ultimately survive. Lymphocyte apoptosis, T cell anergy, increased proportion of T regulatory cells, monocyte deactivation, decreased HLA-DR expression, a T_H2 cytokine profile, and neutrophil impairment are all hallmarks of immunosuppression in sepsis. Diagnostic modalities that will enable the physician to track a patient's immune status and accordingly tailor treatment need to be developed. The goal is to be able to administer immune-stimulating therapies during periods of immune suppression and several promising candidates under development.

AUTHORS' RECOMMENDATIONS

- Septic patients have an immunosuppressed state characterized by loss of delayed hypersensitivity, inability to clear primary infections, and susceptibility to secondary infections.
- Most deaths in sepsis occur late in the course of the syndrome, and survivors show evidence of immune recovery.
- Mechanisms of immunosuppression in sepsis include lymphocyte, dendritic cell, and gut apoptosis; a switch from a T_H1 to a T_H2 cytokine profile; release of anti-inflammatory mediators; lymphocyte anergy; and monocyte deactivation.
- Diagnostic modalities aimed at monitoring the immune response in sepsis may help tailor future therapies intended to modulate the immune system.

REFERENCES

1. Koch R, Cheyne WW. *Investigations into the Etiology of Traumatic Infective Diseases.* London: The New Sydenham Society Publications; 1880. Print.
2. Schweinburg FB, Fine J. Evidence for a lethal endotoxemia as the fundamental feature of irreversibility in three types of traumatic shock. *J Exp Med.* 1960;112:793–800. Print.
3. Cerami A, et al. Weight loss associated with an endotoxin-induced mediator from peritoneal macrophages: the role of cachectin (tumor necrosis factor). *Immunol Lett.* 1985;11(3–4):173–177. Print.
4. Baue AE. The horror autotoxicus and multiple-organ failure. *Arch Surg.* 1992;127(12):1451–1462. Print.
5. Zeni F, Freeman B, Natanson C. Anti-inflammatory therapies to treat sepsis and septic shock: a reassessment. *Crit Care Med.* 1997;25(7):1095–1100. Print.
6. Fisher Jr CJ, et al. Initial evaluation of human recombinant interleukin-1 receptor antagonist in the treatment of sepsis syndrome: a randomized, open-label, placebo-controlled multicenter trial. *Crit Care Med.* 1994;22(1):12–21. Print.
7. Abraham E, et al. Efficacy and safety of monoclonal antibody to human tumor necrosis factor alpha in patients with sepsis syndrome. A randomized, controlled, double-blind, multicenter clinical trial. TNF-alpha MAB Sepsis Study Group. *JAMA.* 1995;273(12):934–941. Print.
8. Ziegler EJ, et al. Treatment of gram-negative bacteremia and septic shock with HA-1A human monoclonal antibody against endotoxin. A randomized, double-blind, placebo-controlled trial. The HA-1A Sepsis Study Group. *N Engl J Med.* 1991;324(7):429–436. Print.
9. Bone RC, et al. A controlled clinical trial of high-dose methylprednisolone in the treatment of severe sepsis and septic shock. *N Engl J Med.* 1987;317(11):653–658. Print.
10. Fisher Jr CJ, et al. Treatment of septic shock with the tumor necrosis factor receptor:Fc fusion protein. The Soluble TNF Receptor Sepsis Study Group. *N Engl J Med.* 1996;334(26):1697–1702. Print.
11. Hotchkiss RS, Karl IE. The pathophysiology and treatment of sepsis. *N Engl J Med.* 2003;348(2):138–150. Print.
12. Hotchkiss RS, Karl IE. Sepsis-induced immunosuppression: from cellular dysfunctions to immunotherapy. *Nat Rev Immunol.* 2013;13(12):862–874. Print.
13. Hotchkiss RS, Monneret G, Payen D. Immunosuppression in sepsis: a novel understanding of the disorder and a new therapeutic approach. *Lancet Infect Dis.* 2013;13(3):260–268. Print.
14. Matzinger P. The danger model: a renewed sense of self. *Science.* 2002;296(5566):301–305. Print.
15. Oberholzer A, Oberholzer C, Moldawer LL. Sepsis syndromes: understanding the role of innate and acquired immunity. *Shock.* 2001;16(2):83–96. Print.
16. Opal SM, DePalo VA. Anti-inflammatory cytokines. *Chest.* 2000;117(4):1162–1172. Print.
17. Serhan CN, Savill J. Resolution of inflammation: the beginning programs the end. *Nat Immunol.* 2005;6(12):1191–1197. Print.
18. Bone RC, et al. Definitions for sepsis and organ failure and guidelines for the use of innovative therapies in sepsis. The ACCP/SCCM Consensus Conference Committee. American College of Chest Physicians/Society of Critical Care Medicine. *Chest.* 1992;101(6):1644–1655. Print.
19. Bone RC. Sir Isaac Newton, sepsis, SIRS, and CARS. *Crit Care Med.* 1996;24(7):1125–1128. Print.
20. Frazier WJ, Hall MW. Immunoparalysis and adverse outcomes from critical illness. *Pediatr Clin North Am.* 2008;55(3):647–668, xi. Print.
21. Lederer JA, Rodrick ML, Mannick JA. The effects of injury on the adaptive immune response. *Shock.* 1999;11(3):153–159. Print.
22. Meakins JL, et al. Delayed hypersensitivity: indicator of acquired failure of host defenses in sepsis and trauma. *Ann Surg.* 1977;186(3):241–250. Print.
23. Torgersen C, et al. Macroscopic postmortem findings in 235 surgical intensive care patients with sepsis. *Anesth Analg.* 2009;108(6):1841–1847. Print.
24. Otto GP, et al. The late phase of sepsis is characterized by an increased microbiological burden and death rate. *Crit Care.* 2011;15(4):R183. Print.
25. Walton AH, et al. Reactivation of multiple viruses in patients with sepsis. *PLoS One.* 2014;9(2):e98819. Print.
26. Hotchkiss RS, et al. Role of apoptosis in Pseudomonas aeruginosa pneumonia. *Science.* 2001;294(5548):1783. Print.
27. Hotchkiss RS, et al. Depletion of dendritic cells, but not macrophages, in patients with sepsis. *J Immunol.* 2002;168(5):2493–2500. Print.
28. Hotchkiss RS, et al. Apoptotic cell death in patients with sepsis, shock, and multiple organ dysfunction. *Crit Care Med.* 1999;27(7):1230–1251. Print.
29. Le Tulzo Y, et al. Early circulating lymphocyte apoptosis in human septic shock is associated with poor outcome. *Shock.* 2002;18(6):487–494. Print.

30. Hotchkiss RS, Nicholson DW. Apoptosis and caspases regulate death and inflammation in sepsis. *Nat Rev Immunol.* 2006;6(11):813–822. Print.

31. Albert ML. Death-defying immunity: do apoptotic cells influence antigen processing and presentation? *Nat Rev Immunol.* 2004;4(3):223–231. Print.

32. Heidecke CD, et al. Selective defects of T lymphocyte function in patients with lethal intraabdominal infection. *Am J Surg.* 1999;178(4):288–292. Print.

33. Hotchkiss RS, et al. Adoptive transfer of apoptotic splenocytes worsens survival, whereas adoptive transfer of necrotic splenocytes improves survival in sepsis. *Proc Natl Acad Sci USA.* 2003;100(11):6724–6729. Print.

34. Hotchkiss RS, et al. Caspase inhibitors improve survival in sepsis: a critical role of the lymphocyte. *Nat Immunol.* 2000;1(6):496–501. Print.

35. Coopersmith CM, et al. Inhibition of intestinal epithelial apoptosis and survival in a murine model of pneumonia-induced sepsis. *JAMA.* 2002;287(13):1716–1721. Print.

36. Hotchkiss RS, et al. Overexpression of Bcl-2 in transgenic mice decreases apoptosis and improves survival in sepsis. *J Immunol.* 1999;162(7):4148–4156. Print.

37. Hotchkiss RS, et al. Sepsis-induced apoptosis causes progressive profound depletion of B and Cd4+ T lymphocytes in humans. *J Immunol.* 2001;166(11):6952–6963. Print.

38. Chang KC, et al. Multiple triggers of cell death in sepsis: death receptor and mitochondrial-mediated apoptosis. *FASEB J.* 2007;21(3):708–719. Print.

39. Venet F, et al. Regulatory T cell populations in sepsis and trauma. *J Leukoc Biol.* 2008;83(3):523–535. Print.

40. Venet F, et al. Increased percentage of Cd4+Cd25+ regulatory T cells during septic shock is due to the decrease of Cd4+Cd25- lymphocytes. *Crit Care Med.* 2004;32(11):2329–2331. Print.

41. MacConmara MP, et al. Increased Cd4+ Cd25+ T regulatory cell activity in trauma patients depresses protective Th1 immunity. *Ann Surg.* 2006;244(4):514–523. Print.

42. Wisnoski N, et al. The contribution of Cd4+ Cd25+ T-regulatory-cells to immune suppression in sepsis. *Shock.* 2007;27(3):251–257. Print.

43. Scumpia PO, et al. Increased natural Cd4+Cd25+ regulatory T cells and their suppressor activity do not contribute to mortality in murine polymicrobial sepsis. *J Immunol.* 2006;177(11):7943–7949. Print.

44. Scumpia PO, et al. Treatment with GITR agonistic antibody corrects adaptive immune dysfunction in sepsis. *Blood.* 2007;110(10):3673–3681. Print.

45. Boomer JS, et al. Immunosuppression in patients who die of sepsis and multiple organ failure. *JAMA.* 2011;306(23):2594–2605. Print.

46. Delano MJ, et al. Myd88-dependent expansion of an immature Gr-1(+)Cd11b(+) population induces T cell suppression and Th2 polarization in sepsis. *J Exp Med.* 2007;204(6):1463–1474. Print.

47. Weighardt H, et al. Sepsis after major visceral surgery is associated with sustained and interferon-gamma-resistant defects of monocyte cytokine production. *Surgery.* 2000;127(3):309–315. Print.

48. Astiz M, et al. Monocyte response to bacterial toxins, expression of cell surface receptors, and release of anti-inflammatory cytokines during sepsis. *J Lab Clin Med.* 1996;128(6):594–600. Print.

49. Manjuck J, et al. Decreased response to recall antigens is associated with depressed costimulatory receptor expression in septic critically ill patients. *J Lab Clin Med.* 2000;135(2):153–160. Print.

50. Oberholzer A, et al. Plasma cytokine measurements augment prognostic scores as indicators of outcome in patients with severe sepsis. *Shock.* 2005;23(6):488–493. Print.

51. Monneret G, et al. The anti-inflammatory response dominates after septic shock: association of low monocyte HLA-DR expression and high interleukin-10 concentration. *Immunol Lett.* 2004;95(2):193–198. Print.

52. Gogos CA, et al. Pro- versus anti-inflammatory cytokine profile in patients with severe sepsis: a marker for prognosis and future therapeutic options. *J Infect Dis.* 2000;181(1):176–180. Print.

53. van Dissel JT, et al. Anti-inflammatory cytokine profile and mortality in febrile patients. *Lancet.* 1998;351(9107):950–953. Print.

54. Lekkou A, et al. Cytokine production and monocyte HLA-DR expression as predictors of outcome for patients with community-acquired severe infections. *Clin Diagn Lab Immunol.* 2004;11(1):161–167. Print.

55. Abcejo AS, et al. Failed interleukin-6 signal transduction in murine sepsis: attenuation of hepatic glycoprotein 130 phosphorylation. *Crit Care Med.* 2009;37(5):1729–1734. Print.

56. Muehlstedt SG, Lyte M, Rodriguez JL. Increased IL-10 production and HLA-DR suppression in the lungs of injured patients precede the development of nosocomial pneumonia. *Shock.* 2002;17(6):443–450. Print.

57. Monneret G, et al. Analytical requirements for measuring monocytic human lymphocyte antigen DR by flow cytometry: application to the monitoring of patients with septic shock. *Clin Chem.* 2002;48(9):1589–1592. Print.

58. Tang BM, et al. Accuracy of procalcitonin for sepsis diagnosis in critically ill patients: systematic review and meta-analysis. *Lancet Infect Dis.* 2007;7(3):210–217. Print.

59. Novotny A, et al. Use of procalcitonin for early prediction of lethal outcome of postoperative sepsis. *Am J Surg.* 2007;194(1):35–39. Print.

60. Jensen JU, et al. Procalcitonin increase in early identification of critically ill patients at high risk of mortality. *Crit Care Med.* 2006;34(10):2596–2602. Print.

61. Pachot A, et al. Longitudinal study of cytokine and immune transcription factor mRNA expression in septic shock. *Clin Immunol.* 2005;114(1):61–69. Print.

62. Meisel C, et al. Granulocyte-macrophage colony-stimulating factor to reverse sepsis-associated immunosuppression: a double-blind, randomized, placebo-controlled multicenter trial. *Am J Respir Crit Care Med.* 2009;180(7):640–648. Print.

63. Docke WD, et al. Monocyte deactivation in septic patients: restoration by IFN-gamma treatment. *Nat Med.* 1997;3(6):678–681. Print.

64. Nalos M, et al. Immune effects of interferon gamma in persistent staphylococcal sepsis. *Am J Respir Crit Care Med.* 2012;185(1):110–112. Print.

65. Radboud, University. *The Effects of Interferon-Gamma on Sepsis-Induced Immunoparalysis;* 2016. Print.

66. Huang X, et al. PD-1 expression by macrophages plays a pathologic role in altering microbial clearance and the innate inflammatory response to sepsis. *Proc Natl Acad Sci USA.* 2009;106(15):6303–6308. Print.

67. Brahmamdam P, et al. Delayed administration of anti-PD-1 antibody reverses immune dysfunction and improves survival during sepsis. *J Leukoc Biol.* 2010;88(2):233–240. Print.

68. Zhang Y, et al. PD-L1 blockade improves survival in experimental sepsis by inhibiting lymphocyte apoptosis and reversing monocyte dysfunction. *Crit Care.* 2010;14(6):R220. Print.

69. Topalian SL, et al. Safety, activity, and immune correlates of anti-PD-1 antibody in cancer. *N Engl J Med.* 2012;366(26):2443–2454. Print.

70. Lundstrom W, Fewkes NM, Mackall CL. IL-7 in human health and disease. *Semin Immunol.* 2012;24(3):218–224. Print.

71. Venet F, et al. IL-7 restores lymphocyte functions in septic patients. *J Immunol.* 2012;189(10):5073–5081. Print.

72. Unsinger J, et al. IL-7 promotes T cell viability, trafficking, and functionality and improves survival in sepsis. *J Immunol.* 2010;184(7):3768–3779. Print.

73. Mackall CL, Fry TJ, Gress RE. Harnessing the biology of IL-7 for therapeutic application. *Nat Rev Immunol.* 2011;11(5):330–342. Print.

74. Hoyert DL, Xu JQ. Deaths: Preliminary Data for 2011. National Vital Statistics Reports vol. 61.6 (2012). Print.

75. Martin GS. Sepsis, severe sepsis and septic shock: changes in incidence, pathogens and outcomes. *Expert Rev Anti Infect Ther.* 2012;10(6):701–706. Print.

76. Martin GS, et al. The epidemiology of sepsis in the United States from 1979 through 2000. *N Engl J Med.* 2003;348(16):1546–1554. Print.

39 What Is the Role of Empirical Antibiotic Therapy in Sepsis?

Fiona Kiernan, Gerard F. Curley

The annual prevalence of sepsis, the systemic inflammatory response to infection, is estimated at 19 million cases worldwide. Over the last 30 years, reported mortality rates in severe sepsis, defined as sepsis plus organ dysfunction, have dropped from over 80% to 20% to 30% because of advances in training, better surveillance and monitoring, prompt initiation of therapy, and organ support.[1]

The timely and correct identification of infection followed by appropriate treatment with antibiotics is crucial to the management of critically ill and injured patients. Antibiotic therapy is founded on principles of appropriate drug selection based on (suspected) susceptibility patterns of the causative pathogen. The goal of antimicrobial administration is to achieve drug concentrations sufficiently effective to exert maximum killing at the infection site and to prevent the emergence of antimicrobial resistance.[2] Selection of empirical antibiotics should be based on the suspected source, such as community-acquired infection or nosocomial infection, medical and culture history, and local microbial susceptibility results.

The latest guidelines for the management of severe sepsis and septic shock provided by the Surviving Sepsis Campaign (SSC) consortium recommend to begin timely appropriate intravenous (IV) broad-spectrum antibiotics after forming a probable diagnosis and obtaining cultures (1B/1C grade recommendations to administer antibiotics within 1 hour after diagnosis of either sepsis or septic shock).[3]

However, accurate infection diagnosis in critically ill patients is confounded by the systemic inflammatory response syndrome (SIRS). Intensivists must use the same criteria (e.g., fever, leukocytosis, tachycardia, tachypnea) supplemented by clinical judgment to distinguish patients with infections from those with SIRS. Because of the devastating consequences of missing a true infection, empirical antibiotic therapy often is initiated when patients are critically ill and physicians are unable to distinguish SIRS from infection. The result is probable overuse of antibiotics.[4,5]

Incorrect use of broad-spectrum antibiotics has potentially serious consequences, including *Clostridium difficile* infection,[6] renal toxicity,[7,8] and encouragement of multidrug-resistant organisms.[9] These events can lead to longer intensive care unit (ICU) stays, greater health-care costs, and a higher mortality rate.[10,11] The full extent of these effects in ICU patients has not been well reported, and antibiotic overuse is inevitable. There currently is no consensus or benchmark for an acceptable rate of overtreatment or for the use of empirical antibiotics in the ICU.

DIAGNOSTIC ISSUES

Clinical Features

Establishing a definitive diagnosis of infection is paramount to the appropriate selection and use of antimicrobials. Once infection is suspected in the ICU patient, a comprehensive workup must be performed to identify the site of infection. The microbial causes of various ICU infections are reasonably predictable once the actual site of infection is known; thus appropriate drug selection properly begins with identification of a known or suspected site of infection. Unfortunately, the site of infection is often unable to be identified with any certainty; studies in septic patients have shown that no source of infection is identified in up to 30% to 40% of patients.[12,13] The clinical manifestations of sepsis are highly variable, depending on the initial site of infection, the causative organism, the pattern of acute organ dysfunction, the underlying health status of the patient, and the interval before initiation of treatment. The signs of both infection and organ dysfunction may be subtle; thus the most recent international consensus guidelines provide a long list of warning signs of incipient sepsis.[14] In particular, clinicians must keep in mind that there are numerous sources of fever in critically ill patients that are not associated with infection. The occurrence of new fever in an ICU patient should prompt a thorough evaluation of noninfectious sources for the fever before initiation of antimicrobial therapy. Patients who have begun receiving antimicrobial therapy and have persistent fever despite the resolution of other signs and symptoms of infection should also be evaluated for noninfectious sources of fever.

Acute organ dysfunction in sepsis most commonly affects the respiratory and cardiovascular systems. Respiratory compromise is classically manifested as the acute respiratory distress syndrome (ARDS), of which sepsis is the most common cause.[15] Cardiovascular compromise may manifest primarily as hypotension or an elevated serum lactate. After adequate volume expansion, hypotension frequently persists, requiring the use of vasopressors, and myocardial dysfunction may occur.[16] Other organ systems are commonly affected. Central nervous system dysfunction is typically manifested as confusion, delirium, or coma. Imaging studies generally show no focal lesions, and findings on electroencephalography are usually consistent with nonfocal encephalopathy.[17] Critical illness polyneuropathy and myopathy are also common, especially in patients with a prolonged ICU stay.[18] Acute kidney injury is manifested as decreasing urine output and an increasing serum creatinine level and frequently requires treatment with renal replacement therapy.[19] Paralytic ileus, elevated bilirubin/aminotransferase levels, altered glycemic control, thrombocytopenia and disseminated intravascular coagulation, adrenal dysfunction, and the nonthyroid illness syndrome are all relatively common in patients with severe sepsis.[20]

Gram Stain and Culture as an Aid to Empirical Therapy

Microbiologists have access to a wide range of invasive and noninvasive diagnostic techniques, and these should be used when appropriate. The institution of antimicrobial therapy should not be delayed for the sake of performing exhaustive diagnostic tests. Gram stain of appropriate specimens from potential sites of infection should be used to help determine appropriate empirical or antimicrobial therapy. Although the yield of useful information from Gram stains is usually not high in critically ill patients, performing this test is nevertheless of value for those patients in whom causative pathogens are identified.[21-23] Gram stains from specimens obtained from certain sites such as the respiratory tract and wounds should be interpreted with caution because of high rates of colonization with nonpathogenic organisms, particularly in patients who have already been hospitalized for several days. Studies have clearly demonstrated the high frequency and rapid time course of microbial colonization of ICU patients.[24-26] Classic studies demonstrated that rates of colonization of the oropharynx and bronchi of critically ill patients with gram-negative organisms reached 45% and 65% within 5 days after ICU admission, respectively, and more than 90% at both sites by day 10.[27] These patients also become highly colonized with gram-positive cocci and particularly yeast soon after ICU admission.

Great care must be taken to differentiate colonizing organisms from true pathogens when evaluating Gram stain and culture results from nonsterile areas of the body or areas that may become colonized after the placement of foreign devices such as catheters (e.g., the urinary tract and respiratory tract). Colonization is often distinguished on the basis of Gram stain results showing multiple morphologic types of bacteria or the absence of clinically relevant signs and symptoms of infection despite the presence of microbial growth. However, in critically ill patients, colonization is often extremely difficult to distinguish from true infection, and antimicrobials are initiated based on a presumptive diagnosis.

Blood Cultures

The role of blood cultures is crucial for the correct fine-tuning of antibiotic therapy in sepsis.[3] Blood cultures are the current "gold standard" of bloodstream infection diagnosis and are based on the detection of viable microorganisms present in blood. Blood cultures have the advantage of allowing for the evaluation of their antimicrobial susceptibility; this characteristic has still not been paralleled by any other technique available to date. This aspect is important because several studies have shown that inadequate antimicrobial therapy is an independent risk factor for mortality or microbiological failure for severely ill patients with life-threatening infections (see later).

However, several factors may still reduce the overall sensitivity of blood cultures. An intrinsic limitation of blood cultures is their low sensitivity to slow-growing and fastidious organisms such as *Bartonella* spp., *Francisella tularensis*, *Mycoplasma* spp., several molds, and *Nocardia* spp.[28] Other uniformly uncultivable pathogens (by the usual bacterial culture systems) such as *Rickettsia* spp., *Coxiella burnetii*, *Chlamydophila pneumoniae*, and *Tropheryma whipplei* are better diagnosed by immunodiagnostic or molecular techniques.[28] The presence of multiple interfering factors such as previous antimicrobial therapy, suboptimal sample collection, or incorrect preanalytic processing may deliver false-negative results even in septic patients with easy-to-culture pathogens such as *Staphylococci* and *Streptococci*.[29]

An important factor influencing blood culture diagnostic yield is blood volume.[30,31] Several studies of adults[32,33] and pediatric patients[34,35] confirmed that the rate of isolation from blood cultures increases with the quantity of blood submitted. Another important variable is the time taken from blood withdrawal to the loading of blood culture bottles into the instrument.[36] Ideally, blood cultures should be loaded immediately into the continuous-monitoring instrument to minimize the time to detection and to reduce the number of false-negative samples caused by delays in loading. A decrease in recovery has been observed when bottles are held at room temperature for more than 12 hours and even more so when they are preincubated at 37° C before being loaded into the automatic instrument.[36]

Role of Rapid Microbiological Diagnostics to Guide Empirical Therapy

The role of the clinical microbiology laboratory in the acute phase of sepsis has traditionally been marginal because at least 24 to 72 hours are necessary for the confirmation of an infectious etiology, identification of the pathogen, and evaluation of its antimicrobial susceptibility. However, with the advent of rapid speciation methods, clinicians are encountering increasing windows of time when they are aware of an infecting organism's species without yet knowing its susceptibilities.[37,38] The most promising techniques are proteomic technologies, including matrix-assisted laser desorption-ionization time-of-flight mass spectrometry.[39] This technique is able to identify bacteria or fungi by determining their proteomic profiles.[40] It has also been used to identify bacterial virulence factors[41] or antibiotic resistance markers.[42] This method has the main advantage of allowing a definitive identification, or typing, of isolated microorganisms in only a few minutes. In addition, several pathogen-specific, broad-range, and multiplex polymerase chain reaction–based amplification strategies have been used to identify positive blood cultures, to aid in rapid speciation, or to diagnose sepsis directly from blood samples.[43] Other molecular methods are being used, including fluorescence in situ hybridization with oligonucleotide probes targeting bacterial or fungal genes (typically ribosomal RNA genes).[44]

With the advent of rapid speciation techniques, there is an opportunity to improve antimicrobial coverage with the added possibility of decreasing unnecessary antimicrobial usage. This will suddenly make institutional species-specific antibiograms much more clinically useful. Moreover, clinicians may be able to more quickly discontinue therapy after identification of obvious culture contaminants (e.g., *Corynebacterium* species) or more rapidly de-escalate therapy after identification of organisms with predictable susceptibilities (e.g., *Listeria monocytogenes*). In some instances, species identification will result in pathogen-guided escalation before susceptibility-guided de-escalation of empirical therapy (e.g., *Enterococcus* species or *Pseudomonas* species).[37]

Despite the remarkable technical advances of nucleic acid testing–based approaches, their widespread use for the microbiological diagnosis of sepsis is still limited by several shortcomings. For example, the detection of circulating microbial DNA (DNAemia) does not necessarily indicate the presence of a viable microorganism responsible for a given infection. The high sensitivity needed for the diagnosis of sepsis may increase the risk of false-positive results due to carryover contamination or due to the detection of environmental DNA contaminating the blood sample. Moreover, DNAemia may be the footprint for transient bacteremia not related to any infection,[45,46] or it may be related to the persistence of circulating DNA still detectable several days after successful anti-infectious therapy has been completed.[47] Another major drawback of the available molecular assays for the diagnosis of sepsis is that they do not provide information on the antimicrobial susceptibility of the detected pathogen.

The rapid detection of a pathogen may allow for better fine-tuning of empirical therapy with possible economic savings, but the lack of a specific susceptibility spectrum, especially with multidrug-resistant pathogens on the rise, may limit the clinical usefulness of these assays. In cases in which the presence of a single gene is always associated with phenotypic resistance (i.e., the mecA gene for oxacillin resistance and van genes for vancomycin resistance), it is relatively simple to design molecular strategies that allow their detection. More troublesome are cases in which the phenotypic resistance is influenced by several concurrent factors, such as the regulatory role of distinct genes that modulate the levels of expression of the gene(s) determining resistance.

Other Assays to Guide Empirical Antibiotic Therapy

Fungi continue to be a major cause of infection-related mortality principally for ICU patients and patients with hematologic malignancies. However, early diagnosis remains a challenge, mainly because of the low specificity of clinical symptoms and the low sensitivity of fungal cultures. The development of an enzyme-linked immunosorbent assay for the detection of galactomannan (GM), an *Aspergillus* sp. cell wall component, has been an important advance for the diagnosis of invasive aspergillosis.[48,49] A positive test confirmed with two sequential samples is considered to be a valid index for invasive aspergillosis diagnosis with European Organisation for Research and Treatment (EORTC) diagnostic criteria.[50] Although the detection of GM in serum is easy to perform, a major disadvantage of the serodiagnosis of invasive aspergillosis is the occurrence of false-positive results.

β-Glucan (BG) is another component of the fungal cell wall present in a wider variety of fungal species, including *Candida* spp.[51] For most patients with confirmed invasive fungal infections, BG levels were elevated several days before clinical diagnosis.[52]

The limitations of blood cultures have also fostered interest in the development of sensitive and rapid laboratory tests aimed at detecting nonspecific biomarkers of sepsis. Assays for C-reactive protein, procalcitonin (PCT), interleukin (IL)–6, and IL-8 have been evaluated for their clinical usefulness. PCT is a propeptide of calcitonin that is ubiquitously expressed as part of the host's inflammatory response to various insults.[53] A growing body of evidence suggests that PCT is a marker of severe bacterial infection[54] and can distinguish patients who have sepsis from patients who have SIRS.[55] In particular, PCT levels in plasma have been correlated with sepsis-related organ failure scores and may be useful in risk assessment.[56] High and persistent elevations in PCT levels have been associated with poor outcomes for ICU patients.[57] Although several studies suggested that PCT is among the most promising biomarkers for sepsis, considerable controversy surrounding its clinical usefulness still remains. A recent meta-analysis[58] indicated that PCT cannot reliably differentiate sepsis from other noninfectious causes of SIRS in critically ill adult patients.

EARLY TREATMENT: THE EVIDENCE

In a well-known study, Rivers et al.[59] demonstrated an impressive absolute reduction of 16% in the in-hospital mortality rate of septic shock and severe sepsis in their single-center, prospective, randomized trial of early goal-directed therapy (EGDT). This was the first study to demonstrate that there was a golden hour (or 4 to 6 hours) for patients with severe sepsis.

The results of the Australasian Resuscitation in Sepsis Evaluation (ARISE) trial[60] and the Protocol-Based Care for Early Septic Shock (ProCESS) study,[61] both of which evaluated the use of resuscitation bundles in sepsis, seem to refute the findings of Rivers et al. These trials failed to show benefit from EGCDT versus controls. One of the criticisms of EGDT as described by Rivers and of other sepsis bundles concerns the uncertain effect that individual parts of the bundle have on survival.[62] EGDT as a whole seems to save lives, but individual parts of the therapy may not be efficacious (central mixed venous oxygen monitoring) or may even be harmful to patients with sepsis (i.e., blood transfusion).[62] The only consistently important factor in several multivariate analyses of the utility of individual elements of the sepsis bundle has been rapid antimicrobial initiation.[62] Indeed, in the ARISE and ProCESS studies, septic shock was recognized early in most patients. Seventy-six percent of the patients in ProCESS received antimicrobial agents by the time they underwent randomization,[61] which occurred a mean of 3 hours after patients' arrival in the emergency department (ED). The rate of antimicrobial administration 6 hours after randomization was approximately 97%, which undoubtedly contributed to the higher rates of survival than projected in this study.

The potential influence of delayed antibiotic therapy was first evaluated in patients with community-acquired pneumonia (CAP). In a study involving 297 U.S. acute care hospitals, Kahn et al.[63] observed a 4% point reduction in 30-day mortality among Medicare patients who received antibiotics within 4 hours of admission and appropriate oxygen therapy. In the early 1990s, McGarvey and Harper[64] demonstrated that care processes that included antibiotic delivery within 4 hours were associated with lower pneumonia mortality at two community hospitals. Meehan and colleagues[65] undertook a multicenter retrospective study of 14,069 patients with CAP treated in 3555 U.S. acute care hospitals and demonstrated that administration of antibiotics within 8 hours of hospital arrival and collecting blood cultures within 24 hours were associated with improved 30-day survival. More recently, Houck et al.[66] described that among 13,771 patients who had not received outpatient antibiotic agents, antibiotic administration within 4 hours of arrival at the hospital was associated with reduced in-hospital mortality (6.8% vs. 7.4%; adjusted odds ratio [AOR], 0.85; 95% confidence interval [CI], 0.74 to 0.98) and mortality within 30 days of admission (11.6% vs. 12.7%; AOR, 0.85; 95% CI, 0.76 to 0.95).

In a study of 261 patients in the ED, Gaieski et al.[67] confirmed the association with timing of antibiotic therapy and mortality in patients with severe sepsis or septic shock.

In addition, Kumar and colleaguers,[68] in a retrospective cohort study of 2154 patients who received empirical antibiotic therapy, observed that the survival was 80% in patients given antibiotics within the first hour of persistent or recurrent hypotension. However, for each hour of delay during the subsequent 6 hours, the chances of survival decreased by 7.6%. In multivariate analysis, the strongest predictor of outcome was time to effective antibiotic administration. Only half the patients received effective antibiotics within 6 hours of hypotension onset, and 30% had delays of more than 12 hours. It is important to point out that this was a retrospective study over 15 years, and recruitment rates were relatively low, with 2154 patients included from 10 sites (14 ICUs). Only 12% of patients had received antibiotics within the first hour. In addition, Kumar et al.[68] focused on septic shock patients with appropriate antibiotic treatment.

In a prospective observational study in 77 ICUs[62] based on propensity scores and adjusting for other treatments, Ferrer et al. reported that among 2796 severe sepsis/septic shock patients, empirical antibiotic treatment reduced mortality (treatment within 1 hour vs. no treatment within first 6 hours of diagnosis; odds ratio [OR] 0.67; 95% CI, 0.50 to 0.90; P = .008).

In a more recent retrospective analysis of a large dataset of 28,150 patients with severe sepsis and septic shock prospectively collected for the SSC in Europe, the United States, and South America, Ferrer and colleagues[69] showed that delay in first antibiotic administration was associated with increased in-hospital mortality. There was a linear increase in mortality risk for each hour of delay in antibiotic administration. Reducing the time to first antibiotic from

more than 6 hours to less than 1 hour may result in a mortality reduction of 9.5% (33.1 to 24.6%). These data demonstrate that the association between timing of antibiotic administration and mortality is true not only for patients with septic shock but also for patients with severe sepsis. Importantly, the beneficial effects of early antibiotic administration reported in this study are based on time from sepsis diagnosis and are not related to onset of hypotension.

On the basis of this evidence, the SSC guidelines recommend that after the recognition of severe sepsis or septic shock, IV broad-spectrum antibiotics should be administered as early as possible and always within 1 hour (for patients identified on the general medical wards) or 3 hours (for patients identified in the ED).[3]

The relationship of prompt antibiotics and better outcomes might represent a surrogate marker for the quality of care in a broader sense. Other important sepsis treatments have shown time dependency, such as quantitative resuscitation[59] or source control.[70] In fact, in a systematic review and meta-analysis, Barochia et al.[71] showed that the implementation of SSC bundles was followed by an improvement in most of the sepsis process-of-care variables, including time-to-antibiotic treatment, followed by a mortality reduction.

APPROPRIATE DRUG SELECTION

Initial selection of adequate or appropriate drug therapy also appears to be of importance in optimizing outcomes of antimicrobial use in critically ill patients. Few would argue with the initial use of broad-spectrum agents. Initial empirical anti-infective therapy should include one or more drugs that have activity against the likely pathogens (bacterial or fungal) and that penetrate into the presumed source of the sepsis. The choice of drugs should be guided by the susceptibility patterns of microorganisms in the community and in the hospital.

Selection of inadequate therapy has been demonstrated in numerous clinical studies to be associated with increased patient mortality,[4,12,21,72-78] and the risk of inadequate therapy is often directly related to rates of antimicrobial resistance in certain pathogens.[4,12,73,76,77] Simply put, adequate therapy is more than a reflection of "sensitive" or "resistant." It needs to be governed by breakpoints that are relevant to the mode of action of an antibiotic and the probability that at any given dose, a drug will exceed either the concentration required for killing most strains of a given bacterial species (concentration-dependent killing) or that the concentration will remain above the minimum inhibitory concentration (MIC) of the strains for certain time periods (time-dependent killing).[79]

Retrospective studies conducted in the 1960s and 1970s have shown that appropriate antimicrobial therapy, defined as the use of at least one antibiotic active in vitro against the causative bacteria, reduced the mortality of gram-negative bacteremia when compared with patients receiving inappropriate therapy.[80-83] In a landmark study of 173 patients with gram-negative bacteremia, who were classified in three categories according to the severity of the underlying disease categories (i.e., rapidly fatal, ultimately fatal, and nonfatal), McCabe et al.[83] observed that appropriate antibiotic therapy reduced mortality from 48% to 22%. Four subsequent studies that included larger numbers of patients yielded similar results.[80-82,84] In a more recent prospective study of 2124 patients with gram-negative bacteremia, mortality was 34% in 670 patients who received inappropriate antibiotics and 18% in 1454 patients who received appropriate antibiotics.[85] Smaller recent studies showed that the appropriateness of the antibiotic regimen favorably influenced the outcome of patients infected with specific gram-negative bacteria, such as *Enterobacter* species,[86] *Pseudomonas aeruginosa*,[87] and ceftazidime-resistant *Klebsiella pneumoniae* or *Escherichia coli*.[88]

Fewer data have been published on the impact of appropriate antibiotic therapy in patients with gram-positive sepsis.[89] Several studies evaluated the impact of appropriate antimicrobials in patients with severe infections due to gram-negative and gram-positive bacteria.[4,12,77,85,90-97] In all but one study,[97] appropriate antibiotic therapy was associated with a better outcome. Such studies are likely to involve special groups of organisms that are known to be less virulent: thus their role as pathogens is difficult to substantiate. This would include organisms such as coagulase-negative staphylococci and enterococci, in which there is controversy concerning either the diagnosis or attributable mortality and which are intrinsically less virulent organisms than gram-negative rods or *Staphylococcus aureus.* The study by Ibrahim et al.[77] of patients with bacteraemia in critical care units showed those treated inadequately with antimicrobials fared far worse than those treated adequately (mortality 61.9% vs. 28.4%, *P* < .001), with almost one third receiving inadequate initial cover. Pathogens inadequately covered included *Candida* species in more than 8%, vancomycin-resistant enterococci, coagulase-negative staphylococci, and *P. aeruginosa*. The presence of fungal infection, prior administration of antibiotics, and central venous catheters each independently increased risk of inadequate cover.[77]

EMPIRICAL ANTIMICROBIAL SELECTION

General Considerations

Because initial selection of adequate drug therapy is of vital importance in optimizing outcomes of antimicrobial use in critically ill patients, several factors are important to consider when choosing initial empirical therapy. These include suspected site(s) of infection (and corresponding potential pathogens), the patient's immunologic status, therapy for a nosocomial- or community-acquired infection, rates of resistance of these pathogens to potentially used drugs, a patient's prior exposure to antimicrobial therapy that may potentially increase the likelihood of antimicrobial resistance, and the results of any pertinent prior diagnostic tests. A reasonable understanding of the pharmacology, pharmacokinetics, pharmacodynamics, potential toxicities, potential drug interactions, and appropriate dosing of individual antimicrobials is also important in the selection of a specific agent once the antimicrobial has been chosen. In general, empirical antimicrobial regimens for critically ill patients should be aggressive (i.e., sufficiently broad spectrum in pharmacologic activity to cover the most likely [rather than all possible] pathogens,

initiated promptly, and given in relatively high doses when the presence of any significant renal or hepatic dysfunction is considered).

Source and Microbiology of Sepsis

In a recent meta-analysis and review, Bochud and colleagues[98] identified the predominant sources of infection in patients with severe sepsis and septic shock, by decreasing order of frequency, as the lungs, the bloodstream (without another identifiable source), the abdomen, the urinary tract, and soft tissues. This is corroborated by a multicenter prospective cohort study by Sands and colleagues,[99] in which, in 866 cases of sepsis syndrome, respiratory infections were the most common, accounting for 42.4% of all infections. This was followed by bloodstream infections of undetermined origin (12.0%). Likewise, in a multicenter prospective study in French public hospitals, the primary source of infection was also pleuropulmonary, with almost half (41%) accounting for total episodes of documented severe sepsis.[100] However, in this cohort, intra-abdominal infections accounted for 32% of episodes of sepsis in which a unique source was identified, whereas primary bacteremia was identified in only 4% of cases. Kumar and colleagues[68,101] similarly found that pleuropulmonary, intra-abdominal, and urinary tract source infection were, in order, the largest contributors to a large (n = 5715), multi-institutional cohort of septic shock cases.

Data from various sources indicate that there have been important changes in the microbial etiology of sepsis over recent decades. The largest survey of sepsis epidemiology reviewed more than 10 million cases of sepsis over a 22-year period (1979 to 2000) from a nationally representative sample of U.S. acute-care hospitals.[102] From 1979 to 1987, gram-negative bacteria were the predominant organisms causing sepsis, but they were overtaken by gram-positive bacteria thereafter. In 2000, among organisms reported to have caused sepsis, gram-positive bacteria accounted for 52.1% of cases, with gram-negative bacteria accounting for 37.6%, polymicrobial infection for 4.7%, anaerobes for 1.0%, and fungi for 4.6%. There was no specific breakdown of causative organisms to species level. A more recent longitudinal study from Spain had similar findings.[103] This study examined 27,419 episodes of significant bloodstream infection in 22,626 patients from a single general hospital in Madrid over a 22-year period (1985 to 2006). There was an increase in the overall incidence of bloodstream infection throughout the study period, from 130.3 per 100,000 population in 1985 to 269.8 per 100,000 population in 2006. Overall, 55% of episodes of bloodstream infections were caused by gram-positive bacteria and 44% by gram-negative bacteria. In a pattern similar to the U.S. study, there was a similar number of episodes caused by both gram-positive and gram-negative bacteria during 1985 to 1987, but gram-positive bacteria became much more predominant thereafter, although the numbers were very similar again for 2004 to 2006. This relative increase in sepsis caused by gram-positive bacteria reflected a general increase in the incidence of all major gram-positive bacteria, although there were marked increases in the incidence of bloodstream infection associated with coagulase-negative staphylococci and *Streptococcus pneumoniae*. The incidence of *S. aureus* bloodstream infection increased steadily throughout the study period, from 24.3 episodes per 100,000 population in 1985 to 30.8 episodes per 100,000 population in 2006. *E. coli* was the most predominant gram-negative bacterial cause of bloodstream infection, with an incidence of 23.5 episodes per 100,000 population in 1985, increasing to 79.1 episodes per 100,000 population in 2006. Bochud et al.[98] identified the gram-positive organisms responsible for sepsis syndromes as predominantly *S. aureus*, coagulase-negative staphylococci, enterococci, and streptococci. In contrast, gram-negative sepsis is commonly caused by members of the family Enterobacteriaceae, especially *E. coli*, *K. pneumoniae*, and *P. aeruginosa*.[98]

There was a 207% increase in the number of cases of sepsis caused by fungal organisms, from 5231 cases in 1979 to 16,042 in 2000.[103] Most causes of fungal sepsis were caused by *Candida* species, which are the fourth most common cause of bloodstream infection and are associated with high mortality.[104] The Madrid study showed a steady increase in fungal bloodstream infections throughout the study period, with a progressive increase in non-albicans *Candida* spp.[103] The overall incidence of fungal bloodstream infection was 1.7 episodes per 100,000 population in 1985 and 12.5 episodes per 100,000 population in 2006.

Anaerobic bacteria are a relatively uncommon cause of sepsis, accounting for 1.0% of cases of sepsis in the United States during 1979 to 2000[102] and 4.1% of episodes of bloodstream infection in Madrid during 1985 to 2006.[103]

Combination Therapy and Monotherapy

There are several potential advantages to using combination anti-infective therapy for serious, life-threatening infections[105]: (1) an increased likelihood that the infective pathogen will be susceptible to at least one of the components of the dual regimen, thereby allowing appropriate initial therapy; (2) prevention of emergence of resistance during therapy; and (3) additive or synergistic effect of the antimicrobials. In contrast, the disadvantages of using a combination of drugs include a greater likelihood of adverse effects, increased cost, possible antagonism between specific drug combinations, and the propagation of antimicrobial resistance.[106]

Although several studies have attempted to address the issue of whether combination antimicrobial therapy improves outcomes in sepsis compared with a single agent, a consensus has not been reached.[107,108] There are several reasons for this. Many studies are observational in nature. In these studies, factors such as selection bias and confounding by indication are difficult to avoid, especially with the use of relatively subjective criteria such as clinical response rather than mortality.[105] Another difficulty is that most randomized studies are designed to assess noninferiority.[109] These studies are explicitly designed with a structural bias in favor of showing equivalence between a newer, more pharmacodynamically potent drug and a combination of two weaker agents. In addition, randomized controlled trials (RCTs) often do not have sufficient numbers of a particular type of microorganism or a particular patient population (such as septic shock) to allow robust

subgroup analyses, and as such, synergy and emergence of resistance cannot be rigorously assessed. Meta-analyses that have combined the results of individual studies allow for critical assessment of the literature, identification of important gaps and limitations, and generation of hypotheses for future trials, but they may also suffer from the heterogeneity and intrinsic weaknesses/deficits of the included studies.[108] The evidence for specific combination versus monotherapy is discussed later.

Community-Acquired Pneumonia

S. pneumoniae remains the most prevalent and lethal cause of CAP.[110] However, in patients with CAP who require admission to the ICU, *Legionella*, gram-negative bacilli, *S. aureus*, and influenza are also important. Risk factors for CAP due to gram-negative bacilli include previous antibiotic therapy, prior hospitalization, immunosuppression, pulmonary comorbidity (e.g., cystic fibrosis, bronchiectasis, or repeated exacerbations of chronic obstructive pulmonary disease that require frequent glucocorticoid or antibiotic use), probable aspiration, and medical comorbidities (e.g., diabetes mellitus, alcoholism).[111,112] Community-associated methicillin-resistant *Staphylococcus aureus* (MRSA) pneumonia remains uncommon,[113] but it typically produces a necrotizing pneumonia with high morbidity and mortality.

The three most frequently recommended initial antibiotic regimens for hospitalized patients with CAP, which have activity against its major causes, include (1) an extended spectrum β-lactam (e.g., amoxicillin/clavulanic acid) with a macrolide, or (2) an extended spectrum β-lactam with a fluoroquinolone, or (3) an antipneumococcal quinolone alone. This last option is increasingly recognized as inferior to combination therapy for severe CAP. Several medical societies have issued guidelines for the treatment of CAP.[111] Recommendations for antibiotic regimens for CAP have been issued by a collaboration between the Infectious Diseases Society of America (IDSA)/American Thoracic Society (ATS) in 2007[111] and separately by the British Thoracic Society (BTS) in 2009.[114] For patients with severe CAP requiring ICU admission, the IDSA/ATS guidelines recommend a β-lactam (ceftriaxone, cefotaxime, ampicillin-sulbactam) plus either IV azithromycin or an antipneumococcal fluoroquinolone unless there is concern for *Pseudomonas* or MRSA infection. If *Pseudomonas* is a concern, an antipseudomonal agent (piperacillin-tazobactam, imipenem, meropenem, or cefepime) plus an antipseudomonal fluoroquinolone (ciprofloxacin or high-dose levofloxacin) should be used. If MRSA is a concern, then either vancomycin or linezolid should be added.

Arguments against dual antibiotic therapy focus on the lack of robust evidence of benefit and the potential harms of such therapy. A recent meta-analysis of randomized clinical trials of antibiotic therapy for CAP failed to find a mortality benefit with dual therapy.[115] Furthermore, the use of broader dual antibiotic coverage increases the risk of antibiotic resistance. For example, macrolide use has been associated with increased risk of macrolide-resistant and penicillin-resistant *S. pneumoniae* isolates in patients with invasive pneumococcal disease.[116] Finally, more antibiotic therapy increases the risk of adverse drug effects.

For example, previous studies[117] have found independent associations between macrolide use and the risk of cardiovascular morbidity.

However, as the guidelines suggest, and despite similar spectra of activity, emerging evidence from mostly retrospective studies suggests the superiority of dual therapy over monotherapy, particularly for patients with severe CAP, or bacteremic pneumococcal pneumonia.[118-124]

In the study by Rodriguez and colleagues,[122] a secondary analysis of a prospective observational cohort was undertaken for patients with CAP who developed shock. Among the 529 patients recruited for the original study, 51% or 270 patients required vasoactive support and were characterized as having shock. Among those patients, combination antibiotic therapy was associated with a significantly higher 28-day adjusted in-ICU survival (hazard ratio [HR] 1.69, CI, 1.09 to 2.6). In addition, even when monotherapy was appropriate in vitro, it still provided a lower 28-day adjusted ICU survival than an adequate antibiotic combination (HR 1.64, CI, 1.01 to 2.64). Of note, combination regimens were further examined to determine whether the difference seen in survival rate with combination or monotherapy was secondary to a specific antibiotic or combination thereof. When compared with monotherapy, survival rates were higher for antibiotic combinations, including β-lactam plus macrolide (HR 1.73, CI, 1.08 to 2.76) and β-lactam plus fluoroquinolones (HR 1.77, CI, 1.01 to 3.15).

More recently, Rodrigo et al.[123] used data from the BTS national audits to retrospectively compare the outcome of CAP for 3239 patients treated with dual β-lactam and macrolide antibiotics with that for 2001 patients treated with β-lactams alone. The authors found that after adjusting for CURB65 scores, age, sex, comorbidities, IV administration of antibiotics, nursing home residency, and admission to ICU, the OR of mortality of patients treated with dual therapy was 0.72 (CI, 0.60 to 0.85) compared with those treated with β-lactams alone. Analyzing the data according to CURB65 score indicated that the beneficial effect of dual therapy was mainly for patients with moderate-severity CAP (CURB65 2) who had a startling mortality OR of 0.54 (CI, 0.41 to 0.72) compared with patients given β-lactams alone. There was also some effect for patients with severe CAP (CURB65 3+; OR, 0.76; CI, 0.60 to 0.96) but none for those with mild CAP (CURB65 0–1; OR, 0.80; CI, 0.56 to 1.16).

A recent meta-analysis[125] of 16 observational studies comparing β-lactam–macrolide combination with a single β-lactam in more than 42,000 patients with all-cause pneumonia found a lower risk of death in favor of the combination treatment (OR, 0.67; 95% CI, 0.61 to 0.73).

Finally, more definitive evidence has been provided by an open-label, multicenter, noninferiority, randomized trial of 580 patients admitted to six hospitals in Switzerland for mildly to moderately severe CAP (Pneumonia Severity Index [PSI] categories I to IV).[109] Patients were randomly allocated to receive monotherapy with a β-lactam or dual therapy with a β-lactam and a macrolide. *Legionella pneumophila* infection was diagnosed with urinary antigen testing, and macrolide therapy was added for patients in the monotherapy arm who had a positive test result. The primary study outcome was the proportion of patients not reaching clinical stability at hospital day 7 with validated criteria. For this outcome, a predefined noninferiority boundary of 8% was assessed with a one-sided 90% CI. Secondary 30- and 90-day outcomes included mortality, readmission, recurrence of pneumonia, and adverse effects to antibiotics. On hospital day 7, more patients in the monotherapy arm compared with the dual therapy arm had not reached clinical stability (41.3% vs. 33.4%; $P = .07$). The upper limit of the one-sided CI for this 7.9% difference was 13.3%, which exceeded the predefined noninferiority boundary. Planned subgroup analyses found a significant delay in reaching clinical stability for patients in the monotherapy arm infected with atypical pathogens (HR, 0.33; 95% CI, 0.13 to 0.85) and a trend toward a delay in PSI category IV (HR, 0.81; 95% CI, 0.59 to 1.10). Although a smaller proportion of patients treated with dual therapy than monotherapy were readmitted at 30 days (3.1% vs. 7.9%; $P = .01$), none of the other secondary outcomes varied between the treatment arms. On the basis of a well-designed noninferiority trial, the authors rejected their primary hypothesis that monotherapy was noninferior to dual therapy.

On the basis of this evidence, it appears that the benefits of combination therapy for CAP may not be limited to those only with severe CAP (PSI category IV/V) or with pneumococcal bacteremia and septic shock but may extend to all patients hospitalized with CAP. Possible explanations for the apparent beneficial effects of combination therapy in CAP include coverage for atypical pathogens (which account for up to 20% of moderate to severe CAP), polymicrobial infections, resistant pathogens, synergistic effects, and the anti-inflammatory immunomodulatory effects of the macrolides.[126] That macrolide antibiotics are unique in that they not only inhibit the production of pneumolysin and other pneumococcal virulence factors but possess neutrophil-directed anti-inflammatory properties may account for the advantage of using them as part of combination therapy for severe CAP.

Ventilator-Associated Pneumonia

Most health-care–associated pneumonia is ventilator-associated pneumonia (VAP), which is the most common nosocomial infection acquired in the ICU. VAP develops in 10% to 20% of patients who undergo mechanical ventilation for longer than 24 hours[127,128] and is associated with longer ICU stays, increased costs, and increased mortality.[129,130]

The type of organism that causes VAP usually depends on the duration of mechanical ventilation. In general, early VAP is caused by pathogens that are sensitive to antibiotics whereas late-onset VAP is caused by multidrug-resistant and more difficult to treat bacteria. Typically, bacteria causing early-onset VAP include *S. pneumoniae* (as well as other *Streptococcus* species), *Hemophilus influenzae*, methicillin-sensitive *S. aureus*, antibiotic-sensitive enteric gram-negative bacilli, *E. coli*, *K. pneumonia*, *Enterobacter* species, *Proteus* species, and *Serratia marcescens*.[131,132] Culprits of late VAP are typically multidrug-resistant bacteria, such as MRSA, *Acinetobacter*, *P. aeruginosa*, and extended-spectrum β-lactamase (ESBL)–producing bacteria.[131,132] Commonly found bacteria in the oropharynx can attain clinically significant numbers in the lower airways. These bacteria include *Streptococcus viridans*, *Corynebacterium*, coagulase-negative

Staphylococcus, and *Neisseria* species. VAP is frequently due to polymicrobial infection. VAP from fungal and viral causes has a very low incidence, especially in the immunocompetent host.[132]

According to the ATS and IDSA treatment guidelines for health-care–associated pneumonia,[132] recommendations for empirical treatment of early VAP are single-agent ceftriaxone, ampicillin/sulbactam, or a fluoroquinolone. In contrast, regimens for late VAP, which is more commonly caused by multiresistant organisms such as *Pseudomonas* spp., *Acinetobacter*, or MRSA, include a carbapenem with or without vancomycin or combination therapy composed of an aminoglycoside or quinolone with an antipseudomonal penicillin, a β-lactam/β-lactamase inhibitor combination, ceftazidime, or cefepime.[132] Guidelines issued by the British Society for Antimicrobial Chemotherapy recommend co-amoxiclav or cefuroxime for patients with early-onset infections who have not previously received antibiotics and have no other risk factors for multidrug-resistant pathogens.[133] In those who have previously received antibiotics or who have other risk factors, a third-generation cephalosporin (cefotaxime or ceftriaxone), a fluoroquinolone, or piperacillin-tazobactam would be appropriate. Acceptable treatment options for late-onset VAP according to these guidelines include ceftazidime, ciprofloxacin, meropenem, and piperacillin-tazobactam.[133] When MRSA is a possibility, vancomycin or linezolid should be included in the antibiotic regimen. Although linezolid penetrates lung tissue better than vancomycin, a recent meta-analysis of RCTs suggest that it is no better than vancomycin.[134]

In a meta-analysis of suspected VAP by Aarts and colleagues[135] comprising 1805 patients, a total of 11 trials compared monotherapy with combination therapy. Eight of the 11 trials, composed of a total of 1459 patients, reported mortality. In a pooled analysis, there was no mortality difference for patients receiving monotherapy in comparison with combination therapy (relative risk [RR], 0.94, 0.76 to 1.16). Likewise, outcomes did not change in a sensitivity analysis of treatment failure (RR, 0.92, 0.72 to 1.17) or in the five trials exclusively enrolling ventilated patients (mortality RR, 0.95, 0.68 to 1.32). The investigators concluded that it did not appear likely that combination therapy was clinically superior to monotherapy.

It appears that the only reason to use combination therapy for VAP that is currently supported by evidence is the increased likelihood of appropriate initial anti-infective therapy. Once the organism is identified, then de-escalation to a single drug should be used if permitted by the susceptibility testing.

Sepsis

The choice of antibiotics in sepsis is largely determined by the source or focus of infection, the patient's immunologic status, whether the infection is nosocomial or community acquired, and knowledge of the local microbiology and sensitivity patterns. Initial empirical anti-infective therapy should include one or more drugs that act against the likely pathogens and that penetrate into the presumed source of sepsis. However, whether the initial regimen in patients with severe sepsis and septic shock should include two or

more antibiotics or an extended spectrum β-lactam antibiotic with the aim of treating all realistically possible microbial causes remains controversial.

In the guidelines for the management of severe sepsis of the SSC, initial combination therapy is recommended,[3] and combination therapy is frequently used in clinical practice. Narrowing the spectrum of coverage after 3 to 5 days is recommended, except for infections caused by *P. aeruginosa* and infections among neutropenic patients for whom continued combination treatment is advised.[3]

Several randomized trials of combination therapy versus monotherapy in serious infections, including endocarditis, gram-negative bacteremia, and neutropenic sepsis,[136-138] and animal models[139,140] have supported the possibility of clinically relevant antimicrobial synergism with appropriate combinations of antibiotics. In a recent large observational Spanish cohort study, Diaz-Martin and colleagues[141] described the effect of empirical combination antimicrobial therapy in patients with severe sepsis and septic shock. Patients who received combination antimicrobial therapy experienced a 15% relative reduction in mortality and a 30% reduction in the odds of death when compared with patients who received single antibiotic therapy.[141]

However, two separate meta-analyses have failed to demonstrate any consistent benefit with combination therapy of β-lactams and aminoglycosides in immunocompetent patients with sepsis, gram-negative bacteremia, or both.[108,142]

Paul and colleagues[108] performed a review and meta-analysis comparing β-lactam–aminoglycoside combination therapy with β-lactam monotherapy for severe infections in nonimmunocompromised patients with sepsis. In this analysis, a total of 69 randomized and quasirandomized trials were included, comprising 7863 patients, of which approximately 1000 had pneumonia. Paul and colleagues[108] concluded there was no difference in all-cause fatality (RR, 0.97; 95% CI, 0.73 to 1.30) and that empirical evidence did not show the synergy effect when adding an aminoglycoside to a β-lactam in the clinical setting. In addition, nephrotoxicity was significantly less frequent with monotherapy (RR, 0.30; 95% CI, 0.23 to 0.39).

In 2004, Safdar and colleagues[142] published a meta-analysis to determine whether a combination of two or more drugs would reduce mortality in patients with gram-negative bacteria. Their study included 17 studies, of which five were prospective cohorts, two were RCTs, and the rest were retrospective. Most studies used β-lactams or aminoglycosides alone and in combination. Overall, they did not observe a mortality benefit with combination therapy (OR, 0.96, 0.7 to 1.32).[142] Several subgroup analyses were also performed to determine whether the findings would differ if trials were separated according to date of publication (i.e., before or after 1990, when more potent antimicrobials were made available) or study design (i.e., retrospective vs. prospective). Regardless of subset analyses, there remained no added benefit to combination therapy.[142] However, in an analysis restricted to five studies of *P. aeruginosa* bacteremia, the summary OR was 0.5 (0.32 to 0.79; *P* <.007), suggesting a 50% relative reduction in mortality with the use of combination therapy. The investigators noted, though, that underlying populations in these studies varied considerably and that a sizable proportion of patients were immunocompromised, making it difficult to apply the results to the general population.

In contrast, a meta-regression study by Kumar et al.[143] suggested that the beneficial effect of combination therapy may be restricted to critically ill patients with septic shock. Kumar and colleagues hypothesized that any beneficial effect of combination (i.e., two antibiotics of different antimicrobial classes active for the isolated pathogen) antimicrobial therapy on the mortality of life-threatening infection is restricted to patients with septic shock or otherwise high risk of death. This hypothesis was tested in a meta-regression study of 50 studies from which 62 evaluable datasets of varying monotherapy mortality were derived. Notably, Kumar and colleagues[143] found the same absence of a significant benefit of combination therapy overall as did Paul and colleagues.[108] However, combination therapy demonstrated a significant advantage over monotherapy when the rate of death/clinical failure exceeded 25% (pooled OR, 0.54; 95% CI, 0.45 to 0.66; $P < .0001$).

Another retrospective, propensity-matched, multicenter cohort study of 4662 patients with culture-positive bacterial septic shock, also by Kumar et al.,[144] demonstrated that combination therapy may decrease 28-day mortality (36.3% vs. 29.0%; HR, 0.77 [95% CI, 0.67 to 0.88]; $P < .001$) and hospital mortality (47.8% vs. 37.4%; OR, 0.69 [95% CI, 0.59 to 0.81]; $P < .001$). Combination therapy was defined as using two or more agents with different mechanisms of action for at least 24 hours after the onset of hypotension, or until death if the patient died in the first 24 hours, and the second agent had to be added within 24 hours of the first agent or within 24 hours of the onset of hypotension. To reach these conclusions, the authors used a complex, propensity-matched method, yielding 1223 matched pairs of patients for analysis. The use of combination therapy also was associated with increased ventilator-free and pressor/inotrope–free days and significant reductions in stay in the ICU. The beneficial effects of combination therapy in the study by Kumar et al.[144] applied to both gram-positive and gram-negative infections, but these findings were restricted to patients treated with β-lactams in combination with aminoglycosides, fluoroquinolones, or macrolides/clindamycin. Carbapenems, extended-spectrum β-lactam or β-lactamase inhibitor combinations, and antipseudomonal cephalosporins, which tend to demonstrate optimal pharmacokinetic indices (with presumably maximal kill rates) for most septic shock pathogens, yielded the weakest evidence of benefit with combination therapy. Notably, the most potent β-lactams including carbapenems failed to exhibit evidence of combination therapy benefit. In this circumstance, the addition of a second drug may have little incremental benefit. In addition, in both groups, mortality was lowest if therapy was given rapidly, and the differences between monotherapy and combination therapy were minimized in the patients who received rapid initiation of therapy.

It is evident from this study that β-lactam/β-lactamase inhibitors (BL/BLIs) and carbapenems are often considered for the treatment of sepsis when the main suspected pathogens are gram-negative bacteria because of their broad spectrum of coverage. Shiber et al.[145] conducted a systematic review and meta-analysis of RCTs that compared BL/BLIs with carbapenems for the treatment of sepsis. They found no differences between BL/BLIs and carbapenems in all-cause mortality (RR, 0.98; 95% CI, 0.79 to 1.20) or clinical failure at the end of treatment (RR, 0.99; 95% CI, 0.89 to 1.11). Subgroup analyses of patients more likely to have had infections caused by ESBL-producing bacteria did not reveal an advantage from using carbapenems. Adverse events requiring discontinuation were more common with BL/BLIs (RR, 1.36; 95% CI, 1.03 to 1.79), most probably related to diarrhea, which was significantly more common with BL/BLIs (RR, 1.46; 95% CI, 1.25 to 1.70). Seizures, vomiting, and *Clostridium difficile*–associated diarrhea (CDAD) were significantly more common with carbapenems. The RR of 0.29 (0.10 to 0.87) for CDAD denotes a 71% lower incidence with BL/BLIs, with 95% CIs ranging from a decrease of 90% to a decrease of 13%.

Finally, in the first randomized trial of its kind, 600 patients with severe sepsis or septic shock at 44 ICUs in Germany were randomized to receive either IV meropenem, 1 g every 8 hours, or meropenem and moxifloxacin, 400 mg per day.[146] Antibiotics were recommended to be provided for 7 days at least, or up to 14 days at the clinician's discretion. Primary outcome was Sequential Organ Failure Assessment (SOFA) score, with secondary outcomes of mortality at 28 and 90 days. There were no statistically significant differences in outcomes between groups. Use of combination antibiotic therapy appeared to decrease the emergence of resistant organisms, albeit to a small extent: eight patients in the meropenem monotherapy group had positive cultures for organisms resistant to meropenem, compared with one in the combination therapy group.

In summary, good quality observational data suggest that early empirical combination antibiotic therapy with two antibiotics of different mechanisms of action is associated with superior outcomes compared with monotherapy in the treatment of bacterial septic shock in patients who have a high baseline risk of mortality.[143,144] However, beneficial effects of combination therapy may be limited to regimens that use less than maximally potent antimicrobials, such as extended penicillins (e.g., ampicillin, ticarcillin, pipercillin); semisynthetic penicillins (e.g., cloxacillin, oxacillin); and first-, second-, and third-generation (nonpseudomonal) cephalosporins. Agents with maximal potency in terms of T > MIC (the time the drug concentration remains above the minimum inhibitory concentration) for most septic shock pathogens (carbapenems, ticarcillin/clavulanate, piperacillin/tazobactam, ceftazidime) may not yield additional benefit with the addition of a supplemental antibiotic.[108,144,146] The key issue may be the ability of combination therapy to augment bacterial clearance compared to monotherapy.[107] If so, then it is likely that augmented bacterial clearance with combination therapy may only be clinically relevant when the β-lactam component of combination therapy is less than maximally potent. Monotherapy is recommended for patients who are not critically ill and at high risk of death.[108] However, further study is clearly needed to definitively address under what circumstances combination therapy may be useful in sepsis and septic shock.

Intra-abdominal Infections

Most intra-abdominal infections (IAIs) are polymicrobial and most commonly involve enteric gram-negative bacilli.

Health-care–associated IAIs, compared with community-acquired IAIs, are significantly more likely to involve resistant pathogens.[147] In vitro susceptibility of organisms isolated from IAIs is documented by the Study for Monitoring Antimicrobial Resistance Trends (SMART), which is a surveillance program that monitors resistance patterns. Over the course of the SMART study, the five most commonly isolated gram-negative pathogens from IAIs were *E. coli, K. pneumoniae, P. aeruginosa. Enterobacter cloacae*, and *Proteus mirabilis*.[148] The incidence of β-lactamase production was 8.8% and 8.9% for *E. coli* and *K. pneumoniae*, respectively. Overall, the most active antimicrobials were amikacin, piperacillin-tazobactam, imipenem, and ertapenem, although β-lactamase production reduced the activity of most agents.[149] Among the ESBL-producing bacteria, the carbapenems retained their activity better than other antimicrobials.[150]

Once adequate source control is obtained, appropriate initial antimicrobial therapy heavily influences outcome in complicated IAIs, as with other severe infections.[151] Evidence-based guidelines regarding selection of antimicrobial therapy for IAIs were formulated by the Surgical Infection Society, the IDSA, the American Society for Microbiology, and the Society of Infectious Disease Pharmacists.[152-154] In the guidelines, the use of either single-drug regimens or combination therapy is recommended. Although it is stated in the guidelines that "antibiotic therapy for such (health-care-associated) infections may require the use of multi-drug regimens (e.g., an aminoglycoside or quinolone or a carbapenem and vancomycin),"[152,154] no specific recommendations are made regarding the use of combination therapy. Alternative guidelines also exist that take into account newer antimicrobials and the treatment of resistant gram-positive and gram-negative infections.[155]

Empirical therapy of community-acquired IAIs should include acylaminopenicillin/BLI or ertapenem or other carbapenems (imipenem/cilastatin, meropenem, doripenem). Alternatively, combinations of metronidazole with group cephalosporins, ciprofloxacin, levofloxacin, or moxifloxacin monotherapy are also appropriate. Antibiotics covering the enterococci are usually not required in community-acquired IAIs. Antibiotic treatment of enterococci is recommended in postoperative IAI or seriously ill patients.[156,157] Microbial causes of postoperative peritonitis tend to be multidrug resistant, including enterococci (including vancomycin-resistant enterococci [VRE]), resistant gram-negative organisms (ESBL or AmpC or carbapenemase-producer), MRSA, and *Candida* species.[155] Appropriate agents may be carbapenems, tigecycline, piperacillin/tazobactam, or moxifloxacin depending on microbial findings. Antifungal treatment is recommended for proven fungal infections (see later).

Several combination regimens have been investigated for treatment of IAIs, including aminoglycoside-based,[153,158,159] cephalosporin-based,[160] or quinolone-based regimens.[161] Some, but not all, of the trials included patients in severe sepsis or septic shock. The systematic review by Bochud and colleagues included five trials that evaluated the use of combination therapy versus monotherapy for the empirical treatment of abdominal sepsis.[98] In all five trials, there was no significant mortality difference between the two treatment arms. Subsequently, two RCTs have examined the use of combination therapy in abdominal infections.[162,163] Yellin and colleagues[162] found that success rates of ertapenem compared with combination therapy using ceftriaxone and metronidazole were similar at 83% (22/29) and 77% (24/31) in the ertapenem and comparator groups, respectively. Solomkin and colleagues[163] compared moxifloxacin monotherapy with ceftriaxone plus metronidazole in patients with complicated community-origin IAI. Moxifloxacin was noninferior to ceftriaxone plus metronidazole in terms of clinical response at test-of-cure in the per protocol population (clinical cure, 90.2% for moxifloxacin vs. 96.5% for ceftriaxone/metronidazole; 95% CI of the difference, −11.7 to −1.7). However, the patients included in these trials were not critically ill. In the study by Yellin and colleagues,[162] 94% of patients in each treatment arm had APACHE (Acute Physiology and Chronic Health Evaluation) scores of 14 or lower, and in the study by Solomkin and colleagues,[163] all patients had community-acquired abdominal infections, none of whom were in severe sepsis or shock. A Cochrane review of antibiotics in secondary peritonitis showed no difference in all-cause mortality between aminoglycosides plus anti-anaerobes and other regimens (OR, 2.03; 95% CI, 0.88 to 4.71), nor was there evidence of an increase in adverse events between the groups (OR, 1.76; 95% CI, 0.87 to 3.53). However, there was evidence of a faster cure rate in the other regimen group, and this resulted in a shorter length of stay.[164] On the basis of limited data, the use of combination therapy in abdominal sepsis does not appear to be advantageous compared with single-drug therapy for as long as the initial antimicrobial drug is appropriate.

Empirical Antifungal Therapy

Candida infections are underrecognized. Culture mechanisms lack sensitivity. This would suggest a possible role for empirical antifungals, particularly in patients with recent exposure to broad-spectrum antibiotics or immunosuppression. However, the SSC recommends against the routine use of empirical antifungals because only a small proportion of septic patients have fungal infections (5% of cases), although this is likely to rise.[13] In the EPIC (Extended Prevalence of Infection in Intensive Care) II study comprising 7087 infected ICU patients in 75 countries, *Candida* spp. was the third most frequent organism cultured, accounting for 19% of all isolates, although it is unclear whether these were the organisms responsible for the sepsis.[165]

A large retrospective study identified delay in administration of antifungal agents as a predictor of hospital mortality in patients subsequently found to have positive cultures for *Candida* spp.[72] With the relatively high morbidity associated with the use of antifungals, it would seem reasonable not to recommend their routine use. However, it is very likely that the timing of antifungal therapy in severe infection is just as critical as that of antibiotic therapy. In high-risk patients, a high index of suspicion for primary or secondary fungal infection and a low threshold for the use of antifungal agents are required.

Fungi are more prevalent as isolates in patients with secondary or tertiary peritonitis, with *Candida* spp. identified in up to 20% of patients with gastrointestinal tract perforation.[166] Risk factors include fecal soiling of the peritoneum, recurrent gastrointestinal perforation, immunosuppressive therapy, inflammatory diseases, and status after transplant. These patients have a high risk of mortality,[167] and some case series suggest benefit from the empirical addition of agents with activity against *Candida* spp.[167,168]

The IDSA has produced guidelines recommending the use of amphotericin B or fluconazole in patients with *Candida* peritonitis for a period of 2 to 3 weeks as a supplement to surgical drainage.[169] However, these guidelines did not offer guidance on the use of prophylactic antifungal agents in patients with peritonitis with risk factors. However, the notion of previous *Candida* colonization is a strong argument in favor of early initiation of antifungal therapy. The increase in frequency of *Candida glabrata* may prompt some units to use echinocandins in preference to azole agents in these high-risk patients.[170,171] In patients with septic shock and suspected *Candida* species, it seems reasonable to promptly initiate treatment with an echinocandin and consider de-escalation as soon as identification and susceptibility results are available.[172]

ANTIBIOTIC RESISTANCE

The continuing emergence of multiresistant gram-positive and gram-negative pathogens as causes of sepsis is a major factor in the appropriate selection and use of antimicrobials in the critical care setting. These changes reflect the emergence of antimicrobial resistance in general and apply not only to sepsis.

The emergence of MRSA is the most significant problem among gram-positive pathogens, and the prevalence of MRSA bloodstream infections reflects the regional prevalence of all MRSA infections, with considerable variation among countries.[173] In Madrid, Spain, the proportion of *S. aureus* bloodstream infections caused by MRSA increased from zero in 1985 to nearly one third in 2006[103] and is a typical pattern in many regions of Europe and in North America. Rates of MRSA and methicillin-resistant coagulase-negative staphylococci have continued to steadily increase over the past decade and are most commonly associated with central catheter-associated bloodstream and wound infections.[174] MRSA has also been increasingly documented as a frequent pathogen in VAPs as well as skin/soft tissue and other infections.[174] The emergence of community-acquired MRSA infections is a problem of growing concern, as is the presence of Panton-Valentine leukocidin–producing strains.

Other worrying trends among gram-positive pathogens are the emergence of vancomycin, ampicillin, and aminoglycoside resistance in enterococci and penicillin nonsusceptibility in *S. pneumoniae*.[173]

Among gram-negative bacteria, the emergence of ESBL-producing Enterobacteriaceae and multidrug-resistant *P. aeruginosa* present major treatment challenges in some regions.[173] In the SENTRY antimicrobial surveillance program from 1997 to 2002, 43% of *Klebsiella* spp. bloodstream

isolates from Latin America had the ESBL phenotype compared with 22% in Europe and 6% in North America.[173] The prevalence of *P. aeruginosa* with the multidrug-resistant phenotype remained relatively low (1.6% to 3.0%) in North America during the surveillance period but increased steadily in Europe (5.1% to 11.5%) and Latin America (12.0% to 18.7%).

Candida albicans is now the fourth most common pathogen associated with nosocomial infections in critically ill patients in the United States. Although *C. albicans* is associated with approximately 7% of all nosocomial infections, it is the second most common cause of nosocomial urinary tract infections (15% of infections), the third most common cause of central-line–associated bloodstream infections (6% of infections), and the fourth most common cause of all nosocomial bloodstream infections.[174] Resistance to antifungal agents among *Candida* species is now a significant problem in many hospitals, with fluconazole resistance being reported in up to 10% of *C. albicans* isolates from bloodstream infections.[175] It is also well documented that the relative frequency of fungal infections with *Candida glabrata*, *Candida krusei*, and other strains with decreased susceptibility to azole antifungals is increasing among certain populations, such as the critically ill and patients with hematologic malignancies,[175] leading to the use of nonazole-type agents such as the echinocandins for empirical therapy of patients at high risk for *Candida* infections.[175]

Infections caused by antimicrobial-resistant bacteria have been demonstrated to be associated with higher mortality rates, longer length of ICU and hospital stays, and higher medical costs.[176,177] However, increased mortality associated with infections caused by resistant bacteria may also be explained by the increased likelihood that patients will receive inadequate empirical antimicrobial treatment. Furthermore, it has been shown in patients with nosocomial pneumonia that changing to more appropriate antibiotics when culture and susceptibility results became available (typically 48 to 72 hours after initiating therapy) did not significantly lower mortality rates compared with patients who received inadequate antibiotics for the entire duration of therapy.[21] Thus the importance of antimicrobial resistance in terms of antimicrobial selection and patient outcomes is difficult to overstate.

Patients with risk factors and local antimicrobial resistance patterns should play a role in empirical antibiotic selection. Previous exposure to antibiotics is also a well-established risk factor for antimicrobial resistance.[174,178] The higher severity of illness found among ICU patients is also related to several other risk factors for antimicrobial resistance, including the presence of invasive devices such as endotracheal tubes and intravascular and urinary catheters, prolonged length of hospital stay, immune suppression, and malnutrition. The increasing prevalence of antimicrobial-resistant pathogens among residents in long-term care facilities is also an increasingly important source for resistant bacteria in ICUs.[174,179] Finally, antimicrobial-resistant pathogens are easily cross-transmitted among patients in ICUs because of poor adherence of hospital personnel to appropriate infection prevention techniques, contamination of equipment, and frequent overcrowding of patients.

DE-ESCALATION

De-escalation of initial empirical broad-spectrum therapy has been advocated to prevent the emergence of resistant organisms, minimize the risk of drug toxicity, and reduce costs, and evidence from observational studies indicates that such an approach is safe.[180] Most observational studies on de-escalation could not find a deleterious effect on outcome, and some studies even suggested that de-escalation is beneficial.[181] However, a recent study by Leone et al.,[182] and the first RCT of de-escalation as a strategy in severe sepsis, raises significant doubt as to whether the reduction of the spectrum of the antibiotic can be considered safe as a routine measure. In their nonblinded randomized noninferiority study, the authors demonstrated that de-escalation, defined as narrowing the spectrum of the antibiotic, was inferior to continuation of the initial antibiotic therapy with length of stay as the primary outcome parameter. Furthermore, antibiotic use was higher in the de-escalation group, presumably driven by the number of superinfections in the de-escalation group.

The results of this study are in contrast with two recent observational studies of de-escalation.[181,183] In a study investigating febrile neutropenia patients, observation was extended to 1 year after ICU discharge, which was the longest recorded follow-up period in the literature.[183] This did not alter the results. Another study demonstrated a protective effect of de-escalation in terms of mortality (OR, 0.54; 95% CI, 0.33 to 0.89).[181]

However, the safety of de-escalation in terms of preserving outcome and reducing antibiotic use has been challenged in an RCT.[182] Despite the limitations of this open-label study, de-escalation should be cautiously applied in patients with severe sepsis, and other strategies to limit antibiotic therapy should be considered.[184]

AUTHORS' RECOMMENDATIONS

- Empirical antibiotic therapy should be administered as soon as possible after diagnosis of sepsis. Reducing time to first antibiotic reduces mortality in observational studies, and this association between timing of antibiotic administration and mortality is true not only for patients with septic shock but also for patients with severe sepsis.
- Selection of inadequate initial antimicrobial therapy has been demonstrated in numerous clinical studies to be associated with increased patient mortality.
- Several factors are important to consider when choosing initial empirical therapy, including suspected site(s) of infection and corresponding potential pathogens, the patient's immunologic status, whether the infection is nosocomial or community acquired, rates of resistance of these pathogens to potentially used drugs, a patient's prior exposure to antimicrobial therapy that may potentially increase the likelihood of antimicrobial resistance, and the results of any pertinent prior diagnostic tests.
- Combination antimicrobial therapy for CAP (e.g., an ESBL with a macrolide or a fluoroquinolone) results in reduced mortality in severe CAP (PSI category IV/V) or with pneumococcal bacteremia and septic shock, and this benefit may extend to all patients hospitalized with CAP.
- Combination therapy does not appear to be superior to monotherapy for VAP.

- Early empirical combination antibiotic therapy with two antibiotics of different mechanisms of action is associated with superior outcomes compared with monotherapy in the treatment of bacterial septic shock in patients who have a high baseline risk of mortality. However, beneficial effects of combination therapy may be limited to regimens that utilize less than maximally potent antimicrobials, whereas agents with maximal potency (e.g., carbapenems, ticarcillin/clavulanate, piperacillin/tazobactam, ceftazidime) may not yield additional benefit with the addition of a supplemental antibiotic.
- In patients with septic shock and suspected *Candida* species, it seems reasonable to promptly initiate treatment with an echinocandin and consider de-escalation as soon as identification and susceptibility results are available.
- De-escalation should be cautiously applied in patients with severe sepsis, and other strategies to limit antibiotic therapy should be considered.

REFERENCES

1. Angus DC, van der Poll T. Severe sepsis and septic shock. *N Engl J Med*. 2013;369(9):840–851.
2. Pinder M, Bellomo R, Lipman J. Pharmacological principles of antibiotic prescription in the critically ill. *Anaesth Intensive Care*. 2002;30(2):134–144.
3. Dellinger RP, Levy MM, Rhodes A, et al. Surviving sepsis campaign: international guidelines for management of severe sepsis and septic shock: 2012. *Crit Care Med*. 2013;41(2):580–637.
4. Kollef MH, Sherman G, Ward S, Fraser VJ. Inadequate antimicrobial treatment of infections: a risk factor for hospital mortality among critically ill patients. *Chest*. 1999;115(2):462–474.
5. Iregui M, Ward S, Sherman G, Fraser VJ, Kollef MH. Clinical importance of delays in the initiation of appropriate antibiotic treatment for ventilator-associated pneumonia. *Chest*. 2002;122(1):262–268.
6. Barbut F, Petit JC. Epidemiology of *Clostridium difficile*-associated infections. *Clin Microbiol Infect*. 2001;7(8):405–410.
7. Harbarth S, Pestotnik SL, Lloyd JF, Burke JP, Samore MH. The epidemiology of nephrotoxicity associated with conventional amphotericin B therapy. *Am J Med*. 2001;111(7):528–534.
8. Lodise TP, Lomaestro B, Graves J, Drusano GL. Larger vancomycin doses (at least four grams per day) are associated with an increased incidence of nephrotoxicity. *Antimicrob Agents Chemother*. 2008;52(4):1330–1336.
9. Peralta G, Sanchez MB, Garrido JC, et al. Impact of antibiotic resistance and of adequate empirical antibiotic treatment in the prognosis of patients with *Escherichia coli* bacteraemia. *J Antimicrob Chemother*. 2007;60(4):855–863.
10. Singh N, Rogers P, Atwood CW, Wagener MM, Yu VL. Short-course empiric antibiotic therapy for patients with pulmonary infiltrates in the intensive care unit. A proposed solution for indiscriminate antibiotic prescription. *Am J Resp Crit Care Med*. 2000;162(2 Pt 1):505–511.
11. Yu VL, Singh N. Excessive antimicrobial usage causes measurable harm to patients with suspected ventilator-associated pneumonia. *Intensive Care Med*. 2004;30(5):735–738.
12. Garnacho-Montero J, Garcia-Garmendia JL, Barrero-Almodovar A, Jimenez-Jimenez FJ, Perez-Paredes C, Ortiz-Leyba C. Impact of adequate empirical antibiotic therapy on the outcome of patients admitted to the intensive care unit with sepsis. *Crit Care Med*. 2003;31(12):2742–2751.
13. Bochud PY, Glauser MP, Calandra T, International Sepsis Forum. Antibiotics in sepsis. *Intensive Care Med*. 2001;27(suppl 1):S33–S48.
14. Levy MM, Fink MP, Marshall JC, et al. 2001 SCCM/ESICM/ACCP/ATS/SIS International sepsis definitions conference. *Crit Care Med*. 2003;31(4):1250–1256.
15. Matthay MA, Ware LB, Zimmerman GA. The acute respiratory distress syndrome. *J Clin Invest*. 2012;122(8):2731–2740.
16. Orde SR, Pulido JN, Masaki M, et al. Outcome prediction in sepsis: speckle tracking echocardiography based assessment of myocardial function. *Crit Care*. 2014;18(4):R149.

17. Papadopoulos MC, Davies DC, Moss RF, Tighe D, Bennett ED. Pathophysiology of septic encephalopathy: a review. *Crit Care Med.* 2000;28(8):3019–3024.

18. Iwashyna TJ, Ely EW, Smith DM, Langa KM. Long-term cognitive impairment and functional disability among survivors of severe sepsis. *JAMA.* 2010;304(16):1787–1794.

19. Zarbock A, Gomez H, Kellum JA. Sepsis-induced acute kidney injury revisited: pathophysiology, prevention and future therapies. *Curr Opin Crit Care.* 2014;20(6):588–595.

20. Cerra FB. The systemic septic response: multiple systems organ failure. *Crit Care Clin.* 1985;1(3):591–607.

21. Luna CM, Vujacich P, Niederman MS, et al. Impact of BAL data on the therapy and outcome of ventilator-associated pneumonia. *Chest.* 1997;111(3):676–685.

22. Bloos F, Hinder F, Becker K, et al. A multicenter trial to compare blood culture with polymerase chain reaction in severe human sepsis. *Intensive Care Med.* 2010;36(2):241–247.

23. Lehmann LE, Hunfeld KP, Steinbrucker M, et al. Improved detection of blood stream pathogens by real-time PCR in severe sepsis. *Intensive Care Med.* 2010;36(1):49–56.

24. Durairaj L, Mohamad Z, Launspach JL, et al. Patterns and density of early tracheal colonization in intensive care unit patients. *J Critical Care.* 2009;24(1):114–121.

25. Nijssen S, Fluit A, van de Vijver D, Top J, Willems R, Bonten MJ. Effects of reducing beta-lactam antibiotic pressure on intestinal colonization of antibiotic-resistant gram-negative bacteria. *Intensive Care Med.* 2010;36(3):512–519.

26. Oostdijk EA, de Smet AM, Blok HE, et al. Ecological effects of selective decontamination on resistant gram-negative bacterial colonization. *Am J Resp Crit Care Med.* 2010;181(5):452–457.

27. Kerver AJ, Rommes JH, Mevissen-Verhage EA, et al. Colonization and infection in surgical intensive care patients–a prospective study. *Intensive Care Med.* 1987;13(5):347–351.

28. Fenollar F, Raoult D. Molecular diagnosis of bloodstream infections caused by non-cultivable bacteria. *Int J Antimicrob Agents.* 2007;30(suppl 1):S7–S15.

29. Breitkopf C, Hammel D, Scheld HH, Peters G, Becker K. Impact of a molecular approach to improve the microbiological diagnosis of infective heart valve endocarditis. *Circ.* 2005;111(11):1415–1421.

30. Hall MM, Ilstrup DM, Washington 2nd JA. Effect of volume of blood cultured on detection of bacteremia. *J Clin Microbiol.* 1976;3(6):643–645.

31. Tenney JH, Reller LB, Mirrett S, Wang WL, Weinstein MP. Controlled evaluation of the volume of blood cultured in detection of bacteremia and fungemia. *J Clin Microbiol.* 1982;15(4):558–561.

32. Arpi M, Bentzon MW, Jensen J, Frederiksen W. Importance of blood volume cultured in the detection of bacteremia. *Eur J Clin Microbiol & Infect Dis.* 1989;8(9):838–842.

33. Bouza E, Sousa D, Rodriguez-Creixems M, Lechuz JG, Munoz P. Is the volume of blood cultured still a significant factor in the diagnosis of bloodstream infections? *J Clin Microbiol.* 2007;45(9):2765–2769.

34. Isaacman DJ, Karasic RB, Reynolds EA, Kost SI. Effect of number of blood cultures and volume of blood on detection of bacteremia in children. *J Pediatr.* 1996;128(2):190–195.

35. Kaditis AG, O'Marcaigh AS, Rhodes KH, Weaver AL, Henry NK. Yield of positive blood cultures in pediatric oncology patients by a new method of blood culture collection. *Pediatr Infect Dis J.* 1996;15(7):615–620.

36. Sautter RL, Bills AR, Lang DL, Ruschell G, Heiter BJ, Bourbeau PP. Effects of delayed-entry conditions on the recovery and detection of microorganisms from BacT/ALERT and BACTEC blood culture bottles. *J Clin Microbiol.* 2006;44(4):1245–1249.

37. Huang AM, Newton D, Kunapuli A, et al. Impact of rapid organism identification via matrix-assisted laser desorption/ionization time-of-flight combined with antimicrobial stewardship team intervention in adult patients with bacteremia and candidemia. *Clin Infect Dis.* 2013;57(9):1237–1245.

38. Nagel JL, Huang AM, Kunapuli A, et al. Impact of antimicrobial stewardship intervention on coagulase-negative *Staphylococcus* blood cultures in conjunction with rapid diagnostic testing. *J Clin Microbiol.* 2014;52(8):2849–2854.

39. Marvin LF, Roberts MA, Fay LB. Matrix-assisted laser desorption/ionization time-of-flight mass spectrometry in clinical chemistry. *Clin Chim Acta.* 2003;337(1–2):11–21.

40. van Baar BL. Characterisation of bacteria by matrix-assisted laser desorption/ionisation and electrospray mass spectrometry. *FEMS Microbiol Rev.* 2000;24(2):193–219.

41. Bernardo K, Fleer S, Pakulat N, Krut O, Hunger F, Kronke M. Identification of *Staphylococcus aureus* exotoxins by combined sodium dodecyl sulfate gel electrophoresis and matrix-assisted laser desorption/ionization-time of flight mass spectrometry. *Proteomics.* 2002;2(6):740–746.

42. Edwards-Jones V, Claydon MA, Evason DJ, Walker J, Fox AJ, Gordon DB. Rapid discrimination between methicillin-sensitive and methicillin-resistant *Staphylococcus aureus* by intact cell mass spectrometry. *J Med Microbiol.* 2000;49(3):295–300.

43. Afshari A, Schrenzel J, Ieven M, Harbarth S. Bench-to-bedside review: rapid molecular diagnostics for bloodstream infection–a new frontier? *Crit Care.* 2012;16(3):222.

44. Kempf VA, Trebesius K, Autenrieth IB. Fluorescent In situ hybridization allows rapid identification of microorganisms in blood cultures. *J Clin Microbiol.* 2000;38(2):830–838.

45. Rodero L, Cuenca-Estrella M, Cordoba S, et al. Transient fungemia caused by an amphotericin B-resistant isolate of *Candida haemulonii*. *J Clin Microbiol.* 2002;40(6):2266–2269.

46. Tomas I, Alvarez M, Limeres J, Potel C, Medina J, Diz P. Prevalence, duration and aetiology of bacteraemia following dental extractions. *Oral Dis.* 2007;13(1):56–62.

47. Mancini N, Clerici D, Diotti R, et al. Molecular diagnosis of sepsis in neutropenic patients with haematological malignancies. *J Med Microbiol.* 2008;57(Pt 5):601–604.

48. Pfeiffer CD, Fine JP, Safdar N. Diagnosis of invasive aspergillosis using a galactomannan assay: a meta-analysis. *Clin Infect Dis.* 2006;42(10):1417–1427.

49. Stynen D, Goris A, Sarfati J, Latge JP. A new sensitive sandwich enzyme-linked immunosorbent assay to detect galactofuran in patients with invasive aspergillosis. *J Clin Microbiol.* 1995;33(2):497–500.

50. Ascioglu S, Rex JH, de Pauw B, et al. Defining opportunistic invasive fungal infections in immunocompromised patients with cancer and hematopoietic stem cell transplants: an international consensus. *Clin Infect Dis.* 2002;34(1):7–14.

51. Odabasi Z, Mattiuzzi G, Estey E, et al. Beta-D-glucan as a diagnostic adjunct for invasive fungal infections: validation, cutoff development, and performance in patients with acute myelogenous leukemia and myelodysplastic syndrome. *Clin Infect Dis.* 2004;39(2):199–205.

52. Almyroudis NG, Segal BH. Prevention and treatment of invasive fungal diseases in neutropenic patients. *Curr Opin Infect Dis.* 2009;22(4):385–393.

53. Becker KL, Nylen ES, White JC, Muller B, Snider Jr RH. Clinical review 167: procalcitonin and the calcitonin gene family of peptides in inflammation, infection, and sepsis: a journey from calcitonin back to its precursors. *J Clin Endocrinol Metab.* 2004;89(4):1512–1525.

54. Jensen JU, Heslet L, Jensen TH, Espersen K, Steffensen P, Tvede M. Procalcitonin increase in early identification of critically ill patients at high risk of mortality. *Crit Care Med.* 2006;34(10):2596–2602.

55. Muller B, Becker KL, Schachinger H, et al. Calcitonin precursors are reliable markers of sepsis in a medical intensive care unit. *Crit Care Med.* 2000;28(4):977–983.

56. Meisner M, Tschaikowsky K, Palmaers T, Schmidt J. Comparison of procalcitonin (PCT) and C-reactive protein (CRP) plasma concentrations at different SOFA scores during the course of sepsis and MODS. *Crit Care.* 1999;3(1):45–50.

57. Wunder C, Eichelbronner O, Roewer N. Are IL-6, IL-10 and PCT plasma concentrations reliable for outcome prediction in severe sepsis? A comparison with APACHE III and SAPS II. *Inflamm Res.* 2004;53(4):158–163.

58. Tang BM, Eslick GD, Craig JC, McLean AS. Accuracy of procalcitonin for sepsis diagnosis in critically ill patients: systematic review and meta-analysis. *Lancet Infect Dis.* 2007;7(3):210–217.

59. Rivers E, Nguyen B, Havstad S, et al. Early goal-directed therapy in the treatment of severe sepsis and septic shock. *N Engl J Med.* 2001;345(19):1368–1377.

60. Peake SL, Delaney A, Bailey M, et al. Goal-directed resuscitation for patients with early septic shock. *N Engl J Med.* 2014;371(16):1496–1506.

61. Yealy DM, Kellum JA, Huang DT, et al. A randomized trial of protocol-based care for early septic shock. *N Engl J Med.* 2014;370(18):1683–1693.
62. Ferrer R, Artigas A, Suarez D, et al. Effectiveness of treatments for severe sepsis: a prospective, multicenter, observational study. *Am J Resp Crit Care Med.* 2009;180(9):861–866.
63. Kahn KL, Rogers WH, Rubenstein LV, et al. Measuring quality of care with explicit process criteria before and after implementation of the DRG-based prospective payment system. *JAMA.* 1990;264(15):1969–1973.
64. McGarvey RN, Harper JJ. Pneumonia mortality reduction and quality improvement in a community hospital. *QRB Qual Rev Bull.* 1993;19(4):124–130.
65. Meehan TP, Fine MJ, Krumholz HM, et al. Quality of care, process, and outcomes in elderly patients with pneumonia. *JAMA.* 1997;278(23):2080–2084.
66. Houck PM, Bratzler DW, Nsa W, Ma A, Bartlett JG. Timing of antibiotic administration and outcomes for Medicare patients hospitalized with community-acquired pneumonia. *Arch Intern Med.* 2004;164(6):637–644.
67. Gaieski DF, Mikkelsen ME, Band RA, et al. Impact of time to antibiotics on survival in patients with severe sepsis or septic shock in whom early goal-directed therapy was initiated in the emergency department. *Crit Care Med.* 2010;38(4):1045–1053.
68. Kumar A, Roberts D, Wood KE, et al. Duration of hypotension before initiation of effective antimicrobial therapy is the critical determinant of survival in human septic shock. *Crit Care Med.* 2006;34(6):1589–1596.
69. Ferrer R, Martin-Loeches I, Phillips G, et al. Empiric antibiotic treatment reduces mortality in severe sepsis and septic shock from the first hour: results from a guideline-based performance improvement program. *Crit Care Med.* 2014;42(8):1749–1755.
70. Wong CH, Chang HC, Pasupathy S, Khin LW, Tan JL, Low CO. Necrotizing fasciitis: clinical presentation, microbiology, and determinants of mortality. *J Bone Jt Surg Am Vol.* 2003;85-A(8):1454–1460.
71. Barochia AV, Cui X, Vitberg D, et al. Bundled care for septic shock: an analysis of clinical trials. *Crit Care Med.* 2010;38(2):668–678.
72. Morrell M, Fraser VJ, Kollef MH. Delaying the empiric treatment of candida bloodstream infection until positive blood culture results are obtained: a potential risk factor for hospital mortality. *Antimicrob Agents Chemother.* 2005;49(9):3640–3645.
73. Shorr AF, Micek ST, Kollef MH. Inappropriate therapy for methicillin-resistant *Staphylococcus aureus:* resource utilization and cost implications. *Crit Care Med.* 2008;36(8):2335–2340.
74. Ortega M, Marco F, Soriano A, et al. *Candida* spp. bloodstream infection: influence of antifungal treatment on outcome. *J Antimicrob Chemother.* 2010;65(3):562–568.
75. Arnold HM, Micek ST, Shorr AF, et al. Hospital resource utilization and costs of inappropriate treatment of candidemia. *Pharmacother.* 2010;30(4):361–368.
76. Alvarez-Lerma F. Modification of empiric antibiotic treatment in patients with pneumonia acquired in the intensive care unit. ICU-Acquired Pneumonia Study Group. *Intensive Care Med.* 1996;22(5):387–394.
77. Ibrahim EH, Ward S, Sherman G, Kollef MH. A comparative analysis of patients with early-onset vs late-onset nosocomial pneumonia in the ICU setting. *Chest.* 2000;117(5):1434–1442.
78. MacArthur RD, Miller M, Albertson T, et al. Adequacy of early empiric antibiotic treatment and survival in severe sepsis: experience from the MONARCS trial. *Clin Infect Dis.* 2004;38(2):284–288.
79. Andes D, Craig WA. Animal model pharmacokinetics and pharmacodynamics: a critical review. *Int J Antimicrob Agents.* 2002;19(4):261–268.
80. Freid MA, Vosti KL. The importance of underlying disease in patients with gram-negative bacteremia. *Arch Intern Med.* 1968;121(5):418–423.
81. Bryant RE, Hood AF, Hood CE, Koenig MG. Factors affecting mortality of gram-negative rod bacteremia. *Arch Intern Med.* 1971;127(1):120–128.
82. Young LS, Martin WJ, Meyer RD, Weinstein RJ, Anderson ET. Gram-negative rod bacteremia: microbiologic, immunologic, and therapeutic considerations. *Ann Intern Med.* 1977;86(4):456–471.
83. Mc CW, Jackson G. Gram-negative bacteremia: I. Etiology and ecology. *Arch Intern Med.* 1962;110(6):847–855.
84. Kreger BE, Craven DE, McCabe WR. Gram-negative bacteremia. IV. Re-evaluation of clinical features and treatment in 612 patients. *Am J Med.* 1980;68(3):344–355.
85. Leibovici L, Paul M, Poznanski O, et al. Monotherapy versus beta-lactam-aminoglycoside combination treatment for gram-negative bacteremia: a prospective, observational study. *Antimicrob Agents Chemother.* 1997;41(5):1127–1133.
86. Chow JW, Fine MJ, Shlaes DM, et al. Enterobacter bacteremia: clinical features and emergence of antibiotic resistance during therapy. *Ann Intern Med.* 1991;115(8):585–590.
87. Vidal F, Mensa J, Almela M, et al. Epidemiology and outcome of *Pseudomonas aeruginosa* bacteremia, with special emphasis on the influence of antibiotic treatment. Analysis of 189 episodes. *Arch Intern Med.* 1996;156(18):2121–2126.
88. Schiappa DA, Hayden MK, Matushek MG, et al. Ceftazidime-resistant *Klebsiella pneumoniae* and *Escherichia coli* bloodstream infection: a case-control and molecular epidemiologic investigation. *J Infect Dis.* 1996;174(3):529–536.
89. Caballero-Granado FJ, Cisneros JM, Luque R, et al. Comparative study of bacteremias caused by *Enterococcus* spp. with and without high-level resistance to gentamicin. The Grupo Andaluz para el estudio de las Enfermedades Infecciosas. *J Clin Microbiol.* 1998;36(2):520–525.
90. Hanon FX, Monnet DL, Sorensen TL, Molbak K, Pedersen G, Schonheyder H. Survival of patients with bacteraemia in relation to initial empirical antimicrobial treatment. *Scand J Infect Dis.* 2002;34(7):520–528.
91. Harbarth S, Ferriere K, Hugonnet S, Ricou B, Suter P, Pittet D. Epidemiology and prognostic determinants of bloodstream infections in surgical intensive care. *Arch Surg.* 2002;137(12):1353–1359; discussion 9.
92. Harbarth S, Garbino J, Pugin J, Romand JA, Lew D, Pittet D. Inappropriate initial antimicrobial therapy and its effect on survival in a clinical trial of immunomodulating therapy for severe sepsis. *Am J Med.* 2003;115(7):529–535.
93. Ispahani P, Pearson NJ, Greenwood D. An analysis of community and hospital-acquired bacteraemia in a large teaching hospital in the United Kingdom. *Q J Med.* 1987;63(241):427–440.
94. Leibovici L, Shraga I, Drucker M, Konigsberger H, Samra Z, Pitlik SD. The benefit of appropriate empirical antibiotic treatment in patients with bloodstream infection. *J Intern Med.* 1998;244(5):379–386.
95. Leone M, Bourgoin A, Cambon S, Dubuc M, Albanese J, Martin C. Empirical antimicrobial therapy of septic shock patients: adequacy and impact on the outcome. *Crit Care Med.* 2003;31(2):462–467.
96. Weinstein MP, Towns ML, Quartey SM, et al. The clinical significance of positive blood cultures in the 1990s: a prospective comprehensive evaluation of the microbiology, epidemiology, and outcome of bacteremia and fungemia in adults. *Clin Infect Dis.* 1997;24(4):584–602.
97. Zaragoza R, Artero A, Camarena JJ, Sancho S, Gonzalez R, Nogueira JM. The influence of inadequate empirical antimicrobial treatment on patients with bloodstream infections in an intensive care unit. *Clin Microbiol Infect.* 2003;9(5):412–418.
98. Bochud PY, Bonten M, Marchetti O, Calandra T. Antimicrobial therapy for patients with severe sepsis and septic shock: an evidence-based review. *Crit Care Med.* 2004;32(suppl 11):S495–S512.
99. Sands KE, Bates DW, Lanken PN, et al. Epidemiology of sepsis syndrome in 8 academic medical centers. *JAMA.* 1997;278(3):234–240.
100. Brun-Buisson C, Doyon F, Carlet J, et al. Incidence, risk factors, and outcome of severe sepsis and septic shock in adults. A multicenter prospective study in intensive care units. French ICU Group for Severe Sepsis. *JAMA.* 1995;274(12):968–974.
101. Kumar A, Ellis P, Arabi Y, et al. Initiation of inappropriate antimicrobial therapy results in a fivefold reduction of survival in human septic shock. *Chest.* 2009;136(5):1237–1248.
102. Martin GS, Mannino DM, Eaton S, Moss M. The epidemiology of sepsis in the United States from 1979 through 2000. *N Engl J Med.* 2003;348(16):1546–1554.
103. Rodriguez-Creixems M, Alcala L, Munoz P, Cercenado E, Vicente T, Bouza E. Bloodstream infections: evolution and trends in the microbiology workload, incidence, and etiology, 1985-2006. *Med.* 2008;87(4):234–249.

104. Pfaller MA, Jones RN, Messer SA, Edmond MB, Wenzel RP. National surveillance of nosocomial blood stream infection due to *Candida albicans*: frequency of occurrence and antifungal susceptibility in the SCOPE Program. *Diagn Microbiol Infect Dis.* 1998;31(1):327–332.

105. Chow JW, Yu VL. Combination antibiotic therapy versus monotherapy for gram-negative bacteraemia: a commentary. *Int J Antimicrob Agents.* 1999;11(1):7–12.

106. Manian FA, Meyer L, Jenne J, Owen A, Taff T. Loss of antimicrobial susceptibility in aerobic gram-negative bacilli repeatedly isolated from patients in intensive-care units. *Infection Control Hosp Epidemiol.* 1996;17(4):222–226.

107. Kumar A, Kethireddy S. Emerging concepts in optimizing antimicrobial therapy of septic shock: speed is life but a hammer helps too. *Crit Care.* 2013;17(1):104.

108. Paul M, Lador A, Grozinsky-Glasberg S, Leibovici L. Beta lactam antibiotic monotherapy versus beta lactam-aminoglycoside antibiotic combination therapy for sepsis. *Cochrane Database Syst Rev.* 2014;1:CD003344.

109. Garin N, Genne D, Carballo S, et al. β-Lactam monotherapy vs β-lactam-macrolide combination treatment in moderately severe community-acquired pneumonia: a randomized noninferiority trial. *JAMA Intern Med.* 2014;174:1894–1901.

110. Blot S, Depuydt P. Antibiotic therapy for community-acquired pneumonia with septic shock: follow the guidelines. *Crit Care Med.* 2007;35(6):1617–1618.

111. Mandell LA, Wunderink RG, Anzueto A, et al. Infectious Diseases Society of America/American Thoracic Society consensus guidelines on the management of community-acquired pneumonia in adults. *Clin Infect Dis.* 2007;44(suppl 2):S27–S72.

112. Arancibia F, Bauer TT, Ewig S, et al. Community-acquired pneumonia due to gram-negative bacteria and *pseudomonas aeruginosa*: incidence, risk, and prognosis. *Arch Intern Med.* 2002;162(16):1849–1858.

113. Moran GJ, Krishnadasan A, Gorwitz RJ, et al. Prevalence of methicillin-resistant *staphylococcus aureus* as an etiology of community-acquired pneumonia. *Clin Infect Dis.* 2012;54(8):1126–1133.

114. Lim WS, Baudouin SV, George RC, et al. BTS guidelines for the management of community acquired pneumonia in adults: update 2009. *Thorax.* 2009;64(suppl 3). iii1-55.

115. Eliakim-Raz N, Robenshtok E, Shefet D, et al. Empiric antibiotic coverage of atypical pathogens for community-acquired pneumonia in hospitalized adults. *Cochrane Database Syst Rev.* 2012;9:CD004418.

116. Vanderkooi OG, Low DE, Green K, Powis JE, McGeer A, Toronto Invasive Bacterial Disease Network. Predicting antimicrobial resistance in invasive pneumococcal infections. *Clini Infect Dis.* 2005;40(9):1288–1297.

117. Ray WA, Murray KT, Hall K, Arbogast PG, Stein CM. Azithromycin and the risk of cardiovascular death. *N Engl J Med.* 2012;366(20):1881–1890.

118. Baddour LM, Yu VL, Klugman KP, et al. Combination antibiotic therapy lowers mortality among severely ill patients with pneumococcal bacteremia. *Am J Res Crit Care Med.* 2004;170(4):440–444.

119. Mufson MA, Stanek RJ. Bacteremic pneumococcal pneumonia in one American City: a 20-year longitudinal study, 1978-1997. *Am J Med.* 1999;107(1A):34S–43S.

120. Waterer GW, Somes GW, Wunderink RG. Monotherapy may be suboptimal for severe bacteremic pneumococcal pneumonia. *Arch Int Med.* 2001;161(15):1837–1842.

121. Weiss K, Low DE, Cortes L, et al. Clinical characteristics at initial presentation and impact of dual therapy on the outcome of bacteremic *Streptococcus pneumoniae* pneumonia in adults. *Can Res J.* 2004;11(8):589–593.

122. Rodriguez A, Mendia A, Sirvent JM, et al. Combination antibiotic therapy improves survival in patients with community-acquired pneumonia and shock. *Crit Care Med.* 2007;35(6):1493–1498.

123. Rodrigo C, McKeever TM, Woodhead M, Lim WS, British Thoracic S. Single versus combination antibiotic therapy in adults hospitalised with community acquired pneumonia. *Thorax.* 2013;68(5):493–495.

124. Lodise TP, Kwa A, Cosler L, Gupta R, Smith RP. Comparison of beta-lactam and macrolide combination therapy versus fluoroquinolone monotherapy in hospitalized Veterans Affairs patients with community-acquired pneumonia. *Antimicrob Agents Chemother.* 2007;51(11):3977–3982.

125. Nie W, Li B, Xiu Q. Beta-lactam/macrolide dual therapy versus beta-lactam monotherapy for the treatment of community-acquired pneumonia in adults: a systematic review and meta-analysis. *J Antimicrob Chemother.* 2014;69(6):1441–1446.

126. Martinez FJ, Curtis JL, Albert R. Role of macrolide therapy in chronic obstructive pulmonary disease. *Int J Chronic obstruct Pulm Dis.* 2008;3(3):331–350.

127. Cook DJ, Kollef MH. Risk factors for ICU-acquired pneumonia. *JAMA.* 1998;279(20):1605–1606.

128. Vincent JL, Bihari DJ, Suter PM, et al. The prevalence of nosocomial infection in intensive care units in Europe. Results of the European Prevalence of Infection in Intensive Care (EPIC) Study. EPIC International Advisory Committee. *JAMA.* 1995;274(8):639–644.

129. Warren DK, Shukla SJ, Olsen MA, et al. Outcome and attributable cost of ventilator-associated pneumonia among intensive care unit patients in a suburban medical center. *Crit Care Med.* 2003;31(5):1312–1317.

130. Heyland DK, Cook DJ, Griffith L, Keenan SP, Brun-Buisson C. The attributable morbidity and mortality of ventilator-associated pneumonia in the critically ill patient. The Canadian Critical Trials Group. *Am J Resp Crit Care Med.* 1999;159(4 Pt 1):1249–1256.

131. Hunter JD. Ventilator associated pneumonia. *BMJ.* 2012;344:e3325.

132. American Thoracic Society. Infectious Diseases Society of A. Guidelines for the management of adults with hospital-acquired, ventilator-associated, and healthcare-associated pneumonia. *Am J Resp Crit Care Med.* 2005;171(4):388–416.

133. Masterton RG, Galloway A, French G, et al. Guidelines for the management of hospital-acquired pneumonia in the UK: report of the working party on hospital-acquired pneumonia of the British Society for Antimicrobial Chemotherapy. *J Antimicrob Chemother.* 2008;62(1):5–34.

134. Walkey AJ, O'Donnell MR, Wiener RS. Linezolid vs glycopeptide antibiotics for the treatment of suspected methicillin-resistant *Staphylococcus aureus* nosocomial pneumonia: a meta-analysis of randomized controlled trials. *Chest.* 2011;139(5):1148–1155.

135. Aarts MA, Hancock JN, Heyland D, McLeod RS, Marshall JC. Empiric antibiotic therapy for suspected ventilator-associated pneumonia: a systematic review and meta-analysis of randomized trials. *Crit Care Med.* 2008;36(1):108–117.

136. Group EIATC. Ceftazidime combined with a short or long course of amikacin for empirical therapy of gram-negative bacteremia in cancer patients with granulocytopenia. The EORTC International Antimicrobial Therapy Cooperative Group. *N Engl J Med.* 1987;317(27):1692–1698.

137. Anderson ET, Young LS, Hewitt WL. Antimicrobial synergism in the therapy of gram-negative rod bacteremia. *Chemother.* 1978;24(1):45–54.

138. Bouza E, Munoz P. Monotherapy versus combination therapy for bacterial infections. *Med Clin North Am.* 2000;84(6):1357–1389; v.

139. Darras-Joly C, Bedos JP, Sauve C, et al. Synergy between amoxicillin and gentamicin in combination against a highly penicillin-resistant and -tolerant strain of *Streptococcus pneumoniae* in a mouse pneumonia model. *Antimicrob Agents Chemother.* 1996;40(9):2147–2151.

140. Calandra T, Glauser MP. Immunocompromised animal models for the study of antibiotic combinations. *Am J Med.* 1986;80(5C):45–52.

141. Diaz-Martin A, Martinez-Gonzalez ML, Ferrer R, et al. Antibiotic prescription patterns in the empiric therapy of severe sepsis: combination of antimicrobials with different mechanisms of action reduces mortality. *Crit Care.* 2012;16(6):R223.

142. Safdar N, Handelsman J, Maki DG. Does combination antimicrobial therapy reduce mortality in Gram-negative bacteraemia? A meta-analysis. *Lancet Infect Dis.* 2004;4(8):519–527.

143. Kumar A, Safdar N, Kethireddy S, Chateau D. A survival benefit of combination antibiotic therapy for serious infections associated with sepsis and septic shock is contingent only on the risk of death: a meta-analytic/meta-regression study. *Crit Care Med.* 2010;38(8):1651–1664.

144. Kumar A, Zarychanski R, Light B, et al. Early combination antibiotic therapy yields improved survival compared with monotherapy in septic shock: a propensity-matched analysis. *Crit Care Med.* 2010;38(9):1773–1785.

145. Shiber S, Yahav D, Avni T, Leibovici L, Paul M. β-Lactam/β-lactamase inhibitors versus carbapenems for the treatment of sepsis: systematic review and meta-analysis of randomized controlled trials. *J Antimicrob Chemother.* 2015;70:41–47.

146. Brunkhorst FM, Oppert M, Marx G, et al. Effect of empirical treatment with moxifloxacin and meropenem vs meropenem on sepsis-related organ dysfunction in patients with severe sepsis: a randomized trial. *JAMA.* 2012;307(22):2390–2399.

147. Nathens AB, Rotstein OD, Marshall JC. Tertiary peritonitis: clinical features of a complex nosocomial infection. *World J Surg.* 1998;22(2):158–163.

148. Morrissey I, Hackel M, Badal R, Bouchillon S, Hawser S, Biedenbach D. A review of ten years of the study for monitoring antimicrobial resistance trends (SMART) from 2002 to 2011. *Pharm.* 2013;6(11):1335–1346.

149. Hoban DJ, Badal R, Bouchillon S, et al. In vitro susceptibility and distribution of beta-lactamases in Enterobacteriaceae causing intra-abdominal infections in North America 2010-2011. *Diagn Microbiol Infect Dis.* 2014;79(3):367–372.

150. Hoban DJ, Bouchillon SK, Hawser SP, Badal RE, Labombardi VJ, DiPersio J. Susceptibility of gram-negative pathogens isolated from patients with complicated intra-abdominal infections in the United States, 2007-2008: results of the Study for Monitoring Antimicrobial Resistance Trends (SMART). *Antimicrob Agents Chemother.* 2010;54(7):3031–3034.

151. Montravers P, Gauzit R, Muller C, Marmuse JP, Fichelle A, Desmonts JM. Emergence of antibiotic-resistant bacteria in cases of peritonitis after intraabdominal surgery affects the efficacy of empirical antimicrobial therapy. *Clin Infect Dis.* 1996;23(3):486–494.

152. Solomkin JS, Mazuski JE, Baron EJ, et al. Guidelines for the selection of anti-infective agents for complicated intra-abdominal infections. *Clin Infect Dis.* 2003;37(8):997–1005.

153. Mazuski JE, Sawyer RG, Nathens AB, et al. The Surgical Infection Society guidelines on antimicrobial therapy for intra-abdominal infections: evidence for the recommendations. *Surg Infect.* 2002;3(3):175–233.

154. Solomkin JS, Mazuski JE, Bradley JS, et al. Diagnosis and management of complicated intra-abdominal infection in adults and children: guidelines by the Surgical Infection Society and the Infectious Diseases Society of America. *Clin Infect Dis.* 2010;50(2):133–164.

155. Eckmann C, Dryden M, Montravers P, Kozlov R, Sganga G. Antimicrobial treatment of "complicated" intra-abdominal infections and the new IDSA guidelines? a commentary and an alternative European approach according to clinical definitions. *Eur J Med Res.* 2011;16(3):115–126.

156. Dupont H. The empiric treatment of nosocomial intra-abdominal infections. *Int J Infect Dis.* 2007;11(suppl 1):S1–S6.

157. Harbarth S, Uckay I. Are there patients with peritonitis who require empiric therapy for *Enterococcus*? *Eur J Clin Microbiol Infect Dis.* 2004;23(2):73–77.

158. Condon RE, Walker AP, Sirinek KR, et al. Meropenem versus tobramycin plus clindamycin for treatment of intraabdominal infections: results of a prospective, randomized, double-blind clinical trial. *Clin Infect Dis.* 1995;21(3):544–550.

159. Dougherty SH, Sirinek KR, Schauer PR, et al. Ticarcillin/clavulanate compared with clindamycin/gentamicin (with or without ampicillin) for the treatment of intra-abdominal infections in pediatric and adult patients. *Am Surg.* 1995;61(4):297–303.

160. Luke M, Iversen J, Sondergaard J, et al. Ceftriaxone/metronidazole is more effective than ampicillin/netilmicin/metronidazole in the treatment of bacterial peritonitis. *Eur J Surg.* 1991;157(6–7):397–401.

161. Cohn SM, Lipsett PA, Buchman TG, et al. Comparison of intravenous/oral ciprofloxacin plus metronidazole versus piperacillin/tazobactam in the treatment of complicated intraabdominal infections. *Ann Surg.* 2000;232(2):254–262.

162. Yellin AE, Hassett JM, Fernandez A, et al. Ertapenem monotherapy versus combination therapy with ceftriaxone plus metronidazole for treatment of complicated intra-abdominal infections in adults. *Int J Antimicrob Agents.* 2002;20(3):165–173.

163. Solomkin J, Zhao YP, Ma EL, Chen MJ, Hampel B, Team DS. Moxifloxacin is non-inferior to combination therapy with ceftriaxone plus metronidazole in patients with community-origin complicated intra-abdominal infections. *Int J Antimicrob Agents.* 2009;34(5):439–445.

164. Wong PF, Gilliam AD, Kumar S, Shenfine J, O'Dair GN, Leaper DJ. Antibiotic regimens for secondary peritonitis of gastrointestinal origin in adults. *Cochrane Database Syst Rev.* 2005; (2): CD004539.

165. Vincent JL, Rello J, Marshall J, et al. International study of the prevalence and outcomes of infection in intensive care units. *JAMA.* 2009;302(21):2323–2329.

166. Solomkin JS, Mazuski J. Intra-abdominal sepsis: newer interventional and antimicrobial therapies. *Infect Dis Clin North Am.* 2009;23(3):593–608.

167. Montravers P, Dupont H, Gauzit R, et al. Candida as a risk factor for mortality in peritonitis. *Crit Care Med.* 2006;34(3):646–652.

168. Eggimann P, Francioli P, Bille J, et al. Fluconazole prophylaxis prevents intra-abdominal candidiasis in high-risk surgical patients. *Crit Care Med.* 1999;27(6):1066–1072.

169. Pappas PG, Rex JH, Sobel JD, et al. Guidelines for treatment of candidiasis. *Clin Infect Dis.* 2004;38(2):161–189.

170. Hof H. Developments in the epidemiolgy of invasive fungal infections - implications for the empiric and targeted antifungal therapy. *Mycoses.* 2008;51(suppl 1):1–6.

171. Pfaller MA, Boyken L, Hollis RJ, et al. In vitro susceptibility of invasive isolates of *Candida* spp. to anidulafungin, caspofungin, and micafungin: six years of global surveillance. *J Clin Microbiol.* 2008;46(1):150–156.

172. Allou N, Allyn J, Montravers P. When and how to cover for fungal infections in patients with severe sepsis and septic shock. *Curr Infect Dis Rep.* 2011;13(5):426–432.

173. Biedenbach DJ, Moet GJ, Jones RN. Occurrence and antimicrobial resistance pattern comparisons among bloodstream infection isolates from the SENTRY Antimicrobial Surveillance Program (1997-2002). *Diagn Microbiol Infect Dis.* 2004;50(1):59–69.

174. Hidron AI, Edwards JR, Patel J, et al. NHSN annual update: antimicrobial-resistant pathogens associated with healthcare-associated infections: annual summary of data reported to the National Healthcare Safety Network at the Centers for Disease Control and Prevention, 2006-2007. *Infect Control Hosp Epidemiol.* 2008;29(11):996–1011.

175. Bassetti M, Righi E, Costa A, et al. Epidemiological trends in nosocomial candidemia in intensive care. *BMC Infect Dis.* 2006;6(21).

176. Roberts RR, Hota B, Ahmad I, et al. Hospital and societal costs of antimicrobial-resistant infections in a Chicago teaching hospital: implications for antibiotic stewardship. *Clin Infect Dis.* 2009;49(8):1175–1184.

177. Engemann JJ, Carmeli Y, Cosgrove SE, et al. Adverse clinical and economic outcomes attributable to methicillin resistance among patients with *Staphylococcus aureus* surgical site infection. *Clin Infect Dis.* 2003;36(5):592–598.

178. Kallen AJ, Hidron AI, Patel J, Srinivasan A. Multidrug resistance among gram-negative pathogens that caused healthcare-associated infections reported to the National Healthcare Safety Network, 2006-2008. *Infect Control Hosp Epidemiol.* 2010;31(5):528–531.

179. Kollef MH, Fraser VJ. Antibiotic resistance in the intensive care unit. *Ann Intern Med.* 2001;134(4):298–314.

180. Heenen S, Jacobs F, Vincent JL. Antibiotic strategies in severe nosocomial sepsis: why do we not de-escalate more often? *Crit Care Med.* 2012;40(5):1404–1409.

181. Garnacho-Montero J, Gutierrez-Pizarraya A, Escoresca-Ortega A, et al. De-escalation of empirical therapy is associated with lower mortality in patients with severe sepsis and septic shock. *Intensive Care Med.* 2014;40(1):32–40.

182. Leone M, Bechis C, Baumstarck K, et al. De-escalation versus continuation of empirical antimicrobial treatment in severe sepsis: a multicenter non-blinded randomized noninferiority trial. *Intensive Care Med.* 2014;40(10):1399–1408.

183. Mokart D, Slehofer G, Lambert J, et al. De-escalation of antimicrobial treatment in neutropenic patients with severe sepsis: results from an observational study. *Intensive Care Med.* 2014;40(1):41–49.

184. De Waele JJ, Bassetti M, Martin-Loeches I. Impact of de-escalation on ICU patients' prognosis. *Intensive Care Med.* 2014;40(10):1583–1585.

40 What MAP Objectives Should Be Targeted in Septic Shock?

François Beloncle, Peter Radermacher, Pierre Asfar

Septic shock is defined by a complex association of cardiovascular dysfunction: decreased systemic vascular resistance, hypovolemia, impaired microcirculation, and depressed myocardial function.[1] This vascular impairment leads to an imbalance between oxygen delivery and demand. Thus, the aim of initial septic shock management is to rebalance this mismatch. Mean arterial pressure (MAP) is one of the hemodynamic targets used to try to ensure that organs are adequately perfused.[2] During initial resuscitation, a MAP level of greater than 65 mm Hg is recommended in the Surviving Sepsis Campaign guidelines (grade 1C: high-grade recommendation based on low-level evidence).[3] Although this goal may be acceptable in a global sense, a target MAP of 65 mm Hg is unlikely to be appropriate for many critically ill patients. However, intervention to achieve a higher MAP carries several risks. In septic shock, we must avoid three risks—underperfusion, tissue edema, and excessive vasoconstriction—that can lead to tissue hypoperfusion. The optimal MAP level (or the optimal vasopressor dose) corresponds to the optimal balance between these risks. The Surviving Sepsis Campaign guidelines suggest that the optimal MAP should be individualized because it may be higher in selected patients such as those with atherosclerosis or previous hypertension.

This review discusses the physiologic rationale and the different clinical studies addressing the question of the optimal MAP in patients with sepsis.

PHYSIOLOGIC RATIONALE

The ultimate goal of septic shock resuscitation is to adapt oxygen (O_2) delivery to each organ's O_2 demand. MAP is commonly considered as a surrogate of global perfusion pressure. Thus, increasing MAP level in septic shock patients might lead to an increase in O_2 delivery to the tissue. However, a better understanding of autoregulatory mechanisms and microcirculation regulation during sepsis is needed to address this question. In addition, increasing MAP level implies increasing vasopressor load, and this raises the question of the side effects of these agents.

Autoregulation

Autoregulation refers to the ability of an organ to maintain a constant blood flow entering the organ irrespective of the perfusion pressure over a range of values called the "autoregulation zone."[4] Below this autoregulation threshold, blood flow is directly dependent on perfusion pressure. Autoregulation is of particular importance in the brain,[5] heart,[6] and kidney.[7] Of note, autoregulation threshold values vary in different organs.[8] The kidney has the highest autoregulation threshold; therefore it may be considered as the first resuscitation objective. Maintenance of a MAP within the renal autoregulatory range allows the organ to be perfused in times of stress. Autoregulation thresholds differ in accordance with patients' age and associated comorbidities (e.g., chronic hypertension). It is unclear whether vascular reactivity impairment in septic patients is associated with changes in the autoregulatory range. In a study by Prowle et al., renal blood flow assessed by cine phase-contrast magnetic resonance imaging was lower in septic patients than in control healthy patients despite a MAP between 70 and 100 mm Hg. These findings suggest that renal autoregulation is disturbed during sepsis.[9] However, in a rat model of sepsis, renal blood flow was altered over a large range of MAP. These findings support the conclusion that autoregulation may be conserved in sepsis.[10] Thus, it is unknown whether autoregulation is maintained during sepsis and whether the autoregulation threshold is unchanged.

It is worth noting that perfusion pressure and MAP differ. Organ perfusion pressure is equal to the difference of the pressure in the artery entering the organ (usually approximated by the MAP) minus the organ venous pressure. The importance of the venous pressure has been shown in particular in the kidney.[11]

Microcirculation

Sepsis is associated with microcirculatory alterations characterized by increased endothelial permeability, leukocyte adhesion, and blood flow heterogeneity that can lead to tissue hypoxia.[12,13] Microcirculatory blood flow may be largely independent of systemic hemodynamics.[14] Consequently, when systemic hemodynamic objectives (in particular MAP target) are achieved, microcirculation abnormalities may persist.[13] Thus, increasing the MAP level above 65 mm Hg may not change microvascular perfusion. However, microcirculation alteration in the early phase of sepsis reflects a low perfusion pressure (i.e., a failure to achieve macrocirculation parameter targets at the beginning of the shock). Thus, although adjusting hemodynamic objectives at the second phase of the septic shock when patients are "hemodynamically stable" is unlikely to improve microcirculation impairment, an early intervention with high MAP levels may prevent microcirculation dysfunction.

Specific Effect of High Vasopressor Load

Increasing the MAP target to high levels may require high doses of vasopressor or inotropic drugs. Norepinephrine is the most commonly used agent in septic patients. It activates both α- and β-adrenergic receptors. Although its main hemodynamic effect is to increase systemic vascular resistance (and thus left ventricle afterload), norepinephrine usually slightly increases cardiac output because of its β-adrenergic stimulation and its effect on venous return.[15] The venous effect of norepinephrine might also affect the perfusion pressure.[11] In addition to the consequences of excessive vasoconstriction, other effects should be taken into account when addressing the question of optimal vasopressor load. Sympathetic overstimulation (or adrenergic stress) may be associated with harmful effects such as diastolic dysfunction; tachyarrythmia; skeletal muscle damage (apoptosis); altered coagulation; or endocrinologic, immunologic, and metabolic disturbances.[16]

OBSERVATIONAL STUDIES

Several observational clinical studies have examined optimal MAP targets in patients with sepsis. Two retrospective studies used MAP recordings and examined the time spent below different threshold values of MAP during early sepsis. Data were correlated with survival and organ dysfunction. In 111 patients with septic shock, Varpula et al.[17] showed that the mean MAP for the first 6 and 48 hours predicted 30-day outcome. With the use of receiver operator characteristic (ROC) curves, the best predictive MAP threshold level for 30-day mortality was 65 mm Hg. In addition, the time spent under this value also correlated with mortality. However, because the MAP level is strongly associated with disease severity, these results may only reflect shock severity. Dünser et al.[18] performed a similar analysis in 274 sepsis or septic shock patients, but they adjusted for disease severity (as assessed by the Simplified Acute Physiology Score [SAPS] II excluding systolic arterial pressure). The authors assessed the association between different arterial blood pressure levels during the first 24 hours after intensive care unit (ICU) admission and 28-day mortality or organ function. A 28-day mortality did not correlate with MAP drops below 60, 65, 70, and 75 mm Hg. However, an hourly time MAP integral that dropped below 55 mm Hg was associated with a significant decrease in the area under the 28-day mortality ROC curve. This suggests that a MAP

level of 60 mm Hg was a sufficient target during the first 24 hours of sepsis. However, the need for renal replacement therapy was best predicted by the ROC curve for the hourly time integral of MAP drops below 75 mm Hg. Thus, a higher MAP level may be required to prevent acute kidney injury (AKI).

In a post hoc analysis of data from a study investigating the effects on mortality of L-NMMA (N-methyl-L-arginine), a nitric oxide inhibitor, there was no association between MAP (or MAP quartiles) and mortality or occurrence of disease-related events in a control group that included 290 septic shock patients.[19] This study used logistic regression models and adjusted for age, the presence of chronic arterial hypertension, disease severity at admission (SAPS II), and vasopressor load.[20] Of note, in this study, age and chronic arterial hypertension did not modify the association between MAP and 28-day mortality or AKI. In addition, the mean vasopressor load correlated with mortality and the number of disease-related events. The authors concluded that "MAP levels of 70 mm Hg or higher do not appear to be associated with improved survival in septic shock" and that "elevating MAP >70 mm Hg by augmenting vasopressor dosages may increase mortality."

In 217 patients with shock (127 or 59% of whom had septic shock), enrolled and followed prospectively, Badin et al.[21] showed that a low MAP averaged over 6 hours or 12 to 24 hours was associated with a high incidence of AKI at 72 hours only in patients with septic shock and AKI at 6 hours. In these patients, the best MAP threshold to predict AKI at 72 hours ranged from 72 to 82 mm Hg. No link between MAP and AKI at 72 hours in the other patients was found. In line with the results of Dünser et al., the authors concluded that a MAP of approximately 72 to 82 mm Hg might be required to avoid AKI in patients with septic shock and initial renal function impairment.

Using the data from the large prospective observational FINNAKI study,[22] Poukkanen et al. identified 423 patients with severe sepsis and showed that those with progression of AKI within the first 5 days of ICU admission (36.2%) had lower time-adjusted MAP than those without progression.[23] The best time-adjusted MAP value to predict progression of AKI was 73 mm Hg. However, as in the study by Badin et al.,[21] the results were not adjusted for severity of disease.

These results are confounded by all of the limitations inherent to the observational studies, but they deserve to be analyzed at the MAP level from ICU admission (closer from the beginning of the disease process than in interventional studies). Although the results are not all consistent and the relationship of disease severity to MAP makes them difficult to interpret, these studies suggest that a MAP target higher than 65 mm Hg may prevent AKI in some septic patients.

INTERVENTIONAL STUDIES

Some prospective interventional studies have attempted to delineate an optimal MAP target in septic patients by modifying the MAP level over a short period of time. In a small randomized controlled trial of 28 patients with septic shock, Bourgoin et al.[24] showed that increasing the MAP level from 65 to 85 mm Hg for 4 hours with norepinephrine increased cardiac index in the experimental arm. However, no change in arterial lactate, oxygen consumption, or renal function variables (urine output, serum creatinine, and creatinine clearance) was detected in either of the groups.

In 10 patients with septic shock, LeDoux et al.[25] found that an increase in the MAP from 65 to 75 and 85 mm Hg using escalating vasopressor doses for less than 2 hours did not significantly alter systemic oxygen metabolism, skin microcirculatory blood flow (assessed by skin capillary blood flow and red blood cell velocity), urine output, or splanchnic perfusion (assessed by gastric mucosal partial pressure of carbon dioxide [Pco_2]). Of note, many of the patients received dopamine and not norepinephrine. In addition, in 20 patients with septic shock, targeting a MAP of 65, 75, or 85 mm Hg did not alter O_2 delivery, consumption, or serum lactate, although the increase in norepinephrine infusion dose was associated with an increase in cardiac index.[26] Furthermore, no change was observed in sublingual capillary microvascular flow index or the percentage of perfused capillaries.

Conversely, in a study including 13 patients with septic shock, Thooft et al.[27] showed that, in comparison with 65 mm Hg, targeting MAP to 85 mm Hg for 30 minutes by increasing norepinephrine increased cardiac output, improved microcirculatory function (assessed by thenar muscle oxygen saturation using near-infrared spectroscopy with serial vaso-occlusive tests on the upper arm and sublingual microcirculation using sidestream dark-field imaging in six patients), and decreased arterial lactate. Interestingly, the microvascular response to MAP changes varied largely from patient to patient, suggesting that the optimal MAP may need to be individualized.

In another study of similar design investigating 16 septic shock patients, raising MAP from 60 to 70, 80, and 90 mm Hg for 45 minutes increased oxygen delivery, cutaneous microvascular flow, and tissue oxygenation (using cutaneous tissue oxygen pressure [Pto_2] measured by a Clark electrode, cutaneous red blood cell flux assessed by laser Doppler flowmetry, and sublingual microvascular flow evaluated by sidestream dark-field imaging).[28] However, as in the study conducted by Dubin et al.,[26] no change in the sublingual microvascular flow abnormalities or lactate or urine output observed at 60 mm Hg were detected when MAP was increased to 90 mm Hg.

In a randomized short-term study comparing the effects of dopamine and norepinephrine in 20 patients, patients were evaluated at baseline (MAP = 65 and 63 mm Hg in the norepinephrine and dopamine group, respectively) and 3 hours after they achieved a MAP greater than 75 mm Hg.[29] Oxygen delivery and consumption (determined by indirect calorimetry) increased in both groups. However, the gastric intramucosal pH (determined by gastric tonometry) increased in the norepinephrine group but decreased in the dopamine group.

Finally, in 11 septic patients, Derrudre et al.[30] showed that increasing MAP from 65 to 75 mm Hg for 2 hours increased urinary output and decreased the renal resistive index measured by echography. However, no changes were detected when MAP was increased from 75 to 85 mm Hg. Importantly, the interpretation of renal resistive index changes is complex because of its numerous determinants.[31]

Nevertheless, this study suggests that for some patients, the optimal balance between the positive effects (i.e., increase in perfusion pressure) and the negative effects of norepinephrine (i.e., excessive vasoconstriction) could correspond to a MAP target of approximately 75 mm Hg. This premise is supported by data from a study on 12 nonseptic, postcardiac surgery patients with vasodilatory shock and AKI.[32] In these individuals, increasing MAP from 60 to 75 mm Hg improved renal oxygen delivery, the renal oxygen delivery/consumption relationship, and glomerular filtration rate, but increasing from 75 to 90 mm Hg did not alter these parameters.

Thus, the data regarding the effects of a MAP of more than 65 mm Hg on organ function and microcirculation are divergent. In addition to the small number of patients and the short observation periods, these differences may be related to differences in cardiac preload and to the point in time at which data were collected. It is of critical importance to note that the inclusion time in all of these studies was very wide and that most of the enrolled patients were already hemodynamically controlled. These human interventional studies are summarized in Table 40-1.

MAP IN LARGE, CONTROLLED RANDOMIZED TRIALS

In clinical practice, safety limits may dictate that the actual MAP be higher than the originally prescribed target. This difference is also observed in large, prospective, randomized controlled trials. In the study by Rivers et al.[33] comparing two strategies of resuscitation in patients with severe sepsis or septic shock (standard therapy vs. early goal-directed therapy [EGDT]), the mean MAP reached in the EGDT group was 95 mm Hg. The MAP was also in excess of the recommended target in the CATS trial from Annane et al.[34] comparing epinephrine with norepinephrine plus dobutamine, in the large trial from De Backer et al.[35] comparing dopamine with norepinephrine in patients with shock, and in the recent ProCESS (Protocolized Care for Early Septic Shock) multicenter study comparing EGDT with usual care.[36] These studies reported any side effects that were suggestive of excessive vasoconstriction (e.g., digital or splanchnic ischemia).[33-36] In the VASST (Vasopressin and Septic Shock Trial), comparing low-dose vasopressin and norepinephrine in addition with conventional catecholamine,[37] the mean MAP level was approximately 80 mm Hg at 3 days in the 2 groups. Although risk factors for ischemic injuries were an exclusion criterion, there was a relatively high rate of digital ischemia (2% in the vasopressin group and 0.5% in the norepinephrine group).

In the study by Lopez et al.,[19] a nitric oxide synthase inhibitor, LNMA, when added to conventional vasopressors, rapidly increased MAP (>90 mm Hg in 25% of the patients). This trial was stopped prematurely because of increased mortality in the LNMA group, primarily as a result of cardiovascular deaths. The association between MAP level and mortality cannot be analyzed in this study because of the very likely direct effect of the LNMA, independent of the MAP effect.

Table 40-1 Clinical Interventional Studies Comparing Different MAP Targets

Reference	Patients (*n*)	Design	MAP Titration (Time/Step)	Main Results of Increase in MAP
Bourgoin et al.[24]	2 × 14	Open-label, randomized controlled study	65 vs. 85 mm Hg (4 hours)	CI ↑ Arterial lactate, Vo_2, and renal function: NS
LeDoux et al.[25]	10	Crossover	65, 75, 85 mm Hg (105 minutes)	CI ↑ Arterial lactate, gastric intramucosal-arterial Pco_2 difference, skin microcirculatory blood flow (skin capillary blood flow and red blood cell velocity), urine output: NS
Dubin et al.[26]	20	Crossover	65, 75, 85 mm Hg (30 minutes)	CI, systemic vascular resistance, left and right ventricular stroke work indexes ↑ Arterial lactate, DO_2, Vo_2, gastric intramucosal-arterial Pco_2 difference, sublingual capillary MFI, and percentage of perfused capillaries (SDF imaging): NS
Thoof et al.[27]	13	Crossover	65, 75, 85 mm Hg (30 minutes)	CI, SvO_2, StO_2, sublingual perfused vessel density, and MFI (SDF imaging) ↑ Vo_2: NS Arterial lactate ↓
Jhanji et al.[28]	16	Crossover	60, 70, 80, 90 mm Hg (45 minutes)	Do_2, cutaneous Pto_2, cutaneous microvascular red blood cell flux (laser Doppler flowmetry) ↑ Sublingual capillary MFI (SDF): NS
Deruddre et al.[30]	11	Crossover	65, 75, 85 mm Hg (120 minutes)	65 to 75 mm Hg: urine output ↑, RRI ↓ 75 to 85 mm Hg: urine output, RRI: NS Creatinine clearance: NS

CI, cardiac index; *Do₂*, oxygen delivery; *MAP*, mean arterial pressure; *MFI*, microvascular flow index; *NS*, not significant; *Pco₂*, partial pressure of carbon dioxide; *Pto₂*, tissue oxygen pressure; *RRI*; R-R interval; *SDF*, sidestream dark-field; *StO₂*, thenar muscle oxygen saturation using near-infrared spectroscopy; *SvO₂*, mixed venous oxygen saturation; *Vo₂*, oxygen consumption.
↑, increase; ↓, decrease.

The large clinical trials in septic patients suggest that a MAP of approximately 80 mm Hg is often reached without overt side effects.

SEPSISPAM

To avoid the limitations described in the previous studies, the SEPSISPAM (Sepsis and Mean Arterial Pressure Trial) study, a randomized, open-label trial, was designed to enroll 800 patients as soon as possible after admission in the ICU (randomization within 6 hours after the initiation of vasopressors) and to target one of two MAP strategies (65 to 70 vs. 80 to 85 mm Hg) from day 1 to day 5 (or until the patient was weaned from vasopressor support).[38] Patients also were stratified to account for chronic hypertension. The high-MAP target group received higher doses of catecholamines over a longer time period than the low-MAP target group. No significant differences in 28-day mortality, in the overall rates of organ dysfunction, or in death at 90 days were identified. However, in a prospectively defined group of patients with previous hypertension (>40% of the patients in the study), the incidence of AKI (defined by doubling of serum creatinine level) and the rate of renal replacement therapy were higher in the low-MAP target group. The overall rate of serious adverse events was not different between the two groups, but there were more episodes of atrial fibrillation, known to be independently associated with an increased risk of stroke, in the high-MAP target group. SEPSISPAM confirms that a MAP of more than 65 mm Hg may be needed

to prevent AKI in patients with a history of arterial hypertension. In addition, this study raises another question: How do fluids and vasopressors have to be used to achieve a target MAP? In SEPSISPAM, the hemodynamic management consisted of the introduction of vasopressor (norepinephrine except in one center where epinephrine was used) after adequate fluid resuscitation (defined as the administration of 30 mL of normal saline per kilogram of body weight or of colloids or determined by clinician's assessment with the method of his or her choice) according to the recommendations of the French Society of Intensive Care Medicine.[39] This strategy led to different "profiles" between fluid and vasopressor loads to obtain the same MAP level in comparison with other large clinical randomized studies.[40] For example, patients received less fluids and more norepinephrine in SEPSISPAM than in some other trials[33,37] but less norepinephrine and more fluids than in the large randomized controlled trial conducted by De Backer et al.[35]

CONCLUSION

Recent studies, especially SEPSISPAM, suggest that a MAP target of 65 mm Hg is usually sufficient in patients with septic shock. However, a higher MAP level (~75 to 85 mm Hg) may prevent the occurrence of AKI in patients with chronic arterial hypertension. This point is of major clinical importance in view of the high prevalence of AKI and the subsequent morbidity of this condition in patients admitted in the ICU for septic shock. In addition, a delay in achieving the target MAP may be as important as the target itself. Finally, the manner in which a MAP target is achieved (amount of fluids, association of vasopressors) requires further investigations, especially in patients with chronic arterial hypertension who may benefit from a high MAP level.

AUTHORS' RECOMMENDATIONS

- Increasing MAP in shocked patients improves perfusion in autoregulated organs and microcirculatory blood flow but implies higher vasopressor load.
- Recent studies suggest that a MAP target of 65 mm Hg is usually sufficient in the patients with septic shock.
- A higher MAP level (around 75 to 85 mm Hg) may prevent the occurrence of AKI in patients with chronic arterial hypertension.
- The microvascular response to MAP changes varies from patient to patient, suggesting that the optimal MAP may need to be individualized.
- A delay in achieving the target MAP may be as important as the target itself.
- The manner in a MAP target is achieved (amount of fluids, association of vasopressors) requires further investigations, especially in patients with chronic arterial hypertension who may benefit from a high MAP level.
- It is unknown whether higher than required MAP targets have either beneficial or detrimental effects.

ACKNOWLEDGMENTS

F.B. was supported by a grant from the University Hospital of Angers.

REFERENCES

1. Angus DC, van der Poll T. Severe sepsis and septic shock. *N Engl J Med*. 2013;369:2063.
2. Augusto J-F, Teboul J-L, Radermacher P, Asfar P. Interpretation of blood pressure signal: physiological bases, clinical relevance, and objectives during shock states. *Intensive Care Med*. 2011;37:411–419.
3. Dellinger RP, Levy MM, Rhodes A, et al. Surviving Sepsis Campaign Guidelines Committee including The Pediatric Subgroup: Surviving Sepsis Campaign: international guidelines for management of severe sepsis and septic shock. *Intensive Care Med*. 2012;2013(39):165–228.
4. Johnson PC. Autoregulation of blood flow. *Circ Res*. 1986;59:483–495.
5. Strandgaard S, Olesen J, Skinhoj E, Lassen NA. Autoregulation of brain circulation in severe arterial hypertension. *Br Med J*. 1973;1:507–510.
6. Berne RM. Regulation of coronary blood flow. *Physiol Rev*. 1964;44:1–29.
7. Cupples WA, Braam B. Assessment of renal autoregulation. *Am J Physiol Renal Physiol*. 2007;292:F1105–F1123.
8. Bellomo R, Wan L, May C. Vasoactive drugs and acute kidney injury. *Crit Care Med*. 2008;36(suppl 4):S179–S186.
9. Prowle JR, Molan MP, Hornsey E, Bellomo R. Measurement of renal blood flow by phase-contrast magnetic resonance imaging during septic acute kidney injury: a pilot investigation. *Crit Care Med*. 2012;40:1768–1776.
10. Burban M, Hamel JF, Tabka M, et al. Renal macro- and microcirculation autoregulatory capacity during early sepsis and norepinephrine infusion in rats. *Crit Care Lond Engl*. 2013;17:R139.
11. Legrand M, Dupuis C, Simon C, et al. Association between systemic hemodynamics and septic acute kidney injury in critically ill patients: a retrospective observational study. *Crit Care Lond Engl*. 2013;17:R278.
12. De Backer D, Donadello K, Taccone FS, Ospina-Tascon G, Salgado D, Vincent J-L. Microcirculatory alterations: potential mechanisms and implications for therapy. *Ann Intensive Care*. 2011;1:27.
13. De Backer D, Creteur J, Preiser J-C, Dubois M-J, Vincent J-L. Microvascular blood flow is altered in patients with sepsis. *Am J Respir Crit Care Med*. 2002;166:98–104.
14. De Backer D, Ortiz JA, Salgado D. Coupling microcirculation to systemic hemodynamics. *Curr Opin Crit Care*. 2010;16:250–254.
15. Hamzaoui O, Georger J-F, Monnet X, et al. Early administration of norepinephrine increases cardiac preload and cardiac output in septic patients with life-threatening hypotension. *Crit Care Lond Engl*. 2010;14:R142.
16. Dünser MW, Hasibeder WR. Sympathetic overstimulation during critical illness: adverse effects of adrenergic stress. *J Intensive Care Med*. 2009;24:293–316.
17. Varpula M, Tallgren M, Saukkonen K, Voipio-Pulkki L-M, Pettilä V. Hemodynamic variables related to outcome in septic shock. *Intensive Care Med*. 2005;31:1066–1071.
18. Dünser MW, Takala J, Ulmer H, et al. Arterial blood pressure during early sepsis and outcome. *Intensive Care Med*. 2009;35:1225–1233.
19. López A, Lorente JA, Steingrub J, et al. Multiple-center, randomized, placebo-controlled, double-blind study of the nitric oxide synthase inhibitor 546C88: effect on survival in patients with septic shock. *Crit Care Med*. 2004;32:21–30.
20. Dünser MW, Ruokonen E, Pettilä V, et al. Association of arterial blood pressure and vasopressor load with septic shock mortality: a post hoc analysis of a multicenter trial. *Crit Care Lond Engl*. 2009;13:R181.
21. Badin J, Boulain T, Ehrmann S, et al. Relation between mean arterial pressure and renal function in the early phase of shock: a prospective, explorative cohort study. *Crit Care Lond Engl*. 2011;15:R135.
22. Nisula S, Kaukonen K-M, Vaara ST, et al. Incidence, risk factors and 90-day mortality of patients with acute kidney injury in Finnish intensive care units: the FINNAKI study. *Intensive Care Med*. 2013;39:420–428.
23. Poukkanen M, Wilkman E, Vaara ST, et al. Hemodynamic variables and progression of acute kidney injury in critically ill patients with severe sepsis: data from the prospective observational FINNAKI study. *Crit Care Lond Engl*. 2013;17:R295.
24. Bourgoin A, Leone M, Delmas A, Garnier F, Albanèse J, Martin C. Increasing mean arterial pressure in patients with septic shock: effects on oxygen variables and renal function. *Crit Care Med*. 2005;33:780–786.
25. LeDoux D, Astiz ME, Carpati CM, Rackow EC. Effects of perfusion pressure on tissue perfusion in septic shock. *Crit Care Med*. 2000;28:2729–2732.
26. Dubin A, Pozo MO, Casabella CA, et al. Increasing arterial blood pressure with norepinephrine does not improve microcirculatory blood flow: a prospective study. *Crit Care Lond Engl*. 2009;13:R92.
27. Thooft A, Favory R, Salgado DR, et al. Effects of changes in arterial pressure on organ perfusion during septic shock. *Crit Care Lond Engl*. 2011;15:R222.
28. Jhanji S, Stirling S, Patel N, Hinds CJ, Pearse RM. The effect of increasing doses of norepinephrine on tissue oxygenation and microvascular flow in patients with septic shock. *Crit Care Med*. 2009;37:1961–1966.
29. Marik PE, Mohedin M. The contrasting effects of dopamine and norepinephrine on systemic and splanchnic oxygen utilization in hyperdynamic sepsis. *JAMA*. 1994;272:1354–1357.
30. Deruddre S, Cheisson G, Mazoit J-X, Vicaut E, Benhamou D, Duranteau J. Renal arterial resistance in septic shock: effects of increasing mean arterial pressure with norepinephrine on the renal resistive index assessed with Doppler ultrasonography. *Intensive Care Med*. 2007;33:1557–1562.
31. Lerolle N. Please don't call me RI anymore; I may not be the one you think I am!. *Crit Care Lond Engl*. 2012;16:174.
32. Redfors B, Bragadottir G, Sellgren J, Swärd K, Ricksten S-E. Effects of norepinephrine on renal perfusion, filtration and oxygenation in vasodilatory shock and acute kidney injury. *Intensive Care Med*. 2011;37:60–67.
33. Rivers E, Nguyen B, Havstad S, et al. Early goal-directed therapy in the treatment of severe sepsis and septic shock. *N Engl J Med*. 2001;345:1368–1377.

34. Annane D, Vignon P, Renault A, et al. CATS Study Group: Norepinephrine plus dobutamine versus epinephrine alone for management of septic shock: a randomised trial. *Lancet*. 2007;370:676–684.

35. De Backer D, Biston P, Devriendt J, et al. SOAP II Investigators: Comparison of dopamine and norepinephrine in the treatment of shock. *N Engl J Med*. 2010;362:779–789.

36. ProCESS Investigators, Yealy DM, Kellum JA, Huang DT, et al. A randomized trial of protocol-based care for early septic shock. *N Engl J Med*. 2014;370:1683–1693.

37. Russell JA, Walley KR, Singer J, et al. Vasopressin versus norepinephrine infusion in patients with septic shock. *N Engl J Med*. 2008;358:877–887.

38. Asfar P, Meziani F, Hamel J-F, et al. High versus low blood-pressure target in patients with septic shock. *N Engl J Med*. 2014;370:1583–1593.

39. Pottecher T, Calvat S, Dupont H, Durand-Gasselin J, Gerbeaux P, SFAR/SRLF Workgroup. Haemodynamic management of severe sepsis: recommendations of the French Intensive Care Societies (SFAR/SRLF) Consensus Conference, 13 October 2005, Paris, France. *Crit Care Lond Engl*. 2006;10:311.

40. Russell JA. Is there a good MAP for septic shock? *N Engl J Med*. 2014;370:1649–1651..

41 What Vasopressor Agent Should Be Used in the Septic Patient?

Colm Keane, Gráinne McDermott, Patrick J. Neligan

This chapter briefly summarizes the hemodynamic derangement associated with sepsis and then sequentially evaluates the various vasopressor agents that have been investigated and are in current use for the treatment of septic shock.

HEMODYNAMIC DERANGEMENT IN SEPSIS

Early sepsis is characterized by hypoperfusion, manifest as cold extremities, oliguria, confusion, lactic acidosis, and increased oxygen extraction, measured by reduced mixed venous oxygen saturation (SvO_2). Current conventional therapy involves early administration of (best-guess) antibiotics and empirical fluid resuscitation of 30 mL/kg.[1] The goal of fluid therapy is to reestablish global blood flow and generate a mean arterial pressure (MAP) of more than 65 mm Hg. Failure to respond to fluid therapy is an indication for vasopressor therapy. Most patients respond to antibiotics and fluids, and vasopressor therapy is usually relatively short.[2,3] A minority of patients become acutely critically ill, consequent of septic shock, because of delayed therapy, failure of source control, or genetic reasons, and require critical care for multiorgan support.[4]

Established (late-stage) septic shock is a complex disease characterized by various cardiovascular and neurohormonal anomalies. Although the hemodynamic consequences are easily described, the underlying mechanisms are incompletely understood. The major features of established septic shock are as follows:

1. Vasoplegia arises from loss of normal sympathetic tone associated with local vasodilator metabolites, which cause activation of adenosine triphosphate–sensitive potassium channels, leading to hyperpolarization of smooth muscle cells. There is increased production of inducible nitric oxide synthetase/nitric oxide synthase-2, resulting in excessive production of nitric oxide. Finally, there is acute depletion of vasopressin. Vasoplegia is associated with relative hypovolemia. Vascular tone is characteristically resistant to catecholamine therapy, but it is very sensitive to vasopressin.
2. Reduced stroke volume is widely thought to be due to the presence of circulating myocardial depressant factors, although it may result from mitochondrial dysfunction. There is reversible biventricular failure, a decreased ejection fraction, myocardial edema, and ischemia. Cardiac output is maintained by a dramatic increase in heart rate.
3. Microcirculatory failure manifests as dysregulation and maldistribution of blood flow, arteriovenous shunting, oxygen utilization defects, and widespread capillary leak. This results in increased sequestration of protein-rich fluid in the extravascular space. These abnormalities are incompletely understood. In addition, there is initial activation of the coagulation system and deposition of intravascular clot, causing ischemia.
4. In mitochondrial dysfunction, the capacity of mitochondria to extract oxygen is impaired. This results in elevated SvO_2 and elevated serum lactate despite adequate oxygen delivery to tissues.

Septic shock should be seen as part of a complex paradigm of multiorgan dysfunction that characterizes acute critical illness. These include kidney injury, hepatic dysfunction, delirium, coagulopathy, and acute hypoxic respiratory failure. The goal of the Surviving Sepsis Campaign[1] is to treat early-phase septic shock and prevent multiorgan failure and chronic critical illness (CCI). This has been remarkably effective,[2,3] despite ongoing controversies regarding components of the bundles. CCI is manifest by failure to liberate from mechanical ventilation, kwashiorkor-like malnutrition, extensive edema, neuromuscular weakness, prolonged dependence on vasopressors/inotropes, and neuroendocrine exhaustion. No interventions currently exist to modulate CCI.

VASOPRESSOR THERAPY

Hypotension and tissue hypoperfusion, unresponsive to intravenous fluid in sepsis, are indications for vasopressor therapy.[4,5] It is generally agreed that fluid resuscitation should precede vasopressor use, although the quantity and type of fluid remain controversial.[6] The question of which vasopressor(s) to use in sepsis has long been debated. Vasopressors are used to target MAP, and inotropes are used to increase cardiac output, stroke volume, and SvO_2. The exact MAP target in patients with septic shock is uncertain because each patient autoregulates within individualized limits. Autoregulation in various vascular beds can be lost below a specific MAP, leading to perfusion becoming linearly dependent on pressure. Often, the patient-specific autoregulation range is unknown. The titration of norepinephrine to a MAP of 65 mm Hg has been shown to preserve tissue perfusion.[6] However, the patient with preexisting hypertension may well require a higher MAP to maintain perfusion. The ideal pressor agent would restore blood pressure while maintaining cardiac output and preferentially perfuse the midline structures of the body (brain, heart, splanchnic organs, and kidneys). Currently, norepinephrine is considered the agent of choice in the fluid-resuscitated patient.

Norepinephrine

Norepinephrine has pharmacologic effects on both α_1- and β_1-adrenergic receptors. In low dosage ranges, the β effect is noticeable, and there is a mild increase in cardiac output. In most dosage ranges, vasoconstriction and increased MAP are evident. Norepinephrine does not increase heart rate. The main beneficial effect of norepinephrine is to increase organ perfusion by increasing vascular tone. Studies that have compared norepinephrine to dopamine head to head have favored the former in terms of overall improvements in oxygen delivery, organ perfusion, and oxygen consumption.[7]

Marik and Mohedin[8] randomized 20 patients with vasoplegic septic shock to dopamine or norepinephrine, titrated to increase the MAP to greater than 75 mm Hg and measured oxygen delivery, oxygen consumption, and gastric mucosal pH (pHi, determined by gastric tonometry) at baseline and after 3 hours of achieving the target MAP. Dopamine increased the MAP largely by increasing the cardiac output, principally by driving up heart rate, whereas norepinephrine increased the MAP by increasing the peripheral vascular resistance while maintaining the cardiac output. Although oxygen delivery and oxygen consumption increased in both groups of patients, the pHi increased significantly in those patients treated with norepinephrine, whereas the pHi decreased significantly in those patients receiving dopamine ($P < .001$, for corrected 3-hour value). Similar data were reported by Ruokenen and associates.[9]

DeBacker and colleagues[7] randomized 1679 patients to receive dopamine (maximum, 20 μg/kg/min) or norepinephrine (maximum, 0.19 μg/kg/min) as first-line vasopressor therapy to restore and maintain blood pressure at a MAP of greater than 65 mm Hg. The primary endpoint was 28-day mortality, and secondary outcomes included organ-support-free days and adverse events. Although 28-day mortality was nonsignificant between dopamine and norepinephrine (52.5% vs. 48.5% respectively, $P = .10$), a significantly higher incidence of arrhythmias—principally atrial fibrillation—occurred in the dopamine group (24.1% vs. 12.4%, $P < .001$). Of note, subgroup analysis of patients with cardiogenic shock showed a significantly higher mortality in the dopamine versus the norepinephrine group ($P = .03$ for cardiogenic shock, $P = .19$ for septic shock, and $P = .84$ for hypovolemic shock).

Norepinephrine is less metabolically active than epinephrine and reduces serum lactate.[7] Norepinephrine significantly improves renal perfusion and splanchnic blood flow in sepsis,[10,11] particularly when combined with dobutamine.[10]

Martin and colleagues[12] undertook a prospective, observational cohort study of 97 patients with septic shock to look at outcome predictors using stepwise logistic regression analysis. The 57 patients treated with norepinephrine had significantly lower hospital mortality rates (62% vs. 82%; $P < .001$; relative risk, 0.68; 95% confidence interval [CI], 0.54 to 0.87) than the 40 patients treated with vasopressors other than norepinephrine (high-dose dopamine, epinephrine, or both). This study was weakened by several factors, including observational nonblinded status, probable selection bias, and a weak endpoint (hospital mortality). However, at the time, the study was significant because many practitioners thought that norepinephrine administration resulted in organ hypoperfusion in critical illness. These data confirmed the work by Goncalves and colleagues.[13]

Does the timing of norepinephrine administration make a difference? Bai and colleagues performed a retrospective analysis of timing of initiation of norepinephrine in 213 patients with septic shock in two intensive care units (ICUs).[14] Patients were divided into two groups: If norepinephrine was started within 2 hours of onset of septic shock, then this was considered early (Early-NE); norepinephrine administered after 2 hours was considered late (Late-NE). The time to initial antimicrobial therapy was not different between the groups. There was significantly higher 28-day mortality in the Late-NE group versus the Early-NE group (for >2 hours delay odds ratio [OR] for death = 1.86; 95% CI, 1.04–3.34; $P = .035$). Every 1-hour delay in norepinephrine initiation during the first 6 hours after septic shock onset was associated with a 5.3% increase in mortality. The duration of hypotension and norepinephrine administration was significantly shorter and the quantity of norepinephrine administered in a 24-hour period was significantly less for the Early-NE group compared with the Late-NE group.

How is this outcome difference explained? Early administration of norepinephrine likely reflects the presence of greater expertise at the bedside. Patients likely reached their resuscitation goals earlier and required less fluid (~500 mL less in the first 24 hours). In the Rivers' study,[5] patients in the late resuscitation group required more fluid over the first 72 hours than in the intervention group, and this may be part of the etiology for poor control group outcomes.

In conclusion, norepinephrine rapidly achieves hemodynamic goals, particularly when administered early in septic shock. It is the agent of choice in septic shock.

Dopamine

Dopamine has predominantly β-adrenergic effects in low to moderate dose ranges (up to 10 μg/kg/min), although there is much interpatient variability. This effect may be due to its conversion to norepinephrine in the myocardium and activation of adrenergic receptors. In higher dose ranges, α-adrenergic receptor activation increases and causes vasoconstriction. Thus the agent is a mixed inotrope and vasoconstrictor. At all dose ranges, dopamine is a potent chronotrope. Dopamine may be a useful agent in patients with compromised systolic function, but it causes more tachycardia and may be more arrhythmogenic than norepinephrine.[7,15] There has been much controversy about the other metabolic functions of this agent. Dopamine is a potent diuretic (i.e., it neither saves nor damages the kidneys).[16] Dopamine has complex neuroendocrine effects; it may interfere with thyroid and pituitary[17] function and may have an immunosuppressive effect.[18] Whether these affect outcomes, in terms of morbidity or mortality, is unknown.

A high-quality prospective trial[16] and a meta-analysis have displayed ample evidence to discourage the use of "renal-dose" dopamine because it does not change mortality, risk for developing renal failure, or the need for renal replacement therapy.[19]

The Sepsis Occurrence in Acutely Ill Patients (SOAP) study was a prospective, multicenter, observational study that was designed to evaluate the epidemiology of sepsis in European countries and was initiated by a working group of the European Society of Intensive Care Medicine. It has been the subject of various database mining exercises, one of which looked at dopamine and outcomes.[20] Of the 3147 patients included in the SOAP study, 1058 (33.6%) had shock at any time; 462 (14.7%) had septic shock. Norepinephrine was the most commonly used vasopressor agent (80.2%), used as a single agent in 31.8% of patients with shock. Dopamine was used in 35.4% of patients with shock, as a single agent in 8.8% of patients, and combined most commonly with norepinephrine (11.6%). Epinephrine was used less commonly (23.3%) but rarely as a single agent (4.5%). Dobutamine was combined with other catecholamines in 33.9% of patients, mostly with norepinephrine (15.4%). All four catecholamines were administered simultaneously in 2.6% of patients. The authors divided patients into those who received dopamine alone or in combination and those who never received dopamine. The dopamine group had higher ICU (42.9% vs. 35.7%; $P = .02$) and hospital (49.9% vs. 41.7%; $P = .01$) mortality rates. A Kaplan-Meier survival curve showed diminished 30-day survival in the dopamine group (log rank, 4.6; $P = .032$). Patients treated with epinephrine had a worse outcome, but this may represent evidence of worse outcomes in patients with more severe shock. This study was observational and nonrandomized, and the original database was not designed to prove that one intervention would be associated with better outcomes than another because of the huge number of confounders.

Finally, why use dopamine? Dopamine is a natural precursor of norepinephrine, converted through β-hydroxylation. When dopamine is administered, serum norepinephrine levels increase. Because dopamine is a neurotransmitter and has metabolic activity in many organ systems, there appears to be little benefit to using dopamine over norepinephrine. Furthermore, a syndrome of dopamine-resistant septic shock (DRSS) has been described, defined as a MAP of less than 70 mm Hg despite administration of dopamine at 20 μg/kg/min.[21]

Levy and colleagues[22] investigated DRSS in a group of 110 patients in septic shock. The incidence of DRSS was 60%, and those patients had a mortality rate of 78%, compared with 16% in the dopamine-sensitive group. Thus, in the highest risk group of patients, the use of dopamine may be associated with delay in achieving hemodynamic goals.

In conclusion, dopamine is an effective inotrope and vasopressor, but it is associated with excess complications and should not be used as first-line therapy in septic shock.

Dobutamine

Dobutamine is a potent β_1-adrenergic receptor agonist, with predominant effects in the heart, where it increases myocardial contractility and thus stroke volume and cardiac output. Dobutamine is less chronotropic than dopamine. In sepsis, dobutamine, although a vasodilator, increases oxygen delivery and consumption. Dobutamine appears particularly effective in splanchnic resuscitation, increasing pHi and improving mucosal perfusion in comparison with dopamine.[23] As part of an early goal-directed resuscitation protocol that combined close medical and nursing attention and aggressive fluid and blood administration, dobutamine was associated with a significant reduction in the risk for mortality.[5] However, it is unclear whether any of this benefit was derived from dobutamine, and the follow-up studies failed to demonstrate outcome benefit with this protocol versus conventional therapy.[6]

Levy and colleagues[24] compared the combination of norepinephrine and dobutamine to epinephrine in septic shock. After 6 hours, the use of epinephrine was associated with an increase in lactate levels (from 3.1 ± 1.5 to 5.9 ± 1.0 mmol/L; $P < .01$), whereas lactate levels decreased in the norepinephrine-dobutamine group (from 3.1 ± 1.5 to 2.7 ± 1.0 mmol/L). The ratio of lactate to pyruvate increased in the epinephrine group (from 15.5 ± 5.4 to 21 ± 5.8; $P < .01$), but it did not change in the norepinephrine-dobutamine group (13.8 ± 5 to 14 ± 5.0). pHi decreased (from 7.29 ± 0.11 to 7.16 ± 0.07; $P < .01$), and the partial pressure of carbon dioxide (P_{CO_2}) gap (tonometer P_{CO_2} – arterial P_{CO_2}) increased (from 10 ± 2.7 to 14 ± 2.7 mm Hg; $P < .01$) in the epinephrine group. In the norepinephrine-dobutamine group, pHi (from 7.30 ± 0.11 to 7.35 ± 0.07) and the P_{CO_2} gap (from 10 ± 3 to 4 ± 2 mm Hg) were normalized within 6 hours ($P < .01$). Thus, compared with epinephrine, dobutamine and norepinephrine were associated, presumably, with better splanchnic blood flow and a reduction in catecholamine-driven lactate production. Whether this is of clinical significance is unclear. Moreover, the decrease in pHi and the increase in the ratio of lactate to pyruvate in the epinephrine group returned to normal within 24 hours. The serum lactate level normalized in 7 hours.

Annane and colleagues[25] performed a multicentre, randomized, double-blind trial that included 330 patients with septic shock. Participants were assigned to receive epinephrine (n = 161) or norepinephrine plus dobutamine (n = 169), titrated to maintain mean blood pressure at 70 mm Hg or more. There was no difference in mortality at 28 days between the groups ($P = .31$; relative risk, 0.86;

95% CI, 0.65 to 1.14), nor was there any difference in serious side effects, time to pressor withdrawal, or time to achieve hemodynamic goals.

Epinephrine

Epinephrine has potent β_1-, β_2-, and α_1-adrenergic activity, although the increase in MAP in sepsis is mainly from an increase in cardiac output (stroke volume). There are three major drawbacks from using this drug: (1) epinephrine increases myocardial oxygen demand; (2) epinephrine increases serum glucose and lactate,[26] which is largely a calorigenic effect (increased release and anaerobic breakdown of glucose); and (3) epinephrine appears to have adverse effects on splanchnic blood flow,[24,27-29] peripherally redirecting blood as part of the fight-and-flight response. As we have seen, factors 2 and 3 are of undetermined significance and are transient. Whether increasing myocardial oxygen consumption in sepsis is a good thing or a bad thing is unknown.

Many data support the hypothesis that epinephrine reduces splanchnic blood flow, at least initially. Seguin and colleagues studied laser Doppler flow in a small group of ICU patients to prospectively determine the effects of different vasopressors on gastric mucosal blood flow (GMBF).[30] The studies showed that a combination of dopexamine-norepinephrine enhanced GMBF more than epineprhine alone did.[30] Conversely, the same group had previously shown that GMBF was increased more with epinephrine than with the combination of dobutamine and norepinephrine.[31] Both studies only looked at GMBF for 6 hours and were unable to demonstrate differences in hepatic blood flow or oxidative stress.

Myburgh and colleagues[32] performed a prospective, multicentered, double-blind, randomized controlled trial of 280 ICU patients comparing epinephrine with norepinephrine. They found no difference in time to achieve target MAP. There was also no difference in the number of vasopressor-free days between the two drugs. However, several patients receiving epinephrine were withdrawn from this study because of a significant but transient tachycardia, increased insulin requirements, and lactic acidosis.

Obi and colleagues[33] performed a meta-analysis of inotropes and vasopressor in patients with septic shock. Fourteen studies with a total of 2811 patients were included in the analysis. Norepinephrine and norepinephrine plus low-dose vasopressin but not epinephrine were associated with significantly reduced mortality compared with dopamine (OR, 0.80 [95% CI, 0.65 to 0.99], 0.69 [0.48 to 0.98], and 0.56 [0.26 to 1.18], respectively).

In summary, epinephrine, although not currently recommended by international organizations[4] as first-line vasopressor therapy in sepsis, is a viable alternative. There are few data to distinguish epinephrine from norepinephrine in achievement of hemodynamic goals, and epinephrine is a superior inotrope. Concern about the effect of epinephrine on splanchnic perfusion may be misguided. It has been assumed that a lower pHi and increased Pco_2 gap correlate with hypoperfusion; however, the opposite may be the case. Epinephrine may increase splanchnic oxygen use and carbon dioxide (CO_2) production through a thermogenic effect, especially if gastric blood flow does not increase to the same extent, inducing a mismatch between splanchnic oxygen delivery and splanchnic oxygen consumption.[34] This is supported by data from Duranteau and colleagues.[35] Concern about the effect of increased serum lactate and hyperglycemia has limited the use of epinephrine. However, it is unclear whether lactate is harmful in sepsis,[34] and concern regarding hyperglycemia appears to be fading.[36]

Phenylephrine

Phenylephrine is an almost pure α_1-adrenergic agonist with moderate potency. Phenylephrine is a less-effective vasoconstrictor than norepinephrine or epinephrine,[37,38] but it is the adrenergic agent least likely to cause tachycardia. Although widely used in anesthesia to treat iatrogenic hypotension, phenylephrine is considered a less-effective agent in sepsis. Previous concerns regarding reduced hepatosplanchnic blood flow[37] appear to have been allayed.[38] Morelli et al.[38] conducted a prospective, randomized controlled trial on 32 septic shock patients using either phenylephrine or norepinephrine as the initial vasopressor. MAP was maintained between 65 and 75 mm Hg and measurements conducted over the first 12 hours. Cardiac output, gastric tonometry, acid base balance, creatinine clearance, and troponin "leaks" were all primary endpoints. Phenylephrine did not worsen hepatosplanchnic perfusion as compared with norepinephrine. It had similar effects as norepinephrine on cardiopulmonary performance and global oxygen transport, but it was less effective than norepinephrine to counteract sepsis-related arterial hypotension as reflected by the higher dosages required to achieve the same goal MAP.

In summary, phenylephrine is not harmful in septic shock, but it is less potent than norepinephrine. Although not addressed by the authors, potential peripheral, rather than central, administration of this agent may increase its utility in early septic shock while central line insertion is planned or taking place.

Vasopressin

Arginine-vasopressin is an endogenous hormone that is released in response to decreased intravascular volume and increased plasma osmolality. Vasopressin directly constricts vascular smooth muscle through V1 receptors. It also increases the responsiveness of the vasculature to catecholamines.[39,40]

Vasopressin has emerged as an additive vasoconstrictor in septic patients who have become resistant to catecholamines.[41] There appears to be a quantitative deficiency of this hormone in sepsis,[42-44] and administration of vasopressin in addition to norepinephrine increases splanchnic blood flow and urinary output.[45] Vasopressin offers theoretical advantages over epinephrine in that it does not significantly increase myocardial oxygen demand and its receptors are relatively unaffected by acidosis.[46]

Early studies demonstrated that the most efficacious dose was 0.04 U/min,[47] and this was not titrated.

This relatively low dose has little or no effect on normotensive patients. Several small early studies demonstrated the potential utility of vasopressin (or its analogs) in sepsis, although there were few compelling supportive data.[45,48-50]

Russell and colleagues[51] performed a multicenter randomized double-blind trial of patients in septic shock who were already receiving 5 μg of norepinephrine per minute (VASST [Vasopressin and Septic Shock Trial]). Three hundred ninety-six patients were randomized to receive vasopressin (0.01 to 0.03 U/min), and 382 were randomized to receive norepinephrine (5 to 15 μg/min) in addition to open-label vasopressors. There was no significant difference between the vasopressin and norepinephrine groups in the 28-day mortality rate (35.4% and 39.3%, respectively; $P = .26$), in 90-day mortality rate (43.9% and 49.6%, respectively; $P = .11$), or in organ dysfunction. Heart rate and total norepinephrine dose, early in the course of critical care, were lower in the vasopressin group. A subgroup analysis suggested a survival benefit for vasopressin in less severe sepsis (i.e., those patients who required a lower overall dose of norepinephrine to achieve MAP targets) at 28 days (35.7% vs. 26.5%; number needed to treat [NNT] 11) and 90 days (46.1% vs. 35.8%; NNT 10) but not for more severe sepsis. In patients whose vasopressin levels were measured, those levels were very low at baseline (median, 3.2 pmol/L; interquartile range, 1.7 to 4.9) and increased in the vasopressin group but not in the norepinephrine group.

Several significant limitations of this study should be noted. This study looked at dose escalation of norepinephrine versus norepinephrine plus complementary vasopressin: the objective was to determine whether the catecholamine-sparing effect of vasopressin improved outcomes. It was not a head-to-head study of vasopressin versus norepinephrine, nor was it a study of vasopressin in early septic shock. There was significant lead-time delay in recruitment (12 hours) before patients were randomized. The VASST study was underpowered; an expected mortality rate of 60% was used for the sample size planning. The actual mortality rate in the control group was 39%. Finally, the dose of vasopressin used in the study (up to 0.03 U/min) may have been inadequate to show a response in the patients with more severe septic shock.

A subsequent retrospective analysis of the VASST study database suggested a beneficial synergy between vasopressin and corticosteroids in patients who had septic shock and were also treated with corticosteroids.[52] Vasopressin, compared with norepinephrine, was associated with significantly decreased mortality (35.9% vs. 44.7%, respectively; $P = .03$) if patients were simultaneously receiving corticosteroids. In patients who received vasopressin infusion, administration of corticosteroids significantly increased plasma vasopressin levels by 33% at 6 hours ($P = .006$) to 67% at 24 hours ($P = .025$) compared with patients who did not receive corticosteroids.

In conclusion, patients in septic shock are depleted of vasopressin. Replacement therapy with arginine vasopressin may be catecholamine sparing in septic shock, particularly in moderate disease.

OTHER VASOPRESSORS

Although this chapter has focused on vasoactive agents that are commonly used and studied in intensive care, various other agents are available and have been used. These include phosphodiesterase inhibitors, such as milrinone and enoximone, and calcium sensitizers, such as levosimendan.[6,53] Phosphodiesterase inhibitors would appear to be an attractive alternative to dobutamine for cardiomyopathy of critical illness[54] and may indeed be efficacious for restoring splanchnic blood flow. However, phosphodiesterase inhibitors are pulmonary and systemic vasodilators and may worsen hypotension in septic shock and venous admixture in acute respiratory distress syndrome. Levosimendan improves sublingual blood flow more effectively than dobutamine at standard doses,[55] and it may have a future role as part of a splanchnic resuscitation strategy. There are currently inadequate data on these agents to recommend their use in septic shock.

Catecholamine Overload

Several investigators have suggested that excessive catecholamine administration may worsen outcomes in septic shock. For example, Dünser and colleagues[56] found that driving MAP above 70 mm Hg by increasing doses of catecholamines appeared to worsen outcomes. This was not confirmed by a multicenter trial of high versus lower blood pressure targets in sepsis.[57] However, persistent tachycardia has been observed to be a negative predictor of outcome in sepsis, and this may be associated with excess β-adrenoceptor activation. Excessive adrenergic activity may lead to myocardial ischemia, tachyarrhythmias, cardiomyopathy, immunosuppression, increased bacterial growth, thrombogenicity, and hyperglycemia.[58,59] In the VASST, there was a significant reduction of heart rate in the vasopressin-treated patients in the less severe shock group, and these patients had a reduction in overall mortality.[51] Morelli and colleagues randomized 77 patients with persistent pressor-dependent septic shock to beta-blockade with esmolol or continued therapy. Esmolol was titrated to maintain heart rate between 80 and 94 beats/min for the duration of ICU stay. It was a phase II study to determine whether heart rate control was indeed possible. All other data represent secondary endpoints. Nonetheless, there was a dramatic reduction in 28-day mortality from 80.5% to 49.4% (absolute risk reduction [ARR] 31%, NNT 3, $P < .001$). Beta-blocked patients required less fluid and had better cardiovascular parameters. The mortality reduction, although significant, was associated with very high mortality in the control group. However, it must be noted that these numbers reflect patients who received treatment such as fluid resuscitation, pressors, and antibiotics for more than 24 hours and remained dependent on norepinephrine to maintain a MAP of 65 mm Hg. We do not have data from other sepsis trials for comparison to this patient population (persistently pressor dependent), and further multicentered studies are awaited.

AUTHORS' RECOMMENDATIONS

- Current standard of care in septic shock involves administration of empiric antibiotics, intravenous fluids, and, if unresponsive, vasopressor agents.
- The goal of vasopressor therapy is to restore MAP to the patient's autoregulation range and restore blood flow to vital organs and the extremities.
- Controversy continues regarding the choice of vasopressor and the method of monitoring the response to therapy. This will continue until adequately powered, multicentered prospective trials are performed.
- Patients should be fluid resuscitated before commencement of vasopressor therapy.
- Norepinephrine appears to be the vasopressor agent of choice in septic shock. It is a potent vasoconstrictor that maintains cardiac output and restores midline blood flow. It is not metabolically active.
- Dopamine is an effective, although unreliable, inotrope, chronotrope, and vasopressor. However, it offers no advantage over norepinephrine in septic shock, it may worsen outcomes in hypovolemic and cardiogenic shock, and it has various nonhemodynamic effects that may affect neurohormonal and immune function.
- Epinephrine is a potent vasoconstrictor and inotrope. When commenced, it causes an early lactic acidosis secondary to aerobic glycolysis and may reduce splanchnic blood flow. The clinical significance of this is unclear, and both of these effects appear to be time limited. Epinephrine should be used as second-line therapy in septic shock.
- Dobutamine is a potent inotrope, but no clear data exist that dobutamine improves outcome in any scenario associated with septic shock. Dobutamine is a powerful splanchnic vasodilator, but the clinical utility of this agent in the setting of splanchnic hypoperfusion is unproven.
- Phenylephrine may be used as initial therapy alongside fluid resuscitation in septic shock, but it is less potent than norepinephrine.
- There is an absolute deficiency of vasopressin in septic shock, and combination therapy with catecholamines should be considered, particularly in early and less severe sepsis. There are no data to support the use of vasopressin as first-line therapy.
- There are inadequate data available to recommend the use of calcium sensitizers or phosphodiesterase inhibitors in septic shock.
- There are emerging data that beta-blocker administration to control the β-adrenergic stress response may improve outcomes in pressor-dependent septic shock.

REFERENCES

1. Dellinger RP, Levy MM, Rhodes A, et al. Surviving Sepsis Campaign: international guidelines for management of severe sepsis and septic shock, 2012. *Intensive Care Med.* February 2013;39(2):165–228.
2. Levy MM, et al. The Surviving Sepsis Campaign: results of an international guideline-based performance improvement program targeting severe sepsis. *Crit Care Med.* February 2010;38(2):367–374.
3. Kaukonen KM, Bailey M, Suzuki S, Pilcher D, Bellomo R. Mortality related to severe sepsis and septic shock among critically ill patients in Australia and New Zealand, 2000-2012. *JAMA.* April 2, 2014;311(13):1308–1316.
4. Angus DG, Van der Poll T. Severe sepsis and septic shock. *N Engl J Med.* 2013;369:840–885.
5. Rivers E, Nguyen B, Havstad S, et al. Early goal-directed therapy in the treatment of severe sepsis and septic shock. *N Engl J Med.* 2001;345:1368–1377.
6. *Trials of Early Goal Directed Resuscitation.* 2014-2015.
   a. The ARISE Investigators and the ANZICS Clinical Trials Group. Goal-directed resuscitation for patients with early septic shock. *N Engl J Med.* 2014;371:1496–1506.
   b. The ProCESS Investigators. A randomized trial of protocol-based care for early septic shock. *N Engl J Med.* 2014;370:1683–1693.
   c. Mouncey PR, et al. Trial of early, goal-directed resuscitation for septic shock (ProMISe Trial). *N Engl J Med.* 2015;372:1301–1311.
7. De Backer D, et al. Comparison of dopamine and norepinephrine in the treatment of shock. *N Engl J Med.* 2010;362:779–789.
8. Marik PE, Mohedin M. The contrasting effects of dopamine and norepinephrine on systemic and splanchnic oxygen utilization in hyperdynamic sepsis. *JAMA.* 1994;272:1354–1357.
9. Ruokonen E, Takala J, Kari A, et al. Regional blood flow and oxygen transport in septic shock. *Crit Care Med.* 1993;21:1296–1303.
10. Hannemann L, Reinhart K, Grenzer O, et al. Comparison of dopamine to dobutamine and norepinephrine for oxygen delivery and uptake in septic shock. *Crit Care Med.* 1995;23:1962–1970.
11. Martin C, Saux P, Eon B, et al. Septic shock: a goal-directed therapy using volume loading, dobutamine and/or norepinephrine. *Acta Anaesthesiol Scand.* 1990;34:413–417.
12. Martin C, Viviand X, Leone M, Thirion X. Effect of norepinephrine on the outcome of septic shock. *Crit Care Med.* 2000;28:2758–2765.
13. Goncalves Jr JA, Hydo LJ, Barie PS. Factors influencing outcome of prolonged norepinephrine therapy for shock in critical surgical illness. *Shock.* 1998;10:231–236.
14. Bai X, Yu W, Ji W, et al. Early versus delayed administration of norepinephrine in patients with septic shock. *Crit Care.* 2014;18:532.
15. Regnier B, Rapin M, Gory G, et al. Haemodynamic effects of dopamine in septic shock. *Intensive Care Med.* 1977;3:47–53.
16. Bellomo R, Chapman M, Finfer S, et al. Low-dose dopamine in patients with early renal dysfunction: a placebo-controlled randomised trial. Australian and New Zealand Intensive Care Society (ANZICS) Clinical Trials Group. *Lancet.* 2000;356:2139–2143.
17. Van den Berghe G, de Zegher F, Lauwers P. Dopamine suppresses pituitary function in infants and children. *Crit Care Med.* 1994;22:1747–1753.
18. Denton R, Slater R. Just how benign is renal dopamine? *Eur J Anaesthesiol.* 1997;14:347–349.
19. Kellum JA. Use of dopamine in acute renal failure: a meta-analysis. *Crit Care Med.* 2001;29:1526–1531.
20. Sakr Y, Reinhart K, Vincent JL, et al. Does dopamine administration in shock influence outcome? Results of the Sepsis Occurrence in Acutely Ill Patients (SOAP) Study. *Crit Care Med.* 2006;34:589–597.
21. Bollaert PE, Bauer P, Audibert G, et al. Effects of epinephrine on hemodynamics and oxygen metabolism in dopamine-resistant septic shock. *Chest.* 1990;98:949–953.
22. Levy B, Dusang B, Annane D, et al. Cardiovascular response to dopamine and early prediction of outcome in septic shock: a prospective multiple-center study. *Crit Care Med.* 2005;33:2172–2177.
23. Neviere R, Mathieu D, Chagnon JL, et al. The contrasting effects of dobutamine and dopamine on gastric mucosal perfusion in septic patients. *Am J Respir Crit Care Med.* 1996;154:1684–1688.
24. Levy B, Bollaert PE, Charpentier C, et al. Comparison of norepinephrine and dobutamine to epinephrine for hemodynamics, lactate metabolism, and gastric tonometric variables in septic shock: a prospective, randomized study. *Intensive Care Med.* 1997;23:282–287.
25. Annane D, et al. Norepinephrine plus dobutamine versus epinephrine alone for management of septic shock: a randomised trial. *Lancet.* 370(9588):676–684.
26. Day NP, Phu NH, Mai NT, et al. Effects of dopamine and epinephrine infusions on renal hemodynamics in severe malaria and severe sepsis. *Crit Care Med.* 2000;28:1353–1362.
27. Zhou SX, Qiu HB, Huang YZ, et al. Effects of norepinephrine, epinephrine, and norepinephrine-dobutamine on systemic and gastric mucosal oxygenation in septic shock. *Acta Pharmacol Sin.* 2002;23:654–658.
28. Meier-Hellmann A, Reinhart K, Bredle DL, et al. Epinephrine impairs splanchnic perfusion in septic shock. *Crit Care Med.* 1997;25:399–404.
29. Martikainen TJ, Tenhunen JJ, Giovannini I, et al. Epinephrine induces tissue perfusion deficit in porcine endotoxin shock: evaluation by regional CO(2) content gradients and lactate-to-pyruvate ratios. *Am J Physiol Gastrointest Liver Physiol.* 2005;288:G586–G592.

30. Seguin P, Laviolle B, Guinet P, et al. Dopamine and norepinephrine versus epinephrine on gastric perfusion in patients with septic shock: a randomized study [NCT00134212]. *Crit Care*. 2006;10:R32.
31. Seguin P, Bellissant E, Le TY, et al. Effects of epinephrine compared with the combination of dobutamine and norepinephrine on gastric perfusion in septic shock. *Clin Pharmacol Ther*. 2002;71:381–388.
32. Myburgh JA, Higgins A, Jovanovska A, et al. A comparison of epinephrine and norepinephrine in critically ill patients. *Intensive Care Med*. 2008;34:2226–2234.
33. Oba Y, Lone NA. Mortality benefit of vasopressor and inotropic agents in septic shock: a Bayesian network meta-analysis of randomized controlled trials. *J Crit Care*. October 2014;29(5):706–710.
34. Levy B. Bench-to-bedside review: Is there a place for epinephrine in septic shock. *Crit Care*. 2005;9:561–565.
35. Duranteau J, Sitbon P, Teboul JL, et al. Effects of epinephrine, norepinephrine, or the combination of norepinephrine and dobutamine on gastric mucosa in septic shock. *Crit Care Med*. 1999;27:893–900.
36. The NICE-SUGAR Study Investigators. Intensive versus conventional glucose control in critically ill patients. *N Engl J Med*. 2009;360:1283–1297.
37. Reinelt H, Radermacher P, Kiefer P, et al. Impact of exogenous beta-adrenergic receptor stimulation on hepatosplanchnic oxygen kinetics and metabolic activity in septic shock. *Crit Care Med*. 1999;27:325–331.
38. Morelli A, Ertmer C, Rehberg S, et al. Phenylephrine versus norepinephrine for initial hemodynamic support of patients with septic shock: a randomized, controlled trial. *Crit Care*. 2008;12:R143.
39. Holmes CL, Patel BM, Russell JA, Walley KR. Physiology of vasopressin relevant to management of septic shock. *Chest*. 2001;120:989–1002.
40. Barrett BJ, Parfrey PS. Clinical practice: preventing nephropathy induced by contrast medium. *N Engl J Med*. 2006;354:379–386.
41. Malay MB, Ashton Jr RC, Landry DW, Townsend RN. Low-dose vasopressin in the treatment of vasodilatory septic shock. *J Trauma*. 1999;47:699–703. discussion 705.
42. Buijk SE, Bruining HA. Vasopressin deficiency contributes to the vasodilation of septic shock. *Circulation*. 1998;98:187.
43. Goldsmith SR. Vasopressin deficiency and vasodilation of septic shock. *Circulation*. 1998;97:292–293.
44. Reid IA. Role of vasopressin deficiency in the vasodilation of septic shock. *Circulation*. 1997;95:1108–1110.
45. Patel BM, Chittock DR, Russell JA, Walley KR. Beneficial effects of short-term vasopressin infusion during severe septic shock. *Anesthesiol*. 2002;96:576–582.
46. Ornato JP. Optimal vasopressor drug therapy during resuscitation. *Crit Care*. 2008;12:123.
47. Tsuneyoshi I, Yamada H, Kakihana Y, et al. Hemodynamic and metabolic effects of low-dose vasopressin infusions in vasodilatory septic shock. *Crit Care Med*. 2001;29:487–493.
48. Albanese J, Leone M, Delmas A, Martin C. Terlipressin or norepinephrine in hyperdynamic septic shock: a prospective, randomized study. *Crit Care Med*. 2005;33:1897–1902.
49. Dunser MW, Mayr AJ, Ulmer H, et al. Arginine vasopressin in advanced vasodilatory shock: a prospective, randomized, controlled study. *Circulation*. 2003;107:2313–2319.
50. Lauzier F, Levy B, Lamarre P, Lesur O. Vasopressin or norepinephrine in early hyperdynamic septic shock: a randomized clinical trial. *Intensive Care Med*. 2006;32:1782–1789.
51. Russell JA, Walley KR, Singer J, et al. Vasopressin versus norepinephrine infusion in patients with septic shock. *N Engl J Med*. 2008;358:877–887.
52. Russell JA, Walley KR, Gordon AC, et al. Interaction of vasopressin infusion, corticosteroid treatment, and mortality of septic shock. *Crit Care Med*. 2009;37:811–818.
53. Ming MJ, Hu D, Chen HS, et al. Effect of MCI-154, a calcium sensitizer, on calcium sensitivity of myocardial fibers in endotoxic shock rats. *Shock*. 2000;14:652–656.
54. Liet JM, Jacqueline C, Orsonneau JL, et al. The effects of milrinone on hemodynamics in an experimental septic shock model. *Pediatr Crit Care Med*. 2005;6:195–199.
55. Morelli A, Donati A, Ertmer C, et al. Levosimendan for resuscitating the microcirculation in patients with septic shock: a randomized controlled study. *Critical Care*. 2010;14:R232.
56. Dunser MW, Takala J, et al. Association of arterial blood pressure and vasopressor load with septic shock mortality: a post hoc analysis of a multicenter trial. *Crit Care*. 2009;13:R181.
57. Asfar P, et al. High versus Low Blood-Pressure Target in Patients with Septic Shock. *N Engl J Med*. 2014;370:1583–1593.
58. Singer M. Catecholamine treatment for shock - equally good or bad? *The Lancet*. 1925;370:636–637.
59. Morelli A, Ertmer C, Westphal M. Effect of heart rate control with esmolol on hemodynamic and clinical outcomes in patients with septic shock: a randomized clinical trial. *JAMA*. 2013;310:1683–1691.

42 How Can We Monitor the Microcirculation in Sepsis? Does It Improve Outcome?

Guillem Gruartmoner, Jaume Mesquida, Can Ince

HOW CAN WE MONITOR THE MICROCIRCULATION IN SEPSIS?

Altered Microcirculation in Sepsis

Sepsis is a clinical condition associated with high morbidity and mortality worldwide, and its management represents a challenge for the clinician in the intensive care unit (ICU). Septic shock is usually characterized by severe hemodynamic alterations. From a macrohemodynamic point of view, it is defined by a decrease in vascular tone with some degree of hypovolemia, with or without concomitant myocardial depression. Of note, even when these global hemodynamic parameters seem to be corrected, signs of tissue hypoperfusion may still persist. Evidence suggests that microcirculatory dysfunction is a fundamental pathologic feature of sepsis.[1] Although until recently examination of the microcirculation has been hampered by technologic limitations, development of microcirculatory evaluation techniques has allowed direct study of this phenomenon. Microcirculatory alterations may produce tissue hypoxia by induction of oxygen supply–demand imbalance at the cellular level. Maintained over time, this situation can lead to cellular and organ dysfunction and ultimately death.[2]

The microcirculation is the final destination of the structures and mechanisms responsible for delivering oxygen to the tissue cells and thus is essential for maintaining adequate organ function. It consists of a complex network of small blood vessels (<100 μm diameter) composed of arterioles, capillaries, and venules. Arterioles are responsible for maintaining vascular tone and are lined by smooth muscle cells. They respond to extrinsic and intrinsic stimuli to match oxygen delivery with local metabolic demand. Capillaries are the primary site of exchange for oxygen and metabolic waste, oxygen diffuses passively along its concentration gradient to the respiring tissue cells, and waste converges on and is taken up by the venules. Far from being just a vessel network, the microcirculation is a complex system that also involves interaction between the different cell types and their subcellular structures to achieve various physiologic functions. These include not just oxygen transport but also hemostasis, hormonal transport,

and host defense. All these elements can interact with each other and are regulated by different complex mechanisms controlling microcirculatory perfusion.[1]

Recently, multiple experimental and clinical studies have reported microcirculatory alterations in severe sepsis and septic shock. These studies observed a decrease in capillary density that likely reflects an alteration in microcirculatory autoregulation. The net effect is an increase in the diffusion distance of oxygen to tissues.[3] Moreover, studies reveal changes in the heterogeneity of microcirculatory perfusion. As a consequence, the number of under- or unperfused capillaries in proximity to well perfused capillaries is increased. This change leads to functionally vulnerable microcirculatory units. Conventional systemic hemodynamic- and oxygen-derived variables may fail to detect this dysfunctional microcirculatory condition.[4] Thus the key hemodynamic deficit in sepsis may well be microcirculatory shunting that results in an oxygen extraction deficit, an alteration that may be a potential target for resuscitation.[4] From this point of view, microcirculatory shunting is considered to play a leading role in the pathophysiology of sepsis and multiorgan failure.[1,3,4]

According to the previously mentioned and current evidence, bedside evaluation of microcirculation may be useful in management of severe sepsis and septic shock patients.[5]

Current Methods to Monitor the Microcirculation in Patients with Sepsis

Evaluation of the microcirculation in critically ill patients presents certain methodological and technical difficulties that have retarded its use at the bedside. By definition, any technique for evaluating the microcirculation can monitor only the tissue bed to which it is applied. Therefore it is necessary to select sites that are easily accessible but that are also representative of the rest of the body. Nevertheless, it is important to understand that the microcirculatory alterations observed in a selected tissue area are a window that is likely to reflect the microcirculation in other areas, provided that there are no local interfering factors.[3]

Current techniques to monitor the microcirculation can be divided into two main groups:

1. Indirect methods to monitor function through evaluation of regional tissue oxygenation.
2. Direct methods to monitor perfusion that allow direct visualization of the microvascular network and of microcirculatory blood flow.

Indirect Methods to Assess Microcirculation: Evaluation of Tissue Oxygenation

Indirect methods based on measures of tissue oxygenation, as surrogates of microcirculatory perfusion, include gastric tonometry, sublingual capnometry, tissue oxygen electrodes, and near-infrared spectroscopy (NIRS). Among these technologies, NIRS has aroused increasing interest in the evaluation of the regional circulation because of its noninvasive nature and easy applicability.

Near-Infrared Spectroscopy

NIRS measures the attenuation of light in the near-infrared spectrum (700 to 1000 nm) to measure chromophores, mainly hemoglobin, present in the sampled tissue. Choosing specific scan lengths minimizes the impact of other tissue chromophores on the NIRS signal. Thus the final signal is derived primarily from oxyhemoglobin and deoxyhemoglobin contained in the microvascular tree (vessels <100 μm) present in the sampled area. Measuring oxy- and deoxyhemoglobin permits calculation of the overall saturation of tissue hemoglobin or tissue oxygen saturation (StO_2). The NIRS system consists of a light source, optical bundles (optodes) for light emission and reception, a processor, and a display system.[6]

Although StO_2 has been evaluated in several organs, skeletal muscle StO_2, which is nonvital and peripheral, may be the optimal early detector of occult hypoperfusion. Because StO_2 measurements can be altered by local factors such as edema and fat thickness, the thenar eminence has been proposed as a reliable site for measurements. In healthy patients under basal conditions, the NIRS signal predominantly reflects the venous oxygenation because an estimated 75% of the blood present in the skeletal muscle is located in the venous compartment. Thus, StO_2 is similar to mixed venous oxygen saturation and reflects the balance between local oxygen supply and consumption. Thus changes in StO_2 can be altered by both changes in local microcirculatory flow and changes in local consumption.[7]

In addition to monitoring the absolute value in the thenar eminence, the StO_2 response to a brief ischemic challenge can provide dynamic information on tissue performance. In the so-called vascular occlusion test (VOT) an artery proximal to the StO_2 probe is occluded until a given ischemic threshold is reached, and the occlusion is then released. This test generates some dynamic parameters: the initial deoxyhemoglobin slope (DeO_2) following ischemia has been proposed as a marker of local oxygen extraction. When the DeO_2 is corrected for the estimated amount of hemoglobin, the result is a parameter of local oxygen consumption, the $nirVo_2$. The reoxygenation slope (ReO_2) that follows the release of the vascular occlusion has been proposed as a marker of endothelial function because it depends on blood inflow and capillary recruitment after the hypoxic stimulus.[8] However, several studies also correlated ReO_2 with perfusion pressure. Thus, the resulting ReO_2 may be derived from the interaction of perfusion pressure with endothelial integrity.[9]

Although septic patients tend to have lower StO_2 values than healthy subjects, there is a huge overlap between these two populations.[10] These observations may be explained by the heterogeneity of microcirculatory alterations in sepsis (ischemic and highly oxygenated areas coexist), with an overall "normal" oxygen content in a given sensed area. The low sensitivity of this approach may be a major limitation of absolute StO_2 in sepsis. However, the use of VOT-derived variables appears to be more promising. Several studies have reported alterations in the StO_2 response to the VOT in sepsis, and the magnitude of these alterations correlated directly with prognostic factors and even with mortality.[9-11]

Direct Methods to Assess Microcirculation: Evaluation of Microvascular Perfusion

Clinical Examination

On the basis of the concept that the peripheral circulation provides an early glimpse into a circulatory disturbance that may lead to shock, some classic clinical findings are used at the bedside as surrogates of the presence of an impaired circulation. This noninvasive peripheral perfusion evaluation includes several easy-to-evaluate bedside measures such as capillary refill time and mottling score and the central-to-toe temperature gradient[12,13] that may be used to relate peripheral tissue hypoperfusion to the severity of organ dysfunction and outcome, independent of systemic hemodynamics.[13] However, these methods have important limitations: they are difficult to quantify and provide relevant information on the peripheral (particularly skin, an organ with independent mechanisms of regulation) rather than the central microcirculation.[14] Therefore these clinical methods, although useful for identifying patients at risk, have limited applications in daily clinical practice.

Videomicroscopy

Developed more than three decades ago, epi-illumination methods were introduced to observe the microcirculation in vivo without the need for transillumination. This approach eliminated one of the main technical issues that limited clinical utility. These methods were later incorporated into handheld microscopes, eventually giving rise to orthogonal polarization spectral (OPS) imaging developed by Slaaf and co-workers[15] and incident dark-field (IDF) illumination developed by Sherman and co-workers.[16] OPS[17] and later sidestream dark-field (SDF, an application of IDF imaging[18]) are videomicroscopic imaging techniques based on similar general principles that filter surface reflections of incident illumination light to allow detection of subsurface microcirculatory structures. After a light source is applied on a surface, the light is reflected by the deeper layers of the tissue, transilluminating superficial tissue layers. Accordingly, this technique can be used only on organs or tissue surfaces covered by a thin epithelial layer because the penetration of the green light used is about 0.5 mm. The selected wavelength (530 nm) of illumination light is absorbed by the hemoglobin in the red blood cells irrespective of its oxygen content. Erythrocytes are seen as black-gray bodies flowing inside capillaries (absorbed light) over a white tissue background (reflected light). Thus, only functional capillaries (with red blood cell flow) would be observed in contrast to physiologic nonfunctional capillaries (without red blood cell flow), which would not be detected.[19] Although the main focus of the technique is evaluation of red blood cell flow and the microvessel network, other microcirculatory elements such as leukocytes can also be identified.

In contrast to animal studies or patients undergoing surgery where several internal organs have been explored with videomicroscopy, in critically ill patients, this technique has been applied in more accessible surfaces, especially the sublingual mucosa. The sublingual area has been the most intensely investigated surface. In this region, different sized venules (25 to 50 μm) and capillaries (<25 μm) can be examined, whereas arterioles (50 to 100 μm) are normally not identified because they are located in deeper layers and the optics in early OPS and SDF devices limit visualization.

The early phase of severe sepsis and septic shock is characterized by a significant decrease in vessel density and in the proportion of perfused capillaries in sublingual videomicroscopy studies.[20,21] In addition, these studies identified an increase in heterogeneity of vascular density and blood velocity between coexisting areas. These alterations were more severe in nonsurvivors, and the rapid resolution of microcirculatory changes after interventional therapy correlated with improved outcome, including mortality.[20,22,23] Conversely, the persistence of microcirculatory alterations after the first 24 hours strongly and independently correlated with early mortality secondary to circulatory failure and with the development of multiorgan dysfunction in the late phase.[24]

Quantification of microcirculatory alterations has been a challenge because these techniques are limited by the hardware and because different scoring systems have been developed. After the conclusions of an expert consensus conference,[25] the ideal microcirculation analysis report should evaluate microvascular blood flow, vascular density, and perfusion heterogeneity. Microcirculatory perfusion is evaluated assessing microvascular flow index (MFI) and the proportion of perfused vessels (PPVs). Vascular density is evaluated by assessing total vessel density and perfused vessel density (PVD). Importantly, tissue perfusion is dependent on functional capillary density (reflected by PVD) and blood velocity (reflected by MFI). Vascular density is thought to be more important than blood velocity in ensuring tissue oxygenation because cells are able to regulate oxygen extraction. Accordingly, homogeneous low flow should be better tolerated than heterogeneous flow even when total blood flow is lower.[26] On the other hand, the presence of very high blood flow may theoretically reduce the time needed for hemoglobin to unload oxygen to cells and also may induce capillary endothelial damage by shear stress.[25] Finally, heterogeneity of perfusion is reflected by PPV in the investigated area and the heterogeneity index (Het Index) in the investigated organ.

Assessing heterogeneity of perfusion is an essential factor for evaluating the shunt fraction in septic shock.[27] Most of these variables are quantitative; flow-related parameters are semiquantitative but are sensitive enough to evaluate microcirculatory performance.

Routine clinical use of handheld microscopes has been sparse because the current first-generation (OPS) and second-generation (SDF) devices are technically limited and because automatic bedside image analysis is problematic. Thus, these approaches have been used primarily for research purposes.[28] Recently, a third-generation handheld microscope with incident dark-field imaging (Cytocam–IDF imaging[29]) has become available. A computer-controlled high-resolution, high pixel–density digital camera permits instant analysis and quantification of images. With this advanced technology, physiologically relevant, functional microcirculatory parameters may be measured and directly related to the clinical setting. This development should allow direct implementation of quantitative microcirculatory imaging monitoring at the bedside and thus open the way for its use in clinical decision making such as titrating fluid resuscitation to achieve microcirculatory endpoints.[30]

Overall, videomicroscopy is considered to be the gold standard technique for assessing microcirculation at the bedside. In the near future, this technique may allow monitoring of the last frontier of tissue perfusion in daily clinical practice.

HOW CAN MONITORING THE MICROCIRCULATION IMPROVE OUTCOME?

Microcirculation Alterations Are Related to Outcome in Sepsis

Over the past 30 years, several studies have indicated that microcirculatory alterations are consistently associated with, and may predict, outcomes from sepsis. From the initial clinical studies with gastric tonometry to the most recent direct microvasculatory visualization with in vivo videomicroscopy, the degree of alteration in local oxygenation, local carbon dioxide (CO_2) production, or capillary perfusion characteristics has been reliably associated with the clinical trajectory of septic patients.[9-11,22-24,31,32] Importantly, microcirculatory abnormalities have been associated with outcome and organ dysfunction even when current international guidelines for resuscitation of the macrocirculation were fully implemented.[33-36] These observations strongly suggest that microcirculatory endpoints must be incorporated into the process of resuscitating septic patients. In addition, microcirculatory monitoring may provide important mechanistic information about the response to therapy.[37-42]

How to Resuscitate the Microcirculation

Current therapeutic interventions in sepsis—fluids, vasopressors, inotropes, blood products—target systemic hemodynamic parameters, with the expectation that increasing global oxygen delivery will improve microvascular perfusion and oxygenation. However, these approaches do not include monitoring of the microcirculation. Given the heterogeneous nature of microcirculatory alterations in sepsis, increasing global organ blood flow may be insufficient to recruit the microcirculation. Indeed, several studies demonstrated that microcirculatory effects of both fluids and/or vasoactive agents were relatively independent of their systemic effects.[38,42-46] Ospina et al.[45] and Pranskunas et al.[38] used videomicroscopy to demonstrate that microcirculatory effects of fluid administration were independent of induced macrocirculatory changes, for example, as enhanced cardiac output. Interestingly, improvements in microcirculatory indices of perfusion were not related to increases in cardiac output. Pranskunas et al. showed clinical parameters indicating that hypovolemia improved only when fluid administration, which resulted in improved microcirculatory flow, resulted in a reduction in clinical parameters of hypovolemia, whereas fluid administration, which did not affect microcirculatory flow, was not effective in correcting clinical parameters of hypovolemia.[38] These observations conflict with the current (Frank-Starling) macrocirculatory-based approach to fluid administration.[47] Current data support targeting microcirculatory variables such as diffusion and convection, in addition to increasing global oxygen delivery. This can be achieved by directly monitoring the microcirculation and using these observations to titrate fluid resuscitation. Using a microcirculatory-monitoring, microcirculatory-guided fluid administration strategy has been proposed whereby microcirculatory convection and diffusion are maximized.[30] Analogous strategies have been envisaged for vasoactive drugs (e.g., for dobutamine infusion).[42,48] Globally, clinical studies evaluating the effect of resuscitation interventions on the microcirculation reinforce the idea that the microcirculatory response is fundamentally best predicted by baseline microcirculatory performance, better than for any macrohemodynamic variable.[38,44] Thus microcirculation evaluation would be mandatory before carrying out any intervention aiming to improve microcirculatory perfusion. Furthermore, interventions that do not appear to alter the circulation globally may significantly affect the microcirculation. These include the administration of hydrocortisone and activated protein C, red cell transfusion, and the use of vasodilatory agents, such as nitroglycerine.[40,49-53] Each of these has been subject to large-scale clinical trials that either have failed to show efficacy or have generated controversy. None of these trials, however, has assessed microcirculatory performance. Given that the microcirculatory effects of activated protein C appear to be independent of its macrocirculatory effects,[51-53] the results might well have been different had the microcirculation been targeted. Randomized trials specifically selecting patients with microcirculatory alterations are needed.

Impact of Targeting the Microcirculation in Sepsis Resuscitation

Despite current efforts to increase our knowledge on how we can evaluate and manipulate the microcirculation, the impact of these efforts remains unclear. To date, there are few prospective trials targeting microcirculatory endpoints in the resuscitation process. In 1992, Gutiérrez et al.[31] reported significant survival benefits when targeting tonometric gastric mucosal pH. The benefit of the intervention was limited to patients who had a normal gastric pH. These results appear to reinforce the interpretation of several large prospective trials with macrocirculatory endpoints that resuscitation interventions led to limited success once tissue or organ damage was present.[54,55] In 2007 Yu and co-workers conducted a prospective interventional trial comparing global resuscitation endpoints with transcutaneous oxygen tension (PtO$_2$) goals. Seventy patients were enrolled, and the PtO$_2$-guided group showed a significant mortality reduction.[56] Regrettably, the results of these trials have not been reproduced afterward. More recently available technologies, such as videomicroscopy or NIRS, have not been included in prospective trials as resuscitation guiding tools in septic shock patients.

Despite its apparent value, the inclusion of microcirculatory variables in the resuscitation process from septic shock appears complex. Some authors have proposed that microcirculatory endpoints be added to the end of the macrocirculatory resuscitation process, once current global endpoints are achieved. Conversely, others propose to "leave behind" current macrocirculatory goals and guide resuscitation with microcirculatory endpoints only.[57] To date, objective data supporting either of these two approaches are lacking, and the arguments remain conjectural. Which strategy offers better results will require future clinical research.

In the end, tools for microcirculation monitoring will be subject to the same concerns that accompanied hemodynamic monitoring devices in the past: No monitoring device, per se, can improve outcome unless coupled to an effective treatment. The advantage of microcirculatory monitoring lies in the insight into basic physiologic mechanisms that it provides. Therapy in critical care medicine too often refers to responders and nonresponders. Monitoring the microcirculation may provide additional depth. Ultimately, monitoring the microcirculation will have to be integrated into routine hemodynamic monitoring for it to truly make a difference.

AUTHORS' RECOMMENDATIONS

- The microcirculation is the ultimate destination of the functional mission of the cardiovascular system to transport oxygen to the tissue cells needed to perform their function in sustaining organ function. That is why monitoring its functional behavior is essential for hemodynamic support of the critically ill patient. Currently there are techniques based on handheld microscopes that allow the microcirculatory determinants of oxygen transport to tissue (convection and diffusion) to be determined.
- Microcirculatory alterations have prognostic implications, regardless of the technology used for its assessment, and independently of global resuscitation endpoints.
- The link between systemic hemodynamics and microcirculatory perfusion is relatively loose, and the current macrocirculatory evaluation approach of the resuscitation process might not always stand for parallel microcirculatory benefits.
- Including microcirculatory endpoints and guiding resuscitation with these technologies might prove beneficial for improving patients' outcomes.

REFERENCES

1. Ince C. The microcirculation is the motor of sepsis. *Crit Care.* 2005;9(suppl 4):S13–S19.
2. De Backer D, Orbegozo D, Donadello K, et al. Pathophysiology of microcirculatory dysfunction and the pathogenesis of septic shock. *Virulence.* 2014;5(1):73–79.
3. De Backer D, Ospina-Tascon G, Salgado D, et al. Monitoring the microcirculation in the critically ill patient: current methods and future approaches. *Intensive Care Med.* 2010;36:1813–1825.
4. Ince C, Sinaasappel M. Microcirculatory oxygenation and shunting in sepsis and shock. *Crit Care Med.* 1999;27:1369–1377.
5. Weil MH, Tang W. Welcoming a new era of hemodynamic monitoring: expanding from the macro to the microcirculation. *Crit Care Med.* 2007;35(4):1204–1205.
6. Boushel R, Piantadosi CA. Near-infrared spectroscopy for monitoring muscle oxygenation. *Acta Physiol Scand.* 2000;168(4):1019–1029.
7. Mesquida J, Espinal C, Gruartmoner G. Skeletal muscle oxygen saturation (StO$_2$) measured by near-infrared spectroscopy in the critically ill patients. *Biomed Res Int.* 2013;2013:502194.
8. Skarda DE, Mulier KE, Myers DE, et al. Dynamic near-infrared spectroscopy measurements in patients with severe sepsis. *Shock.* 2007;27:348–353.
9. Mesquida J, Espinal C, Gruartmoner G, et al. Prognostic implications of tissue oxygen saturation in human septic shock. *Intensive Care Med.* 2012;38:592–597.
10. Creteur J, Carollo T, Soldati G, et al. The prognostic value of muscle StO$_2$ in septic patients. *Intensive Care Med.* 2007;33:1549–1556.
11. Shapiro N, Arnold R, Sherwin R, et al. The association of near-infrared spectroscopy-derived tissue oxygenation measurements with sepsis syndromes, organ dysfunction and mortality in emergency department patients with sepsis. *Crit Care.* 2011;35:456–459.
12. Joly HR, Weil MH. Temperature of the great toe as an indication of the severity of shock. *Circulation.* 1969;39:131–138.
13. Lima A, Jansen TC, van Bommel J, et al. The prognostic value of the subjective assessement of peripheral perfusion in critically ill patients. *Crit Care Med.* 2009;37:934–938.
14. Boerma EC, Kuiper MA, Kingma WP, et al. Disparity between skin perfusion and sublingual microcirculatory alterations in severe sepsis and septic shock: a prospective observational study. *Intensive Care Med.* 2008;34:1294–1298.
15. Slaaf DW, Tangelder GJ, Reneman RS, et al. A versatile incident illuminator for intravital microscopy. *Int J Microcirc Clin Exp.* 1987;6(4):391–397.
16. Sherman H, Klausner S, Cook WA. Incident dark-field illumination: a new method for microcirculatory study. *Angiology.* 1971;22:295–303.
17. Groner W, Winkelman JW, Harris AG, et al. Orthogonal polarization spectral imaging: a new method for study of the microcirculation. *Nat Med.* 1999;5(10):1209–1212.
18. Goedhart PT, Khalilzada M, et al. Sidestream Dark Field (SDF) imaging: a novel stroboscopic LED ring-based imaging modality for clinical assessment of the microcirculation. *Opt Express.* 2007;15(23):15101–15114.
19. Medina ER, Milstein DMJ, Ince C. Monitoring the microcirculation in critically ill patients. In: Ehrenfeld JM, Cannesson M, eds. *Monitoring Technologies in Acute Care Environments: A Comprehensive Guide to Patient Monitoring Technologies.* Springer; 2013. ISBN: 978-1-4614-8557-5:127–137.
20. De Backer D, Creteur J, Preiser JC, et al. Microvascular blood flow is altered in patients with sepsis. *Am J Respir Crit Care Med.* 2002;166:98–104.
21. Edul V, Enrico C, Laviolle B, et al. Quantitative assessment of the microcirculation in healthy volunteers and in patients with septic shock. *Crit Care Med.* 2012;40:1443–1448.
22. Trzeciak S, Dellinger RP, Parrillo JE, et al. Early microcirculatory perfusion derangements in patients with severe sepsis and septic shock: relationship to hemodynamics, oxygen transport, and survival. *Ann Emerg Med.* 2007;49:88–98.
23. De Backer, Donadello A, Sakr Y, et al. Microcirculatory alterations in patients with severe sepsis: impact of time of assessment and relationship to outcome. *Crit Care Med.* 2013;41. 0–0.
24. Sakr Y, Dubois MJ, De Backer D, et al. Persistant microvasculatory alterations are associated with organ failure and death in patients with septic shock. *Crit Care Med.* 2004;32:1825–1831.
25. De Backer D, Hollenberg S, Boerma EC, et al. How to evaluate the microcirculation: report of a round table conference. *Crit Care.* 2007;11:R101.
26. Walley KR. Heterogeneity of oxygen delivery impairs oxygen extraction by peripheral tissues: theory. *J Appl Physiol.* 1996;81:885–894.
27. Ellis CG, Bateman RM, Sharpe MD, et al. Effect of a maldistribution of microvascular blood flow on capillary O2 extraction in sepsis. *Am J Physiol.* 2002;282:H156–H164.
28. Bezemer R, Bartels SA, Bakker J, Ince C. Microcirculation-targeted therapy–almost there. *Crit Care.* 2012;16(3):224–228.5, 19.
29. Aykut G, Ince Y, Ince C. A new generation computer-controlled imaging sensor-based hand-held microscope for quantifying bedside microcirculatory alterations. In: Vincent JL, ed. *Annual Update in Intensive Care and Emergency Medicine 2014.* Heidelberg: Springer; 2014. ISBN: 978-3-319-03745-5:367–381.
30. Ince C. The rationale for microcirculatory-guided fluid therapy. *Curr Opinion in Crit Care.* 2014;20(3):301–308.
31. Gutiérrez G, Palizas F, Doglio G, et al. Gastric intramucosal pH as a therapeutic index of tissue oxygenation in critically ill patients. *Lancet.* 1992;339:195–199.
32. Yu M, Morita SY, Daniel SR, et al. Transcutaneous pressure of oxygen: a noninvasive and early detector of peripheral shock and outcome. *Shock.* 2006;26:450–456.
33. Poeze M, Solberg B, Greve JW, et al. Monitoring global volume-related hemodynamic or regional variables after initial resuscitation: what is a better predictor of outcome in critically ill septic patients? *Crit Care Med.* 2005;33:2494–2500.
34. Lima A, van Bommel J, Jansen TC, et al. Low tissue oxygen saturation at the end of early goal-directed therapy is associated with worse outcome in critically ill patients. *Crit Care.* 2009;13(5):S13.
35. Donati A, Tibboel D, Ince C. Towards integrative physiological monitoring of the critically ill: from cardiovascular to microcirculatory and cellular function monitoring at the bedside. *Crit Care.* 2013;17(suppl 1):S5.
36. Vellinga NA, Boerma EC, Koopmans M, for the microSOAP Study Group, et al. International study on microcirculatory shock occurrence in acutely ill patients. *Crit Care Med.* 2015;43:48–56. PMID: 25126880.
37. Pottecher J, Deruddre S, Teboul JL, et al. Both passive leg raising and intravascular volume expansion improve sublingual microcirculatory perfusion in severe sepsis and septic shock patients. *Intensive Care Med.* 2010;36(11):1867–1874.
38. Pranskunas A, Koopmans M, Koetsier PM, et al. Microcirculatory blood flow as a tool to select ICU patients eligible for fluid therapy. *Intensive Care Med.* 2013;39:612–619.
39. Dubin A, Pozo O, Casabell C, et al. Increasing arterial blood pressure with norepinephrine does not improve microcirculatory blood flow: a prospective study. *Crit Care.* 2009;13:R92.
40. Yuruk K, Goedhart P, Ince C. Blood transfusions recruit the microcirculation during cardiac surgery. *Transfusion.* 2010;51(5):961–967.
41. Sakr Y, Chierego M, Piagnerelli M, et al. Microvascular response to red blood cell transfusion in patients with severe sepsis. *Crit Care Med.* July 2007;35(7):1639–1644.
42. De Backer D, Creteur J, Dubois MJ, et al. The effects of dobutamine on microcirculatory alterations in patients with septic shock are independent of its systemic effects. *Crit Care Med.* 2006;34:403–408.
43. Mesquida J, Borrat X, Lorente JA, Masip J, Baigorri F. Objectives of hemodynamic resuscitation. *Med Intensiva.* 2011;35(8):499–508.
44. Silva E, De Backer D, Creteur J, Vincent JL. Effects of fluid challenge on gastric mucosal pCO$_2$ in septic patients. *Intensive Care Med.* 2004;30:423–429.
45. Ospina-Tascon G, Neves AP, Occhipinti G, et al. Effects of fluids on microvascular perfusion in patients with severe sepsis. *Intensive Care Med.* 2010;36:949–955.
46. Hernandez G, Bruhn A, Luengo C, et al. Effects of dobutamine on systemic, regional and microcirculatory perfusion parameters in septic shock: a randomized, placebo-controlled, double-blind, crossover study. *Intensive Care Med.* 2013;39:1435–1443.
47. Vincent JL, Weil MH. Fluid challenge revisited. *Crit Care Med.* May 2006;34:1333–1337.
48. Enrico C, Kanoore Edul VS, Vazquez AR, et al. Systemic and microcirculatory effects of dobutamine in patients with septic shock. *J Crit Care.* 2012;27(6):630–638.

49. De Backer D, Ortiz JA, Salgado D. Coupling microcirculation to systemic hemodynamics. *Curr Opin Crit Care*. 2010;16:250–254.

50. Spronk PE, Ince C, Gardien MJ, et al. Nitroglycerin in septic shock after intravascular volume resuscitation. *Lancet*. 2002;360:1395–1396.

51. Masip J, Mesquida J, Luengo C, et al. Near-infrared spectroscopy StO$_2$ monitoring to assess the therapeutic effect of drotrecogin alfa (activated) on microcirculation in patients with severe sepsis or septic shock. *Ann Intensive Care*. September 4, 2013;3(1):30.

52. De Backer D, Verdant C, Chierego M, et al. Effects of drotrecogin alfa activated on microcirculatory alterations in patients with severe sepsis. *Crit Care Med*. 2006;34:1918–1924.

53. Donati A, Romanelli M, Botticelli L, et al. Recombinant activated protein C treatment improves tissue perfusion and oxygenation in septic patients measured by near-infrared spectroscopy. *Crit Care*. 2009;13(suppl 5):S12.

54. Gattinoni L, razzi L, Pelosi P, et al. A trial of goal-oriented hemodynamic therapy in critically ill patients. SvO$_2$ Collaborative Group. *N Engl J Med*. 1995;333:1025–1032.

55. Kern JW, Shoemaker WC. Meta-analysis of hemodynamic optimization in high-risk patients. *Crit Care Med*. 2002;30:1686–1692.

56. Yu M, Chapital A, Ho HC, et al. A prospective randomized trial comparing oxygen delivery versus transcutaneous pressure of oxygen values as resuscitative goals. *Shock*. 2007;27:615–622.

57. Dünser MW, Takala J, Brunauer A, et al. Re-thinking resuscitation: leaving blood pressure cosmetics behind and moving forward to permissive hypotension and a tissue perfusion-based approach. *Crit Care*. 2013;17(5):326.

43 Do the Surviving Sepsis Campaign Guidelines Work?

Laura Evans, Amit Uppal, Vikramjit Mukherjee

WHAT ARE BUNDLES?

The development and publication of guidelines seldom lead to changes in clinical behavior, and guidelines are rarely integrated into bedside practice in a timely fashion. Bundles are a group of evidence-based interventions that, when instituted together, may provide an impact greater than any single intervention alone.[1] Ideally, a bundle provides a simple and uniform way to implement best practices.

NEED FOR BUNDLES IN SEVERE SEPSIS AND SEPTIC SHOCK

Sepsis accounts for 20% of all admissions in noncardiac intensive care units (ICUs) and is the leading cause of death in such units.[2] There are approximately 750,000 new sepsis cases in the United States every year, and the overall mortality rate remains close to 30%.[3] It is the single most expensive condition treated in the United States, exceeding $20 billion annually.[4] Mortality and health-care costs associated with sepsis can be reduced by the coordinated and timely application of a group of evidence-based interventions.[5-7] Thus sepsis is a syndrome that is particularly amenable to bundle-based management.

Recognizing the global impact of sepsis and the growing evidence for interventions that would improve outcomes, the Surviving Sepsis Campaign (SSC) Guidelines were published initially in 2004, incorporating the best available evidence at that time. Beyond the guidelines, the SSC developed an international collaborative initiative to increase awareness of sepsis and to apply bundles as a means of translating the available evidence into improved patient outcomes on a global scale.

Over the last 10 years, the SSC has progressed in phases with multiple goals: building awareness, educating healthcare professionals, and improving the management of sepsis. Thus the SSC structured itself into an international practice improvement project, with in-depth collection of performance data and a goal of reducing sepsis mortality by 25% within 5 years (2004-2009).[8] During this time, the bundles themselves have been adapted in response to an evolving evidence base and data collected from the SSC itself (Table 43-1).

Is There Evidence That Application of the SSC Bundles Improves Outcomes?

Although the components of the bundles themselves have generated ample debate since their development, there is little doubt that the SSC bundles have been effective. Ferrer et al.[6] published the results of a national, SSC-based educational effort in Spain. The effort, based on the SSC guidelines, resulted in a reduction of in-hospital and 28-day mortality from severe sepsis or septic shock by 11% and 14%, respectively (Fig. 43-1). Improvement in outcomes was greatest in hospitals with the poorest initial performance. The key to improving outcomes, however, seemed to lie in persistent and penetrating education. The postintervention cohort still had a compliance rate of only 10% to 15%, and during long-term follow-up, compliance with the resuscitation bundle returned to baseline.

The hypothesis that increased bundle compliance would lead to improved outcomes was tested by the Intermountain Healthcare Intensive Medicine Clinical Program. This large, multicenter study involving 11 hospitals and 18 ICUs enrolled nearly 4500 patients and conducted a quality improvement study to evaluate the effects of implementation of sepsis bundles (Fig. 43-2).[9] By the end of the study period, bundle compliance was almost 75%, and in-hospital mortality rate had fallen below 10%.

The SSC itself has collected data from more than 15,000 patients at 165 sites participating in the collaborative. Bundle compliance rates and their association with hospital mortality were examined. Compliance rates with both phases of the bundle improved over the 2-year campaign. Simultaneously, there was a 7% absolute risk reduction in unadjusted hospital mortality over this time period. As the authors noted, by instituting a practice improvement program grounded in evidence-based guidelines, the SSC successfully increased compliance with sepsis bundles, and this change was associated with better patient outcomes.

In 2014, the SSC published the effects of bundle adoption over a 7.5-year period.[10,11] Analysis of nearly 30,000 patients from three different continents and more than 200 hospitals with up to 4 years of data revealed the sustainability of improved outcomes with increasing bundle compliance. Participation in the SSC alone led to an overall decline in mortality. Higher compliance to either resuscitation or management bundles led to improvements in

Table 43-1 Surviving Sepsis Campaign Care Bundles

Original Bundle (2005)	Updated Bundle (2012)
Resuscitation bundle (to be completed within the first 6 hr) • Serum lactate measured • Blood cultures obtained before antibiotic administration • Broad spectrum antibiotics administered within 3 hr for ED admissions, 1 hr for non-ED admissions • If hypotensive or if lactate ≥4 mmol/L, initial bolus of 20 mL/kg crystalloid (or colloid equivalent) administered; if MAP still <65 mm Hg, vasopressors applied • If hypotension or hyperlactemia persists, CVP >8 mm Hg and ScvO₂ of >65% achieved (or MVo₂ >65%)	To be completed within 3 hr • Serum lactate measured • Blood cultures obtained before antibiotic administration • Broad-spectrum antibiotics administered • 30 mL/kg of crystalloids administered for hypotension or lactate ≥4 mmol/L
Management bundle (to be completed within the first 24 hr) • Low-dose steroids administered for septic shock • Drotrecogin alpha (activated) administered • Glucose control maintained between lower limit of normal and <150 mg/dL • Inspiratory plateau pressures maintained <30 cm water for patients who are mechanically ventilated	To be completed within 6 hr • Vasopressors applied for refractory hypotension to maintain MAP≥65 • If initial lactate >4 mmol/L or if hypotension persists after volume resuscitation, measure CVP and ScvO₂ • Remeasure lactate if initial lactate was elevated

Adapted from Dellinger RP, Levy MM, Rhodes A, et al. Surviving sepsis campaign: International guidelines for management of severe sepsis and septic shock: 2012. *Crit Care Med.* 2013;41:580–637; and from Levy MM, Dellinger RP, Townsend SR, et al. The Surviving Sepsis Campaign: results of an international guideline-based performance improvement program targeting severe sepsis. *Crit Care Med.* 2010;38(2):368.[16]

CVP, central venous pressure; *ED*, emergency department; *MAP*, mean arterial pressure; *MVo₂*, myocardial oxygen consumption; *ScvO₂*, central venous oxygen saturation.

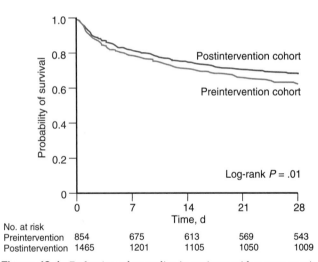

No. at risk				
Preintervention	854	675	613	569	543
Postintervention	1465	1201	1105	1050	1009

Figure 43-1. Reduction of mortality in patients with severe sepsis and septic shock by implementation of the Surviving Sepsis Campaign guidelines. *(Adapted from Ferrer R, Artigas A, Levy MM, et al. Improvement in process of care and outcome after a multicenter severe sepsis educational program in Spain.* JAMA. *2008;299(19):2294–2303.)*

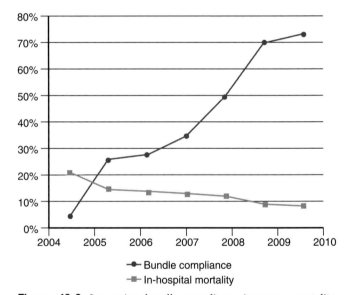

Figure 43-2. Improving bundle compliance improves mortality. *(Adapted from Miller RR 3rd, Dong L, Nelson NC, et al; Intermountain Healthcare Intensive Medicine Clinical Program. Multicenter implementation of a severe sepsis and septic shock treatment bundle.* Am J Respir Crit Care Med. *2013;188(1):77–82.)*

mortality. Continued participation in the SSC led to additional reductions in mortality by 7% per quarter. In addition, for every 10% increase in bundle use, there were significant decreases in hospital and ICU lengths of stay.

Although there are regional differences in bundle compliance and mortality, improved outcomes are not limited to resource-intensive settings when there is adherence to the SSC bundles. Raymond and colleagues showed that bundle compliance in India reduced mortality from 35% to 21%,[1] including reductions in intensive care length of stay

and ventilator-free days. Similar observations have been seen in China and Brazil.[12,13] As of 2014, there are more than 40 studies showing that increased bundle compliance leads to improvements in mortality. As a corollary, noncompliance with these bundles was associated with increases in hospital mortality. In fact, a study in the United Kingdom showed that noncompliance with the 6-hour sepsis bundle was associated with a more than twofold increase in hospital mortality.[14]

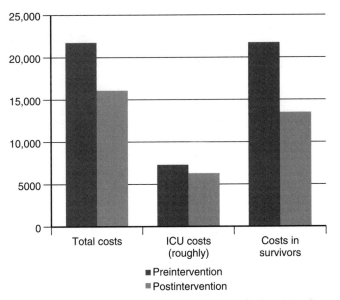

Figure 43-3. Cost savings from implementation of a Surviving Sepsis Campaign bundle. *ICU,* intensive care unit. *(From Shorr AF, Micek ST, Jackson WL Jr, Kollef MH. Economic implications of an evidence-based sepsis protocol: can we improve outcomes and lower costs? Crit Care Med. 2007;35(5):1257–1262.)*

Is There Evidence That the SSC Bundles Are Cost-Effective?

Treatment of severe sepsis and septic shock is resource intensive, with annual costs exceeding $20 billion in the United States alone.[3] Several studies have analyzed the cost-effectiveness, from a health-care perspective, of compliance with the SSC bundle elements. On implementation, the overall mean cost per patient may increase; however, this is driven by improved survival leading to increased length of stay. The incremental cost-effectiveness ratio, a commonly used approach to decision making regarding health interventions, was as low as €4435 per life year gained (LYG) in one such study from Spain.[7] This ratio was significantly lower than the frequently used limit of €30,000 per LYG to gauge cost-effectiveness of an intervention in that country. Data from the United States showed a reduction of nearly $5000/patient when the SSC bundles were implemented.[15] ICU costs fell by nearly 35%, and there was a simultaneous reduction in hospital length of stay by around 5 days. In a subgroup analysis, the cost savings was $8000 per survivor, despite an increase in hospital length of stay (Fig. 43-3).

In a period where health-care spending is being scrutinized, such cost-saving measures have important economic implications. With the extrapolation of the data described previously to all patients with severe sepsis and septic shock, consistent adherence to the SSC bundle elements could potentially save $4 billion annually in the United States.

SUMMARY

There is overwhelming evidence that implementation of the SSC bundles saves lives as well as reduces health-care spending. Through the bundles, the SSC has successfully created a paradigm shift in the approach to severe sepsis and septic shock. Therein lies the strength of bundles: guidelines that may take years to change clinical behavior can now be distilled into something easily implementable at the bedside. As new evidence becomes available, these bundle elements can be adapted and the new evidence quickly translated to improved patient care.

AUTHORS' RECOMMENDATIONS

- The Surviving Sepsis Guidelines consist of a series of bundled interventions that aim to improve outcome by standardizing care.
- When bundled together, evidence-based interventions are thought to have a greater impact on outcomes than the sum of the individual components.
- To date, multiple publications have demonstrated a compelling relationship between improved outcomes and compliance with the SSC bundles. This also has been shown to reduce health care spending.
- Worldwide, the SSC has been associated with reduced mortality in patients diagnosed with sepsis. It is unclear whether this universal benefit arises from bundle implementation, increased awareness of sepsis or both.
- The major benefit of bundles over guidelines is simplicity and plasticity. Bundles can be rapidly rolled out and easily implemented. Compliance is relatively easy to audit. Bundles can be changed quickly as new evidence emerges.

REFERENCES

1. Khan P, Divatia JV. Severe sepsis bundles. *Indian J Crit Care Med.* January 2010;14(1):8–13. http://dx.doi.org/10.4103/0972-5229.63028. PubMed PMID: 20606903; PubMed Central PMCID: PMC2888324.
2. Brun-Buisson C, Doyon F, Carlet J, et al. Incidence, risk factors, and outcome of severe sepsis and septic shock in adults. A multicenter prospective study in intensive care units. French ICU Group for Severe Sepsis. *JAMA.* September 27, 1995;274(12):968–974. PubMed PMID: 7674528.
3. http://www.ihi.org/topics/Sepsis/Pages/default.aspx.
4. Torio CM, Andrews RM. *National Inpatient Hospital Costs: The Most Expensive Conditions by Payer, 2011: Statistical Brief #160*; August 2013. Healthcare Cost and Utilization Project (HCUP) Statistical Briefs [Internet]. Rockville (MD): Agency for Health Care Policy and Research (US); February 2006.
5. Levy MM, Dellinger RP, Townsend SR, et al. The Surviving Sepsis Campaign: results of an international guideline-based performance improvement program targeting severe sepsis. *Intensive Care Med.* February 2010;36(2):222–231. http://dx.doi.org/10.1007/s00134-009-1738-3. Epub 2010 Jan 13. Review. PubMed PMID: 20069275.
6. Ferrer R, Artigas A, Levy MM, Blanco J, Edusepsis Study Group, et al. Improvement in process of care and outcome after a multicenter severe sepsis educational program in Spain. *JAMA.* May 21, 2008;299(19):2294–2303. http://dx.doi.org/10.1001/jama.299.19.2294. PubMed PMID: 18492971.
7. Suarez D, Ferrer R, Artigas A, Edusepsis Study Group, et al. Cost-effectiveness of the Surviving Sepsis Campaign protocol for severe sepsis: a prospective nation-wide study in Spain. *Intensive Care Med.* March 2011;37(3):444–452. http://dx.doi.org/10.1007/s00134-010-2102-3. Epub 2010 Dec 9. PubMed PMID: 21152895.
8. http://www.survivingsepsis.org/Bundles/Pages/default.aspx.
9. Miller 3rd RR, Dong L, Nelson NC, Intermountain Healthcare Intensive Medicine Clinical Program, et al. Multicenter implementation of a severe sepsis and septic shock treatment bundle. *Am J Respir Crit Care Med.* July 1, 2013;188(1):77–82.
10. Levy MM, Rhodes A, Phillips GS, Townsend SR, et al. Surviving Sepsis Campaign:Association Between Performance Metrics and Outcomes in a 7.5-Year Study. *Crit Care Med.* 2015;43:3–12.

11. Levy MM, Rhodes A, Phillips GS, Townsend SR, et al. Surviving Sepsis Campaign: association between performance metrics and outcomes in a 7.5-year study. *Intensive Care Med*. 2014;40:1623–1633.

12. Li ZQ, Xi XM, Luo X, et al. Implementing surviving sepsis campaign bundles in China: a prospective cohort study. *Chin Med J (Engl)*. 2013;126(10):1819–1825. PubMed PMID: 23673093.

13. Shiramizo SC, Marra AR, Durão MS, et al. Decreasing mortality in severe sepsis and septic shock patients by implementing a sepsis bundle in a hospital setting. *PLoS One*. 2011;6(11):e26790. http://dx.doi.org/10.1371/journal.pone.0026790. Epub 2011 Nov 3. PubMed PMID: 22073193.

14. Gao F, Melody T, Daniels DF, et al. The impact of compliance with 6-hour and 24-hour sepsis bundles on hospital mortality in patients with severe sepsis: a prospective observational study. *Crit Care*. 2005;9(6):R764–R770. Epub 2005 Nov 11. PubMed PMID: 16356225; PubMed Central PMCID: PMC1414020.

15. Shorr AF, Micek ST, Jackson Jr WL, et al. Economic implications of an evidence-based sepsis protocol: can we improve outcomes and lower costs?. *Crit Care Med*. May 2007;35(5):1257–1262. PubMed PMID: 17414080.

16. Dellinger RP, Levy MM, Rhodes A, Surviving Sepsis Campaign Guidelines Committee including The Pediatric Subgroup, et al. Surviving Sepsis Campaign: international guidelines for management of severe sepsis and septic shock, 2012. *Intensive Care Med*. February 2013;39(2):165–228. http://dx.doi.org/10.1007/s00134-012-2769-8. Epub 2013 Jan 30. PubMed PMID: 23361625.

44 | Has Outcome in Sepsis Improved? What Has Worked? What Has Not Worked?

Jean-Louis Vincent

Sepsis, defined as some degree of associated organ dysfunction attributed to a dysregulated host response in association with severe infection,[1] remains a common condition affecting 1% to 11% of hospitalized patients[2-4] and about 30% of intensive care unit (ICU) patients.[5,6]

HAVE OUTCOMES FROM SEPSIS IMPROVED?

Recent studies have suggested that outcomes for patients with sepsis have improved over the years.[7] As early as 1998, in a review of studies examining patients with septic shock published between 1958 and 1997, Friedman et al. reported a decrease in hospital mortality rates from about 65% to about 42%.[8] In another early study, Martin et al.[9] reported that in-hospital mortality rates for patients with sepsis admitted to a sample of U.S. hospitals decreased from 28% for the period 1979 to 1984 and 18% for the period 1995 to 2000. More recently, Stevenson et al.[10] used data from the control arms of randomized clinical trials in patients with sepsis published between 1991 and 2009 and reported a 3% annual decrease in 28-day mortality rates ($P = .009$). The same authors and others have reported similar trends for in-hospital mortality when using administrative hospitalization data in the United States[10-13] and other countries.[14,15] Using data from the Australian and New Zealand Intensive Care Society adult ICU patient database, Kaukonen et al.[16] reported an absolute decrease in the hospital mortality rate of sepsis from 35% in 2000 to 18.4% in 2012; after logistic regression analysis, the odds ratio (OR) for mortality was 0.49 (95% confidence interval [CI], 0.46 to 0.52) in 2012 with 2000 as reference.

Taken together, there is, therefore, some evidence of improved outcomes from sepsis over the last couple of decades (Table 44-1). Nevertheless, the apparent extent of the decrease in mortality should be interpreted with some caution. Indeed, increased awareness of sepsis, changes in the code definitions used to classify the disorder, and altered reimbursement strategies have likely led to an inclusion of an increased number of patients with less severe disease and, hence, inherently lower risk of death, in studies on sepsis; this effect certainly accounts for some of the reported temporal increase in the number of septic patients—including less severe cases—with concurrent decrease in mortality.[17-19]

WHAT HAS NOT WORKED?

Over the years, our understanding of the pathophysiology of sepsis has improved so that many of the complex responses to infection and how they interact to cause sepsis are now well detailed and defined.[20] Multiple pathways and molecules have been identified as potential targets for therapeutic intervention; however, despite more than 100 randomized controlled clinical trials of sepsis-modulating therapies, no effective intervention has been identified.[21] Clearly then, this approach to improve survival has not worked. There have been many putative explanations for these apparent "failed" trials, including discrepancies arising when preclinical models and experimental data are translated to the clinical arena; issues with the in vivo efficacy of the intervention under examination; concerns about the dose and timing of the intervention; and problems with clinical trial design, including choice of outcome measures.[21] Perhaps the key problem, though, has been in the selection of patients for these studies. Lack of a clear and specific definition or marker of sepsis has led to the inclusion of very heterogeneous groups of patients. Patients with different degrees of disease severity, different sepsis sources and causative microorganisms, different genetic backgrounds, and different comorbidities and ages have all received the same intervention. Many studies also included multiple centers with an associated variability in standards of care, resource availability, and staff training.[21] Moreover, it has become apparent that patients have different types of immune response—both proinflammatory and anti-inflammatory responses are present simultaneously—and the balance between these two forms may determine a patient's response to treatment.[22] This has rarely been taken into consideration when clinical trials are designed. In a trial that includes such heterogeneous groups of patients, a single intervention may be of benefit in some but harmful

Table 44-1 Some of the Published Studies Reporting Trends in Mortality Rates in Sepsis

First Author (References)	Patients	Type of Data	Year Span	Change in Mortality Rate
Friedman[8]	Septic shock	Systematic review	1958-1997	Hospital mortality decreased from 65% to 42%
Martin[9]	Sepsis	Hospital discharge records, ICD codes	1979/1984-1995/2000	Hospital mortality decreased from 28% to 18%
van Ruler[56]	Severe sepsis	Control arms of randomized trials of sepsis treatment	1990-2000	Hospital mortality decreased from 44% to 35%
Dombrovskiy[57]	Severe sepsis	National inpatient database, ICD codes	1995-2002	Hospital case fatality rate decreased from 51% to 45%
Dombrovskiy[58]	Sepsis	ICD codes	1993-2003	Hospital case fatality rate decreased from 46% to 38%
Harrison[14]	Severe sepsis	National ICU database	1996-2004	Hospital mortality decreased from 48% to 45%
Kumar[11]	Severe sepsis	National inpatient database, ICD codes	2000-2007	Hospital mortality decreased from 39% to 27%
Lagu[12]	Severe sepsis	National inpatient database, ICD codes	2003-2007	Hospital mortality decreased from 37% to 29%
Ani[13]	Severe sepsis	Administrative database, ICD codes	1999-2008	Hospital mortality decreased from 40% to 28%
Dreiher[59]	Sepsis	Retrospective multicenter cohort	2002-2008	Hospital mortality unchanged (53% vs. 55%)
Stevenson[10]	Sepsis	Control arms of randomized trials of sepsis treatment	1991/1995-2006/2009	Hospital mortality decreased from 47% to 29%
Ayala-Ramírez[15]	Sepsis	Administrative database, ICD codes	2003-2011	Hospital mortality decreased from 40% to 32% in males and from 42% to 35% in females only in patients with severe sepsis
Kaukonen[16]	Sepsis	Retrospective, multicenter, observational study	2000-2012	Hospital mortality decreased from 35% to 18%

ICD, International Classification of Diseases; *ICU,* intensive care unit.

in others so that the overall study outcome may not accurately reflect the true efficacy of the therapeutic agent had it been tested in a more select population. For example, a patient with a primarily proinflammatory response is unlikely to respond to an agent that further promotes inflammation; thus administration of granulocyte colony-stimulating factor (G-CSF) to all patients with septic shock was not associated with improved outcomes.[23] Similarly, giving an anti-inflammatory agent to a patient who is already immunosuppressed will probably not be of benefit. Indeed, in many of the studies of immunomodulatory agents that showed no overall improvement in outcome, beneficial effects were identified in certain subgroups.[24-30]

Other specific aspects of patient management have also not consistently been shown to be effective. An early goal-directed therapy protocol reduced mortality in a selected group of patients at a single center[31] but had no beneficial effects on outcomes in two larger, multicenter studies.[32,33] Similarly, tight blood glucose control improved outcomes in a single center study on critically ill surgical patients[34] but not in a more general population of ICU patients.[35] Glucocorticoid therapy reduced the risk of death in one study in patients with septic shock,[36] but these effects were not confirmed in later studies.[37]

Single interventions in heterogeneous groups of "septic" patients have therefore clearly not worked. Improving patient characterization so that those patients who are most

likely to respond to the intervention(s) in question can be identified and studied is necessary for future clinical trials in sepsis therapeutics.[38]

WHAT HAS WORKED?

Despite the lack of specific sepsis treatments and some problems with diluted data, patient outcomes from sepsis have improved over the years. Therefore if single specific interventions have not been effective, what has worked? It is logical to invoke two major factors in these improved outcomes: (1) the enhanced awareness of sepsis as a possible diagnosis and realization of the importance of early recognition and management[39] and (2) a gradual improvement in the general process of care for these, and indeed all, critically ill patients.[40,41] Taking the former aspect first, early effective antibiotic treatment, infectious source removal, adequate fluid administration, and vasopressor and organ support have all been associated with improved outcomes.[39] Guidelines with recommendations for best patient care, stressing the need for rapid institution of these practices, have been written by teams of experts,[39] and bundles of care items (including measurement of blood lactate level, early administration of broad-spectrum antibiotics, administration of fluids when hypotension is present, and administration of vasopressors for hypotension that does not readily respond to initial fluid resuscitation) have been developed.[42] Compliance with these bundles has been associated with improved outcomes in different ICU settings,[43-46] although intensivists should not be restricted by specified time limits and all aspects of these bundles should be performed as rapidly as possible. The use of multidisciplinary sepsis response teams has been suggested to improve the initial stabilization of patients with sepsis, ensuring that all aspects of management can be performed rapidly.[47] A specially equipped and staffed room or "shock lab" could similarly improve early management in these patients.[48]

In terms of process of care, of the many aspects that have seen gradual change over the years and led, in combination, to improved patient outcomes in all critically ill patients, including those with sepsis, four merit specific discussion. The development of intensive care as a specialty in its own right with trained intensivists familiar with the complexities of critical illness has contributed hugely to the ongoing improved process of care. First, intensivists have generally become less invasive and less aggressive in some aspects of their patient management. They have come to understand that many of the seemingly pathophysiologic effects of sepsis are, in fact, beneficial and should not necessarily be "treated" or "normalized." The use of interventions that have been associated with poorer outcome has gradually been reduced and even eliminated. Thus, fewer transfusions are given, patients are fed less, tidal volumes have been reduced, and sedation has been minimized. Second, intensivists have come to appreciate the unique circumstances surrounding each patient and have thus individualized treatment rather than manage all ICU patients in the same way. Conversely, intensivists have standardized critical aspects of care by introducing guidelines and protocols so that key elements are less likely to be forgotten or mismanaged. This dichotomy can, in some circumstances, become problematic. Although protocols can improve the delivery of care when quality is suboptimal, especially when there is a shortage of well-trained staff, they may be too rigid in many centers where care is already optimal and may limit intensivists' ability to account for the importance of individual patient factors; here, checklists may be a better approach.[49] Third, intensivists have realized the importance of multidisciplinary teamwork within the ICU setting, moving from a rather paternal, physician-directed approach to patient management and decision making that is much more inclusive, with input from all members of the ICU team, including nurses, physiotherapists, nutritionists, and pharmacists. Good teamwork can help reduce medical errors and improve job satisfaction, as well as improve patient outcomes.[50,51] One of the key aspects of good teamwork is good communication, and this concept extends also to patients and their relatives. Patients, whenever possible, and next of kin are now informed more openly of patient progress, treatment options, and likely prognosis. End-of-life decisions in particular are now discussed more candidly and clearly with families, and patients increasingly share in the decision-making process.[52,53] Fourth, realization of the importance of early recognition and management of critical illness has led many hospitals to extend the ICU beyond its physical four-wall structure by creating medical emergency teams or ICU outreach teams. These consist of trained intensivists, nursing staff, or both who can assess and initiate management of patients on the general ward before they deteriorate to the point where they require ICU admission.[54] Critical illness generally starts some time before ICU admission, and the severity of illness could potentially be limited by early intervention, thus improving patient outcomes.[55] Similarly, early patient mobilization has largely improved the convalescent phase.

CONCLUSION

Sepsis remains a common condition in critically ill patients. Improvements in the process of care for these patients in general, and in early recognition and management of patients with sepsis in particular, have helped improve survival rates, but further progress is needed. Improvements in diagnostic methods will facilitate more rapid patient management, and better patient characterization will help select more homogeneous patient groups for clinical trials of new specific sepsis therapies. Early administration of appropriate antibiotics, early source control when needed, rapid resuscitation, and hemodynamic stabilization must remain the key focus of patient management, and dedicated sepsis teams can help achieve these targets.

AUTHOR'S RECOMMENDATIONS

- Mortality rates from sepsis have decreased in recent years but likely to a lesser degree than reports suggest.
- There are no specific treatments for sepsis, and management relies on early diagnosis and rapid anti-infective strategies, together with early and complete resuscitation.
- Improvement in the process of care for all critically ill patients is the main reason behind the improved mortality rates in patients with sepsis.

REFERENCES

1. Vincent JL, Opal S, Marshall JC, et al. Sepsis definitions: time for change. *Lancet*. 2013;381:774–775.
2. Sundararajan V, Macisaac CM, Presneill JJ, et al. Epidemiology of sepsis in Victoria, Australia. *Crit Care Med*. 2005;33:71–80.
3. Liu V, Escobar GJ, Greene JD, et al. Hospital deaths in patients with sepsis from 2 independent cohorts. *JAMA*. 2014;312:90–92.
4. Martin GS. Sepsis, severe sepsis and septic shock: changes in incidence, pathogens and outcomes. *Expert Rev Anti Infect Ther*. 2012;10:701–706.
5. Vincent JL, Rello J, Marshall J, et al. International study of the prevalence and outcomes of infection in intensive care units. *JAMA*. 2009;302:2323–2329.
6. Vincent JL, Marshall JC, Namendys-Silva SA, et al. Assessment of the worldwide burden of critical illness: the intensive care over nations (ICON) audit. *Lancet Respir Med*. 2014;2:380–386.
7. Chen YC, Chang SC, Pu C, et al. The impact of nationwide education program on clinical practice in sepsis care and mortality of severe sepsis: a population-based study in Taiwan. *PLoS One*. 2013;8:e77414.
8. Friedman G, Silva E, Vincent JL. Has the mortality of septic shock changed with time? *Crit Care Med*. 1998;26:2078–2086.
9. Martin GS, Mannino DM, Eaton S, et al. The epidemiology of sepsis in the United States from 1979 through 2000. *N Engl J Med*. 2003;348:1546–1554.

10. Stevenson EK, Rubenstein AR, Radin GT, et al. Two decades of mortality trends among patients with severe sepsis: a comparative meta-analysis. *Crit Care Med.* 2014;42:625–631.

11. Kumar G, Kumar N, Taneja A, et al. Nationwide trends of severe sepsis in the 21st century (2000-2007). *Chest.* 2011;140:1223–1231.

12. Lagu T, Rothberg MB, Shieh MS, et al. Hospitalizations, costs, and outcomes of severe sepsis in the United States 2003 to 2007. *Crit Care Med.* 2012;40:754–761.

13. Ani C, Farshidpanah S, Bellinghausen SA, et al. Variations in organism-specific severe sepsis mortality in the United States. *Crit Care Med.* 2015;43:65–77.

14. Harrison DA, Welch CA, Eddleston JM. The epidemiology of severe sepsis in England, Wales and Northern Ireland, 1996 to 2004: secondary analysis of a high quality clinical database, the ICNARC Case Mix Programme Database. *Crit Care.* 2006;10:R42.

15. Ayala-Ramirez OH, Dominguez-Berjon MF, Esteban-Vasallo MD. Trends in hospitalizations of patients with sepsis and factors associated with inpatient mortality in the Region of Madrid, 2003-2011. *Eur J Clin Microbiol Infect Dis.* 2013;33:411–421.

16. Kaukonen KM, Bailey M, Suzuki S, et al. Mortality related to severe sepsis and septic shock among critically ill patients in Australia and New Zealand, 2000-2012. *JAMA.* 2014;311:1308–1316.

17. Lindenauer PK, Lagu T, Shieh MS, et al. Association of diagnostic coding with trends in hospitalizations and mortality of patients with pneumonia, 2003-2009. *JAMA.* 2012;307:1405–1413.

18. Iwashyna TJ, Angus DC. Declining case fatality rates for severe sepsis: good data bring good news with ambiguous implications. *JAMA.* 2014;311:1295–1297.

19. Rhee C, Gohil S, Klompas M. Regulatory mandates for sepsis care–reasons for caution. *N Engl J Med.* 2014;370:1673–1676.

20. Angus DC, van der Poll T. Severe sepsis and septic shock. *N Engl J Med.* 2013;369:840–851.

21. Marshall JC. Why have clinical trials in sepsis failed? *Trends Mol Med.* 2014;20:195–203.

22. Vincent JL. Assessing cellular responses in sepsis. *EBioMedicine.* 2014;1:10–11.

23. Stephens DP, Thomas JH, Higgins A, et al. Randomized, double-blind, placebo-controlled trial of granulocyte colony-stimulating factor in patients with septic shock. *Crit Care Med.* 2008;36:448–454.

24. Greenman RL, Schein RM, Martin MA, et al. A controlled clinical trial of E5 murine monoclonal IgM antibody to endotoxin in the treatment of gram-negative sepsis. The XOMA Sepsis Study Group. *JAMA.* 1991;266:1097–1102.

25. Dhainaut JF, Tenaillon A, Le TY, et al. Platelet-activating factor receptor antagonist BN 52021 in the treatment of severe sepsis: a randomized, double-blind, placebo-controlled, multicenter clinical trial. BN 52021 Sepsis Study Group. *Crit Care Med.* 1994;22:1720–1728.

26. Baudo F, Caimi TM, de Cataldo F, et al. Antithrombin III (ATIII) replacement therapy in patients with sepsis and/or postsurgical complications: a controlled double-blind, randomized, multicenter study. *Intensive Care Med.* 1998;24:336–342.

27. Ziegler EJ, Fisher Jr CJ, Sprung CL, et al. Treatment of gram-negative bacteremia and septic shock with HA-1A human monoclonal antibody against endotoxin. A randomized, double-blind, placebo-controlled trial. The HA-1A Sepsis Study Group. *N Engl J Med.* 1991;324:429–436.

28. Fisher CJ, Dhainaut JF, Opal SM, et al. Recombinant human interleukin 1 receptor antagonist in the treatment of patients with sepsis syndrome. *JAMA.* 1994;271:1836–1843.

29. Kienast J, Juers M, Wiedermann CJ, et al. Treatment effects of high-dose antithrombin without concomitant heparin in patients with severe sepsis with or without disseminated intravascular coagulation. *J Thromb Haemost.* 2006;4:90–97.

30. Laterre PF, Opal SM, Abraham E, et al. A clinical evaluation committee assessment of recombinant human tissue factor pathway inhibitor (tifacogin) in patients with severe community-acquired pneumonia. *Crit Care.* 2009;13:R36.

31. Rivers E, Nguyen B, Havstad S, et al. Early goal-directed therapy in the treatment of severe sepsis and septic shock. *N Engl J Med.* 2001;345:1368–1377.

32. Yealy DM, Kellum JA, Huang DT, et al. A randomized trial of protocol-based care for early septic shock. *N Engl J Med.* 2014;370:1683–1693.

33. Peake SL, Delaney A, Bailey M, et al. Goal-directed resuscitation for patients with early septic shock. *N Engl J Med.* 2014;371:1496–1506.

34. Van den Berghe G, Wouters P, Weekers F, et al. Intensive insulin therapy in critically ill patients. *N Engl J Med.* 2001;345:1359–1367.

35. Finfer S, Chittock DR, Su SY, et al. Intensive versus conventional glucose control in critically ill patients. *N Engl J Med.* 2009;360:1283–1297.

36. Annane D, Sebille V, Charpentier C, et al. Effect of treatment with low doses of hydrocortisone and fludrocortisone on mortality in patients with septic shock. *JAMA.* 2002;288:862–871.

37. Sprung CL, Annane D, Keh D, et al. Hydrocortisone therapy for patients with septic shock. *N Engl J Med.* 2008;358:111–124.

38. Vincent JL, Van Nuffelen M. Septic shock: new pharmacotherapy options or better trial design? *Expert Opin Pharmacother.* 2013;14:561–570.

39. Dellinger RP, Levy MM, Rhodes A, et al. Surviving Sepsis Campaign: international guidelines for management of severe sepsis and septic shock, 2012. *Intensive Care Med.* 2013;39:165–228.

40. Vincent JL, Singer M, Marini JJ, et al. Thirty years of critical care medicine. *Crit Care.* 2010;14:311.

41. Vincent JL. Critical care–where have we been and where are we going? *Crit Care.* 2013;17(suppl 1):S2.

42. Surviving Sepsis Campaign. Bundles. Available at: http://www.survivingsepsis.org/Bundles/Pages/default.aspx

43. Miller III RR, Dong L, Nelson NC, et al. Multicenter implementation of a severe sepsis and septic shock treatment bundle. *Am J Respir Crit Care Med.* 2013;188:77–82.

44. Castellanos-Ortega A, Suberviola B, Garcia-Astudillo LA, et al. Impact of the Surviving Sepsis Campaign protocols on hospital length of stay and mortality in septic shock patients: results of a three-year follow-up quasi-experimental study. *Crit Care Med.* 2010;38:1036–1043.

45. van Zanten AR, Brinkman S, Arbous MS, et al. Guideline bundles adherence and mortality in severe sepsis and septic shock. *Crit Care Med.* 2014;42:1890–1898.

46. Levy MM, Rhodes A, Phillips GS, et al. Surviving Sepsis Campaign: association between performance metrics and outcomes in a 7.5-year study. *Intensive Care Med.* 2014;40:1623–1633.

47. Vincent JL, Pereira AJ, Gleeson J, et al. Early management of sepsis. *Clin Exp Emerg Med.* 2014;1:3–7.

48. Piagnerelli M, Van Nuffelen M, Maetens Y, et al. A 'shock room' for early management of the acutely ill. *Anaesth Intensive Care.* 2009;37:426–431.

49. Vincent JL, Carraso Serrano E, Dimoula A. Current management of sepsis in critically ill adult patients. *Expert Rev Anti Infect Ther.* 2011;9:847–856.

50. Sexton JB, Berenholtz SM, Goeschel CA, et al. Assessing and improving safety climate in a large cohort of intensive care units. *Crit Care Med.* 2011;39:934–939.

51. Dietz AS, Pronovost PJ, Mendez-Tellez PA, et al. A systematic review of teamwork in the intensive care unit: what do we know about teamwork, team tasks, and improvement strategies? *J Crit Care.* 2014;29:908–914.

52. Truog RD, Campbell ML, Curtis JR, et al. Recommendations for end-of-life care in the intensive care unit: a consensus statement by the American College [corrected] of Critical Care Medicine. *Crit Care Med.* 2008;36:953–963.

53. Curtis JR, Vincent JL. Ethics and end-of-life care for adults in the intensive care unit. *Lancet.* 2010;376:1347–1353.

54. Hillman K. Critical care without walls. *Curr Opin Crit Care.* 2002;8:594–599.

55. Beitler JR, Link N, Bails DB, et al. Reduction in hospital-wide mortality after implementation of a rapid response team: a long-term cohort study. *Crit Care.* 2011;15:R269.

56. van Ruler O, Schultz MJ, Reitsma JB, et al. Has mortality from sepsis improved and what to expect from new treatment modalities: review of current insights. *Surg Infect (Larchmt).* 2009;10:339–348.

57. Dombrovskiy VY, Martin AA, Sunderram J, et al. Facing the challenge: decreasing case fatality rates in severe sepsis despite increasing hospitalizations. *Crit Care Med.* 2005;33:2555–2562.

58. Dombrovskiy VY, Martin AA, Sunderram J, et al. Rapid increase in hospitalization and mortality rates for severe sepsis in the United States: a trend analysis from 1993 to 2003. *Crit Care Med.* 2007;35:1244–1250.

59. Dreiher J, Almog Y, Sprung CL, et al. Temporal trends in patient characteristics and survival of intensive care admissions with sepsis: a multicenter analysis. *Crit Care Med.* 2012;40:855–860.

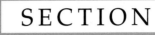
INFECTIONS

45 How Do I Diagnose and Manage Catheter-Related Bloodstream Infections?

Mike Scully

INCIDENCE

Annually in the United States alone, more than 5 million central venous catheters (CVCs) are inserted, and patients are exposed to more than 15 million catheter days in the intensive care unit (ICU).[1] Approximately 250,000 bloodstream infections are reported in hospitals,[2] 80,000 of which are in critical care units.[1] The reported incidence density in the literature is highly variable; in a review by Maki, the reported variance was from 0.1 to 2.7 cases/1000 catheter days.[2] Although some studies have questioned whether catheter-related bloodstream infections (CRBSIs) are associated with mortality,[3] others have reported up to 25% directly attributable deaths.[4] Length of hospital stay and health-care costs are significantly increased by an episode of CRBSI.[5-7] As reported by Shah, on average, affected patients will stay an extra 10 to 20 days in the hospital, with their health-care costs increasing by an additional $4000 to $56,000 per episode of CRBSI.[8] Overall, it is estimated that CRBSI accounts for 11% of health-care–associated infections (HAIs) in the United States.[3,5,9,10] Given the significant impact on patient outcomes, reduction in the incidence of CRBSI has become a priority for health-care providers. However, it is possible to achieve dramatic reductions when institutions have introduced educational programs and policies focused on minimizing their incidence.

DIAGNOSIS

The diagnosis of CRBSI may be established by criteria where the catheter is left in situ and separate criteria where the catheter has been removed. In the clinical context, where a patient manifests signs of sepsis, a CVC is in situ and there is no other focus of sepsis identified, then the likelihood of the catheter being the source is increased. Where the catheter is not removed, the quantitative method to establish the diagnosis is more than 100 colony-forming units (CFUs)/mL of blood drawn through the CVC. It is recommended to pair the sample obtained from the CVC with peripherally obtained cultures. Confirmatory evidence of line infection is indicated when the same species is identified in both CVC and peripherally drawn samples, there is a differential time to positivity of more than 2 hours for CVC drawn samples, and the culture yield is more than

fivefold higher for the blood obtained through the catheter. The criteria for diagnosis where the catheter has been removed are established by a positive culture of a catheter segment; this may be semiquantitative (>15 CFU) or quantitative (>1000 CFU).[1,3]

PATHOGENESIS

Infection of an in-dwelling catheter occurs by a number of mechanisms. Organisms that have colonized the patient's skin may track along the catheter path and infect the catheter tip.[11,12] This is the most likely portal in the short-term (<10 days in situ).[11] Infection of the catheter hub tips may also occur as a result of handling by health-care personnel;[13,14] this appears to be the leading etiology when the catheter has been in situ for a prolonged period.[1] Rarely, CRBSI may result because of hematogenous seeding of the catheter from a remote source of sepsis, such as pneumonia.[15] Finally, contaminated infusions have been implicated in rare instances.[16]

ORGANISMS

Epidemiologic data on organisms frequently identified are compiled in the United States by the National Healthcare Safety Network (NHSN) of the Centers for Disease Control and Prevention (CDC). The most common isolates remain coagulase-negative staphylococci (31%), but *Staphylococcus aureus* (20%) and enterococci (9%) are also frequent isolates.[17,18] Fungi have become more prevalent, and *Candida* species are increasingly implicated as the pathogen involved (currently 9%).[17] Gram-negative organisms now appear to account for approximately 20% of cases, with *Escherichia coli* and *Klebsiella* subspecies accounting for 6% and 5%, respectively.[19] Antimicrobial resistance is also increasing; cases of gram-negative organisms resistant to third-generation cephalosporins and carbapenems are becoming more prevalent.[19] This is also the case with *Candida* infections where fluconazole resistance is becoming more common.[3] However, methicillin-resistant *Staphylococcus aureus* (MRSA) infections appear to be decreasing.[18] However, isolation of *Staphylococcus* infections should prompt a thorough evaluation for endocarditis, including echocardiography.[20]

RISK FACTORS

Several risk factors have been identified, including the following:

1. Inexperience of the physician performing the procedure.[2,3]
2. Failure to adhere to maximum sterile barrier precautions; this requires thorough antisepsis of the insertion site, all health-care–associated personnel in the vicinity to wear protective clothing, and draping of the patient's whole body with sterile covers.
3. Density of flora on the patient's skin surface.[3]
4. Duration of catheter insertion; the risk is magnified fourfold when the catheter is in situ more than 7 days and fivefold when the catheter is in more than 15 days.[11]
5. In the ICU, a high nurse/patient ratio.[21]
6. Patient factors, such as immune status, nutritional state, steroid therapy, and coincidental sepsis.

Other considerations include the antiseptic solution used, the material used to manufacture the catheter, and the pathogenicity of the infecting organism. Chlorhexidine (at least 0.5% in alcohol; ideally 2%) has become the standard antiseptic solution; data from studies suggest that its use may be associated with a 1.6% decrease in CRBSI and 0.23% mortality improvement, with associated cost benefits.[22,23] However, on repeated exposure, patients may become sensitized, and rarely, severe reactions, including anaphylaxis, have been described. Povidone-iodine and 70% alcohol are acceptable alternatives in these cases. In relation to catheter material, devices manufactured with polyvinyl chloride or polyethylene appear to have a higher rate of colonization and CRBSI than those manufactured with polytetrafluoroethylene or polyurethane because they may be intrinsically less resistant to biofilm formation.[24,25]

PREVENTION

Prevention of HAI has become a priority for health-care providers. In relation to CRBSI, Pronovost demonstrated in a large study of 103 ICUs (representing > 375,000 CVC days) a mean reduction in incidence density from 7.7 to 1.4/1000 catheter days at 18 months after the adoption of a specific protocol.[4] The interventions were five straightforward practices: meticulous hand hygiene, sterile barrier precautions, chlorhexidine antisepsis, avoidance of the femoral site, and removal of the catheter when no longer clinically indicated (Table 45-1). Comprehensive

---

Table 45-1 Central Line "Bundle" Shown to Reduce CRBSI[4]

1. Handwashing
2. Full-barrier precautions (during the insertion of CVC)
3. Chlorhexidine (2%) to clean the skin (allow to dry before insertion)
4. Avoiding the femoral site if possible
5. Removing unnecessary catheters

CRBSI, catheter-related bloodstream infection; *CVC,* central venous catheter.

---

guidelines have been published to assist institutions in devising evidence-based programs to reduce their rate of CRBSI.[4]

Meticulous attention to hygiene is a fundamental objective that must be achieved. Investment in education and training in performing CVC insertion is imperative and is required on an institution-wide basis given the prevalence of these infections in the non-ICU environment. Handling of the line after insertion demands strict observation of hand hygiene practices and correct management of infusates, lines, and dressings. Use of two-dimensional (2-D) ultrasound has not definitively demonstrated a reduction in the incidence of CRBSI; however, there is a reduction in technical complications (such as carotid arterial puncture), time to insertion, and possibly reduced colonization at the internal jugular site.[26] Consequently, if the technology is unavailable, ultrasound-guided CVC insertion is recommended. Where possible, a nonsuture-based anchoring device should be used.[3,27] In addition to a chlorhexidine-based antiseptic agent, use of a chlorhexidine-impregnated sponge device placed at the line insertion site has demonstrated efficacy at reducing CRBSI even where the baseline rate of infection was low.[28] Similarly, daily cleansing of the catheter insertion site with a 2% chlorhexidine wash is also beneficial.

The subclavian vein is the recommended site for routine line placement, for example, for total parenteral nutrition (TPN).[3] This is, however, controversial. Studies have shown that, compared with the subclavian site, there are higher rates of colonization of both the internal jugular and the femoral sites (in particular with obese patients).[29-32] Surprisingly, this does not appear to translate to higher rates of infection.[33] The subclavian site is associated with a higher rate of complications—inadvertent arterial puncture or pneumothorax—and is technically more difficult to perform with ultrasound guidance. Therefore, while the subclavian site may appear to be the preferred option, the clinician must consider other factors when deciding on the site for line placement, such as respiratory reserve in the event of pneumothorax or coagulopathy. It is clear, however, that attempting to reduce the burden of skin colonization with prophylactic antibiotics does not reduce the incidence of CRBSI, and their use for this purpose is not indicated. Similarly, although there appears to be a linear relationship between the duration of line insertion and the CRBSI, scheduled line removal and reinsertion expose the patient to the technical hazards of the procedures without the benefit of reducing the CRBSI rate.[3] Instead, a transparent dressing should be applied enabling daily inspection of the site, with prompt removal of the line if any symptoms of sepsis develop in the absence of another focus.

Care of the management of infusion is critical. For nonblood- or nonlipid-containing preparations where the infusions are administered without interruption, it is recommended that the administration sets are changed between 4 and 7 days. For lipid-based preparations, this frequency is typically increased, and on average it is advised to change these sets every 24 hours. Propofol administration sets should be changed every 6 to 12 hours.[3]

As discussed previously, the material used to manufacture the catheter can influence the development of CRBSI. As a further development, catheters coated with antiseptics (typically chlorhexidine/silver sulfadiazine) or antibiotics (minocycline/rifampicin) have been developed.[34,35] The current second generation of antiseptic-coated catheters differs from the earlier version by having triple the amount of antiseptic applied. They are also coated on internal and external lumina, as opposed to the eternal lumen only in the first-generation device.[36] These second-generation antibiotic-coated catheters demonstrated superiority in reducing CRBSI when compared with the first-generation antiseptic-coated lines.[36] A Cochrane Collaboration meta-analysis of studies comparing impregnated with "plain" central lines demonstrated outcome benefit in intensive care (relative risk [RR], 0.68; 95% confidence interval [CI], 0.59 to 0.78) but not in hematology or oncology units and not in long-term TPN patients.[37] It is recommended that impregnated catheters be considered for use in instances where a catheter is expected to be left in situ for more than 5 days and the institutional CRBSI rate remains above an acceptable threshold despite instituting a comprehensive training and education program and adoption of best practices.[3,8]

AUTHOR'S RECOMMENDATIONS

- CRBSIs are common, increase health-care costs, and adversely affect patient outcomes.
- It is possible to achieve extremely low levels of CRBSI by instituting a series of noncomplex interventions supported by an educational and training program (Table 45-1).
- The subclavian route is associated with the lowest incidence of CRBSIs but a higher incidence of technical complications.
- Ultrasound guidance does not reduce the incidence of CRBSI but may reduce the incidence of technical complications during catheter insertion.
- Antibiotic-impregnated catheters reduce CRBSIs in the ICU and are recommended in cases where central catheterization is expected to exceed 5 days.

REFERENCES

1. Mermel LA. Prevention of intravascular catheter-related infections. *Ann Intern Med.* 2000;132:391–402.
2. Maki DG, Kluger DM, Crnich CJ. The risk of bloodstream infection in adults with different intravascular devices: a systematic review of 200 published prospective studies. *Mayo Clin Proc.* 2006;81(9):1159–1171.
3. O'Grady NP, Alexander M, Burns LA, Healthcare Infection Control Practices Advisory Committee, et al. Guidelines for the prevention of intravascular catheter-related infections. *Am J Infect Control.* May 2011;39(4 suppl 1):S1–S34.
4. Pronovost P, Needham D, Berenholtz S, et al. An intervention to decrease catheter-related bloodstream infections in the ICU. *N Engl J Med.* 2006;355(26):2725–2732.
5. Dimick JB, Pelz RK, Consunji R, et al. Increased resource use associated with catheter-related bloodstream infection in the surgical intensive care unit. *Arch Surg.* 2001;136:229–234.
6. Warren DK, Quadir WW, Hollenbeak CS, et al. Attributable cost of catheter-associated bloodstream infections among intensive care patients in a nonteaching hospital. *Crit Care Med.* 2006;34:2084–2089.
7. Blot SI, Depuydt P, Annemans L, et al. Clinical and economic outcomes in critically ill patients with nosocomial catheter-related bloodstream infections. *Clin Infect Dis.* 2005;41:1591–1598.
8. Shah H, Bosch W, Thompson KM, Hellinger WC. Intravascular Catheter-Related Bloodstream Infection. *Neurohospitalist.* 2013;3(3):144–151.
9. Warren DK, Quadir WW, Hollenbeak CS, Elward AM, Cox MJ, Fraser VJ. Attributable cost of catheter-associated bloodstream infections among intensive care patients in a nonteaching hospital. *Crit Care Med.* 2006;34:2084–2089.
10. Blot SI, Depuydt P, Annemans L, et al. Clinical and economic outcomes in critically ill patients with nosocomial catheter-related bloodstream infections. *Clin Infect Dis.* 2005;41:1591–1598.
11. Safdar N, Maki DG. The pathogenesis of catheter-related bloodstream infection with noncuffed short-term central venous catheters. *Intensive Care Med.* 2004;30:62–67.
12. Maki DG, Weise CE, Sarafin HW. A semiquantitative culture method for identifying intravenous-catheter-related infection. *N Engl J Med.* 1977;296:1305–1309.
13. Raad I, Costerton W, Sabharwal U, Sacilowski M, Anaissie E, Bodey GP. Ultrastructural analysis of indwelling vascular catheters: a quantitative relationship between luminal colonization and duration of placement. *J Infect Dis.* 1993;168:400–407.
14. Dobbins BM, Kite P, Kindon A, McMahon MJ, Wilcox MH. DNA fingerprinting analysis of coagulase negative staphylococci implicated in catheter related bloodstream infections. *J Clin Pathol.* 2002;55:824–828.
15. Anaissie E, Samonis G, Kontoyiannis D, et al. Role of catheter colonization and infrequent hematogenous seeding in catheter-related infections. *Eur J Clin Microbiol Infect Dis.* 1995;14:134–137.
16. Raad I, Hanna HA, Awad A, et al. Optimal frequency of changing intravenous administration sets: is it safe to prolong use beyond 72 hours? *Infect Control Hosp Epidemiol.* 2001;22:136–139.
17. Wisplinghoff H, Bischoff T, Tallent SM, Seifert H, Wenzel RP, Edmond MB. Nosocomial bloodstream infections in US hospitals: analysis of 24,179 cases from a prospective nationwide surveillance study. *Clin Infect Dis.* 2004;39:309–317.
18. Burton DC, Edwards JR, Horan TC, Jernigan JA, Fridkin SK. Methicillin-resistant *Staphylococcus aureus* central line-associated bloodstream infections in US intensive care units, 1997–2007. *JAMA.* 2009;301:727–736.
19. Gaynes R, Edwards JR. Overview of nosocomial infections caused by gram-negative bacilli. *Clin Infect Dis.* 2005;41:848–854.
20. Holland TL, Arnold C, Fowler VG. Clinical Management of *Staphylococcus aureus* bacteremia; a review. *JAMA.* 2014;312(13):1330–1341.
21. Fridkin SK, Pear SM, Williamson TH, Galgiani JN, Jarvis WR. The role of understaffing in central venous catheter-associated bloodstream infections. *Infect Control Hosp Epidemiol.* 1996;17:150–158.
22. Maki D, Ringer D, Alvarado CJ. Prospective randomised trial of povidone-iodine, alcohol and chlorhexidine for prevention of infection associated with central venous and arterial catheters. *Lancet.* 1991;338(8763):339–343.
23. Chaiyakunapruk N, Veenstra DL, Lipsky BA, Sullivan SD, Saint S. Vascular catheter site care; the clinical and economic benefits of chlorhexidine-gluconate compared with povidone-iodine. *Clin Infec Dis.* 2003;37(6):764–771.
24. Sheth NK, Franson TR, Rose HD, Buckmire FL, Cooper JA, Sohnle PG. Colonization of bacteria on polyvinyl chloride and Teflon intravascular catheters in hospitalized patients. *J Clin Microbiol.* 1983;18:1061–1063.
25. Maki DG, Ringer M. Evaluation of dressing regimens for prevention of infection with peripheral intravenous catheters. Gauze, a transparent polyurethane dressing, and an iodophor-transparent dressing. *JAMA.* 1987;258:2396–2403.
26. Karakitsos D, Labropoulos N, De Groot E. Ultrasound-guided catheterization of the internal jugular vein; a prospective comparison with the landmark technique in critically ill patients. *Crit Care.* 2006;10(6):R162.
27. Yamamoto AJ, Solomon JA, Soulen MC, et al. Sutureless securement device reduces complications of peripherally inserted central venous catheters. *J Vasc Interv Radiol.* 2002;13:77–81.
28. Timsit JF, Schwebel C, Bouadma L, et al. Chlorhexidine-impregnated sponges and less frequent dressing changes for prevention of catheter-related infections in critically ill adults: a randomized controlled trial. *JAMA.* 2009;301:1231–1241.
29. Goetz AM, Wagener MM, Miller J, Muder RR. Risk of infection due to central venous catheters: effect of site of placement and catheter type. *Infect Control Hosp Epidemiol.* 1998;19(11):842–845.
30. Mermel LA, McCormick RD, Spring SR, Maki DG. The pathogenesis and epidemiology of catheter-related infection with pulmonary artery Swan-Ganz catheters: a prospective study utilizing molecular subtyping. *Am J Med.* 1991;91(3B):197S–205S.

31. Richet H, Hubert B, Nitenberg G. Prospective multi-center study of vascular catheter related complications and risk-factors for positive central culture catheters in intensive care unit patients. *J Clin Microbiol*. 1990;28(11):2520–2525.

32. Gowardmen JR, Robertson IK, Parkes S, Rickard CM. Influence of insertion site on central venous catheter colonization and blood stream infection rates. *Intensive care Med*. 2008;34(6):1038–1045.

33. Parienti JJ, du Cheyron D, Timsit JF, et al. Meta-analysis of subclavian insertion and nontunneled central venous catheter-associated infection risk reduction in critically ill adults. *Crit Care Med*. 2012;40(5):1627–1634.

34. Darouiche RO, Raad II, Heard SO, et al. A comparison of two antimicrobial-impregnated central venous catheters. Catheter Study Group. *N Engl J Med*. 1999;340:1–8.

35. Veenstra DL, Saint S, Sullivan SD. Cost-effectiveness of antiseptic-impregnated central venous catheters for the prevention of catheter-related bloodstream infection. *JAMA*. 1999;282: 554–560.

36. Rupp ME, Lisco SJ, Lipsett PA, et al. Effect of a second-generation venous catheter impregnated with chlorhexidine and silver sulfadiazine on central catheter-related infections: a randomized, controlled trial. *Ann Intern Med*. 2005;143:570–580.

37. Lai NM, Chaiyakunapruk N, Lai NA, O'Riordan E, Pau WSC, Saint S. Catheter impregnation, coating or bonding for reducing central venous catheter-related infections in adults. *Cochrane Database Syst Rev*. 2013;6:CD007878. http://dx.doi.org/10.1002/14651858. CD007878.pub2.

46 | Is Selective Decontamination of the Digestive Tract Useful?

John Lyons, Craig M. Coopersmith

Selective decontamination of the digestive tract (SDD) refers to the administration of prophylactic antibiotics to critically ill patients in the hopes of either preventing or treating airway or digestive tract colonization by organisms that could potentially cause an infection. The rationale behind this practice posits that elimination of selected microorganisms from the oropharynx and upper gastrointestinal (GI) tract will prevent respiratory or bloodstream infections in critically ill patients.

The question of whether to implement SDD on a regular basis is somewhat unique. SDD has been extensively investigated through numerous randomized trials and multiple meta-analyses, with the preponderance of data supporting its use as beneficial. Despite the large literature supporting its use, a consensus on the appropriateness of SDD is lacking among critical care practitioners worldwide, and, in fact, large-scale adoption of SDD has not occurred because of continued concerns about SDD inducing antibiotic resistance.

DETAILS OF SELECTIVE DECONTAMINATION OF THE DIGESTIVE TRACT

The prevention of aerodigestive tract colonization with pathogenic bacteria is the goal of SDD. Theoretically, selectively decreasing the bacterial populations of the upper digestive tract and airway of critically ill patients should decrease the risk of developing ventilator-associated pneumonia.[1,2] As such, SDD protocols aim to selectively limit the presence of potentially harmful bacteria without adversely impacting the overall microbiome of the patient or the intensive care unit (ICU). Antibiotics used in SDD plans are therefore chosen to treat two different groups of microbes: endogenous bacteria already present in patients that could become pathogenic (such as *Staphylococcus aureus* or *Streptococcus pneumoniae*), and gram-negative organisms that may secondarily colonize a patient during acute illness. Therefore SDD typically involves the administration of (1) a short intravenous course of a broad-spectrum cephalosporin aimed at treating existing, potentially pathogenic organisms and (2) ongoing enteral administration of nonabsorbable agents targeted toward gram-negative bacteria.

SDD should be contrasted with *selective oral decontamination,* or SOD, which treats only the oral cavity. Although SOD is frequently a component of broader SDD treatment plans, confusion may arise in interpreting study results because authors may varyingly consider SDD and SOD to be identical or separate interventions. For the purpose of clarity, this chapter distinguishes between the two whenever possible.

Representative examples of treatment strategies for both SDD and SOD are listed in Table 46-1.[3,4] SDD contains three components: (a) third-generation cephalosporins are dosed intravenously during the first 4 to 5 days of ICU admission, (b) nonabsorbable enteral antibiotics are given in a liquid form through a nasoenteric tube, and (c) pastes or gels are given to the oropharynx. The most commonly used enteral and oral agents are amphotericin, colistin, and tobramycin, although several other agents have also been studied.[5-11] Although the term *SDD* is universally used, in actuality, it is a misnomer because there are multiple components to successful treatment regiments, including elements that are not directed at the digestive system per se.

In contrast to SDD, SOD omits parenteral and enteral treatments and uses only oral pastes.[3,12,13]

EVIDENCE ON THE EFFICACY OF SELECTIVE DECONTAMINATION OF THE DIGESTIVE TRACT

SDD has been extensively studied. Investigations include numerous randomized trials and meta-analyses with results that generally indicate benefit in ICU patients. An initial publication from the Netherlands in the early 1980s found that SDD significantly reduced both secondary colonization with pathogenic gram-negative organisms and associated infections in patients with severe trauma.[14] Serial culture data documented decreased airway and GI colonization with pathogenic bacteria, and infection rates fell drastically in the SDD group (16% vs. 81%).

These initial findings prompted a large number of subsequent evaluations. Indeed, SDD is unique in critical illness trials related to the sheer size of the data pool that addresses it. To date, various iterations of SDD or SOD have been analyzed in more than 50 randomized controlled

Table 46-1 Examples of SDD and SOD Treatments

	Oral	Enteral	Parenteral
SDD	Paste of amphotericin, colistin, tobramycin, 2% each, applied to oropharynx q6 hr for duration of ICU stay	Amphotericin (500 mg), colistin (100 mg), tobramycin (80 mg) combined in 10 mL liquid suspension, administered via nasogastric tube q6 hr for duration of ICU stay	Cefotaxime 1 g q6 hr or ceftriaxone 2 g q24 hr for 4 days on ICU admission
SOD	Paste of amphotericin, colistin, tobramycin, 2% each, applied to oropharynx q6 hr for duration of ICU stay	—	—

ICU, intensive care unit; SDD, selective digestive decontamination; SOD, selective oral decontamination.

trials (Table 46-2).[3-13,15-57] As a group, the data almost uniformly demonstrate a significant reduction in infectious complications in patients receiving SDD/SOD treatment, although impact on mortality varies widely among studies. For example, a randomized trial in Dutch ICUs of nearly 1000 patients found that a typical SDD regimen significantly lowered rates of colonization by resistant organisms (16% vs. 26%) and was associated with a decreased ICU mortality (15% vs. 23%).[8] Similarly, a subsequent, even larger Dutch trial (nearly 6000 patients) found that infectious complications were reduced in SDD and SOD treatment groups and although crude mortality rates did not differ from the control group, mortality also decreased modestly after adjustment for varying patient characteristics in experimental arms.[4]

More recent trials from Dutch investigators have continued to indicate positive results seen in prior trials; a 2011 randomized trial composed of more than 5000 patients also indicated reduced risk of colonization or infection, particularly with highly resistant organisms, in groups undergoing SDD.[56] Further subgroup analysis from this same data set suggested that SDD or even SOD alone may be sufficient to reduce 28-day mortality in medical ICU patients.[57] The findings in these and other publications contrast with several smaller studies that showed unchanged mortality.* Although the dominant outcomes typically examined with SDD are infection and mortality, preoperative SDD has also been shown to reduce the incidence of anastomotic leakage in patients undergoing GI surgery.[41]

Multiple reviews and meta-analyses have attempted to synthesize the broad body of literature on SDD (Table 46-3). Similar to the source publications, these studies indicate that SDD decreases rates of infection, although data regarding mortality benefit are at least somewhat conflicting. Meta-analyses from the early 1990s documented a decreased risk of pneumonia with SDD but found that hospital mortality was unaltered.[59-61] Subsequent reviews published later in the decade showed that SDD decreased mortality but only in critically ill surgery patients.[62] Moreover, a 2001 review noted that, as the methodological quality of SDD studies increased, the relative risk reduction for pneumonia decreased, suggesting perhaps that the benefits detailed in early investigations were overstated because of inadequate design or analysis.[63]

More recently, a 2007 meta-analysis that included 51 trials and over 8000 patients determined that SDD does prevent mortality,[64] a finding replicated in a 2009 Cochrane review[65] as well as a large meta-analysis of 29 trials published in 2014.[66] The fact that there are significantly fewer trials in more recent meta-analyses is reflective of different opinions about quality of source data, a potential confounder in assessing the utility of SDD. Of note, recent reviews have also shown a decreased risk of infectious complications when SDD is administered to critically ill pediatric patients or to adult GI surgery patients, although SDD is not associated with a mortality benefit in these populations.[67,68]

COMPARISON OF SELECTIVE DECONTAMINATION OF THE DIGESTIVE TRACT AND SELECTIVE ORAL DECONTAMINATION

SDD is a combination of therapies: parenteral, enteral, and oral. If SDD protocols benefit patients, it seems reasonable to ask which component of SDD is most directly responsible and if simpler protocols provide equivalent benefits. Further, concerns about antibiotic resistance (outlined below) are higher with systemic and enteral antibiotic use than with oral prophylaxis alone. As such, multiple studies have also examined the value of SOD only with oropharyngeal antibiotic paste alone.

In general, published data indicate that SDD is more effective in preventing infection and mortality than SOD, although this is not unequivocally the case. In a large, randomized, crossover study involving 13 ICUs in the Netherlands, SDD and SOD were compared both to standard therapy and to themselves. Adjusted mortality figures indicated a survival benefit for both SDD and SOD, although mortality was 0.6% better with SDD than SOD.[4] Similar results were generated by a follow-up investigation, which found that SOD was slightly less effective at preventing bacteremia with highly resistant organisms.[69] Other analyses of the Dutch data have found that, although SOD is able to reduce mortality in addition to colonization and bacteremia, the mortality benefit is only apparent in nonsurgical patients.[57] Furthermore, although a 2014 meta-analysis concluded that both SDD and SOD are superior to simple oral care, it could not determine how SDD and SOD differed and called for further investigations.[66] In aggregate, the data appear to support the conclusion that both

*References 12, 13, 15, 24, 16, 58

Text continued on p. 319

Table 46-2 **Randomized Trials of SDD**

Year	Author	No. of Subjects (Treatment/ Control)	Patient Population	Treatment	Control	Outcomes
1984	Stoutenbeek	181 (122/59)	Trauma	Amphotericin B (AB), polymyxin E (PE), tobramycin (T)	Controls were historical; nonrandomized trial	Infection rate • 6% vs. 81%
1987	Unertl	39 (19/20)	Mixed	AB, PE, gentamicin	Standard care	Respiratory infections • 1 vs. 14 ($P < .001$) No change in mortality
1988	Kerver	96 (49/47)	Mixed	AB, PE, T, IV cefotaxime	Placebo	Infection • 39% vs. 81% ($P < .001$) Mortality • 28.5% vs. 32% ($P < 0.05$)
1989	Ulrich	100 (48/52)	Mixed	AB, PE, norfloxacin, IV trimethoprim	Standard care	Respiratory infection • 6% vs. 44% UTI • 4% vs. 27% Line infection • 0% vs. 15% Mortality • 31% vs. 54%
1990	Flaherty	107 (51/56)	Cardiac surgery	PE, gentamicin, nystatin	Sucralfate	Infection • 12% vs. 27% ($P = 0.04$) No change in mortality
1990	Rodriguez-Roldan	28 (15/13)	Mixed	AB, PE, T	Placebo	Tracheobronchitis • 3 vs. 3 ($P < .001$) Pneumonia • 0 vs. 11 ($P < .001$) No change in mortality
1990	Tetteroo	114 (56/58)	Esophageal surgery	AB, PE, T, IV cefotaxime	Standard care	Total infections • 18 vs. 58 ($P < .001$)
1991	Aerdts	56 (17/18 + 21)	Mixed	AB, PE, norfloxacin, iv cefotaxime	Standard care	Lower respiratory tract infections • Control: 1:78% • Control: 2:62% • SDD: 6% ($P = .0001$)
1991	Blair	256 (126/130)	Mixed	AB, PE, T, IV cefotaxime	Placebo	Infection • 16.7% vs. 30.8% ($P = .008$) Mortality in patients with APACHE II scores 10-19 • 8 of 76 SDD vs. 15 of 70 controls ($P = .03$)
1991	Pugin	79 (38/41)	Trauma	SOD only: PE, neomycin, vancomycin	Placebo	Pneumonia • 16% vs. 78% ($P < .0001$) No change in mortality
1991	Zobel	50 (25/25)	Pediatric	AB, PE, gentamicin, IV cefotaxime	Standard care	Infection • 8% vs. 36% ($P < .025$) No change in mortality
1992	Cerra	46 (23/23)	Surgical	Norfloxacin, nystatin	Placebo	Total infections • 22 vs. 44 ($P = .002$) No change in mortality
1992	Cockerill	150 (75/75)	Mixed	PE, gentamicin, nystatin	Placebo	Total infections • 36 vs. 12 ($P = .04$) No change in mortality
1992	Gastinne	445 (220/225)	Mixed	AB, PE, T	Placebo	No change in pneumonia or mortality
1992	Hammond	239 (114/125)	Mixed	AB, PE, T, IV cefotaxime	Placebo	No change in infection rate or mortality

Continued

Table 46-2 **Randomized Trials of SDD—cont'd**

Year	Author	No. of Subjects (Treatment/Control)	Patient Population	Treatment	Control	Outcomes
1992	Rocha	101 (47/54)	Mixed	AB, PE, T, IV cefotaxime	Placebo	Overall infection • 26% vs. 63% ($P < .001$) Pneumonia • 15% vs. 46% ($P < .001$) Mortality • 21% vs. 44% ($P < .01$)
1992	Winter	183 (91/92) 84 historic	Medical	AB, PE, T, IV ceftazidime	Standard care	Total infections • 32 in controls vs. 27 historical • 3 in treated group ($P < .01$) No change in mortality
1993	Korinek	123 (63/60)	Neurosurgical	AB, PE, T, vancomycin added to oral solution	Placebo	Pneumonia • 15 vs. 25 ($P < .01$) Mortality • 3 vs. 7 ($P < .01$)
1993	Rolando	Group 1: 21 Group 2: 21 Group 3: 28 Group 4: 31	Hepatic failure	1: IV cefuroxime 2: AB, PE, T, IV cefuroxime 3: AB, PE, T, IV cefuroxime	4: Standard care	Total infections (Group 3 vs. Group 4) • 9 vs. 18 ($P < .05$) No change in mortality between any groups
1994	Bion	59 (27/32)	Liver transplant	AB, PE, T, IV cefotaxime, IV ampicillin	Nystatin, IV cefotaxime, IV ampicillin	Infections • 3 vs. 12 ($P < .49$) No change in endotoxemia No change in multiorgan dysfunction
1994	Ferrer	80 (39/41)	Mixed	AB, PE, T, IV cefotaxime	Placebo, IV cefotaxime	No change in infection rate, pneumonia, or mortality
1994	Laggner	67 (33/34)	Mixed	Oral gentamicin only	Placebo	No change in pneumonia or mortality
1995	Luiten	102 (50/52)	Pancreatitis	AB, PE, enteral norfloxacin	Standard care	Mortality • 22% vs. 35% ($P = .048$)
1995	Wiener	61 (30/31)	Mixed	AB, PE, gentamicin	Placebo	No change in infection rate, pneumonia, or mortality
1996	Arnow	69 (34/35)	Liver transplant	AB, PE, T, IV cefotaxime, IV ampicillin	IV cefotaxime, IV ampicillin	Aerobic gram-negative infections • 0% vs. 7% ($P < .05$)
1996	Quinio	148 (76/72)	Trauma	AB, PE, gentamicin	Placebo	Total infections • 19 vs. 37 ($P < .01$) No change in LOS or mortality
1996	Rolando	108 (47/61)	Hepatic failure	AB, PE, T, IV ceftazidime, flucloxacillin	AB, IV ceftazidime, flucloxacillin	No change in infection rate or mortality
1997	Abele-Horn	88 (58/30)	Surgical	SOD only: AB, PE, T	Placebo	Primary pneumonia • 0% vs. 33% ($P < .05$) No change in mortality
1997	Lingnau	313 Group 1: 83 Group 2: 82 Control: 148	Trauma	Group 1: AB, PE, T, IV ciprofloxacin Group 2: AB, PE, IV ciprofloxacin	Placebo, IV ciprofloxacin	No change in rates of pneumonia, sepsis, organ dysfunction, or mortality
1997	Schardey	205 (102/103)	Surgical	AB, polymyxin B, T, oral vancomycin, IV cefotaxime	Placebo	Anastomotic leak • 2.9 vs. 10.6% ($P = .0492$) Pulmonary infections • 8.8 vs. 22.3% ($P = .02$) No change in mortality

Table 46-2 **Randomized Trials of SDD—cont'd**

Year	Author	No. of Subjects (Treatment/Control)	Patient Population	Treatment	Control	Outcomes
1997	Verwaest	615 Group 1: 195 Group 2: 200 Control: 220	Mixed	Group 1: AB, ofloxacin enteral and IV Group 2: AB, PE, T, IV cefotaxime	Standard care	Group 1 vs. Group 2: Infection • OR: 0.27 (95% CI: 0.27-0.64) Respiratory infections • OR: 0.47 (95% CI: 0.26-0.82) Control vs. Group 2: Resistant organisms • 83% vs. 55% ($P < .05$) Gram-positive bacteremia • OR: 1.22 (95% CI: 0.72-2.08) No change in mortality for all comparisons
1998	Ruza	226 (116/110)	Pediatric	PE, T, nystatin	Standard care	No change in infection rate or mortality
1998	Sanchez Garcia	271 (131/140)	Trauma	AB, PE, oral and enteral gentamicin, IV ceftriaxone	Placebo	VAP • 11% vs. 29.3% ($P < .001$) Other infection • 19.1% vs. 30% ($P < .04$) Cost • $11,926 vs. $16,296 No change in mortality
2001	Barret	23 (11/12)	Pediatric burn	AB, PE, T	Placebo	No difference in pneumonia or sepsis
2001	Begmans	226 87 Control in same ICU: 78 (Group A) Control different setting: 61 (Group B)	Mixed	SOD only: PE, gentamicin, vancomycin	Placebo	VAP • SDD: 10%, Group A: 31%, Group B: 23% ($P = .001$, $P = .04$) No change in LOS or mortality
2002	Bouter	51 (24/27)	Cardiac bypass	PE, neomycin	Placebo	Aerobic gram-negative carriage • 27% vs. 93% ($P < .001$) No change in perioperative endotoxemia, postoperative fever, or LOS
2002	Hellinger	80 (37/43)	Liver transplant	PE, nystatin, gentamicin	Nystatin	No change in infection rate or mortality
2002	Krueger	527 (265/262)	Surgical	PE, gentamicin, IV ciprofloxacin	Placebo	Total infection • OR: 0.477 (95% CI: 0.367-0.620) Pneumonia • 6 vs. 29 ($P = .007$) BSI • 14 vs. 36 ($P = .007$) Organ dysfunction • 63 vs. 96 ($P = .0051$) No change in mortality
2002	Pneumatikos	61 (30/31)	Trauma	AB, PE, T (subglottic decontamination only)	Placebo	Pneumonia • 16.6% vs. 51.6% ($P < .05$) No change in mortality
2002	Rayes	95 Group 1: 32 Group 2: 31 Control: 32	Liver transplant	Group 1: AB, PE, T Group 2: Enteral fiber, *Lactobacillus plantarum* 299	Placebo	Group 1 vs. Group 2: Infection • 48% vs. 13% ($P = .017$) Group 1 vs. Control: No change in infections No change in LOS for all comparisons
2002	Zwaveling	55 (26/29)	Liver transplant	AB, PE, T	Placebo	No change in rate of infection

Continued

Table 46-2 Randomized Trials of SDD—cont'd

Year	Author	No. of Subjects (Treatment/ Control)	Patient Population	Treatment	Control	Outcomes
2003	de Jonge	934 (466/468)	Surgical	AB, PE, T, IV cefotaxime	Standard care	ICU mortality • 15% vs. 23% ($P = .002$) Hospital mortality • 24% vs. 31% ($P = 0.02$) Resistant gram-negative colonization • 16% vs. 26% ($P = .001$)
2005	Camus	515 Group 1: 130 Group 2: 130 Group 3: 129 Control: 126	Mixed	Group 1: PE, T Group 2: Nasal mupirocin, chlorhexidine wash Group 3: Both treatments	Placebo	Group 3 vs. Control: Infections • OR 0.44 (95% CI: 0.26-0.75) No difference between two treatments
2005	de la Cal	107 (53/54)	Burn	AB, PE, T	Placebo	Mortality • 9.4% vs. 27.8%, RR: 0.25 (95% CI: 0.08-0.76) Hospital mortality • RR: 0.28 (95% CI: 0.10-0.8) Pneumonia • 17/1000 vent days vs. 30.8/1000 vent days ($P = .03$)
2006	Gosney	203 (103/100)	Stroke	SOD only: AB, PE	Placebo	Pneumonia • 1 vs. 7 ($P = .029$) No change in mortality
2006	Koeman	385 Group 1: 127 Group 2: 128 Control: 130	Mixed	SOD only: Group 1: Chlorhexidine Group 2: Chlorhexidine, PE	Placebo	Pneumonia Group 1: • OR: 0.352 (95% CI: 0.160-0.791) Group 2: • OR: 0.454 (95% CI: 0.224-0.925) No change in mortality
2007	Stoutenbeek	401 (200/201)	Trauma	AB, PE, T, IV cefotaxime	Standard care	Respiratory infection • 30.9% vs. 50% ($P < .01$) Pneumonia • 9.5% vs. 23% ($P < .01$) BSI, AGNB • 2.5% vs. 7.5% ($P = .02$) No change in organ dysfunction or mortality
2008	Farran	91 (40/51)	Surgical	Erythromycin, gentamicin, nystatin	Placebo	No change in anastomotic leak rate, pneumonia, or mortality
2009	de Smet	6299 Group 1: 1904 Group 2: 2405 Control: 1990	Mixed	Group 1: SOD only, AB, PE, T Group 2: SDD, AB, PE, T, IV cefotaxime	Standard care	Gram-negative infections SOD: • OR: 0.49 (95% CI: 0.27-0.87) SDD: • OR: 0.43 (95% CI: 0.24-0.77) Mortality SOD: • OR: 0.86 (95% CI: 0.74-0.99) SDD: • OR: 0.83 (0.72-0.97)
2011	Roos	289 (143/146)	Surgical	AB, T, polymyxin B	Placebo	Infectious complications • 19.6% vs. 30.8% ($P = .028$) Anastomotic leakage • 6.3% vs. 15.1% ($P = .016$) No change in LOS or mortality

Table 46-2 **Randomized Trials of SDD—cont'd**

Year	Author	No. of Subjects (Treatment/Control)	Patient Population	Treatment	Control	Outcomes
2011	de Smet (post hoc analysis from de Smet, 2009)	5927 Group 1: 1904 Group 2: 2034 Control: 1989	Mixed	Group 1: SOD only, AB, PE, T Group 2: SDD, AB, PE, T, IV cefotaxime	Standard care	Bacteremia SOD: • OR: 0.66 (95% CI: 0.53-0.82) SDD: • OR 0.48 (95% CI: 0.38-0.60) Highly resistant bacteremia SOD: • OR: 0.37 (95% CI: 0.16-0.85) SDD: • OR 0.41 (95% CI: 0.18-0.94) Highly resistant colonization SOD: • OR 0.65 (95% CI: 0.49-0.87) SDD: • OR 0.58 (95% CI: 0.43-0.78)
2012	Melsen (post hoc analysis from de Smet, 2009)	5927 Surgical: Group 1: 866 Group 2: 923 Control: 973 Medical: Group 1: 1038 Group 2: 1111 Control: 1016	Mixed	Group 1: SOD only, AB, PE, T Group 2: SDD, AB, PE, T, IV cefotaxime	Standard care	Mortality in nonsurgical patients SOD: • OR: 0.77 (95% CI: 0.63-0.94) SDD: no change in mortality Mortality in surgical patients SOD: no change in mortality SDD: no change in mortality

AGNB, aerobic gram-negative bacillus; *APACHE*, Acute Physiology and Chronic Health Evaluation; *BSI*, bloodstream infection; *CI*, confidence interval; *ICU*, intensive care unit; *IV*, intravenous; *LOS*, length of stay; *OR*, odds ratio; *RR*, relative risk; *SDD*, selective digestive decontaminant; *SOD*, selective oral decontaminant; *VAP*, ventilator-associated pneumonia.

Table 46-3 **Reviews and Meta-analyses of SDD**

Author, Year	Number of Trials	Number of Subjects (Intervention/No Intervention)	Treatment	Outcomes
SDD Trialists' Group, 1993	22	4142 (2047/2095)	AB, PE, T, IV cefotaxime Some received quinolone and gentamicin	Respiratory tract infection • OR: 0.37 (95% CI: 0.31-0.43) Mortality • OR: 0.9 (95% CI: 0.79-1.04) Mortality in trials giving parenteral and enteral treatment • OR: 0.8 (95% CI: 0.67-0.97)
Kollef, 1994	16	2270 (1105/1165)	Most studies: AB, PE, T, IV cefotaxime	Pneumonia • 7.4% vs. 21.9% (*P* < .0001) Tracheobronchitis • 6.5% vs. 11.7% (*P* = .004) No change in gram-positive pneumonia or mortality
Heyland, 1994	25	Not given	Most studies: AB, PE, T, cefotaxime	Pneumonia • RR: 0.46 (95% CI: 0.39-0.56; *P* = .01) No change in mortality
D'Amico, 1998	16	3361	Most studies: AB, PE, T, enteral antibiotic	Pneumonia • OR: 0.29 (95% CI: 0.29-0.41) Mortality • OR 0.80 (95% CI: 0.69-0.93)
	17	2366	Most studies: AB, PE, T	Pneumonia • OR: 0.56 (95% CI: 0.46-0.68) No change in mortality

Continued

Table 46-3 Reviews and Meta-analyses of SDD—cont'd

Author, Year	Number of Trials	Number of Subjects (Intervention/No Intervention)	Treatment	Outcomes
Nathens, 1999	11 RCTs for surgical	Not given	Most studies: AB, PE, T, IV cefotaxime	Pneumonia • OR 0.19 (95% CI: 0.15-0.26) Mortality • OR: 0.70 (95% CI: 0.52-0.93)
	10 RCTs for medical	Not given	Most studies: AB, PE, T, IV cefotaxime	Pneumonia • OR: 0.45 (95% CI: 0.33-0.62) No change in mortality
Van Nieuwenhoven, 2001	32	4804 (2400/2404)	Varied	RRR for pneumonia • OR: 0.57 (95% CI: 0.49-0.65) RRR for mortality • OR: 0.12 (95% CI: 0.04-0.32)
Safdar, 2004	14 (liver transplant	201 (treated vs. control not given)	Varied	Overall infection • RR: 0.88 (95% CI: 0.07-1.1) Gram-negative infection • OR: 0.16 (95% CI: 0.07-0.37) No change in mortality
Liberati, 2004	17	4295	Varied, topical, systemic antibiotic	Respiratory tract infection • OR 0.35 (95% CI: 0.29-0.41) Mortality • OR 0.78 (95% CI: 0.68-0.89)
	17	2664	Topical antibiotics only	Respiratory tract infection • OR: 0.52 (95% CI: 0.43-0.63) Mortality • OR: 0.97 (95% CI: 0.81-1.16)
Silvestri, 2005	42	6075	Enteral antifungals	Fungal carriage • OR: 0.32 (95% CI: 0.12-0.53) No change in fungemia
Silvestri, 2007	51	8065 (4079/3986)	AB, PE, T, IV cefotaxime	BSI • OR: 0.73 (95% CI: 0.59-0.90) Gram-negative BSI • OR: 0.39 (95% CI: 0.24-0.63) Mortality • OR: 0.80 (95% CI: 0.69-0.94)
	31 (subgroup analysis for BSI)	4753 (2453/2300)		BSI • OR: 0.73 (95% CI: 0.59-0.90)
	30 (subgroup analysis for mortality)	4527 (2337/2190)		Mortality • OR: 0.80 (95% CI: 0.69-0.94)
	16 (subgroup analysis for parenteral vs. enteral)	3331 (1645/1686)		Mortality (parenteral vs. enteral) • OR: 0.74 (95% CI: 0.61-0.91) BSI (parenteral vs. enteral) • OR: 0.63 (95% CI: 0.46-0.87)
Silvestri, 2008	54	9473 (4672/4801)	Varied	Overall gram-negative infection • OR: 0.17 (95% CI: 0.10-0.28) Gram-negative BSI • OR: 0.35 (95% CI: 0.21-0.67) Gram-negative respiratory infection • OR: 0.11 (95% CI: 0.06-0.20) Gram-positive respiratory infection • OR: 0.52 (95% CI: 0.34-0.78) Gram-positive BSI • OR 1.03 (95% CI: 0.75-1.41)

Table 46-3 Reviews and Meta-analyses of SDD—cont'd

Author, Year	Number of Trials	Number of Subjects (Intervention/No Intervention)	Treatment	Outcomes
Silvestri, 2009	21	4902	Most trials: AB, PE, T, iv cefotaxime	Mortality • OR: 0.71 (95% CI: 0.61-0.82)
Silvestri, 2010	7	1270 (637/633)	Varied	MODS • OR: 0.50 (95% CI: 0.34-0.74) No change in MODS-related mortality or overall mortality
Petros, 2013	4 (pediatric)	335	Varied	Pneumonia • OR: 0.31 (95% CI: 0.11-0.87) No change in mortality
Roos, 2013	8 (perioperative SDD)	1668 (828/840)	Varied	Infection • OR: 0.58 (95% CI: 0.42-0.82) Anastomotic leakage • OR: 0.42 (95% CI: 0.24-0.73)
Price, 2014	29	Not given	SOD vs. SDD vs. chlorhexidine	Mortality • SOD OR: 0.85 (95% CI: 0.74-0.97) • SDD OR: 0.73 (95% CI: 0.64-0.84) • Chlorhexidine OR: 1.25 (95% CI: 1.05-1.50)

AB, amphotericin B; *BSI*, bloodstream infection; *CI*, confidence interval; *IV*, intravenous; *MODS*, multiple organ dysfunction syndrome; *OR*, odds ratio; *PE*, polymyxin E; *RCT*, randomized controlled trial; *RR*, relative risk; *RRR*, relative risk reduction; *SDD*, selective digestive decontaminant; *SOD*, selective oral decontaminant; *T*, tobramycin.

SDD and SOD prevent infection and that SDD likely does so more effectively across broader patient groups.

OPPOSITION TO SELECTIVE DECONTAMINATION OF THE DIGESTIVE TRACT

The reluctance to widely adopt SDD is easily understood. In theory, the increased use of antibiotics associated with SDD could lead to the development of drug-resistant organisms, a problem already routinely encountered in modern health-care settings and especially in ICUs. Although patients undergoing SDD may themselves experience a clinical benefit, future patients could fall victim to untreatable infections, eventually yielding a substantial net negative population effect. This concern is understandable, as increased antibiotic usage nearly invariably selects for resistant microorganism. There are data, however, to suggest that the use of SDD/SOD may not have an effect on antibiotic resistance. In fact, a 2014 study encompassing more than 30 Dutch ICUs and spanning 4 years noted that although the levels of antibiotic resistance were unchanged in units using standard antibiotic therapy, those that used SDD were actually able to *decrease* the occurrence of resistant organisms.[70] Another 5-year study revealed that the use of SDD actually reduced proportions of resistant organisms over time.[71] Low levels of antibiotic resistance over 4 years were again noted in a separate Dutch trial of SDD and SOD. The authors did discover that although SDD was able to generate lower rates of bacterial resistance overall, it also was associated with higher rates of aminoglycoside-resistant organisms than SOD.[3]

Despite some data suggesting that SDD may not result in increasing resistance, opponents still fear negative long-term outcomes, and there is information to support such concerns. Modern molecular analysis shows that treatment of a patient with SDD results in a marked upregulation of resistance genes in gut flora.[72] Importantly, these genes appear transferable between species, and changes brought about by SDD therapy may persist long after antibiotic treatment has ceased. Also, composition of the gut microbial populations may be significantly altered after treatment.[55] Of even greater concern, cases of colistin-resistant organisms in association with SDD have now been documented.[73,74] In addition, most of the large trials reporting benefits with SDD have taken place in the Netherlands and, to a lesser degree, other parts of Europe. This geographical distribution has led to wide variance in adoption, with many countries that have higher rates of resistant microorganisms (including the United States) reluctant to adopt the practice.

Ultimately, however, despite the size of the data set addressing SDD—perhaps the largest for any topic in critical care medicine—a global consensus on the practice has not been reached. Survey data indicate that many clinical practitioners are fearful of antibiotic resistance, a concern that has led to poor acceptance of SDD in ICUs outside the Netherlands.[75] Although many may agree on the effectiveness of SDD in preventing pneumonia, skepticism regarding the evidence base is common.[76,77] Further investigation into how the increased antibiotic usage associated with SDD affects bacterial ecology in places with higher endemic rates of resistance is likely necessary before widespread adoption of the practice could potentially occur.[69,78]

For now, the use of SDD remains one of the more divisive issues in critical care. On the one hand, proponents have gone so far as to state that withholding SDD from patients is unethical.[3,79] Conversely, the use of SDD has not gained traction internationally. This ambivalence is reflected in the 2013 Surviving Sepsis Guidelines, which gave SDD a level 2b grade with the statement that "we suggest that SOD and SDD be introduced and investigated as a method to reduce the incidence of ventilator-associated pneumonia; this infection control measure can then be instituted in health-care settings and regions where this method is found to be effective."[80]

AUTHORS' RECOMMENDATIONS

- Selective digestive decontamination (SDD) refers to the administration of prophylactic antibiotics to ICU patients to prevent infection from commensal or acquired organisms. It commonly involves length-of-stay dosing of oral and enteral of nonabsorbable combinations of tobramycin, amphotericin, and colistin, as well as a short course of intravenous cephalosporin.
- Selective oral decontamination (SOD) is similar but involves only treatment of the oral cavity and does not incorporate intravenous or enteral antibiotics.
- There is a substantial body of literature regarding SDD and SOD, and data indicate that the practices are able to prevent infection and may prevent mortality. SDD may be more effective than SOD, although this is not fully clear.
- There is concern regarding the induction of antimicrobial resistance in ICUs where antibiotic resistance levels are high. This fear of worsening resistance has prevented SDD and SOD from gaining widespread global adoption.

REFERENCES

1. Garrouste-Orgeas M, et al. Oropharyngeal or gastric colonization and nosocomial pneumonia in adult intensive care unit patients. A prospective study based on genomic DNA analysis. *Am J Respir Crit Care Med*. 1997;156(5):1647–1655.
2. Johanson Jr WG, et al. Nosocomial respiratory infections with gram-negative bacilli. The significance of colonization of the respiratory tract. *Ann Intern Med*. 1972;77(5):701–706.
3. Oostdijk EA, et al. Effects of decontamination of the oropharynx and intestinal tract on antibiotic resistance in ICUs: a randomized clinical trial. *JAMA*. 2014;312(14):1429–1437.
4. de Smet AM, et al. Decontamination of the digestive tract and oropharynx in ICU patients. *N Engl J Med*. 2009;360(1):20–31.
5. Cerra FB, et al. Selective gut decontamination reduces nosocomial infections and length of stay but not mortality or organ failure in surgical intensive care unit patients. *Arch Surg*. 1992;127(2):163–167. discussion 167-9.
6. Blair P, et al. Selective decontamination of the digestive tract: a stratified, randomized, prospective study in a mixed intensive care unit. *Surgery*. 1991;110(2):303–309. discussion 309-10.
7. Cockerill 3rd FR, et al. Prevention of infection in critically ill patients by selective decontamination of the digestive tract. *Ann Intern Med*. 1992;117(7):545–553.
8. de Jonge E, et al. Effects of selective decontamination of digestive tract on mortality and acquisition of resistant bacteria in intensive care: a randomised controlled trial. *Lancet*. 2003;362(9389):1011–1016.
9. de La Cal MA, et al. Survival benefit in critically ill burned patients receiving selective decontamination of the digestive tract: a randomized, placebo-controlled, double-blind trial. *Ann Surg*. 2005;241(3):424–430.
10. Hellinger WC, et al. A randomized, prospective, double-blinded evaluation of selective bowel decontamination in liver transplantation. *Transplantation*. 2002;73(12):1904–1909.
11. Aerdts SJ, et al. Antibiotic prophylaxis of respiratory tract infection in mechanically ventilated patients. A prospective, blinded, randomized trial of the effect of a novel regimen. *Chest*. 1991;100(3):783–791.
12. Bergmans DC, et al. Prevention of ventilator-associated pneumonia by oral decontamination: a prospective, randomized, double-blind, placebo-controlled study. *Am J Respir Crit Care Med*. 2001;164(3):382–388.
13. Camus C, et al. Prevention of acquired infections in intubated patients with the combination of two decontamination regimens. *Crit Care Med*. 2005;33(2):307–314.
14. Stoutenbeek CP, et al. The effect of selective decontamination of the digestive tract on colonisation and infection rate in multiple trauma patients. *Intensive Care Med*. 1984;10(4):185–192.
15. Abele-Horn M, et al. Decrease in nosocomial pneumonia in ventilated patients by selective oropharyngeal decontamination (SOD). *Intensive Care Med*. 1997;23(2):187–195.
16. Arnow PM, et al. Randomized controlled trial of selective bowel decontamination for prevention of infections following liver transplantation. *Clin Infect Dis*. 1996;22(6):997–1003.
17. Barret JP, Jeschke MG, Herndon DN. Selective decontamination of the digestive tract in severely burned pediatric patients. *Burns*. 2001;27(5):439–445.
18. Bion JF, et al. Selective decontamination of the digestive tract reduces gram-negative pulmonary colonization but not systemic endotoxemia in patients undergoing elective liver transplantation. *Crit Care Med*. 1994;22(1):40–49.
19. Bouter H, et al. No effect of preoperative selective gut decontamination on endotoxemia and cytokine activation during cardiopulmonary bypass: a randomized, placebo-controlled study. *Crit Care Med*. 2002;30(1):38–43.
20. Diepenhorst GM, et al. Influence of prophylactic probiotics and selective decontamination on bacterial translocation in patients undergoing pancreatic surgery: a randomized controlled trial. *Shock*. 2011;35(1):9–16.
21. Farran L, et al. Efficacy of enteral decontamination in the prevention of anastomotic dehiscence and pulmonary infection in esophagogastric surgery. *Dis Esophagus*. 2008;21(2):159–164.
22. Ferrer M, et al. Utility of selective digestive decontamination in mechanically ventilated patients. *Ann Intern Med*. 1994;120(5):389–395.
23. Flaherty J, et al. Pilot trial of selective decontamination for prevention of bacterial infection in an intensive care unit. *J Infect Dis*. 1990;162(6):1393–1397.
24. Gastinne H, et al. A controlled trial in intensive care units of selective decontamination of the digestive tract with nonabsorbable antibiotics. The French Study Group on Selective Decontamination of the Digestive Tract. *N Engl J Med*. 1992;326(9):594–599.
25. Gosney M, Martin MV, Wright AE. The role of selective decontamination of the digestive tract in acute stroke. *Age Ageing*. 2006;35(1):42–47.
26. Hammond JM, et al. Double-blind study of selective decontamination of the digestive tract in intensive care. *Lancet*. 1992;340(8810):5–9.
27. Kerver AJ, et al. Prevention of colonization and infection in critically ill patients: a prospective randomized study. *Crit Care Med*. 1988;16(11):1087–1093.
28. Korinek AM, et al. Selective decontamination of the digestive tract in neurosurgical intensive care unit patients: a double-blind, randomized, placebo-controlled study. *Crit Care Med*. 1993;21(10):1466–1473.
29. Krueger WA, Unertl KE. Selective decontamination of the digestive tract. *Curr Opin Crit Care*. 2002;8(2):139–144.
30. Laggner AN, et al. Oropharyngeal decontamination with gentamicin for long-term ventilated patients on stress ulcer prophylaxis with sucralfate? *Wien Klin Wochenschr*. 1994;106(1):15–19.
31. Lingnau W, et al. Selective intestinal decontamination in multiple trauma patients: prospective, controlled trial. *J Trauma*. 1997;42(4):687–694.
32. Luiten EJ, et al. Controlled clinical trial of selective decontamination for the treatment of severe acute pancreatitis. *Ann Surg*. 1995;222(1):57–65.
33. Oudhuis GJ, et al. Probiotics versus antibiotic decontamination of the digestive tract: infection and mortality. *Intensive Care Med*. 2011;37(1):110–117.
34. Pneumatikos I, et al. Selective decontamination of subglottic area in mechanically ventilated patients with multiple trauma. *Intensive Care Med*. 2002;28(4):432–437.

35. Pugin J, et al. Oropharyngeal decontamination decreases incidence of ventilator-associated pneumonia. A randomized, placebo-controlled, double-blind clinical trial. *JAMA*. 1991;265(20):2704–2710.

36. Quinio B, et al. Selective decontamination of the digestive tract in multiple trauma patients. A prospective double-blind, randomized, placebo-controlled study. *Chest*. 1996;109(3):765–772.

37. Rayes N, et al. Early enteral supply of lactobacillus and fiber versus selective bowel decontamination: a controlled trial in liver transplant recipients. *Transplantation*. 2002;74(1):123–127.

38. Rocha LA, et al. Prevention of nosocomial infection in critically ill patients by selective decontamination of the digestive tract. A randomized, double blind, placebo-controlled study. *Intensive Care Med*. 1992;18(7):398–404.

39. Rodriguez-Roldan JM, et al. Prevention of nosocomial lung infection in ventilated patients: use of an antimicrobial pharyngeal nonabsorbable paste. *Crit Care Med*. 1990;18(11):1239–1242.

40. Rolando N, et al. Prospective study comparing the efficacy of prophylactic parenteral antimicrobials, with or without enteral decontamination, in patients with acute liver failure. *Liver Transpl Surg*. 1996;2(1):8–13.

41. Roos D, et al. Randomized clinical trial of perioperative selective decontamination of the digestive tract versus placebo in elective gastrointestinal surgery. *Br J Surg*. 2011;98(10):1365–1372.

42. Ruza F, et al. Prevention of nosocomial infection in a pediatric intensive care unit (PICU) through the use of selective digestive decontamination. *Eur J Epidemiol*. 1998;14(7):719–727.

43. Sanchez Garcia M, et al. Effectiveness and cost of selective decontamination of the digestive tract in critically ill intubated patients. A randomized, double-blind, placebo-controlled, multicenter trial. *Am J Respir Crit Care Med*. 1998;158(3):908–916.

44. Schardey HM, et al. The prevention of anastomotic leakage after total gastrectomy with local decontamination. A prospective, randomized, double-blind, placebo-controlled multicenter trial. *Ann Surg*. 1997;225(2):172–180.

45. Smith SD, et al. Selective decontamination in pediatric liver transplants. A randomized prospective study. *Transplantation*. 1993;55(6):1306–1309.

46. Stoutenbeek CP, et al. The effect of selective decontamination of the digestive tract on mortality in multiple trauma patients: a multicenter randomized controlled trial. *Intensive Care Med*. 2007;33(2):261–270.

47. Tetteroo GW, et al. Selective decontamination to reduce gram-negative colonisation and infections after oesophageal resection. *Lancet*. 1990;335(8691):704–707.

48. Ulrich C, et al. Selective decontamination of the digestive tract with norfloxacin in the prevention of ICU-acquired infections: a prospective randomized study. *Intensive Care Med*. 1989;15(7):424–431.

49. Unertl K, et al. Prevention of colonization and respiratory infections in long-term ventilated patients by local antimicrobial prophylaxis. *Intensive Care Med*. 1987;13(2):106–113.

50. Verwaest C, et al. Randomized, controlled trial of selective digestive decontamination in 600 mechanically ventilated patients in a multidisciplinary intensive care unit. *Crit Care Med*. 1997;25(1):63–71.

51. Wiener J, et al. A randomized, double-blind, placebo-controlled trial of selective digestive decontamination in a medical-surgical intensive care unit. *Clin Infect Dis*. 1995;20(4):861–867.

52. Winter R, et al. A controlled trial of selective decontamination of the digestive tract in intensive care and its effect on nosocomial infection. *J Antimicrob Chemother*. 1992;30(1):73–87.

53. Zobel G, et al. Reduction of colonization and infection rate during pediatric intensive care by selective decontamination of the digestive tract. *Crit Care Med*. 1991;19(10):1242–1246.

54. Zwaveling JH, et al. Selective decontamination of the digestive tract to prevent postoperative infection: a randomized placebo-controlled trial in liver transplant patients. *Crit Care Med*. 2002;30(6):1204–1209.

55. Benus RF, et al. Impact of digestive and oropharyngeal decontamination on the intestinal microbiota in ICU patients. *Intensive Care Med*. 2010;36(8):1394–1402.

56. de Smet AM, et al. Selective digestive tract decontamination and selective oropharyngeal decontamination and antibiotic resistance in patients in intensive-care units: an open-label, clustered group-randomised, crossover study. *Lancet Infect Dis*. 2011;11(5):372–380.

57. Melsen WG, et al. Selective decontamination of the oral and digestive tract in surgical versus non-surgical patients in intensive care in a cluster-randomized trial. *Br J Surg*. 2012;99(2):232–237.

58. Koeman M, et al. Oral decontamination with chlorhexidine reduces the incidence of ventilator-associated pneumonia. *Am J Respir Crit Care Med*. 2006;173(12):1348–1355.

59. Heyland DK, et al. Selective decontamination of the digestive tract. An overview. *Chest*. 1994;105(4):1221–1229.

60. Kollef MH. The role of selective digestive tract decontamination on mortality and respiratory tract infections. A meta-analysis. *Chest*. 1994;105(4):1101–1108.

61. Meta-analysis of randomised controlled trials of selective decontamination of the digestive tract. Selective Decontamination of the Digestive Tract Trialists' Collaborative Group. *BMJ*. 1993;307(6903):525–532.

62. Nathens AB, Marshall JC. Selective decontamination of the digestive tract in surgical patients: a systematic review of the evidence. *Arch Surg*. 1999;134(2):170–176.

63. van Nieuwenhoven CA, et al. Relationship between methodological trial quality and the effects of selective digestive decontamination on pneumonia and mortality in critically ill patients. *JAMA*. 2001;286(3):335–340.

64. Silvestri L, et al. Selective decontamination of the digestive tract reduces bacterial bloodstream infection and mortality in critically ill patients. Systematic review of randomized, controlled trials. *J Hosp Infect*. 2007;65(3):187–203.

65. Liberati A, et al. Antibiotic prophylaxis to reduce respiratory tract infections and mortality in adults receiving intensive care. *Cochrane Database Syst Rev*. 2009;4:CD000022.

66. Price R, et al. Selective digestive or oropharyngeal decontamination and topical oropharyngeal chlorhexidine for prevention of death in general intensive care: systematic review and network meta-analysis. *BMJ*. 2014;348:g2197.

67. Petros A, et al. Selective decontamination of the digestive tract in critically ill children: systematic review and meta-analysis. *Pediatr Crit Care Med*. 2013;14(1):89–97.

68. Roos D, et al. Systematic review of perioperative selective decontamination of the digestive tract in elective gastrointestinal surgery. *Br J Surg*. 2013;100(12):1579–1588.

69. de Smet AM, Bonten MJ, Kluytmans JA. For whom should we use selective decontamination of the digestive tract? *Curr Opin Infect Dis*. 2012;25(2):211–217.

70. Houben AJ, et al. Selective decontamination of the oropharynx and the digestive tract, and antimicrobial resistance: a 4 year ecological study in 38 intensive care units in the Netherlands. *J Antimicrob Chemother*. 2014;69(3):797–804.

71. Ochoa-Ardila ME, et al. Long-term use of selective decontamination of the digestive tract does not increase antibiotic resistance: a 5-year prospective cohort study. *Intensive Care Med*. 2011;37(9):1458–1465.

72. Buelow E, et al. Effects of selective digestive decontamination (SDD) on the gut resistome. *J Antimicrob Chemother*. 2014;69(8):2215–2223.

73. Brink AJ, et al. Emergence of OXA-48 and OXA-181 carbapenemases among Enterobacteriaceae in South Africa and evidence of in vivo selection of colistin resistance as a consequence of selective decontamination of the gastrointestinal tract. *J Clin Microbiol*. 2013;51(1):369–372.

74. Halaby T, et al. Emergence of colistin resistance in Enterobacteriaceae after the introduction of selective digestive tract decontamination in an intensive care unit. *Antimicrob Agents Chemother*. 2013;57(7):3224–3229.

75. Canter RR, et al. Observational study of current use of selective decontamination of the digestive tract in UK critical care units. *Br J Anaesth*. 2014;113:610–617.

76. Duncan EM, et al. The views of health care professionals about selective decontamination of the digestive tract: an international, theoretically informed interview study. *J Crit Care*. 2014;29(4):634–640.

77. Cuthbertson BH, et al. Clinical stakeholders' opinions on the use of selective decontamination of the digestive tract in critically ill patients in intensive care units: an international Delphi study. *Crit Care*. 2013;17(6):R266.

78. Kollef MH, Micek ST. Rational use of antibiotics in the ICU: balancing stewardship and clinical outcomes. *JAMA*. 2014;312(14):1403–1404.

79. Zandstra DF, et al. Withholding selective decontamination of the digestive tract from critically ill patients must now surely be ethically questionable given the vast evidence base. *Crit Care*. 2010;14(5):443.

80. Dellinger RP, et al. Surviving sepsis campaign: international guidelines for management of severe sepsis and septic shock: 2012. *Crit Care Med*. 2013;41(2):580–637.

PERSISTENT CRITICAL ILLNESS

47 Is Persistent Critical Illness an Iatrogenic Disorder?

John C. Marshall

Medicine is an ancient discipline, but the capacity to avert otherwise certain death is recent. Intravenous fluid therapy was first used in London during the cholera epidemic of 1832; refinements in an understanding of the role of intravascular volume in shock have altered the management of a spectrum of disorders, from multiple trauma to overwhelming infection. The development of dialysis techniques in the 1940s transformed renal failure from a rapidly lethal illness to a chronic condition.[1] Similarly the development of techniques of mechanical ventilator support during the Scandinavian polio epidemic of the 1950s set the stage for intensive care units (ICUs) to become geographic locales capable of providing a spectrum of life-sustaining therapies[2]—therapies whose target was not the specific cause of the illness but rather its life-threatening physiologic consequences.

The ability to avert, or at least delay, death through ICU intervention has fundamentally changed acute illness. It has allowed gravely ill or injured patients to survive conditions that in earlier times would have been lethal, but it has also created an entirely new spectrum of medical disorders that are only possible because death has been averted and whose roots lie solidly in the interventions used to accomplish that goal. Critical illness is a quintessentially iatrogenic disorder: it only arises in patients who in the absence of intervention would have died, but it is also shaped by the inadvertent consequences of that intervention.[3] Understanding and mitigating the harmful effects of life-sustaining therapy have thus become paramount priorities because the consequences can be severe and prolonged.

Consider the following hypothetical, but uncomfortably familiar, scenario:

A previously healthy 72-year-old man is admitted to the ICU after a Hartman procedure for perforated diverticulitis. He remains intubated and paralyzed, and the plan is for overnight mechanical ventilation. He is noted to be tachycardic; 2 L of saline is given to correct a presumed fluid deficit, and the rate of his analgesic infusion is increased. The following morning he is thought to be too obtunded to consider extubation; further sedation is given to keep him comfortable, and a further fluid bolus administered when his blood pressure dips after a bolus of analgesic. Norepinephrine is administered, targeting a mean arterial pressure (MAP) of 65 and titrated up when the pressure drops but not down when it is increased. He continues taking vasopressors the next day, with a MAP of 78, but because of the use of vasopressors, it is deemed preferable to keep him sedated

and ventilated for another day. Because he is receiving vasopressors and is still intubated, antibiotic coverage is broadened and a decision is made to perform a computed tomography (CT) scan to look for an intra-abdominal collection. The result of the scan is negative; he returns from the scanner on a controlled ventilator mode. Gastric residuals are high, perhaps because of ileus secondary to his illness and to the narcotics given for analgesia; bile is suctioned from the oropharynx. On the fourth day, purulent secretions are suctioned from his lung, and he has a low-grade temperature; Pseudomonas is cultured from the sputum. Review of his course so far shows that he is in 9 L positive fluid balance and still ventilator dependent; his creatinine level is twice the normal level. The clinicians decide that recovery will be slow and arrange a tracheostomy. After 32 days, several bouts of ventilator-associated pneumonia, and a short course of dialysis, he is discharged from the ICU. He is profoundly weak and has a sacral pressure ulcer. Two weeks later he is discharged from the hospital to a chronic care facility where he remains an additional 2 months.

Much of his course has been shaped by iatrogenic factors—well-meaning clinical decisions that unnecessarily prolonged his ICU stay—and set him up for new ICU complications. What if he had been extubated in the operating room? None of the individual decisions during his management was necessarily wrong, but in aggregate they increased his dependence on technologies that bring both benefit and harm; even more important, the fact that these technologies were used convinced the clinicians that they were needed. In the ICU, clinicians treat patients who are very ill, but clinicians also make them look ill and make them even more ill through the inadvertent consequences of their support.

ORGAN DYSFUNCTION AS AN IATROGENIC DISORDER

The establishment of the first ICUs in the 1950s and 1960s brought with it the emergence of new clinical syndromes whose development was only possible because patients who would otherwise have died were kept alive through the use of a spectrum of life support technologies. Initially described as syndromes reflecting derangements in a single organ system (e.g., acute respiratory distress syndrome [ARDS], septic shock, acute renal failure, disseminated intravascular coagulation), they came to be conceptualized

325

as the manifestations of a common systemic process initially termed *multiple systems organ failure,*[4] and more recently, the *multiple organ dysfunction syndrome (MODS).*[5] It is only relatively recently that clinicians have begun to realize that MODS is not only a descriptive term for the acute derangements that are the raison d'être for organ support in the ICU but also often a consequence of that support.[6]

The Lung: From Acute Respiratory Distress Syndrome to Ventilator-Induced Lung Injury

The earliest description of pulmonary dysfunction as a consequence of remote organ injury was by Moon who, in 1948, identified congestion and atelectasis in the lungs of a cohort of patients who had died of shock.[7] Burke and colleagues described a condition they termed *high output respiratory failure* that complicated the course of some patients with peritonitis who had been supported by positive pressure mechanical ventilation.[8] In their classic report, Ashbaugh et al. termed this disorder the *adult* (now *acute*) *respiratory distress syndrome (ARDS),*[9] drawing attention to its cardinal features: severe arterial hypoxemia and diffuse bilateral fluffy infiltrates on the chest radiograph in the face of normal left atrial pressures and in association with autopsy findings of hyaline membranes. The cornerstone of the treatment of ARDS has been mechanical ventilation (although 5 of the 12 patients described by Ashbaugh et al. did not undergo ventilation); as this therapeutic modality expanded and evolved, it became not only the treatment for but also increasingly the cause of the clinical syndrome.

The earliest events in ARDS are increased pulmonary capillary permeability and an influx of innate immune cells—largely neutrophils—into the lung. Injury to the pulmonary parenchyma and the influx of inflammatory cells activate both the local microvascular coagulation and the processes of tissue repair, resulting, in conjunction with the debris from a loss of type I pulmonary epithelial cells, in hyaline membrane formation. Although external insults such as pneumonia or contusion or internal insults such as enhanced neutrophil recruitment in the face of an activated systemic inflammatory response play an important role in the evolution of ARDS, it has become evident that readily modifiable iatrogenic factors are equally culpable.

Computerized tomography of the lung of a patient with ARDS reveals that the apparently homogeneous diffuse fluffy infiltrates seen on chest radiograph are actually evidence of a more complex lesion, including dependent atelectasis and antidependent cystic degeneration of the lung (Fig. 47-1). The former changes reflect atelectasis in dependent lung zones of a patient who has been nursed for an extended period of time in the supine position, whereas the latter reflect overdistention of the lung by excessively large tidal volumes. The terminology *ventilator-induced lung injury* was first used in the 1990s[10] and shifted the focus of studies of ARDS from the biochemical mechanisms that underlie lung injury to the potentially modifiable iatrogenic factors that further aggravate the initial injury. Indeed, strategies to limit dependent atelectasis by prone positioning[11] and to minimize lung overdistention

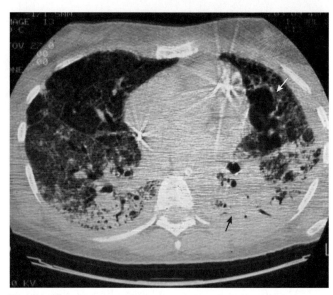

Figure 47-1. Computerized tomography of the lungs of a patient with acute respiratory distress syndrome reveals the importance of iatrogenic factors in lung injury, in particular atelectasis and collapse in dependent lung regions (*dark arrow*) and hyperinflation and cystic degeneration in the antidependent lung zones (*white arrow*).

Table 47-1 Effective Interventions in ARDS Are Those That Address the Sequelae of Mechanical Ventilation Rather Than the Pathophysiology of Lung Injury

Alter Outcomes	Ineffective
Reduced tidal volume	Antioxidants
Prone positioning	Beta-2 agonists
High frequency oscillation	G-CSF
Open lung ventilation	Nitric oxide
Neuromuscular blockade	Ketoconazole
Fluid restriction	Trophic feeding

by reducing tidal volumes[12] have shown impressive effects on reducing the mortality of ARDS. Moreover, it is striking that, of all the clinical trials of interventions for patients with ARDS, only those where the intervention sought to minimize iatrogenic harm, rather than those that sought to modulate the pathologic processes mediating that harm, have significantly affected clinically important outcomes (Table 47-1).

There is, moreover, evidence from human studies demonstrating that reducing tidal volumes attenuates the systemic inflammatory response,[13] whereas animal studies indicate that injurious mechanical ventilation strategies can induce remote organ injury in the kidney.[14]

ARDS is defined as an acute process, but its long-term consequences are profound. In a landmark study of ARDS survivors, Herridge and colleagues reported that disability, manifested as a reduced capacity for physical activity along with residual mild derangements in pulmonary function tests, persists even 5 years after the acute illness.[15]

Fluids and Hemodynamic Support

The capacity to correct intravascular volume deficit through the administration of intravenous fluids and the ability to titrate resuscitation through the measurement of indices of intravascular filling and myocardial function represented major advances in the care of the acutely ill.[16] Along with the provision of invasive respiratory support, advanced hemodynamic support and monitoring represent a major indication for ICU admission. This support also carries inadvertent iatrogenic consequences.

Large volumes of intravenous fluids are characteristically administered to unstable critically ill patients, not only during the initial phases of resuscitation but also over the course of the ICU stay. A cumulatively positive fluid balance is associated with increased ICU mortality[17-19] and with an increased risk of complications such as abdominal compartment syndrome.[20] Conversely there is evidence that more conservative fluid management strategies can attenuate organ dysfunction and improve outcomes.[18,21] Iatrogenic edema contributes to organ dysfunction involving the brain, heart, lung, kidney, and gastrointestinal (GI) tract; it contributes as well to the development of pressure sores.[22] The adverse effects of interstitial edema result from several factors, including a greater distance for oxygen diffusion to reach cells and a loss of tissue compliance.

Vasoactive agents increase blood pressure by virtue of their ability to increase peripheral vascular resistance and so, potentially, to reduce tissue blood flow. For example, it has been shown that vasopressor use is an independent risk factor for anastomotic leak after GI surgery.[23] Similarly, although inotropic agents can increase cardiac output, in large doses they also may increase mortality.[24]

Blood transfusion is similarly a double-edged sword: lifesaving in the face of massive hemorrhage but also potentially injurious. The Transfusion Requirements in Critical Care (TRICC) trial revealed that transfusion to an arbitrary threshold of 10 g/dL resulted in increased organ dysfunction, primarily pulmonary and cardiovascular.[25]

Sedation and Analgesia

Alleviating pain and anxiety for gravely ill patients in an ICU is a clinical and humane priority, but doing so may result in further harm. In a landmark trial, Kress and colleagues showed that daily wakening of critically ill patients enhanced the probability of survival.[26] Others have confirmed that prolonged early sedation is associated with an increased risk of ICU mortality,[27-29] and a randomized clinical trial indicated that withholding sedation resulted in a shorter duration of mechanical ventilation and ICU stay.[30] On the other hand, inadequate control of delirium is also a risk factor for adverse outcome in the ICU.[31,32] The optimal balance between attenuation of anxiety and oversedation has yet to be defined; however, emerging evidence suggests that activity, rather than rest, is central to a successful outcome from critical care.[33]

Anti-infective Strategies

The indigenous microbial flora of the GI tract plays a key role in normal development and immune homeostasis.[34] Conversely, derangements in normal patterns of microbial colonization are both common in critical illness[35-37] and associated with adverse outcome. The normal indigenous flora of the healthy individual comprises in excess of 1000 microbial species and remains remarkably constant over time. Loss of microbial diversity is characteristic of critical illness; the proximal gut in particular shows striking patterns of pathologic colonization with the same microbial flora that predominates in ICU-acquired infections.[35]

The mechanisms underlying normal host-microbial homeostasis in the GI tract are enormously complex. Nonetheless, studies in animal models reveal that disruption of the normal gut flora by the administration of systemic antibiotics is sufficient to induce microbial translocation from the gut lumen into regional mesenteric lymph nodes,[38] and that changes in the composition of the gut flora can induce alterations in systemic immune responsiveness.[39] The extent to which antibiotic-induced changes in gut flora contribute to an increased risk of ICU-acquired infection or to other derangements of critical illness is unknown.

Stress Ulcer Prophylaxis

Acute GI bleeding from gastric erosions was one of the first life-threatening derangements reported in association with care in an ICU[40] and also a risk factor for mortality for those patients in whom it developed. Rates of stress-induced bleeding have declined since these initial reports,[41] likely as a consequence of better resuscitation, earlier initiation of enteral nutrition, and improved diagnosis and management of infection. A legitimate question in the contemporary ICU is whether strategies to prevent stress-induced GI bleeding yield clinical benefit or whether they expose the patient to greater harm by predisposing to nosocomial ICU-acquired pneumonia or *Clostridium difficile* colitis.

Bed Rest

Not only is prolonged bed rest unnatural, but it is also a risk factor for complications such as atelectasis, pneumonia, and deep venous thrombosis and pulmonary embolism. Prone positioning partially corrects some of the adverse effects of prolonged bed rest and improves survival in ARDS.[11] Similarly, a program of physical therapy and mobilization has been shown to reduce the duration of delirium and mechanical ventilation and to improve functional outcomes at the time of hospital discharge.[33]

IS PERSISTENT CRITICAL ILLNESS AN IATROGENIC DISORDER?

Although management of acute life-threatening illness has been the primary focus of intensive care research and education, there is a growing awareness that much more attention must be directed toward the aftermath of initial success, both the factors that prolong stay in the ICU[42] and those that impair long-term quality of life after ICU discharge.[43] In focusing on the resuscitation and initial stabilization of the acutely ill, clinicians have underemphasized the complexities of moving from resuscitated and alive to recovered and independent.

Chronic critical illness has been variously defined as an ongoing need for ICU supportive care for more than 3 weeks[44] or an ICU stay of 8 days or longer in a patient with a diagnosis of prolonged acute mechanical ventilation, tracheostomy, sepsis, severe trauma, stroke, or traumatic brain injury.[45] Approximately 10% of patients admitted to an ICU meet criteria for chronic critical illness; their care generates upward of $26 billion per year in costs.[45] Mortality is substantial and continues to remain high even after ICU discharge.

The influences contributing to chronic critical illness represent a complex matrix of medical, cultural, and religious factors. Nonresolving acute illnesses such as stroke or head injury are important risk factors, as are preexisting comorbid conditions such as chronic lung disease and chronic renal failure. Chronicity is further affected by social factors, including uncertainty or disagreement about the patient's wishes at the end of life or religious beliefs that limit consideration of the withdrawal of life support in the face of evidence that ongoing support is nonbeneficial.[46] However, iatrogenic factors such as those described earlier play a substantial role.

The scientific underpinnings of chronic critical illness are underdeveloped, both because the focus of clinical research has been on acute treatment rather than on mitigation of the adverse consequences of that treatment and because metrics to detect longer term morbidity are poorly developed and inconsistently reported. However, three core principles frame an approach to limit iatrogenesis in the ICU.

First, every intervention has its cost, and it is therefore important to consider both beneficial and detrimental consequences before initiation of any management strategy. A vasopressor infusion can raise the mean arterial pressure to an arbitrary level, but does it help the patient who is producing urine or responding to voice and so showing evidence of adequate end organ perfusion? Are the potential consequences on splanchnic or extremity perfusion outweighed by the presumed benefits on coronary or cerebral perfusion? A patient may grimace when suctioned, but does this transient discomfort justify increasing doses of analgesics or sedation? The hemoglobin level may be low, but will transfusion be beneficial? Often the answers to these questions are unknown, and decisions must be made by integrating available knowledge with clinical judgment and common sense.

Second, in the end, the most important thing the intensivist does is to help the patient get out of the ICU. Stabilizing an unstable patient is an early priority, but once this is accomplished, the next priority is liberation from ICU support. There is no benefit, and only harm, associated with a state of quiet stability—even though this is all too often an end to which we aspire—and a lack of progress translates into an increased risk of adverse outcome.

Finally, despite adequate treatment of the underlying illness and full support in the ICU, many patients do not survive their ICU stay. Although it is often very difficult to know when ICU care is heroic and lifesaving and when it is little more than meddling in the process of dying, the distinction usually becomes clear over a relatively short period. Chronic critical illness may be a reflection of the most unfortunate form of iatrogenesis—a failure of the ICU team to advocate a transition from active support to the acceptance of the end of life. In doing so, the patient is exposed to the harms of support without the possibility of benefit, and the family to the illusion of choice without the possibility of altering outcome.

AUTHOR'S RECOMMENDATIONS

- In the ICU, clinicians treat patients who are very ill, but clinicians also make them look ill and make them more ill by inadvertent effects of their treatment.
- Ventilator-induced lung injury is the most widely recognized iatrogenic injury in the ICU.
- Excessive intravenous fluid therapy, high-dose inotropes, and indiscriminate blood transfusions are known to worsen outcomes.
- Although sedation and analgesia are administered to make patients more comfortable, prolonged sedation has been associated with increased mortality and morbidity. Bed rest, likewise, is associated with prolonged ICU stays.
- Indiscriminate antimicrobial therapy is associated with the proliferation of resistant strains and *Clostridium difficile* colitis.
- Chronic critical illness is multifactorial—a complex matrix of medical, cultural, and religious factors. The degree to which iatrogenic injury contributes to this is underdescribed.
- Chronic critical illness may at times reflect a failure of the ICU team to advocate a transition from active support to the acceptance of the end of life.

REFERENCES

1. Bywaters EG, Joekes AM. The artificial kidney; its clinical application in the treatment of traumatic anuria. *Proc R Soc Med.* 1948;41(7):420–426.
2. Safar P, DeKornfeld T, Pearson J, et al. Intensive care unit. *Anesthesia.* 1961;16:275.
3. Marshall JC. Critical illness is an iatrogenic disorder. *Crit Care Med.* 2010;38(suppl 10):S582–S589.
4. Baue AE. Multiple, progressive, or sequential systems failure. A syndrome of the 1970s. *Arch Surg.* 1975;110:779–781.
5. Bone RC, Balk RA, Cerra FB, et al. ACCP/SCCM CONSENSUS CONFERENCE. Definitions for sepsis and organ failure and guidelines for the use of innovative therapies in sepsis. *Chest.* 1992;101:1644–1655.
6. Slutsky AS, Tremblay LN. Multiple system organ failure. Is mechanical ventilation a contributing factor? *Am J Resp Crit Care Med.* 1998;157(6 Pt 1):1721–1725.
7. MOON VH. The pathology of secondary shock. *Am J Pathol.* 1948;24(2):235–273.
8. Burke JF, Pontoppidan H, Welch CE. High output respiratory failure: an important cause of death ascribed to peritonitis or ileus. *Ann Surg.* 1963;158:581–595.
9. Ashbaugh DG, Bigelow DB, Petty TL, Levine BE. Acute respiratory distress in adults. *Lancet.* 1967;2:319–323.
10. Hickling KG, Henderson SJ, Jackson R. Low mortality associated with low volume pressure limited ventilation with permissive hypercapnia in severe adult respiratory distress syndrome. *Intensive Care Med.* 1990;16:372–377.
11. Guerin C, Reignier J, Richard JC, et al. Prone positioning in severe acute respiratory distress syndrome. *N Engl J Med.* 2013;368(23):2159–2168.
12. Brower RG, Matthay MA, Morris A, et al. Ventilation with lower tidal volumes as compared with traditional tidal volumes for acute lung injury and the acute respiratory distress syndrome. *N Engl J Med.* 2000;342(18):1301–1308.
13. Ranieri VM, Suter PM, Tortorella C, et al. Effect of mechanical ventilation on inflammatory mediators in patients with acute respiratory distress syndrome. A randomized controlled trial. *JAMA.* 1999;282(1):54–61.

14. Imai Y, Parodo J, Kajikawa O, et al. Injurious mechanical ventilation and end-organ epithelial cell apoptosis and organ dysfunction in an experimental model of acute respiratory distress syndrome. *JAMA*. 2003;289(16):2104–2112.
15. Herridge MS, Tansey CM, Matte A, et al. Functional disability 5 years after acute respiratory distress syndrome. *N Engl J Med*. 2011;364(14):1293–1304.
16. Myburgh JA, Mythen MG. Resuscitation fluids. *N Engl J Med*. 2013;369(13):1243–1251.
17. Boyd JH, Forbes J, Nakada TA, Walley KR, Russell JA. Fluid resuscitation in septic shock: a positive fluid balance and elevated central venous pressure are associated with increased mortality. *Crit Care Med*. 2011;39(2):259–265.
18. Murphy CV, Schramm GE, Doherty JA, et al. The importance of fluid management in acute lung injury secondary to septic shock. *Chest*. 2009;136(1):102–109.
19. Payen D, de Pont AC, Sakr Y, Spies C, Reinhart K, Vincent JL. A positive fluid balance is associated with a worse outcome in patients with acute renal failure. *Crit Care*. 2008;12(3):R74.
20. Malbrain ML, Marik PE, Witters I, et al. Fluid overload, de-resuscitation, and outcomes in critically ill or injured patients: a systematic review with suggestions for clinical practice. *Anaesthesiol Intensive Ther*. 2014;46(5):361–380.
21. National Heart Lung, and Blood Institute Acute Respiratory Distress Syndrome (ARDS) Clinical Trials Network, Wiedemann HP, Wheeler AP, et al. Comparison of two fluid-management strategies in acute lung injury. *N Engl J Med*. 2006;354(24):2564–2575.
22. Prowle JR, Echeverri JE, Ligabo EV, Ronco C, Bellomo R. Fluid balance and acute kidney injury. *Nat Rev Nephrol*. 2010;6(2):107–115.
23. Zakrison T, Nascimento Jr BA, Tremblay LN, Kiss A, Rizoli SB. Perioperative vasopressors are associated with an increased risk of gastrointestinal anastomotic leakage. *World J Surg*. 2007;31(8):1627–1634.
24. Hayes MA, Timmins AC, Yau EHS, Palazzo M, Hinds CJ, Watson D. Elevation of systemic oxygen delivery in the treatment of critically ill patients. *N Engl J Med*. 1994;330:1717–1722.
25. Hebert PC, Wells G, Blajchman MA, et al. A multicentre randomized controlled clinical trial of transfusion requirements in critical care. *N Engl J Med*. 1999;340:409–417.
26. Kress JP, Pohlman AS, O'Connor MF, Hall JB. Daily interruption of sedative infusions in critically ill patients undergoing mechanical ventilation. *N Engl J Med*. 2000;342:1471–1477.
27. Shehabi Y, Chan L, Kadiman S, et al. Sedation depth and long-term mortality in mechanically ventilated critically ill adults: a prospective longitudinal multicentre cohort study. *Intensive Care Med*. 2013;39(5):910–918.
28. Lonardo NW, Mone MC, Nirula R, et al. Propofol is associated with favorable outcomes compared with benzodiazepines in ventilated intensive care unit patients. *Am J Respir Crit Care Med*. 2014;189(11):1383–1394.
29. Shehabi Y, Bellomo R, Reade MC, et al. Early intensive care sedation predicts long-term mortality in ventilated critically ill patients. *Am J Respir Crit Care Med*. 2012;186(8):724–731.
30. Strom T, Martinussen T, Toft P. A protocol of no sedation for critically ill patients receiving mechanical ventilation: a randomised trial. *Lancet*. 2010;375(9713):475–480.
31. Salluh JI, Soares M, Teles JM, et al. Delirium epidemiology in critical care (DECCA): an international study. *Crit Care*. 2010;14(6):R210.
32. Mehta S, Cook D, Devlin JW, et al. Prevalence, risk factors, and outcomes of delirium in mechanically ventilated adults. *Crit Care Med*. 2015;43(3):557–566.
33. Schweickert WD, Pohlman MC, Pohlman AS, et al. Early physical and occupational therapy in mechanically ventilated, critically ill patients: a randomised controlled trial. *Lancet*. 2009;373(9678):1874–1882.
34. Marshall JC, Nathens AB. The gut in critical illness: Evidence from human studies. *Shock*. 1996;6:S10–S16.
35. Marshall JC, Christou NV, Meakins JL. The gastrointestinal tract. The "undrained abscess" of multiple organ failure. *Ann Surg*. 1993;218:111–119.
36. Zaborin A, Smith D, Garfield K, et al. Membership and behavior of ultra-low-diversity pathogen communities present in the gut of humans during prolonged critical illness. *MBio*. 2014;5(5):e01361–14.
37. Iapichino G, Callegari ML, Marzorati S, et al. Impact of antibiotics on the gut microbiota of critically ill patients. *J Med Microbiol*. 2008;57(Pt 8):1007–1014.
38. Berg RD. Promotion of the translocation of enteric bacteria from the gastrointestinal tracts of mice by oral treatment with penicillin, clindamycin, or metronidazole. *Infect Immun*. 1981;33:854–861.
39. Marshall JC, Christou NV, Meakins JL. Immunomodulation by altered gastrointestinal tract flora. The effects of orally administered, killed *Staphylococcus epidermidis*, *Candida*, and *Pseudomonas* on systemic immune responses. *Arch Surg*. 1988;123:1465–1469.
40. Skillman JJ, Bushnell LS, Goldman H, Silen W. Respiratory failure, hypotension, sepsis, and jaundice. A clinical syndrome associated with lethal hemorrhage and acute stress ulceration in the stomach. *Am J Surg*. 1969;117:523–530.
41. Cook DJ, Fuller H, Guyatt GH, et al. Risk factors for gastrointestinal bleeding in critically ill patients. *N Engl J Med*. 1994;330:377–381.
42. Martin CM, Hil AD, Burns K, Chen LM. Characteristics and outcomes for critically ill patients with prolonged intensive care unit stays. *Crit Care Med*. 2005;33(9):1922–1927.
43. Needham DM, Davidson J, Cohen H, et al. Improving long-term outcomes after discharge from intensive care unit: report from a stakeholders' conference. *Crit Care Med*. 2012;40(2):502–509.
44. Nelson JE, Cox CE, Hope AA, Carson SS. Chronic critical illness. *Am J Respir Crit Care Med*. 2010;182(4):446–454.
45. Kahn JM, Le T, Angus DC, et al. The epidemiology of chronic critical illness in the United States. *Crit Care Med*. 2015;43(2):282–287.
46. Downar J, You JJ, Bagshaw SM, et al. Nonbeneficial treatment Canada: definitions, causes, and potential solutions from the perspective of healthcare practitioners. *Crit Care Med*. 2015;43(2):270–281.

48 What Is the Role of Autonomic Dysfunction in Critical Illness?

Gareth L. Ackland

The term *autonomic dysfunction* is frequently associated with the syndrome of critical illness. Numerous studies have reported a striking association among depressed autonomic activity (usually measured as reduced heart rate variability), disease severity, and outcome.[1,2] More sophisticated interrogation of various components of the autonomic nervous system also reveals that the loss of chemoreflex[3] or baroreflex[4] responses is associated with higher mortality in critically ill patients. However, the marker versus mediator debate over the significance of these findings is difficult to disentangle—at least from clinical studies. Moreover, much of the literature making an association between the development of critical illness and the autonomic dysfunction is hampered by the variety of techniques used to detect alterations in autonomic control, the lack of population norms, variable analysis techniques, and lack of suitable controls and follow-up.[5] Nevertheless, emerging laboratory and trial data suggest that autonomic dysfunction may be a clinically underappreciated driver of established critical illness. Specifically, the argument put forward here is that critical illness occurs as a direct result of autonomic dysfunction, which also serves as an essential biological precursor for priming pathophysiologic responses that subsequently result in multiorgan failure/dysfunction. As a complementary hypothesis, acquired autonomic dysfunction may also portend worse outcomes following disparate triggers of critical illness.

WHAT IS AUTONOMIC DYSFUNCTION?

From a basic biological perspective, autonomic dysfunction should be considered as the uncoupling of cellular and integrative physiologic control.[6] In other words, autonomic dysfunction may be defined as changes in afferent, integrative (central nervous system [CNS]), or efferent components of sympathetic or parasympathetic neural control, associated with pathologic states. This broadens the scope of its potential impact on understanding the pathophysiology of critical illness. Coordinated and self-limiting sympathetic activation, coupled with the maintenance of parasympathetic tone, appears to be associated with a favorable physiologic response to tissue injury and sepsis. The "uncoupling" of these autonomic control mechanisms, and consequent loss of neurally mediated interorgan feedback pathways, is a feature of the development of

multiorgan dysfunction syndrome. In established critical illness, there is a temporally related association between autonomic dysfunction and derangements in immune, metabolic, and bioenergetic mechanisms that appear to be prognostically linked to outcome. From a neuropathologic viewpoint, postmortem samples of brain tissue, obtained from septic patients, show evidence for neuronal death in autonomic centers.[7] At the molecular level, disruption of normal G-protein–coupled receptor (GPCR) recycling[8] is a feature of neurohormonal dysregulation in disease states where biological variability is disrupted. In many respects, core features of established critical illness may be erroneously attributed to conventional clinical explanations rather than the consequences of autonomic dysfunction alone (Table 48-1).

AT WHAT POINT DOES AUTONOMIC DYSFUNCTION INFLUENCE THE DEVELOPMENT OF CRITICAL ILLNESS?

Many patients who ultimately require critical care have established features of autonomic dysfunction well before the clinical manifestation of critical illness, as a result of various established chronic disease states. The striking observation that several chronic diseases such as cardiac and renal failure confer increased risk for sepsis suggests that an underlying common mechanism contributes to this increased propensity for multiorgan dysfunction.[9] Subclinical changes in autonomic function precede the onset of diabetes and hypertension.[10] Patients with overt or occult heart failure are at particularly high risk of having critical illness, including acquiring infection or sustaining excess postoperative morbidity following cardiac or noncardiac surgery. It has become increasingly apparent that many of the pathophysiologic features of cardiac failure are present in deconditioned patients, with poor aerobic capacity and low anaerobic threshold, yet no formal diagnosis of heart failure.[11] Cardiac failure is characterized by increased sympathetic drive, high levels of circulating catecholamines and cortisol, and withdrawal of parasympathetic activity.[12] Elevated plasma levels of proinflammatory cytokines and deficient immune function are also common features of chronic heart failure.[13] Restoration toward normal autonomic function with conventional or experimental therapies improves cardiac function, as well

Table 48-1 **Common Symptoms/Signs in Critically Ill Patients Mimicked by Features of Aberrant Autonomic Control**

Symptom of Critical Illness	Conventional Explanation	Alternative "Dysautonomia" Hypothesis
Tachycardia	Agitation[55]/fever[56]	Loss of baroreflex diminution of heart rate Cytokine stimulation of peripheral chemoreceptors
Cardiac ischemia	Underlying or acquired coronary disease[57]/ hypercoaguability[58]	Loss of cardioprotective vagal innervation
Loss of inotropic performance	Cardiac ischemic damage	Neurohormonal downregulation of β-adrenoreceptors ± cardiac receptors
Failure to wean	Cardiac failure	All above
Fever of uncertain origin	Undeclared infectious source	Cytokinemia derived from neurohormonal activation of immune cells
Persistently raised inflammatory markers	Undeclared infectious source	Cytokinemia derived from neurohormonal activation of immune cells
Bacterial colonization	Immunosuppression	Adrenergic fuel for microorganism growth

as reduces excess neurohormonal and inflammatory activation.[13] A growing body of evidence in both chronic heart failure[14] and critically ill patients is accumulating, indicating that sympatholysis is associated with a counterintuitive improvement in left ventricular function[15] in addition to reductions in left ventricular remodeling and reduced plasma levels of inflammatory cytokines.[16] Loss of vagal activity in chronic heart failure is a predictor of high mortality.[17] Beyond overt cardiovascular disease, patients with extracardiac disease also show features of established autonomic dysfunction. For example, end-stage renal disease[18] and obstructive jaundice[19] are characterized by impaired baroreflex sensitivity and increased levels of plasma atrial natriuretic peptide.

AUTONOMIC DYSFUNCTION AT THE VERY ONSET OF CRITICAL ILLNESS

The hallmark of the onset of critical illness is tachycardia, frequently accompanied by tachypnea.[20,21] Sepsis, hypoxia, and acidosis are all major stimuli for driving tachypnea/tachycardia through peripheral chemoreceptor-driven autonomic reflexes.[22] Similarly, sterile inflammation, or danger-associated molecular patterns, may also be an important—though underrecognized—additional driver for this physiologic response.[22] Thus, afferent sensors of the autonomic nervous system are hardwired to detect pathologic changes in oxygen, carbon dioxide, acidosis, glucose, electrolytes, neurohormones, and inflammatory mediators (Fig. 48-1). Experimental models of endotoxin infusion illustrate the speed with which neural afferents detect inflammatory changes, in parallel with the rapid and dramatic pathophysiologic features that can appear in otherwise previously well, healthy individuals.[23,24] Typical pathophysiologic changes in respiratory function—beyond tachypnea—include increased airway resistance and secretions. Discrete activation of the peripheral chemoreflex triggers the release of cortisol and vasopressin, prototypical neurohormones of critical illness. These responses may

form part of the protective autonomic response to triggers of critical illness because acute carotid sinus denervation hastens mortality after lethal experimental endotoxemia.[25] Loss of baroreflex control through denervation of the carotid sinus and aortic baroreceptor nerves appears to compromise the compensatory response to hypotension induced by acute sepsis, with lower mean blood pressure, cardiac output, total peripheral resistance, and central venous pressure.[26]

IS AUTONOMIC DYSFUNCTION IN CRITICAL ILLNESS INDUCED BY MODERN CRITICAL CARE STRATEGIES?

By most accounts, many of the therapies used in critically ill patients profoundly alter, if not ablate, autonomic, baroreflex, and chemoreceptor control. Sedation inhibits parasympathetic neuronal activity while reducing sympathetic drive.[27] Neuromuscular blockade agents such as vecuronium inhibit peripheral chemoreceptor sensitivity[28] and conceivably produce immunosuppression through nicotinic receptor blockade.[29] Inotropes dramatically reduce baroreflex control and inhibit parasympathetic activity, as reflected by changes in heart rate variability.[30,31] Furthermore, catecholamines directly fuel infection by promoting bacterial acquisition of normally inaccessible sequestered host iron, which is released by transferrin as a result of catecholamines forming protein complexes with ferric iron.[32]

Perhaps most strikingly, models of enforced bed rest in healthy volunteers show the rapid onset of autonomic dysfunction appearing well before other features of deconditioning. Typically, these changes involve sympathetic activation and parasympathetic withdrawal.[33] The increasingly recognized, though seldom detected, problem of psychological stress induced by the critical care environment reduces baroreflex sensitivity and promotes tachycardia.[34] Experimental models of enforced bed rest demonstrate a mechanistic interaction between dysautonomia and

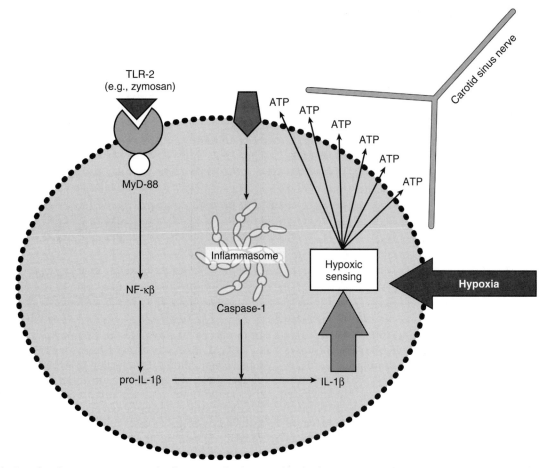

Figure 48-1. Peripheral autonomic sensing of inflammation by the carotid body chemoreceptors. Hypoxic sensing is transduced by the release of adenosine triphosphate (*ATP*) as a neurotransmitter at the carotid sinus nerve; ATP is also required for activation of inflammation (NLRP3 inflammasome by the toll-like receptor 2 [*TLR-2*] agonist zymosan). TLR-2 activation increases production of prointerleukin-1β (*pro-IL-1β*) in a myeloid differentiation primary response gene 88 (*MyD-88*), nuclear factor-κB (NF-κB)–dependent fashion. In turn, concomitant NLRP3 activation by extracellular ATP causes caspase-1 upregulation and cleavage of pro-IL-1β, which mimics hypoxia through the induction of hypoxia-inducible factor 1-α (HIF-1α). *IL-1β,* interleukin 1β.

anhedonia (loss of the capacity to experience pleasure),[35] which may relate to depression being a negative prognosticator of outcome in critical illness.[36] Given the current vogue for early physical, occupational, or behavioral therapy,[37] it is tempting to speculate that restoring autonomic control may be an underappreciated feature of the apparent success of this strategy.

CARDIOVASCULAR DYSFUNCTION IN CRITICAL ILLNESS AS A DIRECT RESULT OF AUTONOMIC DYSFUNCTION

Cardiovascular dysfunction, a hallmark of critical illness, frequently prevents successful liberation from mechanical ventilation.[38] The etiology of cardiac injury during critical illness remains unclear and appears unlikely to be merely attributable to coronary artery disease given the strikingly broad demographic associated with abnormal levels of circulating troponin. Excessive sympathetic activity alone leads to accumulation of intracellular calcium, triggering myocardial necrosis.[39] Acute stress, whether it be psychological or hemodynamic in origin, triggers coagulation and endothelial cell dysfunction through sustained increases in sympathetic activity.[40] Together with persistent tachycardia, endothelial dysfunction and a sympathetic-mediated prothrombotic state may explain in part elevations in troponin frequently seen in critically ill patients. Catecholamine-associated metabolic dysregulation, typified by "stress" hyperglycemia, may further exacerbate myocardial injury.[41] The carefully targeted use of alpha-2 agonists[42] and beta blockers[43] may contribute to a useful therapeutic role in this context.

In the absence of direct myocardial injury, prolonged sympathetic activation results in β-adrenoreceptor downregulation and desensitization. Circulating inflammatory mediators directly disrupt effective coupling of adrenergic receptors from their downstream signaling kinases.[44] As a result, the pathologic failure to recycle GPCRs may explain the impaired cardiometabolic response to exogenous β-adrenoreceptor stimulation. Several clinical studies have repeatedly shown that increased mortality is associated with the loss of the typical cardiometabolic response to exogenous β-adrenergic agonists in established critical illness.[45]

The parasympathetic limb of the autonomic nervous system also plays an important cardioprotective role, through several disparate mechanisms. In addition to the well-recognized hemodynamic effects of increasing diastolic filling time, recent experimental data add important new mechanisms of direct relevance to established critical illness. Remote preconditioning is activated by numerous afferent inputs, including pain and transient ischemia in distant organs. Cardioprotective remote ischemic preconditioning is dependent on intact vagal efferent innervations of the myocardium.[46] Some of these cardioprotective effects may further be mediated through a parasympathetic-mediated anti-inflammatory mechanism, at least in the context of myocardial dysfunction triggered by inflammatory myocarditis.[47]

IMMUNE DYSFUNCTION IN CRITICAL ILLNESS AS A RESULT OF AUTONOMIC DYSFUNCTION

Experimental data show that multiple autonomic mechanisms contribute to immunoparesis and immunosuppression, key features of established critical illness. Monocyte deactivation is associated with increased risk of infection and higher mortality, accompanied by β-adrenergic desensitization.[48] Catecholamines exacerbate the hepatic dysfunction observed during sepsis,[49] which may be reversed by targeted beta-blockade.[50] The parasympathetic nervous system, acting through the vagus nerve, can sense inflammation in the periphery and relay this information to the brain, resulting in fever and activation of the hypothalamic-pituitary-adrenal axis and sympathetic activation.[51] Enhancing efferent vagal activity, at least in animal models, attenuates macrophage release of inflammatory cytokines through nicotinic alpha-7 agonism.[52] Other parasympathetic neurotransmitters,[53] and pathways,[54] may also contribute to neuro-immunomodulation.

CONCLUSIONS

An abnormal cardiometabolic response to sympathoexcitation is robustly associated with key features of chronic critical illness and paralleled by the loss of parasympathetic activity. Emerging clinical data provide some support for these largely experimental concepts. Precedents from the clinical cardiac failure literature suggest that autonomic modulation provides a rational target for preventing/reversing critical illness.

AUTHOR'S RECOMMENDATIONS

- Persistent tachycardia should not automatically be attributed to conventionally thought-of triggers of excess sympathetic activity, such as hypovolemia or pain.
- Early efforts to minimize prolonged immobility may be beneficial through preventing associated autonomic dysfunction.
- Targeted treatments to ameliorate tachycardia, using α2 adrenoceptor agonists, such as dexmedetomidine or clonidine, or titratable beta-blockers, such as esmolol, may also be beneficial.

REFERENCES

1. Hoyer D, Friedrich H, Zwiener U, et al. Prognostic impact of autonomic information flow in multiple organ dysfunction syndrome patients. *Int J Cardiol.* 2006;108:359–369.
2. Schmidt H, Muller-Werdan U, Hoffmann T, et al. Attenuated autonomic function in multiple organ dysfunction syndrome across three age groups. *Biomed Tech (Berl).* 2006;51:264–267.
3. Schmidt H, Muller-Werdan U, Nuding S, et al. Impaired chemoreflex sensitivity in adult patients with multiple organ dysfunction syndrome–the potential role of disease severity. *Intensive Care Med.* 2004;30:665–672.
4. Schmidt H, Muller-Werdan U, Hoffmann T, et al. Autonomic dysfunction predicts mortality in patients with multiple organ dysfunction syndrome of different age groups. *Crit Care Med.* 2005;33:1994–2002.
5. Stein PK. Challenges of heart rate variability research in the ICU. *Crit Care Med.* 2013;41:666–667.
6. Godin PJ, Buchman TG. Uncoupling of biological oscillators: a complementary hypothesis concerning the pathogenesis of multiple organ dysfunction syndrome. *Crit Care Med.* 1996;24:1107–1116.
7. Sharshar T, Gray F, Lorin de la Grandmaison G, et al. Apoptosis of neurons in cardiovascular autonomic centres triggered by inducible nitric oxide synthase after death from septic shock. *Lancet.* 2003;362:1799–1805.
8. Hupfeld CJ, Olefsky JM. Regulation of receptor tyrosine kinase signaling by GRKs and beta-arrestins. *Annu Rev Physiol.* 2007;69:561–577.
9. Phillips JK. Autonomic dysfunction in heart failure and renal disease. *Front Physiol.* 2012;3:219.
10. Davis JT, Rao F, Naqshbandi D, et al. Autonomic and hemodynamic origins of pre-hypertension: central role of heredity. *J Am Coll Cardiol.* 2012;59:2206–2216.
11. Sultan P, Edwards MR, Gutierrez del Arroyo A, et al. Cardiopulmonary exercise capacity and preoperative markers of inflammation. *Mediators Inflamm.* 2014;2014:727451.
12. Schwartz PJ, De Ferrari GM. Sympathetic-parasympathetic interaction in health and disease: abnormalities and relevance in heart failure. *Heart Fail Rev.* 2011;16:101–107.
13. Maisel AS. Beneficial effects of metoprolol treatment in congestive heart failure. Reversal of sympathetic-induced alterations of immunologic function. *Circulation.* 1994;90:1774–1780.
14. McAlister FA, Wiebe N, Ezekowitz JA, Leung AA, Armstrong PW. Meta-analysis: beta-blocker dose, heart rate reduction, and death in patients with heart failure. *Ann Intern Med.* 2009;150:784–794.
15. Gore DC, Wolfe RR. Hemodynamic and metabolic effects of selective beta1 adrenergic blockade during sepsis. *Surgery.* 2006;139:686–694.
16. Felder RB, Yu Y, Zhang ZH, Wei SG. Pharmacological treatment for heart failure: a view from the brain. *Clin Pharmacol Ther.* 2009;86:216–220.
17. Van Wagoner DR. Chronic vagal nerve stimulation for the treatment of human heart failure: progress in translating a vision into reality. *Eur Heart J.* 2011;32:788–790.
18. Chesterton LJ, McIntyre CW. The assessment of baroreflex sensitivity in patients with chronic kidney disease: implications for vasomotor instability. *Curr Opin Nephrol Hypertens.* 2005;14:586–591.
19. Song JG, Cao YF, Sun YM, et al. Baroreflex sensitivity is impaired in patients with obstructive jaundice. *Anesthesiology.* 2009;111:561–565.
20. Rangel-Frausto MS, Pittet D, Costigan M, Hwang T, Davis CS, Wenzel RP. The natural history of the systemic inflammatory response syndrome (SIRS). A prospective study. *JAMA.* 1995;273:117–123.
21. Annane D, Trabold F, Sharshar T, et al. Inappropriate sympathetic activation at onset of septic shock: a spectral analysis approach. *Am J Respir Crit Care Med.* 1999;160:458–465.
22. Ackland GL, Kazymov V, Marina N, Singer M, Gourine AV. Peripheral neural detection of danger-associated and pathogen-associated molecular patterns. *Crit Care Med.* 2013;41:e85–92.
23. Godin PJ, Fleisher LA, Eidsath A, et al. Experimental human endotoxemia increases cardiac regularity: results from a prospective, randomized, crossover trial. *Crit Care Med.* 1996;24:1117–1124.
24. Taylor EW, Jordan D, Coote JH. Central control of the cardiovascular and respiratory systems and their interactions in vertebrates. *Physiol Rev.* 1999;79:855–916.

25. Tang GJ, Kou YR, Lin YS. Peripheral neural modulation of endotoxin-induced hyperventilation. *Crit Care Med*. 1998;26:1558–1563.

26. Koyama S, Terada N, Shiojima Y, Takeuchi T. Baroreflex participation of cardiovascular response to *E. coli* endotoxin. *Jpn J Physiol*. 1986;36:267–275.

27. Bradley BD, Green G, Ramsay T, Seely AJ. Impact of sedation and organ failure on continuous heart and respiratory rate variability monitoring in critically ill patients: a pilot study. *Crit Care Med*. 2013;41:433–444.

28. Eriksson LI, Sato M, Severinghaus JW. Effect of a vecuronium-induced partial neuromuscular block on hypoxic ventilatory response. *Anesthesiology*. 1993;78:693–699.

29. Wang H, Yu M, Ochani M, et al. Nicotinic acetylcholine receptor alpha7 subunit is an essential regulator of inflammation. *Nature*. 2003;421:384–388.

30. Hogue Jr CW, Davila-Roman VG, Stein PK, Feinberg M, Lappas DG, Perez JE. Alterations in heart rate variability in patients undergoing dobutamine stress echocardiography, including patients with neurocardiogenic hypotension. *Am Heart J*. 1995;130:1203–1209.

31. van de Borne P, Heron S, Nguyen H, et al. Arterial baroreflex control of the sinus node during dobutamine exercise stress testing. *Hypertension*. 1999;33:987–991.

32. Lyte M, Freestone PP, Neal CP, et al. Stimulation of *Staphylococcus epidermidis* growth and biofilm formation by catecholamine inotropes. *Lancet*. 2003;361:130–135.

33. Hughson RL, Yamamoto Y, Maillet A, et al. Altered autonomic regulation of cardiac function during head-up tilt after 28-day head-down bed-rest with counter-measures. *Clin Physiol*. 1994;14:291–304.

34. Truijen J, Davis SC, Stok WJ, et al. Baroreflex sensitivity is higher during acute psychological stress in healthy subjects under beta-adrenergic blockade. *Clin Sci*. 2011;120:161–167.

35. Moffitt JA, Grippo AJ, Beltz TG, Johnson AK. Hindlimb unloading elicits anhedonia and sympathovagal imbalance. *J Appl Physiol*. 1985;2008(105):1049–1059.

36. Desai SV, Law TJ, Needham DM. Long-term complications of critical care. *Crit Care Med*. 2011;39:371–379.

37. Schweickert WD, Pohlman MC, Pohlman AS, et al. Early physical and occupational therapy in mechanically ventilated, critically ill patients: a randomised controlled trial. *Lancet*. 2009;373:1874–1882.

38. Lara TM, Hajjar LA, de Almeida JP, et al. High levels of B-type natriuretic peptide predict weaning failure from mechanical ventilation in adult patients after cardiac surgery. *Clinics (Sao Paulo)*. 2013;68:33–38.

39. Ellison GM, Torella D, Karakikes I, et al. Acute beta-adrenergic overload produces myocyte damage through calcium leakage from the ryanodine receptor 2 but spares cardiac stem cells. *J Biol Chem*. 2007;282:11397–11409.

40. Bruno RM, Ghiadoni L, Seravalle G, Dell'oro R, Taddei S, Grassi G. Sympathetic regulation of vascular function in health and disease. *Front Physiol*. 2012;3:284.

41. Weekers F, Giulietti AP, Michalaki M, et al. Metabolic, endocrine, and immune effects of stress hyperglycemia in a rabbit model of prolonged critical illness. *Endocrinology*. 2003;144:5329–5338.

42. MacLaren R. Immunosedation: a consideration for sepsis. *Crit Care*. 2009;13:191.

43. Morelli A, Ertmer C, Westphal M, et al. Effect of heart rate control with esmolol on hemodynamic and clinical outcomes in patients with septic shock: a randomized clinical trial. *JAMA*. 2013;310:1683–1691.

44. Coggins M, Rosenzweig A. The fire within: cardiac inflammatory signaling in health and disease. *Circ Res*. 2012;110:116–125.

45. Collin S, Sennoun N, Levy B. Cardiovascular and metabolic responses to catecholamine and sepsis prognosis: a ubiquitous phenomenon? *Crit Care*. 2008;12:118.

46. Mastitskaya S, Marina N, Gourine A, et al. Cardioprotection evoked by remote ischaemic preconditioning is critically dependent on the activity of vagal pre-ganglionic neurones. *Cardiovasc Res*. 2012;95:487–494.

47. Leib C, Goser S, Luthje D, et al. Role of the cholinergic antiinflammatory pathway in murine autoimmune myocarditis. *Circ Res*. 2011;109:130–140.

48. Link A, Selejan S, Maack C, Lenz M, Bohm M. Phosphodiesterase 4 inhibition but not beta-adrenergic stimulation suppresses tumor necrosis factor-alpha release in peripheral blood mononuclear cells in septic shock. *Crit Care*. 2008;12:R159.

49. Aninat C, Seguin P, Descheemaeker PN, Morel F, Malledant Y, Guillouzo A. Catecholamines induce an inflammatory response in human hepatocytes. *Crit Care Med*. 2008;36:848–854.

50. Ackland GL, Yao ST, Rudiger A, et al. Cardioprotection, attenuated systemic inflammation, and survival benefit of beta1-adrenoceptor blockade in severe sepsis in rats. *Crit Care Med*. 2010;38:388–394.

51. Goehler LE, Gaykema RP, Hansen MK, Anderson K, Maier SF, Watkins LR. Vagal immune-to-brain communication: a visceral chemosensory pathway. *Auton Neurosci*. 2000;85:49–59.

52. Tracey KJ. Understanding immunity requires more than immunology. *Nat Immunol*. 2010;11:561–564.

53. Smalley SG, Barrow PA, Foster N. Immunomodulation of innate immune responses by vasoactive intestinal peptide (VIP): its therapeutic potential in inflammatory disease. *Clin Exp Immunol*. 2009;157:225–234.

54. Cailotto C, Gomez-Pinilla PJ, Costes LM, et al. Neuro-anatomical evidence indicating indirect modulation of macrophages by vagal efferents in the intestine but not in the spleen. *PLoS One*. 2014;9:e87785.

55. Chevrolet JC, Jolliet P. Clinical review: agitation and delirium in the critically ill–significance and management. *Crit Care*. 2007;11:214.

56. Launey Y, Nesseler N, Malledant Y, Seguin P. Clinical review: fever in septic ICU patients–friend or foe? *Crit Care*. 2011;15:222.

57. Lim W, Qushmaq I, Devereaux PJ, et al. Elevated cardiac troponin measurements in critically ill patients. *Arch Intern Med*. 2006;166:2446–2454.

58. Alhazzani W, Lim W, Jaeschke RZ, Murad MH, Cade J, Cook DJ. Heparin thromboprophylaxis in medical-surgical critically ill patients: a systematic review and meta-analysis of randomized trials. *Crit Care Med*. 2013;41:2088–2098.

49 Is Sepsis-Induced Organ Dysfunction an Adaptive Response?

Scott L. Weiss, Richard J. Levy, Clifford S. Deutschman

Organ dysfunction is a hallmark of sepsis.[1] Scientific investigation has focused on identifying potential causes and therapeutic targets of this component of the syndrome. Although various pathways and cellular systems are altered by sepsis and inflammation, to date no unifying or causative etiology has been uncovered. Historically, clinicians and investigators have viewed sepsis-induced organ dysfunction as a pathologic process that is deleterious to the survival of the host.[2] Indeed, multiorgan dysfunction syndrome is the primary antecedent to sepsis-associated mortality.[3,4] Recently, an interesting alternative hypothesis has been proposed: Does organ dysfunction during sepsis represent an adaptive prosurvival response?[5-7] This concept is based on the observation that, despite physiologic and biochemical dysfunction, there is minimal evidence of cell death in affected organ systems, survivors rapidly recover organ function, and the downregulation of metabolism described during sepsis resembles a hibernating or suspended-animation state.[1,8]

In nature, hibernation (torpor) is a protective adaptation to harsh environmental conditions and is a regulated, seasonal response largely coordinated by changes in mitochondrial respiration.[9] This response allows hibernating mammals to reduce their metabolism to promote survival amid decreased substrate availability.[9] Although a profound and prolonged metabolic downregulation can trigger death, the conservation of this physiologic response across models and species suggests that some degree of transient energetic swoon early in sepsis is likely to be adaptive.[10] In this chapter, we review (1) the mechanisms that downregulate metabolism in sepsis, highlighting the role of mitochondria; (2) the evidence supporting the development of a hibernation-like state in during sepsis; and (3) the role for mitochondrial biogenesis to restore organ function and promote survival.

MITOCHONDRIA AS THE MEDIATOR OF METABOLIC DOWNREGULATION IN SEPSIS

It has been proposed that an acquired defect in oxidative phosphorylation prevents cells from using molecular oxygen for adenosine triphosphate (ATP) production and potentially causes sepsis-induced organ dysfunction.[11,12] Most energy production in vertebrate cells occurs in the mitochondria and is generated by aerobic respiration.[13] This process, called "oxidative phosphorylation," couples oxidation of NADH (nicotinamide adenine dinucleotide) and flavin adenine dinucleotide with phosphorylation of adenosine diphosphate (ADP) to form ATP.[12,13] Oxidative phosphorylation is accomplished by a series of enzyme complexes termed the *electron transport system (ETS)*.[13] Located on the mitochondrial inner membrane, these enzymes use energy released during transfer of electrons between complexes to actively pump protons from the mitochondrial matrix into the intermembrane space.[12,13] The resultant proton motive force is then used by ATP synthase (complex V) to synthesize ATP from ADP.[13]

Each mitochondrion contains 2 to 10 copies of a circular, double-stranded DNA called *mitochondrial DNA (mtDNA)*. mtDNA encodes key subunits of the ETS enzyme complexes, whereas structural subunits and the mitochondrial translational machinery primarily arise from nuclear genes.[14] Thus, expression of genes that give rise to the protein complexes of the ETS is under dual control. An acquired defect in gene expression, protein translation, or functional activity of any of the ETS enzymes could impair oxidative phosphorylation and lead to sepsis-induced organ dysfunction.[11,12]

Ultrastructural mitochondrial abnormalities have been recognized across organ systems in in vivo, ex vivo, and in vitro models of sepsis for over 30 years.[8] For example, Crouser et al. demonstrated marked swelling and disruption of mitochondrial architecture in the liver 24 hours after cecal ligation and puncture (CLP) in a cat model.[15] Similar morphologic abnormalities have been noted in mitochondria taken from heart, endothelial cells, intestinal epithelial cells, kidney, and skeletal muscle in animal models of sepsis.[16] In human sepsis, heart and liver biopsies obtained immediately postmortem from adult nonsurvivors showed substantial accumulation of hydropic mitochondria.[17]

Functional changes in mitochondrial respiration have been variably reported as increased, decreased, or unchanged in short-term sepsis models, although longer-term models more consistently demonstrate depressed mitochondrial function. Data about mitochondrial dysfunction in human sepsis remain relatively scant, although most—but not all—studies demonstrate decreased mitochondrial oxygen consumption in immune and nonimmune cells.[8,18,19] When considering bioenergetic impairment in sepsis, investigators have most commonly focused on NADH:ubiquinone oxidoreductase (complex I) and cytochrome oxidase (complex IV). As the largest complex of the ETS (comprising 45 proteins), complex I is subject to impairment from changes in various protein subunits. Multiple studies have demonstrated decreased activity of ETS complex I in sepsis models and in humans.[20,21] Complex IV is composed of only 13 subunits, many of which have been investigated in sepsis. Subunits 1, 2, and 3 make up the catalytic center and are encoded by mtDNA.[13] The other 10 subunits arise from nuclear DNA.[13] Subunit 1, the active site, houses the heme $aa3$ binuclear center.[13] Numerous studies have demonstrated abnormalities in expression and function of cytochrome oxidase during sepsis and in related models.[22-26] For example, steady-state levels of cytochrome oxidase subunit I messenger RNA (mRNA) and protein are decreased in the murine heart after CLP and in endotoxin-stimulated macrophages.[22,23] Injection of LPS into healthy human volunteers also resulted in widespread suppression of genes regulating mitochondrial energy production and protein synthesis.[27] Reductions in ETS complex mRNA expression and protein translation result in reduced enzyme content and could affect the bioenergetic capacity of the cell.

Changes in mRNA and protein levels of key enzyme complex subunits are only functionally significant if they lead to or contribute to enzyme dysfunction. To this point, myocardial cytochrome oxidase activity decreased to 51% of baseline in baboons after *Escherichia coli* infusion.[28] In murine sepsis, myocardial cytochrome oxidase inhibition was reported after CLP.[22] This inhibition was initially competitive but later became noncompetitive. This change occurred at a time when cardiac function was markedly impaired and when mortality was high.[22] Cytochrome oxidase dysfunction also has been shown in septic liver and in the medulla of the endotoxemic rat.[29,30] Furthermore, reduced state 3 mitochondrial oxygen consumption has been demonstrated in the neonatal rat heart, feline liver, and rat diaphragm during endotoxemia.[24,31,32]

Complex IV contains two heme subgroups (cytochrome a and $a3$) that assist in the transfer of electrons and reduction of oxygen to water. A reduced cytochrome $aa3$ redox state in the absence of tissue hypoxia indicates a defect in mitochondrial oxygen use and suggests impaired oxidative phosphorylation. Several investigators have demonstrated reduced redox status during endotoxemia and gram-negative bacteremia in the heart, brain, skeletal muscle, and intestine in various animals.[33-37] In addition, diminished heme $aa3$ content in heart and skeletal muscle has also been shown in experimental sepsis.[22,38]

Bioenergetic failure as a potential cause of sepsis-induced organ failure is not a new concept. With regard to sepsis-associated myocardial depression, early investigation extensively evaluated oxygen delivery, global myocardial perfusion, and high-energy phosphate levels.[39-45] These studies clearly demonstrated that coronary blood flow and global cardiac perfusion were maintained and often increased during sepsis.[39-41,46] In addition, there is evidence to suggest that tissue oxygen tension was unchanged in the dysfunctional septic heart.[43] These findings argue strongly against decreased oxygen availability as a cause of myocardial depression in sepsis and support a defect in oxygen utilization. Organ-specific impairment of oxygen utilization is further supported by a progressive decline in whole-body oxygen consumption and resting metabolic rate with increasing severity of sepsis.[47] Although other studies have reported oxygen consumption to be unchanged or increased in sepsis, it has been postulated that this may be due to an uncoupling of mitochondrial respiration leading to inefficient electron flux and heat generation.[8]

However, the literature is less clear regarding ATP availability. In many studies, preserved ATP levels were demonstrated in dysfunctional septic myocardium. Other investigations reported decreased high-energy phosphates in experimental sepsis and endotoxemia.[26,42-45,48] In a study of 28 adults with severe sepsis, 12 (43%) of whom died of sepsis-related multiple organ dysfunction syndrome, nonsurvivors were distinguished from sepsis survivors and nonseptic controls by lower levels of ATP in skeletal muscle.[20] However, even preservation of ATP does not imply an absence of mitochondrial dysfunction in sepsis.[44,49] During reduced oxygen delivery and cellular hypoxia, cells can adapt to maintain viability by downregulating oxygen consumption, energy requirements, and ATP demand.[50,51] Thus, although ATP content may remain unchanged, ATP use can be decreased dramatically. In the heart, this response is called *myocardial hibernation* and classically occurs during myocardial ischemia.[50] This adaptive, prosurvival response results in cardiomyocyte hypocontractility with preserved cellular ATP.[50] If cellular metabolic activity continued unchanged despite mitochondrial dysfunction, then ATP levels would inevitably diminish and cell death pathways would be activated. Because cell death does not appear to be a primary feature of sepsis-induced organ dysfunction, it follows that cells may instead adapt to cope with the falling energy supply.[8] Thus, finding preserved ATP during sepsis reveals little about the integrity of oxidative phosphorylation and may support the notion of a similar prosurvival response.

Development of a Hibernation-Like State in Sepsis

Metabolic downregulation is a crucial response that facilitates tolerance to a lack of energetic substrates during harsh environmental conditions and promotes survival during true hibernation.[10] The hibernating state prevents a cellular bioenergetic crisis by reducing demand for ATP when substrate and/or oxygen supply are low and decreases mitochondrial oxidative stress.[10] Central to this response are reduced oxygen consumption and cytochrome oxidase activity. In the hibernating frog, whole-body oxygen consumption decreases by 50% in normoxic 3°C water.[52] Whole-body oxygen consumption and respiration of isolated skeletal muscle mitochondria decreased further when hibernating frogs were placed in hypoxic cold water.[52] Furthermore, cytochrome oxidase activity in frog skeletal muscle progressively decreases during different stages of hibernation.[52] In the hibernating ground squirrel, state 3 respiration decreased by approximately 70% in liver mitochondria.[53] In squirrels that fail to hibernate, though, the changes observed in kidney cytochrome oxidase within their hibernating counterparts do not occur.[10] Thus, it is clear that metabolic downregulation, in part because of reversible cytochrome oxidase inhibition and reduced activity, is key to initiating and maintaining the hibernating phenotype in various species. Importantly, the reduction in cytochrome oxidase activity and mitochondrial respiration characteristic of hibernation are similar to the changes seen during early sepsis.

Pharmacologic inhibition of cytochrome oxidase has been shown to induce a hibernation-like or suspended-animation state.[54,55] Reversible inhibition of cytochrome oxidase with carbon monoxide (CO) arrests embryogenesis in *Caenorhabditis elegans* embryos yet preserves their viability in hypoxic conditions.[54] In addition, noncompetitive cytochrome oxidase inhibition with inhaled hydrogen sulfide (H₂S) induces a suspended-animation state in nonhibernating mice.[55] On exposure to H_2S, mice dramatically reduced their core body temperature and metabolic rate in a dose-dependent and reversible manner.[55] At the cellular level, noncompetitive inhibition of cytochrome oxidase with sodium azide causes a rapid and reversible reduction in cardiomyocyte contraction and metabolic demand, mimicking myocardial hibernation.[50]

Similar to hibernation and exposure to certain compounds, cytochrome oxidase inhibition is well described during sepsis.[22] For example, in the heart, cytochrome oxidase was competitively inhibited during the early phase of sepsis and progressed to become noncompetitively inhibited during the late, hypodynamic phase.[22] This specific pattern of enzyme inhibition is known to induce metabolic downregulation and a suspended-animation state. In addition, these biochemical changes coincide with the time course and progression of myocardial depression in humans, in which an early depression of cardiac contractility is compensated for by ventricular dilation and increased stroke volume with subsequent diastolic dysfunction and reduced cardiac output over time.[56-59] The decrease in cardiac contractility seen early in sepsis is similar to the reduced systolic function characteristic of hibernation in grizzly bears and marmots[60,61] and may reflect the decreased total-body oxygen requirement to produce ATP observed in sepsis and hibernation. However, the interval development of reduced diastolic relaxation later in sepsis is not observed in hibernating animals and may underlie a transition point during which metabolic downregulation becomes maladaptive and pathologic in sepsis compared with natural hibernation. When sepsis-induced mitochondrial and cellular defects become irreversible, as is the case with cytochrome oxidase inhibition over time, organ dysfunction may also become irreversible and lead to death. If this is true, then the challenges for clinicians will be to differentiate reversible adaptive organ "hibernation" from pathologic organ "failure," to recognize when this switch has occurred, and to intervene to prevent the alteration.

Several different mediators may be responsible for metabolic downregulation and mitochondrial dysfunction in sepsis. The most likely offenders include nitric oxide (NO), CO, H₂S, peroxynitrite, and reactive oxygen species. Certainly, all of these agents are endogenously produced in various tissues during sepsis, largely in response to an upregulation of the proinflammatory cytokines tumor necrosis factor-α (TNF-α), interleukin-1β (IL-1β), high-mobility group protein-1, and others.[62-66] The high levels of NO observed in sepsis may assist antimicrobial defense, but they are also cytotoxic to host cell oxidative phosphorylation at several postulated sites.[9] Notably, the impairment in cytochrome oxidase activity during sepsis mimics that of true hibernation, suggesting that, at least early on, such impairment may be an adaptive response to an inflammatory insult. As discussed later, the failure to restore mitochondrial function and recover organ function after acute inflammation separates sepsis-induced organ dysfunction from true hibernation.

MITOCHONDRIAL BIOGENESIS TO RESTORE ORGAN FUNCTION AND PROMOTE SURVIVAL

From an evolutionary perspective, it may be adaptive to reduce metabolic demands when oxygen and substrate availability are low to protect cells from a bioenergetic crisis and limit exposure to oxidative stress. Such a shutdown is manifest clinically as organ dysfunction. As with recovery from hibernation, though, once the infectious/inflammatory stimulus has abated, functional mitochondria are needed to restore cellular energy supply. All cells that undergo oxidative phosphorylation have robust quality control mechanisms to ensure a full complement of healthy mitochondria. Cells optimize the overall mitochondrial number, distribution, and function through a network of interrelated processes of biogenesis, fission, fusion, and mitophagy.[9]

Mitochondrial biogenesis is the process of synthesizing new functional mitochondria and can be induced by exercise, fasting, exposure to cold temperatures, oxidative stress, and inflammation.[9] Depending on the stimulus, mitochondrial biogenesis is executed through several signaling pathways that converge on a common set of coactivators and transcription factors. The nuclear-encoded factors include peroxisome proliferator-activated receptor γ-1 coactivator-α (PGC-1α), nuclear respiratory factors (NRF-1 and NRF-2), nuclear factor erythroid-2-related factor 2 (Nrf2), and mitochondrial transcription factor A (TFAM).[9] These proteins either increase transcription of nuclear-encoded mitochondrial proteins or are imported into the mitochondria to directly upregulate expression of mtDNA to promote ETS complex assembly.

Common inflammatory mediators of the innate immune response, including TNF-α, IL-6, and interferon-γ (IFN-γ), can activate one or several well-defined pathways of mitochondrial biogenesis. These cytokines/chemokines are produced in response to the presence of microbial antigens (pathogen-associated molecular patterns) that are sensed by cellular pattern recognition receptors such as toll-like receptors (TLRs). Subsequent activation of the nuclear factor-κB (NF-κB), mitogen-activated protein kinases, and protein kinase B (Akt) pathways lead to increased expression of the factors regulating mitochondrial biosynthesis.[9]

Upregulation of NO also stimulates mitochondrial biogenesis through increased PGC-1α activity.[67] Finally, stimulation of heme metabolism in sepsis due to hypoxia and inflammation leads to a heme oxygenase-1 (HO-1)–mediated production of CO that increases Nrf2 activation, thereby further increasing mitochondrial biogenesis.[68] Notably, despite elevated blood levels of cytokines, intracellular signaling may be impaired in severe sepsis and may be a mechanism leading to insufficient mitochondrial recovery in nonsurvivors.[69]

The inhibition of oxidative phosphorylation and mitochondrial damage in sepsis also provide potent stimuli for mitochondrial quality control mechanisms. For example, an increase in the adenosine monophosphate/ATP or oxidized NAD (NAD+)/NADH ratios induces PGC-1α through several pathways.[9] Mitochondrial damage due to oxidative stress results in mtDNA translocation to the cytoplasm, which upregulates NF-κB through TLR-9 signaling and acts as a danger-associated molecular pathogen to further promote inflammatory mediates that affect mitochondrial biogenesis.[70] In this regard, removal of dysfunctional mitochondria—termed *mitophagy*—has also been shown to be protective in sepsis.[71,72] For example, in the liver and kidney of hyperglycemic critically ill rabbits, biochemical markers indicating insufficient mitophagy were more pronounced in nonsurviving animals.[72] Interestingly, after 3 and 7 days of illness, mitophagy was better preserved in animals treated with insulin to preserve normoglycemia, which correlated with improved mitochondrial function and less organ damage. Moreover, stimulation of mitophagy in the kidney with rapamycin correlated with protection of renal function in this study.[72]

Data from animal studies and septic patients provide key evidence that mitochondrial recovery is predictive of or associated with recovery of organ function and survival. Haden et al. showed that mitochondrial biogenesis is evident over 1 to 3 days after a nonlethal exposure to *Staphylococcus aureus* in a rodent model, with a subsequent recovery of oxidative phosphorylation.[73] The same group further showed that sepsis survival could be improved in rodents treated with daily exposure to a low dose of CO and demonstrated a mechanistic link to induction of HO-1, Nrf2, and Akt signaling.[68] In humans, Carre demonstrated a significant association in the upregulation of the mitochondrial biogenesis factors PGC-1α and NRF-1 with survival in sepsis.[74]

Evidence of mitochondrial recovery—and biogenesis in particular—is also present in hibernating animals. Ground squirrels in torpor exhibited a shift to slow-twitch type I muscle fibers that was accompanied by activation of PGC-1α and enhanced mitochondrial abundance and metabolism.[75] Pharmacologic agents that induce mitochondrial biogenesis, such as pioglitazone,[76] resveratrol,[77] and recombinant human TFAM,[78] may hold promise as a novel therapeutic strategy in sepsis-induced organ dysfunction that fails to recover after an initial "hibernation-like" phase.

Recent evidence clearly suggests that the resolution of inflammation is an active process driven by a group of specialized and unique mediators.[79] These compounds are derived from polyunsaturated fatty acids that include lipoxins, E- and D-series resolvins, protectins, and maresins. These lipids, alone or in combination, suppress activated leukocytes and macrophage activity, inhibit proinflammatory cytokine production, attenuate inappropriate inflammatory responses, enhance bacterial clearance, and improve survival.[79,80] Their importance to the current discussion lies in recent demonstration of a biosynthesis pathway for these lipid mediators in mitochondria that is activated after tissue injury.[81] Although the role of these proresolving mediators in sepsis is unknown, the presence of a responsive pathway within mitochondria suggests their potential importance and identifies an area for future investigation.

CONCLUSION

Sepsis and hibernation have similarities that suggest that sepsis-induced organ dysfunction may represent an adaptive response. Mitochondrial dysfunction and cytochrome oxidase inhibition are likely central to the process. As in hibernation, it is possible that reversible cytochrome oxidase inhibition initiates metabolic downregulation during sepsis, leading to clinical organ dysfunction. Although it is possible that the reduction in metabolism during sepsis may initially be adaptive, it is clear that this can progress to become maladaptive and pathologic with a failure to recover mitochondrial oxidative phosphorylation as metabolic demand increases. Substantial progress has been made in the general understanding of signal transduction pathways that regulate metabolic changes in sepsis, including mitochondrial biogenesis and mitophagy. Future investigation will need to focus on the dynamic nature of these processes and attempt to identify the key mechanisms underlying the switch from reversible to irreversible mitochondrial inhibition that may lead to progressive organ dysfunction and death. With further understanding, clinicians may be able to identify when and how to intervene at critical time points in the disease process to restore the metabolic capacity of the cell.

AUTHORS' RECOMMENDATIONS

- Sepsis and hibernation share biochemical and physiologic features that suggest that sepsis-induced organ dysfunction may represent an adaptive response, at least early in the disease course. Mitochondrial dysfunction and cytochrome oxidase inhibition are likely central to the process.
- Although the reduction in metabolism during sepsis may initially be adaptive, a state of insufficient cellular bioenergetics can progress to become maladaptive and pathologic if mitochondrial oxidative phosphorylation is not restored concurrently with increased metabolic demand.
- Mitochondrial quality control mechanisms, especially mitochondrial biogenesis and mitophagy, are active in the later phases of sepsis to restore cellular ATP and remove dysfunctional mitochondria in survivors in animal models and human studies. Pharmacologic agents that induce mitochondrial biogenesis and mitophagy may hold promise as a novel therapeutic strategy in sepsis-induced organ dysfunction that fails to recover after an initial hibernation-like phase.
- Future investigation will need to focus on temporal changes in cellular metabolism and attempt to identify the key mechanisms involved in the switch from reversible to irreversible mitochondrial inhibition and organ dysfunction.

REFERENCES

1. Hotchkiss RS, Karl IE. The pathophysiology and treatment of sepsis. *N Engl J Med*. 2003;348:138–150.
2. Marshall JC. Inflammation, coagulopathy, and the pathogenesis of the multiple organ dysfunction syndrome. *Crit Care Med*. 2001;29:S99–S106.
3. Proulx F, Joyal JS, Mariscalco MM, et al. The pediatric multiple organ dysfunction syndrome. *Pediatr Crit Care Med*. 2009;10:12–22.
4. Vincent JL, Sakr Y, Sprung CL, et al. Sepsis in European intensive care units: results of the SOAP study. *Crit Care Med*. 2006;34:344–353.
5. Protti A, Singer M. Bench-to-bedside review: potential strategies to protect or reverse mitochondrial dysfunction in sepsis-induced organ failure. *Crit Care*. 2006;10:228.
6. Levy RJ. Mitochondrial dysfunction, bioenergetic impairment, and metabolic down-regulation in sepsis. *Shock*. 2007;28:24–28.
7. Singer M. Mitochondrial function in sepsis: acute phase versus multiple organ failure. *Crit Care Med*. 2007;35:S441–S448.
8. Singer M. The role of mitochondrial dysfunction in sepsis-induced multi-organ failure. *Virulence*. 2014;5:66–72.
9. Cherry AD, Piantadosi CA. Regulation of mitochondrial biogenesis and its intersection with inflammatory responses. *Antiox Redox Signal*. 2015;22:965–976.
10. Hittel DS, Storey KB. Differential expression of mitochondria-encoded genes in a hibernating mammal. *J Exp Biol*. 2002;205:1625–1631.
11. Fink MP. Bench-to-bedside review: cytopathic hypoxia. *Crit Care*. 2001;6:491–499.
12. Fink MP. Cytopathic hypoxia: is oxygen use impaired in sepsis as a result of an acquired intrinsic derangement in cellular respiration. *Crit Care Clin*. 2002;18:165–175.
13. Saraste M. Oxidative phosphorylation at the fin de siecle. *Science*. 1999;283:1488–1493.
14. Wallace DC. Mitochondrial diseases in man and mouse. *Science*. 1999;283:1482–1488.
15. Crouser ED. Mitochondrial dysfunction in septic shock and multiple organ dysfunction syndrome. *Mitochondrion*. 2004;4:729–741.
16. Singer M, Brealey D. Mitochondrial dysfunction in sepsis. *Biochem Soc Symp*. 66:149-166.
17. Takasu O, Gault JP, Watanabe E, et al. Mechanisms of cardiac and renal dysfunction in patients dying of sepsis. *Am J Respir Crit Care Med*. 2013;187:509–517.
18. Weiss SL, Selak MA, Tuluc F, et al. Mitochondrial dysfunction in peripheral blood mononuclear cells in pediatric septic shock. *Pediatr Crit Care Med*. 2015;16:e4–e12.
19. Sjovall F, Morota S, Persson J, et al. Patients with sepsis exhibit increased mitochondrial respiratory capacity in peripheral blood immune cells. *Crit Care*. 2013;17:R152.
20. Brealey D, Brand M, Hargreaves I, et al. Association between mitochondrial dysfunction and severity and outcome of septic shock. *Lancet*. 2002;20:219–223.
21. Brealey D, Karyampudi S, Jacqeues TS, et al. Mitochondrial dysfunction in a long-term rodent model of sepsis and organ failure. *Am J Physiol Regul Integr Comp Physiol*. 2004;286:R491–R497.
22. Levy RJ, Vijayasarathy C, Raj NR, et al. Competitive and noncompetitive inhibition of myocardial cytochrome c oxidase in sepsis. *Shock*. 2004;21:110–114.
23. Wei J, Guo H, Kuo PC. Endotoxin-stimulated nitric oxide production inhibits expression of cytochrome C oxidase in ANA-1 murine macrophages. *J Immunol*. 2002;168:4721–4727.
24. Callahan LA, Supinski GS. Sepsis induces diaphragm electron transport chain dysfunction and protein depletion. *Am J Respir Crit Care Med*. 2005;172:861–868.
25. Callahan LA, Supinski GS. Downregulation of diaphragm electron transport chain and glycolytic enzyme gene expression in sepsis. *J Appl Physiol*. 2005;99:1120–1126.
26. Chen HW, Hsu C, Lu TS, et al. Heat shock pretreatment prevents cardiac mitochondrial dysfunction during sepsis. *Shock*. 2003;20:274–279.
27. Calvano SE, Xiao W, Richards DR, et al. A network-based analysis of systemic inflammation in humans. *Nature*. 2005;13:1032–1037.
28. Gellerich FN, Trumbeckaite S, Hertel K, et al. Impaired energy metabolism in hearts of septic baboons: diminished activities of complex I and complex II of the mitochondrial respiratory chain. *Shock*. 1999;11:336–341.
29. Chuang YC, Tsai JL, Chang AY, et al. Dysfunction of the mitochondrial respiratory chain in the rostral ventrolateral medulla during experimental endotoxemia in the rat. *J Biomed Sci*. 2002;9:542–548.
30. Chen HW, Kuo HT, Lu TS, et al. Cytochrome C oxidase as the target of the heat shock protective effect in septic liver. *Int J Exp Pathol*. 2004;85:249–256.
31. Crouser ED, Julian MW, Blaho DV, Pfeiffer DR. Endotoxin-induced mitochondrial damage correlates with impaired respiratory activity. *Crit Care Med*. 2002;30:276–284.
32. Fukumoto K, Pierro A, Spitz L, Eaton S. Neonatal endotoxemia affects heart but not kidney bioenergetics. *J Pediatr Surg*. 2003;38:690–693.
33. Snow TR, Dickey DT, Tapp T, et al. Early myocardial dysfunction induced with endotoxin in rhesus monkeys. *Can J Cardiol*. 1990;6:130–136.
34. Schaefer CF, Biber B, Lerner MR, et al. Rapid reduction of intestinal cytochrome a,a3 during lethal endotoxemia. *J Surg Res*. 1991;51:382–391.
35. Simonson SG, Welty-Wolf K, Huang YT, et al. Altered mitochondrial redox responses in gram negative septic shock in primates. *Circ Shock*. 1994;43:34–43.
36. Forget AP, Mangalaboyi J, Mordon S, et al. *Escherichia coli* endotoxin reduces cytochrome aa3 redox status in pig skeletal muscle. *Crit Care Med*. 2000;28:3491–3497.
37. Schaefer CF, Biber B. Effects of endotoxemia on the redox level of brain cytochrome a,a3 in rats. *Circ Shock*. 1993;40:1–8.
38. Tavakoli H, Mela L. Alterations of mitochondrial metabolism and protein concentrations in subacute septicemia. *Infect Immun*. 1982;38:536–541.
39. Cunnion RE, Schaer GL, Parker MM, et al. The coronary circulation in human septic shock. *Circulation*. 1986;73:637–644.
40. Dhainaut JF, Huyghebaert MF, Monsallier JF, et al. Coronary hemodynamics and myocardial metabolism of lactate, free fatty acids, glucose, and ketones in patients with septic shock. *Circulation*. 1987;75:533–541.
41. Lang CH, Bagby GJ, Ferguson JL, Spitzer JJ. Cardiac output and redistribution of organ blood flow in hypermetabolic sepsis. *Am J Physiol*. 1984;246:R331–R337.
42. Hotchkiss RS, Karl IE. Reevaluation of the role of cellular hypoxia and bioenergetic failure in sepsis. *JAMA*. 1992;267:1503–1510.
43. Hotchkiss RS, Rust RS, Dence CS, et al. Evaluation of the role of cellular hypoxia in sepsis by the hypoxic marker [18F]fluoromisonidazole. *Am J Physiol*. 1991;261:R965–R972.
44. Solomon MA, Correa R, Alexander HR, et al. Myocardial energy metabolism and morphology in a canine model of sepsis. *Am J Physiol*. 1994;266:H757–H768.
45. Levy B, Mansart A, Bollaert PE, et al. Effects of epinephrine and norepinephrine on hemodynamics, oxidative metabolism, and organ energetics in endotoxemic rats. *Intensive Care Med*. 2003;29:292–300.
46. Levy RJ, Piel DA, Acton PD, et al. Evidence of myocardial hibernation in the septic heart. *Crit Care Med*. 2005;33:2752–2756.
47. Kreyman G, Grosser S, Buggisch P, et al. Oxygen consumption and reseting metabolic rate in sepsis, sepsis syndrome, and septic shock. *Crit Care Med*. 1993;21:1012–1019.
48. Mutschler DK, Eriksson MB, Wikstrom BG, et al. Microdialysis-evaluated myocardial cyclooxygenase-mediated inflammation and early circulatory depression in porcine endotoxemia. *Crit Care Med*. 2003;31:1780–1785.
49. Hotchkiss RS, Song SK, Neil JJ, et al. Sepsis does not impair tricarboxylic acid cycle in the heart. *Am J Physiol*. 1991;260:C50–C57.
50. Budinger GR, Duranteau J, Chandel NS, Schumacker PT. Hibernation during hypoxia in cardiomyocytes: role of mitochondria as the O_2 sensor. *J Biol Chem*. 1998;273:3320–3326.
51. Schumacker PT, Chandel N, Agusti AG. Oxygen conformance of cellular respiration in hepatocytes. *Am J Physiol*. 1993;265:L395–L402.
52. St-Pierre J, Boutilier RG. Aerobic capacity of frog skeletal muscle during hibernation. *Physiol Biochem Zool*. 2001;74:390–397.
53. Lerner E, Shug AL, Elson C, Shrago E. Reversible inhibition of adenosine nucleotide translocation by long chain fatty acyl coenzyme A esters in liver mitochondria of diabetic and hibernating animals. *J Biol Chem*. 1972;247:1513–1519.
54. Nystul TG, Roth MB. Carbon monoxide-induced suspended animation protects against hypoxic damage in *Caenorhabditis elegans*. *Proc Natl Acad Sci USA*. 2004;101:9133–9136.

55. Blackstone E, Morrison M, Roth MB. H2S induces a suspended animation-like state in mice. *Science*. 2005;308:518.
56. Kumar A, Haery C, Parrillo JE. Myocardial dysfunction in septic shock. *Crit Care Clin*. 2000;16:251–287.
57. Parrillo JE, Parker MM, Natanson C, et al. Septic shock in humans: advances in the understanding of pathogenesis, cardiovascular dysfunction, and therapy. *Ann Intern Med*. 1990;113:227–242.
58. Parker MM, Shelhamer JH, Natanson C, et al. Serial cardiovascular variables in survivors and nonsurvivors of human septic shock: heart rate as an early predictor of prognosis. *Crit Care Med*. 1987;15:923–929.
59. Natanson C. Studies using a canine model to investigate the cardiovascular abnormality of and potential therapies for septic shock. *Clin Res*. 1990;38:206–214.
60. Zatzman ML, Thornhill GV. Seasonal variation of cardiovascular function in the marmot, *Marmota flaviventris*. *Cryobiology*. 1987;24:376–385.
61. Nelson OL, McEwen MM, Robbins CT, et al. Evaluation of cardiac function in active and hibernating grizzly bears. *J Am Vet Med Assoc*. 2003;223:1170–1175.
62. Barth E, Radermacher P, Thiemermann C, et al. Role of inducible nitric oxide synthase in the reduced responsiveness of the myocardium to catecholamines in a hyperdynamic, murine model of septic shock. *Crit Care Med*. 2006;34:307–313.
63. Yuan S, Huaqiang L, Jie P, et al. Role of endogenous carbon monoxide in endotoxin shock. *Chin Med Sci J*. 2000;15:98–102.
64. Lancel S, Tissier S, Mordon S, et al. Peroxynitrite decomposition catalysts prevent myocardial dysfunction and inflammation in endotoxemic rats. *J Am Coll Cardiol*. 2004;43:2348–2358.
65. Victor VM, Rocha M, Esplugues JV, De la Fuente M. Role of free radicals in sepsis: antioxidant therapy. *Curr Pharm Des*. 2005;11:3141–3158.
66. Schumacker P, Gillespie MN, Nakahira K, et al. Mitochondria in lung biology and pathology: more than just a powerhouse. *Am J Physiol Lung Cell Mold Physiol*. 2014;306:L962–L974.
67. Nisoli E, Clementi E, Paolucci C, et al. Mitochondrial biogenesis in mammals: the role of endogenous nitric oxide. *Science*. 2003;299:896–899.
68. MacGarvey NC, Suliman HB, Bartz RR, et al. Activation of mitochondrial biogenesis by heme oxygenzse-1-mediated NF-E2-related factor-2 induction rescues mice form lethal *Staphylococus aureus* sepsis. *Am J Respir Crit Care Med*. 2012;185:851–861.
69. Abcejo AS, Andrejko KM, Raj NR, Deutschman CS. Failed interleukin-6 signal transduction in murine sepsis: attenuation of hepatic glycoprotein 130 phosphorylation. *Crit Care Med*. 2009;37:1729–1734.
70. Zhang JZ, Liu Z, Liu J, Ren JX, Sun TS. Mitochondrial DNA induces inflammation and increases TLR9/NF-kappaB expression in lung tissue. *Int J Mol Med*. 2014;33:817–824.
71. Hsiao HW, Tsai KL, Wang LF, et al. The decline of autophagy contributes to proximal tubular dysfunction during sepsis. *Shock*. 2012;37:289–296.
72. Gunst J, DereseI A, Aertgeerts A, et al. Insufficient autophagy contributes to mitochondrial dysfunction, organ failure, and adverse outcome in an animal model of critical illness. *Crit Care Med*. 2013;41:182–194.
73. Haden DW, Sulliman HB, Carraway MS, et al. Mitochondrial biogenesis restores oxidative metabolism during *Staphylococcus aureus* sepsis. *Am J Respir Crit Care Med*. 2007;15:768–777.
74. Carre JE, Orban JC, Re L, et al. Survival in critical illness is associated with early activation of mitochondrial biogenesis. *Am J Respir Crit Care Med*. 182:745-751.
75. Xu R, Andres-Mateos E, Mejias R, et al. Hibernating squirrel muscle activates the endurance exercise pathway despite prolonged immobilization. *Exp Neurol*. 2013;247:392–401.
76. Bogacka I, Xie H, Bray GA, Smith SR. Pioglitazone induces mitochondrial biogenesis in human subcutaneous adipose tissue in vivo. *Diabetes*. 2005;54:1392–1399.
77. Baur J, Pearson KJ, Price NL, et al. Resveratrol improves health and survival of mice on a high-calorie diet. *Nature*. 2006;16:337–342.
78. Thomas RR, Khan SM, Portell FR, Smigrodzki RM, Bennett JP. Recombinant human mitochondrial transcription factor A sitmulates mitochondrial biogenesis and ATP synthesis, improves motor function after MPTP, reduces oxidative stress and increases survival after endotoxin. *Mitochondrion*. 2011;11:108–118.
79. Serhan CN, Petasis NA. Resolvins and protectins in inflammation-resolution. *Chem Rev*. 2011;111:5922–5943.
80. Das U. HLA-DR expression, cytokines and bioreactive lipids in sepsis. *Arch Med Sci*. 2014;10:325–335.
81. Tyurina YY, Poloyac SM, Tyurin VA, et al. A mitochondrial pathway for biosynthesis of lipid mediators. *Nat Chem*. 2014;6:542–552.

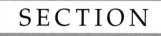

CARDIOVASCULAR CRITICAL CARE

50 How Do I Manage Acute Heart Failure?

Shiro Ishihara, Naoki Sato, Alexandre Mebazaa

The vast majority of patients with acute heart failure (AHF) are hospitalized with signs and symptoms of volume overload.[1,2] Therefore the most important treatment strategy is to alleviate organ congestion, including lung congestion, renal congestion, and liver congestion.

Because elevation of left-sided filling pressure leads to lung congestion, and elevation of right-sided filling pressure leads to liver and renal congestion, alleviating organ congestion requires a reduction of cardiac filling pressures. Among pharmacologic agents that may reduce filling pressures, vasodilators are the most powerful and fastest acting drugs.

HOW TO UNLOAD THE HEART WITH VASODILATORS

Vasodilators can reduce the pulmonary capillary wedged pressure and systemic vascular resistance (SVR), which decreases both the preload and the afterload and is likely to increase cardiac output (CO). These favorable effects will appear soon after starting these agents. The European Society of Cardiology guideline[3] and practical recommendation[4] for the management of AHF recommend vasodilator use with normal to high blood pressure (BP) in acute settings. Table 50-1 details the currently recommended agents doses and side effects, and Table 50-2 indicates the mechanisms and hemodynamic effects of each drug. Although vasodilators have many favorable effects, they should be avoided in patients with low admission BP because they may lead to an excessive early drop in systolic BP, which is problematic because vasodilator-induced hypotension has been associated with poor outcomes.[5]

Importantly, while vasodilator therapy has been extensively used to treat heart failure, its value has never been demonstrated in a prospective clinical trial. Such studies that have been performed have not provided a significant alteration in mortality or readmission rates.

Nitroglycerin

Nitroglycerin is a powerful venodilator and a mild arterial dilator. Its immediate effects occur primarily through venodilation, which lowers preload and, to a lesser extent, afterload, and increases CO. Because of its favorable effect on hemodynamic profiles in patients with AHF, nitroglycerin is widely used in acute settings throughout the world. When BP is adequate, nitroglycerin can be administered sublingually while preparing for intravenous treatment. Intravenous nitroglycerin is usually started at ≈ 5 to 10 μg/min and is titrated until symptoms improve (i.e., when a favorable hemodynamic response is observed) or until the patient has side effects or reaches the maximum dose (200 μg/min). Tachyphylaxis can develop within 24 hours, which can lead to an escalation in dose to achieve the desired effect.

Sodium Nitroprusside

The use of sodium nitroprusside has decreased in recent years. This agent can unload the heart through balanced venodilation and arteriodilation, lowering left and right heart filling pressures (preload and afterload) and increasing CO. Nitroprusside is particularly useful in the acute setting, which includes hypertensive crisis and acute valvular regurgitation. Invasive hemodynamic monitoring is recommended to avoid hypotension. Nitroprusside should be avoided in patients with active ischemia because it dilates resistance vessels in nonischemic myocardium, which can lead to the coronary steal phenomenon.[6] In general, a nitroprusside infusion is started at 0.3 μg/kg/min and titrated gradually until symptoms improve. Long-term use, high doses, or renal dysfunction have been associated with the risk of isocyanate toxicity. For rebound vasoconstriction to be avoided, nitroprusside must be tapered gradually.

Nesiritide

Nesiritide is a recombinant form of human B-type natriuretic peptide and has variable effects. Through its main activity, vasodilation, nesiritide can reduce SVR, increase CO, and increase sodium urinary excretion. However, in the Renal Optimization Strategies Evaluation in Acute Heart Failure (ROSE) trial, nesiritide was not found to be superior to placebo with respect to urine output (see later section on dopamine).[7] Nesiritide infusions can be started at 0.01 μg/kg/min without need for a bolus. If hypotension occurs during infusion, the dose should be reduced or discontinued and, after BP is restored, restarted at a 30% lower dose. Nesiritide does not cause tachyphylaxis.[8]

HOW TO REDUCE EXTRACELLULAR VOLUME

Loop Diuretics

Loop diuretics are the most widely used agents worldwide and are commonly used to treat heart failure (Table 50-3). Loop diuretics inhibit sodium/potassium/chloride cotransporters at the luminal membrane, so they should be secreted into tubular lumen by the organic acid transporter (OAT).[9] Intravenous administration of loop diuretics can cause mild venodilation with a decrease in cardiac preload before diuretic response, an action that also contributes to rapid improvement of symptoms.[10] Loop diuretics induce the formation of urine that contains 0.45% sodium chloride (natriuresis). The effects of loop diuretics are powerful, and urine substantially comes from the intravascular space, indicating that excessive and sudden urine output could lead to deleterious hemodynamic changes and also adversely affect the renin angiotensin aldosterone system. There are a significant number of patients who exhibit diuretic resistance.[11] The etiology of this phenomenon is multifactorial and complex, but renal dysfunction is the most important cause. The dose of agent secreted into the tubular lumen will be decreased in patients with renal dysfunction and may require titration of the dose. In addition, loop diuretics compete with other organic acids for access to the OAT receptor. The accumulation of these acids in renal impairment could therefore lead to diuretic resistance.[9]

Vasopressin Antagonists

Vasopressin antagonists induce aquaresis (Table 50-3).[12] In contrast to loop diuretics, water excreted in response to vasopressin antagonists comes from both the extracellular (1/3) and the intracellular (2/3) spaces. Thus aquaresis could contribute to less neurohormonal activation, fewer hemodynamic changes, and fewer changes in renal function.[13] Vasopressin antagonists block vasopressin 2 receptors throughout the entire collecting duct. Interestingly, vasopressin antagonists act on the basolateral membrane. Thus, in contrast to loop diuretics, they do not need to be secreted into tubular lumen, perhaps providing an advantage over loop diuretics in patients with renal dysfunction. When vasopressin antagonists are used, loop diuretics can be coadministered to obtain an additive increase in urine output. Importantly, vasopressin antagonists are also vasodilators.

Mineralocorticoid Receptor Antagonists

Although mineralocorticoid receptor antagonists (MRAs) are recommended in patients with New York Heart Association class II to IV and who have left ventricular systolic dysfunction, there is little evidence to support their use in AHF patients. Because the vast majority of patients with AHF are hospitalized with signs and symptoms of volume overload, diuretic doses (e.g., 50 to 100 mg/day furosemide) may be appropriate.[14] When MRAs are prescribed, attention should be paid to renal dysfunction and potassium levels to avoid hyperkalemia-related arrhythmias.

Hemofiltration

Hemofiltration (HF) is an alternative method for removing excess fluid in patients with AHF (Table 50-3). Several small studies have shown that this approach offers several advantages over diuretics. Because fluid removed by HF is isotonic, with HF more fluid can be removed than with diuretics.[15] In addition, hypokalemia can be avoided. Importantly, the use of HF provides control over the rate

Table 50-1 Recommended Doses and Side Effects of Vasodilators

Drug	Dose	Major Limitations
Nitroglycerin	Start with 10-20 µg/min, 200 µg/min	Hypotension, headache, tachyphylaxis
Sodium nitroprusside	Start with 0.3 µg/kg/min and increase up to 5 µg/kg/min	Hypotension, isocyanate toxicity, coronary steal, rebound vasoconstriction
Nesiritide	Bolus 2 µg/kg + infusion 0.01 µg/kg/min*	Hypotension

*Nerisitide can be initiated without bolus.

Table 50-2 Mechanism of Actions and Hemodynamic Effects in AHF

Drugs	Mechanisms	HEMODYNAMIC EFFECTS						
		CI/CO	PCWP	MAP	HR	SVR	PVR	CBF
Nitroglycerin	NO-mediated vasodilation (vein > artery)	↑	↓	↓	→	↓	↓	↑
Nitroprusside	NO-mediated vasodilation (vein = artery)	↑	↓	↓	→	↓	↓	↓
Nesiritide	cGMP-mediated vasodilation in both endothelial and vascular smooth muscle cells	↑	↓	↓	→	↓	↓	↑

AHF, acute heart failure; *CBF*, cerebral blood flow; *CI*, cardiac index; *cGMP*, cyclic 3″,5′-guanosine monophosphate; *CO*, cardiac output; *HR*, heart rate; *MAP*, mean atrial pressure; *NO*, nitric oxide; *PCWP*, pulmonary capillary wedged pressure; *PVR*, peripheral vascular resistance; *SVR*, systemic vascular resistance.

at which fluid is removed. This advantage prevents fluid removal from exceeding the rate at which interstitial fluid is mobilized, thus maintaining intravascular blood volume and avoiding hypotension. Despite these favorable findings, there is no clear evidence that HF is superior to conventional diuretics.

HOW TO DIRECTLY AND TRANSIENTLY IMPROVE CARDIAC FUNCTION

Inotropes

Inotropic drugs improve short-term outcome in patients with signs and symptoms of hypoperfusion-associated organ dysfunction secondary to severely depressed contractility. Although there is evidence that use of inotropic agents is associated with poor prognosis,[16-18] administration of inotropic agents such as dobutamine, dopamine, milrinone, levosimendan, and norepinephrine can dramatically improve hemodynamic parameters in patients with cardiogenic shock. Inotropic agents should be strongly considered in patients with profound hemodynamic disturbances. Similarly, they should be withdrawn without hesitation at the earliest point possible to avoid side effects.

Dopamine

Despite the fact that low-dose dopamine causes vasodilation of renal arteries and increases renal blood flow, clinical use of "renal dose" dopamine is no longer acceptable. The ROSE trial[7] enrolled patients who were hospitalized with AHF and renal dysfunction (glomerular filtration rate of 15 to 60 mL/min/1.73 m^2 as estimated by the Modification of Diet in Renal Disease equation) and evaluated the efficacy of low-dose dopamine (2 µg/kg/min for 72 hours) and low-dose nesiritide (0.005 µg/kg/min for 72 hours). There were no differences in total urine volume, change in cystatin C, plasma creatinine, weight, or NT-proBNP (N-terminal pro-brain natriuretic peptide) from baseline to 72 hours between the drugs. Thus dopamine is not superior to a simple vasodilator, which can be used without concomitant effects (for example, tachycardia) on the heart itself. Thus the routine use of low-dose dopamine is no longer accepted.

Dobutamine

There is no clear evidence that dobutamine offers an advantage over other agents in the treatment of AHF. However, dobutamine can increase CO with only a modest increase in heart rate. Most patients respond to doses of 2 to 20 µg/kg/min,[3] but tachycardia, myocardial ischemia, and arrhythmias appear frequently when doses exceed 15 µg/kg/min. Although tolerance to dobutamine has been observed after 72 hours,[19] the plasma half-life is only 2.4 ± 0.7 minutes,[20] indicating that almost all dobutamine could be eliminated within 15 min.

Norepinephrine

Norepinephrine functions as a potent vasoconstrictor. It acts on all three groups of adrenergic receptors, but, while it has a strong affinity for alpha-1 and beta-1 receptors, it is a much weaker beta-2 agonist. Therefore it increases peripheral vascular resistance primarily because it causes less intense vasodilation (beta-2 activity) than other agents such as epinephrine. At high doses, it can cause limb ischemia. Norepinephrine is most often used in conjunction with inotropes like dobutamine to treat patients with cardiogenic shock. It is usually started at ≈ 0.1 to 0.15 µg/kg/min and titrated until the hemodynamic response becomes favorable.[3]

Nonadrenergic Inotropic Agents

Milrinone

Milrinone is a phosphodiesterase inhibitor approved for use in the United States, Europe, and Japan. It increases CO by inhibiting cyclic adenosine monophosphate (cAMP) breakdown in cardiomyocytes. In vascular muscle cells, increases in cAMP enhance calcium removal, reducing tone. Milrinone can also decrease pulmonary vascular resistance (PVR). Because of its inotropic and vasodilatory effects, it is usually referred to as an "inodilator." There is no clear evidence that milrinone offers advantages over other agents such as dobutamine. However, its mechanism of action may offer an advantage over β-adrenergic drugs in patients taking beta blockers. Caution is required when milrinone is administered to patients with coronary artery disease

Table 50-3 **Characteristics of Decongestive Agents**

Modality	Urine Na Excretion	RAA Activation	IV Volume	eGFR	CO	PCWP	RAP	PAP	SVR	PVR	Amount of Urine	Bioavailability
Intravenous diuretic	Hypotonic with plasma (half normal saline)	↑↑↑	↓	→,↓	↓	↓	↓	↓	↑	↑	Unpredictable	10-100 (%)
Tolvaptan	None*	→,↑	?	→	→	↓	↓	↓	→	→,↓	Unpredictable	42-80 (%)
Ultrafiltration	Isotonic with plasma	↓	→	→	→,↑	↓	↓	↓	→	→,↓	Controllable, adjustable	(-)

*Na excretion can be increased when it is combined with loop diuretics.

CO, cardiac output; *eGFR,* estimated glomerular filtration fraction; *IV,* intravenous Na, sodium; *PAP,* pulmonary artery pressure; *PCWP,* pulmonary capillary wedge pressure; *PVR,* pulmonary vascular resistance; *RAA,* renin angiotensin aldosterone; *RAP,* right arterial pressure; *SVR,* systemic vascular resistance.

because its use has been reported to increase mortality.[21] Low-dose milrinone can be combined with low-dose dobutamine because the different sites of actions may provide a synergistic effect. Milrinone should not be bolused because this practice may cause hypotension. Milrinone is renally cleared and thus should be used cautiously in patients with renal dysfunction.

Levosimendan

Levosimendan enhances cardiac troponin C (TnC) sensitivity to intracellular calcium, increasing CO.[22] Because levosimendan detaches from TnC during diastole, it acts during systole and therefore does not affect diastolic relaxation. Levosimendan can also activate potassium channels in vascular smooth muscle, leading to a reduction in SVR and PVR.[23] Despite its favorable effects on hemodynamics, a large randomized, double-blind, multicenter trial in patients with AHF (Survival of Patients with Acute Heart Failure in Need of Intravenous Inotropic Support [SURVIVE] trial) did not demonstrate an improvement in 180-day all-cause mortality relative to dobutamine; however, there was a benefit at 30 days and in patients on beta blockers.[24]

Intra-aortic Balloon Pumping

Although intra-aortic balloon pumping (IABP) has been used in critical settings for nearly 50 years, recent clinical trials have been unable to demonstrate a reduction in mortality.[25] However, IABP is a powerful device that can support the failing heart, increase coronary flow and CO, and decrease myocardial oxygen demand. There is no clear evidence to support IABP introduction in patients with AHF; therefore routine placement is not recommended.

AUTHORS' RECOMMENDATIONS

In summary, vasodilators should be used often early in AHF, especially when associated with normal or high BP. Diuretics or vasopressin antagonists should be used only when there are clear clinical signs of congestion. Inotropes should be restricted to cardiogenic shock in the presence of clear signs of organ dysfunction.

REFERENCES

1. Adams Jr KF, Fonarow GC, Emerman CL, et al. Characteristics and outcomes of patients hospitalized for heart failure in the United States: rationale, design, and preliminary observations from the first 100,000 cases in the Acute Decompensated Heart Failure National Registry (ADHERE). *Am Heart J.* 2005;149(2):209–216.
2. Harjola VP, Follath F, Nieminen MS, et al. Characteristics, outcomes, and predictors of mortality at 3 months and 1 year in patients hospitalized for acute heart failure. *Eur J Heart Fail.* 2010; 12(3):239–248.
3. McMurray JJ, Adamopoulos S, Anker SD, et al. ESC Guidelines for the diagnosis and treatment of acute and chronic heart failure 2012: The Task Force for the Diagnosis and Treatment of Acute and Chronic Heart Failure 2012 of the European Society of Cardiology. Developed in collaboration with the Heart Failure Association (HFA) of the ESC. *Eur Heart J.* 2012;33(14):1787–1847.
4. Mebazaa A, Gheorghiade M, Pina IL, et al. Practical recommendations for prehospital and early in-hospital management of patients presenting with acute heart failure syndromes. *Crit Care Med.* 2008;36(suppl 1):S129–S139.
5. Voors AA, Davison BA, Felker GM, et al. Early drop in systolic blood pressure and worsening renal function in acute heart failure: renal results of Pre-RELAX-AHF. *Eur J Heart Fail.* 2011;13(9): 961–967.
6. Flaherty JT. Role of nitroglycerin in acute myocardial infarction. *Cardiology.* 1989;76(2):122–131.
7. Chen HH, Anstrom KJ, Givertz MM, et al. Low-dose dopamine or low-dose nesiritide in acute heart failure with renal dysfunction: the ROSE acute heart failure randomized trial. *JAMA.* 2013;310(23):2533–2543.
8. Publication Committee for the VI. Intravenous nesiritide vs nitroglycerin for treatment of decompensated congestive heart failure: a randomized controlled trial. *JAMA.* 2002;287(12):1531–1540.
9. Wilcox CS. New insights into diuretic use in patients with chronic renal disease. *J Am Soc Nephrol.* 2002;13(3):798–805.
10. Dormans TP, Pickkers P, Russel FG, Smits P. Vascular effects of loop diuretics. *Cardiovasc Res.* 1996;32(6):988–997.
11. Metra M, Cotter G, Gheorghiade M, Dei Cas L, Voors AA. The role of the kidney in heart failure. *Eur Heart J.* 2012;33(17):2135–2142.
12. Costello-Boerrigter LC, Smith WB, Boerrigter G, et al. Vasopressin-2-receptor antagonism augments water excretion without changes in renal hemodynamics or sodium and potassium excretion in human heart failure. *Am J Physiol Renal Physiol.* 2006;290(2): F273–F278.
13. Ambrosy A, Goldsmith SR, Gheorghiade M. Tolvaptan for the treatment of heart failure: a review of the literature. *Expert Opin Pharmacother.* 2011;12(6):961–976.
14. Schrier RW, Gheorghiade M. Challenge of rehospitalizations for heart failure: potential of natriuretic doses of mineralocorticoid receptor antagonists. *Am Heart J.* 2011;161(2):221–223.
15. Costanzo MR, Guglin ME, Saltzberg MT, et al. Ultrafiltration versus intravenous diuretics for patients hospitalized for acute decompensated heart failure. *J Am Coll Cardiol.* 2007;49(6):675–683.
16. De Backer D, Biston P, Devriendt J, et al. Comparison of dopamine and norepinephrine in the treatment of shock. *N Engl J Med.* 2010;362(9):779–789.
17. O'Connor CM, Gattis WA, Uretsky BF, et al. Continuous intravenous dobutamine is associated with an increased risk of death in patients with advanced heart failure: insights from the Flolan International Randomized Survival Trial (FIRST). *Am Heart J.* 1999;138(1 Pt 1):78–86.
18. Abraham WT, Adams KF, Fonarow GC, et al. In-hospital mortality in patients with acute decompensated heart failure requiring intravenous vasoactive medications: an analysis from the Acute Decompensated Heart Failure National Registry (ADHERE). *J Am Coll Cardiol.* 2005;46(1):57–64.
19. Akhtar N, Mikulic E, Cohn JN, Chaudhry MH. Hemodynamic effect of dobutamine in patients with severe heart failure. *Am J Cardiol.* 1975;36(2):202–205.
20. Leier CV, Unverferth DV. Drugs five years later: Dobutamine. *Ann Intern Med.* 1983;99(4):490–496.
21. Felker GM, Benza RL, Chandler AB, et al. Heart failure etiology and response to milrinone in decompensated heart failure: results from the OPTIME-CHF study. *J Am Coll Cardiol.* 2003;41(6): 997–1003.
22. Givertz MM, Andreou C, Conrad CH, Colucci WS. Direct myocardial effects of levosimendan in humans with left ventricular dysfunction: alteration of force-frequency and relaxation-frequency relationships. *Circulation.* 2007;115(10):1218–1224.
23. Slawsky MT, Colucci WS, Gottlieb SS, et al. Acute hemodynamic and clinical effects of levosimendan in patients with severe heart failure. Study Investigators. *Circulation.* 2000;102(18): 2222–2227.
24. Mebazaa A, Nieminen MS, Packer M, et al. Levosimendan vs dobutamine for patients with acute decompensated heart failure: the SURVIVE Randomized Trial. *JAMA.* 2007;297(17):1883–1891.
25. Thiele H, Zeymer U, Neumann FJ, et al. Intraaortic balloon support for myocardial infarction with cardiogenic shock. *N Engl J Med.* 2012;367(14):1287–1296.

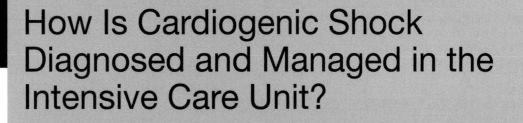

51 How Is Cardiogenic Shock Diagnosed and Managed in the Intensive Care Unit?

Benjamin A. Kohl

Cardiogenic shock (CS) is defined as an inability of the heart to provide adequate blood flow to maintain the metabolic demands of tissue despite adequate intravascular volume. This definition, and similar variants, has been used for decades in numerous textbooks despite its inherent vagaries. For practical purposes, most would agree that CS exists when a patient exhibits sustained hypotension with evidence of impaired cardiac function. With few exceptions, CS is an emergency that requires prompt diagnosis and appropriate therapy. This chapter reviews how to best diagnose and manage CS in the intensive care unit (ICU).

EPIDEMIOLOGY AND ETIOLOGY

Although there are a plethora of theoretical causes of CS in the ICU (Table 51-1), the most frequent cause of CS in the ICU is acute coronary syndrome (ACS) resulting in acute left ventricular dysfunction.[1,2] Autopsy studies have shown that more than 40% of left ventricular myocardium must be sacrificed for CS to ensue.[3,4] Other relatively common causes, usually as a result of acute myocardial infarction (AMI), include acute mitral regurgitation, cardiac tamponade (from ventricular free-wall rupture), and ventricular septal rupture.[5] Finally, a rare though increasingly recognized cause of CS in the ICU (particularly in the postoperative setting) is a stress-induced (so-called Takotsubo) cardiomyopathy.[6] CS occurs in 8.6% of patients sustaining ST-elevation myocardial infarction (STEMI) and in roughly 2.5% of patients with sustained non-ST-elevation myocardial infarction (NSTEMI).[7,8] Rarely, drugs have been shown to incite CS. In the Clopidogrel and Metoprolol in Myocardial Infarction Trial (COMMIT), the incidence of CS was 5% in patients receiving early metoprolol (roughly 30% greater than those who did not receive metoprolol).[9] Finally, all of these scenarios incite an acute inflammatory response that augments the initial insult and results in a vicious cycle that, if left untreated, culminates in death (Fig. 51-1).[10] Mortality rates for patients who sustain STEMI *with* CS are approximately 68% over 30 days compared with approximately 10% in those patients who did not have CS.[11-14] Evaluation of mortality trends within the United States reveals that a changing management scheme has decreased the mortality of this disease significantly (60.3% in 1995 vs. 47.9% in 2004).[7] Although this change in mortality is undoubtedly multifactorial, few would argue that an increased rate of cardiac catheterization (51.5% in 1995 vs. 74.4% in 2004) and of percutaneous cardiac intervention (27.4% in 1995 vs. 54.4% in 2004) had a major impact. Of note, during this registry period (that included more than 250,000 patients in more than 750 U.S. hospitals), there was no change in the use of intraaortic balloon pumps (IABPs) (39%) or in immediate coronary artery bypass graft (CABG) surgery (3%). Although prognostication can be difficult in this population, recent evidence suggests that hemodynamic variables in the first 24 hours may be useful.[15]

DIAGNOSIS

What is evident from almost all studies is that rapid diagnosis of CS is imperative. Hemodynamic criteria consistent with a diagnosis of CS include sustained (≥30 minutes) hypotension with systolic blood pressure less than 90 mm Hg, depressed cardiac index (CI) (<2.2 L/min/m²), and elevated pulmonary artery occlusion pressure (PAOP) (>15 mm Hg).[16] From the aforementioned indices, it would appear that one should be able to rapidly identify this entity if CI is known. Many patients with CS have a distributive shock, though, which lowers their systemic vascular resistance (SVR) and normalizes their CI.[17] Thus it is necessary that the clinician have a systematic method of diagnosing CS.

In the absence of more objective data, a critically ill patient in shock usually has hypovolemia, sepsis, pulmonary embolism, or myocardial ischemia. As with most ailments, diagnosis begins with the physical examination. Often, the diagnosis can be made simply by placing one's hands on the patient's extremities. Frequently, CS manifests with cold and clammy extremities as the body attempts to maintain adequate perfusion to vital organs by peripheral vasoconstriction. With impaired myocardial contraction, auscultation of the lungs frequently reveals crackles due to an elevated left ventricular end-diastolic pressure (LVEDP) with exudate filling the pulmonary interstitium. Obviously, however, most physical examination findings, although supportive of a diagnosis, are nonspecific.

Therefore additional information is frequently needed. A chest radiograph should be ordered in any patient presenting with symptoms of shock. Signs of interstitial edema (often in the absence of physical examination findings) are suggestive of CS. An electrocardiogram should be ordered and examined for signs of myocardial ischemia. If CS remains a consideration, cardiac enzymes should be sent.

Table 51-1 Causes of Cardiogenic Shock

Acute myocardial infarction
- Pump failure
- Large infarction
- Smaller infarction with preexisting left ventricular dysfunction
- Infarction extension
- Severe recurrent ischemia
- Mechanical complications
- Acute mitral regurgitation caused by papillary muscle rupture
- Ventricular septal defect
- Free-wall rupture
- Pericardial tamponade
- Right ventricular infarction

Other conditions
- End-stage cardiomyopathy
- Myocarditis
- Myocardial contusion (blunt cardiac injury)
- Prolonged cardiopulmonary bypass
- Septic shock with myocardial depression
- Aortic stenosis
- Left ventricular outflow tract obstruction
- Obstruction to left ventricular filling (e.g., mitral stenosis)
- Acute aortic insufficiency
- Pulmonary embolism
- Pheochromocytoma

From Topalian S, Ginsberg F, Parrillo JE. Cardiogenic shock. *Crit Care Med.* 2008; 36:S66–S74.

Echocardiography is the test of choice to diagnose CS and should be ordered promptly. The sensitivity of this modality approaches 100%, whereas the specificity is roughly 95%.[18,19] If transesophageal imaging is unavailable, contraindicated, or too cumbersome, transthoracic echocardiography should be ordered. A quick examination should allow rapid assessment of any left or right ventricular dysfunction, new valvular regurgitation, pericardial effusion, and ventricular septal rupture.[18] Rapid availability of this imaging modality may preclude the need for further invasive monitors because pulmonary artery systolic pressure and PAOP can be estimated by Doppler echocardiography.[20] Precise physiologic parameters are frequently necessary both to diagnose and to manage patients with CS. Invasive monitoring is probably warranted if there are persistent signs of hypoperfusion despite adequate volume therapy. The American College of Cardiology and American Heart Association (ACC/AHA) gives a class IIa (weight of evidence and opinion is in favor of usefulness and efficacy) recommendation for placement of a pulmonary artery catheter (PAC) in patients with CS.[21] PACs can aid in diagnosis and can be helpful with subsequent management, although data showing a mortality benefit are equivocal.[22-24] There are data to suggest that certain calculated indices, such as cardiac power and stroke work index, may have short-term prognostic value.[25] Interpretation of PAC data requires a detailed knowledge of pathophysiology. A quick look at the numbers will rarely yield the diagnosis. Most causes of cardiogenic shock result in elevated central venous and pulmonary arterial pressures (the exception being isolated right ventricular ischemia). For the various causes to be differentiated, a detailed understanding of the various waveforms is necessary.

The central venous pressure (CVP) is probably the most underused physiologic parameter. A plethora of

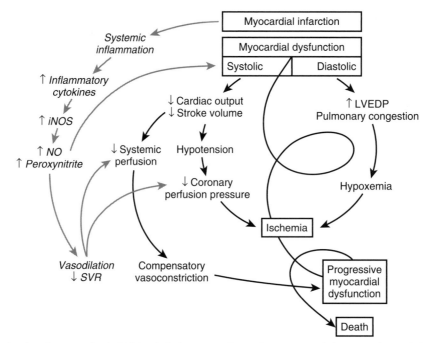

Figure 51-1. Vicious cycle of cardiogenic shock. *iNOS,* inhaled nitric oxide synthase; *LVEDP,* left ventricular end-diastolic pressure; *NO,* nitric oxide; *SVR,* systemic vascular resistance. *From Antman EM, Braunwald E. Acute myocardial infarction. In: Braunwald ED, Fauci E, Kasper D, eds. Harrison's Principles of Internal Medicine, 15th ed. New York: McGraw-Hill; 2001:1395.*

information can be obtained with proper analysis. For the interpretation of the various waves, the scale must be set so that all portions of the wave can be seen (usually a scale with 20 to 30 mm Hg maximum is optimal). The various components of the CVP can be seen in Fig. 51-2. By breaking the waveform into various cardiac events, it becomes apparent that not all elevated venous pressures are equal. Cardiac tamponade will cause a monophasic CVP with a very small *x*-descent and often complete loss of the *y*-descent, whereas right ventricular ischemia with tricuspid regurgitation will yield a very large, fused *c-v* wave. The *c-v* wave is a fused *c* and *v* wave resulting from severe tricuspid regurgitation. Because of the regurgitant flow, there is an inability to differentiate the slight increased atrial pressure generated from closure of the tricuspid valve and atrial filling during atrial diastole. A complete analysis of CVP waveform is beyond the scope of this chapter, and the reader is referred to other texts.[26, 27]

The equivalent CVP for the left side of the heart is the PAOP. Similarly, with correct identification of the waves and translation of the waves into a portion of the cardiac cycle, various diseases become unmasked.[28-30] Acute mitral regurgitation is associated with very large *v* waves on PAOP. Acute cardiac ischemia often first manifests as left ventricular diastolic dysfunction. This, in turn, leads to a higher left ventricular end-diastolic volume (LVEDV) that causes an elevated LVEDP. Although this culminates in an elevated PAOP, through evaluation of the waveform, an exaggerated *a* wave is consistent with diastolic dysfunction.

MANAGEMENT: AN EVIDENCE-BASED APPROACH

Management of CS should focus on augmentation of oxygen delivery and blood pressure to restore microcirculatory function and maximize tissue perfusion. A delay in diagnosis or therapy will have a direct impact on mortality.

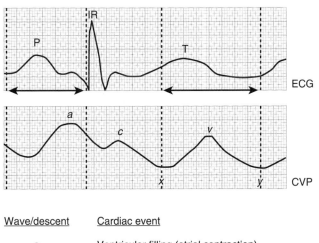

Wave/descent	Cardiac event
a	Ventricular filling (atrial contraction)
c	Tricuspid valve (isovolemic contraction)
v	Atrial filling (ventricular contraction)
x	Atrial relaxation (start of atrial filling)
y	Tricuspid valve opening (rapid ventricular filling)

Figure 51-2. Components of the central venous pressure (*CVP*) waveform. *ECG*, electrocardiogram.

Management of CS can be pharmacologic therapy, mechanical therapy, or revascularization.

Pharmacologic Therapy

It should be stated at the outset that there have been very few large controlled trials evaluating the efficacy of different vasopressor or inotrope therapies in CS, none of which have confirmed any outcome difference with any particular agent.[31]

Initial treatment for patients with CS should focus on restoration of normal hemodynamics, oxygenation, and avoidance of arrhythmia. In patients without significant pulmonary edema, it is reasonable to administer a fluid challenge before vasopressor therapy. If pulmonary edema is present or there is no response to a fluid challenge, pharmacologic therapy should be initiated. Pharmacologic therapy for CS initially should focus on those compounds that have both inotropic and vasopressor activity.[32,33] Drugs to consider as first-line treatment include norepinephrine, dopamine, dobutamine, and epinephrine. There is some evidence, however, that dopamine administration for CS may in fact increase mortality[34]; however, this has not been validated in randomized controlled studies. In addition, in patients with heart failure, a 2002 meta-analysis showed a trend (not statistically significant) with increased mortality in patients given adrenergic inotropic agents.[35] Part of the reason for these observations may be that the improved hemodynamics seen with these agents come at a cost of increased myocardial oxygen consumption. More recently, vasopressin was used in place of norepinephrine and showed similar hemodynamic effects.[36] Although phosphodiesterase inhibitors (e.g., milrinone) may be considered (particularly with right ventricular dysfunction), the resultant decrease in SVR is often not well tolerated by the hemodynamically unstable patient. Finally, levosimendan, an investigational calcium sensitizer that also promotes coronary vasodilation, continues to show promise as a novel treatment for CS.[37-39] These studies highlight the need for randomized controlled trials to confirm the efficacy of one therapy over another. In general, maintenance of normal physiologic parameters (e.g., mean arterial pressure, CI) should be the goal. Although high-dose vasopressors have been associated with poorer survival, this finding may be an epiphenomenon representing only those patients who have greater hemodynamic instability.[40]

Mechanical Therapy

In patients who are unresponsive to conventional pharmacologic therapy, mechanical augmentation of flow may be of benefit.[41] The ACCF/AHA guidelines have recently downgraded the recommendation of an IABP for CS from a class I ("is recommended") to a class IIa ("can be useful").[42] The only randomized trial to evaluate the efficacy of IABP (with or without thrombolysis) in patients with CS was able to show a dramatic decrease in 6-month mortality rate (39% vs. 80%; *P* < .05) in patients with severe shock who received an IABP.[43] Nonrandomized trials also have shown decreased mortality. More recent observational studies, however, have been fraught with greater equipoise.[44] The use of this device, though, is frequently associated with more aggressive therapies such as revascularization.[45] One of the inherent benefits of IABP counterpulsation devices is that they can be placed at the bedside to augment diastolic pressure and reduce left ventricular afterload (without increasing myocardial oxygen demand). The incidence of major complications (e.g., arterial injury and perforation, limb ischemia, visceral ischemia) with IABP insertion is 2.5% to 3.0%.[45,46] If an IABP is contraindicated (e.g., severe aortic insufficiency, severe peripheral vascular disease, aortic aneurysm, and dissection) or unavailable or the patient is unresponsive to its effects, ventricular assist device (VAD) placement may be considered.[47,48] A variety of other devices, including institution of extracorporeal membrane oxygenation and placement of the CardioWest total artificial heart, also have been tried with varying success.[49-51] Newer percutaneous VADs are making this option more feasible in smaller centers.[52] A 2005 investigation randomized patients with CS to IABP or TandemHeart (a percutaneous left ventricular assist device [LVAD]).[53] Although there were no significant differences in 30-day mortality between the two groups, patients in the LVAD subgroup had a significant improvement in hemodynamics, renal function, and clearance of serum lactate compared with the IABP cohort. A more recent multicenter randomized trial comparing TandemHeart with IABP in 42 patients with CS revealed similar improvements in hemodynamics with the LVAD without a statistically significant difference in 30-day mortality.[54] Although many of these newer devices appear promising, there will clearly be a limited number of centers that will have access to such technology. Experience with device placement and hemodynamic management is necessary for optimal benefit. In the National Registry of Myocardial Infarction, IABP use was independently associated with survival in those centers with experience in their use.[55] Finally, many of these devices are placed as a bridge to cardiac transplantation, and resources must be available to continue this often lengthy, workup.

Revascularization Therapy

Although management of AMI is beyond the scope of this chapter, a brief synopsis is provided here. Because AMI is frequently the inciting event culminating in CS, reestablishing blood flow to the affected myocardial territory is of utmost importance.[56] It has become evident that prompt revascularization reduces the mortality of this disease. One method of reestablishing coronary arterial flow is by the administration of thrombolytic agents. In a randomized trial involving more than 40,000 patients with AMI, the GUSTO-I (Global Utilization of Tissue Plasminogen Activator and Streptokinase for Occluded Coronary Arteries) trial demonstrated a survival advantage with the use of tissue plasminogen activator (tPA) over streptokinase.[57] Since these results have been published, a number of other thrombolytics have been developed; however, randomized trials have been unable to show a difference with respect to CS progression between the tPA and these newer agents.[58] Moreover, once CS has been established, no studies have shown an improvement in mortality with the administration of thrombolytic agents. The preferred modality of revascularization remains either percutaneous coronary intervention (PCI) or CABG.[14,32,59-62] Although a facilitated PCI strategy (i.e., planned immediate PCI after fibrinolytic administration) has not been shown to be effective,[63,64] fibrinolytics may still be considered in those situations in which PCI is not attainable for more than 90 minutes, the patient is within 3 hours of his or her infarction, and there are no contraindications.[65] The Should We Emergently Revascularize Occluded Coronaries for Cardiogenic Shock (SHOCK) trial emphasized this aspect, showing that early revascularization reduced mortality by 22% in those patients who presented with CS and by 16% in those who had CS subsequent to admission.[58] The question of how and when it is best to achieve reperfusion has been evaluated. The SHOCK trial prospectively randomized 302 patients with CS due to AMI to either emergency revascularization (either CABG or PCI) or medical stabilization.[59] Although 30-day mortality was similar for both groups, there was a significant survival advantage in the early revascularization group at 6 months, 1 year, and 6 years. This trial did not demonstrate an advantage of one revascularization therapy over another. Given these results and others, early revascularization (either with PCI or CABG surgery) therapy is a class I recommendation by the ACC/AHA for patients younger than 75 years with CS complicated by ACS.[7] Although there are few data to support revascularization in the non–ST-segment elevation CS population, the SHOCK registry did find a nonsignificant decrease in mortality among those patients who underwent early revascularization.[1]

AUTHOR'S RECOMMENDATIONS

Cardiogenic shock requires rapid diagnosis and appropriate therapy to significantly affect mortality. ICU patients often have multiple-organ failure, and differentiating CS from other forms of shock can often be difficult. In patients in whom a diagnosis of CS is being entertained, I recommend the following:

- Maximize oxygen delivery, immediately obtain an electrocardiogram, place invasive monitoring (at least arterial and central venous monitoring), and undertake laboratory (including cardiac enzymes) evaluation.
- Rapid echocardiography may not only confirm the diagnosis but may aid in management.
- If echocardiography is not immediately available and there are no signs of pulmonary edema, I recommend giving an initial intravenous fluid challenge with 500 mL of crystalloid. Repeat fluid challenge may be necessary if there is no increase in blood pressure or right atrial pressure.
- If the patient remains in CS despite adequate intravascular volume, I recommend dobutamine or epinephrine as first-line vasopressor therapy to maintain mean arterial pressure higher than 60 mm Hg. Vasopressin or norepinephrine can be added if there is not rapid improvement in mean arterial pressure.
- If there is not a dramatic improvement in perfusion within 1 hour, placement of an IABP should be *considered*.
- In patients with electrocardiographic changes suggestive of myocardial ischemia, an immediate search for a culprit vessel should be sought, and early revascularization should be considered.
- It is important to recognize that the treatment of CS often crosses multiple disciplines. Communication among the intensivist, invasive cardiologist, and cardiac surgeon is often necessary to ensure optimal care with optimal timing. As bedside echocardiography becomes more commonplace in ICUs, there is no doubt that intensivists will be diagnosing this entity more frequently and in a more timely manner.

REFERENCES

1. Jacobs AK, French JK, Col J, et al. Cardiogenic shock with non-ST-segment elevation myocardial infarction: a report from the SHOCK Trial Registry. SHould we emergently revascularize Occluded coronaries for Cardiogenic shocK? *J Am Coll Cardiol.* 2000;36:1091–1096.
2. Topalian S, Ginsberg F, Parrillo JE. Cardiogenic shock. *Crit Care Med.* 2008;36:S66S74.
3. Alonso DR, Scheidt S, Post M, Killip T. Pathophysiology of cardiogenic shock: quantification of myocardial necrosis, clinical, pathologic and electrocardiographic correlations. *Circulation.* 1973;48:588–596.
4. Harnarayan C, Bennett MA, Pentecost BL, Brewer DB. Quantitative study of infarcted myocardium in cardiogenic shock. *Br Heart J.* 1970;32:728–732.
5. Hochman JS, Buller CE, Sleeper LA, et al. Cardiogenic shock complicating acute myocardial infarction—etiologies, management and outcome: A report from the SHOCK Trial Registry. SHould we emergently revascularize Occluded coronaries for Cardiogenic shocK? *J Am Coll Cardiol.* 2000;36:1063–1070.
6. Chockalingam A, Mehra A, Dorairajan S, Dellsperger KC. Acute left ventricular dysfunction in the critically ill. *Chest.* 2010;138(1):198–207.
7. Babaev A, Frederick PD, Pasta DJ, et al. Trends in management and outcomes of patients with acute myocardial infarction complicated by cardiogenic shock. *JAMA.* 2005;294:448–454.
8. Holmes Jr DR, Berger PB, Hochman JS, et al. Cardiogenic shock in patients with acute ischemic syndromes with and without ST-segment elevation. *Circulation.* 1999;100:2067–2073.
9. Chen ZM, Pan HC, Chen YP, et al. Early intravenous then oral metoprolol in 45,852 patients with acute myocardial infarction: randomised placebo-controlled trial. *Lancet.* 2005;366:1622–1632.
10. Antman EM, Braunwald E. Acute myocardial infarction. In: Braunwald ED, Fauci E, Kasper D, eds. *Harrison's Principles of Internal Medicine.* 15th ed. New York: McGraw-Hill; 2001:1395.
11. Mehta SR, Yusuf S, Diaz R, et al. Effect of glucose-insulin-potassium infusion on mortality in patients with acute ST-segment elevation myocardial infarction: the CREATE-ECLA randomized controlled trial. *JAMA.* 2005;293:437–446.
12. Goldberg RJ, Gore JM, Alpert JS, et al. Cardiogenic shock after acute myocardial infarction. Incidence and mortality from a community-wide perspective, 1975 to 1988. *N Engl J Med.* 1991;325:1117–1122.
13. Singh M, White J, Hasdai D, et al. Long-term outcome and its predictors among patients with ST-segment elevation myocardial infarction complicated by shock: insights from the GUSTO-I trial. *J Am Coll Cardiol.* 2007;50:1752–1758.
14. Hochman JS, Sleeper LA, Webb JG, et al. Early revascularization and long-term survival in cardiogenic shock complicating acute myocardial infarction. *JAMA.* 2006;295:2511–2515.
15. Rigamonti F, Graf G, Merlani P, Bendjelid K. The short-term prognosis of cardiogenic shock can be determined using hemodynamic variables: a retrospective cohort study. *Crit Care Med.* 2014;41(11):2484–2491.
16. Hollenberg SM, Kavinsky CJ, Parrillo JE. Cardiogenic shock. *Ann Intern Med.* 1999;131:47–59.
17. Lim N, Dubois MJ, De Backer D, Vincent JL. Do all nonsurvivors of cardiogenic shock die with a low cardiac index? *Chest.* 2003;124:1885–1891.
18. Berkowitz MJ, Picard MH, Harkness S, et al. Echocardiographic and angiographic correlations in patients with cardiogenic shock secondary to acute myocardial infarction. *Am J Cardiol.* 2006;98:1004–1008.
19. Joseph MX, Disney PJ, Da Costa R, Hutchison SJ. Transthoracic echocardiography to identify or exclude cardiac cause of shock. *Chest.* 2004;126:1592–1597.
20. Reynolds HR, Anand SK, Fox JM, et al. Restrictive physiology in cardiogenic shock: observations from echocardiography. *Am Heart J.* 2006;151:890e9–15.
21. Richard C, Warszawski J, Anguel N, et al. Early use of the pulmonary artery catheter and outcomes in patients with shock and acute respiratory distress syndrome: a randomized controlled trial. *JAMA.* 2003;290:2713–2720.
22. Mimoz O, Rauss A, Rekik N, et al. Pulmonary artery catheterization in critically ill patients: a prospective analysis of outcome changes associated with catheter-prompted changes in therapy. *Crit Care Med.* 1994;22:573–579.
23. Porter A, Iakobishvili Z, Haim M, et al. Balloon-floating right heart catheter monitoring for acute coronary syndromes complicated by heart failure: discordance between guidelines and reality. *Cardiology.* 2005;104:186–190.
24. Fincke R, Hochman JS, Lowe AM, et al. Cardiac power is the strongest hemodynamic correlate of mortality in cardiogenic shock: a report from the SHOCK trial registry. *J Am Coll Cardiol.* 2004;44:340–348.
25. Magder S. Central venous pressure: a useful but not so simple measurement. *Crit Care Med.* 2006;34:2224–2227.
26. Magder S. Central venous pressure monitoring. *Curr Opin Crit Care.* 2006;12:219–227.
27. Pinsky MR. Clinical significance of pulmonary artery occlusion pressure. *Intensive Care Med.* 2003;29:175–178.
28. Pinsky MR. Pulmonary artery occlusion pressure. *Intensive Care Med.* 2003;29:19–22.
29. O'Quin R, Marini JJ. Pulmonary artery occlusion pressure: clinical physiology, measurement, and interpretation. *Am Rev Respir Dis.* 1983;128:319–326.
30. Antman EM, Anbe DT, Armstrong PW, et al. ACC/AHA guidelines for the management of patients with ST-elevation myocardial infarction. A report of the American College of Cardiology/American Heart Association Task Force on Practice Guidelines (Committee to Revise the 1999 Guidelines for the Management of Patients with Acute Myocardial Infarction). *Circulation.* 2004;10:e82–1292.
31. De Backer D, Biston P, Devriendt J, et al. Comparison of dopamine and norepinephrine in the treatment of shock. *N Engl J Med.* 2010;362:779–789.
32. Reynolds HR, Hochman JS. Cardiogenic shock: Current concepts and improving outcomes. *Circulation.* 2008;117:686–697.
33. Sakr Y, Reinhart K, Vincent JL, et al. Does dopamine administration in shock influence outcome? Results of the Sepsis Occurrence in Acutely Ill Patients (SOAP) Study. *Crit Care Med.* 2006;34:589–597.
34. Thackray S, Easthaugh J, Freemantle N, Cleland JG. The effectiveness and relative effectiveness of intravenous inotropic drugs acting through the adrenergic pathway in patients with heart failure: a meta-regression analysis. *Eur J Heart Fail.* 2002;4:515–529.
35. Jolly S, Newton G, Horlick E, et al. Effect of vasopressin on hemodynamics in patients with refractory cardiogenic shock complicating acute myocardial infarction. *Am J Cardiol.* 2005;96:1617–1620.
36. Garcia-Gonzalez MJ, Dominguez-Rodriguez A, Ferrer-Hita JJ. Utility of levosimendan, a new calcium sensitizing agent, in the treatment of cardiogenic shock due to myocardial stunning in patients with ST-elevation myocardial infarction: a series of cases. *J Clin Pharmacol.* 2005;45:704–708.
37. Rokyta Jr R, Pechman V. The effects of levosimendan on global haemodynamics in patients with cardiogenic shock. *Neuro Endocrinol Lett.* 2006;27:121–127.
38. Follath F, Cleland JG, Just H, et al. Efficacy and safety of intravenous levosimendan compared with dobutamine in severe low-output heart failure (the LIDO study): a randomised double-blind trial. *Lancet.* 2002;360:196–202.
39. Valente S, Lazzeri C, Vecchio S, et al. Predictors of in-hospital mortality after percutaneous coronary intervention for cardiogenic shock. *Int J Cardiol.* 2007;114:176–182.
40. Ohman EM, Nanas J, Stomel RJ, et al. Thrombolysis and counterpulsation to improve survival in myocardial infarction complicated by hypotension and suspected cardiogenic shock or heart failure: results of the TACTICS trial. *J Thromb Thrombolysis.* 2005;19:33–39.
41. Pitsis AA, Visouli AN. Mechanical assistance of the circulation during cardiogenic shock. *Curr Opin Crit Care.* 2011;17(5):425–438.
42. O'Gara PT, Kushner FG, Ascheim DD, et al. ACCF/AHA guideline for the management of ST-elevation myocardial infarction: a report of the American College of Cardiology Foundation/American Heart Association Task Force on Practice Guidelines. *J Am Coll Cardiol.* 2013;61:e78–e140.
43. Trost JC, Hillis LD. Intra-aortic balloon counterpulsation. *Am J Cardiol.* 2006;97:1391–1398.
44. Taylor J. ESC guidelines on acute myocardial infarction (STEMI). *Eur Heart J.* 2012;33:2501–2502.

45. Stone GW, Ohman EM, Miller MF, et al. Contemporary utilization and outcomes of intra-aortic balloon counterpulsation in acute myocardial infarction: the benchmark registry. *J Am Coll Cardiol.* 2003;41:1940–1945.

46. Leshnower BG, Gleason TG, O'Hara ML, et al. Safety and efficacy of left ventricular assist device support in postmyocardial infarction cardiogenic shock. *Ann Thorac Surg.* 2006;81:1365–1370. discussion 70–71.

47. Tayara W, Starling RC, Yamani MH, et al. Improved survival after acute myocardial infarction complicated by cardiogenic shock with circulatory support and transplantation: comparing aggressive intervention with conservative treatment. *J Heart Lung Transplant.* 2006;25:504–509.

48. Chen YS, Yu HY, Huang SC, et al. Experience and result of extracorporeal membrane oxygenation in treating fulminant myocarditis with shock: what mechanical support should be considered first? *J Heart Lung Transplant.* 2005;24:81–87.

49. Dang NC, Topkara VK, Leacche M, et al. Left ventricular assist device implantation after acute anterior wall myocardial infarction and cardiogenic shock: a two-center study. *J Thorac Cardiovasc Surg.* 2005;130:693–698.

50. El-Banayosy A, Arusoglu L, Morshuis M, et al. CardioWest total artificial heart: Bad Oeynhausen experience. *Ann Thorac Surg.* 2005;80:548–552.

51. White HD, Assmann SF, Sanborn TA, et al. Comparison of percutaneous coronary intervention and coronary artery bypass grafting after acute myocardial infarction complicated by cardiogenic shock. Results from the Should We Emergently Revascularize Occluded Coronaries for Cardiogenic Shock (SHOCK) trial. *Circulation.* 2005;112:1992–2001.

52. Thiele H, Sick P, Boudriot E, et al. Randomized comparison of intra-aortic balloon support with a percutaneous left ventricular assist device in patients with revascularized acute myocardial infarction complicated by cardiogenic shock. *Eur Heart J.* 2005;26:1276–1283.

53. Burkhoff D, Cohen H, Brunckhorst C, O'Neill WW. A randomized multicenter clinical study to evaluate the safety and efficacy of the TandemHeart percutaneous ventricular assist device versus conventional therapy with intraaortic balloon pumping for treatment of cardiogenic shock. *Am Heart J.* 2006;152:469e1–469e8.

54. Chen EW, Canto JG, Parsons LS, et al. Relation between hospital intra-aortic balloon counterpulsation volume and mortality in acute myocardial infarction complicated by cardiogenic shock. *Circulation.* 2003;108:951–957.

55. Bengtson JR, Kaplan AJ, Pieper KS, et al. Prognosis in cardiogenic shock after acute myocardial infarction in the interventional era. *J Am Coll Cardiol.* 1992;20:1482–1489.

56. The GUSTO Investigators. An international randomized trial comparing four thrombolytic strategies for acute myocardial infarction. *N Engl J Med.* 1993;329:673–682.

57. Hasdai D, Holmes Jr DR, Topol EJ, et al. Frequency and clinical outcome of cardiogenic shock during acute myocardial infarction among patients receiving reteplase or alteplase. Results from GUSTO-III. Global Use of Strategies to Open Occluded Coronary Arteries. *Eur Heart J.* 1999;20:128–135.

58. Hochman JS, Sleeper LA, Webb JG, et al. Early revascularization in acute myocardial infarction complicated by cardiogenic shock. SHOCK Investigators: Should We Emergently Revascularize Occluded Coronaries for Cardiogenic Shock. *N Engl J Med.* 1999;341:625–634.

59. Keeley EC, Boura JA, Grines CL. Primary angioplasty versus intravenous thrombolytic therapy for acute myocardial infarction: a quantitative review of 23 randomised trials. *Lancet.* 2003;361:13–20.

60. Hochman JS, Sleeper LA, White HD, et al. One-year survival following early revascularization for cardiogenic shock. *JAMA.* 2001;285:190–192.

61. Antman EM, Hand M, Armstrong PW, et al. 2007 Focused update of the ACC/AHA 2004 guidelines for the management of patients with ST-elevation myocardial infarction. A report of the American College of Cardiology/American Heart Association Task Force on Practice Guidelines. Developed in collaboration with the Canadian Cardiovascular Society endorsed by the American Academy of Family Physicians: 2007 Writing Group to Review New Evidence and Update the ACC/AHA 2004 Guidelines for the Management of Patients with ST-Elevation Myocardial Infarction, Writing on Behalf of the 2004 Writing Committee. *Circulation.* 2008;117:296–329.

62. Primary versus tenecteplase-facilitated percutaneous coronary intervention in patients with ST-segment elevation acute myocardial infarction (ASSENT-4 PCI): randomised trial. *Lancet.* 2006;367:569–578.

63. Cantor WJ, Brunet F, Ziegler CP, et al. Immediate angioplasty after thrombolysis: a systematic review. *CMAJ.* 2005;173:1473–1481.

64. Hochman JS. Cardiogenic shock complicating acute myocardial infarction: expanding the paradigm. *Circulation.* 2003;107:2998–3002.

65. Jeger RV, Harkness SM, Ramanathan K, et al. Emergency revascularization in patients with cardiogenic shock on admission: a report from the SHOCK trial and registry. *Eur Heart J.* 2006;27:664–670.

52 When Is Hypertension a True Crisis, and How Should It Be Managed in the Intensive Care Unit?

Emily K. Gordon, Jacob T. Gutsche, John G. Augoustides, Clifford S. Deutschman

Systemic hypertension remains a global priority because it is common and serious.[1,2] Hypertension affects approximately 1 billion people worldwide and is responsible for over 9 million deaths each year.[1-3] It is estimated that systemic hypertension accounts for approximately 50% of deaths due to cardiovascular disease and stroke.[1-3] A hypertensive crisis is typically defined as acute severe hypertension characterized by a diastolic blood pressure (BP) of 110 mm Hg or higher or a systolic BP of 180 mm Hg or higher.[4,5] New or worsening end-organ dysfunction was observed in 59% of patients with hypertensive crises requiring hospitalization, and the associated mortality at 90 days was 11%.[6]

Since the advent of effective antihypertensive therapy, the prevalence of hypertensive crises has significantly declined.[4,5,7,8] Although the incidence of hypertensive crises in the intensive care unit (ICU) has not been precisely measured, it remains common in medical and perioperative patients in the hospital.[9,10] In light of the above considerations, it follows that a hypertensive crisis is an often-encountered ICU complication. This chapter outlines a clinical approach to the diagnosis and management of this hemodynamic emergency in the ICU.

CLINICAL CLASSIFICATION OF AN ACUTE HYPERTENSIVE CRISIS: EMERGENCY VERSUS URGENCY

Hypertensive crises may be divided into hypertensive emergencies or hypertensive urgencies. A hypertensive urgency lacks apparent or threatened end-organ damage. Nonetheless, treatment is indicated. An approach to the management of hypertensive urgencies is outlined in Table 52-1.[14] In contrast, a *hypertensive emergency*, the focus of this chapter, is severe hypertension with actual or threatened acute end-organ damage (Table 52-2) and is, by definition, life threatening, mandating immediate therapy in an ICU with titratable, short-acting intravenous vasodilators (Table 52-3).

CLINICAL FEATURES OF SELECTED HYPERTENSIVE EMERGENCIES

Neurologic Hypertensive Emergencies

Neurologic hypertensive emergencies may have overlapping features (Table 52-4). Hypertensive encephalopathy is often the most difficult to diagnose.[15,16] There is apparent disruption of the blood–brain barrier and loss of cerebral autoregulation, resulting in diffuse cerebral edema and neurologic dysfunction. The diagnosis of hypertensive encephalopathy requires exclusion of stroke, intracranial hemorrhage, seizures, and mass lesions, usually through neuroimaging.[3-5,15,16] There are no large clinical trials examining the optimal treatment for hypertensive encephalopathy. Expert opinion suggests that therapy for hypertensive encephalopathy includes careful titration of a vasodilator in an ICU setting.[14-16] Recommendations for first-line vasodilator drugs and BP goals for neurologic hypertensive emergencies are summarized in Table 52-5.[15,16] It has been observed that pharmacologic relief is associated with significant neurologic improvement.[15,16] The patient requires close clinical observation because changes in the neurologic examination may reflect a secondary process—a new stroke or hypotensive overshoot—requiring immediate intervention.[15,16]

In patients with acute ischemic or hemorrhagic strokes, hypertension can be viewed as an adaptive or compensatory response to enhance perfusion pressure and thus maintain blood flow to the affected area. Nonetheless, current guidelines suggest that correction of BP elevation be modest and gradual.[15,16] A recent randomized trial in patients with acute intracerebral hemorrhage (N=2839) demonstrated that reducing systolic BP to 140 mm Hg within 1 hour significantly improved functional outcomes but did not reduce the risks of death or severe disability.[17] Post hoc analysis suggested that smooth and sustained control of excessive hypertension in acute intracerebral hemorrhage would further enhance the outcome benefits of vasodilator therapy.[18]

Table 52-1 Suggested Clinical Approach to a Hypertensive Urgency*

Step 1: Confirm that the BP elevation is truly severe

Step 2: Confirm that there are no clinical indications of threatened or actual end-organ damage

Step 3: Detect and manage triggering factors such as
- Pain—administer analgesia
- Anxiety and stress—consider anxiolytics
- Delirium—consider antipsychotics
- Drug withdrawal—treat accordingly
- Intracranial hypertension
- Urinary retention—drain bladder
- Hypoxia/hypercapnia—treat cause, administer oxygen, support ventilation
- Hypoglycemia—treat cause, administer glucose

Step 4: If still hypertensive after above measures, then consider antihypertensive therapy to lower BP to desired range in a gradual fashion

Adapted from: Salgado DR, Silva E, Vincent JL. Control of hypertension in the critically ill: a pathophysiologic approach. *Ann Intensive Care.* 2013;3:17.

*Defined as severe hypertension with no real or threatened end-organ damage.

BP, blood pressure.

Table 52-2 Clinical Scenarios in Which Severe Hypertension Is an Emergency

NEUROLOGIC
Hypertensive encephalopathy
Intracranial hemorrhage
Subarachnoid hemorrhage
Thrombotic stroke with severe hypertension

CARDIOVASCULAR
Left ventricular failure
Unstable angina
Myocardial infarction
Aortic dissection
Postoperative period after cardiac or vascular surgery (threatened suture lines)

RENAL
Gross hematuria
Acute renal injury/failure

SEVERE CATECHOLAMINE EXCESS
Pheochromocytoma
Recreational drug exposure
Drug withdrawal (e.g., beta blockers, clonidine)
Interactions with MAOIs

MAOIs, monoamine oxidase inhibitors.

Table 52-3 Drugs for Intravenous Management of a Hypertensive Crisis

Agent	Dose	Onset	Duration	Adverse Effects	Comments
Nitroglycerin	25 to 200 µg/min	2 to 5 min	5 to 10 min	Headache, vomiting, tolerance, methemoglobinemia	Consider in myocardial ischemia and cocaine intoxication
Sodium nitroprusside	1 to 10 µg/kg/min	Immediate	1 to 2 min	Vomiting, cyanide poisoning	Caution in raised intracranial pressure, spinal cord ischemia, and azotemia
Nicardipine (calcium channel blocker)	5 to 15 mg/h	5 to 10 min	15 to 30 min but may last 4 h	Headache, vomiting, tachycardia	Caution in acute heart failure
Clevidipine (calcium channel blocker)	2 to 16 mg/h	1 to 2 min	5 to 10 min	Tachycardia	Intralipid vehicle limits total dose in 24 h
Diltiazem (calcium channel blocker)	5 to 15 mg/h	5 to 10 min	2 to 4 h but may persist past 6 h	Hypotension, heart failure, bradycardia, heart block	Caution in bradycardia, heart block, and heart failure
Esmolol (beta-blocker)	50 to 100 µg/kg/min	1 to 2 min	10 to 30 min	Bronchospasm, heart block, and heart failure	Consider in aortic dissection; avoid in cocaine intoxication
Labetalol (beta-blocker)	1 to 5 mg/min	5 to 10 min	3 to 6 h	Bronchospasm, heart block, and heart failure	Caution in acute heart failure; avoid in cocaine intoxication
Enalapril (angiotensin converting enzyme inhibitor)	1.25 to 5 mg every 6 to 8 h	15 to 30 min	6 to 12 h	Hypotension in high rennin states	Acute ventricular failure; caution in azotemia and renal artery stenosis
Fenoldopam (dopamine-1 agonist)	0.1 to 0.3 µg/kg/min	2 to 5 min	30 min	Headache, vomiting, and tachycardia	Caution with glaucoma
Hydralazine	10 to 20 mg	10 to 20 min	1 to 4 h	Headache, vomiting, and tachycardia	Consider in eclampsia
Phentolamine	5 to 15 mg bolus	1 to 2 min	10 to 30 min	Headache, vomiting, and tachycardia	Consider in catecholamine excess states

Adapted from: Marik PE, Rivera R. Hypertensive emergencies: an update. *Curr Opin Crit Care.* 2011;17:569–580.

Table 52-4 **Clinical Features of Selected Neurologic Hypertensive Emergencies**

Clinical Feature	Hypertensive Encephalopathy	Subarachnoid Hemorrhage	Intraparenchymal Hemorrhage	Acute Infarction
History of hypertension	Universal	Common	Common	Common
Symptom duration	Usually subacute	Acute	Acute	Acute
Headache	Severe	Severe	Variable	Variable
Focal neurologic deficit	Unusual	Variable	Depends on location of hemorrhage	Depends on location of infarction
Retinopathy	Universal	Variable	Variable	Variable
Brain imaging	Typically normal	May show hemorrhage	Often demonstrates site and extent of hemorrhage	Frequently delineates site and extent of infarction
Lumbar puncture (if performed)	Typically normal—may have high opening pressure	Frank blood initially; xanthochromic later	Frank blood initially; xanthochromic later	Typically normal—may have high opening pressure
Acute treatment	ICU—vasodilator therapy	ICU—therapy with vasodilators; may require neurosurgical intervention	ICU—vasodilator therapy	ICU—cautious vasodilator therapy

Adapted from: Manning L, Robinson TG, Anderson CS. Control of blood pressure in hypertensive neurological emergencies. *Curr Hypertens Rep.* 2014;16:436.
ICU, intensive care unit.

Table 52-5 **Recommended Vasodilator Management in Neurologic Hypertensive Emergencies**

Hypertensive Emergency	Suitable Vasodilators	BP Goals	Comments
Hypertensive encephalopathy	Labetalol, clevidipine, nicardipine, sodium nitroprusside	25% decrease in mean arterial pressure over 4 to 8 hr	Consider anticonvulsants for control of seizures to tighten control of BP. Caution with sodium nitroprusside because it may increase intracranial pressure.
Acute cerebral infarction with BP>220/120 mm Hg	Labetalol, clevidipine, nicardipine, sodium nitroprusside	15% decrease in mean arterial pressure over 1 to 2 hr	Monitor closely for neurologic deterioration.
Acute cerebral infarction with indication for thrombolytic therapy and BP>185/110 mm Hg	Labetalol, clevidipine, nicardipine, sodium nitroprusside	15% decrease in mean arterial pressure over 1 to 2 hr	Monitor closely for neurologic deterioration.
Cerebral hemorrhage with normal intracranial pressure and systolic BP>180 mm Hg or mean arterial pressure >130 mm Hg	Labetalol, clevidipine, nicardipine, sodium nitroprusside	Modest decrease in mean arterial pressure over 1 to 2 hr with a goal BP of ~160/90 mm Hg, if tolerated clinically	Monitor closely for neurologic deterioration.
Cerebral hemorrhage with raised intracranial pressure and systolic BP>180 mm Hg or mean arterial pressure >130 mm Hg	Labetalol, clevidipine, nicardipine, sodium nitroprusside	Modest decrease in mean arterial pressure over 1 to 2 hr with a goal BP of ~160/90 mm Hg, if tolerated clinically	Monitor closely for neurologic deterioration. Consider monitoring of intracranial pressure and maintain cerebral perfusion pressure >60 mm Hg. Caution with sodium nitroprusside because it may increase intracranial pressure.
Subarachnoid hemorrhage	Labetalol, clevidipine, nicardipine	Modest decrease in mean arterial pressure over 1 to 2 hr with a goal BP of ~140 to 160/90 mm Hg, if tolerated clinically	Caution with sodium nitroprusside because it may increase intracranial pressure. Maintain mean arterial pressure >90 mm Hg.
Hypertension after craniotomy	Labetalol, clevidipine, nicardipine, sodium nitroprusside	Modest decrease in mean arterial pressure over 1 to 2 hr with a goal BP of <160/90 mm Hg, if tolerated clinically	Monitor closely for neurologic deterioration.

Adapted from: Manning L, Robinson TG, Anderson CS. Control of blood pressure in hypertensive neurological emergencies. *Curr Hypertens Rep.* 2014;16:436.
BP, blood pressure.

Table 52-6 Recommendations for Cardiovascular Hypertension Emergencies

ACUTE CORONARY SYNDROME

BP goal is <140/90 mm Hg
First-line agents include beta blockers and nitroglycerin
Caution with thrombolysis in severe hypertension

ACUTE HEART FAILURE

BP goal is systolic BP <140 mm Hg
First-line agents include nitroglycerin and angiotensin blockers
Reduce drug doses as hypertension resolves

ACUTE AORTIC DISSECTION

Goal BP is systolic BP <120 mm Hg
Adequate analgesia is important
First-line agents include beta blockers and nicardipine
Caution with beta blockade in aortic regurgitation

PERIOPERATIVE HYPERTENSION

Goal BP is typically within 20% of baseline
High-risk scenarios call for BP goal for systolic BP <140 mm Hg (e.g., after craniotomy; fresh vascular suture lines)
Note latest guidelines about beta blockers

HYPERTENSION AFTER CAROTID REVASCULARIZATION

Goal BP is typically systolic BP <140 mm Hg
Neurologic deficits require serial neurologic examination and imaging
Cerebral hyperperfusion may require systolic BP <120 mm Hg

BP, blood pressure.

Table 52-7 Recommendations for Hypertension Emergencies Due to Catecholamine Excess

PHEOCHROMOCYTOMA

Control hypertensive crisis with phentolamine, sodium nitroprusside, and nicardipine
Prepare for surgery with alpha blockade titrated to effect
Consider beta blockade only in setting of adequate alpha blockade
Consider metyrosine for suppression of tumor catecholamine synthesis
Vasopressor therapy may be required after tumor resection in the postoperative period

DRUG INTOXICATION (E.G., COCAINE)

Control hypertensive crisis with fenoldopam, sodium nitroprusside, and nicardipine
Avoid beta blockade
Supportive therapy includes titrated benzodiazepine for sedation

MAOIS

Control hypertensive crisis with phentolamine, sodium nitroprusside, and nicardipine
Avoid trigger agents
Consider serotonin blockade with cyproheptadine in the serotonin syndrome

DRUG WITHDRAWAL

Control hypertensive crisis with phentolamine, sodium nitroprusside, and nicardipine
Titrate replacement therapy to effect (e.g., beta blocker, clonidine)

Hypertension after craniotomy is also classified as an emergency because of the risk of devastating intracranial hemorrhage.[19,20] In a retrospective single-center case-controlled study of 11,214 adult craniotomy patients between 1976 and 1992, intracranial hemorrhage was frequently preceded by either a systolic BP greater than 159 mm Hg or a diastolic BP over 89 mm Hg.[19] Patients with intracranial hemorrhage had an 11.4-fold increase in mortality (18.2% vs. 1.6%; $P < .05$) and a 2.2-fold increase in median hospital stay (24.5 days vs. 11.0 days; $P < .05$).[19] Multiple studies have since confirmed these findings.[20,21] A BP target below 160/90 mm Hg would appear reasonable in this setting.[20,21] A small randomized trial (N=52) demonstrated that nicardipine infusion was more effective in treating postcraniotomy hypertension than esmolol.[22]

Cardiovascular Hypertensive Emergencies (Table 52-6)

Hypertension with an Acute Coronary Syndrome

The goal of therapy in the hypertensive patient with acute coronary syndrome is to reduce the risk of ischemia induced by increased left ventricular wall stress.[23,24] In patients with a history of mild or no hypertension, vasodilator therapy can be titrated for symptom relief. There are no data identifying an "optimal" BP. Thus therapy is determined by individual clinical feature, although normalization may not be clinically tolerated. In patients with long-standing uncontrolled hypertension, organ ischemia

may develop when BP is reduced too rapidly.[14] In patients with coronary artery disease and hypertension, expert opinion recommends the use of vasodilator therapy when the BP is greater than 140/90 mm Hg.[24]

The treatment of hypertension may require the use of more than one agent. Current guidelines recommend nitroglycerin and beta blockers for the acute management of hypertension in an acute coronary syndrome.[14,15]

The presence of severe hypertension may profoundly influence clinical decision making in acute coronary syndrome. Expert opinion suggests that thrombolytic therapy is contraindicated for myocardial infarction with ST segment elevation when hypertension remains poorly controlled despite immediate vasodilator therapy or when the BP exceeds 185/110 mm Hg.[25] Furthermore, it is recommended that thrombolytic agents be applied cautiously in patients with severe hypertension and altered mental status until the neurologic evaluation is completed because cerebral hemorrhage may be extended.[25]

Hypertension with Left Heart Failure

Hypertension is common in patients who have acute heart failure.[26] The presenting systolic BP is an independent predictor of mortality in this patient group.[26] Beyond this, there are few hard data, and most recommendations reflect expert opinion. It is suggested that patients with acute heart failure, pulmonary edema, and a systolic BP over 140 mm Hg receive vasodilator therapy.[27] Nitroglycerin, administered either sublingually or intravenously, is the preferred vasodilator, although data to support its value relative to other choices do not exist. Second-line vasodilator agents include intravenous nitroprusside and angiotensin-converting enzyme inhibitors.[27] Importantly, none of these agents has been subjected to randomized controlled trials. BP should be titrated to clinical effect for both symptom relief and control of hypertension. Because hypertension may resolve quickly in this scenario, it is reasonable to reduce the vasodilator therapy after 24 hours.[27]

Ongoing clinical trials are investigating new candidate vasodilators for use in acute heart failure. The RELAX-AHF (Relaxin in Acute Heart Failure) study looked at the effects of recombinant human relaxin-2 (serelaxin) that increases nitric oxide production by vascular smooth muscle. Although serelaxin did improve dyspnea, it had no effect on cardiovascular death or readmission endpoints. In addition to randomized trials, comparative effectiveness trials will be essential.

Hypertension with Aortic Dissection

Acute aortic dissection is both a hypertensive and a surgical emergency that requires perioperative intervention.[4,5,7,8,28] Guidelines based on expert opinion recommended initial analgesia for control of aortic pain and then titration of vasodilators to a systolic BP below 120 mm Hg, although these goals are not based on evidence.[29,30] Beta blockade is also recommended in this setting, in the absence of aortic regurgitation, in which optimal cardiac output requires relative tachycardia.[29,30]

Hypertension After Carotid Revascularization

Carotid endarterectomy (CEA) or stenting may be associated with postprocedural hypertension that can adversely affect clinical outcome.[33,34] In a retrospective analysis of 291 patients, severe postoperative hypertension (systolic BP > 220 mm Hg) after CEA was associated with death and stroke.[34] Tan et al. retrospectively reviewed data from 7677 patients after CEA and found that postoperative hypertension requiring intravenous vasoactive medication was associated with increased perioperative mortality (0.7% vs. 0.1%; $P < .001$), stroke (1.9% vs. 1%; $P = .018$) and cardiac complications (1.9% vs. 0.5%; $P < .001$).[35] This study is limited by the large database used, which did not specifically define the BP criteria necessitating intervention or the intravenous medications used to treat those patients with perioperative hypertension. Hypertension rarely complicates endovascular carotid stenting.[33,36,37]

Severe vascular complications after carotid surgery include cerebral hyperperfusion syndrome (ipsilateral headache with or without nausea and vomiting, seizures, focal neurologic deficit, or computed tomography evidence of edema on the side of the CEA) and intracranial hemorrhage.[33] Three recent large series (cumulative N > 5000) reported a 1.05% incidence of cerebral hyperperfusion and a 0.6% incidence of intracerebral hemorrhage after carotid revascularization, whether CEA or carotid stenting.[38-40] Although these complications are rare, they are associated with significant periprocedural mortality and morbidity.[38-40] Ogasawara et al. demonstrated that poor postoperative control of BP was associated with development of intracranial hemorrhage in patients with cerebral hyperperfusion syndrome after CEA.[40]

Aggressive management of BP (systolic BP < 140 mm Hg in general, <120 mm Hg for hyperperfusion or hemorrhage) after carotid intervention seems logical and is recommended.[33,40,41] However, data demonstrating that BP control reduces the incidence of neurologic complication are limited. In a "before-and-after" study of 836 (266 before and 570 after) patients undergoing carotid stenting, the application of a strict BP management protocol was associated with significant reductions in both cerebral hyperperfusion (29.4% to 4.2%; $P = .006$) and intracerebral hemorrhage (17.6% to 0%; $P = .006$).[41]

Hypertension in the Perioperative Period

Uncontrolled hypertension in the perioperative period may become life threatening.[28] Potential adverse events include hemorrhagic shock, airway compromise after CEA or neck surgery,[42] or serious intracranial hemorrhage.[33] Conversely, impaired blood flow to key organs has been implicated in the pathogenesis of the postoperative organ dysfunction syndrome. Therefore the medical management of perioperative hypertension must balance the risks for surgical hemorrhage with the risks for end-organ hypoperfusion.[3-5]

Several recent studies have demonstrated an association between "spikes" in pulse pressure and poor perioperative outcome, including coronary ischemic events, stroke and other cerebral events, congestive heart failure, renal dysfunction, and death.[43-45] However, there are no data demonstrating that intervening to control BP improved outcome.

Renal Hypertensive Emergencies

Patients with true hypertensive emergencies may have acute kidney injury (AKI). Conversely, patients with AKI may have acute severe hypertension.[14,15] Pharmacologic therapy for a hypertensive crisis with AKI is usually managed through titration of intravenous vasodilators such as labetalol, nicardipine, clevidipine, or sodium nitroprusside, targeting a 25% reduction in mean arterial pressure over several hours.[15] Again, data demonstrating efficacy are minimal.

Severe Catecholamine Excess Resulting in Hypertensive Emergencies

True hypertensive emergencies due to catecholamine excess are rare. Actual causes are listed in Table 52-2. Current recommendations for hypertensive emergencies characterized by catecholamine excess are summarized in Table 52-7.

Pheochromocytoma

Although unusual, approximately 7% of patients with previously undiagnosed pheochromocytoma present in hypertensive crisis or after a stroke, requiring aggressive management in the ICU for hemodynamic stabilization.[53-55] Elective surgical resection is indicated after medical stabilization has been achieved.[56]

Recreational Drug Use

Certain recreational drugs such as cocaine, amphetamines, or phencyclidine have sympathomimetic effects, and users may present in hypertensive crisis or with myocardial ischemia. The primary cause is norepinephrine overload, usually secondary to impaired reuptake. β-Adrenergic antagonists should be avoided because unopposed α-adrenergic activity can actually exacerbate coronary vasoconstriction, can increase heart rate and BP, and can even decrease survival.[57,58] Although labetalol had been the drug of choice because of its combined α- and β-adrenergic blockade, experimental studies do not support its use.[59,60] Anxiolysis with benzodiazepines may help decrease sympathetic stimulation secondary to cocaine use and is recommended by the American Heart Association, although there are no data to support this approach. Bauman et al. and Honderick et al. found that treatment of cocaine intoxication with a combination of benzodiazepines and nitroglycerin improves chest pain but did not affect outcome. Two studies have examined use of calcium channel blockers for cocaine-associated chest pain. This approach improved hemodynamics without any adverse outcome. Current recommendations are for nicardipine, fenoldapam, or verapamil plus a benzodiazepine as best for BP control, although there are no data of outcome.[58,61]

Monoamine Oxidase Inhibitors

Monoamine oxidase inhibitors (MAOIs), such as phenelzine, tranylcypromine, isocarboxazid, and selegiline, have been used for management of depression since the 1950s.[62] Their popularity has diminished because of the acute hypertensive crisis precipitated by tyramine-containing foods such as aged cheeses, bananas, soy condiments, and red wine.[62]

Monoamine oxidases inactivate neurotransmitters such as dopamine, epinephrine, norepinephrine, serotonin, and tyramine (a precursor of dopamine). These enzymes are present in the nervous system, in the liver, in the gastrointestinal tract, and in mitochondria. In addition, MAOIs interact with indirectly acting sympathomimetics such as ephedrine, pseudoephedrine, and phenylpropanolamine. These agents are often present in over-the-counter nasal decongestants.[63] In severe cases, hypertensive control has required ICU admission for titration of intravenous vasodilators such as nitroprusside or nicardipine.

MAOIs also adversely interact with meperidine.[64,65] This drug combination may precipitate the serotonin syndrome, a potentially fatal complication characterized by mental status changes, autonomic hyperreactivity, and neuromuscular abnormalities.[64,65] The management of the serotonin syndrome includes avoidance of pharmacologic triggers, supportive care, and administration of serotonin receptor blockers such as cyproheptadine.[64,65] Hypertension from the serotonin syndrome can be managed with short-acting intravenous agents such as nitroprusside and esmolol. In severe cases, hyperthermia due to excessive muscular activity may require sedation, neuromuscular blockade with cisatracurium, and mechanical ventilation.[64,65]

Drug Withdrawal

Discontinuation of beta blockers in the perioperative period can lead to tachycardia; hypertension; and, in severe cases, cardiac arrhythmias and myocardial ischemia that have been associated with increased mortality and morbidity.[66-69] A recent study by Wallace et al. (N = 38,779) showed that beta blockade withdrawal after surgery was associated with an increase in 30-day (odds ratio [OR], 3.93; 95% confidence interval [CI], 2.57 to 6.01; P < .0001) and 1-year mortality (OR, 1.96; 95% CI, 1.49 to 2.58; P < .0001).[70] Management involves reinstitution of beta blockade and may require ICU admission.

Withdrawal from clonidine, a centrally acting alpha agonist available in oral, transdermal, and parenteral formulations, has been associated with delirium, headache, hypertension, and myocardial ischemia that may result in ICU admission.[48,71,72]

AUTHORS' RECOMMENDATIONS

Our recommendations are based on current multidisciplinary guidelines, including those from the American Heart Association, American College of Cardiology, and the European Society of Cardiology. However, most are not based on evidence; rather, they reflect expert opinion, including our own.

- The prompt and effective management of hypertension in the ICU depends on differentiating hypertensive urgency from true hypertensive emergency.
- In the absence of true evidence, the management of a hypertensive emergency should be based on a working knowledge of current guidelines.
- The management of severe hypertension in a clinical emergency should be based on selection of recommended intravenous vasodilators at therapeutic doses titrated to recommended goals.
- The correction of severe hypertension in a clinical emergency should be integrated with the management of the associated disease state.

REFERENCES

1. James PA, Oparil S, Carter BL, et al. Evidence-based guideline for the management of high blood pressure in adults. *JAMA*. 2014;311:507–520.
2. Go AS, Bauman MA, Coleman King SM, et al. An effective approach to high blood pressure control: a science advisory from the American Heart Association, the American College of Cardiology, and the Centers for Disease Control and Prevention. *Hypertension*. 2014;63:878–885.
3. Kielsen S, Feldman RD, Lisheng L, et al. Updated national and international hypertension guidelines: a review of current recommendations. *Drugs*. 2014;74:2033–2051.
4. Fontes M, Varon J. Perioperative hypertensive crisis: newer concepts. *Int Anesthesiol Clin*. 2012;50:40–58.
5. Marik PE, Rivera R. Hypertensive emergencies: an update. *Curr Opin Crit Care*. 2011;17:569–580.
6. Katz JN, Gore JM, Amin A, Anderson FA, et al. Practice patterns, outcomes, and end-organ dysfunction for patients with acute severe hypertension: the Studying the Treatment of Acute hyperTension (STAT) registry. *Am Heart J*. 2009;158:599–606.
7. Pappadopoulos DP, Mourouzis I, Thomopoulos C, et al. Hypertension crisis. *Blood Press*. 2010;19:328–336.
8. Rodrigues MA, Kumar SK, De Care M. Hypertensive crisis. *Cardiol Rev*. 2010;18:102–107.
9. Axon RN, Cousineau I, Egan RM. Prevalence and management of hypertension in the inpatient setting: a systematic review. *J Hosp Med*. 2011;6:417–422.
10. Tulman DB, Stawicki SP, Papadimos TJ, et al. Advances in management of acute hypertension: a concise review. *Discov Med*. 2012;13:375–383.
11. Deleted in review.
12. Deleted in review.
13. Deleted in review.

14. Salgado DR, Silva E, Vincent JL. Control of hypertension in the critically ill: a pathophysiologic approach. *Ann Intensive Care.* 2013;3:17.

15. van den Born BJ, Beutler JJ, Gaillard CA, et al. Dutch guidelines for the management of hypertensive crisis. *Neth J Med.* 2011;69: 248–255.

16. Manning L, Robinson TG, Anderson CS. Control of blood pressure in hypertensive neurological emergencies. *Curr Hypertens Rep.* 2014;16:436.

17. Anderson CS, Heeley E, Huang Y, et al. Rapid blood-pressure lowering in patients with acute intracerebral hemorrhage. *N Engl J Med.* 2013;368:2355–2365.

18. Manning L, Hirakawa Y, Arima H, et al. Blood pressure variability and outcome after acute intracerebralhaemorrhage: a post-hoc analysis of INTERACT2, a randomized controlled trial. *Lancet Neurol.* 2014;13:364–373.

19. Basall A, Mascha EJ, Kalfas I, et al. Relation between perioperative hypertension and intracranial hemorrhage after craniotomy. *Anesthesiology.* 2000;93:48–54.

20. Seifman MA, Lewis PM, Rosenfeld JV, et al. Postoperative intracranial hemorrhage: a review. *Neurosurg Rev.* 2011;34:393–407.

21. Jian M, Li X, Wang A, et al. Flurbiprofen and hypertension but not hydroxyehtylstarch are associated with post-craniotomy intracranial haematoma requiring surgery. *Br J Anaesth.* 2014;113:832–839.

22. Bebawy JF, Houston CC, Kosky JL, et al. Nicardipine is superior to esmolol for the management of postcraniotomy emergence hypertension: a randomized open-label study. *Anesth Analg.* 2015;120:186–192.

23. Nadir SK, Tayebee MH, Messendi F, et al. Target organ damage in hypertension: pathophysiology and implications for drug therapy. *Curr Pharm Des.* 2006;12:1581–1592.

24. Fihn SD, Gardin JM, Abrams J, et al. 2012 ACCF/AHA/ACP/AATS/PCNA/SCA/STS guideline for the management of patients with stable ischemic heart disease: a report of the American College of Cardiology Foundation/American heart Association Task Force on Practice Guidelines, and the American College of Physicians, American Association for Thoracic Surgery, preventive cardiovascular Nurses Association, Society for Cardiovascular Angiography and Interventions, and Society of Thoracic Surgeons. *J Am Coll Cardiol.* 2012;60:e44–e164.

25. O'Gara PT, Kushner FG, Ascheim DD, et al. 2013 ACCF/AHA guideline for the management of ST-elevation myocardial infarction: a report of the American College of Cardiology Foundation/American Heart Association Task Force on Practice Guidelines. *J Am CollCardiol.* 2013;61:e78–e140.

26. Gheorghiade M, Abraham WT, Albert NM, et al. Systolic blood pressure at admission; clinical characteristics; and outcomes in patients hospitalized for acute heart failure. *JAMA.* 2006;296: 2217–2226.

27. Fermann GJ, Collins SP. Initial management of patients with acute heart failure. *Heart Fail Clin.* 2013;9:291–301.

28. Aronson S. Perioperative hypertensive emergencies. *Curr Hypertens Rep.* 2014;16:448.

29. Erbel R, Aboyans V, Boileau C, et al. 2014 ESC guidelines on the diagnosis and treatment of aortic diseases. *Eur Heart J.* 2014;35: 2873–2926.

30. Hiratzka LF, Bakris GL, Beckman JA, et al. 2010 ACCF/AHA/AATS/ACR/ASA/SCA/SCAI/SIR/STS/SVM guidelines for the diagnosis and management of patients with thoracic aortic disease: a report of the American College of Cardiology Foundation/American Heart Association Task Force on Practice Guidelines/American Association for Thoracic Surgery/American College of Radiology/American Stroke Association/Society of Cardiovascular Anesthesiologists/Society for Cardiovascular Angiography and Interventions/Society for Interventional Radiology/Society of Thoracic Surgeons, and Society for Vascular Medicine. *J Am Coll Cardiol.* 2010;55:e27–e129.

31. Deleted in review.

32. Deleted in review.

33. Augoustides J, Gutsche JT. Anesthesia for carotid endarterectomy and carotid stenting. UpToDate Topic 90608 Available at: www.uptodate.com [last updated October 21st 2014].

34. Wong JH, Findlay JM, Suarez-Almazor ME. Hemodynamic instability after carotid endarterectomy: risk factors and associations with operative complications. *Neurosurgery.* 1997;41:35–41.

35. Tan TW, Eslami MH, Kalish JA, et al. The need for treatment of hemodynamic instability following carotid endarterectomy is associated with increased perioperative and 1-year morbidity and mortality. *J Vasc Surg.* 2014;59:16–24.

36. Taha MM, Toma N, Sakaida H, et al. Periprocedural hemodynamic instability with carotid angioplasty and stenting. *Surg Neurol.* 2008;70:279–285.

37. Gupta R, Abou-Chebl A, Bajzer CT, et al. Rate, predictors and consequences of hemodynamic depression after carotid artery stenting. *J Am Coll Cardiol.* 2006;47:1538–1543.

38. Brantley HP, Kiessling JL, Milteer Jr HB, et al. Hyperperfusion syndrome following carotid artery stenting: the largest single-operator series to date. *J Invasive Cardiol.* 2009;21:27–30.

39. Abou-Chebl A, Yadav JS, Reginelli JP, et al. Intracranial hemorrhage and hyperperfusion syndrome following carotid artery stenting: risk factors, prevention and treatment. *J Am Coll Cardiol.* 2004;43:1596–1601.

40. Ogasawara K, Sakai N, Kuroiwa T, et al. Intracranial hemorrhage associated with cerebral hyperperfusion syndrome following carotid endarterectomy and carotid artery stenting: retrospective review of 4494 patients. *J Neurosurg.* 2007;107:1130–1136.

41. Abou-Chebl A, Reginelli J, Bajzer CT, et al. Intensive treatment of hypertension decreases the risk of hyperperfusion and intracerebral hemorrhage following carotid artery stenting. *Catheter Cardiovasc Interv.* 2007;69:690–696.

42. Augoustides JG, Groff BE, Mann DG, et al. Difficult airway management after carotid endarterectomy: utility and limitations of the laryngeal mask airway. *J Clin Anesth.* 2007;19:218–221.

43. Fontes ML, Aronson S, Mathew JP, et al. for the Multicenter Study of Perioperative Ischemia (McSPI) Research Group and the Ischemia Research and Education Foundation (IREF) investigators. Risk of adverse outcomes in coronary bypass surgery. *Anesth Analg.* 2008;107:1123–1130.

44. Franklin SS, Khan SA, Wong ND, et al. Is pulse pressure useful in predicting risk for coronary heart disease? The Framingham Heart Study. *Circulation.* 1999;100:353–360.

45. Aronson S, Fontes ML, Miao Y, et al. Risk index for perioperative renal dysfunction/failure: critical dependence on pulse pressure hypertension. *Circulation.* 2007;115:733–742.

46. Deleted in review.

47. Deleted in review.

48. Fleisher LA, Fleischmann KE, Auerbach AD, et al. 2014 ACC/AHA guideline on perioperative cardiovascular evaluation and management of patients undergoing noncardiac surgery: executive summary: a report of the American College of Cardiology/American Heart Association Task Force on Practice Guidelines. *Circulation.* 2014;130:2215–2245.

49. Deleted in review.

50. Deleted in review.

51. Deleted in review.

52. Deleted in review.

53. Lenders JWM, Eisenhofer G, Mannelli M, et al. Phaeochromocytoma. *Lancet.* 2005;366:665–675.

54. Kinney MA, Narr BJ, Warner MA. Perioperative management of pheochromocytoma. *J Cardiothorac Vasc Anesth.* 2002;10:359–369.

55. Augoustides JG, Abrams M, Berkowitz D, et al. Vasopressin for hemodynamic rescue in catecholamine-resistant vasoplegic shock after resection of massive pheochromocytoma. *Anesthesiology.* 2004;10:1022–1024.

56. Lord MS, Augoustides JG. Perioperative management of pheochromocytoma: focus on magnesium, clevidipine, and vasopressin. *J Cardiothorac Vasc Anesth.* 2012;26:526–531.

57. Lange RA, Cigarroa RG, Flores ED, et al. Potentiation of cocaine-induced coronary vasoconstriction by beta-adrenergic blockade. *Ann Intern Med.* 1990;112:897–903.

58. Hollander JE. The management of cocaine-associated myocardial ischemia. *N Engl J Med.* 1995;333:1267–1272.

59. Dusenberry SJ, Hicks MJ, Mariani PJ. Labetalol treatment of cocaine toxicity. *Ann Emerg Med.* February 1987;16(2):235.

60. Boehrer JD, Moliterno DJ, Willard JE, et al. Influence of labetalol on cocaine-induced coronary vasoconstriction in humans. *Am J Med.* 1993;94:608–610.

61. Negus BH, Willard JE, Hillis LD, et al. Alleviation off cocaine-induced coronary vasoconstriction with intravenous verapamil. *Am J Cardiol.* 1994;73:510–513.

62. Rapaport MH. Dietary restrictions and drug interactions with monoamine oxidase inhibitors: the state of the art. *J Clin Psych.* 2007;68:42–46.

63. Aggarwal M, Kahn IA. Hypertensive crisis: hypertensive emergencies and urgencies. *Cardiol Clin.* 2006;24:135–146.

64. Boyer EW, Shannon M. The serotonin syndrome. *N Engl J Med.* 2005;352:1112–1120.

65. Rastogi R, Swarm RA, Patel TA. Case scenario: opioid association with serotonin syndrome: implications to the practitioners. *Anesthesiology.* 2011;115:1291–1298.

66. Hoeks SE, Scholte Op Reimer WJM, van Urk H, et al. Increase of 1-year mortality after perioperative beta-blocker withdrawal in endovascular and vascular surgery patients. *Eur J Vasc Endovasc Surg.* 2007;33:13–19.

67. Shammash JB, Trost JC, Gold JM, et al. Perioperative beta-blocker withdrawal and mortality in vascular surgical patients. *Am Heart J.* 2001;141:148–153.

68. Goldman L. Noncardiac surgery in patients receiving propranolol: case reports and recommended approach. *Arch Intern Med.* 1981;141:193–196.

69. Teichert M, Smet PA, Hofman A, et al. Discontinuation of beta-blockers and the risk of myocardial infarction in the elderly. *Drug Saf.* 2007;30:541–549.

70. Wallace AW, Au S, Cason BA. Association of the pattern of use of perioperative beta-blockade and postoperative mortality. *Anesthesiology.* 2010;112:794–805.

71. Brenner WI, Lieberman AN. Acute clonidine withdrawal syndrome following open heart operation. *Ann Thorac Surg.* 1977;24:80–82.

72. Simic J, Kishineff S, Goldberg R, et al. Acute myocardial infarction as a complication of clonidine withdrawal. *J Emerg Med.* 2003;25:399–402.

53 How Does One Prevent or Treat Atrial Fibrillation in Postoperative Critically Ill Patients?

Jonathan K. Frogel, Stuart J. Weiss

Supraventricular arrhythmias are the most common rhythm disturbance encountered in postsurgical patients.[1] The incidence of postoperative atrial fibrillation may be as high as 50% after cardiac surgery,[2] 40% after pneumonectomy,[3] and 20% after lung resection.[4] In addition, other postsurgical patients have an incidence of new-onset supraventricular arrhythmias approaching 10%.[5]

Patients who have supraventricular arrhythmias after major noncardiac surgery are at increased risk for stroke and have significantly higher early and late mortality.[5] After cardiac surgery, atrial fibrillation may herald a prolonged intensive care unit (ICU) course,[2] increased risk of stroke, and increased risk of early and late mortality.[6] Cost of care in a patient who has postoperative atrial fibrillation is increased by an average of $10,000.[7] Thus the human and economic toll of this disease entity in the postsurgical patient population is substantial.

WHAT ARE THE PATIENT RISK FACTORS AND PERIOPERATIVE CONDITIONS THAT INCREASE THE RISK OF ATRIAL FIBRILLATION?

Multiple risk factors that predispose patients to atrial fibrillation have been identified (Table 53-1).[8-10] Every 10-year increase in age beyond 30 years is associated with a 75% increase in risk after cardiac surgery.[8] Thus the risk for development of atrial fibrillation in octogenarians may be greater than 50%.[9] A history of cardiac disease (atrial fibrillation, hypertension, valvular disease, and cardiomyopathy) and chronic pulmonary disease are significant factors that predispose to all postoperative dysrhythmias. In addition, obesity and increased body mass index have also been shown to be predictors of postoperative atrial fibrillation.[10] Preoperative consideration of these factors can prompt clinicians to alter the perioperative medical and surgical management in hope of mitigating some of this increased risk.

WHAT IS THE PATHOGENESIS OF POSTOPERATIVE ATRIAL FIBRILLATION?

The pathogenesis of atrial fibrillation in the postoperative period is complex and multifactorial. Several disease processes and conditions predispose to atrial enlargement and fibrosis, which provide the substrate for conduction abnormalities.[11] The inflammatory response induced by surgery is associated with increased release of endogenous catecholamines. Elevated levels may be increased further by the administration of exogenous inotropes and vasopressors. These and other factors (Table 53-2) trigger supraventricular arrhythmias by altering atrial refractoriness and conductivity, thereby predisposing to increased automaticity and reentrant rhythms.[12]

The type of surgery performed has a marked impact on the incidence of perioperative atrial fibrillation. In patients undergoing intrathoracic procedures, direct surgical manipulation or compression of the atria and/or pulmonary veins contributes to the pathogenesis.[13] During cardiac surgery, myocardial ischemia and ventricular dysfunction can lead to atrial dilation and elevation of atrial pressures that further contribute to atrial irritability.[13] Although the data in general surgery patients are not as robust as in cardiac surgical patients, minimally invasive laparoscopic techniques may decrease the risk for postoperative atrial fibrillation when compared with open approaches.[13,14] This finding has been taken to imply that attenuation of the inflammatory and stress responses after surgery may decrease the risk of developing postoperative supraventricular arrhythmias, but this hypothesis is not currently supported by data.

WHAT STRATEGIES ARE EFFECTIVE FOR THE PREVENTION OF POSTOPERATIVE ATRIAL FIBRILLATION?

Although atrial fibrillation in postsurgical patients has long been recognized, the implementation of prophylactic

Table 53-1 Comparison of the Risk Factors for Permanent Atrial Fibrillation and Postoperative Atrial Fibrillation

Risk Factor	Permanent	Cardiac	Noncardiac
EPIDEMIOLOGIC			
Advanced age	X	X	X
Male gender	X	X	X
Height	X		
MEDICAL CONDITIONS			
CAD	X		
HTN	X	X	
LAE/LVH	X		
CHF	X	X	X
Cardiomyopathy	X		
Valvular disease	X	X	X
Prior AF	N/A	X	X
Myocarditis	X		
CHD	X		
OLD	X	X	X
OSA	X		
PVD	X	X	X
Obesity	X	X	
DM	X		
Hyperthyroidism	X		
Alcohol	X		

From Mayson SE, Greenspon AJ, Adams S et al. The changing face of postoperative atrial fibrillation prevention: A review of current medical therapy. *Cardiol Rev.* 2007;15:232.

Alcohol, significant alcohol use; *CAD,* coronary artery disease; *Cardiac,* postoperative atrial fibrillation (POAF) after cardiac surgery; *CHF,* congestive heart failure; *CHD,* congenital heart disease; DM, diabetes mellitus; Height, tall stature; *HTN,* hypertension; *LAE/LVH,* left atrial enlargement/left ventricular hypertrophy; *Noncardiac, POAF* after noncardiac surgery; *OLD,* obstructive lung disease; *OSA,* obstructive sleep apnea; *Permanent,* permanent atrial fibrillation; *Prior AF,* history of prior atrial fibrillation; *PVD,* peripheral vascular disease; *X,* risk factor present.

Table 53-2 Stressors of the Perioperative and Intensive Care Periods

Induction and emergence of general anesthesia
Hemodynamic shifts
Surgical trauma
Manipulation of the heart and pulmonary veins
Pain
Electrolyte abnormalities (hypokalemia, hypomagnesemia)
Hypervolemia (distension of the atria)
Subtherapeutic levels of antiarrhythmics (i.e., beta blockers)
Administration of catecholamine inotropes
Pulmonary insufficiency (dyspnea, weaning from ventilator)

ANTIARRHYTHMIC AGENTS

Beta Blockers

Considering the inciting role of increased sympathetic tone in the pathogenesis of atrial fibrillation, it is not surprising that beta-blocker administration for postoperative prevention has been extensively examined. Many studies have confirmed the utility of prophylactic beta blockers to limit the occurrence of postoperative atrial fibrillation. In a meta-analysis of 27 randomized trials published in 2002, Crystal et al. found that beta blockers reduced the risk for development of atrial fibrillation after cardiac surgery by more than 60% (relative risk [RR], 0.39; 95% confidence interval [CI], 0.28 to 0.52).[15] These findings were reaffirmed in a 2004 meta-analysis of 58 trials by the same author.[16] The antiarrhythmic benefit was observed when beta antagonists were started before or immediately after surgery and was independent of the agent or dose used. More recently, a meta-analysis comprising 33 studies and 4698 subjects demonstrated a significant atrial fibrillation risk reduction in cardiac surgical patients receiving perioperative beta blockers.[17] On the basis of this evidence, the most recent American College of Cardiology Foundation (ACCF)/ American Heart Association (AHA) guidelines for patients undergoing coronary artery bypass graft (CABG) surgery recommend that all such patients receive perioperative beta blockers from 24 hours before surgery onward.[18]

In the postgeneral thoracic (noncardiac) surgery patient population, a meta-analysis of two studies totaling 129 subjects demonstrated that perioperative beta blockade significantly reduced the incidence of postoperative atrial tachyarrhythmias (RR, 0.40; 95% CI, 0.17 to 0.95) but also increased the risk for hypotension and pulmonary edema.[19] The calculated protective effect of beta blockers in some of these trials (and by extension in the meta-analysis) may have been overestimated by failure to adequately account for beta blocker withdrawal in the control groups. Of greater concern, more recent data have uncovered potential adverse outcomes associated with perioperative beta blockade. The PeriOperative Ischemia Evaluation (POISE) trial, a large randomized controlled study (8351 patients) in a noncardiac surgical population, found that perioperative beta blockers

strategies to prevent new or recurrent arrhythmias has just recently gained traction. As knowledge of causative factors and the resulting pathophysiology continues to evolve, the pool of potentially beneficial interventions has broadened. Conceptually, prophylactic strategies against atrial fibrillation fall into one of five categories: antiarrhythmic agents, electrolyte repletion or maintenance, atrial pacing, modulation of the inflammatory response to surgery, and alterations of surgical technique. In general, the utility of prophylactic strategies has been most thoroughly evaluated in patients after cardiac surgery. Therefore considerations pertaining to specific risk and pathophysiology in this population must be considered before extrapolating data to the general surgical population.

decreased the incidence of cardiac arrest (3.6% vs. 5.1%) and myocardial infarction (4.2% vs. 5.7%) but increased the risk of perioperative hypotension, bradycardia, stroke (1.0% vs. 0.5%), and all-course mortality.[20] A post hoc analysis suggested that the increased incidence of clinically significant hypotension, bradycardia, and stroke may contribute to the increased risk for death observed in the treatment group. A meta-analysis of 33 randomized controlled trials totaling 12,306 patients confirmed these findings, in particular further documenting the increased risk of bradycardia, hypotension, and nonfatal stroke observed in the experimental group.[21]

The most recent guidelines from the American Association for Thoracic Surgery on the prevention of postoperative atrial fibrillation in patients undergoing noncardiac thoracic surgery recommend continuation of beta blockers in patients already receiving them. They do not, though, recommend initiation of beta blockers in naïve patients.[22] For patients undergoing noncardiac, nonthoracic surgery, the risk of adverse effects of beta blockers would also appear to outweigh any theoretical reduction in the incidence of postoperative atrial fibrillation in beta blocker naïve patients. However, continuation of long-standing beta blocker therapy through the perioperative period is recommended for cardiac, thoracic, and general surgery patients. Initiation of beta blocker therapy for atrial fibrillation prophylaxis should be reserved for patients undergoing surgical coronary revascularization.

Amiodarone

Amiodarone, one of the most commonly used antiarrhythmic agents in the ICU setting, is frequently the antiarrhythmic of choice in patients with obstructive lung disease or cardiomyopathy. The prophylactic use of amiodarone to prevent postoperative atrial fibrillation has been extensively studied. A recent meta-analysis comprising 33 studies and 5402 subjects demonstrated a significant reduction in the risk for postoperative atrial fibrillation in amiodarone-treated patients undergoing cardiac surgery.[17] However, use of amiodarone is not benign; long-term use of this drug has been associated with hepatic, pulmonary, and endocrine toxicity. In addition, amiodarone administration can cause significant bradycardia, heart block, and hypotension. A meta-analysis of 18 trials (3408 patients) performed to assess the safety of amiodarone to prevent atrial fibrillation after cardiac surgery found an increased risk for bradycardia and hypotension in the amiodarone-treated group but no statistically significant differences in any other measured endpoints (heart block, myocardial infarction, stroke, and death).[23] These findings were most apparent in patients treated with high doses (>1 g per day), with intravenous formulations and in those in whom the drug was initiated in the postoperative period.

The most recent American College of Cardiology (ACC)/AHA guidelines ascribe a class IIA recommendation for postcardiac surgery atrial fibrillation prophylaxis with amiodarone,[18] whereas American College of Chest Physicians (ACCP) guidelines recommend consideration of amiodarone prophylaxis for patients in whom beta blockers are contraindicated.[24] There are insufficient data available to recommend amiodarone prophylaxis for patients undergoing noncardiac surgery.

Sotalol

Sotalol is a class III antiarrhythmic agent that has both beta- and potassium channel–blocking activity. A Cochrane database review of 11 studies with 1609 subjects found significant reductions in the incidence of postoperative atrial fibrillation in patients undergoing cardiac surgery who received sotalol in the perioperative period.[17] Despite these findings, potentially dangerous side effects (QT prolongation, torsade de pointes, hypotension, and bradycardia) have limited the use of this agent in the post–cardiac surgical population. These same concerns make the adoption of sotalol for prophylaxis during noncardiac surgery unlikely at this time.

Calcium Channel Blockers and Digoxin

Few data support the use of other antiarrhythmic drugs for atrial fibrillation prophylaxis. Early data regarding the use of nondihydropyridine calcium channel antagonists in preventing postoperative atrial fibrillation were inconclusive, and an early meta-analysis could not demonstrate benefit.[25] However, a more recent meta-analysis suggests that they may be of some use. A review of four studies in patients undergoing general thoracic surgery found that calcium channel blockers were effective in preventing postoperative atrial fibrillation[19] whereas the most recent randomized controlled trial failed to demonstrate efficacy.[26] Currently, neither the ACCP nor the ACC/AHA guidelines recommend calcium channel blockers for the prevention of atrial fibrillation after cardiac surgery.

Digoxin was at one time advocated as effective prophylaxis against postoperative atrial fibrillation. However, the literature does not support its use as detailed in a meta-analysis that could not document that digoxin significantly altered the incidence of postoperative atrial fibrillation after cardiac surgery.[25] In fact, one study noted an increased risk for postoperative atrial fibrillation after thoracic surgery in patients who received digoxin.[19] Although it can be effectively used for rate control of atrial fibrillation, no consensus guidelines recommend the use of digoxin for postoperative atrial fibrillation prophylaxis.

ELECTROLYTE REPLETION AND MAINTENANCE

Magnesium

Electrolyte derangements and membrane instability are postulated to play important roles in the pathogenesis of atrial fibrillation, particularly in the postoperative setting. The importance of the magnesium depletion that typically occurs during cardiopulmonary bypass and after diuretic administration has been studied in patients after cardiac surgery. In a meta-analysis, 16 trials including 2029 patients evaluating the use of prophylactic magnesium were identified. Supraventricular arrhythmias occurred significantly less often in patients treated with magnesium compared with controls (23% vs. 31%).[27] A more recent Cochrane review of 19 studies and 2988 subjects demonstrated similar reductions in patients treated with supplemental magnesium during or after cardiac surgery.[17] It remains unclear whether avoidance of hypomagnesemia or achievement of supernormal magnesium levels was responsible for the observed benefit. Nonetheless, current guidelines of the ACCP recommend maintenance of serum magnesium levels in the normal range after cardiac surgery and suggest that empirical supplementation be considered in this high-risk population.[28]

ATRIAL PACING

Atrial pacing has been proposed as a strategy to decrease the incidence of atrial fibrillation after cardiac surgery. It is theorized that overdrive suppression of supraventricular foci may retard the development of atrial fibrillation in the immediate postsurgical period. Heterogeneity within the literature examining pacing for atrial fibrillation prophylaxis makes interpretation of the data challenging. Nonetheless, several meta-analyses have been published. In a review of 13 prospective randomized controlled trials in which right atrial pacing, left atrial pacing, or biatrial pacing was used, Archbold and Schilling found that the most significant reduction in postoperative atrial fibrillation occurred in patients receiving biatrial pacing (RR, 0.46; 95% CI, 0.30 to 0.71).[29] Pacing protocols varied but usually were set 10 to 20 beats above the intrinsic rate for a period ranging from 1 to 5 days. Atrial pacing after cardiac surgery appears to be efficacious in preserving sinus rhythm, but identification of the optimal site and pacing algorithm is limited by the lack of large, well-controlled studies.

Although potentially advantageous, this strategy has not been explored in the non–cardiac surgery population. Pacing is limited to patients with implanted pacemakers and those with transvenous or temporary epicardial pacing wires placed after cardiac surgery.

MODULATION OF THE INFLAMMATORY RESPONSE TO SURGERY

Given the role that the inflammatory response seems to play in the pathogenesis of postoperative atrial fibrillation, various interventions targeting this response have been used in efforts to reduce risk.

Corticosteroids

A meta-analysis of 50 randomized controlled trials of prophylactic steroid administration for patients undergoing cardiac surgery demonstrated a significant reduction in postoperative atrial fibrillation in patients receiving steroids (25.1% vs. 35.1% incidence).[30] Conversely, the Dexamethasone in Cardiac Surgery (DECS) study, a large, multicenter, randomized controlled trial of dexamethasone versus placebo, failed to demonstrate a similar response in patients receiving 1 mg/kg of dexamethasone.[31] The Steroids In caRdiac Surgery (SIRS) trial currently underway across 82 centers in 18 countries may help clarify the risks and benefits of methylprednisolone administration for cardiac surgical patients.[32] Given the potential risks of routine administration of corticosteroids (hyperglycemia, increased risk of infection), they are not currently recommended for postoperative atrial fibrillation prophylaxis.

Statins

In addition to their effects on lipid profiles, statins have known anti-inflammatory effects that are thought to contribute to the observed reduction in new-onset atrial fibrillation. A meta-analysis of 3 randomized controlled trials and 16 observational studies comprising 31,725 patients found that the incidence of postoperative atrial fibrillation after cardiac surgery was significantly reduced by statins (odds ratio [OR], 0.67; 95% CI, 0.51 to 0.88).[33] Interestingly, a meta-analysis examining data on patients undergoing either isolated CABG or isolated aortic valve replacement (AVR) demonstrated a reduction in atrial fibrillation in the CABG group but not in the AVR group.[34] Current ACCF/AHA recommendations call for perioperative statins in all patients with CABG regardless of baseline lipid profile.[18] Evidence is currently lacking to recommend statins for atrial fibrillation prophylaxis for patients undergoing non-CABG surgery.

Epidural Analgesia

Epidural analgesia modulates the sympathetic nervous system and the inflammatory response to surgery. There is some evidence that use of epidural analgesia in patients undergoing noncardiac surgery under general anesthesia reduces the risk of postoperative atrial fibrillation. For example, a meta-analysis of 9 studies and 2016 subjects demonstrated a statistically significant reduction in the incidence of atrial fibrillation in patients receiving epidural analgesia for noncardiac surgery when compared with controls (20.1% vs. 25.4%).[35] Although these limited data are of interest, more robust evidence is required before recommending perioperative epidural analgesia for routine prophylaxis of atrial fibrillation before general or thoracic surgery.

Colchicine

Colchicine is a powerful anti-inflammatory drug that inhibits neutrophil activity. The COPPS-1 (COlchicine for Prevention of Postcardiotomy Syndrome) trial demonstrated a significant reduction in postoperative atrial fibrillation in patients receiving the drug 3 days after undergoing cardiac surgery.[36] Because of study design, efficacy in preventing early-onset (postoperative days 1 to 2) atrial fibrillation was not demonstrated. The recently published COPPS-2 trial failed to show a statistically significant reduction in early postoperative atrial fibrillation in patients receiving colchicine but demonstrated an increased risk of gastrointestinal complications of the drug.[37] Although current AHA/ACC/Heart Rhythm Society (HRS) guidelines ascribe a class IIb recommendation for the use of colchicine for atrial fibrillation prophylaxis in cardiac surgical patients,[24] the COPPS-2 data suggest that colchicine should not be used for this indication.

WHAT IS APPROPRIATE THERAPY FOR POSTOPERATIVE ATRIAL FIBRILLATION IN A HEMODYNAMICALLY STABLE PATIENT: RATE CONTROL OR RHYTHM CONTROL?

The initial approach to the development of postoperative atrial fibrillation in the patient who is not hemodynamically compromised is to control the ventricular response rate. After this has been accomplished, electrical or pharmacologic cardioversion can be attempted. Early restoration of sinus rhythm theoretically avoids the need for anticoagulation, improves quality of life, decreases the risk for thromboembolic events, improves hemodynamics, and decreases the incidence of future episodes of atrial fibrillation. However, regardless of how intuitively attractive the concept, the data supporting the advantages of chronic rhythm control over rate control in the outpatient population have failed to demonstrate the superiority of rhythm control. No studies have shown definitively that rhythm control is superior to rate control or vice versa for the primary outcome measure of mortality in outpatients. These conclusions are based on several large randomized controlled trials.

The Atrial Fibrillation Follow-up Investigation of Rhythm Management (AFFIRM) trial was the largest of these studies, enrolling 4060 patients. The mean follow-up in the study was 3.5 years, and no significant mortality difference between the rate control and rhythm control groups was found.[40] However, there was a slightly higher incidence of noncardiovascular death, stroke (7.3% vs. 5.7%), and hospitalization (80% vs. 73%) in the rhythm control group. Other smaller studies were initially interpreted to exhibit similar findings. The strategy of rhythm control offered no overall mortality benefit and may have contributed to an increased incidence of noncardiac death.

Reevaluation of the data from the rate versus rhythm trials suggests that remaining in sinus rhythm may confer several advantages. These include improved hemodynamics, reduction of thromboembolic events, lower mortality, improved quality of life, and improved exercise tolerance.[41,42] A good discussion supporting the early restoration and maintenance of sinus rhythm was presented by van Gelder and Hemels.[43] A post hoc analysis of the AFFIRM trial, Congestive Heart Failure Survival Trial of Antiarrhythmic Therapy (CHF-STA) trial, and Danish Investigators of Arrhythmia and Mortality on Dofetilide (DIAMOND) trial concluded that restoration of sinus rhythm is a marker for improved survival.[40,44,45] The largest multicenter randomized study of 4060 patients found sinus rhythm to be a predictor of survival, with a 47% reduction in mortality.

The premise that maintenance of sinus rhythm improves outcome remains controversial and awaits further clarification. In addition, a multimodal approach with wider application of angiotensin-receptor blockers (ARBs), angiotensin-converting enzyme (ACE) inhibitors, and statins may potentially affect success in restoring and maintaining sinus rhythm.

Postoperative atrial fibrillation should be considered an entity distinct from chronic atrial fibrillation. More than 90% of patients who develop post-CABG atrial fibrillation revert to sinus rhythm within 6 to 8 weeks.[46] Although not demonstrated in the noncardiac surgical patient population, cardioversion to sinus rhythm after the stressors of the

Table 53-3 Common Medication Dosage for Rate Control of AF

	Intravenous Administration	Usual Oral Maintenance Dose
BETA BLOCKERS		
Metoprolol tartrate	2.5-5.0 mg IV bolus over 2 min; up to 3 doses	25-100 mg BID
Metoprolol XL (succinate)	N/A	50-400 mg QD
Atenolol	N/A	25-100 mg QD
Esmolol	500 µg/kg IV bolus over 1 min, then 50-300 µg/kg/min IV	N/A
Propranolol	1 mg IV over 1 min, up to 3 doses at 2-min intervals	10-40 mg TID or QID
Nadolol	N/A	10-240 mg QD
Carvedilol	N/A	3.125-25 mg BID
Bisoprolol	N/A	2.5-10 mg QD
NONDIHYDROPYRIDINE CALCIUM CHANNEL ANTAGONISTS		
Verapamil	0.075-0.15 mg/kg IV bolus over 2 min; may give an additional 10.0 mg after 30 min if no response, then 0.005-mg/kg/min infusion	180-480 mg QD (ER)
Diltiazem	0.25 mg/kg IV bolus over 2 min, then 5-15 mg/hr	120-360 mg QD (ER)
DIGITALIS GLYCOSIDES		
Digoxin	0.25 mg IV with repeat dosing to a maximum of 1.5 mg over 24 hr	0.125-0.25 mg QD
OTHERS		
Amiodarone*	300 mg IV over 1 hr, then 10-50 mg/hr over 24 hr	100-200 mg QD

From 2014 AHA/ACC/HRS Guideline for Management of Patients with Atrial Fibrillation. *J Am Coll Cardiol.* 2014;64(21):e1–e76.
*Multiple dosing schemes exist for the use of amiodarone.
AF, atrial fibrillation; *BID,* twice daily; *ER,* extended release; *IV,* intravenous; *N/A,* not applicable; *QD,* once daily; *QID,* 4 times a day; *TID,* 3 times a day.

postoperative period have abetted seems to be a reasonable but as yet unproven strategy.

Rate Control

Beta blockers, with their ability to modulate the hyperadrenergic tone encountered in the postoperative patient, are considered first-line agents for rate control in the ACC/AHA guidelines section on postoperative atrial fibrillation[24] and the ACCP guidelines on the management of postoperative atrial fibrillation after cardiac surgery (Table 53-3).[28] The non-dihydropyridine calcium channel blockers are recommended as second-line agents.

Rhythm Control

Despite the self-limited nature of most cases of postoperative atrial fibrillation, the current ACC/AHA guidelines ascribe a class IIa recommendation for pharmacologic or electrical cardioversion in this patient population. The ACCP guidelines recommend the use of amiodarone, particularly for patients with depressed left ventricular function. Antiarrhythmic use for postoperative atrial fibrillation should be continued for 4 to 6 weeks after surgery.[47]

ANTICOAGULATION STRATEGY BEFORE RESTORATION OF SINUS RHYTHM: ATRIAL FIBRILLATION FOR LESS THAN 48 HOURS

It is common practice for patients with new onset of atrial fibrillation of less than 48 hours' duration to proceed to cardioversion without transesophageal echocardiography or anticoagulation. There is evidence in the literature that new-onset atrial fibrillation (duration <48 hours) may be associated with an incidence of left atrial thrombus formation of up to 4%.[48] Prospective data after cardioversion of 3143 patients found a 0.7% incidence of thromboembolic complications during a 30-day follow-up period but a significantly higher incidence in patients with increased stroke risk factors.[50] Since 2010, the European Society of Cardiology (ESC) has recommended consideration of anticoagulation with unfractionated or low-molecular-weight heparin for all patients with new-onset atrial fibrillation undergoing cardioversion.[51] In addition, the ESC recommends lifelong anticoagulation after cardioversion of new-onset atrial fibrillation for patients at high risk for stroke as assessed by the CHADS$_2$ (Congestive heart failure, Hypertension, Age ≥75 years, Diabetes mellitus, Prior Stroke or TIA or Thromboembolism [doubled]) and CHA$_2$DS$_2$-VASc (Congestive heart failure, Hypertension, Age ≥75 years, Diabetes mellitus, Prior Stroke or TIA or Thromboembolism [doubled], Vascular disease, Age 65 to 74 years, Sex thromboembolic) Risk Stratification Scoring Systems (Table 53-4).[51]

Although these recommendations were based on studies of nonsurgical patients, the guidelines have been applied to the postsurgical patients as the inflammatory response to surgery induces a hypercoagulable state that may increase the risk for an early thromboembolic event. Therefore it may be prudent to selectively anticoagulate before cardioversion of high-risk patients with atrial fibrillation of less than 48 hours' duration. However, it is clear that in the postoperative setting, the risk of thrombotic events in the absence of anticoagulation must be weighed against the risk of bleeding from fresh surgical sites after anticoagulation administration.

ANTICOAGULATION STRATEGY BEFORE RESTORATION OF SINUS RHYTHM: ATRIAL FIBRILLATION FOR MORE THAN 48 HOURS

At times, patients enter the ICU with atrial fibrillation for more than 48 hours. In these individuals, anticoagulation before cardioversion is the accepted standard. ACC/AHA

Table 53-4 Comparison of the CHADS$_2$ and CHA$_2$DS$_2$-VASc Risk Stratification Scores for Subjects with Nonvalvular AF

DEFINITION AND SCORES FOR CHADS$_2$ AND CHA$_2$DS$_2$-VASc		STROKE RISK STRATIFICATION WITH THE CHADS$_2$ AND CHA$_2$DS$_2$-VASc SCORES	
Score		Adjusted Stroke Rate (%/yr)	
CHADS$_2$ acronym		*CHADS$_2$ acronym**	
Congestive HF	1	0	1.9
Hypertension	1	1	2.8
Age ≥75 yr	1	2	4.0
Diabetes mellitus	1	3	5.9
Stroke/TIA/TE	2	4	8.5
Maximum score	6	5	12.5
		6	18.2
CHA$_2$DS$_2$-VASc acronym		*CHA$_2$DS$_2$-VASc acronym*†	
Congestive HF	1	0	0
Hypertension	1	1	1.3
Age ≥75 yr	2	2	2.2
Diabetes mellitus	1	3	3.2
Stroke/TIA/TE	2	4	4.0
Vascular disease (prior MI, PAD, or aortic plaque)	1	5	6.7
Age 65-74 yr	1	6	9.8
Sex category (i.e., female sex)	1	7	9.6
Maximum score	9	8	6.7
		9	15.20

From 2014 AHA/ACC/HRS Guideline for management of patients with atrial fibrillation. *J Am Coll Cardiol.* 2014; 64(21):e1–e76.[24]

*These adjusted-stroke rates are based on data for hospitalized patients with AF and were published by Shepard and colleagues in 2001. Because stroke rates are decreasing, actual stroke rates in contemporary, nonhospitalized cohorts might vary from these estimates.

†Adjusted-stroke rate scores are based on data from Lip and colleagues. Actual rates of stroke in contemporary cohorts might vary from these estimates.

AF, atrial fibrillation; *CHADS$_2$,* Congestive heart failure, Hypertension, Age ≥75 years, Diabetes mellitus, Prior Stroke or TIA or Thromboembolism (doubled); *CHA$_2$DS$_2$-VASc,* Congestive heart failure, Hypertension, Age ≥75 years, Diabetes mellitus, Prior Stroke or TIA or Thromboembolism (doubled), Vascular disease, Age 65 to 74 years, Sex thromboembolic; *HF,* heart failure; *MI,* myocardial infarction; *PAD,* peripheral artery disease; *TE,* thromboembolism; *TIA,* transient ischemic attack.

and ACCP guidelines recommend 3 weeks of anticoagulation before cardioversion of patients with chronic atrial fibrillation.[24,40] However, in cases of hemodynamic instability, cardioversion should not be delayed for initiation of anticoagulation. Timing for initiation of anticoagulation therapy (heparin as a bridge to an oral agent) in the postoperative patient must account for the potential for bleeding complications.

Selection of an antithrombotic regimen must balance the risks of harm and potential benefit of avoiding ischemic stroke or other embolic complications. Platelet inhibitors, alone or in combination (aspirin and clopidodrel), are less effective than warfarin in preventing strokes.[12] Administration of a direct thrombin inhibitor (dabigatran) or factor Xa inhibitors (rivaroxaban apixaban) are gaining wider use for in-hospital and outpatient settings. Although these agents are more convenient, they are more costly and difficult to reverse in cases of bleeding or if the need to perform emergency invasive procedures arises. Data from a European observational study found that a greater international normalized ratio (INR) produced better outcomes. The incidence of thromboembolic events was 0.8% (4 of 530 patients) when the INR was 2.0 to 2.4 compared with no events when the INR was 2.5 or greater.[52] In addition, reversal of warfarin anticoagulation has the benefit of being dependably achieved by the administration of vitamin K or fresh frozen plasma. It is the opinion of these authors that the newer agents are not superior to warfarin for stroke prevention and may pose a significantly higher risk to the postsurgical patient population.

SHOULD ANTICOAGULATION BE INSTITUTED OR CONTINUED AFTER ELECTRICAL CARDIOVERSION TO SINUS RHYTHM?

The period after conversion to sinus rhythm is associated with an increased risk of thrombus formation and subsequent embolization. The recurrence of asymptomatic atrial fibrillation ranges from 40% to 60%,[41,55] and other predisposing factors such as atheromatous disease and poor ventricular function also may increase the risk for thromboembolism.[56] Perhaps the most significant factor is the transient decrease in atrial mechanical function that occurs after cardioversion to sinus rhythm.[57] Mechanical dysfunction after cardioversion appears to last 24 hours in patients having atrial fibrillation of less than 2 weeks' duration, 1 week in patients with atrial fibrillation of 2 to 6 weeks' duration, and 1 month for more prolonged precardioversion atrial fibrillation.[57] To date, there is no pharmacologic intervention to hasten the return of atrial mechanical activity.

Support for continued anticoagulation can be gleaned from the AFFIRM and RACE (Rate Control versus Electrical Cardioversion) trials.[43,58] Anticoagulation during these studies was often discontinued after restoration of sinus rhythm. Ischemic events occurred at equal frequency in both arms of the trials (rate control and rhythm control). Review of the data showed that such complications occurred most often after anticoagulation was terminated (rhythm control group) or when the INR was subtherapeutic (rate control group). Although the patients in these studies had chronic (not postoperative) atrial fibrillation, restoration of sinus rhythm in subtherapeutic or nonanticoagulated patients was associated with the increased incidence of thromboembolic events. Furthermore, the literature that provides the basis for these recommendations in general does not distinguish between patients who required electric cardioversion and those who spontaneously or pharmacologically converted to sinus rhythm. It seems prudent that guidelines for electrical and pharmacologic cardioversion be followed in a similar manner.

Current guidelines of the ACCP recommend 4 weeks of anticoagulation for patients who undergo cardioversion after an episode of atrial fibrillation lasting more than 48 hours. For episodes less than 48 hours in duration, the ACCP guidelines do not recommend postcardioversion anticoagulation.[59] The ESC and ACC/AHA guidelines add that the decision to initiate postcardioversion anticoagulation for patients with atrial fibrillation of less than 48 hours' duration should be based on the patients' risk for development of thromboembolism.[51] Although neither the ACCP nor ACC/AHA guidelines specifically address postcardioversion anticoagulation for postoperative atrial fibrillation, it seems prudent to follow these recommendations, provided that the risk for bleeding does not outweigh the risk for a thromboembolic event.

AUTHORS' RECOMMENDATIONS

- The pathogenesis of atrial fibrillation in the postoperative period is complex and multifactorial. The inflammatory response and increased levels of circulating catecholamines induced by surgery trigger supraventricular arrhythmias by altering atrial refractoriness and conductivity, predisposing to automaticity and re-entrant rhythms.
- The type of surgery performed has a significant impact on the incidence of perioperative atrial fibrillation. Direct surgical manipulation or compression of the atria or pulmonary veins is associated with postoperative atrial fibrillation.
- Prophylactic strategies against atrial fibrillation include maintenance of electrolytes (magnesium), atrial pacing, and administration of antiarrhythmic agents (beta blockers). Other strategies that include a role for anti-inflammatory agents have been proposed and are under active investigation.
- β-Adrenergic antagonists and alternative agents (such as amiodarone) are recommended for prophylaxis against atrial fibrillation by the ACC/AHA guidelines. Patients taking beta blockers on an outpatient basis should continue receiving them during the perioperative period. However, the prophylactic use of such agents in patients with low cardiac risk is controversial.
- Postoperative atrial fibrillation associated with hemodynamic instability should be treated with biphasic cardioversion at 200 J.
- Postoperative atrial fibrillation is often an acute event with a high conversion rate to sinus rhythm. The premise that maintenance of sinus rhythm improves outcome remains controversial. Rate and rhythm control are acceptable approaches to treating chronic atrial fibrillation.
- Patients with new onset of atrial fibrillation of longer than 48 hours' duration are at increased risk for thromboembolic events and should receive anticoagulant therapy. Anticoagulation should be temporarily continued after restoration of sinus rhythm because of a transient decrease in atrial mechanical function that increases the risk for thromboembolic events. Potential benefits of anticoagulation must be weighed against the risks for postoperative bleeding.
- After cardioversion, anticoagulation may be considered for patients at high risk for stroke. The decision to initiate anticoagulation in this setting should balance the risk of thromboembolic event with that of bleeding complications in postsurgical patients.

REFERENCES

1. Seguin P, Signouret T, Laviolle B, Branger B, Malledant Y. Incidence and risk factors of atrial fibrillation in a surgical intensive care unit. *Crit Care Med.* 2004;32(3):722–726.
2. Creswell LL, Schuessler RB, Rosenbloom M, Cox JL. Hazards of postoperative atrial arrhythmias. *Ann Thorac Surg.* 1993;56(3):539–549.
3. Harpole DH, Liptay MJ, DeCamp Jr MM, Mentzer SJ, Swanson SJ, Sugarbaker DJ. Prospective analysis of pneumonectomy: risk factors for major morbidity and cardiac dysrhythmias. *Ann Thorac Surg.* 1996;61(3):977–982.
4. Roselli EE, Murthy SC, Rice TW, et al. Atrial fibrillation complicating lung cancer resection. *J Thorac Cardiovasc Surg.* 2005;130(2):438–444.
5. Brathwaite D, Weissman C. The new onset of atrial arrhythmias following major noncardiothoracic surgery is associated with increased mortality. *Chest.* 1998;114(2):462–468.
6. Mariscalco G, Klersy C, Zanobini M, et al. Atrial fibrillation after isolated coronary surgery affects late survival. *Circulation.* 2008;118(16):1612–1618.
7. Villareal RP, Hariharan R, Liu BC, et al. Postoperative atrial fibrillation and mortality after coronary artery bypass surgery. *J Am Coll Cardiol.* 2004;43(5):742–748.
8. Mathew JP, Fontes ML, Tudor IC, et al. A multicenter risk index for atrial fibrillation after cardiac surgery. *JAMA.* 2004;291(14):1720–1729.
9. Aranki SF, Shaw DP, Adams DH, et al. Predictors of atrial fibrillation after coronary artery surgery. Current trends and impact on hospital resources. *Circulation.* 1996;94(3):390–397.
10. Zacharias A, Schwann TA, Riordan CJ, Durham SJ, Shah AS, Habib RH. Obesity and risk of new-onset atrial fibrillation after cardiac surgery. *Circulation.* 2005;112(21):3247–3255.
11. Fuster V, Ryden LE, Cannom DS, Heart Rhythm Association and the Heart Rhythm Society, et al. ACC/AHA/ESC 2006 guidelines for the management of patients with atrial fibrillation: a report of the American College of Cardiology/American Heart Association Task Force on Practice Guidelines and the European Society of Cardiology Committee for Practice Guidelines (Writing Committee to Revise the 2001 Guidelines for the Management of Patients With Atrial Fibrillation). *Circulation.* 2006;114(7):e257–354.
12. Hogue Jr CW, Creswell LL, Gutterman DD, Fleisher LA, American College of Chest Physicians. Epidemiology, mechanisms, and risks: American College of Chest Physicians guidelines for the prevention and management of postoperative atrial fibrillation after cardiac surgery. *Chest.* 2005;128(suppl 2):9S–16S.
13. Siu CW, Tung HM, Chu KW, Jim MH, Lau CP, Tse HF. Prevalence and predictors of new-onset atrial fibrillation after elective surgery for colorectal cancer. *Pacing Clin Electrophysiol.* 2005;28(suppl 1):S120–S123.
14. Friscia ME, Zhu J, Kolff JW, et al. Cytokine response is lower after lung volume reduction through bilateral thoracoscopy versus sternotomy. *Ann Thorac Surg.* 2007;83(1):252–256.
15. Crystal E, Connolly SJ, Sleik K, Ginger TJ, Yusuf S. Interventions on prevention of postoperative atrial fibrillation in patients undergoing heart surgery: a meta-analysis. *Circulation.* 2002;106(1):75–80.
16. Crystal E, Garfinkle MS, Connolly SS, Ginger TT, Sleik K, Yusuf SS. Interventions for preventing post-operative atrial fibrillation in patients undergoing heart surgery. *Cochrane Database Syst Rev.* 2004;(4):CD003611.
17. Arsenault KA, Yusuf AM, Crystal E, et al. Interventions for preventing post-operative atrial fibrillation in patients undergoing heart surgery. *Cochrane Database Syst Rev.* 2013;1:CD003611.
18. Hillis LD, Smith PK, Anderson JL, et al. 2011 ACCF/AHA Guideline for Coronary Artery Bypass Graft Surgery: executive summary: a report of the American College of Cardiology Foundation/American Heart Association Task Force on Practice Guidelines. *Circulation.* 2011;124(23):2610–2642.
19. Sedrakyan A, Treasure T, Browne J, Krumholz H, Sharpin C, van der Meulen J. Pharmacologic prophylaxis for postoperative atrial tachyarrhythmia in general thoracic surgery: evidence from randomized clinical trials. *J Thorac Cardiovasc Surg.* 2005;129(5):997–1005.
20. Group PS, Devereaux PJ, Yang H, et al. Effects of extended-release metoprolol succinate in patients undergoing non-cardiac surgery (POISE trial): a randomised controlled trial. *Lancet.* 2008;371(9627):1839–1847.
21. Bangalore S, Wetterslev J, Pranesh S, Sawhney S, Gluud C, Messerli FH. Perioperative beta blockers in patients having non-cardiac surgery: a meta-analysis. *Lancet.* 2008;372(9654):1962–1976.
22. Frendl G, Sodickson AC, Chung MK, et al. 2014 AATS guidelines for the prevention and management of perioperative atrial fibrillation and flutter for thoracic surgical procedures. Executive summary. *J Thorac Cardiovasc Surg.* 2014;148(3):772–791.
23. Patel AA, White CM, Gillespie EL, Kluger J, Coleman CI. Safety of amiodarone in the prevention of postoperative atrial fibrillation: a meta-analysis. *Am J Health Syst Pharm.* 2006;63(9):829–837.
24. January CT, Wann LS, Alpert JS, et al. 2014 AHA/ACC/HRS guideline for the management of patients with atrial fibrillation: a report of the American College of Cardiology/American Heart Association Task Force on practice guidelines and the Heart Rhythm Society. *J Am Coll Cardiol.* 2014;64(21):e1–e76.
25. Andrews TC, Reimold SC, Berlin JA, Antman EM. Prevention of supraventricular arrhythmias after coronary artery bypass surgery. A meta-analysis of randomized control trials. *Circulation.* 1991;84(suppl 5):III236–244.
26. Ciszewski P, Tyczka J, Nadolski J, Roszak M, Dyszkiewicz W. Comparative efficacy and usefulness of acebutolol and diltiazem for the prevention of atrial fibrillation during perioperative time in patients undergoing pulmonary resection. *Thorac Cardiovasc Surg.* 2013;61(4):365–372.
27. Shiga T, Wajima Z, Inoue T, Ogawa R. Magnesium prophylaxis for arrhythmias after cardiac surgery: a meta-analysis of randomized controlled trials. *Am J Med.* 2004;117(5):325–333.
28. Martinez EA, Epstein AE, Bass EB, American College of Chest Physicians. Pharmacologic control of ventricular rate: American College of Chest Physicians guidelines for the prevention and management of postoperative atrial fibrillation after cardiac surgery. *Chest.* 2005;128(suppl 2):56S–60S.
29. Archbold RA, Schilling RJ. Atrial pacing for the prevention of atrial fibrillation after coronary artery bypass graft surgery: a review of the literature. *Heart.* 2004;90(2):129–133.
30. Ho KM, Tan JA. Benefits and risks of corticosteroid prophylaxis in adult cardiac surgery: a dose-response meta-analysis. *Circulation.* 2009;119(14):1853–1866.
31. Dieleman JM, Nierich AP, Rosseel PM, et al. Intraoperative high-dose dexamethasone for cardiac surgery: a randomized controlled trial. *JAMA.* 2012;308(17):1761–1767.
32. Whitlock R, Teoh K, Vincent J, et al. Rationale and design of the steroids in cardiac surgery trial. *Am Heart J.* 2014;167(5):660–665.
33. Liakopoulos OJ, Choi YH, Haldenwang PL, et al. Impact of preoperative statin therapy on adverse postoperative outcomes in patients undergoing cardiac surgery: a meta-analysis of over 30,000 patients. *Eur Heart J.* 2008;29(12):1548–1559.
34. Kuhn EW, Liakopoulos OJ, Stange S, et al. Meta-analysis of patients taking statins before revascularization and aortic valve surgery. *Ann Thorac Surg.* 2013;96(4):1508–1516.
35. Popping DM, Elia N, Van Aken HK, et al. Impact of epidural analgesia on mortality and morbidity after surgery: systematic review and meta-analysis of randomized controlled trials. *Ann Surg.* 2014;259(6):1056–1067.
36. Imazio M, Brucato A, Ferrazzi P, et al. Colchicine reduces postoperative atrial fibrillation: results of the Colchicine for the Prevention of the Postpericardiotomy Syndrome (COPPS) atrial fibrillation substudy. *Circulation.* 2011;124(21):2290–2295.
37. Imazio M, Brucato A, Ferrazzi P, et al. Colchicine for prevention of postpericardiotomy syndrome and postoperative atrial fibrillation: the COPPS-2 randomized clinical trial. *JAMA.* 2014;312(10):1016–1023.
38. Deleted in review.
39. Deleted in review.
40. Corley SD, Epstein AE, DiMarco JP, et al. Relationships between sinus rhythm, treatment, and survival in the Atrial Fibrillation Follow-Up Investigation of Rhythm Management (AFFIRM) Study. *Circulation.* 2004;109(12):1509–1513.
41. Singh SN, Tang XC, Singh BN, et al. Quality of life and exercise performance in patients in sinus rhythm versus persistent atrial fibrillation: a Veterans Affairs Cooperative Studies Program Substudy. *J Am Coll Cardiol.* 2006;48(4):721–730.
42. Chung MK, Shemanski L, Sherman DG, et al. Functional status in rate- versus rhythm-control strategies for atrial fibrillation: results of the Atrial Fibrillation Follow-Up Investigation of Rhythm Management (AFFIRM) Functional Status Substudy. *J Am Coll Cardiol.* 2005;46(10):1891–1899.

43. Van Gelder IC, Hemels ME. The progressive nature of atrial fibrillation: a rationale for early restoration and maintenance of sinus rhythm. *Europace*. 2006;8(11):943–949.

44. Deedwania PC, Singh BN, Ellenbogen K, Fisher S, Fletcher R, Singh SN. Spontaneous conversion and maintenance of sinus rhythm by amiodarone in patients with heart failure and atrial fibrillation: observations from the veterans affairs congestive heart failure survival trial of antiarrhythmic therapy (CHF-STAT). The Department of Veterans Affairs CHF-STAT Investigators. *Circulation*. 1998;98(23):2574–2579.

45. Pedersen OD, Bagger H, Keller N, Marchant B, Kober L, Torp-Pedersen C. Efficacy of dofetilide in the treatment of atrial fibrillation-flutter in patients with reduced left ventricular function: a Danish investigations of arrhythmia and mortality on dofetilide (diamond) substudy. *Circulation*. 2001;104(3):292–296.

46. Kowey PR, Stebbins D, Igidbashian L, et al. Clinical outcome of patients who develop PAF after CABG surgery. *Pacing Clin Electrophysiol*. 2001;24(2):191–193.

47. Martinez EA, Bass EB, Zimetbaum P, American College of Chest Physicians. Pharmacologic control of rhythm: American College of Chest Physicians guidelines for the prevention and management of postoperative atrial fibrillation after cardiac surgery. *Chest*. 2005;128(suppl 2):48S–55S.

48. Kleemann T, Becker T, Strauss M, Schneider S, Seidl K. Prevalence of left atrial thrombus and dense spontaneous echo contrast in patients with short-term atrial fibrillation <48 hours undergoing cardioversion: value of transesophageal echocardiography to guide cardioversion. *J Am Soc Echocardiogr*. 2009;22(12):1403–1408.

49. Deleted in review.

50. Airaksinen KE, Gronberg T, Nuotio I, et al. Thromboembolic complications after cardioversion of acute atrial fibrillation: the FinCV (Finnish CardioVersion) study. *J Am Coll Cardiol*. 2013;62(13):1187–1192.

51. European Heart Rhythm Association, European Association for Cardio-Thoracic Surgery, Camm AJ, et al. Guidelines for the management of atrial fibrillation: the Task Force for the Management of Atrial Fibrillation of the European Society of Cardiology (ESC). *Eur Heart J*. 2010;31(19):2369–2429.

52. Gallagher MM, Hennessy BJ, Edvardsson N, et al. Embolic complications of direct current cardioversion of atrial arrhythmias: association with low intensity of anticoagulation at the time of cardioversion. *J Am Coll Cardiol*. 2002;40(5):926–933.

53. Deleted in review.

54. Deleted in review.

55. Antonielli E, Pizzuti A, Palinkas A, et al. Clinical value of left atrial appendage flow for prediction of long-term sinus rhythm maintenance in patients with nonvalvular atrial fibrillation. *J Am Coll Cardiol*. 2002;39(9):1443–1449.

56. Echocardiographic predictors of stroke in patients with atrial fibrillation: a prospective study of 1066 patients from 3 clinical trials. *Arch Intern Med*. 1998;158(12):1316–1320.

57. Manning WJ, Silverman DI, Katz SE, et al. Impaired left atrial mechanical function after cardioversion: relation to the duration of atrial fibrillation. *J Am Coll Cardiol*. 1994;23(7):1535–1540.

58. Wyse DG, Waldo AL, DiMarco JP, et al. A comparison of rate control and rhythm control in patients with atrial fibrillation. *N Engl J Med*. 2002;347(23):1825–1833.

59. Singer DE, Albers GW, Dalen JE, et al. Antithrombotic therapy in atrial fibrillation: American College of Chest Physicians Evidence-Based Clinical Practice Guidelines (8th edition). *Chest*. 2008;133(suppl 6):546S–592S.

54 Is Right Ventricular Failure Common in the Intensive Care Unit? How Should It Be Managed?

Evin Yucel, Steven M. Hollenberg

In 1616, William Harvey described the relationship of the right ventricle (RV) to the pulmonary circulation.[1] For many years after that, this cardiac chamber has been underappreciated. Indeed, in 1943, after demonstrating that ablation of the RV free wall in dogs had little effect on central venous pressure (CVP), Starr concluded that the RV was merely a passive conduit.[2]

In 1974, the RV's importance reemerged when Cohn and colleagues[3] noticed that RV myocardial infarction (MI) was common and difficult to manage. We now appreciate that RV involvement in inferior MI increases mortality eightfold,[4] and RV dysfunction in acute pulmonary embolism (PE) is a predictor of mortality.[5]

RV failure is defined as the inability of that chamber to provide adequate blood flow through the pulmonary circulation at a normal CVP. Right ventricular failure is common and coexists with a broad range of critical illnesses, including respiratory failure, sepsis, PE, and right ventricular MI. Nonetheless, the RV still remains poorly studied when compared with the left ventricle (LV). Cardiologists focus on the LV, pulmonologists tend to concentrate on the causes and treatment of pulmonary arterial hypertension (PAH), and both neglect the RV. In fact, the RV is barely mentioned in American College of Cardiology (ACC)/American Heart Association (AHA) practice guidelines, and no guidance is provided for management of RV dysfunction.[6]

The heterogeneity of illnesses and varying degrees of disease severity make randomized controlled trials difficult to conduct in the critically ill patient with RV dysfunction. Most intensive care unit (ICU) therapies are instituted on the basis of pathophysiologic considerations and extrapolation from trials in other settings. Because of these difficulties, this review begins with brief consideration of normal and abnormal RV function.

PHYSIOLOGY

The physiology of the RV differs dramatically from that of the LV. The RV is not simply a weak LV. The RV wall is 3 to 4 times thinner than the normal LV wall. RV contraction moves from the apex to its outflow tract in a peristaltic-like motion. The normal RV generates one sixth of the work of the LV while moving the same volume of blood. The easily distensible RV pumps blood into the low-pressure pulmonary circuit, allowing the chamber to accommodate dramatic variations in venous return while maintaining constant cardiac output. Global function of the RV depends on contributions from the interventricular septum and the RV free wall.[7]

PATHOPHYSIOLOGY

The RV first responds to increased afterload by increasing contractility and later by dilating according to the Frank-Starling mechanism. Guyton[8] showed that, with progressive constriction of the pulmonary artery, generated RV pressure increases until the RV can no longer compensate, at which point systemic pressure (SP) and cardiac output fall (see Fig. 54-1). As RV SP increases, ischemia may ensue.

When RV failure occurs, either due to excessive contractile demand or impaired contractile function, CVP will increase. RV dilation ultimately occurs. Eventually, as increased wall stress impairs contraction and impinges on the LV through the interventricular septum, the process becomes maladaptive (Fig. 54-2).

DIAGNOSIS

No one sign, symptom, or laboratory test perfectly identifies RV failure. However, RV failure is not present if the jugular venous pressure is normal. A parasternal heave, right third heart sound, loud P_2, tricuspid regurgitation murmur, hepatomegaly, ascites, and peripheral edema may be present in RV failure. Electrocardiography (ECG) findings are nonspecific, but right axis deviation, R/S greater than 1 in V_1, or P-pulmonale may be seen. Absence of pulmonary congestion with elevated CVP has been considered most

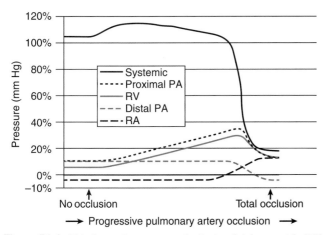

Figure 54-1. This figure demonstrates the limits of right ventricle (*RV*) contractile function in the setting of increasing pulmonary artery outflow obstruction, which results in an abrupt and catastrophic collapse in systemic hemodynamics once RV compensatory mechanisms are exhausted. *PA,* pulmonary artery; *RA,* right atrium. (*Modified from Guyton.*[8])

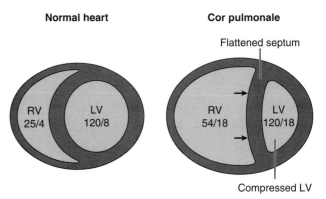

Figure 54-2. Ventricular interdependence. Right ventricle (*RV*) failure and dilation can lead to encroachment of the interventricular septum on the left ventricle (*LV*), causing increased left ventricular end diastolic pressure (*LVEDP*).[75]

specific for RV failure. However, severe RV failure can shift the interventricular septum and increase left ventricular end diastolic pressure (LVEDP), which may cause pulmonary congestion (see Fig. 54-2). Even in the absence of LV dysfunction, serum brain natriuretic peptide (BNP) level may be increased with RV volume overload or RV pressure overload, although lower values are lower than those observed in LV failure.[9] BNP levels are predictive of survival in acute RV failure from PAH.[10] In one study of patients with chronic thromboembolic PAH, BNP levels greater than 168 ng/mL identified patients with RV dysfunction with a sensitivity of 88% and specificity of 86%.[11]

Assessment of RV function can be challenging because of the ventricle's complex geometry. Cardiac magnetic resonance imaging (MRI) is now an accepted standard because the attendant spatial resolution may demonstrate the RV's complex geometry. However, MRI is limited in the ICU setting because it may not be available and because it is difficult to continuously monitor critically ill patients in the scanner. Radionuclide scanning is limited by poor spatial resolution, the need for background radiation correction, and lack of portability. Contrast ventriculography is invasive and provides limited incremental information when compared with echocardiography.[12]

Echocardiography is a noninvasive, portable modality that can be used to assess the size and function of the RV. With transthoracic echocardiography (TTE), RV linear dimensions can be measured in end-diastole from the focused four-chamber view. One quantitative approach involves determination of the volumes at end-systole and end-diastole, but this method is limited by the fallacious assumption that the RV is a cylindrical structure. Three-dimensional echocardiography (3D echo) is now recommended to overcome these limitations of two-dimensional echocardiography (2D echo), but in critically ill patients, 3D echo has its own limitations because it relies on excellent image quality and absence of arrhythmias.[13] A good rule of thumb is that the normal-sized RV should be two thirds the size of the LV. When it is larger, the RV is considered dilated.

Right and left heart hemodynamics can be estimated with Doppler techniques. Key measurements include the systolic

excursion of the tricuspid annular plane (TAPSE), the fractional area change (FAC), or longitudinal strain. RV function can be visually estimated by examining the contractility of the RV free wall and interventricular septum using TAPSE.[14] Abnormal TAPSE has been shown to have prognostic value, especially in patients with PAH.[15,16] Although TAPSE has been shown to be the most accurate measurement of RV function in PAH,[17,18] it may overestimate RV function when there is significant cardiac translation (e.g., because of a large pericardial effusion). Alternatively, TAPSE may underestimate RV function after cardiac surgery, when the pericardium may be inflamed. RV FAC gives an estimate of global RV function; values below 35% indicate RV dysfunction.[13] RV global longitudinal strain has been shown to provide prognostic value in various disease states such as heart failure, acute MI, and pulmonary hypertension. Although they appear to be reproducible and feasible in clinical practice, there currently exists a need for normative data. 3D echo can also provide an RV ejection fraction (EF), with a normal value more than 45%. RV wall thickness, which increases in chronic states, can be measured by either M-mode or 2D echo.[13,19]

Distinct echocardiographic patterns have been described in patients with RV failure with different causes. RV free wall hypokinesia that spares the apex is known as McConnell's sign and was originally described in patients with massive or submassive PE; it was thought to be specific for that disorder.[19] However, a retrospective study cast doubt on the specificity of McConnell's sign; in PE, its sensitivity was 70%, its specificity was 33%, and the sign was present in 67% of patients with RV infarction.[20] A D-shaped, flattened septum during diastole is seen in RV volume overload. Conversely, pressure overload causes right ventricular hypertrophy (RVH) and septal flattening throughout the entire cardiac cycle.[21]

The main pitfall of TTE in ventilated critically ill patients is that the images are often suboptimal and technically limited. Transesophageal echocardiography can be used when TTE images are not interpretable.

CAUSES OF RIGHT VENTRICLE DYSFUNCTION

The causes of RV failure can be divided into RV pressure overload, RV volume overload, decreased RV contractility,

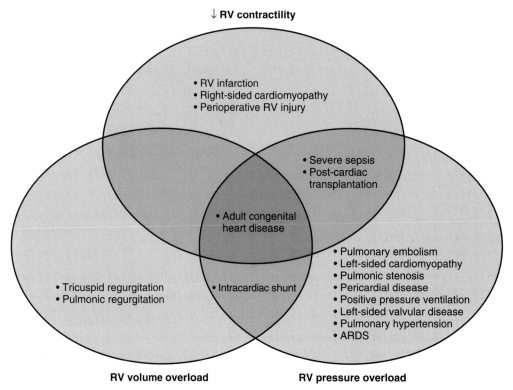

Figure 54-3. Causes of right ventricular failure. *ARDS,* acute respiratory distress syndrome; *RV,* right ventricle.

or a combination of these (Fig. 54-3). Sepsis is a disease process that has two potential mechanisms of RV dysfunction: myocardial depression and increased pulmonary vascular resistance (PVR).[22]

MANAGEMENT OF RIGHT VENTRICLE FAILURE

Definitive therapy for acutely decompensated RV failure requires primary treatment of the underlying condition in addition to hemodynamic support. The RV is very resilient and can recover substantial function if the underlying condition is successfully addressed.[23] Examples include percutaneous coronary intervention for RV MI and thrombolysis or open surgical embolectomy for massive PE.

RIGHT VENTRICLE MYOCARDIAL INFARCTION

RV MI is a distinct clinical entity, and there is a reasonable evidence base regarding its management. One third of inferior wall MIs are accompanied by RV MI. This typically occurs when there is acute thrombotic occlusion of the right coronary artery (RCA) proximal to the RV marginal branches.[24] In acute RV injury, chamber enlargement, depressed contractility, and impaired ventricular emptying lead to elevated right-sided volume and pressure. RV compliance also decreases, further raising pressures. This leads to conformational change of the RV and affects the LV through ventricular interdependence.

The classic clinical features of RV MI are hypotension, systemic venous congestion, and clear lungs. ECG findings

of ST elevation greater than 1 mm in right-sided lead V_{4R} in the presence of inferior wall injury are reliable and predictive of RV MI (88% sensitive, 78% specific).[4] Other ECG findings include atrioventricular (AV) nodal block and right bundle branch block. Hemodynamic findings include elevated right atrium (RA) pressure in relation to left-sided filling pressures. Equalization of diastolic filling pressures among the RA, RV, and pulmonary capillary wedge (PCW) pressures can also be seen. The steep *y* descent of the RA pressure tracing and the characteristic dip and plateau of the RV pressure tracing make this entity more hemodynamically similar to constrictive pericarditis and differentiate RV MI from cardiac tamponade. 2D echo is useful in identifying RV chamber enlargement and wall motion abnormalities of the free wall. Paradoxical septal motion can be seen in the presence of RV pressure/volume overload.

RV MI may be complicated by cardiogenic shock and high-grade AV block, both of which affect mortality.[25,26] RA dilation can lead to atrial fibrillation, which may further affect hemodynamics.

Treatment of RV MI includes close monitoring in a specialized cardiac unit. Unlike LV infarction, the initial treatment is volume expansion. In general, nitrates, morphine, diuretics, and other vasodilators should be avoided. Although patients with RV failure are often preload dependent, volume loading has the potential to overdistend the ventricles and increase wall tension, decrease contractility, increase ventricular interdependence, impair LV filling, and reduce systemic cardiac output.[23] The utility of volume loading appears to depend on various factors, including the baseline cardiovascular function of the patient, the degree of RV afterload, and volume status.[27] A clinical study of fluid resuscitation in patients with RV MI[28] showed that the RV achieves its maximum stroke work with RA pressure from 0 to 14 mm Hg; the optimal PCW pressure was 17 mm Hg in this study. An initial trial of volume may be appropriate for patients with decompensated RV failure, provided there is no evidence of pulmonary edema or increased right-sided preload conditions.[23] If signs of RV volume overload, including a CVP of greater than 15 mm Hg, or septal shift is noted on echocardiography, then the initiation of inotropic support without additional volume administration may be prudent. Pulmonary artery catheterization may be helpful in determining the ideal volume loading conditions.[23]

Hemodynamic support of the patient with decompensated RV failure may require combinations of vasopressors and inotropes. The normotensive patient with evidence of decreased cardiac output should be started on inotropic therapy, with vasopressors added if hypotension develops. The hypotensive patient with decreased cardiac output should receive vasopressors along with inotropes. Dobutamine has been shown to have beneficial effects on RV contractile function in pulmonary hypertension without affecting PVR. Milrinone, a selective phosphodiesterase (PDE)-3 inhibitor, has inotropic and vasodilatory effects, decreasing PVR and increasing RV EF in acute and chronic pulmonary hypertension,[29] but its use may be limited by hypotension. Norepinephrine has inotropic effects through β_1 agonism, but concomitant α_1 stimulation causes vasoconstriction and increased RV afterload. Levosimendan is a calcium sensitizer that increases cardiac contractility and has vasodilatory effects by activating the adenosine triphosphate (ATP)-sensitive potassium channels in vascular smooth muscle.[30] In an animal model of RV failure, levosimendan decreased afterload and increased RV contractility better than dobutamine because of its additional pulmonary vasodilatory effects.[31] Levosimendan is currently not approved in the United States, but it is used in Europe.

One study examined the effects of inhaled nitric oxide (NO) in 13 patients with right ventricular infarction and cardiogenic shock.[32] Acute hemodynamic improvement was seen, with a 24% increase in cardiac output along with a 12% decrease in RA pressure, a 13% decrease in pulmonary artery pressure, and a 36% decrease in PVR. Systemic blood pressure and PCW pressure were unchanged.[32] The presumed mechanism was selective pulmonary vasodilation.

Maintenance of sinus rhythm and AV synchrony can also be crucial in maximizing RV preload and function. Intra-aortic balloon pump counterpulsation may be considered when there is ongoing ischemia or refractory hemodynamic instability.

Fibrinolytic therapy has demonstrated limited benefit in acute inferior MI with RV involvement for various reasons. First, reocclusion has been shown to be more common when the RCA is the infarct-related artery. Second, mortality from acute inferior MI is considerably less than for anterior MI. Finally, RV function has been shown to improve spontaneously over time even in the absence of reperfusion therapy.[33]

A retrospective analysis of 1110 patients enrolled in phase II of the Thrombolysis in Myocardial Infarction trial showed that fibrinolysis reduced the frequency of RV dysfunction in patients with inferior infarction as demonstrated by radionuclide ventriculography. In a prospective trial, tissue plasminogen activator (t-PA) was administered along with antithrombotic and antiplatelet therapy within 4 hours of symptom onset to 90 patients presenting with inferior MI with or without RV involvement.[34] Coronary angiography performed later in the hospital course found that normal coronary flow was more likely in those without RV MI. In RV MI, complications were higher and late vessel patency was only 29% at 12 days after t-PA administration.[34]

The advantages of percutaneous transluminal coronary angioplasty (PTCA) over fibrinolysis include better infarct-related artery patency rates, lower incidence of intracranial hemorrhage, and decreased recurrent ischemia. In a study of 53 patients with inferior and RV MI taken for emergent PTCA, restoration of flow to the major RV branches was achieved in 77% of patients, and those with successful reperfusion had early recovery of RV function, sometimes as early as 1 hour.[35] Those who had unsuccessful reperfusion had protracted hemodynamic compromise requiring inotropic support, with a mortality rate of 58% compared with 2% in the reperfused group. Emergency revascularization efforts in these patients with RV MI is a class I recommendation in ACC/AHA guidelines for the treatment of acute MI.[36]

Mechanical ventilatory support for patients with acute RV failure should aim to improve oxygenation and ventilation without worsening RV impedance, venous return, or diastolic function. Hypoxemia and acidosis should be reversed because they can contribute to increased PVR.[37,38] A low respiratory rate and low tidal volume should be used to limit air trapping, which may increase PVR. Lower positive end-expiratory pressure settings may also moderate the effect of mechanical ventilation on PVR.[29,39]

VASODILATOR THERAPY

The goal of vasodilator use in RV failure is to improve right-sided cardiac output by reducing afterload. There is substantial evidence concerning vasodilator therapy in PAH and fewer data in secondary pulmonary hypertension (Table 54-1). Available therapies include NO, prostaglandins, PDE inhibitors, and endothelin (ET) antagonists.

Nitric Oxide

In acute RV failure, most of the data concern pulmonary vasodilation with inhaled nitric oxide (iNO).[40] iNO is rapidly inactivated; therefore it has minimal effects on systemic blood pressure. Its effects are limited to ventilated areas of the lung, which theoretically will improve ventilation/perfusion matching. Caution should be exhibited in patients with LV dysfunction because iNO can precipitate acute pulmonary edema. Other risks include platelet dysfunction and the formation of toxic compounds such as peroxynitrites.[40] iNO is usually well tolerated. Its use is mostly limited by its high cost and significant rebound effects on discontinuation.

Several randomized studies[41-43] have tested iNO in acute respiratory distress syndrome (ARDS). The results (shown in Table 54-2) are consistent and show a significant improvement in hypoxemia and PVR in patients with ARDS who were treated with iNO between 1 and 80 ppm but no

Table 54-1 Prospective Studies of Vasodilator Therapy in Chronic Pulmonary Hypertension

Authors Drug	Descriptor	Number of Patients NYHA Class Etiology	Results
Barst et al.[51] Epoprostenol IV (1996)	Multicenter open comparison conventional therapy alone vs. conventional therapy along with an intravenous infusion of epoprostenol	81 Class III-IV PPH	At 12 weeks: • Improvement on a 6-min walk test and hemodynamics. • 8 patients in the conventional therapy group died during the study, whereas no deaths occurred in the epoprostenol group ($P = .003$).
Badesch et al.[50] Epoprostenol IV (2000)	Multicenter open comparison conventional therapy alone vs. conventional therapy along with an intravenous infusion of epoprostenol	111 Class II-IV scleroderma and mod PHTN	At 12 weeks: • Improvement on a 6-min walk test and hemodynamics. • No mortality benefit.
Simonneau et al.[56] Treprostinil SQ (2000)	Double blind Placebo vs. treprostinil	470 Class II-IV PPH, connective tissue disease, congenital left-to-right shunt	At 12 weeks: • Modest but significant median increase of 16 m on the 6-min walk test. • Treprostinil appeared to significantly improve indexes of dyspnea, signs and symptoms of pulmonary hypertension, and hemodynamic measures.
Galie et al.[76] Beraprost PO (2002)	Double blind Placebo controlled	130 Class II-III All PAH	At 12 weeks: • Minimal improvement in 6-min walk test. • No change in hemodynamics. • Frequent side effects.
Barst et al.[77] Beraprost PO (2003)	Double blind Placebo controlled	116 Class II-III PPH, PAH related to either collagen vascular diseases or congenital systemic to pulmonary shunts	• Improved 6-min walk scores at 3 and 6 mo. • Effect not sustained at 9 and 12 mo.
Olschewski et al.[78] Iloprost INH (2002)	Multicenter placebo controlled Used a combined endpoint of a 10% increase in patients' scores on a 6-min walk test and improvement in NYHA functional class	207 Class III-IV PPH, CTD, chronic thromboembolic	At 12 weeks: • 17% of treated patients reached this endpoint, as compared with 4% of the placebo group ($P = .007$). • Hemodynamic values measured after inhalation were better in the iloprost group. • Short half-life requires multiple doses (6-12) because of short duration of action.
Channick et al.[63] Bosentan PO (2001)	Double blind Placebo	33 Class III PPH or associated with scleroderma	• Patients receiving bosentan had a mean gain of 76 m in the 6-min walk test ($P = .02$). • Significant improvements in pulmonary artery pressure, cardiac output, and PVR.
Rubin et al.[62] Bosentan PO (2002)	Double blind Placebo	213 Class III-IV PPH or associated with connective tissue disease	• On 6-min walk test, a gain of 44 m among patients in the overall study population ($P < .001$). • Patients receiving bosentan also had improvement in the time to clinical worsening. • High incidence of serum aminotransferase increases.
Galie et al.[79] Ambrisentan PO (2005)	Double blind Placebo	64 Class II-III PPH or associated with collagen vascular disease, anorexigen use, or HIV	At 12 weeks: • Ambrisentan increased 6-min walk duration. • Improvements were also observed in Borg dyspnea index, WHO functional class, subjective global assessment, and mean pulmonary arterial pressure.

Table 54-1 Prospective Studies of Vasodilator Therapy in Chronic Pulmonary Hypertension—cont'd

Authors Drug	Descriptor	Number of Patients NYHA Class Etiology	Results
Pulido et al.[64] Macitentan (2013)	Multicenter Double blind, placebo controlled Macitentan (3 and 10 mg) Primary endpoint: time to occurrence of a composite endpoint of death, AS, lung transplantation, initiation of treatment with prostanoids, or worsening of PAH	742 Class II-IV PPH or related to connective tissue disease, repaired congenital systemic-to-pulmonary shunts, HIV, or drug use/toxin exposure	• Mean duration of follow-up 85-104 weeks. • Primary endpoint occurred in 31.4% with 10-mg dose vs. 38% with 3-mg dose vs. 46.4% with placebo. • HR of 10-mg dose compared with placebo was 0.55.
Galie et al.[57] Sildenafil (2005)	Double blind, placebo controlled Sildenafil (20, 40, 80 mg)	278 Class II-IV PPH, CTD, and repaired congenital disease	At 12 weeks: • Improvement of 45-60 m on 6-min walk. • Improved hemodynamics. • No dose-response relationship.
Galie et al.[59] Taladafil (2009)	Double blind, placebo controlled Taladafil (2.5, 10, 20, 40 mg)	405 Class II-IV Idiopathic/heritable or related to anorexigen use, connective tissue disease, HIV infection, or congenital systemic-to-pulmonary shunts	At 16 weeks: • Dose response: only 40-mg dose met statistical significance. • Improvement of 44 m in bosentan-naïve group, 23 m in patients receiving bosentan therapy. • Improved time to clinical worsening, incidence of clinical worsening, and HRQOL. • No change in WHO functional class. • 52-week follow-up study showed sustained effects.[60]

AS, atrial septostomy; CTD, connective tissue disease; HIV, human immunodeficiency virus; HR, heart rate; HRQOL, health-related quality of life; INH, inhalation; NYHA, New York Heart Association; PAH, pulmonary arterial hypertension; PHTN, pulmonary hypertension; PPH, primary pulmonary hypertension; PO, by mouth; PVR, pulmonary vascular resistance; SQ, subcutaneously; WHO, World Health Organization.

Table 54-2 Randomized Controlled Trials of iNO in ARDS

Authors	Descriptor	Number of Patients and Etiology	Results
Dellinger et al.[38] (1997)*	Prospective, multicenter, randomized, double-blind, placebo-controlled study Placebo (nitrogen gas) or iNO at concentrations of 1.25, 5, 20, 40, or 80 ppm	177 patients Disease onset within 72 hr of randomization	• An acute response to treatment gas, defined as a Pao_2 increase >20%, was seen in 60% of the patients receiving iNO with no significant differences between dose groups compared with 24% of placebo patients. • The initial increase in oxygenation translated into a reduction in the Fio_2 over the first day and in the intensity of mechanical ventilation over the first 4 days of treatment, as measured by the oxygenation index. • There were no differences in mortality, the number of days alive and off mechanical ventilation, or the number of days alive after meeting oxygenation criteria for extubation.
Lundin et al.[39] (1999)	Prospective, open, randomized, multicenter, Phase III trial NO responders: Patients whose Pao_2 increased by more than 20% when receiving 0, 2, 10, and 40 ppm of iNO for 10 min within 96 hr of study entry NO responders were randomized to conventional treatment with/without iNO (1-40 ppm)	180 of 268 patients were NO responders	• Frequency of reversal of ARDS was no different in iNO patients (61%) and controls (54%; $P > .2$). • Development of severe respiratory failure was lower in the iNO patients (2.2%) than in controls (10.3%; $P < .05$). • There was no significant difference in mortality.
Taylor and Dellinger et al.[50] (2004)	Multicenter, randomized, placebo-controlled triple-blinded study Placebo (nitrogen gas) or iNO at 5 ppm until 28 days, discontinuation of assisted breathing, or death	385 patients with ALI	• iNO at 5 ppm did not increase the number of days patients were alive and off assisted breathing. • This lack of effect on clinical outcomes was seen despite a statistically significant increase in Pao_2 that resolved by 48 hr. • Mortality was similar between groups.

*In patients receiving 5 iNO 5 ppm, there was a post hoc difference in the percentage of patients alive and off mechanical ventilation at day 28.
ALI, acute lung injury; ARDS, acute respiratory distress syndrome; Fio_2, fraction of inspired oxygen; iNO, inhaled nitric oxide; NO, nitric oxide; Pao_2, partial pressure of oxygen in arterial blood.

improvement in mortality. The physiologic benefits demonstrated in patients with ARDS have led to the use of iNO as a supportive treatment for acute right ventricular dysfunction in other settings. A nonrandomized study[44] evaluated iNO in critically ill patients with pulmonary hypertension and echocardiographically diagnosed acute RV failure. The causes of RV failure included ARDS, PAH, chronic obstructive pulmonary disease, PE, and obstructive sleep apnea. In responders, iNO significantly reduced the pulmonary artery pressures and PVR and consequently increased cardiac output, stroke volume, and mixed venous oxygen saturation. No mortality benefit was demonstrated. Other studies have demonstrated a hemodynamic improvement in patients with RV dysfunction after cardiac surgery,[45,46] acute massive PE,[47,48] and right ventricular failure after insertion of a left ventricular assist device (LVAD).[49]

Prostanoids

Prostacyclin has vasodilatory and antiplatelet properties.[50-53] Intravenous epoprostenol is limited by its systemic hypotensive effects. Furthermore, a very short half-life mandates delivery by continuous central infusion. Inhaled epoprostenol has an effect on hemodynamics and oxygenation similar to that of NO in patients with ARDS without systemic side effects.[40] Epoprostenol has a longer half-life than NO (3 to 6 minutes), causing recirculation and thereby a greater pulmonary and systemic hypotensive effect, but it causes less improvement in oxygenation.[40] iNO and nebulized prostacyclin have been observed to have additive effects (e.g., after lung transplantation and after cardiac surgery). An alternative prostacyclin formulation, treprostinil, has a half-life of approximately 4 hours and can be administered either intravenously or subcutaneously. Treprostinil has been approved for inhaled administration.[54-56] Another alternative, iloprost, has a half-life of 20 to 30 minutes and can be injected or inhaled. Although iloprost and inhaled treprostinil have fewer systemic side effects, epoprostenol is the preferred prostacyclin in a critical care setting because of its short half-life and greater selective vasodilatory effects.

Phosphodiesterase Inhibitors

NO mediates its effects by increasing cyclic guanosine monophosphate (cyclic GMP) in vascular smooth muscle cells. Inhibition of PDEs that inactivate cyclic GMP augments the pulmonary vasodilatory response of endogenous NO or iNO in PAH. Sildenafil is an inhibitor of PDE-5, the isoform most abundant in the lung. Open-label and crossover trials have shown that sildenafil can prolong the effects of iNO and improve hemodynamics.[57,58] Sildenafil can act synergistically with inhaled iloprost without significant adverse hemodynamic effects.[57] An alternative, taladafil, may be viable, but it has not been used in the critically ill.[59,60]

Endothelin Receptor Antagonists

ET-1 is a potent vasoconstrictor that is found in high concentrations in the lungs of patients with PAH.[61] There are two distinct ET receptors: ET_A, which is found on smooth muscle cells and mediates vasoconstriction and hypertrophy, and ET_B, which is found on endothelial cells and mediates release of NO and prostacyclin. Bosentan is a competitive antagonist of ET-1 at the ET_A and ET_B receptors that has been shown in randomized trials to improve hemodynamics, symptoms, and functional class in patients with PAH.[62,63] Macitentan is another oral ET receptor antagonist that has been studied in patients with patients with primary PAH.[64] Neither bosentan nor macitentan has been studied in critical care.

Given the opposing effects of ET_A and ET_B receptors, selective ET_A receptor blockade would appear to be a promising strategy. Ambrisentan, an oral agent that selectively blocks ET_A, has been used in ambulatory patients, but it has not been studied in the ICU.[65,66]

MECHANICAL SUPPORT, ATRIAL SEPTOSTOMY, AND TRANSPLANTATION

Intra-aortic balloon pumps have been used in RV failure to augment RCA perfusion, reduce ischemia, and allow for the weaning of vasopressors that may have adverse effects on PVR. Right ventricular assist devices (RVADs) may improve hemodynamics and act as bridges to cardiac transplantation in patients with RV failure secondary to disease intrinsic to the ventricle. Timing of RVAD insertion is crucial. In the setting of increased afterload, RVAD may not be sufficient, and extracorporeal membrane oxygenation should be considered for patients with potentially reversible RV failure. When the cause of RV failure is LV failure, LVADs may be used to decrease PA pressures; however, this may exacerbate the RV failure in some cases.

Atrial septostomy (AS) has been used in severe pulmonary hypertension with concomitant RV failure when maximal medical therapy has failed. The creation of a shunt at the atrial level allows for right-sided decompression, a reduction in RV end-diastolic pressure, decreased wall tension, and improved contractility. Although the right-to-left shunt leads to oxygen desaturation, an increased left-sided filling augments cardiac output and appears to improve oxygen delivery.[67] The defect may close over time, requiring a repeat procedure. The procedural mortality is high (~15%).[68] Contraindications include severe right ventricular failure on cardiorespiratory support, mean right atrial pressure (mRAP) greater than 20 mm Hg, and pulmonary vascular resistance index (PVRI) greater than 55 U/m^2.[67] The use of RVADs can be considered if significant organ dysfunction has not yet occurred.[69,70]

Heart and heart-lung transplantation may be considered as a final option in patients with RV failure, although patients are often unsuitable candidates. Severe RV failure itself is a risk factor for unsuccessful bridging to transplantation.[23] RV failure secondary to recurrent PE causing chronic thromboembolic pulmonary hypertension may be treated with surgical pulmonary thromboendarterectomy.

MISCELLANEOUS THERAPIES

Diuretics should be used judiciously when appropriate to decrease volume load on the distended RV. Venovenous ultrafiltration has been used for decompensated left-sided heart failure in patients refractory to aggressive diuretic therapy, but its utility has not been formally investigated. The use of digoxin in patients with RV dysfunction is controversial. In a study of the short-term effects of digoxin in 17 patients with severe primary pulmonary hypertension,[71] cardiac index improved mildly and catecholamine levels decreased, but PVR did not change and mean pulmonary artery pressure (PAP) increased. In a retrospective study, digoxin did not have any survival benefit.[72] Because there are more effective drugs to treat RV dysfunction and supraventricular arrhythmias, digoxin is not commonly used in the ICU in this setting. There are no studies of calcium channel blockers in critically ill patients with PAH, and the negative inotropic effects of these agents may precipitate fatal worsening of right ventricular failure.[70] Aside from treatment of acute and chronic thromboembolic diseases, several observational and subanalysis studies suggest improved survival with anticoagulation in patients with pulmonary hypertension.[72-74]

PROGNOSIS

RV failure is often a marker of the severity of the underlying disease process and a poor prognostic sign. Cardiogenic shock because of RV failure is associated with a high mortality rate similar to shock from LV failure. The presence of RV infarction affects the prognosis in inferior MI. The underlying disorder and its degree of reversibility also influence the prognosis among patients with RV failure.

CONCLUSION

In summary, evidence-based data concerning treatment of right ventricular failure in the ICU are relatively sparse. Few randomized controlled trials focus on the treatment of this clinical entity. Nonetheless, RV failure accompanies many of the disease processes encountered in the ICU. Furthermore, many of the therapies commonly used for critically ill patients with RV dysfunction, such as volume resuscitation and mechanical ventilation, can worsen their clinical state. The dearth of studies on RV failure in the ICU can be attributed to several factors, including (1) the heterogeneity of causes, (2) the heterogeneity of disease severities, (3) the lack of a portable gold standard imaging modality, and (4) underestimation of the importance of the RV. Most ICU therapies are currently based on pathophysiologic considerations and extrapolation from trials in other settings.

AUTHORS' RECOMMENDATIONS

- RV failure is defined as the inability of the RV to provide adequate blood flow through the pulmonary circulation at a normal CVP.
- RV failure can be divided into RV pressure overload, RV volume overload, decreased RV contractility, or a combination of these.
- RV function is best evaluated by echocardiography: transthoracic echocardiography, initially, or transesophageal if views are inadequate.
- Definitive therapy for an acutely decompensated RV requires primary treatment of the underlying condition (e.g., percutaneous coronary intervention, thrombolysis) in addition to hemodynamic support.

- Hemodynamic support of the patient with decompensated RV failure may require combinations of vasopressors (norepinephrine) and inotropes (dobutamine or milrinone).
- Other interventions that may be used include inhaled nitric oxide, prostacyclin, and diuretics.
- The RV is very resilient and can recover substantially if the underlying condition is successfully addressed.

REFERENCES

1. Harvey W. *On the Motion of the Heart and Blood in Animals.* Reprinted. Buffalo, NY: Prometheus Books; 1993.
2. Starr IJW, Meade RH. The absence of conspicuous increments of venous pressure after severe damage to the right ventricle of the dog, with a discussion of the relation between clinical congestive failure and heart disease. *Am Heart J.* 1943;26:291–301.
3. Cohn JN, Guiha NH, Broder MI, Limas CJ. Right ventricular infarction. Clinical and hemodynamic features. *Am J Cardiol.* 1974;33:209–214.
4. Zehender M, Kasper W, Kauder E, et al. Right ventricular infarction as an independent predictor of prognosis after acute inferior myocardial infarction. *N Engl J Med.* 1993;328:981–988.
5. Goldhaber SZ, Visani L, De Rosa M. Acute pulmonary embolism: clinical outcomes in the International Cooperative Pulmonary Embolism Registry (ICOPER). *Lancet.* 1999;353:1386–1389.
6. Writing Committee M, Yancy CW, Jessup M, et al. American College of Cardiology Foundation/American Heart Association Task Force on Practice G. 2013 ACCF/AHA guideline for the management of heart failure: A report of the American College of Cardiology Foundation/American Heart Association Task Force on practice guidelines. *Circulation.* 2013;128:e240–e327.
7. Greyson CR. Pathophysiology of right ventricular failure. *Crit Care Med.* 2008;36:S57–S65.
8. Guyton AC, Lindsey AW, Gilluly JJ. The limits of right ventricular compensation following acute increase in pulmonary circulatory resistance. *Circ Res.* 1954;2:326–332.
9. Nagaya N, Nishikimi T, Okano Y, et al. Plasma brain natriuretic peptide levels increase in proportion to the extent of right ventricular dysfunction in pulmonary hypertension. *J Am Coll Cardiol.* 1998;31:202–208.
10. Sztrymf B, Souza R, Bertoletti L, et al. Prognostic factors of acute heart failure in patients with pulmonary arterial hypertension. *Eur Respir J.* 2010;35:1286–1293.
11. Reesink HJ, Tulevski II, Marcus JT, et al. Brain natriuretic peptide as noninvasive marker of the severity of right ventricular dysfunction in chronic thromboembolic pulmonary hypertension. *Ann Thorac Surg.* 2007;84:537–543.
12. Woods J, Monteiro P, Rhodes A. Right ventricular dysfunction. *Curr Opin Crit Care.* 2007;13:532–540.
13. Lang RM, Badano LP, Mor-Avi V, et al. Recommendations for cardiac chamber quantification by echocardiography in adults: An update from the American Society of Echocardiography and the European Association of Cardiovascular Imaging. *Eur Heart J Cardiovasc Imaging.* 2015;16:233–270.
14. Lopez-Candales A, Rajagopalan N, Saxena N, Gulyasy B, Edelman K, Bazaz R. Right ventricular systolic function is not the sole determinant of tricuspid annular motion. *Am J Cardiol.* 2006;98:973–977.
15. Forfia PR, Fisher MR, Mathai SC, et al. Tricuspid annular displacement predicts survival in pulmonary hypertension. *Am J Respir Crit Care Med.* 2006;174:1034–1041.
16. Mathai SC, Sibley CT, Forfia PR, et al. Tricuspid annular plane systolic excursion is a robust outcome measure in systemic sclerosis-associated pulmonary arterial hypertension. *J Rheumatol.* 2011;38:2410–2418.
17. Sato T, Tsujino I, Ohira H, et al. Validation study on the accuracy of echocardiographic measurements of right ventricular systolic function in pulmonary hypertension. *J Am Soc Echocardiogr.* 2012;25:280–286.
18. Sato T, Tsujino I, Oyama-Manabe N, et al. Simple prediction of right ventricular ejection fraction using tricuspid annular plane systolic excursion in pulmonary hypertension. *Int J Cardiovasc Imaging.* 2013;29:1799–1805.

19. McConnell MV, Solomon SD, Rayan ME, Come PC, Goldhaber SZ, Lee RT. Regional right ventricular dysfunction detected by echocardiography in acute pulmonary embolism. *Am J Cardiol.* 1996;78:469–473.

20. Casazza F, Bongarzoni A, Capozi A, Agostoni O. Regional right ventricular dysfunction in acute pulmonary embolism and right ventricular infarction. *Eur J Echocardiogr.* 2005;6:11–14.

21. Feigenbaum HA, Armstrong WF, Ryan T. *Feigenbaum's Echocardiography.* Lippincott Williams & Wilkins; 2004.

22. Dhainaut JF, Lanore JJ, de Gournay JM, et al. Right ventricular dysfunction in patients with septic shock. *Intensive Care Med.* 1988;14(suppl 2):488–491.

23. Piazza G, Goldhaber SZ. The acutely decompensated right ventricle: pathways for diagnosis and management. *Chest.* 2005;128:1836–1852.

24. Bowers TR, O'Neill WW, Pica M, Goldstein JA. Patterns of coronary compromise resulting in acute right ventricular ischemic dysfunction. *Circulation.* 2002;106:1104–1109.

25. Jacobs AK, Leopold JA, Bates E, et al. Cardiogenic shock caused by right ventricular infarction: a report from the shock registry. *J Am Coll Cardiol.* 2003;41:1273–1279.

26. Nedeljkovic SZ, Ryan TJ. Right ventricular infarction. In: Hollenberg SM, ed. *Cardiogenic Shock.* Armonk, NY: Futura Publishing; 2002:161–186.

27. Dell'Italia LJ, Starling MR, Blumhardt R, Lasher JC, O'Rourke RA. Comparative effects of volume loading, dobutamine, and nitroprusside in patients with predominant right ventricular infarction. *Circulation.* 1985;72:1327–1335.

28. Berisha S, Kastrati A, Goda A, Popa Y. Optimal value of filling pressure in the right side of the heart in acute right ventricular infarction. *Br Heart J.* 1990;63:98–102.

29. Mekontso Dessap A, Charron C, Devaquet J, et al. Impact of acute hypercapnia and augmented positive end-expiratory pressure on right ventricle function in severe acute respiratory distress syndrome. *Intensive Care Med.* 2009;35:1850–1858.

30. Pathak A, Lebrin M, Vaccaro A, Senard JM, Despas F. Pharmacology of levosimendan: inotropic, vasodilatory and cardioprotective effects. *J Clin Pharm Ther.* 2013;38:341–349.

31. Kerbaul F, Rondelet B, Demester JP, et al. Effects of levosimendan versus dobutamine on pressure load-induced right ventricular failure. *Crit Care Med.* 2006;34:2814–2819.

32. Inglessis I, Shin JT, Lepore JJ, et al. Hemodynamic effects of inhaled nitric oxide in right ventricular myocardial infarction and cardiogenic shock. *J Am Coll Cardiol.* 2004;44:793–798.

33. Nedeljkovic ZS, Ryan TJ, Hollenberg SM, Bates ER, eds. *Right Ventricular Infarction in Cardiogenic Shock.* Armonk, NY: Futura Publishing; 2002.

34. Giannitsis E, Potratz J, Wiegand U, Stierle U, Djonlagic H, Sheikhzadeh A. Impact of early accelerated dose tissue plasminogen activator on in-hospital patency of the infarcted vessel in patients with acute right ventricular infarction. *Heart.* 1997;77:512–516.

35. Bowers TR, O'Neill WW, Grines C, Pica MC, Safian RD, Goldstein JA. Effect of reperfusion on biventricular function and survival after right ventricular infarction. *N Engl J Med.* 1998;338:933–940.

36. Kushner FG, Hand M, Smith Jr SC, et al. 2009 focused updates: ACC/AHA guidelines for the management of patients with st-elevation myocardial infarction (updating the 2004 guideline and 2007 focused update) and ACC/AHA/SCAI guidelines on percutaneous coronary intervention (updating the 2005 guideline and 2007 focused update) a report of the American College of Cardiology Foundation/American Heart Association Task Force on practice guidelines. *J Am Coll Cardiol.* 2009;54:2205–2241.

37. Moudgil R, Michelakis ED, Archer SL. Hypoxic pulmonary vasoconstriction. *J Appl Physiol (1985).* 2005;98:390–403.

38. Fischer LG, Van Aken H, Burkle H. Management of pulmonary hypertension: Physiological and pharmacological considerations for anesthesiologists. *Anesth Analg.* 2003;96:1603–1616.

39. Bouferrache K, Vieillard-Baron A. Acute respiratory distress syndrome, mechanical ventilation, and right ventricular function. *Curr Opin Crit Care.* 2011;17:30–35.

40. Griffiths MJ, Evans TW. Inhaled nitric oxide therapy in adults. *N Engl J Med.* 2005;353:2683–2695.

41. Dellinger RP, Zimmerman JL, Taylor RW, et al. Effects of inhaled nitric oxide in patients with acute respiratory distress syndrome: results of a randomized phase II trial. Inhaled nitric oxide in ARDS study group. *Crit Care Med.* 1998;26:15–23.

42. Lundin S, Mang H, Smithies M, Stenqvist O, Frostell C. Inhalation of nitric oxide in acute lung injury: results of a European multicentre study. The European Study Group of Inhaled Nitric Oxide. *Intensive Care Med.* 1999;25:911–919.

43. Taylor RW, Zimmerman JL, Dellinger RP, et al. Inhaled Nitric Oxide in ASG. low-dose inhaled nitric oxide in patients with acute lung injury: a randomized controlled trial. *JAMA.* 2004;291:1603–1609.

44. Bhorade S, Christenson J, O'Connor M, Lavoie A, Pohlman A, Hall JB. Response to inhaled nitric oxide in patients with acute right heart syndrome. *Am J Respir Crit Care Med.* 1999;159:571–579.

45. De Wet CJ, Affleck DG, Jacobsohn E, et al. Inhaled prostacyclin is safe, effective, and affordable in patients with pulmonary hypertension, right heart dysfunction, and refractory hypoxemia after cardiothoracic surgery. *J Thorac Cardiovasc Surg.* 2004;127:1058–1067.

46. Fattouch K, Sbraga F, Bianco G, et al. Inhaled prostacyclin, nitric oxide, and nitroprusside in pulmonary hypertension after mitral valve replacement. *J Card Surg.* 2005;20:171–176.

47. Capellier G, Jacques T, Balvay P, Blasco G, Belle E, Barale F. Inhaled nitric oxide in patients with pulmonary embolism. *Intensive Care Med.* 1997;23:1089–1092.

48. Szold O, Khoury W, Biderman P, Klausner JM, Halpern P, Weinbroum AA. Inhaled nitric oxide improves pulmonary functions following massive pulmonary embolism: a report of four patients and review of the literature. *Lung.* 2006;184:1–5.

49. Wagner F, Dandel M, Gunther G, et al. Nitric oxide inhalation in the treatment of right ventricular dysfunction following left ventricular assist device implantation. *Circulation.* 1997;96:II-291–296.

50. Badesch DB, Tapson VF, McGoon MD, et al. Continuous intravenous epoprostenol for pulmonary hypertension due to the scleroderma spectrum of disease. A randomized, controlled trial. *Ann Intern Med.* 2000;132:425–434.

51. Barst RJ, Rubin LJ, Long WA, Primary Pulmonary Hypertension Study Group, et al. A comparison of continuous intravenous epoprostenol (prostacyclin) with conventional therapy for primary pulmonary hypertension. *N Engl J Med.* 1996;334:296–301.

52. Barst RJ, Rubin LJ, McGoon MD, Caldwell EJ, Long WA, Levy PS. Survival in primary pulmonary hypertension with long-term continuous intravenous prostacyclin. *Ann Intern Med.* 1994;121:409–415.

53. McLaughlin VV, Shillington A, Rich S. Survival in primary pulmonary hypertension: the impact of epoprostenol therapy. *Circulation.* 2002;106:1477–1482.

54. Voswinckel R, Ghofrani HA, Grimminger F, Seeger W, Olschewski H. Inhaled treprostinil [corrected] for treatment of chronic pulmonary arterial hypertension. *Ann Intern Med.* 2006;144:149–150.

55. Tapson VF, Gomberg-Maitland M, McLaughlin VV, et al. Safety and efficacy of IV treprostinil for pulmonary arterial hypertension: a prospective, multicenter, open-label, 12-week trial. *Chest.* 2006;129:683–688.

56. Simonneau G, Barst RJ, Galie N, Treprostinil Study Group, et al. Continuous subcutaneous infusion of treprostinil, a prostacyclin analogue, in patients with pulmonary arterial hypertension: A double-blind, randomized, placebo-controlled trial. *Am J Respir Crit Care Med.* 2002;165:800–804.

57. Galie N, Ghofrani HA, Torbicki A, Sildenafil Use in Pulmonary Arterial Hypertension Study Group, et al. Sildenafil citrate therapy for pulmonary arterial hypertension. *N Engl J Med.* 2005;353:2148–2157.

58. Pepke-Zaba J, Gilbert C, Collings L, Brown MC. Sildenafil improves health-related quality of life in patients with pulmonary arterial hypertension. *Chest.* 2008;133:183–189.

59. Galie N, Brundage BH, Ghofrani HA, et al. Tadalafil therapy for pulmonary arterial hypertension. *Circulation.* 2009;119:2894–2903.

60. Oudiz RJ, Brundage BH, Galie N, et al. Tadalafil for the treatment of pulmonary arterial hypertension: a double-blind 52-week uncontrolled extension study. *J Am Coll Cardiol.* 2012;60:768–774.

61. Channick RN, Sitbon O, Barst RJ, Manes A, Rubin LJ. Endothelin receptor antagonists in pulmonary arterial hypertension. *J Am Coll Cardiol.* 2004;43:62S–67S.

62. Rubin LJ, Badesch DB, Barst RJ, et al. Bosentan therapy for pulmonary arterial hypertension. *N Engl J Med.* 2002;346:896–903.

63. Channick RN, Simonneau G, Sitbon O, et al. Effects of the dual endothelin-receptor antagonist bosentan in patients with pulmonary hypertension: a randomised placebo-controlled study. *Lancet.* 2001;358:1119–1123.

64. Pulido T, Adzerikho I, Channick RN, et al. Macitentan and morbidity and mortality in pulmonary arterial hypertension. *N Engl J Med*. 2013;369:809–818.

65. Galie N, Olschewski H, Oudiz RJ, et al. Ambrisentan in Pulmonary Arterial Hypertension RD-BP-CMESG. Ambrisentan for the treatment of pulmonary arterial hypertension: results of the ambrisentan in pulmonary arterial hypertension, randomized, double-blind, placebo-controlled, multicenter, efficacy (ARIES) study 1 and 2. *Circulation*. 2008;117:3010–3019.

66. Oudiz RJ, Galie N, Olschewski H, et al. Long-term ambrisentan therapy for the treatment of pulmonary arterial hypertension. *J Am Coll Cardiol*. 2009;54:1971–1981.

67. Keogh AM, Mayer E, Benza RL, et al. Interventional and surgical modalities of treatment in pulmonary hypertension. *J Am Coll Cardiol*. 2009;54:S67–S77.

68. McLaughlin VV, Archer SL, Badesch DB, et al. ACCF/AHA 2009 expert consensus document on pulmonary hypertension a report of the American College of Cardiology Foundation Task Force on Expert Consensus Documents and the American Heart Association developed in collaboration with the American College of Chest Physicians; American Thoracic Society, Inc.; and the Pulmonary Hypertension Association. *J Am Coll Cardiol*. 2009;53:1573–1619.

69. McNeil K, Dunning J, Morrell NW. The pulmonary physician in critical care. 13: The pulmonary circulation and right ventricular failure in the ITU. *Thorax*. 2003;58:157–162.

70. Zamanian RT, Haddad F, Doyle RL, Weinacker AB. Management strategies for patients with pulmonary hypertension in the intensive care unit. *Crit Care Med*. 2007;35:2037–2050.

71. Rich S, Seidlitz M, Dodin E, et al. The short-term effects of digoxin in patients with right ventricular dysfunction from pulmonary hypertension. *Chest*. 1998;114:787–792.

72. Kawut SM, Horn EM, Berekashvili KK, et al. New predictors of outcome in idiopathic pulmonary arterial hypertension. *Am J Cardiol*. 2005;95:199–203.

73. Fuster V, Steele PM, Edwards WD, Gersh BJ, McGoon MD, Frye RL. Primary pulmonary hypertension: natural history and the importance of thrombosis. *Circulation*. 1984;70:580–587.

74. Frank H, Mlczoch J, Huber K, Schuster E, Gurtner HP, Kneussl M. The effect of anticoagulant therapy in primary and anorectic drug-induced pulmonary hypertension. *Chest*. 1997;112:714–721.

75. Marino P. *ICU Book*. Lippincott Williams & Wilkins; 2006.

76. Galie N, Humbert M, Vachiery JL, Arterial Pulmonary Hypertension, Beraprost European Study Group, et al. Effects of beraprost sodium, an oral prostacyclin analogue, in patients with pulmonary arterial hypertension: a randomized, double-blind, placebo-controlled trial. *J Am Coll Cardiol*. 2002;39:1496–1502.

77. Barst RJ, McGoon M, McLaughlin V, Beraprost Study Group, et al. Beraprost therapy for pulmonary arterial hypertension. *J Am Coll Cardiol*. 2003;41:2119–2125.

78. Olschewski H, Simonneau G, Galie N, Aerosolized Iloprost Randomized Study Group, et al. Inhaled iloprost for severe pulmonary hypertension. *N Engl J Med*. 2002;347:322–329.

79. Galie N, Badesch D, Oudiz R, et al. Ambrisentan therapy for pulmonary arterial hypertension. *J Am Coll Cardiol*. 2005;46:529–535.

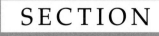
KIDNEY INJURY AND CRITICAL ILLNESS

55 How Does One Rapidly and Correctly Identify Acute Kidney Injury?

Gianluca Villa, Zaccaria Ricci, Claudio Ronco

Acute kidney injury (AKI) is a syndrome that is frequently and commonly observed among hospitalized and especially critically ill patients. The incidence of AKI varies based on the criteria used to diagnose the disorder, but it ranges from 4% to 20%[1] and reaches 60% among patients in the intensive care unit (ICU).[2] Patients affected by AKI usually require admission to the ICU and are often burdened by long ICU and in-hospital lengths of stay as well as poor short- and long-term outcomes. Although many advances have been made in understanding the pathophysiology of AKI and in the development of renal replacement therapy (RRT), significant morbidity and mortality rates (up to 80%) have been reported.[3]

Diagnosis of AKI is often complicated by the heterogeneity of etiology and onset and by the heterogeneity of disease severity and comorbidities.[1] Moreover, for some time, the absence of a consensus definition of AKI further complicated the diagnosis and staging of this syndrome.[2]

Avoiding AKI is probably the best way to improve outcomes of critically ill patients with renal dysfunction.[4] However, if AKI occurs, improved renal support (pharmacologic and nonpharmacologic) and the avoidance of further nephron insults (e.g., the use of nephrotoxic drugs) may reduce the progression of AKI and the development of complications, and it may also improve outcome. An early identification of AKI is essential to define prognosis and to guide clinical decision-making in these patients.

CLINICAL ACUTE KIDNEY INJURY

The definition, diagnosis, and staging of AKI are currently based on indices that estimate the glomerular filtration rate (GFR). The GFR is widely accepted as the best overall index of renal function in health and disease. However, it is difficult to measure; thus it is usually estimated from the serum level of endogenous filtration markers, such as creatinine.[5]

Risk, Injury, Failure, Loss, and End-Stage Renal Disease Classification

The first widely accepted AKI definition, validated in more than half a million patients worldwide, was proposed in

2004.[6] The Acute Dialysis Quality Initiative (ADQI) first suggested the use of serum creatinine (SCr) and urinary output (UOP) to univocally define AKI and summarize different stages of severity and outcome into the RIFLE classification[7] (see Table 55-1). The RIFLE classification had the unquestioned advantage of providing a uniform and broadly accepted definition of AKI. The acronym RIFLE delineates classes of increasing severity (Risk, Injury, and Failure) and outcome (Loss and End-Stage Renal Disease [ESRD]). The three severity grades are defined on the basis of the changes in SCr or UOP, in which the worst measurement is used. The two outcome criteria, Loss and ESRD, are defined by the duration of loss of kidney function[5] (see Table 55-1).

This classification system primarily considers the change in some measure of renal function from baseline. In a patient without known chronic kidney disease and in whom the baseline value of SCr is unknown, the Modification of Diet in Renal Disease formula with a creatinine clearance of 75 mL/min per 1.73 m[2] provides an estimated baseline.[2] The UOP, often unreliably measured outside of the ICU, has been discarded in several studies. However, comparing the results obtained with RIFLE classification with and without UOP data indicates that elimination of UOP delays or completely misses the diagnosis of AKI and is associated with a higher rate of AKI-associated mortality.[6]

Acute Kidney Injury Network Classification

In 2007, the Acute Kidney Injury Network (AKIN) introduced small but important modifications to the RIFLE classification, suggesting that use of less profound changes in SCr would make the RIFLE criteria more sensitive and reliable[8] (see Table 55-1). Increasing evidence from different settings has suggested that even modest changes in SCr levels can be associated with increased mortality. In particular, a creatinine increase of 0.3 mg/dL (26.4 μmol/L) constitutes an independent risk factor for death in several different studies.[9,10] Moreover, the AKIN classification introduced a temporal dimension into the definition of AKI. Thus progressive and modest changes in SCr were not considered for AKI definition. In particular, an acute increase of SCr over a threshold value within a 48-hour period could be used to define AKI.

Table 55-1 Comparison Among RIFLE, AKIN, and KDIGO Classifications

	SCR CRITERIA		
RIFLE	AKIN	KDIGO	UOP Criteria
Risk Increase in SCr 1.5-fold from baseline or GFR decrease >25%	**Stage 1** Increase of ≥0.3 mg/dL (≥26.5 µmol/L) or increase to ≥150%-200% (1.5- to 2-fold) from baseline	**Stage 1** Increase in SCr 1.5- to 1.9-fold from baseline or ≥0.3 mg/dL (≥26.5 µmol/L)	<0.5 mL/kg/hr for >6 hr
Injury Increase in SCr 2-fold from baseline or GFR decrease >50%	**Stage 2** Increase to >200-300% (>2- to 3-fold) from baseline	**Stage 2** Increase in SCr 2- to 2.9-fold from baseline	<0.5 mL/kg/hr for >12 hr
Failure Increase in SCr 3-fold from baseline, or SCr >4 mg/dL (>354 µmol/L) with an acute increase >0.5 mg/dL (>44 µmol/L) or GFR decrease >75%	**Stage 3** Increase to >300% (>3-fold) from baseline, or ≥4.0 mg/dL (≥354 µmol/L) with an acute increase of at least 0.5 mg/dL (44 µmol/L), or on RRT	**Stage 3** Increase in SCr 3- fold from baseline *or* increase in SCr to ≥4.0 mg/dL (≥353.6 µmol/L) *or* initiation of RRT In patients <18 yr, decrease in estimated GFR to <35 mL/min/1.73 m²	<0.3 mL/kg/hr for 24 hr or anuria for 12 hr
Loss Complete loss of kidney function >4 weeks			
ESRD ESRD >3 months			

AKIN, Acute Kidney Injury Network; *ESRD*, end-stage renal disease; *GFR*, glomerular filtration rate; *KDIGO*, Kidney Disease: Improving Global Outcomes; *RIFLE*, Risk, Injury, Failure, Loss, and End-stage renal disease; *RRT*, renal replacement therapy; *Scr*, serum creatinine; *UOP*, urinary output.

In contrast to RIFLE, in AKIN an individual's baseline SCr is not estimated. Indeed, the AKIN classification requires two SCr measurements: one initial (corresponding to the baseline in RIFLE) and a second obtained after 48 hours.[11] Finally, patients who received RRT were included in the highest level of the staging system, regardless of their SCr or UOP at the time that RRT was started.[2]

Kidney Disease: Improving Global Outcomes Classification

More recently, the Kidney Disease: Improving Global Outcomes (KDIGO) AKIN group[5] proposed additional changes in AKI staging (see Table 55-1). This classification covers the AKIN and RIFLE criteria, incorporating changes in SCr within 48 hours or a decline in the GFR over 7 days. Moreover, to simplify the staging of AKI for patients reaching Stage 3 with SCr criteria (SCr >4.0 mg/dL [>354 µmol/L]), KDIGO requires that the patient first achieve the change in SCr specified in the AKI definition (either >0.3 mg/dL [>26.5 µmol/L] within a 48-hour time window or an increase of >1.5 times baseline). For pediatric patients, including infants and children with low muscle mass who may not reach an SCr of 4.0 mg/dL (354 µmol/L), the criteria used a change in estimated creatinine clearance (eCrCl) based on the Schwartz formula. These patients automatically reach Stage 3 if they have an eCrCl < 35 mL/min per 1.73 m².[5]

Limitations of Clinical Classifications

Although the definition, diagnosis, and staging of AKI is currently as detailed as previously mentioned, several confounding factors may affect the clinical reliability of these markers. In particular, drugs such as diuretics and the concomitant presence of tubular damage may reduce the sensitivity and specificity of UOP. Hydration status may highly affect UOP and SCr in critical care patients. Indeed, fluid loading may dilute SCr, delaying diagnosis [1] or producing an "atypical AKI."[5] Moreover, SCr mainly depends on nonrenal factors such as age, gender, and muscle mass. Creatinine metabolism varies widely during AKI, and clearance is altered by treatment with several drugs (e.g., cimetidine).[12] Creatinine is freely filtered through the glomerulus and partially secreted in the proximal tubules (10% to 20% of the urinary excreted load). Thus use of creatinine clearance will overestimate GFR. The contribution of tubular creatinine secretion to clearance may reach 50% when GFR is reduced, and this process is highly variable among individuals. In contrast, the tubules increase reabsorption of creatinine in clinical settings, such as decompensated heart failure and uncontrolled diabetes.[1]

In addition, the renal functional reserve maintains SCr within the normal range until at least 50% of nephrons have been lost, mainly through recruitment and hyperfiltration of undamaged nephrons. Finally, in the RIFLE, AKIN, and KDIGO classifications, the SCr and UOP criteria require specific changes over a specific period of time. Major clinical repercussions may lead to deviations that hamper these specific characteristics, making the diagnosis and staging of AKI through these clinical classifications retrospective[12] (see Fig. 55-1).

SUBCLINICAL ACUTE KIDNEY INJURY

Only recently has kidney damage without glomerular function loss been identified and its presence associated with worse renal and overall outcomes. This condition

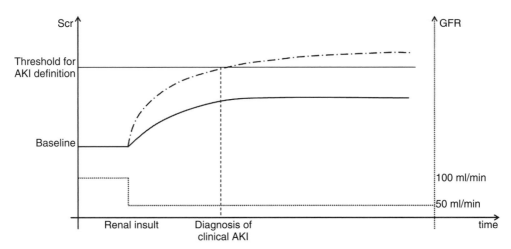

Figure 55-1. Clinical and subclinical acute kidney injury (*AKI*) diagnosis after an acute decrease of glomerular filtration rate (*GFR*) (*dotted line*) from 100 to 50 mL/min because of a renal insult. The subsequent increase in serum creatinine (*SCr*) concentration (*dot-dashed line*) requires a specific period of time to reach the threshold value to diagnose AKI, and the clinical identification of this syndrome is practically delayed. Moreover, if a patient who undergoes fluid resuscitation is considered (*continuous line*), the dilution of SCr may further delay the diagnosis of clinical AKI or may avoid reaching the threshold value to diagnose AKI ("atypical AKI").

has been termed *subclinical AKI,* and it has challenged the traditional view that kidney dysfunction is clinically relevant only when there is loss of filtration (i.e., kidney dysfunction),[13] making diagnosis with the RIFLE, AKIN, or KDIGO classifications possible. Conversely, if a metabolic stressor (e.g., iodinated contrast media, nephrotoxic drugs, mediators of systemic inflammation during sepsis, etc.) is applied, kidney damage that is not reflected in SCr or UOP may occur, especially in the early phase. Damage that does not alter SCr or UOP has been termed "subclinical AKI." Prolonged stress may increase kidney damage until the condition reduces GFR and thus becomes clinically manifest as kidney dysfunction.[14]

Subclinical AKI may also lead to the development of complications and worse outcome. If subclinical AKI cannot be prevented, then it should be identified and treated as early as possible. This process requires the measurement of specific biomarkers of kidney damage.[15] The use of biomarkers could more fully delineate an acute kidney syndrome, the entire spectrum of which would encompass subclinical kidney damage and clinical kidney dysfunction.[16] A recently proposed, more generic term, *kidney attack,* highlights the importance of all clinical and subclinical presentations of AKI, including loss of nephrons and functional reserve and their relation to the patient outcome.[17]

BIOMARKERS OF KIDNEY DAMAGE

Transcriptomic and proteomic techniques have identified several potential biomarkers of AKI. These include, but are not limited to, neutrophil gelatinase-associated lipocalin (NGAL), cystatin-C (Cys-C), kidney injury molecule-1 (KIM-1), interleukin-18 (IL-18), liver-type fatty acid binding protein, or *N*-acetyl-β-D-glucosaminidase (NAG). These molecules or proteins are produced primarily outside of the kidney and may be released into the systemic circulation during an insult to the renal parenchyma.[18] The biological roles of these biomarkers may be enzymatic, inflammatory, or structural. Biomarkers may be low molecular weight

molecules that are physiologically filtered through the glomerular barrier and catabolized in the healthy tubular epithelium (as Cys-C).[12]

Specific Biomarkers

NGAL is a protein derived from human neutrophils and exists as a 25-kDa monomer, a 45-kDa homodimer, or conjugated to gelatinase as a 135-kDa heterodimer.[19] The monomeric and heterodimeric forms are produced primarily by tubular epithelial cells, whereas the homodimeric forms are mainly synthesized by activated neutrophils.[20] The circulating NGAL is filtered through the glomerular barrier and reabsorbed through megalin-facilitated endocytosis. Urinary albumin may act as a competitive inhibitor, reducing the effectiveness of reabsorption and falsely increasing the biomarker's urine concentrations.[21] A similar effect is observed in other biomarkers (e.g., Cys-C or KIM-1) that are reabsorbed through the megalin receptor.

Cys-C is a 13-kDa protein produced by all nucleated cells. It is not bound by plasma proteins and is completely filtered at the glomerulus; thus, it is reabsorbed in the proximal tubules. In contrast to creatinine, it is not secreted into the urine by the tubules.[21] Consequently, higher urinary values during AKI mainly reflect the Cys-C glomerular filtration and a reduced reabsorption by damaged proximal tubules.[22] Urine Cys-C appears to be an earlier and more sensitive marker of AKI when compared with serum Cys-C. However, the blood concentration of Cys-C correlates with GFR in a range in which SCr is insensitive (60 to 90 mL/min).[23]

KIM-1 is a type I cell membrane glycoprotein of which soluble ectodomain (~90 kDa) is shed by a metalloproteinase-dependent process; thus, it becomes detectable in the urine during AKI.[21] During kidney injury, KIM-1 may facilitate remodeling of injured epithelia by increasing phagocytosis of apoptotic cells.[21]

IL-18 is an 18-kDa molecule produced by mononuclear cells, macrophages, and nonimmune cells including proximal tubule cells, its presumed source during acute ischemic AKI.[21] In an obstructive AKI model, IL-18 activated epithelial FasL, increasing expression of caspase-3 and caspase-8.[24]

NAG is a large (~140 kDa) protein that originates from lysosomes in proximal tubule cells. Its high molecular weight precludes glomerular filtration; therefore high urinary levels are unlikely to originate from a nonrenal source. NAG correlates with histologic evidence of proximal tubule injury and with renal recovery during treatment. Urinary NAG at ICU admission correlates with outcome in critically ill patients.[21]

Clinical Uses

Several studies have examined AKI detection, differential diagnosis, staging, and follow-up using biomarkers. Most of these studies were performed in patients undergoing cardiac surgery, in which the timing of the major insult is clear. In the TRIBE (Translational Research Investigating Biomarker Endpoints) study, performed on more than 1200 patients mainly undergoing elective on-pump coronary revascularization, authors reported higher concentrations of urinary IL-18 and of urinary and plasmatic NGAL in patients who went on to have clinical AKI within 6 hours of ICU admission. These biomarkers identified AKI at least 24 hours before it could be diagnosed clinically (receiver operator characteristic area under the curve [ROC-AUC] of 0.74, 0.67, and 0.7, respectively, for urinary IL-18 and urinary and plasma NGAL).[25,26] Similar results were obtained in critically ill patients. Biomarkers also predicted the need for RRT at ICU admission or in the emergency department. In this context, the tenth ADQI consensus conferences suggested that high-risk patients have biomarkers measured at ICU admission and followed over the course of care.[12] Several studies indicate that biomarkers of kidney damage also provide information above and beyond the simple prediction of AKI. Indeed, biomarkers provide additional prognostic information on the severity and duration of AKI, the need for RRT, the occurrence of delayed or nonrecovery of kidney function, and mortality.[26]

The combined use of clinical classification and biomarkers of AKI enables a more accurate and useful differential diagnosis on etiology and mechanisms leading to AKI.[14] For example, a functional reduction without evidence of kidney damage (biomarkers negative) may be used to improve clinical categorization in what is currently called "prerenal azotemia" (i.e., a volume-responsive and reversible alteration in kidney function).[27] Isolated kidney dysfunction without evidence of kidney damage is also recognized early in "postrenal" obstructive disease. Use of biomarkers could focus attention on the time-sensitive reversibility of this condition before actual damage.[14] Indeed, renal biomarkers might effectively identify the underlying pathophysiology and sequence of events during AKI, without restricting the differential diagnosis to merely anatomic prerenal, intrarenal, and postrenal categories.[14] However, it is important to note that threshold values for these biomarkers are lacking; thus further testing and validation are required.[14] Indeed, the recent ADQI Consensus Conference suggestions, as well as KDIGO recommendations, clearly affirm that SCr and UOP remain the best markers of renal injury.[12]

It has been suggested that biomarkers could be used to inform the decision to initiate renal support therapy.[28] However, this process remains challenging[29] because consensus criteria do not exist and there are methodological concerns with most studies. Considering that different biomarkers may have varying kinetics after AKI, timing of specimen collection with respect to the main kidney insult may significantly affect their predictive value. Moreover, the number of days between the increase in biomarkers and RRT initiation has not been reported in several studies, and among studies reporting these data, a broad difference has usually been shown. Finally, there are no cutoff values for individual biomarkers that specifically suggest the need for RRT in different clinical settings. Thus, to date, no recommendations or suggestions regarding the use of biomarkers for early and appropriate initiation of RRT have been advanced.[29]

For misinterpretations of results to be avoided and for management of patients with AKI to be improved, variables that may alter biomarker sensitivity and specificity (e.g., chronic kidney disease,[30] albuminuria,[31] or the concomitant presence of systemic illness[32]) should be considered in clinical practice.

BIOMARKERS OF CELL-CYCLE ARREST

Urinary insulin-like growth factor binding protein-7 (IGFBP-7) and urinary tissue inhibitor of metalloproteinase-2 (TIMP-2) are recently identified biomarkers of AKI.[33] Both of these molecules are involved in G1 cell-cycle arrest during the early phases of cell injury. As in other cell types, renal tubular cells enter a short period of cell-cycle arrest after injury in experimental models of sepsis[34] or ischemia.[35] This process should stop cells from dividing when their DNA is damaged. Existing biomarkers that identify damage to renal cells include TIMP-2 and IGFBP-7. In these conditions, the cell may be still able to recover without permanent injury if stressor mechanisms are removed.[33]

Kashani et al. validated the combination of these biomarkers in a prospective cohort of 728 critically ill patients (the Sapphir study) and compared their predictive value to other biomarkers. They found an ROC-AUC of 0.80 for development of AKI, a value significantly better than any previously examined biomarker ($P < .002$). Moreover, the performance of cell-cycle arrest biomarkers was independent of concomitant severe systemic conditions such as sepsis or comorbidities such as chronic kidney disease. Moreover, in an observational study on patients undergoing cardiac surgery, Meersch et al. demonstrated that cell-cycle biomarkers correlated with renal recovery (ROC-AUC = 0.79).[36]

CONCLUSIONS

- AKI is a frequently observed condition associated with poor outcome in critically ill patients. Early diagnosis and appropriate treatment of AKI may improve outcome.
- The diagnosis of AKI is currently based on clinical identification of a reduction in GFR, most often reflected in an increase in SCr and/or a reduction in UOP. However,

there are significant limitations in these parameters that may impair the diagnosis of AKI.

- Kidney dysfunction may involve only a functional alteration or it may be associated with anatomical alterations in nephrons (i.e., kidney damage). However, even clinically undetectable (subclinical) AKI may be associated with poorer outcome, a fact that should be taken into account in clinical practice.
- Biomarkers of kidney damage are currently the only indices capable of recognizing subclinical AKI.
- Evidence in the literature indicates that biomarkers of AKI may be present 24 to 48 hours before clinical diagnosis of AKI is possible. Thus, we propose that they be used for early diagnosis of this clinical syndrome. However, although several studies demonstrated a correlation between these biomarkers and adverse outcomes, both renal and nonrenal, current limitations prevent their routine use in clinical decision-making.

AUTHORS' RECOMMENDATIONS

- It is important to recognize that several factors can reduce the sensitivity and specificity of SCr and UOP to detect AKI. Therefore it is prudent to assume that a critically ill patient has already developed AKI and manage accordingly rather than wait for overt clinical manifestations.
- Use of biomarkers of kidney damage to identify subclinical AKI should be considered in all high-risk patients.
- During clinical AKI, measurement of specific biomarkers is necessary to determine if kidney dysfunction is associated with kidney damage.

REFERENCES

1. Endre ZH, Pickering JW, Walker RJ. Clearance and beyond: the complementary roles of GFR measurement and injury biomarkers in acute kidney injury (AKI). *Am J Physiol Renal Physiol.* 2011;301:F697–F707.
2. Valette X, du Cheyron D. A critical appraisal of the accuracy of the RIFLE and AKIN classifications in defining "acute kidney insufficiency" in critically ill patients. *J Crit Care.* 2013;28:116–125.
3. Thadhani R, Pascual M, Bonventre J. Acute renal failure. *N Engl J Med.* 1996;334:1448–1460.
4. Ricci Z, Ronco C. New insights in acute kidney failure in the critically ill. *Swiss Med Wkly.* 2012;142.
5. Kidney Disease: Improving Global Outcomes (KDIGO). Acute Kidney Injury Work Group: KDIGO clinical practice guideline for acute kidney injury. *Kidney Int Suppl.* 2012;2:1–138.
6. Wlodzimirow K, Abu-Hanna A, Slabbekoorn M, et al. A comparison of RIFLE with and without urine output criteria for acute kidney injury in critically ills. *Crit Care.* 2012;16:R200.
7. Bellomo R, Ronco C, Kellum J, et al. Acute renal failure - definition, outcome measures, animal models, fluid therapy and information technology needs: the Second International Consensus Conference of the Acute Dialysis Quality Initiative (ADQI) Group. *Crit Care.* 2004;8:R204–R212.
8. Mehta RL, Kellum J, Shah SV, et al. Acute Kidney Injury Network: report of an initiative to improve outcomes in acute kidney injury. *Crit Care.* 2007;11:R31.
9. Lassnigg A, Schmidlin D, Mouhieddine M, et al. Minimal changes of serum creatinine predict prognosis in patients after cardiothoracic surgery: a prospective cohort study. *J Am Soc Nephrol.* 2004;15:1597–1605.
10. Chertow GM, Burdick E, Honour M, et al. Acute kidney injury, mortality, length of stay, and costs in hospitalized patients. *J Am Soc Nephrol.* 2005;16:3365–3370.
11. Levi TM, de Souza SP, de Magalhães JG, et al. Comparison of the RIFLE, AKIN and KDIGO criteria to predict mortality in critically ill patients. *Rev Bras Ter intensiva.* 2013;25:290–296.
12. McCullough P, Shaw A, Haase M, et al. Diagnosis of acute kidney injury using functional and injury biomarkers: workgroup statements from the tenth Acute Dialysis Quality Initiative Consensus Conference. *Contrib Nephrol.* 2013;182:13–29.
13. Ronco C, Kellum J, Haase M. Subclinical AKI is still AKI. *Crit Care.* 2012;16:313.
14. Murray P, Mehta R, Shaw A, et al. Potential use of biomarkers in acute kidney injury: report and summary of recommendations from the 10th Acute Dialysis Quality Initiative consensus conference. *Kidney Int.* 2014;85:513–521.
15. Ronco C. Kidney attack: overdiagnosis of acute kidney injury or comprehensive definition of acute kidney syndromes. *Blood Purif.* 2013;36:65–68.
16. Ronco C, McCullough P, Chawla L. Kidney attack versus heart attack: evolution of classification and diagnostic criteria. *Lancet.* 2013;382:939–940.
17. Kellum JA, Bellomo R, Ronco C. Kidney Attack. *JAMA.* 2012;307:2265–2266.
18. McIlroy D, Wagener G, Lee H. Biomarkers of acute kidney injury: an evolving domain. *Anesthesiology.* 2010;112:998–1004.
19. Kjeldsen L, Johnsen A, Sengeløv H, et al. Isolation and primary structure of NGAL, a novel protein associated with human neutrophil gelatinase. *J Biol Chem.* 1993;268:10425–10432.
20. Mårtensson J, Bellomo R. The rise and fall of NGAL in acute kidney injury. *Blood Purif.* 2014;37:304–310.
21. Charlton JR, Portilla D, Okusa MD. A basic science view of acute kidney injury biomarkers. *Nephrol Dial Transplant.* 2014;29:1301–1311.
22. Vanmassenhove J, Vanholder R, Nagler E, et al. Urinary and serum biomarkers for the diagnosis of acute kidney injury: an in-depth review of the literature. *Nephrol Dial Transplant.* 2013;28:254–273.
23. Herget-rosenthal S, Bökenkamp A, Hofmann W. How to estimate GFR-serum creatinine, serum cystatin C or equations? *Clin Biochem.* 2007;40:153–161.
24. Zhang H, Hile KL, Asanuma H, et al. IL-18 mediates proapoptotic signaling in renal tubular cells through a Fas ligand-dependent mechanism. *Am J Physiol Ren Physiol.* 2011;310:F171–F178.
25. Parikh CR, Coca SG, Thiessen-philbrook H, et al. Postoperative biomarkers predict acute kidney injury and poor outcomes after adult cardiac surgery. *J Am Soc Nephrol.* 2011;22:1748–1757.
26. Parikh CR, Devarajan P, Zappitelli M, et al. Postoperative biomarkers predict acute kidney injury and poor outcomes after pediatric cardiac surgery. *J Am Soc Nephrol.* 2011;22:1737–1747.
27. Himmelfarb J, Ikizler T. Acute kidney injury: changing lexicography, definitions, and epidemiology. *Kidney Int.* 2007;71:971–976.
28. Cruz D, Bagshaw S, Maisel A, et al. Use of biomarkers to assess prognosis and guide management of patients with acute kidney injury. *Contrib Nephrol.* 2013;182:45–64.
29. Cruz DN, Geus De HR, Bagshaw SM. Biomarker strategies to predict need for renal replacement therapy in acute kidney injury. *Semin Dial.* 2011;24:124–131.
30. Mcilroy DR, Wagener G, Lee HT. Neutrophil gelatinase-associated lipocalin and acute kidney injury after cardiac surgery: the effect of baseline renal function on diagnostic performance. *Clin J Am Soc Nephrol.* 2010;5:211–219.
31. Nejat M, Hill JV, Pickering JW, et al. Albuminuria increases cystatin C excretion: implications for urinary biomarkers. *Nephrol Dial Transplant.* 2012;27:96–103.
32. Doi K, Negishi K, Ishizu T, et al. Evaluation of new acute kidney injury biomarkers in a mixed intensive care unit. *Crit Care Med.* November 2011;39:2464–2469.
33. Kashani K, Al-khafaji A, Ardiles T, et al. Discovery and validation of cell cycle arrest biomarkers in human acute kidney injury. *Crit Care.* 2013;17:R25.
34. Yang Q, Liu D, Long Y, et al. Acute renal failure during sepsis: potential role of cell cycle regulation. *J Infect.* 2009;58:459–464.
35. Witzgall R, Brown D, Schwarz C, et al. Localization of proliferating cell nuclear antigen, vimentin, c-Fos, and clusterin in the postischemic kidney. *J Clin Invest.* 1994;93:2175–2188.
36. Meersch M, Schmidt C, Van Aken H, et al. Urinary TIMP-2 and IGFBP7 as early biomarkers of acute kidney injury and renal recovery following cardiac surgery. *PLoS One.* 2014;9. http://dx.doi.org/10.1371/journal.pone.0093460.

How Does One Optimize Care in Patients at Risk for or Presenting with Acute Kidney Injury?

Celina D. Cepeda, Josée Bouchard, Ravindra L. Mehta

Acute kidney injury (AKI) is common in the intensive care unit (ICU) and is associated with poor outcomes. There is evidence that even minor short-term changes in serum creatinine (i.e., ≥0.3 mg/dL or 26 μmol/L) are linked to increased morbidity and mortality, and early intervention may be of benefit.[1,2] It is important for ICU physicians to recognize AKI, assess its reversibility, and institute timely interventions to prevent further kidney damage and facilitate complete recovery. This chapter provides an overview of current and emerging strategies to optimize care for patients with AKI with an ultimate goal to improve outcomes from this disease.

EVALUATION

History and Physical Examination

A careful history and physical examination are keystones for evaluating patients suspected to have AKI. Underlying risk factors for AKI should be documented, including chronic kidney disease (CKD), heart failure, cirrhosis, pulmonary disease, and diabetes mellitus.[3] In the pediatric population, risk factors for AKI include being in the ICU, multiorgan dysfunction, exposure to nephrotoxic agents, hypoxemia, thrombocytopenia, and neurologic dysfunction.[3] Recent studies have designated a renal angina index (RAI) as a method to identify patients who are at high risk for AKI (Table 56-1). In combination with acute events, the RAI has a good performance in predicting the development and severity of AKI. Basu et al. have validated the RAI, and more recently have incorporated AKI biomarkers, including neutrophil gelatinase-associated lipocalin (NGAL), into the RAI and found improvement in discrimination for severe AKI.[4-6] Precipitating factors for AKI should be identified (Table 56-2). Imaging with radiocontrast, surgery, trauma, recent illnesses, and systemic complaints should be specifically documented.

As the movement toward electronic health records continues, it is feasible to use electronic reporting to identify and monitor patients at risk of or who have AKI. Selby et al. reported the implementation of a hospital-wide electronic reporting system to aid in the early recognition of AKI based on Acute Kidney Injury Network (AKIN) criteria (Table 56-3). Along with alerts to physicians about elevations in creatinine, AKI stages, AKI clinical guidelines, and AKIN diagnostic criteria were provided. The authors believe implementation of such an alert system could help raise the standard of care across all acute specialties involved in the care of patients with AKI.[7] Colpaert et al. were able to implement an electronic alert based on RIFLE (Risk, Injury, Failure, Loss of kidney function, and End-stage kidney disease) criteria in a single ICU where physicians were notified of patients' worsening kidney function (Table 56-3).[9] A multicenter Italian study to look at the epidemiology of AKI in the ICU developed a data collection tool with a RIFLE class alert system. The authors believe it could be used to help physicians gather AKI data and guide decision-making for institution of renal replacement therapy (RRT).[10]

Laboratory Studies

Laboratory studies are useful to recognize and confirm AKI, assess functional changes and kidney damage, and

Table 56-1 Renal Angina Index

RISK		INJURY		
Risk	Score	↓ eCCl	% FO	Score
Moderate (PICU admission)	1	No change	<5%	1
High (solid-organ or bone marrow transplant)	2	↓ 0%-25%	≥5%	2
Ventilation and inotropy (intubation + at least one vasopressor or inotrope)	3	↓ 25%-50%	≥10%	4
		↓ ≥50%	≥15%	8

Renal angina is the risk of AKI × signs of injury. Injury score is based on the worst parameter, either ↓ eCCl or % FO.
Score ranges from 1 to 40. AKI rates are higher in patients with a score of ≥8.
AKI, acute kidney injury; *eCCl,* estimated creatinine clearance; *FO,* fluid overload; *PICU,* pediatric intensive care unit.

aid with the differential diagnosis. Oliguria has been validated as a diagnostic criterion for AKI, and its magnitude and duration are used to classify and stratify the severity of AKI.[11,12] A study by Mandelbaum et al. in ICU patients observed for 1 to 7 days found that mortality increased quickly as urine output (UO) decreased below 0.5 mL/kg/hr and was higher when oliguria was prolonged.[13,14] Currently in development are electronic monitoring sensors of urine flow that could aid clinicians to use UO as tool to improve AKI management. One caveat is to recognize that oliguria can be a normal response to a prerenal state and may not be due to kidney damage.[14] Anuria is a relatively late event and occurs when glomerular filtration ceases or if there is complete urinary obstruction.[3]

Urinalysis (UA) and microscopy are helpful to determine the cause of AKI (see Table 56-4). With reversible renal functional changes, a concentrated urine with high specific gravity and acidic pH are usually noted and cellular elements and casts are generally lacking. An abnormal UA with proteinuria, hematuria, and/or casts suggests an intrinsic renal cause for AKI.[3]

If the UA reveals protein, then a urine protein-to-urine creatinine ratio or a 24-hour urine sample for protein should be checked. The ratio can be used to rule out significant proteinuria because it is not affected by a patient's hydration status and correlates well with a 24-hour urine sample for protein. In general, a cutoff ratio greater than 0.2 would signify the need for a 24-hour urine sample for quantification of protein.[15,16] A 24-hour urine protein greater than 2 g/day in adults and 4 mg/m²/hr in children suggests a glomerular cause for AKI.[3,17] Measurement of urine creatinine and urine urea nitrogen should be simultaneously obtained to calculate urinary clearances in addition to proteinuria.

Urine microscopy is helpful by revealing the presence of cells, casts, and/or crystals. Blood detected on UA in the absence of red blood cells (RBCs) supports pigment nephropathy diagnosis. Muddy brown granular casts are associated with acute tubular necrosis (ATN), but there could be another cause for AKI in addition, such as vasculitis. Pyelonephritis is usually associated with numerous white blood cells (WBCs). Acute or allergic interstitial nephritis (AIN) can also lead to WBCs and WBC casts in the urine.[3] Classically, greater than 1% eosinophils in the urine has been used to diagnose AIN, but a recent study by Muriithi et al. found that urine eosinophils were present in practically all causes of AKI. The 1% cutoff value has poor sensitivity and likelihood ratios, and even a cutoff of 5% did not readily distinguish AIN from ATN or other kidney diseases.[18] In 2008, Chawla et al. developed an AKI cast scoring index (CSI) based on the number and percentage of granular casts or epithelial cell casts seen per low-power field and found that CSI was higher in patients without renal recovery versus those with recovery, suggesting CSI could aid in predicting renal outcome.[19] In the study by Perazella et al., a urinary sediment

Table 56-2 Factors Precipitating AKI

Patient Factors/Exposures	Procedures
Volume depletion	Cardiopulmonary bypass
Sepsis	Surgery involving aortic clamp
Nephrotoxins/contrast material	Increased intra-abdominal pressure
Hypertension	Large arterial catheter placement with risk for atheroembolization
Hypotension	Liver transplantation
Multiorgan failure	Kidney transplantation
Invasive mechanical ventilation	Stem cell transplantation
Neurologic dysfunction	

AKI, acute kidney injury.

Table 56-3 AKI Staging Criteria

Stage		RIFLE	AKIN	KDIGO
1 (Risk in RIFLE)	SCr	↑ × 1.5 or GFR >25%	↑ × 1.5-2 or ↑ ≥0.3 mg/dL	1.5-1.9 × baseline or ↑ ≥ 0.3 mg/dL
	UO	<0.5 mL/kg/hr × 6-12 hr		
2 (Injury in RIFLE)	SCr	↑ × 2 or GFR >50%	↑ SCr × > 2-3	2-2.9 baseline
	UO	<0.5 mL/kg/hr × ≥12 hr		
3 (Failure in RIFLE)	SCr	↑ × 3 or GFR >75% or if baseline SCr ≥4 mg/dL ↑ >0.5 mg/dL	↑ SCr × >3 or if baseline SCr ≥4 mg/dL ↑ ≥0.5 mg/dL	3 × baseline or ↑ ≥4 mg/dL or in patients <18 yr ↓ in estimated GFR to <35 mL/min/1.73 m²
			Patients receiving RRT are considered to have met stage 3 criteria, irrespective of stage they are in at time of RRT	
	UO	<0.3 mL/kg/hr × ≥ 24 hr or anuria ×12 hr		
4 (Loss in RIFLE)		Complete loss of renal function >4 weeks		
5 (End-stage in RIFLE)		Complete loss of kidney function >3 months		

AKI, acute kidney injury; *AKIN,* Acute Kidney Injury Network; *KDIGO,* Kidney Disease: Improving Global Outcomes; *RIFLE,* Risk, Injury, Failure, Loss of kidney function, and End-stage kidney disease; *RRT,* renal replacement therapy; *SCr,* serum creatinine; *UO,* urine output.

scoring system was devised based on the number of renal tubular epithelial cells and granular casts. Scores correlated with AKIN stages of AKI and may be able to predict worsening of AKI due to ATN or prerenal AKI during hospitalization.[20] Limitations to using scoring systems such as these include standardization of the approach and reproducibility across various users.

Urine sodium concentration, fractional excretion of sodium (FeNa), and fractional excretion of urea (FeUN) are common tools to differentiate between prerenal disease and ATN (Table 56-1). FeNa helps differentiate between prerenal AKI and AKI due to ATN (intrinsic renal problem, as opposed to prerenal problem). An FeNa value below 1% is suggestive of prerenal AKI, and a value higher than 2% typically indicates ATN. A marked decrease in FeNa in patients with ATN can suggest superimposed prerenal disease.

However, FeNa can be falsely elevated by diuretics and preexisting CKD, and it may be falsely low in congestive heart failure, hepatic failure, severe burns, sepsis, rhabdomyolysis, and contrast nephropathy, among others. FeUN is not altered by prior diuretic use, and a cutoff value of 35% or less is usually consistent with a prerenal state. Dewitte et al. found FeUN to be a sensitive and specific index for distinguishing between transient and persistent AKI, but other studies have not found it or FeNa to be helpful.[22-24]

Serum creatinine often used in conjunction with blood urea nitrogen (BUN) is the standard biomarker that is used to detect AKI. A BUN-to-creatinine ratio greater than 20:1 often suggests a prerenal cause for AKI and therefore better prognosis. However, Rachoin et al. found that a ratio greater than 20 was associated with increased mortality; they surmised the higher BUN was likely due to increased protein

Table 56-4 Urinary Findings

UA	Components	Sensitivity/Specificity (S/S)	Comments
Hematuria	Eumorphic RBC		Lower urinary tract source, malignancy
Hematuria	Dysmorphic RBC or RBC casts		Glomerular source of bleeding
Hematuria	No RBC Muddy brown granular casts		Pigment nephropathy ATN, vasculitis
Leukocyte esterase	WBC		Pyelonephritis
Leukocyte esterase	WBC and/or WBC casts (eosinophils)	Differentiating AIN from ATN[18]: • 30.8%/71% Differentiating drug-induced AIN from ATN[18]: • 35.6%/71%	Classically >1% eosinophils suggests AIN
	FeNa, % $\dfrac{\text{Urine sodium concentration} \times \text{plasma creatinine}}{\text{Plasma sodium concentration} \times \text{urine creatinine concentration}} \times 100$	Predicting transient AKI in ICU FeNa <1%[22]: • No diuretics 39%/71% • With diuretics 27%/69% Predicting persistent AKI in ICU FeNa >1%[24]: • No diuretics 48%/70% • With diuretics 75%/56%	Usual cutoff: <1% prerenal >2% ATN Falsely elevated: Diuretic use, CKD Falsely low: congestive heart failure, hepatic failure, severe burns, sepsis, rhabdomyolysis, contrast nephropathy
	FeUN, % $\dfrac{\text{Urine urea nitrogen concentration} \times \text{plasma creatinine}}{\text{Blood urea nitrogen concentration} \times \text{urine creatinine concentration}} \times 100$	S/S predicting transient AKI in ICU FeUN <40%[22]: • No diuretics 83%/75% • With diuretics 80%/85% S/S detecting persistent AKI in ICU FeUN <35%[24]: • No diuretics 63%/54% • With diuretics 61%/56% S/S detecting persistent AKI in ICU FeUN <40%[23]: • 24%/56%	Usual cutoff: <35% prerenal Not affected by diuretic use
Protein	Urine protein/creatinine ratio	For abnormal urine protein excretion In adults[15]: • 69%-96%/41%-97% In children[16]: • 96.6%/96.3%	>0.21 abnormal
Protein	24-hr urine protein		2 g/day adult, 4 mg/m²/hr child suggest glomerular disease

AIN, acute or allergic interstitial nephritis; *AKI*, acute kidney injury; *ATN*, acute tubular necrosis; *CKD*, chronic kidney disease; *FeNA*, fractional excretion of sodium; *FeUN*, fractional excretion of urea; *ICU*, intensive care unit; *RBC*, red blood cells; *UA*, urinalysis; *WBC*, white blood cells.

catabolism and lower serum creatinine from decreased muscle mass in the older female patients studied.[25] BUN is affected by nutrition (protein intake and catabolism) and may be elevated by bleeding and steroid treatment or low in advanced liver disease. Creatinine is affected by muscle mass, age, race, and gender. Lower values in children, the elderly, and those with disabilities may fall within a laboratory's normal range but still be "abnormal" compared with baseline values.[26] In addition, creatinine is affected by the volume of distribution. Macedo et al. evaluated the effect of fluid accumulation on serum creatinine to estimate AKI severity in ICU patients and found that dilution due to net positive fluid balance led to underestimation of AKI severity. Serum creatinine should be corrected for the accumulated fluid using the simple formula for a more accurate determination of AKI severity in ICU patients.[27] More recently, Pickering et al. combined creatinine and volume kinetics to quantify changes in glomerular filtration rate (GFR) in ICU patients. Serum creatinine underestimation was influenced by fluid infusion rate, crystalloid versus colloid fluid, serum creatinine sample timing in relation to fluid infusion timing, and excess fluid urine excretion rate. They suggest delaying blood sampling to an hour after a large bolus and obtaining kidney injury biomarkers if serum creatinine does not decrease after 4 hours in clinical practice.[28]

Cystatin C is a cysteine protease inhibitor produced by all nucleated cells. Unlike creatinine, it is not affected by muscle mass, age, race, or gender, and its urinary excretion marks renal dysfunction that correlates with the severity of acute tubular injury. Studies have shown that cystatin C increases occur up to 2 days before creatinine increases. Cystatin C is also better at picking up smaller changes in GFR than creatinine. However, its levels are affected by thyroid dysfunction, obesity, inflammation, and steroid use.[26,29]

Because creatinine is a late marker of renal dysfunction, other biomarkers have been sought.[26,29,30] In a meta-analysis of 19 studies that included adults and children in different settings, NGAL was a useful early marker of AKI and in predicting the need for dialysis and mortality. However, its limitations include its abundant extrarenal expression in systemic stress without the presence of AKI, its higher level in patients with underlying CKD, malignancies, and systemic bacterial infections. NGAL also seems to be less sensitive and specific in cases in which AKI is due to multiple factors.[26,29,30]

Another biomarker being studied is human kidney injury molecule-1. This transmembrane protein is not found in the normal kidney, but it is quickly and highly expressed and excreted by the proximal tubular epithelium when there is ischemic or toxic damage; it persists in cells until their full recovery.[26] Its expression has also been found to be associated with the need for dialysis and death.[26,29,30]

Interleukin-18 (IL-18) is a proinflammatory cytokine continually expressed by cells in the distal tubule and collecting duct of healthy kidneys. It has been shown to be a marker for AKI and in predicting mortality during mechanical ventilation. However, because it is a proinflammatory cytokine, the concentration of IL-18 can be influenced by endotoxemia, inflammatory diseases, and autoimmune diseases.[26,29,30]

In September 2014, the U.S. Food and Drug Administration (FDA) approved the use of a new test, *NephroCheck* (Astute Medical), to assess the risk of ICU patients with moderate to severe AKI. The levels of two proteins in the urine, insulin-like growth-factor binding protein-7 and tissue inhibitor of metalloproteinases-2, predict the risk of a patient with AKI in the 12 hours after testing. Both markers are involved in cell cycle arrest during the early phase of cell injury, a key mechanism implicated in AKI. Kashani et al. studied more than 1000 ICU patients and showed that these two biomarkers performed better than previously known biomarkers for predicting AKI and improved risk stratification in a nine-variable clinical model.[31]

Imaging Studies

According to the American College of Radiology's Appropriateness Criteria, renal ultrasound with Doppler is the most reasonable imaging modality to evaluate patients with AKI.[32] Renal parenchymal disease can be distinguished on ultrasound by increased echogenicity (96% specificity).[33] This finding alone cannot distinguish between AKI and CKD; however, the finding along with that of small kidneys correlates well with CKD.[34] One to three percent of AKI cases in the ICU are due to obstruction, and ultrasound is the imaging choice in the evaluation for this. Most patients with obstruction will have hydronephrosis; sensitivity is nearly 100% when moderate to severe hydronephrosis is noted.[33]

Ultrasound with Doppler imaging is helpful to look at blood flow velocity by way of resistive index (RI); the larger the RI, the more resistance to blood flow during diastole.[33] Increased RI is seen in AKI due to obstruction, sepsis, and hepatorenal syndrome, among other reasons, and portends worse outcomes. Prerenal azotemia and glomerular diseases do not affect RI.[33] Vessel wall compliance, systemic vascular resistance, and heart rate are factors that can affect the RI.[33]

Contrast-enhanced ultrasound is imaging that uses microbubble-based contrast agents to look at vascular structures and detect blood flow down to the level of the capillaries.[37,38] This technique is especially sensitive and specific in detecting infarction and cortical necrosis in ischemic renal transplants, but its use in the early diagnosis of AKI remains to be determined.[37,39]

PREVENTION OF ACUTE KIDNEY INJURY

General Measures

The primary goal is to correct any reversible detrimental factors that could contribute to AKI. Detrimental factors include volume depletion, hypotension, decreased cardiac output and renal perfusion, sepsis, obstruction, high intra-abdominal pressure, and nephrotoxic agents (Table 56-5). The most common nephrotoxic agents are radiocontrast, nonsteroidal anti-inflammatory drugs (NSAIDs), and antibiotics (aminoglycosides, amphotericin, and vancomycin). These agents should be avoided if possible in patients at risk for AKI. The use of diuretics, angiotensin-receptor blockers, and angiotensin-converting enzyme inhibitors should be avoided in prerenal settings.

Table 56-5 Common Nephrotoxic Agents

- Contrast dye
- NSAIDs
- Antimicrobials
  - Acyclovir
  - Aminoglycosides
  - Amphotericin
  - Beta-lactams (penicillins, cephalosporins)
  - Vancomycin
- Angiotensin-converting enzyme inhibitors
- Angiotensin receptor blockers
- Chemotherapy drugs
  - Cisplatin
  - Methotrexate
- Diuretics
  - Loop
  - Thiazides
- Proton-pump inhibitors
  - Lansoprazole
  - Omeprazole
  - Pantoprazole
- Miscellaneous
  - Allopurinol
  - Phenytoin
  - Ranitidine

Specific Interventions (Table 56-6)

Optimizing Volume Status and Treating Hypotension

The effect of fluid expansion on hemodynamic status and renal function is often assessed by trial and error because clinical parameters are unreliable to assess volume status. In prerenal states, fluid administration can improve organ perfusion and renal function. In ischemic ATN, experimental data suggest that autoregulation is lost and that renal blood flow becomes linearly pressure dependent so that subsequent hypoperfusion due to volume depletion or vasodilatation can cause new kidney lesions.[43] In severe congestive heart failure or diastolic dysfunction, renal perfusion is inadequate despite normal volume status or volume overload. In these patients, fluid expansion can lead to worsening of cardiac function and pulmonary edema.

Unfortunately, there are no absolute guidelines on how hemodynamic and fluid status can be used to optimize renal function. Recommendations from the Surviving Sepsis Campaign can be helpful.[44] The recent randomized trial of protocol-based care for early septic shock (ProCESS), designed to examine the effects of early therapy with intravenous fluids, vasopressors, inotropes, and blood transfusions on 60-day in-hospital mortality, found incidence of renal failure (new need for RRT) to be higher in the standard protocol group, but duration of therapy was not significantly different. Overall, there was no significant advantage in morbidity or mortality and no significant benefit of central hemodynamic monitoring.[45]

Volume Expanders

There have been several studies published on the effect of different types of fluids on outcomes over the last years. The Kidney Disease: Improving Global Outcomes (KDIGO) AKI guidelines suggest that isotonic crystalloids should be used instead of synthetic (hydroxyethyl starch [HES]) and nonsynthetic colloids (albumin) for intracellular volume expansion in patients at risk or presenting with AKI in the absence of hemorrhagic shock.[3] For HES, these recommendations are supported by two large randomized controlled trials (RCTs) in severe sepsis and critically ill patients showing that HES was detrimental to kidney function and survival and increased the need for RRT.[46,47]

For albumin, the Saline versus Albumin Fluid Evaluation (SAFE) RCT, which included 6997 critically ill patients, did not demonstrate any difference in either mortality or duration of RRT with 4% (iso-oncotic) albumin versus saline.[48] However, kidney function was not independently reported, and only severe cases of AKI were collected.[49] The recently published ALBIOS (Albumin Italian Outcome Sepsis) RCT on the effect of hyperoncotic albumin (20%) versus crystalloids in hypoalbuminemic patients with severe sepsis and septic shock did not show any difference in mortality and severe AKI between the groups.[50] Importantly, the ALBIOS study differed from other studies because albumin was administered not according to the clinical context but on a daily basis if the albumin level was less than 30 g/L. The cumulative fluid balance was also lower in the albumin group. The only group in which albumin seems to be beneficial is patients with cirrhosis.[51]

Regarding crystalloids, saline infusions have been proven of benefit in RCTs to prevent the nephrotoxicity of radiocontrasts, cisplatin, and amphotericin.[52-54] Lower levels of evidence support a prompt use of saline for rhabdomyolysis.[55,56] However, in ICU patients, a retrospective study has shown that chloride-restrictive fluids (lactated solution with balanced buffer–chloride concentration of 98 mmol/L or chloride-poor 20% albumin–chloride concentration of 19 mmol/L) compared with chloride-rich intravenous fluids (0.9% saline, gelatin, or 4% albumin) were associated with a significant decrease in AKI incidence and RRT requirement.[56] These results will need to be confirmed with other studies.

Loop Diuretics, Natriuretics, and Vasoactive Agents

A few small single-center studies on the use of diuretics to prevent AKI have failed to demonstrate benefit.[3] A small RCT in high-risk cardiac surgery patients treated with prophylactic nesiritide, a B-type natriuretic peptide, did not show any effect on RRT requirement or lengths of stay, although AKI rates were lower with nesiritide.[57] Additional studies are needed on this topic. Meta-analyses including RCTs have confirmed that so-called "renal-dose" dopamine (0.5 to 3 µg/kg/min) increases UO but does not prevent AKI.[58-60] In a meta-analysis, fenoldopam, a pure dopamine type-1 receptor agonist, was shown to reduce the risk of AKI in critically ill patients.[61] However, several concerns present in this study limit confidence in the results.[61] Large RCTs are required to confirm these findings before this agent can be recommended to prevent AKI.

Statins

Statins have recently been studied in several RCTs to prevent contrast-induced acute kidney injury (CI-AKI).[62,63] In a recent meta-analysis, statins were shown to prevent CI-AKI (relative risk [RR], 0.54; 95% confidence interval [CI], 0.38 to 0.78) in patients with a glomerular filtration below and above 60 mL/min.[64] However, technical issues have raised concerns. Therefore it is unclear if statins should be prescribed to prevent CI-AKI in the absence of other indications. In a recent meta-analysis, statins did not reduce postoperative AKI when restricting the analysis to the RCTs.[65] Future RCTs are warranted to assess the role of statins to prevent postoperative AKI.

Table 56-6 **Strategies Used for Prevention of AKI**

Strategy	Effect	Comments
Crystalloids	Volume expansion	KDIGO recommendation; in absence of hemorrhagic shock[3]
Saline	Prevent nephrotoxicity due to radiocontrast, cisplatin, amphotericin[52-54]	In RCTs
Lactated Ringer's solution	Decrease in AKI incidence and RRT requirement	Retrospective study in ICU patients; fluids with lower chloride concentrations vs. higher concentrations[56]
HES	Detrimental to kidney function Increased RRT need	In severe sepsis; compared to Ringer's acetate In ICU patients[46,47]
Albumin	No difference in mortality or duration of RRT No difference in mortality or severity of AKI	SAFE RCT involved 4% albumin vs. saline[48] ALBIOS RCT used 20% albumin vs. crystalloid in hypoalbuminemic patients with severe sepsis/septic shock[50]
Loop diuretics	No effect on kidney function	Few small single-center studies[3]
Nesiritide	Lower rates of AKI; no effect on RRT requirement or hospital length of stay	Small RCT in high-risk cardiac surgery patients[57]
Dopamine	Increases UO; does not prevent AKI	Meta-analyses using "renal dose" (0.5-3 µg/kg/min)[58-60]
Fenoldopam	Reduce the risk of AKI	Meta-analysis in critically ill patients but limitations in studies[61]
Statins	Prevent CK-AKI Did not reduce AKI after major surgery	Meta-analysis in patients with GFR below and above 60 mL/min but limitations in studies[64] Meta-analysis of RCTs[65]
Insulin	Decrease AKI incidence	In medical and surgical ICU settings[66] KDIGO recommends target blood glucose 110-149 mg/dL (6.1-8.3 mmol/L)[3]
N-Acetylcysteine	Does not prevent AKI	In patients at risk or with early ATN[67-72] Used in prevention of radiocontrast AKI
Sodium bicarbonate	Does not prevent perioperative AKI after cardiac surgery	Meta-analysis[73]
Calcium-channel blockers	Some benefits on renal clearance	Demonstrated in small RCTs[75]
Multipotent mesenchymal stem cells	Maintained stable renal function after surgery	Phase I clinical trial of on-pump cardiac surgery[76]
RIPC	No effect on frequency of AKI May be beneficial to prevent AKI	RCT of patients with CKD and cardiac surgery[77] Meta-analysis in patients having cardiac/vascular surgery or percutaneous coronary interventions[78]

AKI, acute kidney injury; *ALBIOS,* Albumin Italian Outcome Sepsis; *ATN,* acute tubular necrosis; *CK-AKI,* contrast-induced acute kidney injury; *CKD,* chronic kidney disease; *GFR,* glomerular filtration rate; *ICU,* intensive care unit; *KDIGO,* Kidney Disease: Improving Global Outcomes; *RCT,* randomized controlled trial; *RIPC,* remote ischemic preconditioning; *RRT,* renal replacement therapy; *SAFE,* Saline versus Albumin Fluid Evaluation; *UO,* urine output.

Other Agents

In 2007, a meta-analysis examining the effect of insulin on the prevention of AKI pointed toward a reduction in the incidence of AKI in medical and surgical ICUs.[66] The KDIGO guidelines suggest insulin therapy targeting plasma glucose 110 to 149 mg/dL (6.1 to 8.3 mmol/L).[3] Multiple RCTs that included patients at risk for or with early ATN indicate that N-acetylcysteine is not effective in preventing AKI.[67-72] In a systematic review and meta-analysis, Tie et al. found that sodium bicarbonate did not prevent cardiac surgery–associated AKI and increased the length of ventilation and ICU stay and the risk of alkalemia.[73] A large multicenter RCT, Prevention of Serious Adverse Events

Following Angiography (PRESERVE), is currently ongoing to compare the effectiveness of intravenous isotonic sodium bicarbonate with intravenous isotonic sodium chloride and oral N-acetylcysteine with oral placebo for the prevention of serious adverse outcomes after angiographic procedures in high-risk patients.[74] Calcium channel blockers were studied in small RCTs that demonstrated some benefits on renal clearance, although no convincing data are available for the incidence of AKI.[75] Multipotent mesenchymal stem cells were assessed in a phase I clinical trial in patients undergoing on-pump cardiac surgery and seemed a promising agent because postoperative kidney function remained stable in the treatment group whereas 20% of controls had AKI.[76]

Remote Ischemic Preconditioning

In remote ischemic preconditioning (RIPC), mild and nonlethal ischemia and reperfusion to an organ or tissue protects a different organ or tissue from subsequent lethal ischemia and reperfusion injury. In a recent RCT including 86 patients with CKD undergoing cardiac surgery, RIPC had no effect on the frequency of AKI.[77] A recent meta-analysis has concluded that RIPC may be beneficial to prevent AKI in patients undergoing cardiac or vascular surgery or percutaneous coronary interventions; however, larger trials will be necessary before making any firm recommendation on the use of RIPC to prevent AKI.[78]

MANAGEMENT OF ACUTE KIDNEY INJURY

Measures used in the prevention of AKI are also applicable to established AKI. In addition, the Vasopressin in Septic Shock Trial (VASST) trial found no differences in mortality or organ dysfunction when comparing vasopressin to norepinephrine, although a post hoc analysis showed that vasopressin may reduce AKI severity in patients with AKI stage 1.[79,80]

Late and prolonged aggressive fluid resuscitation in critically ill patients with AKI has been associated with worse kidney outcomes and increased mortality in large observational studies, but no RCTs have been performed on this subject in AKI.[81,82] Nevertheless, fluid expansion should probably be stopped when patients are no longer fluid responsive.

Loop Diuretics

A meta-analysis did not support the use of loop diuretics to reduce mortality or improve renal recovery, but it did demonstrate a need for a shorter course of RRT in the setting of AKI.[83] Two meta-analyses have confirmed the lack of benefit for in-hospital mortality, the need for RRT, or a reduction in the number of dialysis sessions required, although a trend was seen in one study.[84,85] An initial cohort study of 552 patients suggested that the use of diuretics was associated with increased mortality, but a prospective multicenter epidemiologic study of 1743 patients failed to confirm this finding despite hazard ratios greater than 1.[86,87] An increased risk for ototoxicity may occur with high doses of diuretics.[84] Despite controversial data, a multinational survey on the clinical use of diuretics in AKI concluded that diuretics are often prescribed in this setting (67.1%) and are most commonly delivered intravenously in bolus.[88] Two RCTs are currently underway, but they are probably too small to provide a definite answer.

Natriuretics

Atrial natriuretic peptide (ANP) has been studied as a treatment for AKI in four RCTs.[89-92] The largest study showed that ANP did not improve overall dialysis-free survival except in oliguric patients.[90] A subsequent trial in 222 oliguric patients failed to confirm the earlier findings. Both trials used ANP for 24 hours and at high doses, which could have influenced the results. The most recent study,

which included only 61 patients after cardiac surgery and used a longer treatment period (5.3 ± 0.8 days), found a decreased probability of dialysis and an improvement in dialysis-free survival.[91] Further studies in a larger number of patients are required to determine the value of ANP in AKI. The KDIGO AKI guidelines do not support the use of nesiritide to treat AKI because there is no current evidence that its use decreases RRT requirement or mortality.[3]

Vasoactive Agents

The current evidence does not support the use of dopamine to treat AKI. In a meta-analysis published in 2005, low-dose dopamine was shown to increase UO but did not have any effect on renal dysfunction or mortality.[58] Two previous meta-analyses had confirmed these findings.[59,60]

Vasopressors are often considered detrimental to organ perfusion. A small prospective study in 14 septic patients revealed that norepinephrine had beneficial effects on creatinine clearance when raising mean arterial pressure over 70 mm Hg.[93] However, another small RCT including 28 patients did not demonstrate any benefit on creatinine or creatinine clearance by increasing mean arterial pressure from 65 to 85 mm Hg.[94]

A meta-analysis found that fenoldopam, a dopamine receptor-1 agonist that increases blood flow to the renal cortex and outer medulla, reduced the risk for AKI as previously mentioned, the need for RRT (6.5% vs. 10.4%; 95% CI, 0.34 to 0.84), and in-hospital mortality (15.1% vs. 18.9%; 95% CI, 0.45 to 0.91) in postoperative or ICU patients.[61] No single prospective study has shown that fenoldopam can reduce the need for RRT. These results need to be confirmed with an adequately powered trial before the use of fenoldopam is promoted in this setting. In an RCT, the use of fenoldopam has not been shown to reduce contrast-induced nephropathy.[96] Targeted renal delivery of fenoldopam may benefit kidney function in patients undergoing contrast procedures compared with intravenous fenoldopam.[97] RCTs are needed to support these preliminary results.

Other Agents

In a secondary outcome of an often-cited 2001 study on the use of intensive insulin therapy, the need for RRT was reduced by 41%. However, a more recent meta-analysis showed that tight glucose control did not improve mortality or new need for dialysis.[98] There are no convincing data that calcium-channel blockers can reduce the need for RRT.[75] Neither thyroid hormone nor insulin-like growth factor-1 provided benefit in AKI patients in RCTs.[99,100]

Correction of Electrolytes and Acid-Base Status

AKI limits the ability of the kidneys to maintain electrolyte and acid-base balance. In oliguric states, this equilibrium is even more difficult to achieve, justifying frequent monitoring of electrolytes to avoid severe and sometimes fatal hyperkalemia. A Cochrane meta-analysis supported the use of salbutamol and intravenous insulin and glucose alone or in combination.[101] Although there are no RCTs to support the use of ion-exchange resins and chloride calcium, ion-exchange resins were recommended in the absence of gastrointestinal disease and intravenous calcium in the presence of electrocardiogram changes or arrhythmias.[101]

Hypocalcemia and hyperphosphatemia are common in AKI. However, no randomized study has evaluated the benefits of treating these disorders. Hyperphosphatemia caused by oral phosphorus-containing medications and tumor lysis syndrome have been proposed as etiologic factors for AKI.[102,103] Thus, severe hyperphosphatemia (>6 mg/dL) should be avoided to prevent further damage. Calcium-based phosphate binders and other phosphate binders can be used in this setting along with a low-phosphate diet.

Metabolic acidosis is the most frequent acid-base disturbance in critically ill patients suffering from AKI.[104] The treatment of metabolic acidosis in AKI has never been the subject of randomized trials, and the consequences of metabolic acidosis in AKI patients are not clear. Therefore, the bicarbonate level to target is unknown. Most acid-base authorities have recommended that a pH value below 7.1 serve as a threshold to administer bicarbonate.[105,106] An online survey by Kraut and Kurtz found that 40% of intensivists would not administer bicarbonate unless pH was less than 7, whereas only 6% of nephrologists would do this. In addition, more than 80% of nephrologists considered the level of partial pressure of carbon dioxide in deciding when to treat with bicarbonate; only 59% of intensivists did this.[107] It has been suggested to administer bicarbonate to achieve an arterial pH of 7.2, but treatment should be individualized and potential complications (e.g., cardiac dysfunction, hypocalcemia, hypernatremia, volume overload) should be kept in mind.[105,106] In patients with CKD, it is recommended to maintain serum bicarbonate levels above 22 mEq/L because of the detrimental effects of acidosis on protein catabolism.[108]

Medication Dose Adjustments

In AKI, doses of drugs that are metabolized and excreted by the kidneys may need to be adjusted to prevent accumulation and toxicity.[109] One key but often misunderstood concept is that it is inappropriate to use the Cockcroft-Gault (CG) equation to estimate the GFR in the presence of AKI.[110] For example, with total renal shutdown, the creatinine level will increase by 1 to 1.5 mg/dL per day. Therefore a normal creatinine might increase from 1 to 2.5 mg/dL.[111] The calculated GFR with the CG equation would be 30 mL/min. However, the "true" GFR in this condition is 0 mL/min. Thus, when medications are adjusted for a patient with progressive AKI, the predicted GFR should be minimized to reflect the real GFR.

Other pharmacokinetic parameters are altered in renal failure. These include drug absorption, volume of distribution, protein binding, and hepatic biotransformation.[110] Thus, dosage may be altered by factors other than GFR, and adjustments must reflect this.

Gadolinium-Based Contrast Agents

Gadolinium-based contrast agents are commonly used for magnetic resonance imaging. These agents have been linked to nephrogenic systemic fibrosis.[112] In addition, gadolinium chelates may cause pseudohypocalcemia and may be nephrotoxic, especially in CKD.[113] At the present time, we do not know whether gadolinium nephrotoxicity is related to free gadolinium or gadolinium chelates. In May 2007, the FDA cautioned that gadolinium be avoided in patients with acute or chronic renal insufficiency (defined as GFR <30 mL/min/1.73 m^2) unless the diagnostic information to be obtained is essential. In addition, the FDA advised that gadolinium be avoided in patients with AKI due to hepatorenal syndrome or in the perioperative liver transplantation period irrespective of the GFR value. Updated information is available on the FDA website at www.fda.gov.

PROGNOSIS

There is increasing interest in the effect of AKI on the development of end-stage renal disease (ESRD). The U.S. Renal Data System listed ATN as the cause of ESRD in 1.7% of patients from 1999 to 2003.[119,120] It is known that in-hospital mortality for AKI patients requiring RRT is greater than 50% and 48% in adults and children, respectively, but long-term outcomes are not as well described.[120,121] In their review of adult literature, Goldberg and Dennen found that 12.5% of AKI survivors who required RRT were dialysis dependent at 1 to 10 years of follow-up and that approximately 25% have CKD; nearly 40% of patients who had AKI and required RRT have CKD or ESRD.[120] Studies in children with AKI have also noted progression to dialysis dependence or CKD.[121] Therefore improving the prognosis of AKI patients might reduce the incidence of CKD and ESRD. No study has evaluated the use of drugs to reduce the incidence of progressive CKD after AKI, although three cohort trials showed that the use of continuous renal replacement therapy (CRRT) reduced dialysis dependence when compared with intermittent hemodialysis.[122-124] However, in four RCTs and one recent meta-analysis, the use of CRRT did not reduce the rate of dialysis dependence at hospital discharge.[125-129] Thus it is important to have survivors of AKI see nephrologists for follow-up because there is a 40% risk of death in the 2 years after hospitalization.[130] Currently, only approximately 8% of patients see a nephrologist within the first year after hospital discharge.[131] KDIGO guidelines recommend follow-up within 90 days of an AKI event[3]; follow-up within this time period was associated with a 24% lower hazard ratio at 2 years by Harel et al.[132]

CONCLUSION

Evidence-based management of AKI is compromised by the heterogeneity of patients and underlying conditions as well as a lack of clear endpoints for trials. However, given that minor short-term changes in serum creatinine are linked to increased morbidity and mortality, any reversible detrimental factor contributing to AKI should be promptly corrected. Many different drugs have been tried to prevent or treat AKI with mixed results. The consequences of acute renal dysfunction on other organs, drug elimination, and progression of CKD should also be considered in the management of patients suffering from AKI.

AUTHORS' RECOMMENDATIONS

- Minor short-term changes in serum creatinine are related to increased morbidity and mortality. Therefore preventive and treatment measures should be applied as soon as there is a significant increase in creatinine.
- High-risk patients can be identified with clinical features and electronic medical records can be programmed for surveillance to alert physicians for changes in serum creatinine and UO.
- Serum creatinine levels should be adjusted for fluid accumulation and UO should be monitored as early parameters for AKI.
- The first goal of therapy is to correct any reversible detrimental factor contributing to AKI. These include volume depletion, hypotension, decreased cardiac output, obstruction, high intra-abdominal pressure, and nephrotoxic agents.
- Neither loop diuretics nor dopamine should be used to prevent AKI, reduce mortality, or improve renal recovery during AKI.
- RRT should be initiated based on clinical context, trends of laboratory values, and presence of conditions that can be modified with RRT.
- A high suspicion of infection, adjustments in drug dosing, and avoiding gadolinium use in severe AKI are essential parts of the management of AKI to avoid harmful complications.
- AKI survivors should have repeat renal functional studies within 2 weeks and nephrology follow-up within 90 days of an AKI event to improve long-term outcomes.

REFERENCES

1. Chertow GM, Burdick E, Honour M, Bonventre JV, Bates DW. Acute kidney injury, mortality, length of stay, and costs in hospitalized patients. *J Am Soc Nephrol*. November 2005;16(11): 3365–3370.
2. Hoste EA, Clermont G, Kersten A, et al. RIFLE criteria for acute kidney injury are associated with hospital mortality in critically ill patients: a cohort analysis. *Crit Care*. 2006;10(3):R73.
3. Khwaja A. KDIGO clinical practice guidelines for acute kidney injury. *Nephron Clin Pract*. 2012;120(4):c1279–c184.
4. Basu RK, Wang Y, Wong HR, Chawla LS, Wheeler DS, Goldstein SL. Incorporation of biomarkers with the renal angina index for prediction of severe AKI in critically ill children. *Clin J Am Soc Nephrol*. April 2014;9(4):654–662.
5. Basu RK, Zappitelli M, Brunner L, et al. Derivation and validation of the renal angina index to improve the prediction of acute kidney injury in critically ill children. *Kidney Int*. March 2014;85(3):659–667.
6. Goldstein SL, Chawla LS. Renal angina. *Clin J Am Soc Nephrol*. May 2010;5(5):943–949.
7. Selby NM, Crowley L, Fluck RJ, et al. Use of electronic results reporting to diagnose and monitor AKI in hospitalized patients. *Clin J Am Soc Nephrol*. April 2012;7(4):533–540.
8. Deleted in review.
9. Colpaert K, Hoste E, Van Hoecke S, et al. Implementation of a real-time electronic alert based on the RIFLE criteria for acute kidney injury in ICU patients. *Acta Clin Belg Suppl*. 2007;(2):322–325.
10. Garzotto F, Piccinni P, Cruz D, et al. RIFLE-based data collection/management system applied to a prospective cohort multicenter Italian study on the epidemiology of acute kidney injury in the intensive care unit. *Blood Purif*. 2011;31(1–3):159–171.
11. Prowle JR, Liu YL, Licari E, et al. Oliguria as predictive biomarker of acute kidney injury in critically ill patients. *Crit Care*. 2011;15(4):R172.
12. Macedo E, Malhotra R, Bouchard J, Wynn SK, Mehta RL. Oliguria is an early predictor of higher mortality in critically ill patients. *Kidney Int*. 2011;80(7):760–767.
13. Mandelbaum T, Lee J, Scott DJ, et al. Empirical relationships among oliguria, creatinine, mortality, and renal replacement therapy in the critically ill. *Intensive Care Med*. March 2013; 39(3):414–419.
14. Cruz DN, Mehta RL. Acute kidney injury in 2013: breaking barriers for biomarkers in AKI–progress at last. *Nat Rev Nephrol*. February 2014;10(2):74–76.
15. Price CP, Newall RG, Boyd JC. Use of protein:creatinine ratio measurements on random urine samples for prediction of significant proteinuria: a systematic review. *Clin Chem*. September 2005;51(9):1577–1586.
16. Morgenstern BZ, Butani L, Wollan P, Wilson DM, Larson TS. Validity of protein-osmolality versus protein-creatinine ratios in the estimation of quantitative proteinuria from random samples of urine in children. *Am J Kidney Dis*. April 2003;41(4):760–766.
17. Edelmann CM, Meadow SR. *Pediatric Kidney Disease*. 2nd ed. Boston: Little, Brown; 1992.
18. Muriithi AK, Nasr SH, Leung N. Utility of urine eosinophils in the diagnosis of acute interstitial nephritis. *Clin J Am Soc Nephrol*. November 2013;8(11):1857–1862.
19. Chawla LS, Dommu A, Berger A, Shih S, Patel SS. Urinary sediment cast scoring index for acute kidney injury: a pilot study. *Nephron Clin Pract*. 2008;110(3):c145–150.
20. Perazella MA, Coca SG, Hall IE, Iyanam U, Koraishy M, Parikh CR. Urine microscopy is associated with severity and worsening of acute kidney injury in hospitalized patients. *Clin J Am Soc Nephrol*. March 2010;5(3):402–408.
21. Deleted in review.
22. Dewitte A, Biais M, Petit L, et al. Fractional excretion of urea as a diagnostic index in acute kidney injury in intensive care patients. *J Crit Care*. October 2012;27(5):505–510.
23. Wlodzimirow KA, Abu-Hanna A, Royakkers AA, et al. Transient versus persistent acute kidney injury and the diagnostic performance of fractional excretion of urea in critically ill patients. *Nephron Clin Pract*. 2014;126(1):8–13.
24. Darmon M, Vincent F, Dellamonica J, et al. Diagnostic performance of fractional excretion of urea in the evaluation of critically ill patients with acute kidney injury: a multicenter cohort study. *Crit Care*. 2011;15(4):R178.
25. Rachoin JS, Daher R, Moussallem C, et al. The fallacy of the BUN:creatinine ratio in critically ill patients. *Nephrol Dial Transplant*. June 2012;27(6):2248–2254.
26. Peres LA, Cunha Junior AD, Schafer AJ, et al. Biomarkers of acute kidney injury. *Jornal Bras Nefrol*. July–September 2013;35(3): 229–236.
27. Macedo E, Bouchard J, Soroko SH, et al. Fluid accumulation, recognition and staging of acute kidney injury in critically-ill patients. *Crit Care*. May 6, 2010;14(3):R82.
28. Pickering JW, Ralib AM, Endre ZH. Combining creatinine and volume kinetics identifies missed cases of acute kidney injury following cardiac arrest. *Crit Care*. January 17, 2013; 17(1):R7.
29. Soni SS, Ronco C, Katz N, Cruz DN. Early diagnosis of acute kidney injury: the promise of novel biomarkers. *Blood Purif*. 2009;28(3):165–174.
30. Obermuller N, Geiger H, Weipert C, Urbschat A. Current developments in early diagnosis of acute kidney injury. *Int Urol Nephrol*. January 2014;46(1):1–7.
31. Kashani K, Al-Khafaji A, Ardiles T, et al. Discovery and validation of cell cycle arrest biomarkers in human acute kidney injury. *Crit Care*. 2013;17(1):R25.
32. Remer EM, Papanicolaou N, Casalino DD, et al. ACR Appropriateness Criteria on renal failure. *Am J Med*. 2014;127: 1041–1048.
33. Faubel S, Patel NU, Lockhart ME, Cadnapaphornchai MA. Renal relevant radiology: use of ultrasonography in patients with AKI. *Clin J Am Soc Nephrol*. February 2014;9(2):382–394.
34. Chen JJ, Pugach J, Patel M, Luisiri A, Steinhardt GF. The renal length nomogram: multivariable approach. *J Urol*. November 2002;168(5):2149–2152.
35. Deleted in review.
36. Deleted in review.
37. Schneider A, Johnson L, Goodwin M, Schelleman A, Bellomo R. Bench-to-bedside review: contrast enhanced ultrasonography–a promising technique to assess renal perfusion in the ICU. *Crit Care*. 2011;15(3):157.
38. Cokkinos DD, Antypa EG, Skilakaki M, Kriketou D, Tavernaraki E, Piperopoulos PN. Contrast enhanced ultrasound of the kidneys: what is it capable of? *BioMed Res Int*. 2013;2013:595873.

39. Sharfuddin A. Renal relevant radiology: imaging in kidney transplantation. *Clin J Am Soc Nephrol*. February 2014;9(2):416–429.
40. Deleted in review.
41. Deleted in review.
42. Deleted in review.
43. Devarajan P. Update on mechanisms of ischemic acute kidney injury. *J Am Soc Nephrol*. June 2006;17(6):1503–1520.
44. Dellinger RP, Levy MM, Carlet JM, et al. Surviving Sepsis Campaign: international guidelines for management of severe sepsis and septic shock: 2008. *Crit Care Med*. January 2008; 36(1):296–327.
45. Yealy DM, Kellum JA, Huang DT, et al. A Randomized Trial of Protocol-Based Care for Early Septic Shock. *N Engl J Med*. May 1, 2014;370(18):1683–1693.
46. Perner A, Haase N, Guttormsen AB, et al. Hydroxyethyl starch 130/0.42 versus Ringer's acetate in severe sepsis. *N Engl J Med*. July 12, 2012;367(2):124–134.
47. Myburgh JA, Finfer S, Bellomo R, et al. Hydroxyethyl starch or saline for fluid resuscitation in intensive care. *N Engl J Med*. November 15, 2012;367(20):1901–1911.
48. Finfer S, Bellomo R, Boyce N, French J, Myburgh J, Norton R. A comparison of albumin and saline for fluid resuscitation in the intensive care unit. *N Engl J Med*. May 27, 2004;350(22):2247–2256.
49. Finfer S, Bellomo R, McEvoy S, et al. Effect of baseline serum albumin concentration on outcome of resuscitation with albumin or saline in patients in intensive care units: analysis of data from the saline versus albumin fluid evaluation (SAFE) study. *BMJ*. November 18, 2006;333(7577):1044.
50. Caironi P, Tognoni G, Gattinoni L. Albumin replacement in severe sepsis or septic shock. *N Engl J Med*. July 3, 2014;371(1):84.
51. Wiedermann CJ, Dunzendorfer S, Gaioni LU, Zaraca F, Joannidis M. Hyperoncotic colloids and acute kidney injury: a meta-analysis of randomized trials. *Crit Care*. 2010;14(5):R191.
52. Mueller C, Buerkle G, Buettner HJ, et al. Prevention of contrast media-associated nephropathy: randomized comparison of 2 hydration regimens in 1620 patients undergoing coronary angioplasty. *Arch Intern Med*. February 11, 2002;162(3):329–336.
53. Santoso JT, Lucci 3rd JA, Coleman RL, Schafer I, Hannigan EV. Saline, mannitol, and furosemide hydration in acute cisplatin nephrotoxicity: a randomized trial. *Cancer Chemother Pharmacol*. July 2003;52(1):13–18.
54. Llanos A, Cieza J, Bernardo J, et al. Effect of salt supplementation on amphotericin B nephrotoxicity. *Kidney Int*. August 1991;40(2):302–308.
55. Gunal AI, Celiker H, Dogukan A, et al. Early and vigorous fluid resuscitation prevents acute renal failure in the crush victims of catastrophic earthquakes. *J Am Soc Nephrol*. July 2004;15(7):1862–1867.
56. Yunos NM, Bellomo R, Hegarty C, Story D, Ho L, Bailey M. Association between a chloride-liberal vs chloride-restrictive intravenous fluid administration strategy and kidney injury in critically ill adults. *JAMA*. October 17, 2012;308(15):1566–1572.
57. Ejaz AA, Martin TD, Johnson RJ, et al. Prophylactic nesiritide does not prevent dialysis or all-cause mortality in patients undergoing high-risk cardiac surgery. *J Thorac Cardiovasc Surg*. October 2009;138(4):959–964.
58. Friedrich JO, Adhikari N, Herridge MS, Beyene J. Meta-analysis: low-dose dopamine increases urine output but does not prevent renal dysfunction or death. *Ann Intern Med*. April 5, 2005;142(7):510–524.
59. Kellum JA, Decker J M. Use of dopamine in acute renal failure: a meta-analysis. *Crit Care Med*. August 2001;29(8):1526–1531.
60. Marik PE. Low-dose dopamine: a systematic review. *Intensive Care Med*. July 2002;28(7):877–883.
61. Landoni G, Biondi-Zoccai GG, Tumlin JA, et al. Beneficial impact of fenoldopam in critically ill patients with or at risk for acute renal failure: a meta-analysis of randomized clinical trials. *Am J Kidney Dis*. January 2007;49(1):56–68.
62. Leoncini M, Toso A, Maioli M, Tropeano F, Villani S, Bellandi F. Early high-dose rosuvastatin for contrast-induced nephropathy prevention in acute coronary syndrome: Results from the PRATO-ACS Study (Protective Effect of Rosuvastatin and Antiplatelet Therapy On contrast-induced acute kidney injury and myocardial damage in patients with Acute Coronary Syndrome). *J Am Coll Cardiol*. January 7–14, 2014;63(1):71–79.
63. Han Y. Reply: Intravenous hydration (with or without rosuvastatin) should remain the cornerstone of the prevention of contrast-induced acute kidney injury in patients with diabetes and chronic kidney disease. *J Am Coll Cardiol*. July 22, 2014;64(3):332–333.
64. Giacoppo D, Capodanno D, Capranzano P, Aruta P, Tamburino C. Meta-analysis of randomized controlled trials of preprocedural statin administration for reducing contrast-induced acute kidney injury in patients undergoing coronary catheterization. *Am J Cardiol*. August 15, 2014;114(4):541–548.
65. Pan SY, Wu VC, Huang TM, et al. effect of preoperative statin therapy on postoperative acute kidney injury in patients undergoing major surgery: systemic review and meta-analysis. *Nephrology (Carlton)*. 2014;19:750–763.
66. Thomas G, Rojas MC, Epstein SK, Balk EM, Liangos O, Jaber BL. Insulin therapy and acute kidney injury in critically ill patients a systematic review. *Nephrol Dial Transplant*. October 2007;22(10):2849–2855.
67. Haase M, Haase-Fielitz A, Bagshaw SM, et al. Phase II, randomized, controlled trial of high-dose N-acetylcysteine in high-risk cardiac surgery patients. *Crit Care Med*. May 2007;35(5):1324–1331.
68. Komisarof JA, Gilkey GM, Peters DM, Koudelka CW, Meyer MM, Smith SM. N-acetylcysteine for patients with prolonged hypotension as prophylaxis for acute renal failure (NEPHRON). *Crit Care Med*. February 2007;35(2):435–441.
69. Burns KE, Chu MW, Novick RJ, et al. Perioperative N-acetylcysteine to prevent renal dysfunction in high-risk patients undergoing cabg surgery: a randomized controlled trial. *JAMA*. July 20, 2005;294(3):342–350.
70. Ristikankare A, Kuitunen T, Kuitunen A, et al. Lack of renoprotective effect of i.v. N-acetylcysteine in patients with chronic renal failure undergoing cardiac surgery. *Br J Anaesth*. November 2006;97(5):611–616.
71. Hynninen MS, Niemi TT, Poyhia R, et al. N-acetylcysteine for the prevention of kidney injury in abdominal aortic surgery: a randomized, double-blind, placebo-controlled trial. *Anesth Analg*. June 2006;102(6):1638–1645.
72. Macedo E, Abdulkader R, Castro I, Sobrinho AC, Yu L, Vieira Jr JM. Lack of protection of N-acetylcysteine (NAC) in acute renal failure related to elective aortic aneurysm repair-a randomized controlled trial. *Nephrol Dial Transplant*. July 2006;21(7):1863–1869.
73. Tie HT, Luo MZ, Luo MJ, Zhang M, Wu QC, Wan JY. Sodium bicarbonate in the prevention of cardiac surgery-associated acute kidney injury: a systematic review and meta-analysis. *Crit Care*. September 12, 2014;18(5):517.
74. Clinical Trials gov. *Prevention of Serious Adverse Events Following Angiography (PRESERVE)*; 2014. http://clinicaltrials.gov/show/NCT01467466. Accessed 14.10.14.
75. Amar D, Fleisher M. Diltiazem treatment does not alter renal function after thoracic surgery. *Chest*. May 2001;119(5):1476–1479.
76. Togel FE, Westenfelder C. Mesenchymal stem cells: a new therapeutic tool for AKI. *Nat Rev Nephrol*. March 2010;6(3):179–183.
77. Gallagher SM, Jones DA, Kapur A, et al. Remote ischemic preconditioning has a neutral effect on the incidence of kidney injury after coronary artery bypass graft surgery. *Kidney Int*. 2015;87:473–481.
78. Yang Y, Lang XB, Zhang P, Lv R, Wang YF, Chen JH. Remote ischemic preconditioning for prevention of acute kidney injury: a meta-analysis of randomized controlled trials. *Am J Kidney Dis*. October 2014;64(4):574–583.
79. Russell JA, Walley KR, Singer J, et al. Vasopressin versus norepinephrine infusion in patients with septic shock. *N Engl J Med*. February 28, 2008;358(9):877–887.
80. Gordon AC, Russell JA, Walley KR, et al. The effects of vasopressin on acute kidney injury in septic shock. *Intensive Care Med*. January 2010;36(1):83–91.
81. Bouchard J, Soroko SB, Chertow GM, et al. Fluid accumulation, survival and recovery of kidney function in critically ill patients with acute kidney injury. *Kidney Int*. May 13, 2009;76(4):422–427.
82. Heung M, Wolfgram DF, Kommareddi M, Hu Y, Song PX, Ojo AO. Fluid overload at initiation of renal replacement therapy is associated with lack of renal recovery in patients with acute kidney injury. *Nephrol Dial Transplant*. March 2012;27(3):956–961.

83. Bagshaw SM, Delaney A, Haase M, Ghali WA, Bellomo R. Loop diuretics in the management of acute renal failure: a systematic review and meta-analysis. *Crit Care Resusc.* March 2007;9(1):60–68.

84. Ho KM, Sheridan DJ. Meta-analysis of frusemide to prevent or treat acute renal failure. *BMJ.* August 26, 2006;333(7565):420.

85. Sampath S, Moran JL, Graham PL, Rockliff S, Bersten AD, Abrams KR. The efficacy of loop diuretics in acute renal failure: Assessment using Bayesian evidence synthesis techniques. *Crit Care Med.* August 14, 2007;35(11):2516–2524.

86. Mehta RL, Pascual MT, Soroko S, Chertow GM. Diuretics, mortality, and nonrecovery of renal function in acute renal failure. *JAMA.* November 27, 2002;288(20):2547–2553.

87. Uchino S, Doig GS, Bellomo R, et al. Diuretics and mortality in acute renal failure. *Crit Care Med.* August 2004;32(8):1669–1677.

88. Bagshaw SM, Delaney A, Jones D, Ronco C, Bellomo R. Diuretics in the management of acute kidney injury: a multinational survey. *Contrib Nephrol.* 2007;156:236–249.

89. Rahman SN, Kim GE, Mathew AS, et al. Effects of atrial natriuretic peptide in clinical acute renal failure. *Kidney Int.* June 1994;45(6):1731–1738.

90. Allgren RL, Marbury TC, Rahman SN, et al. Anaritide in acute tubular necrosis. Auriculin Anaritide Acute Renal Failure Study Group. *N Engl J Med.* March 20, 1997;336(12):828–834.

91. Sward K, Valsson F, Odencrants P, Samuelsson O, Ricksten SE. Recombinant human atrial natriuretic peptide in ischemic acute renal failure: a randomized placebo-controlled trial. *Crit Care Med.* June 2004;32(6):1310–1315.

92. Lewis J, Salem MM, Chertow GM, et al. Atrial natriuretic factor in oliguric acute renal failure. Anaritide Acute Renal Failure Study Group. *Am J Kidney Dis.* October 2000;36(4):767–774.

93. Albanese J, Leone M, Garnier F, Bourgoin A, Antonini F, Martin C. Renal effects of norepinephrine in septic and nonseptic patients. *Chest.* August 2004;126(2):534–539.

94. Bourgoin A, Leone M, Delmas A, Garnier F, Albanese J, Martin C. Increasing mean arterial pressure in patients with septic shock: effects on oxygen variables and renal function. *Crit Care Med.* April 2005;33(4):780–786.

95. Deleted in review.

96. Stone GW, McCullough PA, Tumlin JA, et al. Fenoldopam mesylate for the prevention of contrast-induced nephropathy: a randomized controlled trial. *JAMA.* November 5, 2003;290(17):2284–2291.

97. Teirstein PS, Price MJ, Mathur VS, Madyoon H, Sawhney N, Baim DS. Differential effects between intravenous and targeted renal delivery of fenoldopam on renal function and blood pressure in patients undergoing cardiac catheterization. *Am J Cardiol.* April 1, 2006;97(7):1076–1081.

98. Wiener RS, Wiener DC, Larson RJ. Benefits and risks of tight glucose control in critically ill adults: a meta-analysis. *JAMA.* August 27, 2008;300(8):933–944.

99. Acker CG, Singh AR, Flick RP, Bernardini J, Greenberg A, Johnson JP. A trial of thyroxine in acute renal failure. *Kidney Int.* January 2000;57(1):293–298.

100. Hirschberg R, Kopple J, Lipsett P, et al. Multicenter clinical trial of recombinant human insulin-like growth factor I in patients with acute renal failure. *Kidney Int.* June 1999;55(6):2423–2432.

101. Mahoney BA, Smith WA, Lo DS, Tsoi K, Tonelli M, Clase CM. Emergency interventions for hyperkalaemia. *Cochrane Database Syst Rev.* 2005;18(2):CD003235.

102. Desmeules S, Bergeron MJ, Isenring P. Acute phosphate nephropathy and renal failure. *N Engl J Med.* September 4, 2003;349(10):1006–1007.

103. Wilson FP, Berns JS. Onco-nephrology: tumor lysis syndrome. *Clin J Am Soc Nephrol.* October 2012;7(10):1730–1739.

104. Rocktaeschel J, Morimatsu H, Uchino S, et al. Acid-base status of critically ill patients with acute renal failure: analysis based on Stewart-Figge methodology. *Crit Care.* August 2003;7(4):R60.

105. Sabatini S, Kurtzman NA. Bicarbonate therapy in severe metabolic acidosis. *J Am Soc Nephrol.* April 2009;20(4):692–695.

106. Kraut JA, Madias NE. Treatment of acute metabolic acidosis: a pathophysiologic approach. *Nat Rev Nephrol.* October 2012;8(10):589–601.

107. Kraut JA, Kurtz I. Use of base in the treatment of acute severe organic acidosis by nephrologists and critical care physicians: results of an online survey. *Clin Exp Nephrol.* June 2006;10(2):111–117.

108. Kopple JD, Kalantar-Zadeh K, Mehrotra R. Risks of chronic metabolic acidosis in patients with chronic kidney disease. *Kidney Int Suppl.* June 2005;(95):S21–S27.

109. Swan SK, Bennett WM. Drug dosing guidelines in patients with renal failure. *West J Med.* June 1992;156(6):633–638.

110. Cockcroft DW, Gault MH. Prediction of creatinine clearance from serum creatinine. *Nephron.* 1976;16(1):31–41.

111. Lameire N, Van Biesen W, Vanholder R. Epidemiology, clinical evaluation, and prevention of acute renal failure. In: Feehally J, Floege J, Johnson RJ, eds. *Comprehensive Clinical Nephrology.* Philadelphia: Mosby Elsevier; 2007:771–785.

112. Othersen JB, Maize JC, Woolson RF, Budisavljevic MN. Nephrogenic systemic fibrosis after exposure to gadolinium in patients with renal failure. *Nephrol Dial Transplant.* November 2007;22(11):3179–3185.

113. Penfield JG, Reilly Jr RF. What nephrologists need to know about gadolinium. *Nat Clin Pract Nephrol.* December 2007;3(12):654–668.

114. Deleted in review.

115. Deleted in review.

116. Deleted in review.

117. Deleted in review.

118. Deleted in review.

119. Block CA, Schoolwerth AC. The epidemiology and outcome of acute renal failure and the impact on chronic kidney disease. *Semin Dial.* November–December 2006;19(6):450–454.

120. Goldberg R, Dennen P. Long-term outcomes of acute kidney injury. *Adv Chronic Kidney Dis.* July 2008;15(3):297–307.

121. Goldstein SL, Devarajan P. Progression from acute kidney injury to chronic kidney disease: a pediatric perspective. *Adv Chronic Kidney Dis.* July 2008;15(3):278–283.

122. Bell M, Granath F, Schon S, Ekbom A, Martling CR. Continuous renal replacement therapy is associated with less chronic renal failure than intermittent haemodialysis after acute renal failure. *Intensive Care Med.* May 2007;33(5):773–780.

123. Uchino S, Bellomo R, Kellum JA, et al. Patient and kidney survival by dialysis modality in critically ill patients with acute kidney injury. *Int J Artif Organs.* April 2007;30(4):281–292.

124. Jacka MJ, Ivancinova X, Gibney RT. Continuous renal replacement therapy improves renal recovery from acute renal failure. *Can J Anaesth.* March 2005;52(3):327–332.

125. Mehta RL, McDonald B, Gabbai FB, et al. A randomized clinical trial of continuous versus intermittent dialysis for acute renal failure. *Kidney Int.* September 2001;60(3):1154–1163.

126. Uehlinger DE, Jakob SM, Ferrari P, et al. Comparison of continuous and intermittent renal replacement therapy for acute renal failure. *Nephrol Dial Transplant.* August 2005;20(8):1630–1637.

127. Augustine JJ, Sandy D, Seifert TH, Paganini EP. A randomized controlled trial comparing intermittent with continuous dialysis in patients with ARF. *Am J Kidney Dis.* December 2004;44(6):1000–1007.

128. Vinsonneau C, Camus C, Combes A, et al. Continuous venovenous haemodiafiltration versus intermittent haemodialysis for acute renal failure in patients with multiple-organ dysfunction syndrome: a multicentre randomised trial. *Lancet.* July 29, 2006;368(9533):379–385.

129. Rabindranath K, Adams J, Macleod AM, Muirhead N. Intermittent versus continuous renal replacement therapy for acute renal failure in adults. *Cochrane Database Syst Rev.* 2007;(3):CD003773.

130. Lafrance JP, Miller DR. Acute kidney injury associates with increased long-term mortality. *J Am Soc Nephrol.* February 2010;21(2):345–352.

131. Siew ED, Peterson JF, Eden SK, et al. Outpatient nephrology referral rates after acute kidney injury. *J Am Soc Nephrol.* February 2012;23(2):305–312.

132. Harel Z, Wald R, Bargman JM, et al. Nephrologist follow-up improves all-cause mortality of severe acute kidney injury survivors. *Kidney Int.* May 2013;83(5):901–908.

57

What Is the Role of Renal Replacement Therapy in the Intensive Care Unit?

Michelle O'Shaughnessy, John O'Regan, David Lappin

The aim of this chapter is to review the evidence surrounding the use of renal replacement therapy (RRT) in the intensive care unit (ICU) setting. It examines the conventional indications for emergency RRT and assesses the emerging evidence for earlier commencement of RRT and the expanded role of RRT in the management of sepsis and multiorgan failure (MOF).

WHAT ARE THE CONVENTIONAL INDICATIONS FOR COMMENCING RENAL REPLACEMENT IN ACUTE KIDNEY INJURY?

There is a paucity of consensus guidelines internationally with regard to RRT use in the ICU, and this has resulted in variable prescribing practices for continuous dialysis. However, some pathophysiologic states are generally considered absolute indications for this intervention (Table 57-1).

Intravascular Volume Overload and Pulmonary Edema Refractory to Diuretic Therapy

The role of negative or neutral fluid balance in acute kidney injury (AKI) with pulmonary edema but without lung injury is unclear. Studies performed in critically ill children with AKI after cardiac surgery have suggested that early institution of continuous renal replacement therapy (CRRT) improves respiratory parameters with an associated improvement in multiple clinical outcomes.[1-3] Randomized controlled trials (RCTs) in adults are lacking, although observational data indicate that a positive fluid balance in critically ill patients with AKI is independently associated with a higher 60-day mortality rate (hazard ratio [HR], 1.21; $P < .001$).[4]

There is no evidence to support the common practice of trial of diuresis in AKI-associated pulmonary edema. Indeed, the use of diuretic therapy may increase the probability of nonrecovery of renal function.[5-8] In addition, studies in animal models suggest that ultrafiltration is more effective than diuresis in reducing extravascular lung water in ARDS.[9]

In conclusion, RRT should be considered early in patients with AKI complicated by refractory pulmonary edema.

Metabolic Acidosis Refractory to Medical Management

Metabolic acidosis is a common complication of AKI, resulting from a combination of chloride-rich fluid resuscitation and the accumulation of lactate, phosphate, and unexcreted metabolic acids. RRT can be highly effective in correcting this acidosis.[10,11] CRRT as a modality may be superior to intermittent hemodiafiltration (IHD) in terms of duration of treatment effect.[12] Importantly, RRT avoids systemic administration of sodium bicarbonate therapy with its associated risk for exacerbating fluid overload and hypernatremia. The threshold pH or base deficit at which to commence RRT has not been established. Because a pH lower than 7.1 is associated with negative inotropic and metabolic effects, in general, one would consider intervening before this level is reached.

Hyperkalemia Refractory to Medical Management

No specific treatment threshold has been established for when to treat hyperkalemia with RRT. In general, myocardial toxicity is considered unlikely when the serum potassium concentration is less than 6.5 mmol/L. Potassium excretion by diuresis is generally ineffective in renal failure. For this reason, the threshold for commencing RRT in AKI might be lowered further, particularly if there is minimal response to initial emergency treatment (insulin-glucose, inhaled beta-agonist, exchange resins).[13]

The Uremic State

Manifestations of the "uremic state" include encephalopathy, pericarditis, and bleeding diathesis. Mental status changes and bleeding propensity can be multifactorial in the septic, critically ill patient, and they can be difficult to attribute solely to renal failure. Uremic pericarditis requires urgent initiation of renal support once it is detected because

Table 57-1 **Conventional Indications for Renal Replacement Therapy**
• Intravascular volume overload unresponsive to diuretic therapy
• Metabolic acidosis (pH < 7.1) refractory to medical management
• Hyperkalemia (K > 6.5 mEq/L) refractory to medical management
• Uremic state (encephalopathy, pericarditis, bleeding diathesis)
• Intoxication with a dialyzable drug or toxin
• Hyperthermia refractory to conventional cooling techniques
• Severe electrolyte derangements in the setting of AKI
• Progressive azotemia or oliguria unresponsive to fluid administration

it carries a high risk for intrapericardial hemorrhage and tamponade.

Intoxication with a Dialyzable Drug or Toxin

Toxins of low molecular weight residing in the extracellular space, which have little or no protein-binding properties, can be effectively removed by RRT. In general, IHD is preferable to CRRT for this purpose because it more rapidly clears solute. A review of the U.S. Poison Center's "Toxic Exposure Surveillance System" records from 1985 to 2005 found that 19,351 cases received extracorporeal toxin removal over this time period.[14] IHD was most commonly used for the treatment of lithium, ethylene glycol, salicylate, valproate, acetaminophen, methanol, ethanol, and theophylline poisoning, although some cases of IHD, used for removal of methotrexate and phenobarbital, were reported. Hemoperfusion techniques are used in the enhanced elimination of toxic levels of lipid-soluble or highly protein-bound substances when intervention will remove the substance more rapidly than endogenous clearance. An important consideration is the platelet-depleting effect of hemoperfusion.

Severe Electrolyte Derangements

AKI can be associated with an array of electrolyte disturbances, including hyponatremia, hypernatremia, hyperphosphatemia, hypercalcemia, hypocalcemia, and hypermagnesemia. CRRT may be helpful in the management of many of these disorders.[12]

Progressive Azotemia or Oliguria Unresponsive to Fluid Administration

In the modern era, RRT is most often initiated before sufficient time has passed for the previously discussed scenarios to develop. Instead, the decision to commence treatment is made when urea and creatinine levels climb, or urine output falls, despite conservative measures.

The threshold values of these parameters that should trigger a decision to commence RRT have not been established and are discussed later.

SHOULD RENAL REPLACEMENT THERAPY BE INITIATED IN ACUTE KIDNEY INJURY BEFORE COMPLICATIONS HAVE DEVELOPED?

Although undisputed indications generally point to RRT as being a "rescue remedy" used when other measures have failed, several studies have examined the value of earlier commencement of therapy in improving patient outcomes (Table 57-2).

It should be noted that there is no clear consensus on what is meant by "earlier" initiation of RRT; initiation at lower urea and creatinine levels,[15,16] initiation closer to the time of renal injury,[17] initiation sooner after urine output is noted to fall,[18,19] and initiation sooner after admission to the ICU have all been studied (see Table 57-2). This makes study comparison and meta-analysis difficult. In addition, the effect of earlier initiation of RRT is likely to be influenced by the etiology of the AKI; thus, the heterogeneity of the populations studied renders meaningful meta-analysis even more difficult.

A small and retrospective study in post-traumatic AKI using a blood urea nitrogen (BUN) threshold for early initiation of RRT of 60 mg/dL demonstrated a significantly lower mortality rate for the early compared with the delayed RRT cohort (relative risk [RR] for death, 0.77; 95% confidence interval [CI], 0.58 to 1.0; $P = .04$).[15] These results suggest that the BUN threshold for considering the initiation of RRT should be lowered to at least 60 mg/dL.

Further support for a strategy of earlier initiation of RRT was provided by retrospective studies in the postoperative coronary artery bypass graft (CABG) patient population.[18,19] These studies used reduced urine output (<100 mL within 8 hours consecutively after surgery, despite frusemide administration) as their criterion for early initiation of CRRT. The attainment of specified BUN, serum creatinine, or potassium thresholds was the trigger for late commencement of therapy. The first of these studies examined the outcomes of 64 patients with a high baseline prevalence of class 3 or 4 heart failure and chronic kidney disease. It reported a survival rate of 78% in the early initiation group compared with 57% in the late initiation group ($P < .05$).[18] The early initiation group was also found to have had a significantly shorter ICU stay (12.5 vs. 8.5 days; $P < .05$), shorter hospital stay (20.9 vs. 15.4 days; $P < .05$), and lower rate of MOF (19% vs. 29%; $P = .01$). The second study, a retrospective analysis of post-CABG AKI using a historical control group, again showed significantly improved survival (77% vs. 45%; $P = .016$), shorter length of ICU stay (12 vs. 8 days; $P = .0001$), and shorter length of hospital stay (30 vs. 15 days) in the early treatment group.[19]

Clinical benefit of early initiation of RRT was also reported in a secondary analysis of a prospectively collected AKI database.[16] Despite there being, on average, more failed organ systems in the early intervention group, the RR for death associated with delayed initiation was

Table 57-2 Studies Evaluating the Timing of Initiation of RRT

Study	Mode	Design	Number of Patients	GROUP DEFINITION Early	Late	SURVIVAL Early	Late
Teschan, 1960[53]	IHD	Case series	15	<100 mg/dL	—	33%	—
Parsons, 1961[54]	IHD	Single-arm (historical control)	33	BUN reaching 120-150 mg/dL	Clinical deterioration or BUN 200 mg/dL	75%	12%
Fischer, 1966[55]	IHD	Retrospective cohort study	162	Clinical deterioration or BUN increase to ~150 mg/dL	Hyperkalemia BUN ~200 mg/dL	43%	26%
Kleinknecht, 1972[56]	IHD	Retrospective cohort study	500	To maintain BUN <93 mg/dL (blood urea <200 mg/dL)	BUN >163 mg/dL (blood urea >350 mg/dL) or severe electrolyte disturbance	73%	58%
Conger, 1975[57]	IHD	RCT	18	BUN <70 mg/dL or SCr <5 mg/dL	BUN ~150 mg/dL, SCr 10 mg/dL, or clinical indication	64%	20%
Gillum, 1986[58]	IHD	RCT	34	Maintenance of BUN <60 mg/dL	Maintenance of BUN ~100 mg/dL	41%	53%
Gettings et al., 1999[15]	CRRT	Retrospective cohort study	100	BUN <60 mg/dL (mean 42.6 mg/dL)	BUN ≥60 mg/dL (mean, 94.5 mg/dL)	39%	20%
Bouman et al., 2002[17]	CVVH	RCT	106	Within 12 hours of developing UO <20 mL/h and Cr clearance <20 mL/min	Urea >40 mmol/L (BUN >112 mg/dL), SK >6.5 mEq/L (>6.5 mmol/L) or severe pulmonary edema	69%	75%
Demirkilic et al., 2004[19]	CVVHDF	Retrospective cohort study	61	UO <100 mL over 8 hours after surgery, despite furosemide bolus	SCr >5 mg/dL or SK >5.5 mEq/L	77%	45%
Elahi et al., 2004[18]	CVVH	Retrospective cohort study	64	UO <100 mL over 8 hours after surgery, despite furosemide infusion	BUN >84 mg/dL, SCr >2.8 mg/dL, or SK >6 mEq/L	57% / 78%	—
Liu et al., 2006[16]	IHD, CRRT	Prospective cohort study	243	BUN <76 mg/dL	BUN >76 mg/dL	65%	59%

BUN, blood urea nitrogen; *Cr*, creatinine; *CRRT*, continuous renal replacement therapy; *CVVH*, continuous venovenous hemofiltration; *CVVHDF*, continuous venovenous-hemodiafiltration; *IHD*, intermittent hemodiafiltration; *RCT*, randomized controlled trial; *SCr*, serum creatinine; *SK*, serum potassium; *UO*, urine output.

1.85 (95% CI, 1.16 to 2.96) after covariate adjustment for age, hepatic failure, sepsis, thrombocytopenia, serum creatinine, study site, and initial dialysis modality.

Although these observational studies generally support earlier commencement of RRT, available higher-level evidence is less convincing. In a prospective RCT of 106 patients examining the effects of timing of initiation of dialysis and dose of dialysis on 28-day survival rates in AKI, there was no survival advantage to early initiation of RRT (survival 69% in the early low-volume group vs. 75% in the late low-volume group, nonsignificant).[17] In addition, and of particular interest, the authors did not find a survival advantage to higher-dose therapy compared with lower-dose therapy (survival 74% in the high-volume group vs. 69% in the low-volume group, nonsignificant). In this trial, patients were randomized to three different treatment groups: an early high-volume hemofiltration group, an early low-volume hemofiltration group, and a late low-volume hemofiltration group. "Early treatment" was defined by treatment initiation within 12 hours of meeting the study's AKI definition, whereas "late treatment" was initiated only when the patient's BUN was higher than 112 mg/dL or hyperkalemia (>6.5 mmol/L) or pulmonary edema developed. Mean BUN in the early treatment group was 48 mg/dL, compared with a mean BUN of 105 mg/dL in the late treatment group. Unfortunately, this study was underpowered to detect a clinically significant treatment effect; six patients in the late group did not require dialysis because they recovered renal function or died.

A recent meta-analysis evaluated the evidence for and against early initiation of RRT in AKI.[20] Two main questions were asked: (1) Does early RRT improve survival? and (2) Is early initiation of RRT associated with improved renal recovery? Marked heterogeneity was noted among study groups in terms of population

Table 57-3 Renal Association Clinical Practice Guidelines on Acute Kidney Injury: Timing of Initiation of Renal Replacement Treatment

Guideline 11.1 – AKI: Timing of initiation of renal replacement treatment

We recommend that the decision to start RRT in patients with AKI should remain a clinical decision based on the fluid, electrolyte, and metabolic status of each individual patient. (1C)

Guideline 11.2 – AKI: Timing of initiation of renal replacement treatment

We recommend that RRT should be initiated once AKI is established and unavoidable but before overt complications have developed. (1B)

Guideline 11.3 – AKI: Timing of initiation of renal replacement treatment

We recommend that the threshold for initiating RRT should be lowered when AKI occurs as part of MOF. (1C)

Guideline 11.4 – AKI: Timing of initiation of renal replacement treatment

We recommend that the initiation of RRT may be deferred if the underlying clinical condition is improving and there are early signs of renal recovery. (1D)

Guideline 11.5 – AKI: Timing of discontinuation of renal replacement treatment

We recommend that an improvement in the patient's clinical condition and urine output would justify temporary discontinuation of ongoing renal support to see if AKI is recovering. (1D)

Renal Association Clinical Practice Guidelines—Acute Kidney Injury. From Dr. Andrew Lewington, Dr. Suren Kanagasundaram. http://www.renal.org/guidelines/modules/acute-kidney-injury.

settings, baseline disease severity, cutoff value definitions of early compared with late initiation, dialysis technique, and duration of study follow-up. The overall study method quality scores were low, and most trials (78%) were observational in nature. Primary analysis of the five included randomized trials that concluded that early RRT was associated with a 36% mortality risk reduction (not significant, $P = .08$). A secondary analysis of nonrandomized trials supported this hypothesis (26% mortality risk reduction; $P < .001$). The meta-analysis of renal recovery included two RCTs and five comparative cohort studies—there was no significant difference in outcomes.

There is clearly a need for a large, multicenter RCT to confirm or refute these hypotheses. The development of novel biomarkers that might estimate the severity of renal injury more accurately than current methods (creatinine, urea, urine output) and better predict likelihood of spontaneous renal recovery would assist greatly in informing the decision to commence early RRT.

Until such time as more definitive evidence is available to confirm the role of earlier initiation of RRT in improving outcome, clinicians must perform a risk-to-benefit analysis for each patient on a case-by-case basis. Decisions can be aided by expert-derived management guidelines, such as the U.K. Renal Association Clinical Practice Guidelines, relating to timing of initiation of renal replacement treatment in AKI (Table 57-3).

WHAT IS THE ROLE OF RENAL REPLACEMENT THERAPY IN THE MANAGEMENT OF PATIENTS WITH THE SYSTEMIC INFLAMMATORY RESPONSE SYNDROME IN THE SETTING OF SEPSIS OR MULTIORGAN FAILURE?

The most common contributing factor to AKI in the modern ICU setting is septic shock.[21] Septic AKI carries a significantly increased mortality when compared with other forms of AKI[21,22] and is often associated with concurrent MOF.[21,22] For these reasons, a significant amount of research has been performed to specifically investigate the role of RRT in managing the patient with sepsis or MOF. Several key questions have been raised:

- Can extracorporeal "blood purification" alter the systemic inflammatory response?
- Should higher doses of ultrafiltration than are conventionally used be prescribed in cases of septic AKI?
- Is CRRT superior to IHD when AKI occurs in the setting of sepsis or MOF?
- Can ultrafiltration serve as a means of support for organs other than the kidney?

CAN EXTRACORPOREAL BLOOD PURIFICATION ALTER THE SYSTEMIC INFLAMMATORY RESPONSE THAT OCCURS IN SEPSIS AND MULTIORGAN FAILURE?

It is widely believed that hemofiltration removes, or alters the production of, inflammatory mediators and thereby restores immune homeostasis.[23] Adsorption of inflammatory mediators onto the surface of hemofilters, in particular polyacrylonitrile filters,[24] plays a complementary role to simple convection in this process. Furthermore, the molecular weight of many inflammatory mediators exceeds the cutoff value of standard hemofilters, "high-flux" membranes have been developed to further enhance clearance, and their use has been associated with positive hemodynamic effects.[25] The IVOIRE (hIgh VOlume in Intensive caRE) study aimed to evaluate the early effects of higher volume hemofiltration (70 mL/kg/h) versus the conventional prescription in septic shock patients. This multicenter RCT was stopped prematurely, but analysis of the data does not demonstrate a benefit in 28-day mortality in the intervention arm.[26]

SHOULD HIGHER DOSES OF ULTRAFILTRATION THAN ARE CONVENTIONALLY USED BE PRESCRIBED IN CASES OF SEPTIC ACUTE KIDNEY INJURY?

The question of whether higher-intensity RRT is associated with improved AKI outcomes when compared with standard-intensity RRT has been a matter of debate for many years. Two studies, the Veterans Affairs/National

Institutes of Health (VA/NIH) Acute Renal Failure Trial Network study[27] and the RENAL (Renal Replacement Therapy) study,[28] addressed this question. The VA study group defined high-intensity RRT as (1) IHD or slow, low-efficiency dialysis 6 times per week in hemodynamically stable patients or (2) continuous veno-venous-hemodiafiltration (CVVHDF) at a rate of 35 mL/kg/h in hemodynamically unstable patients. Standard-intensity treatment was defined as three intermittent treatment sessions per week or CVVHDF at 20 mL/kg/h, respectively. This study found that higher-intensity treatment was not associated with reduced mortality (the mortality rate by day 60 was 53.6% with high-intensity therapy and 51.5% with lower intensity therapy [$P = .47$]), improved renal recovery, or reduced rate of nonrenal organ failure when compared with less-intensive therapy.

The RENAL study, performed in Australia and New Zealand, enrolled 1508 critically ill patients with AKI: 747 to a high-intensity approach involving CVVHDF and 40 mL/kg/h effluent dose (high-volume ultrafiltration) and 761 to a lower-intensity approach of CVVHDF plus 25 mL/kg/h effluent dose (standard approach). At 90 days, 322 deaths had occurred in the high-intensity group and 332 deaths in the standard-intensity group: There was no statistical significance in outcomes (the mortality rate was of 44.7% in each group [odds ratio 1.00; 95% CI, 0.81 to 1.23; $P = .99$]). There was no difference in the need for continued RRT at 90 days.

Although outcomes in the VA study[27] appear to have been worse than in the RENAL study,[28] the populations were unlikely to have been comparable. However, specific to AKI in the setting of sepsis and MOF, an argument may still be made that higher-dose ultrafiltration can clear inflammatory mediators better than standard-dose ultrafiltration. Although this may not necessarily hasten renal recovery, or even improve survival, it may have a positive effect on the patient's overall clinical condition and vasopressor requirement.[29] For this reason, despite the findings of the VA/NIH trial, a strategy of somewhat higher-volume ultrafiltration than is conventionally prescribed may be reasonable when specifically treating sepsis-associated AKI.

There has been no convincing evidence to date to support the use of RRT in the management of sepsis in the absence of coexisting AKI. Therefore its use, at present, cannot be advocated.

IS CONTINUOUS RENAL REPLACEMENT THERAPY SUPERIOR TO INTERMITTENT HEMODIALYSIS WHEN ACUTE KIDNEY INJURY OCCURS IN THE SETTING OF SEPSIS OR MULTIORGAN FAILURE?

Advocates of CRRT propose that its use is associated with less hemodynamic instability than is seen with IHD, an important consideration in the septic patient with MOF. A second potential advantage to this method is that it may increase rates of dialysis independence at hospital discharge when compared with IHD,[30,31] although all reported studies supporting this association have been observational in nature. To date, RCTs exploring this issue have failed to find any significant difference in terms of hemodynamic effects or survival between the two methods.[32-34] Meta-analyses have found both IHD and CRRT to have comparable mortality outcomes.[35,36] It is likely that critically ill patients can be safely treated with IHD.[35]

On balance, it appears that CRRT and IHD are equally effective in the management of AKI in terms of patient survival and renal recovery; the theoretical concern for increased hemodynamic instability during IHD has not been confirmed in clinical trials. Nevertheless, in some specific clinical scenarios, CRRT may still be preferable to IHD:

- AKI in the setting of cerebral edema: The slower and more gradual reduction in plasma osmolality seen with CRRT can prevent dialysis dysequilibrium and has been associated with improved hemodynamic stability and better preserved cerebral perfusion pressure in patients with AKI and cerebral edema.[37]
- AKI in the setting of hypercatabolism: CRRT facilitates delivery of full-dose nutrition. CRRT may also be preferable for patients requiring high-volume intravenous fluids (blood products, antibiotics). These are nearly universal scenarios in the ICU, where CRRT ensures tight hour-by-hour control of volume.
- AKI in the setting of congestive heart failure: Although CRRT has been shown to improve cardiac function (see earlier), it has not been proved to be superior to IHD in this context. However, CRRT does have the theoretical advantage of being associated with fewer hemodynamic alterations, which may be preferable in the individual patient in cardiogenic shock.

CAN ULTRAFILTRATION SERVE AS A MEANS OF SUPPORT FOR ORGANS OTHER THAN THE KIDNEY?

In the intensive care setting, AKI occurs in 20% to 40% of patients with ARDS,[38] 33% of patients with cardiogenic shock,[39] and 55% of patients with fulminant hepatic failure.[40] Experience using CRRT in the management of these patients has generated interest in whether this intervention can improve outcomes even in patients without AKI; that is, whether CRRT has a supportive role in the management of heart, lung, or liver failure.

Cardiac Support

In an RCT of patients with decompensated heart failure, continuous ultrafiltration was reported to produce greater weight and fluid loss than intravenous diuretics, in addition to reducing patient rehospitalization rates.[41] Another older study, this time observational, found that, in patients with diuretic-resistant congestive cardiac failure, hemofiltration can restore dry body weight, improve urinary output, decrease neurohumoral activation, and prolong symptom-free and edema-free time.[42] This benefit appears greater than would be expected due to fluid removal alone and may be related to the removal of myocardial depressant factors from the circulation.[43]

Lung Support

Ultrafiltration with continuous arteriovenous hemofiltration for oleic acid-induced pulmonary edema in dogs was more effective than diuresis in reducing extravascular lung water.[2] This was despite significantly less overall fluid loss, suggesting an additional role of RRT over and above simple fluid removal. ARDS is often secondary to systemic inflammation, associated with increased levels of tumor necrosis factor-α, interleukin (IL)-1β, and IL-6 found in the bronchoalveolar lavage fluid of affected patients. Hence, there is a potential unproven advantage of CRRT over diuretics associated with the removal of humoral mediators of lung injury from the circulation. Presently, CRRT is only indicated for patients with ARDS who have coexisting AKI.

Liver Support

Application of blood purification strategies to humans with liver failure has mainly occurred in trial settings and is not yet common practice. Experimental approaches have included hemodiabsorption[44] and the molecular adsorbent recirculating system.[45,46] Small studies using these techniques in the management of hepatic failure showed benefit in patients with acute-on-chronic hepatic failure,[44] the hepatorenal syndrome,[45] and even fulminant hepatic failure.[46] However, in the absence of more robust evidence to confirm these findings, no recommendation can be given to support their routine use in clinical practice.

WHAT TYPES OF ANTICOAGULATION ARE AVAILABLE FOR CONTINUOUS RENAL REPLACEMENT THERAPY?

There are two primary approaches to achieving anticoagulation during CRRT: (1) systemic anticoagulation (with unfractionated heparin) and (2) regional anticoagulation in the extracorporeal circuit with the use of a citrate-based regime. Although widely used worldwide, citrate is not currently approved by the U.S. Food and Drug Administration for anticoagulation in continuous venovenous hemofiltration therapy. Two multicenter randomized control trials have compared these regimens with regard to patient survival, safety, and cost. No difference was seen in terms of mortality between the two regimens, and citrate-based anticoagulation was associated with longer filter survival times, lower cost, and fewer bleeding complications.[47,48] A further single-center randomized trial comparing both regimes also found superior filter survival times with a citrate-based regimen.[49] Longer filter survival times reduce underdosing of RRT. Citrate has also been compared to low molecular weight heparin (nadroparin) and was associated with superior survival outcomes and fewer bleeding events.[50] Relative contraindications with systemic heparin include bleeding risk on a case-by-case basis. Relative contraindications to citrate use include advanced liver failure and lactic acidosis. Less commonly used regimens with limited evidence include prostacyclin,[51] which antagonizes platelets, thereby reducing anticoagulation use, or direct thrombin inhibitors such as argatroban.[52]

REFERENCES

1. Goldstein SL, Currier H, Graf CD, et al. Outcome in children receiving continuous venovenous hemofiltration. *Pediatrics.* 2001;107:1309–1312.
2. Gillespie RS, Seidel K, Symons JM. Effect of fluid overload and dose of replacement fluid on survival in hemofiltration. *Pediatr Nephrol.* 2004;19:1394–1399.
3. Foland JA, Fortenberry JD, Warshaw BL, et al. Fluid overload before continuous hemofiltration and survival in critically ill children: a retrospective analysis. *Crit Care Med.* 2004;32:1771–1776.
4. Payen D, de Pont AC, Sakr Y, et al. Sepsis Occurrence in Acutely Ill Patients (SOAP) investigators: a positive fluid balance is associated with a worse outcome in patients with acute renal failure. *Crit Care.* 2008;12:R74.
5. Mehta RL, Pascual MT, Soroko S, Chertow GM, PICARD Study Group. Diuretics, mortality, and nonrecovery of renal function in acute renal failure. *JAMA.* 2002;288:2547–2553.
6. Uchino S, Doig GS, Bellomo R, et al. Beginning and Ending Supportive Therapy for the Kidney (B.E.S.T. Kidney) Investigators: diuretics and mortality in acute renal failure. *Crit Care Med.* 2004;32:1669–1677.
7. Cantarovich F, Rangoonwala B, Lorenz H, High-Dose Furosemide in Acute Renal Failure Study Group, et al. High-dose furosemide for established ARF: a prospective, randomized, double-blind, placebo-controlled, multicenter trial. *Am J Kidney Dis.* 2004;44:402–409.
8. Bagshaw SM, Delaney A, Haase M, et al. Loop diuretics in the management of acute renal failure: a systematic review and meta-analysis. *Crit Care Resusc.* 2007;9:60–68.
9. Sivak ED, Tita J, Meden G, et al. Effects of furosemide versus isolated ultrafiltration on extravascular lung water in oleic acid-induced pulmonary edema. *Crit Care Med.* 1986;14:48–51.
10. Bouchard J, Mehta RL. Acid-base disturbances in the intensive care unit: current issues and the use of continuous renal replacement therapy as a customized treatment tool. *Int J Artif Organs.* 2008;31:6–14.
11. Naka T, Bellomo R. Bench-to-bedside review. Treating acid-base abnormalities in the intensive care unit: the role of renal replacement therapy. *Crit Care.* 2004;8:108–114.
12. Uchino S, Bellomo R, Ronco C. Intermittent versus continuous renal replacement therapy in the ICU: impact on electrolyte and acid-base balance. *Intensive Care Med.* 2001;27:1037–1043.
13. Mahoney BA, Smith WA, Lo DS, et al. Emergency interventions for hyperkalaemia. *Cochrane Database Syst Rev.* 2005;18:CD003235.
14. Holubek WJ, Hoffman RS, Goldfarb DS, Nelson LS. Use of hemodialysis and hemoperfusion in poisoned patients. *Kidney Int.* 2008;74:1327–1334.

15. Gettings LG, Reynolds HN, Scalea T. Outcome in post-traumatic acute renal failure when continuous renal replacement therapy is applied early vs late. *Intensive Care Med*. 1999;25:805–813.

16. Liu KD, Himmelfarb J, Paganini E, et al. Timing of initiation of dialysis in critically ill patients with acute kidney injury. *Clin J Am Soc Nephrol*. 2006;1:915–919.

17. Bouman CS, Oudemans-Van Straaten HM, Tijssen JG, et al. Effects of early high-volume continuous venovenous hemofiltration on survival and recovery of renal function in intensive care patients with acute renal failure: a prospective, randomized trial. *Crit Care Med*. 2002;30:2205–2211.

18. Elahi MM, Lim MY, Joseph RN, et al. Early hemofiltration improves survival in post-cardiotomy patients with acute renal failure. *Eur J Cardiothorac Surg*. 2004;26:1027–1031.

19. Demirkiliç U, Kuralay E, Yenicesu M, et al. Timing of replacement therapy for acute renal failure after cardiac surgery. *J Card Surg*. 2004;19:17–20.

20. Seabra VF, Balk EM, Liangos O, et al. Timing of renal replacement therapy initiation in acute renal failure: a meta-analysis. *Am J Kidney Dis*. 2008;52:272–284.

21. Bagshaw SM, Uchino S, Bellomo R, et al. Beginning and Ending Supportive Therapy for the Kidney (BEST Kidney) Investigators. Septic acute kidney injury in critically ill patients: clinical characteristics and outcomes. *Clin J Am Soc Nephrol*. 2007;2:431–439.

22. Bagshaw SM, George C, Bellomo R, for the ANZICS Database Management Committee. Early acute kidney injury and sepsis: a multicentre evaluation. *Crit Care*. 2008;12:R47.

23. Honoré PM, Joannes-Boyau O, Gressens B. Blood and plasma treatments: the rationale of high-volume hemofiltration. *Contrib Nephrol*. 2007;156:387–395.

24. Kellum JA, Song M, Venkataraman R. Hemoadsorption removes tumor necrosis factor, interleukin-6, and interleukin-10, reduces nuclear factor-kappaB DNA binding, and improves short-term survival in lethal endotoxemia. *Crit Care Med*. 2004;32:801–805.

25. Morgera S, Haase M, Kuss T, et al. Pilot study on the effects of high cutoff hemofiltration on the need for norepinephrine in septic patients with acute renal failure. *Crit Care Med*. 2006;34:2099–2104.

26. Joannes-Boyau O, Honoré PM, Perez P, Bagshaw SM, et al. High-volume versus standard-volume haemofiltration for septic shock patients with acute kidney injury (IVOIRE study): a multicentre randomized controlled trial. *Intensive Care Med*. September 2013;39(9):1535–1546.

27. Palevsky PM, Zhang JH, O'Connor TZ, for the VA/NIH Acute Renal Failure Trial Network, et al. Intensity of renal support in critically ill patients with acute kidney injury. *N Engl J Med*. 2008;359:7–20.

28. Bellomo R, et al. Intensity of continuous renal-replacement therapy in critically ill patients. *N Engl J Med*. 2009;361(17): 1627–1638.

29. Boussekey N, Chiche A, Faure K, et al. A pilot randomized study comparing high and low volume hemofiltration on vasopressor use in septic shock. *Intensive Care Med*. 2008;34:1646–1653.

30. Bell M, Granath F, Schön S, et al. Continuous renal replacement therapy is associated with less chronic renal failure than intermittent haemodialysis after acute renal failure. *Intensive Care Med*. 2007;33:773–780.

31. Uchino S, Bellomo R, Kellum JA, for the Beginning and Ending Supportive Therapy for the Kidney (B.E.S.T. Kidney) Investigators Writing Committee, et al. Patient and kidney survival by dialysis modality in critically ill patients with acute kidney injury. *Int J Artif Organs*. 2007;30:281–292.

32. Mehta RL, McDonald B, Gabbai FB, for the Collaborative Group for Treatment of ARF in the ICU, et al. A randomized clinical trial of continuous versus intermittent dialysis for acute renal failure. *Kidney Int*. 2001;60:1154–1163.

33. Uehlinger DE, Jakob SM, Ferrari P, et al. Comparison of continuous and intermittent renal replacement therapy for acute renal failure. *Nephrol Dial Transplant*. 2005;20:1630–1637.

34. Vinsonneau C, Camus C, Combes A, for the Hemodiafe Study Group, et al. Continuous venovenoushaemodiafiltration versus intermittent haemodialysis for acute renal failure in patients with multiple-organ dysfunction syndrome: a multicentre randomised trial. *Lancet*. 2006;368:379–385.

35. Kellum JA, Angus DC, Johnson JP, et al. Continuous versus intermittent renal replacement therapy: a meta-analysis. *Intensive Care Med*. 2002;28:29–37.

36. Tonelli M, Manns B, Feller-Kopman D. Acute renal failure in the intensive care unit: a systematic review of the impact of dialytic modality on mortality and renal recovery. *Am J Kidney Dis*. 2002;40:875–885.

37. Davenport A, Finn R, Goldsmith SJ. Management of patients with acute renal failure complicated by cerebral edema. *Blood Purif*. 1989;7:203–209.

38. Valta P, Uusaro A, Nunes S, et al. Acute respiratory distress syndrome: frequency, clinical course, and costs of care. *Crit Care Med*. 1999;27:2367–2374.

39. Koreny M, Karth GD, Geppert A, et al. Prognosis of patients who develop acute renal failure during the first 24 hours of cardiogenic shock after myocardial infarction. *Am J Med*. 2002;112:115–119.

40. Ring-Larsen H, Palazzo U. Renal failure in fulminant hepatic failure and terminal cirrhosis: a comparison between incidence, types, and prognosis. *Gut*. 1981;22:585–591.

41. Costanzo MR, Guglin ME, Saltzberg MT, for the UNLOAD Trial Investigators, et al. Ultrafiltration versus intravenous diuretics for patients hospitalized for acute decompensated heart failure. *J Am Coll Cardiol*. 2007;49:675–683.

42. Cipolla CM, Grazi S, Rimondini A. Changes in circulating norepinephrine with haemofiltration in advanced congestive cardiac failure. *Am J Cardiol*. 1990;66:987–994.

43. Blake P, Hasegawa Y, Khosla MC, et al. Isolation of myocardial depressant factors from the ultrafiltrate of heart failure patients with acute renal failure. *ASAIO J*. 1996;42:M911–M915.

44. Ash SR. Powdered sorbent liver dialysis and pheresis in treatment of hepatic failure. *Ther Apher*. 2001;5:404–416.

45. Mitzner SR, Stange J, Klammt S, et al. Improvement of hepatorenal syndrome with extracorporeal albumin dialysis MARS: results of a prospective, randomized, controlled clinical trial. *Liver Transpl*. 2000;6:277–286.

46. Novelli G, Rossi M, Pretagostini M, et al. One hundred sixteen cases of acute liver failure treated with MARS. *Transplant Proc*. 2005;37:2557–2559.

47. Schilder L, Nurmohamed S, Bosch FH, et al. Citrate anticoagulation versus systemic heparinisation in continuous venovenous hemofiltration in critically ill patients with acute kidney injury: a multi-center randomized clinical trial. *Crit Care*. 2014;18(4):472.

48. Hetzel GR, Schmitz M, Wissing H, et al. Regional citrate versus systemic heparin for anticoagulation in critically ill patients on continuous venovenoushaemofiltration: a prospective randomized multicentre trial. *Nephrol Dial Transplant*. 2011;26(1):232–239.

49. Monchi M, Berghmans D, Ledoux D, Canivet JL, Dubois B, Damas P. Citrate vs heparin for anticoagulation in continuous venovenous hemofiltration: a prospective randomized study. *Intensive Care Med*. 2004;30(2):260–265.

50. Oudemans-van Straaten HM1, Bosman RJ, Koopmans M, et al. Citrate anticoagulation for continuous venovenous hemofiltration. *Crit Care Med*. 2009;37(2):545–552.

51. Langenecker SA, Felfernig M, Werba A, Mueller CM, Chiari A, Zimpfer M. Anticoagulation with prostacyclin and heparin during continuous venovenous hemofiltration. *Crit Care Med*. 1994;22(11):1774–1781.

52. Tang IY, Cox DS, Patel K, et al. Argatroban and renal replacement therapy in patients with heparin-induced thrombocytopenia. *Ann Pharmacother*. 2005;39(2):231–236.

53. Teschan P, Baxter C, O'Brian T, et al. Prophylactic haemodialysis in the treatment of acute renal failure. *Ann Intern Med*. 1960;53:992–1016.

54. Parsons FM, Hobson SM, Blagg CR, McCracken BH. Optimum time for dialysis in acute reversible renal failure. Description and value of an improved dialyser with large surface area. *Lancet*. 1961;1:129–134.

55. Fischer RP, Griffen Jr WO, Reiser M, Clark DS. Early dialysis in the treatment of acute renal failure. *Surg Gynecol Obstet*. 1966;123: 1019–1023.

56. Kleinknecht D, Jungers P, Chanard J, Barbanel C, Ganeval D. Uremic and non-uremic complications in acute renal failure: evaluation of early and frequent dialysis on prognosis. *Kidney Int*. 1972;1:190–196.

57. Conger JD. A controlled evaluation of prophylactic dialysis in post-traumatic acute renal failure. *J Trauma*. 1975;15:1056–1063.

58. Gillum DM, Dixon BS, Yanover MJ, et al. The role of intensive dialysis in acute renal failure. *Clin Nephrol*. 1986;25:249–255.

Chapter 17

METABOLIC ABNORMALITIES IN CRITICAL ILLNESS

58 How Should Acid-Base Disorders Be Diagnosed and Managed?

Patrick J. Neligan

Arterial blood gas (ABG) analysis, a core component of critical care monitoring, provides immediate information on the status of the patient's respiratory system and whether a state of acidosis or alkalosis is present. With a variety of empiric "rules" applied, the information contained in an ABG is often sufficient to allow one to identify the presence, cause, and progression of a disease. The diagnostic sensitivity of blood gas analysis is augmented when a serum chemistry panel and glucose, lactate, and ketone measurements are added. Unlike abnormalities of serum and urinary electrolytes, radiographic or electrocardiographic changes, there is no clear agreement between intensive care specialists regarding the optimal method of evaluating acid base balance.

Several different approaches to acid–base balance are in widespread use.[1] These can be described as descriptive, based on changes in the Henderson-Hasselbalch equation; semiquantitative, based on calculations and nomograms; or quantitative, based on physical chemistry. The descriptive approach uses the interrelationship between partial pressure of carbon dioxide in arterial blood ($Paco_2$) and bicarbonate [HCO_3^-] to detect and diagnose acid base abnormalities. An extension of this is the anion gap (AG). The semiquantitative approach includes the buffer base concept, the standardized base deficit–excess, and the base-deficit gap (BDG). The quantitative approach uses strong ion difference (SID) and total weak acid concentration (A_{TOT}) and is quantified with the strong ion gap (SIG).

SCIENTIFIC BACKGROUND

In the early part of the twentieth century it was widely known that, in critical illness, the carbon dioxide (CO_2) content of the blood fell. As early as 1831 O'Shaughnessy identified loss of "carbonate of soda" from the blood as a fundamental disturbance in patients dying of cholera.[2] L. J. Henderson, in 1909, coined the term "acid base" balance.[3] He was able to define this process in terms of carbonic acid equilibrium. This work was later refined by Hasselbalch in 1916.[4] Their method described acid-base balance in terms of the hydration equation for CO_2, the only clinical chemistry test available at that time.

$$CO_2 + H_2O \rightarrow H_2CO_3 \rightarrow H^+ + HCO_3^-$$

$$pH = pKa + \log[HCO_3^-] / [H_2CO_3]$$

$$\text{Total } CO_2 = [HCO_3^-] + [\text{Dissolved } CO_2] + [\text{Carbamino } CO_2] + [H_2CO_3]$$

$$\approx PCO_2 \times 0.03 \text{mmol } CO_2/L/mm \text{ Hg}$$

thus, substituting into the equation above:

$$pH = 6.1 + \log[HCO_3^-] / PCO_2 \times 0.03:$$
The Henderson-Hasselbalch equation

Svante Arrhenius (1859-1927) in 1903 established the foundations of acid–base chemistry. In an aqueous solution, an Arrhenius acid is any substance that delivers a hydrogen ion into the solution.[2] A base is any substance that delivers a hydroxyl ion into the solution. Water is a highly ionizing amphiprotic solution, so substances with polar bonds will dissociate into their component part in it. Water may act as an acid or a base.

The degree of dissociation of substances in water determines whether they are strong acids or strong bases. Thus lactic acid, which has an ion dissociation constant (pKa) of 3.4, is completely dissociated at physiologic pH, and is a strong acid. Conversely, carbonic acid, which has a pKa of 6.4, is incompletely dissociated, and is a weak acid. Similarly, ions, such as sodium, potassium, and chloride, which do not easily bind to other molecules, are considered strong ions—they exist free in solution.

In any solution, the ion dissociation constant for water, Kw', dictates that the relative ratio of [H^+] to [OH^-] must always be constant, and electrical neutrality must always hold. Consequently, strong cations, Na^+, K^+, Ca^{2+}, Mg^{2+}, will act as Arrhenius bases (they deliver hydroxide into the aqueous solution), and strong anions, Cl^-, LA^-, ketones, sulfate, and formate, will act as Arrhenius acids (they deliver hydrogen ions into the aqueous solution).

The Arrhenius theory was superseded in 1923 by Brønsted and Lowry. They defined acids as proton donors and bases as proton acceptors.

$$NH_3 + H_2O \leftrightarrow NH_4^+ + OH^-$$

In this situation, water is the proton donor, the Brønsted-Lowry acid, and ammonia the proton acceptor, the Brønsted-Lowry (BL) base. Conversely, consider the following reaction:

$$HCL + H_2O \rightarrow H_3O^+ + Cl^-$$

In this reaction, hydrogen chloride acts as a Brønsted-Lowry (BL) acid and water as a BL base.

$$CO_2 + H_2O \leftrightarrow H_2CO_3 \leftrightarrow H^+ + HCO_3^-$$

In this reaction, CO_2 is hydrated to carbonic acid, a BL acid that subsequently dissociates to hydrogen and bicarbonate.

STRONG IONS

Strong ions are completely dissociated at physiologic pH. The most abundant strong ions in the extracellular space are sodium (Na^+) and chloride (Cl^-). Other important strong ions include K^+, SO_4^{2-}, Mg^{2+}, and Ca^{2+}. Each applies a direct electrochemical and osmotic effect.

In the extracellular space the difference between the charge carried on strong cations and strong anions is calculated by

$$SID = ([Na^+] + [K^+] + [Ca^{2+}] + [Mg^{2+}])$$
$$- ([Cl^-] + [Other\ strong\ anions: A^-]) = 40\text{-}44\ mEq$$

This excess of positive charge, called the strong ion difference, by Peter Stewart,[5] is always positive, and is balanced by an equal amount of "buffer base," principally in the form of phosphate, albumin, and bicarbonate.[6] SID independently influences water dissociation, determined by electrical neutrality and mass conservation. If all other factors (Pco_2, albumin, and phosphate) are kept constant, an increase in SID, due to a relative increase in the ratio of strong cations to strong anions, will decrease hydrogen ion availability causing alkalosis. A decrease in SID, due to a relative decrease in the relative ratio of strong cations to strong anions, results in greater accumulation of hydrogen ions causing acidosis.

The chief determinant of SID is the relationship between the relative concentrations of sodium, chloride, and free water in extracellular fluid (ECF). The normal ratio of sodium to chloride is approximately 1.4:1. Any process that reduces that ratio reduces SID and leads to acidosis (sodium loss, chloride gain, or free water gain). Any process that increases that ratio increases SID and leads to alkalosis (sodium gain, chloride loss, or free water gain).

WEAK ACIDS

Albumin and phosphate are weak acids, in which the degree of dissociation is related to temperature and pH. Weak acids, represented by the symbol A_{TOT}, independently influence acid base balance, depending on absolute quantity and dissociation equilibria.[5,7]

The principal limitation of traditional approaches to acid base balance has been the limited attention paid to changes in A_{TOT}.[8] Although this may be valid in otherwise healthy patients, perioperative care and critical illness cause hypoalbuminemia due to crystalloid administration, hepatic reprioritization, and capillary leak.[9] A reduction in serum albumin or phosphate leads to metabolic alkalosis.[10] Hypophosphatemia is associated with malnutrition, refeeding, diuresis, and hemodilution. Hyperphosphatemia occurs in renal failure. Hyperphosphatemia leads to metabolic acidosis.

CARBON DIOXIDE

Aerobic metabolism results in the production of large quantities of CO_2. CO_2 is hydrated by carbonic anhydrase in red cell erythrocytes to carbonic acid. This liberates the equivalent of 12,500 mEq of H^+ per day. Hydrogen ions bind to histidine residues on deoxyhemoglobin, and bicarbonate is actively pumped out of the cell. CO_2 exists in four forms: CO_2 [denoted $CO_2(d)$], carbonic acid (H_2CO_3), bicarbonate ions (HCO_3^-) and carbonate ions CO_3^{2-}. The principal mechanism of excretion is via alveolar ventilation, although some CO_2 is excreted from the kidney as bicarbonate as part of a sodium-chloride cotransporter.

Chronic respiratory acidosis is associated with increase in total body CO_2 content, reflected principally by an increase in serum bicarbonate. Mathematically $\Delta HCO_3^- = 0.5\ \Delta PaCO_2$.[11] It is important that this is not confused with "metabolic compensation for hypercarbia," a relatively slow process that reduces SID by increased urinary chloride excretion.[12]

ACID-BASE DISTURBANCES

Acid-base disturbances are an important part of clinical and laboratory investigation of perioperative and critically ill patients.

There are six primary acid-base abnormalities (Table 58-1):

1. Acidosis due to increased $Paco_2$
2. Acidosis due to decreased SID
   - Increased chloride (hyperchloremic), reduced sodium (dilutional)/increased free water
   - Acidosis due to the increased presence of lactate, ketones, or unmeasured anions (UMA)
3. Acidosis due to increased A_{TOT}
   - Hyperphosphatemia, hyperproteinemia
4. Alkalosis due to decreased $Paco_2$
5. Alkalosis due to increased SID
   - Decreased chloride (hypochloremic), increased sodium/decreased free water (contraction)
6. Alkalosis due to decreased A_{TOT}
   - Hypophosphatemia, hypoalbuminemia

ACUTE RESPIRATORY ACIDOSIS AND ALKALOSIS

Acute respiratory acidosis results from hypoventilation, due to loss of respiratory drive, neuromuscular or

Table 58-1 **Classification of Acid-Base Abnormalities**		
	Acidosis	**Alkalosis**
Respiratory	Increased P_{CO_2}	Decreased P_{CO_2} $\uparrow SID^+ + \downarrow [Cl^-]$
METABOLIC		
1. Abnormal SID^+		
a. Due to water	Water excess = dilution $\downarrow SID^+ \downarrow [Na+]$	Water deficit = contraction $\uparrow SID^+ \uparrow [Na+]$
b. Due to electrolytes Chloride (measured)	Chloride excess $\downarrow SID^+ \uparrow [Cl^-]$	Chloride deficit $\uparrow SID^+ + \downarrow [Cl^-]$
Others (Unmeasured anions) e.g., lactate, keto acids	$\downarrow SID^+ \uparrow [A^-]$	-
2. Abnormal A_{TOT}		
a. Albumin [alb]	$\uparrow [Alb^-]$ (intravenous albumin)	$\downarrow [Alb^-]$
b. Phosphate [Pi]	$\uparrow [Pi^-]$	$\downarrow [Pi^-]$

$A-$, abnormal A_{TOT}; A_{TOT}, total weak acid concentration; Cl^-, chloride; P_{CO_2}, partial pressure of carbon dioxide; *Na*, sodium; *SID*, strong ion difference.

chest wall disorders, or rapid-shallow breathing, which increases the fraction of dead space ventilation. Acute respiratory acidosis is often associated with a precipitous reduction in pH due to the absence of a rapid buffering system for large quantities of CO_2. Acute respiratory alkalosis (pH > 7.5) is caused by hyperventilation due to anxiety, central respiratory stimulation (as occurs early in salicylate poisoning), or excessive artificial ventilation. Acute respiratory alkalosis usually accompanies acute metabolic acidosis (pH < 7.35). A useful rule of thumb in this case is that the reduction in P_{CO_2} from baseline (usually 40 mm Hg) is equal to the magnitude of the base deficit (see later). For example, in a patient with lactic acidosis, with a lactate of 10 mEq/L, the base deficit should be −10, and the P_{CO_2} 30 mm Hg. If the P_{CO_2} is higher than expected, then there is a problem with the respiratory apparatus. This is seen, for example, in a multitrauma patient in which there is massive blood loss, causing lactic acidosis, plus a flail chest, causing respiratory acidosis.

ACUTE METABOLIC ACIDOSIS

Acute metabolic acidosis is caused by an alteration in SID or A_{TOT}. SID is changed by an alteration in the relative quantity of strong anions to strong cations. This can be caused by anion gain, as occurs with lactic acidosis, renal acidosis, ketoacidosis, and hyperchloremic acidosis, or cation loss, as occurs with severe diarrhea. Acidosis also results from increased free water relative to strong ions—dilutional acidosis, which results from excessive hypotonic fluid intake, certain poisonings (methanol, ethylene glycol, or isopropyl alcohol), or hyperglycemia.

Metabolic Acidosis Due to Unmeasured Anions

In acute metabolic acidosis, three diagnoses should be immediately investigated: lactic acidosis, ketoacidosis due to diabetes (hyperglycemic) or starvation (normoglycemia), and acute kidney injury, demonstrated by high serum urea and creatinine and low total P_{aCO_2}. The presence of a low serum sodium (<135 mEq/L), or an otherwise unexplained metabolic acidosis in a comatose patient, should alert the clinician to the possibility of a dilutional acidosis, caused by alcohol poisoning. Alcohols such as ethanol, methanol, isopropyl alcohol, and ethylene glycol are osmotically active molecules that expand extracellular water (glucose and mannitol have the same effect but also promote diuresis, as the molecules are small enough to be filtered by the kidney). Alcohol poisoning is suspected by the presence of an osmolar gap: a difference between the measured and calculated serum osmolality of greater than 12 mOsm demonstrates the presence of unmeasured osmoles. Toxicology laboratories can investigate for the presence of various toxic alcohols.

Hyperchloremic and Dilutional Acidosis Associated with Intravenous Fluids

The administration of intravenous fluids to patients has significant impact on acid-base balance. There are changes in free water volume, SID, and A_{TOT} (principally albumin). "Dilutional acidosis" results from administration of pure water to extracellular fluid (which is alkaline).[13] This can occur with large volume administration of any fluid whose SID is 0: 5% dextrose, 0.9% saline (NS, contains 154 mEq of both Na^+ and Cl^+), or other hypotonic saline infusions.[14] Hence the administration of each liter of NS results in a net ECF gain of 50 mEq/L chloride, or, put another way, hydrochloric acid. Hyperchloremic acidosis is frequently seen in perioperative patients after large volume administration of 0.9% saline solution,[15] or 6% hetastarch (both formulated in normal saline), hypertonic saline, or gelatin-based solutions.[16-22] The administration of albumin results in metabolic acidosis due to an increase in A_{TOT}.[23,24]

Renal Tubular Acidosis

In metabolic acidosis, chloride is preferentially excreted by the kidney. Indeed this is the resting state of renal physiology because sodium and chloride are absorbed in the diet in relatively equal quantities.[25] In metabolic acidosis chloride is preferentially excreted.[26] In metabolic alkalosis, chloride is retained, and sodium and potassium are excreted. Acetazolamide corrects metabolic alkalosis by increasing SID secondary to reduced chloride excretion.[27]

Abnormalities in the renal handling of chloride may be responsible for several inherited and acquired acid-base disturbances. In critical illness, acquired renal tubular acidosis appears to be quite common.[28] In inherited renal tubular acidosis, there is an inability to excrete Cl^- in proportion to Na^+.[29] Similarly, pseudohypoaldosteronism appears to be due to high reabsorption of chloride.[30] Bartter syndrome is caused by a mutation in the gene encoding the chloride channel, CLCNKB, which regulates the Na-K-2Cl cotransporter (NKCC2).[31]

Clinical Relevance of Hyperchloremic Acidosis

What is the clinical relevance of hyperchloremic acidosis? The most common cause of hyperchloremia in clinical medicine is fluid resuscitation with 0.9% saline; the relative addition of hydrochloric acid in this fluid results in hyperchloremic acidosis. Although hyperchloremia is often dismissed as less relevant to "pathologic" acidosis, lactic acidosis or ketoacidosis,[32] it is important to note that metabolic acidosis regardless of origin can depress myocardial contractility and reduce cardiac output and tissue perfusion. Acidosis inactivates membrane calcium channels and inhibits the release of norepinephrine from sympathetic nerve fibers, leading to vasodilatation and maldistribution of blood flow.

There are emerging data that hyperchloremia, per se, may negatively affect splanchnic[33] and renal function. In the human diet, sodium and chloride are ingested in roughly equimolar concentrations. A major component of renal function is the excretion of relatively more chloride than sodium. Hence chloride in and of itself, when delivered to an injured or ischemic kidney, may potentially act as a nephrotoxin. Plasma chloride levels affect afferent arteriolar tone through calcium-activated chloride channels and modulate the release of renin.[34] Hyperchloremia can reduce renal blood flow and glomerular filtration rate.[35] Hyperchloremia reduces overall splanchnic blood flow.[36] In a study of healthy volunteers, normal saline was associated with reduced urinary output compared with lactated Ringer's solution.[37] A crossover trial of 12 healthy male volunteers that received 2-L intravenous infusions of 0.9% saline or PlasmaLyte 148 over 1 hour demonstrated a significant reduction in mean renal artery flow velocity ($P = .045$) and renal cortical tissue perfusion ($P = .008$) from baseline after saline, but not after PlasmaLyte 148 (a balanced salt solution).[38]

In a study of fluid prehydration to prevent contrast nephropathy, the use of (chloride free) sodium bicarbonate was associated with a 11.9% absolute reduction in the risk of renal injury (defined as a 25% increase in creatinine).[39] Haase and colleagues compared perioperative $NaHCO_3$ or NS (4 mmol/kg over 24 hours) in patients undergoing cardiac surgery.[40] There was a 20% absolute risk increase of renal dysfunction in the patients receiving NS (odds ratio, 0.43; 95% confidence interval [CI], 0.19 to 0.98) ($P = .043$). After liver transplantation, perioperative administration of more than 3200 mL chloride liberal fluids (resulting in hyperchloremia) resulted in a substantial increase in the risk of acute kidney injury (hazard ratio, 6.25; 95% CI, 2.69, 14.5; $P < .000$).[41]

An observational study of 31,000 surgical patients comparing intravenous saline to intravenous balanced salt solutions (BSS) demonstrated significant outcome differences, favoring BSS.[42] Complications that were increased by the use of 0.9% saline included postoperative infections, blood transfusions, and kidney injury requiring dialysis. Patients with perioperative metabolic acidosis, either hyperchloremic acidosis or lactic acidosis, have prolonged duration of hospital stay.[43] In a relatively large before-and-after cohort study of patients treated in an Australian intensive care unit (ICU), the use of chloride-rich fluids was associated with a 3.7% absolute increase in the risk for need in renal replacement therapy relative to balanced salt solution.[44]

Renal Acidosis and the Impact of Dialysis

Renal acidosis is widely thought to be caused by accumulation of strong ion products of metabolism excreted exclusively by the kidney. Although "renal acids" such as sulfate and formate are usually considered the cause of "renal acidosis," hyperchloremia is the major cause of strong ion gain.[26,45-47] In addition, there is accumulation of a weak acid, phosphate. Moreover, free water gain may result in a concomitant hyponatremic dilutional acidosis.[48]

Continuous renal replacement therapy (CRRT) is used in critical illness to hemofiltrate and hemodialyze patients who are hemodynamically unstable. Rocktaschel[49] and colleagues have demonstrated that CRRT resolves the acidosis of acute kidney injury by removing strong ions and phosphate, but metabolic alkalosis was unmasked because of hypoalbuminemia. Serum lactate may increase (depending on the dialysis fluid), but this does not result in acidosis.[22] In the setting of severe hepatic failure, weak acids are no longer effectively removed by the liver, and metabolic acidosis will require more aggressive dialysis to resolve.[50]

ACUTE METABOLIC ALKALOSIS

Hyperventilation of patients with chronic respiratory failure results in acute metabolic alkalosis, due to chronic compensatory alkalosis associated with chloride loss in urine. More frequently, metabolic alkalosis is associated with increased SID due to sodium gain. This occurs because of administration of fluids in which sodium is "buffered" by weak ions, citrate (in blood products),[51] acetate (in parenteral nutrition), and, of course, bicarbonate.[52,53] In each of these situations, the anion is converted to CO_2 (usually by hepatic metabolism) and excreted through respiration; net sodium gain follows because of mass conservation.

The most frequent single disturbance in acid-base chemistry in critically ill patients is hypoalbuminemia.[54] This is ubiquitous and causes an unpredictable metabolic alkalosis. Hypoalbuminemia may mask significant alterations in SID, such as lactic acidemia. All intravenous fluids that do not contain albumin are alkalizing. Thus, all patients that receive significant volumes of intravenous fluid in the operating room develop a hypoalbuminemic alkalosis. It is unknown whether this anomaly has any clinical significance. Morgan and colleagues, in a series of elegant studies, have determined that the optimal SID of resuscitation fluid should be 24 mEq/L, rather than 40 mEq/L.[13,55] Progressive dilution of albumin is alkalinizing; thus net chloride gain is required to maintain the normal balance between SID and A_{TOT}.[56]

Other Acid-Base Problems in Critical Illness

Critically ill patients are vulnerable to significant changes in SID and free water. Nasogastric suctioning causes chloride loss; diarrhea leads to sodium and potassium loss.[57] Surgical drains placed in tissue beds may remove fluids with varying electrolyte concentrations (the pancreatic bed, for example, secretes fluid rich in sodium). Fever, sweating, oozing tissues, and inadequately humidified ventilator circuits lead to large volume insensible loss and contraction alkalosis.[58] Loop diuretics and polyuric renal failure may be associated with significant contraction alkalosis, due to loss of chloride and free water.

Parenteral infusions may be responsible for stealth alterations in serum chemistry. Many antibiotics, such as piperacillin–tazobactam, are diluted in sodium-rich solutions. Others, such as vancomycin, are administered in large volumes of free water (5% dextrose). Lorazepam is diluted in propylene glycol, large volumes of which will cause metabolic acidosis similar to that seen with ethylene glycol.[59] Mannitol may cause metabolic acidosis by the same mechanism.[60]

ANALYTICAL TOOLS USED IN ACID–BASE CHEMISTRY

In this section, some of the tools that have evolved over the past 60 years to assist in the interpretation of acid–base conundrums are considered. None are entirely accurate,[61] and each has a dedicated group of followers.[62] The approaches can be described as descriptive, based on changes in the in the Henderson-Hasselbalch equation; semiquantitative, based on calculations and nomograms; or quantitative, based on physical chemistry.

DESCRIPTIVE CARBON DIOXIDE–BICARBONATE (BOSTON) APPROACH

In the early 1960s, Schwartz, Relman, and colleagues, at Tufts University in Boston, developed an approach to acid–base chemistry, based on a large series of observational data that derived nomograms and mathematical constructs that related $Paco_2$ to $[HCO_3^-]$.[63] A number of patients with known acid–base disturbances, at steady states of compensation, were evaluated. The degree of compensation, from what was considered normal, was measured for each disease state. The investigators were able to describe six primary states of acid–base imbalance, using linear equations or maps, relating hydrogen ion concentration to $Paco_2$ for respiratory disturbances, and $Paco_2$ to HCO_3^- concentration, for metabolic disturbances (Table 58-2). For any given acid–base disturbance, an expected $[HCO_3^-]$ was determined. This resulted in the development of several simple "rules of thumb" (see Table 58-2). For example, in acute respiratory acidosis, the $[HCO_3^-]$ will increase by 1 mEq/L for every 10 mm Hg elevation in $Paco_2$ above 40 mm Hg. In chronic respiratory acidosis, the $[HCO_3^-]$ will increase by 4 mEq/L for every 10 mm Hg elevation in $Paco_2$ above 40 mm Hg. In metabolic acidosis, the expected $Paco_2$ follows the $1.5 \times HCO_3^- + 8$ (range: $+/-2$) rule.

In general, this approach has remained very popular with pulmonologists and nephrologists, particularly in North America, in clinical situations where acid-base abnormalities are relatively straightforward. There are several inherent pitfalls to the $PCO_2 - HCO_3^-$ approach,

Table 58-2 **Rules of Thumb for Boston Approach to Acid–Base Balance**

Disturbance	HCO_3^- vs. $Paco_2$
Acute respiratory acidosis	Expected $[HCO_3^-] = 24 + Paco_2 - 40)/10$
Acute respiratory alkalosis	Expected $[HCO_3^-] = 24 - 2(40 - Paco_2)/10$
Chronic respiratory acidosis	Expected $[HCO_3^-] = 24 + 4(Paco_2 - 40)/10$
Metabolic acidosis	Expected $Paco_2 = 1.5 \times [HCO_3^-] + 8$
Metabolic alkalosis	Expected $Paco_2 = 0.7[HCO_3^-] + 20$

HCO_3^-, bicarbonate; $Paco_2$, partial pressure of carbon dioxide in arterial blood.

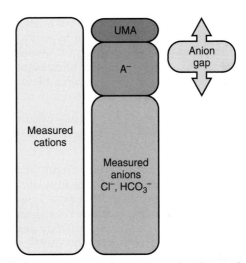

Figure 58-1. The anion gap. A^- represents phosphate and albumin; A^- refers to the charge carried on albumin and phosphate. *UMA,* unmeasured anions.

particularly in relation to the metabolic component. The system neither explains nor accounts for many of the complex acid–base abnormalities seen in perioperative and critically ill patients, such as those with acute acidosis in the setting of hypoalbuminemia, hyperchloremic acidosis, or dilutional acidosis or with lactic acidosis in the setting of chronic respiratory acidosis.

ANION GAP APPROACH

For the primary limitation of the Boston approach to be addressed, the AG was developed by Emmit and Narins in 1975[64] to deal with metabolic acidosis. The AG is based on the law of electrical neutrality. The sum of the difference in charge of the common extracellular ions reveals an unaccounted for "gap" of –12 to –16 mEq/L (the original anion gap = $[Na^+] - ([CL^-] + [HCO_3^-])$ (Fig. 58-1). If the patient has a metabolic acidosis and the gap "widens" to, for example, −20 mEq/L (because of consumption of bicarbonate), then the acidosis is caused by UMA—lactate or ketones or "renal acids." If the gap does not widen, then the anions *are* being measured, and the acidosis has been caused by hyperchloremia (bicarbonate cannot independently influence acid-base status).

There are three widely used variants of the AG, depending on whether potassium and lactate are included:

$$Anion\ Gap\ (simple) = ([Na^+] - ([CL^-] + [HCO_3^-]))$$
$$= 12\ to\ 14\ mEq/L$$

$$Anion\ Gap\ (conventional) = ([Na^+] + [K^+]$$
$$- ([CL^-] + [HCO_3^-]))$$
$$= 14\ to\ 18\ mEq/L$$

$$Anion\ Gap\ (modern) = ([Na^+] + [K^+]$$
$$- ([CL^-] + [HCO_3^-] + [lactate^-]))$$
$$= 14\ to\ 18\ mEq/L$$

The AG frequently underestimates the extent of the metabolic disturbance.[65] Although this is a useful tool, it is weakened by the assumption of what is or is not a "normal gap."[66] Most critically ill patients are hypoalbuminemic, and many are also hypophosphatemic.[67] Consequently, the gap may be normal in the presence of unmeasured anions. Fencl and Figge developed a useful variant known as the corrected anion gap (AGC)[68]:

$$Anion\ Gap\ Corrected\ (for\ albumin) = calculated$$
$$anion\ gap + 2.5\ (normal\ albumin\ [g/dL] - observed$$
$$albumin\ [g/dL]).$$

The AG remains a very simple, useful, and reliable screening tool in acute illness and it usefully distinguishes metabolic acidosis due to hyperchloremia from acidosis due to UMA. Moviat and colleagues have demonstrated that the AG corrected for albumin accurately detects complex acid-base abnormalities in intensive care.[69]

Another version of the AG is the delta AG—an approach that has successfully been used to predict adverse outcomes in critical illness—where prehospital and following admission AGs were compared.[70] Confusingly, other clinicians use the delta ratio (delta Δ/Δ)[71]:

$$Delta\ Ratio = \Delta\ Anion\ gap / \Delta\ [HCO_3^-]$$

Simply, if the AG is normal, or unchanged and the bicarbonate level falls, then the delta ratio will be less than 0.4, and a hyperchloremic acidosis is present. A delta ratio between 1 and 2 is what one would expect from metabolic acidosis due to unmeasured anions or lactate. If the ratio is greater than 2, mixed acid-base abnormalities are present.

SEMIQUANTITATIVE (BASE DEFICIT/EXCESS [COPENHAGEN]) APPROACH

In metabolic acidosis, additional anions introduced to the extracellular fluid result in a net gain of one hydrogen ion for each anion. This is "buffered," principally by bicarbonate, such that each anion gained results in an equivalent fall in the bicarbonate concentration (and the generation of CO_2). Adherents to the descriptive approach to acid base refer to this as the "delta" bicarbonate. This is problematic, though,

Table 58-3 Changes in Standardized Base Deficit or Excess in Response to Acute and Chronic Acid-Base Disturbances

Disturbance	BDE vs. Paco₂
Acute respiratory acidosis	$\Delta BDE = 0$
Acute respiratory alkalosis	$\Delta BDE = 0$
Chronic respiratory acidosis	$\Delta BDE = 0.4\ \Delta Paco_2$
Metabolic acidosis	$\Delta Paco_2 = \Delta BDE$
Metabolic alkalosis	$\Delta Paco_2 = 0.6\ \Delta BDE$

Modified from Narins RB, Emmett M. Simple and mixed acid–base disorders: a practical approach. *Medicine.* 1980;59:161–187.[11]
BDE, base deficit–excess; *Paco₂,* partial pressure of carbon dioxide in arterial blood.

because it does not separate out the effect of CO_2 metabolism on the $[HCO_3^-]$. Singer and Hastings, in 1948, decided to look at acid-base abnormalities from a different angle, Henderson-Hasselbalch, by quantifying the metabolic component.[6] They proposed that changes in whole blood buffer base (BB) could be used to quantify metabolic abnormalities. The BB represented the sum of the bicarbonate and the nonvolatile buffer ions (essentially the serum albumin, phosphate, and hemoglobin). With the law of electrical neutrality applied, the buffer base was forced to equal the electrical charge difference between strong (fully dissociated) ions. Thus, normally $BB = [Na^+] + [K^+] - [Cl^-]$. Alterations in BB represented changes, essentially, in strong ion concentrations (which could not be easily measured in 1948). BB increases in metabolic alkalosis, and decreases in metabolic acidosis. The major drawback of the use of BB measurements is the potential for changes in buffering capacity associated with alterations in hemoglobin concentration.

Siggard-Anderson and colleagues developed this concept further by providing a simpler measure of metabolic acid-base activity, the base deficit–excess (BDE).[72] This, they defined, is the amount of strong acid or base required to return the pH of 1 L of blood in vitro to 7.4, assuming a Paco₂ of 40 mm Hg and temperature of 38° C. The initial use of whole blood BDE was criticized because of the dynamic activity of red cells within the acid–base paradigm—gas and electrolyte exchange. This approach was modified in the 1960s to use only serum BDE and the calculation became the *standardized* base excess (SBE). Current algorithms for computing the SBE are derived from the Van Slyke equation (1977).[73] The BDE approach to acid-base chemistry has been successfully validated by Schlichtig[74] and Morgan.[75]

Simple mathematic rules can be applied with the BDE approach in each of the common acid–base disturbances (Table 58-3). For example, in acute respiratory acidosis or alkalosis, BDE does not change. Conversely, in acute metabolic acidosis, the magnitude of change of the Pco₂ (in millimeters of mercury) is the same as that of the BDE (in milliequivalents per liter), and the change in BDE represents the overall sum total of all acidifying and alkalinizing effects. This makes interpretation of acid-base abnormalities simple but misleading.

The major advantage of the BDE approach is that it allows a simple "eyeballing" of a blood gas result to indicate

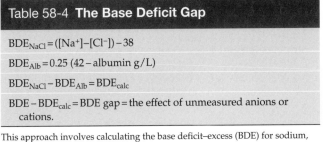

Table 58-4 The Base Deficit Gap

$BDE_{NaCl} = ([Na^+] - [Cl^-]) - 38$

$BDE_{Alb} = 0.25 (42 - albumin\ g/L)$

$BDE_{NaCl} - BDE_{Alb} = BDE_{calc}$

$BDE - BDE_{calc} = BDE\ gap = $ the effect of unmeasured anions or cations.

This approach involves calculating the base deficit–excess (BDE) for sodium, chloride, and free water (BDE_{NaCl}) and the BDE for albumin (BDE_{Alb}). The result is the calculated BDE (BDE_{calc}). This is subtracted from the measured BDE to find the BDE gap.

to the clinician the presence of a metabolic acidosis *or* alkalosis. The BDE has, however, two significant limitations. The first problem is that BDE does not account for changes in acid-base chemistry associated with hypoproteinemia (A_{TOT}); indeed, the Van Slyke equation assumes normal serum proteins, which is not the case in critical illness.[10] The second limitation is that this approach does not distinguish between metabolic acidosis associated with hyperchloremia and that associated with unmeasured anions.

To address the problem of A_{TOT} Wooten corrected SBE for weak acids (albumin and phosphate) and produced an accurate multicompartment model (SBE_c)[76]:

$$SBE_c = \left(\begin{array}{c} (HCO_3 - 24.4) \\ + \left(\begin{array}{c} [8.3 \times albumin\ g/dL \times 0.15] + \\ [0.29 \times phosphate\ mg/dL \times 0.32] \end{array} \right) \\ \times [pH - 7.4] \end{array} \right)$$

With Wooten's multicompartment model,[76] it can be seen that the SBE is the quantity of strong anions or strong cations required to bring SID back to normal, with the pH corrected to 7.4 and the P_{CO_2} at 40 mm Hg.

For the second problem to be addressed, the BDG was developed by Gilfix and colleagues,[77] evaluated by Balasubramanyan et al.,[78] and simplified by Story and Bellomo (Table 58-4).[79] This allows the physician, at the bedside, to recalculate the BDE for strong ions, free water, and albumin. Subtracting the measured BDE from the calculated BDE provides a BDG, and this represents the quantity of strong anions or cations in the system (it can be used for metabolic acidosis and alkalosis). Acid-base abnormalities that are undetected with either the bicarbonate or the base deficit–excess approach may be found with this approach.[80] In addition, this approach teases out the components of BDE represented by Na^+, Cl^-, and albumin. The BDG should mirror the SIG and, indeed, corrected AG. Caution is advised, though, because in cardiac surgical patients, the BDG does not correlate well with SIG.[81]

STEWART–FENCL (QUANTITATIVE) APPROACH

A more accurate reflection of true acid-base status can be derived with the Stewart–Fencl approach. This, like the AG, is based on the concept of electrical neutrality. There exists, in plasma, an SID $[(Na^+ + Mg^{2+} + Ca^{2+} = K^+) - (Cl^- + A^-)]$ of 40 to −44 mEq/L, balanced by the negative charge on bicarbonate and A_{TOT} (the buffer base). There is a small difference

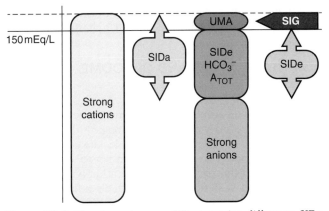

Figure 58-2. The strong ion gap. *SID*, strong ion difference; *SIDa*, apparent SID; *SIDe*, effective SID; *SIG*, strong ion gap; A_{TOT}, total weak acid concentration; *UMA*, unmeasured anions.

between SIDa (apparent SID) and weak acid buffers (SIDe [effective SID]). This represents an SIG that quantifies the amount of unmeasured anion present (Fig. 58-2).

The SIDa (apparent SID) = $([Na^+] + [K^+] + [Mg^{2+}] + [Ca^{2+}]) - [Cl^-]$.

The SIDe (effective SID) is $[HCO_3^-] + $ [charge on albumin] + [charge on Pi] (in mmol/L)

Weak acids' degree of ionization is pH dependent, so one must calculate for this:

$[alb-] = [alb\ g/L] \times (0.123 \times pH - 0.631)$

$[Pi]\ (in\ mg/dL) = [Pi]/10 \times pH - 0.47$

$SIG = SIDa - SIDe.$

The BDE and SIG approaches are consistent with one another, and can be derived from a master equation.[82] The Stewart approach,[83] refined by Figge,[10,84] Fencl,[2,65] and others, more accurately measures the contribution of charge from weak acids, which change with temperature and pH.

The weakness of this system is that the SIG does not necessarily represent unmeasured strong anions, merely all anions that are unmeasured. Furthermore, SID changes quantitatively in absolute and relative terms, when there are changes in plasma water concentration. Fencl[65] has addressed this by correcting the chloride concentration for free water ($Cl^-\ corr$) using the following equation:

$[Cl^-]corr = [Cl^-]observed \times ([Na^+]normal/[Na^+]observed.$

This corrected chloride concentration may then be inserted into the SIDa equation above. Likewise, the derived value for UMA should also be corrected for free water with UMA instead of Cl^- in this equation.[65] In a series of nine normal subjects, Fencl estimated the "normal" SIG as 8 ± 2 mEq/L.[65]

Although few refute the accuracy of the SID–SIG approach as a new gold standard for addressing, in particular, metabolic acidosis, calculation of SIG is cumbersome. The data required are more extensive and thus more expensive than other approaches and there is much confusion about the normal range of SIG. It is unclear, in standard clinical practice, that SIG has any advantage over AGc (which is SIG without calcium, magnesium, and phosphate, which usually cancel each other's charges out).[85,86]

ACID-BASE TOOLS AND OUTCOME PREDICTION

Lactic acidosis on admission to the emergency department is a marker of severity of illness. The magnitude of acidosis and the degree of elevation of serum lactate correlate well with patient outcomes.[87-89] Also, the speed of clearance of lactate from the circulation is also a known prognostic indicator.[89-92] Base deficit does not reliably reflect lactate in the emergency setting.[93-95] Kaplan and Kellum looked at a variety of acid-base measurements in the acute trauma setting. SIG was superior at predicting outcome versus all other measures.[96] Only one (2%) survivor had an SIG greater than 5 mEq/L, and only two (7%) nonsurvivors had an SIG less than 5 mEq/L. Admission pH, HCO_3^-, and lactate were poor predictors of hospital mortality after trauma. Similar data have been reported by a variety of groups in emergency settings.[97-99]

To date, studies of critically ill patients have failed to demonstrate that SIG predicts outcomes.[100,101] This may be due to the complexity of the medley of acid-base disturbances that are going on simultaneously. For example, Moviat and colleagues found that unmeasured strong anions were present in 98%, hyperchloremia was present in 80%, and elevated lactate levels were present in 62% of patients.[102]

CONCLUSIONS

Much of the confusion regarding acid–base chemistry relates to the attempt to apply observational approaches, such as that of Henderson-Hasselbalch and Schwartz and Relman, to the entire spectrum of pathophysiologic processes. The use of physical chemistry principles has improved our ability to teach, understand, and diagnose acid-base abnormalities. All acid-base disorders can be explained in terms of SID, A_{TOT}, and Pco_2. This is important to intensivists, who are routinely faced with complex acid-base abnormalities in practice.

AUTHOR'S RECOMMENDATIONS

- A significant acid–base abnormality may be an early indicator of a sinister underlying disease process resulting in early and aggressive intervention (for example, lactic acidosis in sepsis and trauma).
- All acid–base abnormalities result from alterations in the dissociation of water.
- Only three factors independently affect acid–base balance: $Paco_2$, SID, and A_{TOT}.
- Respiratory acidosis and alkalosis are caused by hypercarbia and hypocarbia, respectively.
- Metabolic acidosis is caused by decreased SID or increased A_{TOT}. Decreased SID results from accumulation of metabolic anions (i.e., shock, ketoacidosis, and renal failure), hyperchloremia, and free water excess. Increased A_{TOT} results from hyperphosphatemia.
- Metabolic alkalosis is caused by increased SID or decreased A_{TOT}. The SID increases because of sodium gain, chloride loss, or free water deficit. A_{TOT} decreases in hypoalbuminemia and hypophosphatemia. This condition is particularly common in critical illness.
- Several analytical tools have been used in acid-base chemistry. The mathematic relation between bicarbonate concentration and partial pressure of carbon dioxide is universally accepted by bedside clinicians.
- For metabolic disturbances the strong ion gap approach is potentially a new gold standard but is cumbersome to use. The corrected AG and base deficit gap are, in most cases, effective at determining the nature of metabolic disturbances and are relatively simple to use at the bedside.

REFERENCES

1. Kellum JA. Reunification of acid-base physiology. *Crit Care.* 2005;9:500–507.
2. Fencl V, Leith DE. Stewart's quantitative acid-base chemistry: applications in biology and medicine. *Respir Physiol.* 1993;91:1–16.
3. Henderson LJ. Das Gleichgewicht zwischen Sauren und Bases im tierischen Organismus. *Ergebn Physiol.* 1909;8:254–325.
4. Hasselbalch KA. Die Berechnung der Wasserstoffzahl des Blutes aus der freien und gebundenen Kohlensaure desselben, und die Sauerstoffbindung des Blutes als Funktion der Wasserstoffzahl. *Biochem Z.* 1916;78:112–144.
5. Stewart PA. Independent and dependent variables of acid-base control. *Respir Physiol.* 1978;33:9–26.
6. Singer RB, Hastings AB. An improved clinical method for the estimation of disturbances of the acid-base balance of human blood. *Medicine.* 1948;10:242.
7. Rossing TH, Maffeo N, Fencl V. Acid-base effects of altering plasma protein concentration in human blood in vitro. *J Appl Physiol.* 1986;61:2260–2265.
8. Corey HE. Stewart and beyond: new models of acid-base balance. *Kidney Int.* 2003;64:777–787.
9. Goldwasser P, Feldman J. Association of serum albumin and mortality risk. *J Clin Epidemiol.* 1997;50:693–703.
10. Figge J, Rossing TH, Fencl V. The role of serum proteins in acid-base equilibria. *J Lab Clin Med.* 1991;117:453–467.
11. Narins R, Emmett M. Simple and mixed acid-base disorders: a practical approach. *Medicine (Baltimore).* 1980;59:161–187.
12. Alfaro V, Torras R, Ibanez J, Palacios L. A physical-chemical analysis of the acid-base response to chronic obstructive pulmonary disease. *Can J Physiol Pharmacol.* 11-11-1996;11(74):1229–1235.
13. Morgan TJ, Venkatesh B. Designing 'balanced' crystalloids. *Crit Care Resusc.* 2003;5:284–291.
14. Gattinoni L, Carlesso E, Cadringher P, Caironi P. Strong ion difference in urine: new perspectives in acid-base assessment. *Crit Care.* 2006;10:137.
15. Park CM, Chun HK, Jeon K, Suh GY, Choi DW, Kim S. Factors related to post-operative metabolic acidosis following major abdominal surgery. *ANZ J Surg.* 2014;84:574–580.
16. Rehm M, O V, Scheingraber S, Kreimeier U, Brechtelsbauer H, Finsterer U. Acid-base changes caused by 5% albumin versus 6% hydroxyethyl starch solution in patients undergoing acute normovolemic hemodilution: a randomized prospective study. *Anesthesiology.* 2000;93:1174–1183.
17. Waters J, Gottlieb A, Schoenwald P, Popovich M. Normal saline versus lactated Ringer's solution for intraoperative fluid management in patients undergoing abdominal aortic aneurysm repair: an outcome study. *Anesth Analg.* 2001;93:817–822.
18. Kim JY, Lee D, Lee KC, Choi JJ, Kwak HJ. Stewart's physicochemical approach in neurosurgical patients with hyperchloremic metabolic acidosis during propofol anesthesia. *J Neurosurg Anesthesiol.* 2008;20:1–7.
19. Alston RP, Cormack L, Collinson C. Metabolic acidosis developing during cardiopulmonary bypass is related to a decrease in strong ion difference. *Perfusion.* 2004;19:145–152.

20. Gueret G, Rossignol B, Kiss G, et al. Metabolic acidosis after cardiac surgery with cardiopulmonary bypass revisited with the use of the Stewart acid-base approach. *Ann Fr Anesth Reanim.* 2007;26:10–16.

21. Witt L, Osthaus WA, Juttner B, Heimbucher C, Sumpelmann R. Alteration of anion gap and strong ion difference caused by hydroxyethyl starch 6% (130/0.42) and gelatin 4% in children. *Paediatr Anaesth.* 2008;18:934–939.

22. Bruegger D, Bauer A, Rehm M, et al. Effect of hypertonic saline dextran on acid-base balance in patients undergoing surgery of abdominal aortic aneurysm. *Crit Care Med.* 2005;33:556–563.

23. Bruegger D, Jacob M, Scheingraber S, et al. Changes in acid-base balance following bolus infusion of 20% albumin solution in humans. *Intensive Care Med.* 2005;31:1123–1127.

24. Rehm M, Orth V, Scheingraber S, Kreimeier U, Brechtelsbauer H, Finsterer U. Acid-base changes caused by 5% albumin versus 6% hydroxyethyl starch solution in patients undergoing acute normovolemic hemodilution: a randomized prospective study. *Anesthesiology.* 2000;93:1174–1183.

25. Kellum JA. In: Shoemaker, ed. *Diagnosis and Treatment of Acid Base Disorders, Textbook of Critical Care Medicine.* 4th ed. Saunders; 2000. pp. 839–53.

26. Moviat M, Terpstra AM, van der Hoeven JG, Pickkers P. Impaired renal function is associated with greater urinary strong ion differences in critically ill patients with metabolic acidosis. *J Crit Care.* 2012;27:255–260.

27. Moviat M, Pickkers P, van der Voort PH, van der Hoeven JG. Acetazolamide-mediated decrease in strong ion difference accounts for the correction of metabolic alkalosis in critically ill patients. *Crit Care.* 2006;10:R14.

28. Brunner R, Drolz A, Scherzer TM, et al. Renal tubular acidosis is highly prevalent in critically ill patients. *Crit Care.* 2015;19:148.

29. Rodriguez-Soriano J. New insights into the pathogenesis of renal tubular acidosis–from functional to molecular studies. *Pediatr Nephrol.* 2000;14:1121–1136.

30. Choate KA, Kahle KT, Wilson FH, Nelson-Williams C, Lifton RP. WNK1, a kinase mutated in inherited hypertension with hyperkalemia, localizes to diverse Cl- -transporting epithelia. *Proc Natl Acad Sci USA.* 2003;100:663–668.

31. Shaer AJ. Inherited primary renal tubular hypokalemic alkalosis: a review of Gitelman and Bartter syndromes. *Am J Med Sci.* 2001;322:316–332.

32. Brill SA, Stewart TR, Brundage SI, Schreiber MA. Base deficit does not predict mortality when secondary to hyperchloremic acidosis. *Shock.* 2002;17:459–462.

33. Tournadre JP, Allaouchiche B, Malbert CH, Chassard D. Metabolic acidosis and respiratory acidosis impair gastro-pyloric motility in anesthetized pigs. *Anesth Analg.* 2000;90:74–79.

34. Hansen PB, Jensen BL, Skott O. Chloride regulates afferent arteriolar contraction in response to depolarization. *Hypertension.* 1998;32:1066–1070.

35. Wilcox CS. Regulation of renal blood flow by plasma chloride. *J Clin Invest.* 1983;71:726–735.

36. Wilkes NJ, Woolf R, Mutch M, et al. The effects of balanced versus saline-based hetastarch and crystalloid solutions on acid-base and electrolyte status and gastric mucosal perfusion in elderly surgical patients. *Anesth Analg.* 2001;93:811–816.

37. Williams EL, Hildebrand KL, McCormick SA, Bedel MJ. The effect of intravenous lactated Ringer's solution versus 0.9% sodium chloride solution on serum osmolality in human volunteers. *Anesth Analg.* 1999;88:999–1003.

38. Chowdhury AH, Cox EF, Francis ST, Lobo DN. A randomized, controlled, double-blind crossover study on the effects of 2-L infusions of 0.9% saline and plasma-lyte-« 148 on renal blood flow velocity and renal cortical tissue perfusion in healthy volunteers. *Ann Surg.* 2012;256.

39. Merten GJ, Burgess WP, Gray LV, et al. Prevention of contrast-induced nephropathy with sodium bicarbonate: a randomized controlled trial. *JAMA.* 2004;291:2328–2334.

40. Haase M, Haase-Fielitz A, Bellomo R, et al. Sodium bicarbonate to prevent increases in serum creatinine after cardiac surgery: a pilot double-blind, randomized controlled trial. *Crit Care Med.* 2009;37:39–47.

41. Nadeem A, Salahuddin N, El Hazmi A, et al. Chloride-liberal fluids are associated with acute kidney injury after liver transplantation. *Crit Care.* 2014;18:625.

42. Shaw AD, Bagshaw SM, Goldstein SL, et al. Major complications, mortality, and resource utilization after open abdominal surgery: 0.9% saline compared to Plasma-Lyte. *Ann Surg.* 2012;255.

43. Park CM, Chun HK, Jeon K, Suh GY, Choi DW, Kim S. Factors related to post-operative metabolic acidosis following major abdominal surgery. *ANZ J Surg.* 2014;84:574–580.

44. Yunos N. Association between a chloride-liberal vs chloride-restrictive intravenous fluid administration strategy and kidney injury in critically ill adults. *JAMA.* 2012;308:1566–1572.

45. Havlin J, Matousovic K, Schuck O, et al. Pathophysiology of metabolic acidosis in patients with reduced glomerular filtration rate according to Stewart-Fencl theory. *Vnitr Lek.* 2009;55:97–104.

46. Liborio AB, da Silva AC, Noritomi DT, Andrade L, Seguro AC. Impact of chloride balance in acidosis control: the Stewart approach in hemodialysis critically ill patients. *J Crit Care.* 2006;21:333–338.

47. Maciel A, Park M, Macedo E. Physicochemical analysis of blood and urine in the course of acute kidney injury in critically ill patients: a prospective, observational study. *BMC Anesthesiol.* 2013;13:31.

48. Story DA, Tosolini A, Bellomo R, Leblanc M, Bragantini L, Ronco C. Plasma acid-base changes in chronic renal failure: a Stewart analysis. *Int J Artif Organs.* 2005;28:961–965.

49. Rocktaschel J, Morimatsu H, Uchino S, Ronco C, Bellomo R. *Int J Artif Organs.* 2003;26:19–25.

50. Naka T, Bellomo R, Morimatsu H, et al. Acid-base balance during continuous veno-venous hemofiltration: the impact of severe hepatic failure. *Int J Artif Organs.* 2006;29:668–674.

51. Morgan TJ. The meaning of acid-base abnormalities in the intensive care unit: part III – effects of fluid administration. *Crit Care.* 2005;9:204–211.

52. Gattinoni L, Taccone P, Carlesso E. Respiratory acidosis: is the correction with bicarbonate worth? *Minerva Anestesiol.* 2006;72:551–557.

53. Sen I, Altunok V, Ok M, Coskun A, Constable PD. Efficacy of oral rehydration therapy solutions containing sodium bicarbonate or sodium acetate for treatment of calves with naturally acquired diarrhea, moderate dehydration, and strong ion acidosis. *J Am Vet Med Assoc.* 2009;234:926–934.

54. Story DA, Poustie S, Bellomo R. Quantitative physical chemistry analysis of acid-base disorders in critically ill patients. *Anaesthesia.* 2001;56:530–533.

55. Morgan TJ, Venkatesh B, Hall J. Crystalloid strong ion difference determines metabolic acid-base change during acute normovolaemic haemodilution. *Intensive Care Med.* 2004;30:1432–1437.

56. Morgan TJ, Venkatesh B, Beindorf A, Andrew I, Hall J. Acid-base and bio-energetics during balanced versus unbalanced normovolaemic haemodilution. *Anaesth Intensive Care.* 2007;35:173–179.

57. Navarro M, Monreal L, Segura D, Armengou L, Anor S. A comparison of traditional and quantitative analysis of acid-base and electrolyte imbalances in horses with gastrointestinal disorders. *J Vet Intern Med.* 2005;19:871–877.

58. Haskins SC, Hopper K, Rezende ML. The acid-base impact of free water removal from, and addition to, plasma. *J Lab Clin Med.* 2006;147:114–120.

59. Tayar J, Jabbour G, Saggi SJ. Severe hyperosmolar metabolic acidosis due to a large dose of intravenous lorazepam. *N Engl J Med.* 2002;346:1253–1254.

60. Flynn BC. Hyperkalemic cardiac arrest with hypertonic mannitol infusion: the strong ion difference revisited. *Anesth Analg.* 2007;104:225–226.

61. Zander R, Lang W. Base excess and strong ion difference: clinical limitations related to inaccuracy. *Anesthesiology.* 2004;100:459–460.

62. Severinghaus JW. Acid-base balance nomogram–a Boston-Copenhagen detente. *Anesthesiology.* 1976;45:539–541.

63. Schwarts WB, Relman AS. A critique of the parameters used in the evaluation of acid-base disorders. "Severe hyperosmolar metabolic acidosis due to a large dose of intravenous Lorazepam-Whole-blood buffer base" and "standard bicarbonate" compared with blood pH and plasma bicarbonate concentration. *N Engl J Med.* 1963;268:1382–1388.

64. Emmett M, Narins RG. Clinical use of the anion gap. *Medicine (Baltimore).* 1977;56:38–54.

65. Fencl V, Jabor A, Kazda A, Figge J. Diagnosis of metabolic acid-base disturbances in critically ill patients. *Am J Respir Crit Care Med.* 2000;162:2246–2251.

66. Salem MM, Mujais SK. Gaps in the anion gap. *Arch Intern Med.* 1992;152:1625–1629.
67. Wilkes P. Hypoproteinemia, strong-ion difference, and acid-base status in critically ill patients. *J Appl Physiol.* 1998;84:1740–1748.
68. Figge J, Jabor A, Kazda A, Fencl V. Anion gap and hypoalbuminemia. *Crit Care Med.* 1998;26:1807–1810.
69. Moviat M, van Haren F, van der Hoeven H. Conventional or physicochemical approach in intensive care unit patients with metabolic acidosis. *Crit Care.* 2003;7:R41–R45.
70. Lipnick MS, Braun AB, Cheung JT-W, Gibbons FK, Christopher KB. The difference between critical care initiation anion gap and prehospital ddmission anion gap is predictive of mortality in critical illness. *Crit Care Med.* 2013;41:49–59.
71. Rastegar A. Use of the ΔAG/ΔHCO3 ratio in the diagnosis of mixed acid-base disorders. *J Am Soc Nephrol.* 2007;18:2429–2431.
72. Siggaard-Anderson O. *The Acid Base Status of the Blood.* 1st ed. Copenhagen: Munksgard; 1963. p. 134.
73. Siggaard-Andersen O. The van Slyke equation. *Scand J Clin Lab Invest Suppl.* 1977;37:15–20.
74. Schlichtig R, Grogono AW, Severinghaus JW. Human $PaCO_2$ and standard base excess compensation for acid-base imbalance. *Crit Care Med.* 1998;26:1173–1179.
75. Morgan TJ, Clark C, Endre ZH. Accuracy of base excess: an in vitro evaluation of the Van Slyke equation. *Crit Care Med.* 2003;28:2932–2936.
76. Wooten EW. Calculation of physiological acid-base parameters in multicompartment systems with application to human blood. *J Appl Physiol.* 2003;95:2333–2344.
77. Gilfix BM, Bique M, Magder S. A physical chemical approach to the analysis of acid-base balance in the clinical setting. *J Crit Care.* 1993;8:187–197.
78. Balasubramanyan N, Havens PL, Hoffman GM. Unmeasured anions identified by the Fencl-Stewart method predict mortality better than base excess, anion gap, and lactate in patients in the pediatric intensive care unit. *Crit Care Med.* 1999;27:1577–1581.
79. Story DA, Morimatsu H, Bellomo R. Strong ions, weak acids and base excess: a simplified Fencl-Stewart approach to clinical acid-base disorders{dagger}. *Br J Anaesth.* 2004;92:54–60.
80. Ahmed SM, Maheshwari P, Agarwal S, Nadeem A, Singh L. Evaluation of the efficacy of simplified Fencl-Stewart equation in analyzing the changes in acid base status following resuscitation with two different fluids. *Int J Crit Illness Inj Sci.* 2013;3:206–210.
81. Agrafiotis M, Sileli M, Ampatzidou F, Keklikoglou I, Panousis P. The base excess gap is not a valid tool for the quantification of unmeasured ions in cardiac surgical patients: a retrospective observational study. *Eur J Anaesthesiol.* 2013;30.
82. Wooten EW. Analytic calculation of physiological acid-base parameters in plasma. *J Appl Physiol.* 1999;86:326–334.
83. Stewart PA. Modern quantitative acid-base chemistry. *Can J Physiol Pharmacol.* 1983;61:1444–1461.
84. Figge J, Mydosh T, Fencl V. Serum proteins and acid-base equilibria: a follow-up. *J Lab Clin Med.* 1992;120:713–719.
85. Antonogiannaki EM, Mitrouska I, Amargianitakis V, Georgopoulos D. Evaluation of acid-base status in patients admitted to ED: pphysicochemical vs traditional approaches. *Am J Emerg Med.* 2015;33:378–382.
86. Mallat J, Michel D, Salaun P, Thevenin D, Tronchon L. Defining metabolic acidosis in patients with septic shock using Stewart approach. *Am J Emerg Med.* 2012;30:391–398.
87. Vitek V, Cowley RA. Blood lactate in the prognosis of various forms of shock. *Ann Surg.* 1971;173:308–313.
88. Eddy VA, Morris Jr JA, Cullinane DC. Hypothermia, coagulopathy, and acidosis. *Surg Clin North Am.* 2000;80:845–854.
89. Husain FA, Martin MJ, Mullenix PS, Steele SR, Elliott DC. Serum lactate and base deficit as predictors of mortality and morbidity. *Am J Surg.* 2003;185:485–491.
90. Abramson D, Scalea TM, Hitchcock R, Trooskin SZ, Henry SM, Greenspan J. Lactate clearance and survival following injury. *J Trauma.* 1993;35:584–588.
91. McNelis J, Marini CP, Jurkiewicz A, et al. Prolonged lactate clearance is associated with increased mortality in the surgical intensive care unit. *Am J Surg.* 2001;182:481–485.
92. Nguyen HB, Rivers EP, Knoblich BP, et al. Early lactate clearance is associated with improved outcome in severe sepsis and septic shock. *Crit Care Med.* 2004;32:1637–1642.
93. Brill SA, Stewart TR, Brundage SI, Schreiber MA. Base deficit does not predict mortality when secondary to hyperchloremic acidosis. *Shock.* 2002;17:459–462.
94. Kaplan LJ, Kellum JA. Initial pH, base deficit, lactate, anion gap, strong ion difference, and strong ion gap predict outcome from major vascular injury. *Crit Care Med.* 2004;32:1120–1124.
95. Martin MJ, FitzSullivan E, Salim A, Brown CV, Demetriades D, Long W. Discordance between lactate and base deficit in the surgical intensive care unit: which one do you trust? *Am J Surg.* 2006;191:625–630.
96. Kaplan LJ, Kellum JA. Comparison of acid-base models for prediction of hospital mortality after trauma. *Shock.* 2008;29:662–666.
97. Zehtabchi S, Soghoian S, Sinert R. Utility of Stewart's strong ion difference as a predictor of major injury after trauma in the ED. *Am J Emerg Med.* 2007;25:938–941.
98. Omron EM. Comparative quantitative acid-base analysis in coronary artery bypass, severe sepsis, and diabetic ketoacidosis. *J Intensive Care Med.* 2005;20:317–326.
99. Martin M, Murray J, Berne T, Demetriades D, Belzberg H. Diagnosis of acid-base derangements and mortality prediction in the trauma intensive care unit: the physiochemical approach. *J Trauma.* 2005;58:238–243.
100. Rocktaeschel J, Morimatsu H, Uchino S, Bellomo R. Unmeasured anions in critically ill patients: can they predict mortality? *Crit Care Med.* 2003;31:2131–2136.
101. Cusack RJ, Rhodes A, Lochhead P, et al. The strong ion gap does not have prognostic value in critically ill patients in a mixed medical/surgical adult ICU. *Intensive Care Med.* 2002;28:864–869.
102. Moviat M, van H F, van der H H. Conventional or physicochemical approach in intensive care unit patients with metabolic acidosis. *Crit Care.* 2003;7:R41–R45.

59 What Is the Meaning of a High Lactate? What Are the Implications of Lactic Acidosis?

Stephen R. Odom, Daniel Talmor

An imbalance of oxygen delivery and demand with resultant organ dysfunction is the hallmark of critical illness. Measuring oxygen delivery, recognizing tissue hypoperfusion, and monitoring the response to therapeutic interventions on clinical grounds can be frustrating and unreliable.[1,2] To this end, the use of serum lactate as a surrogate for tissue hypoperfusion and stress has been studied in many states of critical illness.

Here, we review the current data related to the use of lactate as an objective measure of tissue hypoperfusion; as a tool for screening, diagnosis, and risk stratification; and as a marker for monitoring the progression of resuscitation and interventions in critical illness.

PRODUCTION OF LACTATE

Under basal conditions, lactate is produced by muscle, skin, brain, red blood cells, and intestine. In critical illness, additional sources include the lungs, white blood cells, and splanchnic organs.[1] Importantly, activated white blood cells have relatively few mitochondria; thus, they favor anaerobic metabolism. When oxygen is present, glucose is most often metabolized to pyruvate and enters the citric acid cycle to produce adenosine triphosphate, essentially bypassing lactate production. When oxygen supply to tissue is limited, lactate is produced and shunted to the liver as a substrate for gluconeogenesis. Under some circumstances, such as exercise and some states of critical illness, pyruvate may accumulate despite abundant oxygen availability and can be shunted to lactate production.[3]

Other measures of acid-base balance in the critically ill patient may be misleading. Anion gap and base excess are associated with lactate production, but they do not always accurately predict lactate concentration. Both are generally regarded as inferior screening tools for tissue hypoperfusion because they do not account for unmeasured ions and hypoalbuminemia, a common occurrence.[4] In addition, "cryptic" or "occult" shock may be present in the critically ill and may be identified only by lactate elevations in the absence of other indicators generally associated with this state.[5-8]

MEASUREMENT OF LACTATE

Only the L-lactate isomer is clinically measured. D-Lactate is a bacterial product only rarely relevant to human acid-base balance.[9]

Arterial and venous lactate are generally regarded as equivalent,[10] although recent evidence suggests that venous and arterial peripheral lactates may vary widely in patients with an initially elevated lactate.[11] Future research on this topic is required because it is in these patients that discrimination is most important.

Elevated serum lactate can be a function of increased production, decreased clearance, or both. Myocardial depression, relative hypovolemia (i.e., vascular dilation and fluid loss from capillary leak), mitochondrial dysfunction,[12] excessive adrenergic stimulation,[3,13,14] and microcirculatory insufficiency[15] all contribute to decreased oxygen delivery or utilization in shock. Research into hyperlactatemia basically focuses on the use of lactate as a "biomarker" or screening tool to stratify risk and characterize the severity of injury in critical illness and trauma. Additional studies have attempted to characterize lactate as an endpoint of resuscitation in many forms of critical illness.

PREHOPSITAL MEASUREMENT OF LACTATE

Capillary lactate in the prehospital setting is associated with injury severity in trauma patients.[16] Coates and colleagues demonstrated that elevated capiillary lactate levels, in the prehospital setting, equate with injury severity in trauma patients. The investigators also determined that lactate was helpful in the triage of patients with normal vital signs despite evidence of tissue hypoperfusion. Additional evaluation in the prehospital setting has demonstrated that lactate is associated with hospital mortality even in patients with initially normal vital signs.[17] In addition, lactate is significantly different in shocked versus nonshocked patients, and elevated lactate is associated with increased hospital length of stay (LOS), intensive care unit (ICU) LOS, and increased mortality (12.2% vs. 44.3%), especially in patients with normal vital signs on admission (mortality of 35% vs. 7%, $P < .001$).[18] Thus the prehospital use of lactate as a screening and triage tool may be useful to uncover subtle organ hypoperfusion.

MEASUREMENT OF LACTATE IN THE EMERGENCY DEPARTMENT

Many studies have been performed assessing presenting lactate levels in the emergency department (ED). Shapiro and colleagues[19] examined 1278 consecutive ED patients with an infection-related diagnosis and uncovered a linear relationship between mortality and lactate. In addition, they found that initial lactate was 36% sensitive and 92% specific for any death within 28 days, whereas lactate was 55% sensitive and 91% specific for early death (within 72 hours of presentation). The same group[7] found a 15% mortality rate in septic patients with a lactate greater than 4.0 mmol/L and normal admission systolic blood pressure. In a multivariate analysis, the odds ratio (OR) of death was 2.1 in patients with lactate between 2.5 and 4 mmol/L and was 7.1 when lactate was greater than 4 mmol/L. The initial lactate level is associated with increased mortality in patients with normal vital signs ("occult" shock) as well as those with overt shock.[20]

LACTATE MEASUREMENT IN THE INTENSIVE CARE UNIT

Investigations into the prognostic value of lactate levels in the ICU have yielded variable results because of unevenness in patient populations, diagnoses, time course of treatment, and the complexity of evolving critical illness. In a well-designed retrospective analysis of 134 mixed ICU patients, receiver-operator analysis was used to investigate the relationship between elevated lactate and Sequential Organ Failure Assessment scores.[21] The risk of organ failure or death increased in patients with a prolonged elevation of lactate. This effect was most profound early in the ICU stay, suggesting that early resuscitation improves mortality in critical illness. In a prospective observational study of 394 consecutive patients, the same group[22] found that mortality decreased in septic patients whose lactate decreased within 12 hours of admission. This difference was independent of hemodynamic status.

GOAL-DIRECTED THERAPY AND LACTATE CLEARANCE

It has been proposed that measurement of lactate levels provides a simple point-of-care test to determine an endpoint of resuscitation in critical illness. Recent large prospective randomized trials have confirmed that early goal-directed therapy (EGDT) provides no survival benefit over standard care. The ProCESS (Protocolized Care for Early Septic Shock) investigators randomized 1341 patients with septic shock at 31 centers to protocol-based EGDT, protocol-based standard therapy, or usual care.[23] Although there was

significant variability in the use of hemodynamic monitors, as well as blood, fluid, and vasopressor use, there was no difference in 60-day or 1-year mortality and no difference in the need for organ support. Supplemental data from this study suggested that EGDT may provide a survival benefit in patients with an initial lactate level greater than 5 mmol/L. Likewise, the ARISE (Australasian Resuscitation in Sepsis Evaluation) investigators found no difference in survival time, in-hospital mortality, or duration of organ support in 1600 randomized patients with septic shock to either EGDT versus standard care.[24] Neither study used lactate level as a goal of resuscitation; rather, they used it as a marker for tissue hypoperfusion and as a means of inclusion in the study. With this information, it cannot be suggested that lactate be used as a target of resuscitation for shocked patients. The results of another large prospective evaluation of EGDT, the ProMISe (The Protocolised Management in Sepsis Trial) study from the United Kingdom, were similar. Again the investigators did not use lactate as a goal of resuscitation.[24a]

Other investigators have found that the early use of physiologic targets in resuscitation is associated with improved survival and decreased organ failure in several clinical shock scenarios, including trauma[25] and sepsis.[26] This effect has been most thoroughly studied in septic shock. To prevent morbidity and overcome obstacles to placement of invasive monitors in septic shock, the use of lactate and its clearance has been proposed as a less invasive measure of the progress of resuscitation.[27]

In a randomized trial by Jansen and colleagues,[28] 348 septic patients were allocated to a lactate-driven protocol versus a lactate-blinded treatment. The study was underpowered, and mortality was not statistically different between the groups (33.9% in the lactate group vs. 43.5% in the control group [$P = .067$]); however, a post hoc multivariate analysis demonstrated an observed 9.6% reduction in hospital mortality. In addition, multiple retrospective observational studies have suggested lactate as a monitor of the therapeutic response during EGDT.[29-31] A randomized prospective trial of septic patients randomly chosen to receive therapy guided by central venous oxygen or lactate showed no difference in outcome, although mortality was lower in the lactate group (23% vs. 17%).[32]

Assuming proper hepatic and renal function, serum lactate should be rapidly cleared. Clearance of lactate has been associated with increased survival in various clinical settings, including trauma,[30,33,34] mixed populations of critically ill patients,[35,36] sepsis,[2,37-40] and after myocardial infarction.[41]

Recent experience suggests that lactate clearance may function as a more robust resuscitative endpoint than central venous oxygen saturation or other traditional oxygen-derived variables.[28,32] The ability to achieve only a central venous oxygen saturation goal was associated with 41% mortality in septic shock, whereas lactate clearance was associated with only 8% mortality.[42] A recent meta-analysis that reviewed 15 original studies examining lactate clearance in critically ill patients found that lactate clearance predicted mortality with 75% sensitivity and 72% specificity.[6]

In summary, the promise of lactate as a goal of resuscitation remains unanswered. It cannot be recommended with current data that lactate be used as the sole endpoint of resuscitation, but it appears to be a reasonable marker for success of resuscitation in shock, particularly in patients with infections and after trauma. If lactate clearance has a role as a goal of resuscitation, then more study is needed.

CLINICAL APPROACH TO ELEVATED LACTATE IN VARIOUS CLINICAL SCENARIOS

Shock—cardiogenic: Several studies have demonstrated the utility of lactate measurement in the identification of acute coronary syndromes[41,42] and to predict the development of shock after acute coronary syndrome.[43] In addition, high lactate levels have been associated with 30-day mortality after percutaneous interventions for myocardial infarction[44,45] and death in the ICU after admission for myocardial infarction.[46]

Attana[47] studied 51 consecutive patients in cardiogenic shock after ST-elevation myocardial infarction and determined that lactate clearance was higher in survivors. Lactate clearance less than 10% was associated with particularly poor survival. Park and colleagues[48] found a mortality of 53% in 96 consecutive patients with cardiogenic shock requiring percutaneous cardiopulmonary support. Multivariate analysis found that a lactate clearance less than 70% at 48 hours was associated with death.

Shock—after arrest: Mullner et al.[49] studied 167 out-of-hospital witnessed cardiac arrest patients and found that lactate levels greater than 16.3 mmol/L were 100% specific for death or poor neurologic recovery. In a review of 394 cardiac arrest patients, multivariate analysis revealed that lactate was an independent predictor of mortality (OR 1.49 per 1 mmol/L increase). Lactate levels greater than 2 mmol/L at 48 hours predicted mortality with a specificity of 86% and predicted poor neurologic outcome with a specificity of 87%. Lactate correlates with good neurologic outcome in out-of-hospital cardiac arrest patients treated with therapeutic hypothermia.[50]

Trauma: Initial serum lactate has been shown in several studies to predict outcome in trauma patients. In a recent study,[51] 1941 patients were retrospectively reviewed. Initial serum lactate (drawn within 35 minutes of admission) was lower in survivors (21 vs. 32 mg/dL, *P* < .001). In multivariate analysis, initial lactate was a significant predictor of mortality and of the need for operative intervention.

In a broad cohort of trauma patients, initial lactate and clearance of lactate at 6 hours was associated with decreased mortality.[34] In patients with an initial lactate level greater than 4 mmol/L, lactate clearance of greater than 60% was associated with a mortality of 7.5% whereas a lactate clearance of less than 30% was associated with a mortality rate of 28.1% (*P* = .001).

Burns: In a study of 166 burn patients,[52] a high initial lactate and an inability to clear lactate at 24 hours were predictive of death (68% survival in lactate clearers vs. 32% in patients whose lactate remained above normal after 24 hours).

Drugs/alcohol: Despite being metabolized via pathways that can produce lactate, alcohol and drugs do not appear to influence the significance of lactate measurement or alter its clinical utility.[53]

Postoperative: Li and colleagues[54] found that elevated lactate after major abdominal surgery was associated with complications. They studied 114 consecutive patients undergoing elective surgery with a Physiologic and Operative Severity Score for the enumeration of Mortality and Morbidity (POSSUM) score of 4 or greater. The degree of lactate elevation and the time-weighted average of lactate over the first 24 hours after surgery correlated with the severity of complications. Lactate clearance at 24 hours was significantly associated with better outcome. They suggested the use of lactate as a therapeutic target in early resuscitation after major abdominal surgery.

In one study of postoperative patients, mortality was increased from 3.9% if lactate cleared in the first 24 hours after surgery to 13.3% if lactate cleared in 48 hours, 42.5% if cleared in the first 96 hours, and 100% if not cleared by 96 hours.[36] Other studies have highlighted the phenomenon of lactate as a marker for poor outcome in surgical ICU patients,[55] in whom mortality was 10% if lactate normalized in the first day after admission versus 67% mortality if lactate did not normalize.

LIMITATIONS IN THE USE OF LACTATE MEASUREMENTS

There are several studies indicating that lactate levels may not be helpful in caring for the critically ill. Between 20% and 30% of patients in overt septic shock have initial lactate values less than 2 mmol/L.[56] A study of vasopressor-dependent patients in septic shock found that lactate did not exceed 2.4 mmol/L in 45% of patients, many of whom went on to die.[57] Lactate levels were normal in 11.1% of patients with mesenteric ischemia.[58] Lactate levels can be misleading in patients with hepatic disease or in those who are taking medications such as metformin, which interferes with the metabolism of lactate and may impair mitochondria. The optimal use of lactate clearance in many settings remains to be defined. Future research should focus on an appropriate level of lactate clearance or if normalization of lactate is the appropriate early goal of resuscitation or remains only a marker of severity in critical illness.

CONCLUSION

Serum lactate levels can function as a surrogate measure of tissue hypoperfusion and severity of stress in critical illness. In addition, they can serve as a screening or diagnostic tool for occult hypoperfusion, they can be useful for risk stratification and prognosis, and they may be useful for monitoring the progression of resuscitation. The value of lactate clearance has yet to be fully defined in the management of critical illness. Despite some notable limitations, lactate is a readily available and interpretable piece of data in the management of these complex patients.

AUTHORS' RECOMMENDATIONS

- Prehospital lactate can potentially be used to stratify and triage patients in the early phases of shock.
- Initial lactate levels can predict mortality and can determine the presence of occult shock, especially in patients with sepsis or after polytrauma.
- Lactate clearance may be useful in the management of resuscitation in shock or after cardiac arrest, and it may be more accurate than other markers of perfusion (vital signs, other markers of acid-base status, or oxygen-derived variables such as central venous oxygen saturation).
- Lactate measurement and clearance can be confusing in patients with other sources of lactate or poor renal or liver function.

REFERENCES

1. Okorie ON, Dellinger P. Lactate: biomarker and potential therapeutic target. *Crit Care Clin*. April 2011;27(2):299–326.
2. Arnold RC, Sherwin R, Shapiro NI, et al. Multicenter observational study of the development of progressive organ dysfunction and therapeutic interventions in normotensive sepsis patients in the emergency department. *Acad Emerg Med*. May 2013;20(5):433–440.
3. Gore DC, Jahoor F, Hibbert JM, DeMaria EJ. Lactic acidosis during sepsis is related to increased pyruvate production, not deficits in tissue oxygen availability. *Ann Surg*. July 1996;224(1):97–102.
4. Chawla LS, Shih S, Davison D, Junker C, Seneff MG. Anion gap, anion gap corrected for albumin, base deficit and unmeasured anions in critically ill patients: implications on the assessment of metabolic acidosis and the diagnosis of hyperlactatemia. *BMC Emerg Med*. December 16, 2008;8:18.
5. Salottolo KM, Mains CW, Offner PJ, Bourg PW, Bar-Or D. A retrospective analysis of geriatric trauma patients: venous lactate is a better predictor of mortality than traditional vital signs. *Scand J Trauma Resusc Emerg Med*. February 14, 2013;21:7.
6. Zhang Z, Xu X. Lactate clearance is a useful biomarker for the prediction of all-cause mortality in critically ill patients: a systematic review and meta-analysis. *Crit Care Med*. September 2014;42(9):2118–2125.
7. Howell MD, Donnino M, Clardy P, Talmor D, Shapiro NI. Occult hypoperfusion and mortality in patients with suspected infection. *Intensive Care Med*. November 2007;33(11):1892–1899. Epub July 6, 2006.
8. Martin JT, Alkhoury F, O'Connor JA, Kyriakides TC, Bonadies JA. 'Normal' vital signs belie occult hypoperfusion in geriatric trauma patients. *Am Surg*. January 2010;76(1):65–69.
9. Kang KP, Lee S, Kang SK. D-lactic acidosis in humans: review of update. *Electrolyte Blood Press*. March 2006;4(1):53–56.
10. Kruse O, Grunnet N, Barfod C. Blood lactate as a predictor for in-hospital mortality in patients admitted acutely to hospital: a systematic review. *Scand J Trauma Resusc Emerg Med*. December 28, 2011;19:74.
11. Bloom B, Pott J, Freund Y, Grundlingh J, Harris T. The agreement between abnormal venous lactate and arterial lactate in the ED: a retrospective chart review. *Am J Emerg Med*. June 2014;32(6):596–600.
12. Watts JA, Kline JA. Bench to bedside: the role of mitochondrial medicine in the pathogenesis and treatment of cellular injury. *Acad Emerg Med*. September 2003;10(9):985–997.
13. Jones AE, Trzeciak S, Kline JA. The Sequential Organ Failure Assessment score for predicting outcome in patients with severe sepsis and evidence of hypoperfusion at the time of emergency department presentation. *Crit Care Med*. May 2009;37(5):1649–1654.
14. Andersen LW, Mackenhauer J, Roberts JC, Berg KM, Cocchi MN, Donnino MW. Etiology and therapeutic approach to elevated lactate levels. *Mayo Clin Proc*. October 2013;88(10):1127–1140.
15. Trzeciak S, Dellinger RP, Chansky ME, et al. Serum lactate as a predictor of mortality in patients with infection. *Intensive Care Med*. June 2007;33(6):970–977.
16. Coats TJ, Smith JE, Lockey D, Russell M. Early increases in blood lactate following injury. *J R Army Med Corps*. June 2002;148(2):140–143.
17. Jansen TC, van Bommel J, Mulder PG, Rommes JH, Schieveld SJ, Bakker J. The prognostic value of blood lactate levels relative to that of vital signs in the pre-hospital setting: a pilot study. *Crit Care*. 2008;12(6):R160.
18. van Beest PA, Brander L, Jansen SP, Rommes JH, Kuiper MA, Spronk PE. Cumulative lactate and hospital mortality in ICU patients. *Ann Intensive Care*. February 27, 2013;3(1):6.
19. Shapiro NI, Howell MD, Talmor D, et al. Serum lactate as a predictor of mortality in emergency department patients with infection. *Ann Emerg Med*. May 2005;45(5):524–528.
20. Mikkelsen ME, Miltiades AN, Gaieski DF, et al. Serum lactate is associated with mortality in severe sepsis independent of organ failure and shock. *Crit Care Med*. May 2009;37(5):1670–1677.
21. Jansen TC, van Bommel J, Bakker J. Blood lactate monitoring in critically ill patients: a systematic health technology assessment. *Crit Care Med*. October 2009;37(10):2827–2839.
22. Jansen TC, van Bommel J, Mulder PG, et al. Prognostic value of blood lactate levels: does the clinical diagnosis at admission matter? *J Trauma*. February 2009;66(2):377–385.
23. ProCESS Investigators, Yealy DM, Kellum JA, Huang DT, Barnato AE, Weissfeld LA, Pike F, Terndrup T, Wang HE, Hou PC, LoVecchio F, Filbin MR, Shapiro NI, Angus DC. A randomized trial of protocol-based care for early septic shock. *N Engl J Med*. May 1, 2014;370(18):1683–1693.
24. ARISE Investigators; ANZICS Clinical Trials Group, Peake SL, Delaney A, Bailey M, Bellomo R, Cameron PA, Cooper DJ, Higgins AM, Holdgate A, Howe BD, Webb SA, Williams P. Goal-directed resuscitation for patients with early septic shock. *N Engl J Med*. October 16, 2014;371(16):1496–1506.
24a. Mouncey PR, et al. ProMISe Trial Investigators. Trial of early, goal-directed resuscitation for septic shock. *N Engl J Med*. 2015;372(14):1301–1311.
25. Ghneim MH, Regner JL, Jupiter DC, et al. Goal directed fluid resuscitation decreases time for lactate clearance and facilitates early fascial closure in damage control surgery. *Am J Surg*. December 2013;206(6):995–999.
26. Rivers E, Nguyen B, Havstad S, et al. Early goal-directed therapy in the treatment of severe sepsis and septic shock. *N Engl J Med*. November 8, 2001;345(19):1368–1377.
27. Coen D, Cortellaro F, Pasini S, et al. Towards a less invasive approach to the early goal-directed treatment of septic shock in the ED. *Am J Emerg Med*. June 2014;32(6):563–568.
28. Jansen TC, van Bommel J, Schoonderbeek FJ, et al. Early lactate-guided therapy in intensive care unit patients: a multicenter, open-label, randomized controlled trial. *Am J Respir Crit Care Med*. September 15, 2010;182(6):752–761.
29. Rady MY, Rivers EP, Nowak RM. Resuscitation of the critically ill in the ED: responses of blood pressure, heart rate, shock index, central venous oxygen saturation, and lactate. *Am J Emerg Med*. March 1996;14(2):218–225.
30. Claridge JA, Crabtree TD, Pelletier SJ, Butler K, Sawyer RG, Young JS. Persistent occult hypoperfusion is associated with a significant increase in infection rate and mortality in major trauma patients. *J Trauma*. January 2000;48(1):8–14.
31. Rossi AF, Khan DM, Hannan R, Bolivar J, Zaidenweber M, Burke R. Goal-directed medical therapy and point-of-care testing improve outcomes after congenital heart surgery. *Intensive Care Med*. January 2005;31(1):98–104.
32. Jones AE, Shapiro NI, Trzeciak S, et al. Lactate clearance vs central venous oxygen saturation as goals of early sepsis therapy: a randomized clinical trial. *JAMA*. February 24, 2010;303(8):739–746.
33. Crowl AC, Young JS, Kahler DM, Claridge JA, Chrzanowski DS, Pomphrey M. Occult hypoperfusion is associated with increased morbidity in patients undergoing early femur fracture fixation. *J Trauma*. February 2000;48(2):260–267.
34. Odom SR, Howell MD, Silva GS, et al. Lactate clearance as a predictor of mortality in trauma patients. *J Trauma Acute Care Surg*. April 2013;74(4):999–1004.
35. Suistomaa M, Uusaro A, Parviainen I, Ruokonen E. Resolution and outcome of acute circulatory failure does not correlate with hemodynamics. *Crit Care*. August 2003;7(4):R52.

36. McNelis J, Marini CP, Jurkiewicz A, et al. Prolonged lactate clearance is associated with increased mortality in the surgical intensive care unit. *Am J Surg*. November 2001;182(5):481–485.

37. Ouellette DR, Shah SZ. Comparison of outcomes from sepsis between patients with and without pre-existing left ventricular dysfunction: a case-control analysis. *Crit Care*. April 23, 2014;18(2):R79.

38. Permpikul C, Sringam P, Tongyoo S. Therapeutic goal achievements during severe sepsis and septic shock resuscitation and their association with patients' outcomes. *J Med Assoc Thai*. March 2014;97(suppl 3):S176–S183.

39. Bakker J, Gris P, Coffernils M, Kahn RJ, Vincent JL. Serial blood lactate levels can predict the development of multiple organ failure following septic shock. *Am J Surg*. February 1996;171(2):221–226.

40. Nguyen HB, Loomba M, Yang JJ, et al. Early lactate clearance is associated with biomarkers of inflammation, coagulation, apoptosis, organ dysfunction and mortality in severe sepsis and septic shock. *J Inflamm (Lond)*. January 28, 2010;7:6.

41. Gatien M, Stiell I, Wielgosz A, Ooi D, Lee JS. Diagnostic performance of venous lactate on arrival at the emergency department for myocardial infarction. *Acad Emerg Med*. February 2005;12(2):106–113.

42. Schmiechen NJ, Han C, Milzman DP. ED use of rapid lactate to evaluate patients with acute chest pain. *Ann Emerg Med*. November 1997;30(5):571–577.

43. Mavrić Z, Zaputović L, Zagar D, Matana A, Smokvina D. Usefulness of blood lactate as a predictor of shock development in acute myocardial infarction. *Am J Cardiol*. March 15, 1991;67(7):565–568.

44. Vermeulen RP, Hoekstra M, Nijsten MW, et al. Clinical correlates of arterial lactate levels in patients with ST-segment elevation myocardial infarction at admission: a descriptive study. *Crit Care*. 2010;14(5):R164.

45. Lazzeri C, Valente S, Chiostri M, Picariello C, Gensini GF. Lactate in the acute phase of ST-elevation myocardial infarction treated with mechanical revascularization: a single-center experience. *Am J Emerg Med*. January 2012;30(1):92–96.

46. Lazzeri C, Sori A, Chiostri M, Gensini GF, Valente S. Prognostic role of insulin resistance as assessed by homeostatic model assessment index in the acute phase of myocardial infarction in nondiabetic patients submitted to percutaneous coronary intervention. *Eur J Anaesthesiol*. October 2009;26(10):856–862.

47. Attaná P, Lazzeri C, Chiostri M, Picariello C, Gensini GF, Valente S. Lactate clearance in cardiogenic shock following ST elevation myocardial infarction: a pilot study. *Acute Card Care*. March 2012;14(1):20–26.

48. Park TK, Yang JH, Choi SH, et al. Clinical outcomes of patients with acute myocardial infarction complicated by severe refractory cardiogenic shock assisted with percutaneous cardiopulmonary support. *Yonsei Med J*. July 2014;55(4):920–927.

49. Müllner M, Sterz F, Domanovits H, Behringer W, Binder M, Laggner AN. The association between blood lactate concentration on admission, duration of cardiac arrest, and functional neurological recovery in patients resuscitated from ventricular fibrillation. *Intensive Care Med*. November 1997;23(11):1138–1143.

50. Lee TR, Kang MJ, Cha WC, et al. Better lactate clearance associated with good neurologic outcome in survivors who treated with therapeutic hypothermia after out-of-hospital cardiac arrest. *Crit Care*. October 31, 2013;17(5):R260.

51. Parsikia A, Bones K, Kaplan M, et al. The predictive value of initial serum lactate in trauma patients. *Shock*. September 2014;42(3):199–204.

52. Kamolz LP, Andel H, Schramm W, Meissl G, Herndon DN, Frey M. Lactate: early predictor of morbidity and mortality in patients with severe burns. *Burns*. December 2005;31(8):986–990.

53. Dunne JR, Tracy JK, Scalea TM, Napolitano LM. Lactate and base deficit in trauma: does alcohol or drug use impair their predictive accuracy? *J Trauma*. May 2005;58(5):959–966.

54. Li S, Peng K, Liu F, Yu Y, Xu T, Zhang Y. Changes in blood lactate levels after major elective abdominal surgery and the association with outcomes: a prospective observational study. *J Surg Res*. October 2013;184(2):1059–1069.

55. Husain FA, Martin MJ, Mullenix PS, Steele SR, Elliott DC. Serum lactate and base deficit as predictors of mortality and morbidity. *Am J Surg*. May 2003;185(5):485–491.

56. Jones AE, Shapiro NI, Trzeciak S, Arnold RC, Claremont HA, Kline JA, Emergency Medicine Shock Research Network (EMShockNet) Investigators. Goal directed fluid resuscitation decreases time for lactate clearance and facilitates early fascial closure in damage control surgery. *Am J Surg*. December 2013;206(6):995–999.

57. Dugas AF, Mackenhauer J, Salciccioli JD, Cocchi MN, Gautam S, Donnino MW. Prevalence and characteristics of nonlactate and lactate expressors in septic shock. *J Crit Care*. August 2012;27(4):344–350.

58. Acosta S, Nilsson T. Current status on plasma biomarkers for acute mesenteric ischemia. *J Thromb Thrombolysis*. May 2012;33(4):355–361.

60 How Does Critical Illness Alter Metabolism?

Mark E. Nunnally

Globally increased metabolism fuels critical illness. The body provides and consumes basic substrates taken from its own structures to run at an accelerated metabolic rate, a rate that cannot be indefinitely sustained. Clinicians in the critical care setting are familiar with the long-term consequences of catabolic processes in patients whose illness is not alleviated; outcomes are poor and mortality is high. This archetype contrasts with a stress response that transitions to a later period of recovery and anabolism with recovery. Patterns vary, but all critically ill patients experience increased metabolism in a neurologic, hormonal, and immunologic milieu that reprioritizes many functions of the healing process. This process is adaptive and, in prolonged and uncontrolled situations, pathogenic.

Cuthbertson was among the first to describe and explain the stress response, a pattern of metabolic changes in injured patients.[1] In his framework, the physiology of response was viewed as adaptive. Metabolic changes from "normal" were thought to be necessary to heal serious injury. As part of this process, patients might become ill enough to require aggressive therapy. Indeed, in patients with underlying comorbidities, intervention to correct or reverse the stress response might be helpful. Unfortunately, although the metabolic changes induced by "stress" have been described, their meaning remains subject to interpretation, and intervention must be undertaken with trepidation. Our understanding of most aspects of the metabolic response to injury is, by and large, characterized by a dearth of clear evidence, a glut of theory, and an absence of consensus. This chapter considers the predictable pattern in response to injury, the interventions that alter this pattern, and the diagnostic utility of comparing a patient's clinical data to a generalized stress response pattern.

PATHOPHYSIOLOGY AND MECHANISM OF ACTION

Cells metabolize glucose, lactate, amino acids, fatty acids, ketones, and their derivatives. They assemble these components into larger carbohydrates (glycogen), proteins, and triglycerides for energy storage and cellular function. Anabolic processes assemble small molecules into larger ones and consume energy. Catabolic processes deconstruct these larger molecules and release energy. Thus, large molecules can be viewed as sites of stored energy.

Catabolism, the hypermetabolic recovery period of "flow" that follows the "ebb" of shock in Cuthbertson's original description,[2] is the trademark of critical illness. These two phases are followed by a third: an anabolic recovery phase that commences after resolution of the stress response and persists for weeks to months (Fig. 60-1). Changes affect the entire body, alter activity in each organ system, and are reflected in secondary dysfunction in these systems. Available evidence supports the theory that this adaptive response enables tissue healing.

Resting energy expenditure increases in critical illness. Glucose and fatty acids are consumed at accelerated rates. Serum levels of both exceed the normal range. Proteins are catabolized to amino acids, which in turn are converted by the liver to glucose. Patients develop hyperglycemia. Levels of lactate increase because of a metabolic shift and do not necessarily reflect tissue hypoperfusion, as is the case in acute shock. The catabolism of stress is not the same as that of starvation. In the former tissue, protein is consumed preferentially rather than spared. The liver produces acute phase reactants, such as C-reactive protein, immunoglobulins, fibrinogen, and haptoglobin, often at the expense of other proteins such as prealbumin, albumin, and transferrin. Muscle tissue provides most of the amino acids for fuel and protein synthesis. Ketosis is rare because hyperglycemia stimulates insulin release and insulin suppresses ketogenesis. Provision of exogenous substrate cannot completely attenuate the loss of body proteins. The intestines continue to absorb glutamine, but conversion to citrulline drops, suggesting nutritional reprioritization.[3] Serum amino acid profiles change in septic patients with their illness trajectory.[4] These findings underscore the fact that nutrient use is altered during critical illness and that metabolic priorities are changed. Critically ill patients will not respond to endocrine, nutritional, or metabolic therapies in the same way that unstressed patients do.

Some end-organ cells lose part of their ability to oxidize fuels in the mitochondria.[5] For these cells, metabolism and oxygen use decrease, leading to a metabolic "shunt" and organ dysfunction. This bioenergetic failure correlates with illness severity. It may be adaptive, and recovery is sometimes possible, but the resulting organ dysfunctions frequently require supportive interventions.

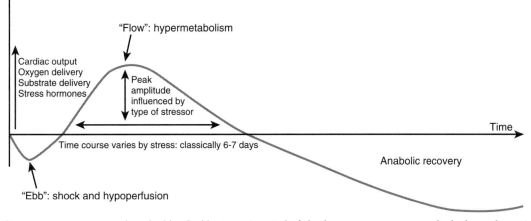

Figure 60-1. Stress response curve, as described by Cuthbertson. A period of shock may or may not precede the hyperdynamic phase during which nutrient and oxygen delivery are increased to peripheral tissues. For details on organ-specific alterations, see chapter text.

Endocrine and neurologic axes drive part of the change in metabolism. The anterior pituitary releases large amounts of growth hormone, thyroid-stimulating hormone, luteinizing hormone, and prolactin, but there is peripheral resistance to normal metabolic effects.[6-10] Metabolism and cardiovascular function change as a consequence of elevated levels of catecholamines and vasopressin. Although insulin, glucagon, and cortisol levels are increased, their anabolic effects are attenuated.

Changes in organ systems function characterize the acute phase of critical illness. Recognition of these findings sometimes heralds a new diagnosis, such as sepsis, and should provoke clinicians to increase monitoring and perhaps begin empiric therapy.

Neurologic. Brain tissue uses a wide variety of metabolic fuel. During stress, glucose, amino acid, and lactate metabolism increases. Encephalopathy frequently develops, possibly related to the presence of elevated levels of aromatic amino acids and their metabolites.[11-13] Global cerebral function declines, manifested as alterations ranging from delirium to overt coma.

Cardiovascular. Stress accelerates oxygen consumption in the periphery. To compensate, cardiac output increases and peripheral vascular tone decreases, augmenting blood flow to peripheral tissues, possibly at the expense of flow to other vascular beds. That oxygen consumption is highest in leukocyte-dense tissues suggests that heightened oxygen delivery is destined for cells that repair tissue and control infection.[14,15] Capillary beds leak because of alterations in glycocalyx function.[16] The balance between fluid extravasation and reabsorption favors the formation of edema because plasma proteins accumulate outside vessel walls, pulling fluid and electrolytes with them.

The result of these changes is a hyperdynamic circulation and accumulation of edema. In some patients, myocardial injury may ensue. Damage may lead to a failure to supplement oxygen delivery, which is associated with a high mortality in critical illness lung injury.[17] Although adaptive, there is little associated benefit from attempts to enhance this response by supplementing oxygen delivery.[18,19]

Fluids, Electrolytes, and Nutrition. Tissue edema and intravascular resuscitation increase body water, and patients characteristically gain weight. The distribution of water during the stress response was explored by Moore and colleagues.[20] The extracellular and vascular compartments expand,[20-23] but intracellular water is lost. This effect suggests that water shifts from the intracellular space to the extracellular space and back again as edema resolves, which has implications for electrolyte balance.

Insensible water loss and diuretic use produce hypernatremia. Sometimes renal water retention dominates, causing hyponatremia. As the stress response abates, water shifts back into the intracellular space, stimulating a concomitant inward flux of potassium, magnesium, phosphate, and proteins from the plasma. Thus hypokalemia, hypomagnesemia, and hyperphosphatemia are common. Hypermetabolism or the refeeding syndrome also may cause hypophosphatemia.[24,25]

Whole-body glucose delivery increases as a consequence of decreased peripheral uptake[26,27] and increased production. Hepatic gluconeogenesis converts amino acids and glycerol to glucose, even during hyperglycemia.[28,29] Amino acids, freed from peripheral protein stores, feed this process. It is likely that the driving force for increased glucose production and decreased utilization is leukocyte demand in injured areas. Hyperglycemia and edema formation deliver glucose to relatively avascular injured areas. Lipid metabolism increases in the stress response, but not as much as triglyceride hydrolysis and re-esterification, resulting in elevated serum triglycerides.[30,31] Many fat stores undergo mobilization and subsequent recomposition.

Pulmonary. Pulmonary insufficiency accompanies the stress response. Enhanced oxygen consumption and carbon dioxide production put greater demand on the pulmonary system. Tachypnea and type I (oxygenation) and type II (ventilation) failure occur. Perivascular flux forces fluids and proteins into alveoli. Inflammatory infiltration exacerbates extravasation in certain patients. Altered immune function and risk for aspiration foment pulmonary infection. Such changes culminate in pulmonary dysfunction, including the adult respiratory distress syndrome.

Gastrointestinal. Intestinal villi atrophy and the gut swells.[32] Ileus heralds worsening stress. These changes confound attempts to provide enteric nutrition and increase the risk of bowel obstruction. Hepatic metabolic changes include impaired excretion of bilirubin and other metabolites.

Renal. Peripheral vasodilatation steals blood flow from the kidneys. Reduced perfusion and circulating mediators produce a syndrome of oliguria. Metabolically active tubular cells suspend function and become quiescent until the stress has long resolved. The extreme example of this condition is acute kidney injury. With recovery, renal function usually returns.[33]

Immunologic. Cell-mediated immunity is classically suppressed during inflammation.[34] Susceptibility to infection increases as systemic inflammatory signals are elevated.

Endocrine. Cortisol, catecholamines, and glucagon drive part of stress hyperglycemia.[27] Relative cortisol deficiency worsens vasodilatory shock and stalls recovery.[35] The peripheral response to insulin changes with immunologic signaling in peripheral muscle and fat.[36-39] Changes in endocrine signaling include the euthyroid sick syndrome, disorders of sleep cycles, and altered immunologic function. Eventually, pituitary hypersecretion and altered peripheral sensitivity may give way to exhaustion.

If critical illness continues unabated, then metabolic signaling changes. Adiponectin levels decrease with acute critical illness, but they then normalize as illness continues,[40] suggesting changing immune and metabolic signaling. In this setting, catabolism continues and may be increased. Anterior pituitary hormone levels decline in a functional state of neuroendocrine exhaustion.

Ongoing stress leads to a state of persistent critical illness. In this state, neuroendocrine exhaustion is compounded by widespread bioenergetics/mitochondrial failure, organ dysfunction, kwashiorkor-like protein malnutrition, and a stymied immune response. Regular biologic oscillators lose their signaling,[41] adiponectin levels increase again, and tissue macrophages adopt an "anti-inflammatory" phenotype.[40] These patients are susceptible to infection and are dependent on life-sustaining organ support therapies.

Recovery from any of these phases entails source control followed by prolonged anabolism. Tissue protein stores slowly recover. It takes time to replete proteins, endocrine axes, and immune responses to their normal function. Myopathies, neuropathies, and wound healing are the most visible manifestations of the slow recovery.

AVAILABLE DATA

Several clinical trials suggest ways in which the physiology of critical illness is mediated and how attempts to interfere with it might help or harm. Herndon et al.[42] studied the use of beta-blockade in burned children to reduce the loss of muscle mass. They found that large doses of propranolol (average 6.3 mg/kg/day) produced a 6% absolute difference in lean body mass after 2 weeks of hospitalization. This trial examined the role of catecholamines in stress hypermetabolism and showed that blockade of rampant protein catabolism might improve outcomes in certain settings.

Adrenal hormone replacement may treat septic shock and other forms of acute critical illness, but the metabolic and immunologic consequences of this therapy are difficult to disentangle. Large doses of cortisol worsened mortality.[43]

One study reported increased survival with selective administration of lower doses of cortisol in patients in whom a cosyntropin stimulation test signaled impaired response.[35] Other investigators[44] have found no survival benefit. The value of diagnostic tests for adrenal insufficiency has been questioned because protein binding is so variable among critically ill patients.[45] Current evidence shows little benefit from therapeutic administration of steroids to patients during the stress response. This volume contains a comprehensive discussion of the topic elsewhere.

The amount of nutrition needed during critical illness is an ongoing source of debate. Nutritional support modestly prevents excessive protein loss, hyperglycemia, or hyperlipidemia and may improve organ and immune function. The available literature is highly prone to bias. A few findings are consistent. Very high levels of nutrients are associated with worse outcomes, "underfeeding" may be beneficial, and parenteral nutrients do not have the same effects as enteric nutrition.[46] Nutritional topics are treated elsewhere in this text.

Attempts to alter stress metabolism can have adverse consequences. Although administration of anabolic hormones might attenuate loss of lean muscle mass and improve outcomes in critical illness, studies of androgen supplementation show mixed results.[47] In one study, growth hormone supplementation increased mortality.[48] In a surgical population, aggressive insulin therapy improved survival and reduced organ dysfunction when serum glucose was driven to nonstress levels.[49] A subsequent study of patients in a medical intensive care unit by the same investigators[50] and studies by others[51-53] failed to replicate these results. The original study was criticized for its large proportion of cardiac surgery patients, the restriction of benefit to patients who stayed in the ICU longer, and the aggressive nutrition given to the patients.[54] Given the changes and variability in stress metabolism during critical illness, it is conceivable that the goals of insulin therapy should vary with a patient's position on the stress curve such that catabolism is not overly suppressed early and anabolism is supported late. This concept remains unstudied.

INTERPRETATION OF DATA

Stress metabolism is incompletely characterized, variable, and multifaceted. Attempts to regulate specific elements on the arc of inflammation have been largely unsuccessful, but available data do provide useful tools for the care of critically ill patients. The original model proposed by Cuthbertson is a template on which a patient's progress can be mapped. Signs of increased metabolism and neurohormonal stress should prompt a search for a cause and aggressive, sometimes empiric, therapy. As an example, the triad of encephalopathy, hyperglycemia, and impaired intestinal motility may herald the onset of sepsis. Conversely, signs that stress is abating, such as a spontaneous negative fluid balance and hypokalemia, can inform decisions to de-escalate monitoring and therapy, reducing iatrogenic risk. In the future, aminograms, lipograms, and even biograms of endogenous flora may help inform clinicians about these transitions. Given that bacteria outnumber somatic cells and mostly fulfill commensal roles, cultivating and monitoring a healthy resident flora is justifiably the subject of ongoing investigation.

Nutrition goals are incompletely characterized and should be tailored to patient response. Clinicians should consider decreasing or even eliminating exogenous dextrose if it worsens hyperglycemia. Protein and fat goals, and the best way to provide them, require further study. Using lactate as a marker for adequate resuscitation may be helpful in early shock, but lactate has a limited effect once the stress response commences. Therapies must be tested in patients with acute, prolonged, and persistent critical illness because improved outcomes are desperately needed.[55-57] The evidence suggests that preventing the transition to persistent critical illness with aggressive source control is the best available strategy.

SUMMARY

Metabolism increases with critical illness. The pattern of increase and decline is predictable, affects every organ system, and is known as the stress response. Increased oxygen and nutrient delivery underlies the observed physiologic changes. The stress response pattern is a useful tool to guide clinical therapy.

AUTHOR'S RECOMMENDATIONS

- Critical illness increases global metabolism.
- The process of elevated global metabolism can be thought of as an adaptive response to facilitate tissue healing.
- Critically ill patients undergo a predictable pattern of metabolic and physiologic changes in the stress response. After injury (with or without initial shock), metabolism accelerates with gradual (days to week) recovery followed by a longer (weeks to months) period of anabolic recovery of proteins. The response is manifested in every organ system in the body.
- Astute clinicians can exploit their knowledge of the stress response by predicting the pattern, mapping patient physiology to the expected changes, and making diagnostic and therapeutic decisions based on the expected trajectory or unexpected variation from the common stress response pattern.

REFERENCES

1. Cuthbertson DP. The disturbance of metabolism produced by bony and non-bony injury, with notes on certain abnormal conditions of bone. *Biochem J.* 1930;24:1244–1263.
2. Cuthbertson D, Tilstone WJ. Metabolism during the postinjury period. *Adv Clin Chem.* 1969;12:1–55.
3. Kao C, Hsu J, Bandi V, et al. Alteration in glutamine metabolism and its conversion to citrulline in sepsis. *Am J Physiol Endocrinol Metab.* 2013;304:E1359–E1364.
4. Hiroso T, Shimizu K, Ogura H, et al. Altered balance of the angiogram in patients with sepsis – the relation to mortality. *Clin Nutr.* 2013;33:179–182.
5. Azevedo LCP. Mitochondrial dysfunction during sepsis. *Endocr Metab Immune Disord Drug Targets.* 2010;10:214–223.
6. Van den Berghe G, de Zegher F, Bouillon R. The somatotrophic axis in critical illness: effects of growth hormone secretagogues. *Growth Horm IGF Res.* 1998;8(suppl B):153–155.
7. Noel GL, Suh HK, Stone JG, et al. Human prolactin and growth hormone release during surgery and other conditions of stress. *J Clin Endocrinol Metab.* 1972;35:840–851.
8. Landry DW, Levin HR, Gallant EM, et al. Vasopressin deficiency contributes to the vasodilation of septic shock. *Circulation.* 1997;95:1122–1125.
9. Kakucska I, Romero LI, Clark BD, et al. Suppression of thyrotropin-releasing hormone gene expression by interleukin-1-beta in the rat: implications for nonthyroidal illness. *Neuroendocrinology.* 1994;59:129–137.
10. Bacci V, Schussler GC, Kaplan TB. The relationship between serum triiodothyronine and thyrotropin during systemic illness. *J Clin Endocrinol Metab.* 1982;54:1229–1235.
11. Stevens RD, Pronovost PJ. The spectrum of encephalopathy in critical illness. *Semin Neurol.* 2006;26:440–451.
12. Takezawa J, Taenake N, Nishijima MK, et al. Amino acids and thiobarbituric acid reactive substances in cerebrospinal fluid and plasma of patients with septic encephalopathy. *Crit Care Med.* 1983;11:876–879.
13. Freund HR, Muggia-Sullam M, Peiser J, et al. Brain neurotransmitter profile is deranged during sepsis and septic encephalopathy in the rat. *J Surg Res.* 1985;28:267–271.
14. Meszaros K, Lang CH, Bagby GJ, et al. Contribution of different organs to increased glucose consumption after endotoxin administration. *J Bio Chem.* 1997;262:10965–10970.
15. Meszaros K, Bojta J, Bautista AP, et al. Glucose utilization by Kupffer cells, endothelial cells, and granulocytes in endotoxemic rat liver. *Am J Physiol.* 1991;260:G7–G12.
16. Woodcock TE, Woodcock TM. Revised Starling equation and the glycocalyx model of transvascular fluid exchange: an improved paradigm for prescribing intravenous fluid therapy. *Br J Anaesth.* 2012;108:384–394.
17. Bajwa EK, Boyce PD, Januzzi JL, et al. Biomarker evidence of myocardial cell injury is associated with mortality in acute respiratory distress syndrome. *Crit Care Med.* 2007;25:2484–2490.
18. Hayes MA, Timmins AC, Yau EH, et al. Elevation of systemic oxygen delivery in the treatment of critically ill patients. *N Engl J Med.* 1994;330:1717–1722.
19. Shoemaker WC, Appel PL, Kram HB, et al. Prospective trial of supranormal values of survivors as therapeutic goals in high-risk surgical patients. *Chest.* 1988;94:1176–1186.
20. Moore FD, Dagher FJ, Boyden CM, et al. Hemorrhage in normal man: I. distribution and dispersal of saline infusions following acute blood loss: clinical kinetics of blood volume support. *Ann Surg.* 1966;163:485–504.
21. Flexner LB, Gellhorn A, Merrell M. Studies on rates of exchange of substances between the blood and extravascular fluid. I. The exchange of water in the guinea pig. *J Biol Chem.* 1942;144:35–40.
22. Flexner LB, Cowie DB, Vosburgh GJ. Studies on capillary permeability with tracer substances. *Symp Quant Biol Cold Spring Harbor.* 1948;13:88–98.
23. Stewart JD, Rourke GM. Intracellular fluid loss in hemorrhage. *J Clin Invest.* 1936;15:697–702.
24. Crook MA, Hally V, Panteli JV. The importance of the refeeding syndrome. *Nutrition.* 2001;17:632–6377.
25. Subramanian R, Khardori R. Severe hypophosphatemia. Pathophysiologic implications, clinical presentations, and treatment. *Medicine.* 2000;79:1–8.
26. Clemens MG, Chaudry IH, Daigneau N, et al. Insulin resistance and depressed gluconeogenic capability during early hyperglycemic sepsis. *J Trauma.* 1984;24:701–708.
27. Lang CH. Beta-adrenergic blockade attenuates insulin resistance induced by tumor necrosis factor. *Am J Physiol.* 1993;264:R984–R991.
28. Jeevanandam M, Young DH, Schiller WR. Glucose turnover, oxidation, and indices of recycling in severely traumatized patients. *J Trauma.* 1990;30:582–589.
29. Shaw JH, Klein S, Wolfe RR. Assessment of alanine, urea and glucose interrelationships in normal subjects and in patients with sepsis with stable isotope tracers. *Surgery.* 1985;97:557–568.
30. Hardardottir I, Grunfeld C, Feingold KR. Effects of endotoxin and cytokines on lipid metabolism. *Curr Opin Lipidol.* 1994;5:207–215.
31. Robin AP, Askanazi J, Greenwood MR, et al. Lipoprotein lipase activity in surgical patients: influence of trauma and infection. *Surgery.* 1981;90:401–408.
32. Hernandez G, Velasco N, Wainstein C, et al. Gut mucosal atrophy after a short enteral fasting period in critically ill patients. *J Crit Care.* 1999;14:73–77.

33. Bagshaw SM, Laupland KB, Doig CJ, et al. Prognosis for long-term survival and renal recovery in critically ill patients with severe acute renal failure: a population-based study. *Crit Care.* 2005;9:R700–R709.

34. Hotchkiss RS, Karl IE. The pathophysiology and treatment of sepsis. *N Eng J Med.* 2003;348:138–150.

35. Annane D, Sebille V, Charpentier C, et al. Effect of treatment with low doses of hydrocortisone and fludrocortisone on mortality in patients with septic shock. *JAMA.* 2002;288:862–871.

36. Vary TC, Drnevich D, Jurasinski C, et al. Mechanisms regulating skeletal muscle glucose metabolism in sepsis. *Shock.* 1995;3:403–410.

37. Wolfe RR, Durkot MJ, Alldop JR, et al. Glucose metabolism in severely burned patients. *Metabolism.* 1979;28:1031–1039.

38. Shangraw RE, Jahoor F, Myoski H, et al. Differentiation between septic and postburn insulin resistance. *Metabolism.* 1989;38:983–989.

39. Virkamaki A, Puhakainen I, Koivisto VA, et al. Mechanisms of hepatic and peripheral insulin resistance during acute infections in humans. *J Clin Endocrinol Metab.* 1992;74:673–679.

40. Marques MB, Langouche L. Endocrine, metabolic and morphologic alterations of adipose tissue during critical illness. *Crit Care Med.* 2013;41:317–325.

41. Godin PJ, Buchman TG. Uncoupling of biological oscillators: a complementary hypothesis concerning the pathogenesis of multiple organ dysfunction syndrome. *Crit Care Med.* 1996;24:1107–1116.

42. Herndon DN, Hart DW, Wolf SE, et al. Reversal of catabolism by beta-blockade after severe burns. *N Engl J Med.* 2001;345:1223–1229.

43. Bone RC, Fisher CJ, Clemmer TP, et al. A controlled clinical trial of high-dose methylprednisolone in the treatment of severe sepsis and septic shock. *N Engl J Med.* 1987;317:653–658.

44. Sprung CL, Annane D, Keh D, et al. Hydrocortisone therapy for patients with septic shock. *N Engl J Med.* 2008;358:111–124.

45. Arafah BM. Hypothalamic pituitary adrenal function during critical illness: limitations of current assessment methods. *J Clin Endocrinol Metab.* 2006;91:3725–3745.

46. Stapleton RD, Jones N, Heyland DK. Feeding critically ill patients: what is the optimal amount of energy? *Crit Care Med.* 2007;35:S535–S540.

47. Herndon DN, Tompkins RG. Support of the metabolic response to burn injury. *Lancet.* 2004;363:1895–1902.

48. Takala J, Ruokonen E, Webster NR, et al. Increased mortality associated with growth hormone treatment in critically ill adults. *N Engl J Med.* 1999;341:785–792.

49. Van den Berghe G, Wouters P, Weekers F, et al. Intensive insulin therapy in critically ill patients. *N Engl J Med.* 2001;345:1359–1367.

50. Van den Berghe G, Wilmer A, Hermans G, et al. Intensive insulin therapy in the medical ICU. *N Engl J Med.* 2006;354:449–461.

51. Arabi YM, Dabbagh OC, Tamim HM, et al. Intensive versus conventional insulin therapy: a randomized control trial in medical and surgical critically ill patients. *Crit Care Med.* 2008;36:3190–3197.

52. Gandhi GY, Nuttall GA, Abel MA, et al. Intensive intraoperative insulin therapy versus conventional glucose management during cardiac surgery. *Ann Intern Med.* 2007;146:233–243.

53. Finfer S, Chitlock DR, Blair D, the NICE-SUGAR Investigators, et al. Intensive versus conventional glucose control in critically ill patients. *N Engl J Med.* 2009;360:1283–1297.

54. Nunnally ME. Con: tight perioperative glycemic control: poorly supported and risky. *J Cardiothorac Vasc Anesth.* 2005;19:689–690.

55. Nunnally ME, Neligan P, Deutschman CS. Metabolism in acute and chronic illness. In: Rolandelli RH, Bankhead R, Boullata JI, Compher CW, eds. *Clinical Nutrition, 4th Edition: Enteral and Tube Feeding.* Philadelphia: Elsevier; 2008:80–94.

56. Vanhorebeek I, Langouche L, Van den Berghe G. Endocrine aspects of acute and prolonged critical illness. *Nat Clin Pract Endocrinol Metab.* 2006;2:20–31.

57. Van den Berghe G. Neuroendocrine pathobiology of chronic critical illness. *Crit Care Clin.* 2002;18:509–528.

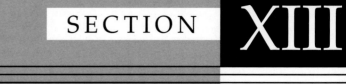
NEUROLOGIC CRITICAL CARE

61 Is It Really Necessary to Measure Intracranial Pressure in Brain-Injured Patients?

Randall M. Chesnut

A search of the literature on the management of severe traumatic brain injury (sTBI) will reveal evidence-based guidelines[1] and consensus-based recommendations[2] supporting intracranial pressure (ICP) monitoring (Table 61-1). These documents support the predominant position of academic neurotraumatologists in highly resourced medical environments that successfully lowering elevated ICP improves recovery by attenuating the morbidity associated with intracranial hypertension. The publication of a randomized controlled trial (RCT)[3] that questions the efficacy of our current use of monitored ICP, as well as the economic and clinical challenges associated with ICP monitoring in less affluent environments, invites a review of the current evidence surrounding the necessity and utility of monitoring ICP in managing sTBI.

The utility of any monitor lies in its interpretation. Most ICP data are treated as end-hour ICP, reflecting the prior 60 minutes, although few studies actually specify their collection technique. End-hour ICP may be the instantaneous ICP value; a nurse's subjectively derived value representing the prior hour; or, more rarely, an average that is based on some algorithm (often unspecified). None of these represent the way ICP is used clinically, which generally reflects instantaneous values, trends, responses to stimulation, spontaneous fluctuations, and the effect of treatment. More recently, higher resolution (real-time) ICP data have been collected, allowing averaging and trending as well as alternative analytic methods (e.g., area under the curve [AUC], ICP variability). The overall lack of rigor in the current literature has greatly hampered studies of the prognostic value of ICP, its optimal treatment threshold(s), the efficacy of treatment on altering outcome, and the definition of a "dose" of intracranial hypertension. Finally, the lack of natural history studies means that all ICP studies are performed with data from patients concomitantly treated at some threshold (most frequently 20 mm Hg). This confounds toxicities of treatment with the detrimental effects of intracranial hypertension, in particular greatly hampering analysis of the predictive value on ICP elevation and the determination of physiologic treatment thresholds. This is the evidentiary environment within which one approaches an analysis of the role of ICP monitoring in sTBI management.

INTRACRANIAL PRESSURE AND PROGNOSIS

In addition to the previously mentioned standardization considerations and the lack of natural history studies, the analysis of ICP as a predictive variable is confounded by irregularities in populations studied (e.g., excluding patients for "futility"), uncontrolled variability in management approaches, treatment toxicities, and mixed injury types.

Most studies evaluate the prognostic utility of ICP based on a set threshold. In general, such analyses support that intracranial hypertension is predictive of increased mortality.[4-17] When morbidity is evaluated with mortality included, intracranial hypertension correlates with poor outcome (e.g., Glasgow Outcome Scale score [GOS] 1 to 3 or Extended GOS [GOS-E] 1 to 4), although this correlation appears to hold better for diffuse injuries than mass lesions.[18,19] If morbidity is analyzed separately from mortality, then intracranial hypertension is frequently not predictive of poor-grade survival.[5,6,11,17,20-22] A recent systematic review of ICP and outcome reported that the degree of intracranial hypertension (especially >40 mm Hg) was associated with unfavorable outcome if death was included but not for survivors alone.[23] It was concluded that the pattern of ICP elevation and ICP that is refractory to treatment were more powerful predictors than peak values or threshold violations.

Analyzing the "refractoriness" of ICP involves evaluating the correlation between outcome and the response of intracranial hypertension to treatment. All such studies have used a 20–mm Hg treatment threshold and have reported significantly higher mortality for intracranial hypertension refractory to treatment.[19,24-27] The systematic

Table 61-1 Published Indications for ICP Monitoring

BTF GUIDELINES FOR ADULTS[1]

- Level II recommendations (based on Class II evidence):
  - ICP should be monitored in all salvageable patients with an sTBI (GCS of 3-8 after resuscitation) and an abnormal CT scan (one that reveals hematomas, contusions, swelling, herniation, or compressed basal cisterns).
- Level III recommendations (based on Class III evidence):
  - ICP monitoring is indicated in patients with sTBI with a normal CT scan if two or more of the following features are noted at admission:
    - Age older than 40 years
    - Unilateral or bilateral motor posturing
    - Systolic blood pressure <90 mm Hg

MILAN CONSENSUS CONFERENCE[2]

Diffuse brain damage

- ICP monitoring recommended:
  - Comatose patients* with initial CT scan demonstrating diffuse damage with signs of brain swelling (e.g., compressed/absent basal cisterns)
- No indication for monitoring:
  - Comatose patients* with clinically available examinations and a normal initial CT scan
  - Comatose patients* with clinically available examinations and abnormal initial CT scan showing minimal signs of injury (e.g., SAH, petechial hemorrhages)
    - ICP monitoring should be started for CT worsening
    - Recommend second CT within 6-12 hr in stable patients
    - Recommend urgent CT for neurologic worsening

Traumatic brain contusions

- ICP monitoring may not be indicated:
  - Older patients despite large-sized traumatic contusions
- ICP monitoring should be considered:
  - Noncomatose patients with large bifrontal contusions and/or hemorrhagic mass lesions near the brainstem
- ICP monitoring recommended:
  - Comatose patients* with an initial CT showing traumatic contusions in whom the interruption of sedation to check neurologic status is dangerous or when the clinical examination is not completely reliable (e.g., severe maxillofacial trauma, spinal cord injury)
  - Patients with large bifrontal contusions and/or hemorrhagic mass lesions near the brainstem regardless of the initial GCS

After decompressive craniectomy for intracranial hypertension (secondary DC)

- ICP monitoring is generally recommended after a secondary DC to assess the effectiveness of DC in terms of ICP control and to guide further therapy.

After evacuation of intracranial traumatic hematomas (primary DC)

- ICP monitoring should be considered for salvageable patients after evacuation of an acute supratentorial intracranial hematoma in the presence of the following features associated with an increased risk of intracranial hypertension:
  - Preoperative clinical findings/imaging data:
    - GCS motor score ≤ 5
    - Pupillary abnormalities (anisocoria or bilateral mydriasis)
    - Prolonged/severe hypoxia and/or hypotension
    - Compressed or obliterated basal cisterns
    - Midline shift exceeds 5 mm
    - Midline shift exceeds thickness of the extra-axial clot
    - Additional extra-axial hematomas, parenchymal injuries (e.g., contusions), or swelling
  - Intraoperative clinical findings:
    - Brain swelling

*Comatose patients defined as patients without eye opening, not obeying commands, and not speaking understandable words after hemodynamic and respiratory stabilization and in the absence of anesthetic or paralyzing agents.
BTF, Brain Trauma Foundation; *CT*, computed tomography; *DC*, decompressive craniectomy; *GCS*, Glasgow Coma Scale; *ICP*, intracranial pressure; *SAH*, subarachnoid hemorrhage; *sTBI*, severe traumatic brain injury.

review of Treggiari et al. concluded that the odds ratios (ORs) of mortality and poor survivorship were significantly associated with intracranial hypertension refractory to treatment.[23]

Overall, the absolute value of ICP appears to be of marginal utility as a prognostic variable, primarily acting as a marker of disease severity in terms of mortality. The pattern of resistance to treatment, particularly a refractory course, offers more prognostic power and is relevant to the critical value of quality of survival. However, its value as an independent predictive value remains unclear.

USE OF INTRACRANIAL PRESSURE MONITORING AND OUTCOME

Intracranial Pressure-Monitor-Based Management Protocols

The association between monitoring ICP and outcome has been evaluated as validation of its use. Studies from single centers not using monitoring showing no associated difference versus historical controls from monitoring centers have been too flawed to be conclusive.[28,29] Small prospective[30] and larger retrospective[16,31,32] single-center reports of the influence of instituting sTBI protocols focused around ICP and cerebral perfusion pressure (CPP) management have uniformly demonstrated increased efficiency (e.g., decreased ventilator days, decreased number of treatments) and generally supported associated improvements in short-term outcomes. Care system modifications ranged from preprinted orders, through explicit algorithms, to formal care pathways. However, one small prospective study reported that initiating an sTBI protocol was not associated with improved outcome and that the significant benefits on management efficiency were statistically independent of whether patients underwent ICP monitoring.[33] A similar, larger, two-paper retrospective series reported that the significant improvements in mortality associated with protocol initiation were independent of ICP monitoring, which was significantly associated with increased use of treatment modalities and intensive care unit (ICU) length of stay.[34,35]

In aggregate, it appears that, if associated with adequate attention to protocol compliance, monitoring of deviations, and definition of the interventions (preprinted orders, flowcharts, management protocols, care pathways), the literature supports that the establishment and enforcement of protocols/care pathways focused on ICP-monitor-based management of sTBI patients can be expected to generally result in decreased resource use and improvements in short-term patient outcome. However, the degree and even direction of the specific contribution of ICP monitoring to these improvements is unclear.

CENTER-BASED STUDIES

Multicenter studies of the association between ICP monitoring and outcome can be divided into center-based and patient-based approaches. Center-based studies focus on "aggressive care" as associated with more frequent ICP monitoring. Bulger et al. analyzed prospective data from 33 level I/II trauma centers, classifying those who monitored ICP in more than 50% of patients that met the Brain Trauma Foundation (BTF) guidelines monitoring criteria[1] (GCS ≤ 8 and an abnormal admission computed tomography [CT] scan) as aggressive.[36] Only 36% of centers met these criteria. This designation strongly covaried with the availability of traumatic brain injury (TBI)-related resources and personnel and with treatment intensity. Overall hospital mortality was significantly lower at "aggressive" centers, suggesting that this ICP monitoring frequency-based definition of aggressive care strongly covaries with practices supportive of improved survival.

This study contrasts with the report of Cremer et al., which retrospectively compared two level I trauma centers, one of which treated suspected intracranial hypertension based on imaging and clinical examination (ICE), the other predominantly directing care based on ICP monitoring (67% of studied patients).[37] The monitoring center used significantly more resources, but there was no difference in survival-to-discharge between centers.

The contrasting results of these two frequently quoted, center-based studies suggest that, although the frequency of ICP monitoring may be a useful index of beneficially attentive care in multicenter studies, it should not be used in isolation as a marker of effective care of sTBI patients. Mauritz et al. found that the frequency of ICP monitoring varied according to center size (increasing from small to medium centers, then decreasing for larger institutions) and severity of injury (increasing, then decreasing as severity increased).[38] It also varied by age. If aggressiveness of care is to be usefully studied, then it clearly warrants a more complex definition derived via multivariate analysis.

PATIENT-BASED STUDIES

Multicenter, patient-based studies have analyzed large databases to investigate the association between ICP monitor insertion and outcomes. Two large studies have been reported based on general trauma databases. An analysis of 5507 patients with abbreviated injury scale (AIS) head scores greater than 3 from the Ontario Trauma Registry found that 9.8% were monitored, with a very wide center-specific range (0.5% to 21.4%). Multivariate analyses controlling for AIS head score, injury severity score (ISS), and injury mechanism indicated that ICP monitoring was associated with significantly improved survival.[39] However, different results were gleaned from sTBI patients (GCS ≤ 8 and an abnormal CT) with ICU stays of 3 or more days from the National Trauma Data Bank.[40] Worse risk-adjusted hospital mortality and discharge functional status as well as increased complications (pneumonia, renal failure, and infections) were reported for 708 monitored patients as compared with 938 nonmonitored patients. Only 43% of patients meeting the BTF guidelines criteria for ICP monitoring were actually monitored.

Although these reports presumably reflect "real-life" treatment of TBI patients at general trauma centers, they lack the neurologic indices necessary for rigorous adjustment for TBI severity. Their disparate findings under these conditions suggest that the use of ICP monitoring as a quality benchmark should be considered relative, not absolute.

Prospective, TBI-specific databases provide the best data for rigorous risk adjustment. Farahvar et al. prospectively analyzed collected data from 1307 sTBI patients who received treatment for intracranial hypertension within 48 hours of injury, 1083 (83%) of who were monitored.[41] Nonmonitored patients were significantly older and had significantly more pupillary abnormalities. Controlling for age, GCS score, CT abnormalities, pupil abnormalities, and hypotension, multivariate logistic regression modeling of 2-week mortality in adults revealed a strong trend toward reduced risk for patients having ICP monitoring (OR, 0.64, 95%; confidence interval [CI], 0.41 to 1.00; $P = .05$).

Mauritz et al. attempted to model the decision to monitor by creating an ICP-monitoring propensity score derived on the basis of severity of injury indices.[38] They applied this score to 1856 prospectively studied sTBI patients from 32 ICUs. When adjusted based on this model, they found no significant independent association between ICP monitoring and risk-adjusted discharge mortality. As noted previously, the frequency of ICP monitoring in this study varied according to age, center size, and severity of injury.

META-ANALYSIS OF PATIENT-BASED STUDIES

Stein et al. performed a meta-analysis of 127 sTBI patient-based studies, analyzing the influence on outcome of aggressive treatment based on ICP monitoring frequency.[42] Their analysis was study-based; they did not use pooled data. They reported significant independent associations of improved outcome and decreased recovery associated with aggressive treatment.

RANDOMIZED CONTROLLED TRIALS

The BEST TRIP (Benchmark Evidence from South American Trials: Treatment of Intracranial Pressure) trial, a recent RCT, compared the outcomes of patients managed according to a protocol based on monitored ICP versus a group treated for intracranial hypertension based on serial ICE without implanted monitors.[3] Both groups were aggressively resuscitated and managed in small ICUs according to specified protocols by intensivists with special interest in neurotrauma, who did the serial examinations themselves. They reported no significant difference at 6 months in a composite outcome score combining mortality, morbidity, functional outcome, and neuropsychological testing. ICP monitor-based treatment was associated with significantly fewer ICU days of treatment for intracranial hypertension and 50% fewer individual ICP treatments. Both groups had equal incidences of neurologic deterioration.

Smith et al. performed a smaller RCT in which patients with ICP monitors were randomized to ICP-based mannitol administration with escalation to high-dose pentobarbital for refractory intracranial hypertension versus scheduled mannitol regardless of monitored ICP, escalated only for neurologic worsening.[43] There was no difference between groups in dichotomized GOS scores at 1 year. ICP was 5.5 mm Hg higher in the group treated based on monitored ICP.

All of these nonrandomized studies analyzing the association between ICP monitoring and outcome suffer from the inability to describe and control for the individual decision making related to the insertion of an ICP monitor in a particular patient. Each such decision reflects an unquantified admixture of individual evaluations, physician preferences, physician policies, institutional policies, and other approaches. The wide center-specific monitoring range in the Lane study,[39] the low compliance with the BTF monitoring guidelines in the Shafi paper,[40] and the low fraction (36%) of level I and II centers that inserted ICP monitors in more than 50% of patients meeting the BTF guidelines criteria for monitoring in the Bulger report[36] highlight the variations

in practice associated with this decision making. Age and severity of injury have been reported to be greater in patients treated for intracranial hypertension but not monitored when compared with those monitored.[8,38] The size of the managing center may also influence monitoring decisions.[38] The critical relationship between the decision to monitor, the perceived prognosis, and the intention to manage intracranial hypertension is uncontrolled in these studies. For instance, it should not be expected that an sTBI patient who is not monitored (and therefore managed expectantly) because of a perceived poor prognosis would have the same outcome as an intensively managed patient who is not monitored based on institutional practices. The vagaries in the association between ICP monitoring and outcome reflected in these studies likely reflects their inability to control for such decision making.

The process of randomizing the use of ICP monitoring removes the above decision making-related vagaries from the study. In addition, the specification of treatment protocols for all randomized groups defines the level of aggressiveness independent of the monitor. Neither of the RCTs supports an association between improved outcome and implantation of an ICP monitor if all patients receive intensive treatment of intracranial hypertension.

Of note, all of these studies examine ICP monitoring in the composite group of patients with sTBI rather than just the subset with established intracranial hypertension. Nevertheless, if aggressiveness of care is actually beneficial to improving outcome from sTBI in general, it does not appear that ICP monitor insertion is a sensitive or specific benchmark or quality assurance indicator.

DOES SUCCESSFUL MANAGEMENT OF INTRACRANIAL PRESSURE IMPROVE OUTCOME?

Whether acting as an indicator of disease severity or as a treatable entity, uncontrolled intracranial hypertension is strongly associated with poor outcome. Therefore, for ethical reasons, modern natural history data or randomized investigations into whether treating elevated ICP improves outcome are lacking. As a proxy, the association between treatment response and outcome is used to address this question.

INTRACRANIAL PRESSURE RESPONSIVE TO ROUTINE TREATMENT

Because the prior individual studies lacked patient numbers sufficient to allow for differentiating the outcomes of patients with elevated ICP who responded to treatment from those with normal ICP or refractory intracranial hypertension, Treggiari et al. combined the available data into a systematic review.[23] They reported that patients with elevated ICP who responded to treatment represented a distinct group with better outcome and lower morbidity and mortality than those with refractory intracranial hypertension, but poorer outcomes than those with normal ICP throughout their course. They concluded that ICP response patterns were more powerful predictors of outcome than ICP values. Their inability to perform thorough risk adjustment prevented them from determining if the intermediate group benefited from ICP manipulation versus simply represented an injury subpopulation with a higher probability of survival.

Subsequently, Farahvar et al. examined ICP response patterns and short-term mortality in 369 prospectively studied patients with ICP greater than 25 mm Hg for 1 hour or more.[8] They defined nonresponders as patients having ICP greater than 25 mm Hg for 1 hour or more within 2 consecutive days after initial treatment. The 25.7% who met their definition of responders had a significantly lower risk of 14-day mortality by multivariate modeling. They did not report outcome for survivors. They concluded that this paper demonstrated that successful treatment of intracranial hypertension improves outcome. Their interpretation is confounded by their finding that there was a 20% greater likelihood of responding to treatment for every 1-hour decrease in the number of hours of ICP over 25 mm Hg during the first 24 hours. In addition, their conclusion is very sensitive to their definition of nonresponders, which represents a very low threshold and renders it very difficult to estimate what percentage of the mortality difference might be due simply to severity of injury.

REFRACTORY INTRACRANIAL PRESSURE RESPONDING TO "SECOND-TIER" THERAPIES

Recognizing the correlation between outcome and the degree of intracranial hypertension and the pattern of ICP response to treatment, it is useful to examine studies of "resistant" ICP.

Eisenberg et al. randomized patients with intracranial hypertension refractory to conventional medical therapy to high-dose pentobarbital versus continued "first-tier" treatment.[44] Mortality was strongly correlated with ICP control for both randomization groups as well as for patients who crossed over into the barbiturate group after failure of continued first-tier treatment. It is interesting to note that 13% of patients whose ICP did not respond to treatment survived, although further detail is lacking on their recovery.

Shiozaki et al. randomized patients with intracranial hypertension resistant to high-dose barbiturates to hypothermia versus continued normothermic management.[45] Six-month mortality was significantly correlated with ICP response to treatment. Sixteen (76%) of 21 patients with persistently resistant intracranial hypertension died of intracranial hypertension. ICP remained above 20 mm Hg in all 17 normothermia patients, although 3 of the 4 whose ICP decreased after 4 to 7 days survived, 1 with good outcome. Fifty percent of the hypothermia patients whose ICP responded to cooling had a good or moderate outcome.

These studies strongly suggest that the mortality associated with elevated ICP, particularly resistant intracranial hypertension, can be reduced by successful treatment. Unfortunately, small study populations and a focus on mortality prevent drawing reliable conclusions regarding the effect of treatment on morbidity, although the systematic review by Treggiari et al. suggest that response to treatment may be associated with improved survivorship.

In the Eisenberg trial, it was noted that patients randomized before 52 hours after injury had only a quarter chance of responding to either therapy versus those assigned later despite the ratio of barbiturate versus control therapy efficacy being the same for both time epochs. In the Shiozaki trial, in which ICP remained uncontrolled in all of those randomized to normothermia, 18% of those patients survived (one with good outcome) whereas all of those randomized to hypothermia whose ICP remained high died. These findings underscore that, in addition to the magnitude of intracranial hypertension, the pattern of ICP response and degree of resistance to treatment are important prognostic attributes. Differentiating which patients with intracranial hypertension will benefit from treatment from those in which their ICP values and course are simply indicators of mortal disease remains a major clinical problem.

Both of these studies reveal that not all patients with "uncontrollable ICP" die, and some may survive to have good outcomes. It is clear that our current clinical interpretation of ICP data remains primitive.

INTRACRANIAL PRESSURE THRESHOLD

Is there an ICP threshold the violation of which represents a detrimental "dose" of intracranial hypertension or where keeping sTBI patients below such a level is beneficial to recovery? The origin of the threshold values currently most widely used for treatment (20, or, less frequently, 25 mm Hg) is unclear, likely representing a desire to prevent ICP values above those accepted as the upper limit of normal ICP. However, the value of a well-validated treatment threshold is the ability to balance the risks and complications of overtreatment (e.g., longer ICU stay, more interventions with their associated toxicities) against the physical hazards of threshold violation. Therefore knowing whether there is a general threshold value or, if not, whether it is possible to define patient-specific thresholds is critical to understanding the value of monitoring.

In the absence of natural history studies, the effects of ICP-threshold-driven treatment on physiologic variables and outcome of all sTBI study populations have confounded attempts at determining an ICP threshold. Smith et al. placed ICP monitors into all sTBI patients (admission GCS < 8) and randomized them to either treatment triggered at 20 mm Hg or scheduled mannitol without ICP-based treatment.[43] Only neurologic worsening prompted treatment escalation in the threshold-free group. There was no significant difference between groups in 1-year dichotomized GOS. Although this study presents acceptable outcomes without a specific treatment threshold, such patients were treated for anticipated intracranial hypertension and, indeed, their mean ICP was 5.5 mm Hg less than that of the threshold group.

Saul and Ducker attempted to study the effects of changing their treatment threshold from 20 to 25 mm Hg to 15 mm Hg in a sequential cohort study and reported significantly better outcome associated with the latter. Unfortunately, their inability to control for the numerous other changes that occurred concomitantly with the threshold variation prevent attributing any degree of causality to the observed decrease in mortality associated with the lower threshold.[16]

Ratanalert et al. randomized patients with ICP of 20 mm Hg or higher to treatment at 20 or 25 mm Hg using the same protocol, which included CPP and jugular venous oxygen saturation control.[46] They found no significant difference in GOS at 6 months. However, with only 27 patients, this study was underpowered and little design or management detail is provided.

Marmarou et al. looked at the magnitude of ICP elevations above levels from 0 to 80 mm Hg as variables in a multivariate outcome model in 428 sTBI patients from the Traumatic Coma Data Bank.[47] They found the percentage of monitored time above 20 mm Hg to be the fourth most powerful predictor, whereas the average of ICP values above individual thresholds did not merit inclusion in the model. Of note, ICP was treated at 20 mm Hg and CPP was not a therapeutic variable during that study. This analysis does support that attempts to incorporate time-based magnitude calculations into the analysis of ICP strengthen its predictive value.

Chambers et al. used receiver operating curve analysis to evaluate optimal predictive thresholds for ICP and CPP in 213 sTBI patients.[48] They analyzed hourly average maximal ICP and minimal CPP values against 6-month dichotomized GOS scores. In adults, mathematically optimal predictive thresholds appeared to be 55 mm Hg for CPP and 35 mm Hg for ICP, with CPP being the predominant variable. The clinical relevance of this analytic approach is unclear, although these values likely represent injury thresholds for the variables as defined.

SURVIVORS DESPITE REFRACTORY INTRACRANIAL HYPERTENSION

As noted in the discussion of the Eisenberg study,[44] not all patients with intracranial hypertension resistant to treatment die or have poor outcomes. Another report on 37 patients with resistant intracranial hypertension (ICP > 20 mm Hg for ≥96 hours) reported 38% favorable outcome (GOS 4 to 5) at 6 months.[49] Age was strongly correlated with favorable outcome in this group. Low admission GCS did not preclude acceptable recovery. Although peak ICP and minimal CPP values did not differ between groups, little additional data on secondary insults were reported. Another case series of nine patients with persistent ICP over 25 mm Hg reported a survival rate of 44%, all with GOS scores of 4 (mild disability).[50] All were vigorously managed, including attempts at maintaining CPP above 60 mm Hg, despite intracranial hypertension.

Although lacking detail on the intracranial hypertension magnitude or its interaction with CPP or other secondary insults, these studies remind us that the ICP thresholds currently commonly used are not absolute and that patients with intracranial hypertension resistant to such values may have satisfactory outcomes if aggressive support is maintained.

ALTERNATIVE APPROACHES TO INTRACRANIAL PRESSURE INTERPRETATION

The traditional method of recording ICP is to have the nurse record the end-hour value. Whether the actual value is truly that on the monitor at the hour or is an "estimated average" of the prior hour seems to depend on the nurse. Until recently, these are the data points used in studies of intracranial hypertension. Automated data recording increases consistency and possibly accuracy in addition to facilitating higher resolution analysis. Several studies comparing "traditional" with automated methods have demonstrated systematically higher rates of intracranial hypertension associated with automated recording methods.[51-53] In their analysis of automated versus manual data, Kahraman et al. compared mean values versus the ICP AUC above a set threshold (20 mm Hg).[51] In addition to demonstrating improved sensitivity of continuously collected data to threshold violations, they found that the AUC was significantly more powerful as an outcome predictor.

Vik et al. suggested that a "dose" of intracranial hypertension might be estimated by the ICP AUC above a set threshold (20 mm Hg) over the course of the monitoring period.[54] Dividing their patients' AUC values into four dosage categories, they found a strong correlation between the probabilities of death or poor outcome and the dose of ICP at 6 months.

Lazaridis et al. used automated data collection and AUC analysis to examine the possibility of individualizing the ICP thresholds used to calculate the AUC estimates of intracranial hypertension.[55] They determined the ICP value associated with an index value of cerebrovascular pressure autoregulation status (pressure reactivity index [PRx] <0.2) that had previously been found associated with increased mortality.[56] The mean ICP threshold values based on PRx was 26 ± 10, ranging from 20 to 32. They reported that the AUC-based dosage measurements based on the individualized ICP thresholds were stronger predictors of 6-month mortality than dosages based on universal thresholds of 20 or 25 mm Hg.

These studies suggest that the traditional methods of recording and analyzing ICP are insufficiently developed. Alternative methods of recording, displaying, and analyzing ICP appear to hold promise toward improving the clinical relevance of ICP in general and adapting treatment thresholds for individual patients. Such developments should improve our ability to use ICP in treating patients and improve the poor signal-to-noise ratio that currently plagues our ability to strongly demonstrate the role of ICP in sTBI management. The concept of determining individual patient "dosages" of intracranial-hypertension-related insults is particularly attractive.

CONSIDERATIONS GERMANE TO SEVERE TRAUMATIC BRAIN INJURY MANAGEMENT WITHOUT MONITORING INTRACRANIAL PRESSURE

Although it has not been rigorously established that ICP monitoring is required to provide superior outcome from sTBI, the large amount of circumstantial evidence in support suggests that the decision not to monitor ICP mandates providing an optimized management environment. As noted above, ICP frequently strongly covaries with the availability of resources (e.g., neurosurgical consultation, prehospital intubation, CT scan use) and the aggressiveness of overall trauma management that is associated with improved outcome from sTBI in general.[3,36,42] Although the precise contribution of ICP monitoring to these relationships has not been established, it would be expected that centers choosing to manage sTBI patients without routine ICP monitoring should provide all of these other aspects of attentive sTBI care if they are to expect similar levels of recovery.

Because it appears that the development, adoption, and enforcement of treatment protocols is associated with improved outcome from sTBI (vide supra), it is notable that there is a severe dearth of evidence-based treatment algorithms to guide management in the absence of monitoring. The only explicit protocol that has been rigorously evaluated is that of the ICE protocol from the BEST TRIP ICP RCT.[3] The ICE protocol was developed ad hoc for this study, in the absence of alternatives from the literature. Although apparently effective in this study, it has not been tested in other studies or outside of the specific environment in which that study was performed. Whether the ICE protocol now serves as a *forme fruste* practice standard is undetermined.

Overall, it should not be expected that the decision not to monitor ICP in sTBI patients would lessen the workload associated with their care. Uncertainty as to whether the decreased monitoring cost would increase overall ICU resource use renders the economic effects of such a decision unclear.

REAL AND POTENTIAL ADVANTAGES OF INTRACRANIAL PRESSURE MONITORING

The RCT demonstrated increased patient care efficiency associated with ICP monitoring, including fewer ICU days directed at brain-specific care, and half of the number of overall ICP-directed interventions.[3] The relative value of such efficiencies in achieving similar outcomes should be considered against the benefits, expenses, and risks associated with ICP monitoring in individual care environments.

The BEST TRIP ICP RCT was performed in small ICUs continuously staffed by intensivists with special interest in neurocritical care. Serial examinations were personally performed by these physicians, using study protocols, which included explicit definitions of neurologic worsening criteria that required documented interventions within 1 hour of occurrence. In situations that do not afford as high a level of personal neurointensivist scrutiny as was practiced in the BEST TRIP trial, ICP monitoring may be considered to potentially serve as a "backup system" toward identifying patients at risk of deterioration.

To date, the value of ICP monitoring has generally been studied in the aggregate of sTBI patients as a whole. The value of ICP monitoring in directing care of that subset of sTBI patients who manifest established intracranial hypertension has not been rigorously evaluated. If it is true that successful ICP management in those specific patients improves outcome, then it is likely that the availability of accurate, quantitative ICP data would be valuable. Performing such a study would be difficult and would greatly benefit from the availability of a reliable, noninvasive means of identifying this patient subgroup.

CONCLUSIONS

There is no clear evidence that ICP-monitor-based treatment of sTBI patients in aggregate is required to provide optimal recovery if aggressive, attentive care is offered in an environment where other critical resources are available (e.g., neurosurgical consultation, ready access to imaging, well-executed prehospital care, expeditious resuscitation). However, the many remarkable shortcomings in our current clinical application of ICP (e.g., optimizing analysis and display, personalized threshold determination based on multimodality monitoring) suggest that much of the problem may be that those methods that have been tested are "undercooked" (Table 61-2). In particular, insufficient knowledge exists regarding whether there is an identifiable subset of patients with established intracranial hypertension whose outcome depends on successful ICP management. In addition, the utility of ICP in facilitating the understanding of other monitored values (e.g., brain tissue oxygen tension, microdialysis, cerebral blood flow pressure autoregulation) is only now starting to be addressed. Finally, there is almost no information available to guide modern acute management of sTBI in the absence of ICP monitoring. Therefore the balance of evidence would seem to support monitoring ICP in patients felt to be at risk of intracranial hypertension. However, the interpretation and application of the ICP data so derived is less clear.

There are critical aspects of ICP-based care that are indeterminate. There is no evidence-based ICP management algorithm and, indeed, many feel that there should not be a single such protocol for all patients. Treating intracranial hypertension requires balancing the toxicity of treatment against the risk of elevated pressures; however, there are no well-defined methods for setting an individual patient's treatment threshold or determining a dangerous dose of intracranial hypertension. Currently, most of these decisions are made by the management teams, in which the benefits of experience and frequent contact with sTBI patients become paramount. In this light, the author strongly supports sTBI management being done at regional neurotrauma centers, where intensivists and neurologic surgeons with special interest and training in neurotrauma can deal with the uncertainties surrounding our most basic TBI monitor.

From a research viewpoint, it is unlikely that interest in ICP will disappear from TBI care in the future. The true value of the BEST TRIP ICP RCT is to illustrate how much of what we have taken for granted in ICP management is questionable. A redefinition of ICP and its proper role in the multimodality-based approach to targeted therapy that appears to be slowly emerging in the neurocritical care of sTBI is needed.

Table 61-2 **Shortcomings of Current Understanding of ICP**

Problem	Manifestation	Solution/Work Around
Limited prognostic value	Overreliance on ICP for prognostic decision-making	Cautiously use "intermediate" ICP values Focus on prediction of mortality above morbidity Consider ICP resistance and trending as prognostic tools
Limited value of end-hour ICP	Inexact understanding of "dosage" of intracranial hypertension	Use high-resolution, automated ICP analysis, including trending Improve bedside displays to include trending Develop alternative methods of analyzing ICP (e.g., AUC)
Variable utility of ICP monitoring as a quality-assurance benchmark	Inexact assessment of quality of care in sTBI Inability to rigorously determine the independent role of ICP monitoring as a practice option, recommendation, or standard	If used, then analyze in parallel with other indices of "aggressiveness" (e.g., time to OR, time to first CT, absence of hypotension, lack of neurologic worsening) Refine decision pathways and improve explicit documentation regarding decisions to monitor ICP in individual patients Add TBI-specific data points to general trauma databases (e.g., pupillary examination, CT classification) Develop noninvasive methods of estimating ICP as indicator for invasive monitoring
Unclear treatment thresholds	Overtreatment (toxicity) Undertreatment?	Cautiously adjust the ICP treatment threshold from 20 to 25 mm Hg based on serial examination and imaging and other monitors as the ICU course develops Develop algorithms to assist in determining and following individual treatment thresholds Be aware that "resistant ICP" is not inconsistent with reasonable survival in all cases if aggressive management is maintained
Uncertainty of which patients specifically benefit from ICP management	Undertreatment and overtreatment Treating all ICP elevations in all patients in a similar fashion	Improve the taxonomy of sTBI patients regarding treatment categories Correlate changes in other variables (e.g., examination, imaging, other monitors) with ICP parameters and response to treatment Target ICP treatment toward the pathophysiology underlying the intracranial hypertension

AUC, area under the curve; *CT*, computed tomography; *ICP*, intracranial pressure; *ICU*, intensive care unit; *OR*, operating room; *sTBI*, severe traumatic brain injury; *TBI*, traumatic brain injury.

AUTHOR'S RECOMMENDATIONS

- There are no clear data to support ICU monitor-based therapy in sTBI.
- A non-ICP monitoring approach to sTBI requires meticulous clinical and radiologic attention.
- There are many problems associated with the methodology of measuring and recording ICP and with interventions performed based on the data derived.
- There may be a subset of patients with established intracranial hypertension whose outcome depends on successful ICP management.
- The utility of ICP in facilitating the understanding of other monitored values (e.g., brain tissue oxygen tension, microdialysis, cerebral blood flow pressure autoregulation) is only now starting to be addressed.
- There is almost no information available to guide modern acute management of sTBI in the absence of ICP monitoring.
- Therefore the balance of evidence would seem to support monitoring ICP in patients thought to be at risk of intracranial hypertension.
- Treating intracranial hypertension requires balancing the toxicity of treatment against the risk of elevated pressures.
- Management of sTBI patients is best performed at regional neurotrauma centers.

REFERENCES

1. Bratton S, Bullock R, Carney N, et al. Guidelines for the management of severe brain injury: 2007 revision. *J Neurotrauma.* 2007;24(suppl 1):S1–S106.
2. Stocchetti N, Picetti E, Berardino M, et al. Clinical applications of intracranial pressure monitoring in traumatic brain injury : report of the Milan consensus conference. *Acta Neurochir.* 2014;156(8):1615–1622.
3. Chesnut RM, Temkin N, Carney N, et al. A trial of intracranial-pressure monitoring in traumatic brain injury. *N Engl J Med.* 2012;367(26):2471–2481.
4. Andrews PJ, Sleeman DH, Statham PF, et al. Predicting recovery in patients suffering from traumatic brain injury by using admission variables and physiological data: a comparison between decision tree analysis and logistic regression. *J Neurosurg.* 2002;97(2):326–336.
5. Badri S, Chen J, Barber J, et al. Mortality and long-term functional outcome associated with intracranial pressure after traumatic brain injury. *Intensive Care Med.* 2012;38(11):1800–1809.
6. Balestreri M, Czosnyka M, Hutchinson P, et al. Impact of intracranial pressure and cerebral perfusion pressure on severe disability and mortality after head injury. *Neurocrit Care.* 2006;4(1):8–13.
7. Budohoski KP, Schmidt B, Smielewski P, et al. Non-invasively estimated ICP pulse amplitude strongly correlates with outcome after TBI. *Acta Neurochir Suppl.* 2012;114:121–125.
8. Farahvar A, Gerber LM, Chiu YL, et al. Response to intracranial hypertension treatment as a predictor of death in patients with severe traumatic brain injury. *J Neurosurg.* 2011;114(5):1471–1478.

9. Fearnside MR, Cook RJ, McDougall P, McNeil RJ. The Westmead Head Injury Project outcome in severe head injury. A comparative analysis of pre-hospital, clinical and CT variables. *Br J Neurosurg.* 1993;7(3):267–279.

10. Kostic A, Stefanovic I, Novak V, Veselinovic D, Ivanov G, Veselinovic A. Prognostic significance of intracranial pressure monitoring and intracranial hypertension in severe brain trauma patients. *Med Pregl.* 2011;64(9–10):461–465.

11. Lannoo E, Van Rietvelde F, Colardyn F, et al. Early predictors of mortality and morbidity after severe closed head injury. *J Neurotrauma.* 2000;17(5):403–414.

12. Papo I, Caruselli G. Long-term intracranial pressure monitoring in comatose patients suffering from head injuries. A critical survey. *Acta Neurochir.* 1977;39(3–4):187–200.

13. Papo I, Caruselli G, Scarpelli M, Luongo A. Intracranial hypertension in severe head injuries. *Acta Neurochir.* 1980;52(3–4):249–263.

14. Richard KE, Frowein RA. Significance of intracranial pressure and neurological deficit as prognostic factors in acute severe brain lesions. *Acta Neurochir Suppl.* 1979;28(1):66–69.

15. Ross AM, Pitts LH, Kobayashi S. Prognosticators of outcome after major head injury in the elderly. *J Neurosci Nurs.* 1992;24(2):88–93.

16. Saul TG, Ducker TB. Intracranial pressure monitoring in patients with severe head injury. *Am Surg.* 1982;48(9):477–480.

17. Vapalahti M, Troupp H. Prognosis for patients with severe brain injuries. *Br Med J.* 1971;3(5771):404–407.

18. Fleischer AS, Payne NS, Tindall GT. Continuous monitoring of intracranial pressure in severe closed head injury without mass lesions. *Surg Neurol.* 1976;6(1):31–34.

19. Miller JD, Becker DP, Ward JD, Sullivan HG, Adams WE, Rosner MJ. Significance of intracranial hypertension in severe head injury. *J Neurosurg.* 1977;47(4):503–516.

20. Czosnyka M, Hutchinson PJ, Balestreri M, Hiler M, Smielewski P, Pickard JD. Monitoring and interpretation of intracranial pressure after head injury. *Acta Neurochir Suppl.* 2006;96:114–118.

21. Struchen MA, Hannay HJ, Contant CF, Robertson CS. The relation between acute physiological variables and outcome on the Glasgow Outcome Scale and Disability Rating Scale following severe traumatic brain injury. *J Neurotrauma.* 2001;18(2):115–125.

22. Levin HS, Eisenberg HM, Gary HE, et al. Intracranial hypertension in relation to memory functioning during the first year after severe head injury. *Neurosurgery.* 1991;28(2):196–199. discussion 200.

23. Treggiari MM, Schutz N, Yanez ND, Romand JA. Role of intracranial pressure values and patterns in predicting outcome in traumatic brain injury: a systematic review. *Neurocrit Care.* 2007;6(2):104–112.

24. Kobayashi S, Nakazawa S, Yano M, Yamamoto Y, Otsuka T. The value of Intracranial Pressure (ICP) measurement in acute severe head injury showing diffuse cerebral swelling. In: Ishi S, Nagai H, Brock M, eds. *Intracranial Pressure V.* Berlin-Heidelberg-New York: Springer Verlag; 1983:527–531.

25. Miller JD, Butterworth JF, Gudeman SK, et al. Further experience in the management of severe head injury. *J Neurosurg.* 1981;54(3):289–299.

26. Narayan RK, Greenberg RP, Miller JD, et al. Improved confidence of outcome prediction in severe head injury. A comparative analysis of the clinical examination, multimodality evoked potentials, CT scanning, and intracranial pressure. *J Neurosurg.* 1981;54(6):751–762.

27. Narayan RK, Kishore PR, Becker DP, et al. Intracranial pressure: to monitor or not to monitor? A review of our experience with severe head injury. *J Neurosurg.* 1982;56(5):650–659.

28. Akopian G, Gaspard DJ, Alexander M. Outcomes of blunt head trauma without intracranial pressure monitoring. *Am Surg.* 2007;73(5):447–450.

29. Stuart GG, Merry GS, Smith JA, Yelland JD. Severe head injury managed without intracranial pressure monitoring. *J Neurosurg.* 1983;59(4):601–605.

30. Vukic M, Negovetic L, Kovac D, Ghajar J, Glavic Z, Gopcevic A. The effect of implementation of guidelines for the management of severe head injury on patient treatment and outcome. *Acta Neurochir.* 1999;141(11):1203–1208.

31. Clayton TJ, Nelson RJ, Manara AR. Reduction in mortality from severe head injury following introduction of a protocol for intensive care management. *Br J Anaesthesia.* 2004;93(6):761–767.

32. Fakhry SM, Trask AL, Waller MA, Watts DD. Management of brain-injured patients by an evidence-based medicine protocol improves outcomes and decreases hospital charges. *J Trauma.* 2004;56(3):492–499. discussion 499–500.

33. Spain DA, McIlvoy LH, Fix SE, et al. Effect of a clinical pathway for severe traumatic brain injury on resource utilization. *J Trauma.* 1998;45(1):101–104. discussion 104–105.

34. Arabi YM, Haddad S, Tamim HM, et al. Mortality reduction after implementing a clinical practice guidelines-based management protocol for severe traumatic brain injury. *J Crit Care.* 2010;25(2):190–195.

35. Haddad S, Aldawood AS, Alferayan A, Russell NA, Tamim HM, Arabi YM. Relationship between intracranial pressure monitoring and outcomes in severe traumatic brain injury patients. *Anaesth Intensive Care.* 2011;39(6):1043–1050.

36. Bulger EM, Nathens AB, Rivara FP, et al. Management of severe head injury: institutional variations in care and effect on outcome. *Crit Care Med.* 2002;30(8):1870–1876.

37. Cremer OL, van Dijk GW, van Wensen E, et al. Effect of intracranial pressure monitoring and targeted intensive care on functional outcome after severe head injury. *Crit Care Med.* 2005;33(10):2207–2213.

38. Mauritz W, Steltzer H, Bauer P, Dolanski-Aghamanoukjan L, Metnitz P. Monitoring of intracranial pressure in patients with severe traumatic brain injury: an Austrian prospective multicenter study. *Intensive Care Med.* 2008;34(7):1208–1215.

39. Lane PL, Skoretz TG, Doig G, Girotti MJ. Intracranial pressure monitoring and outcomes after traumatic brain injury. *Can J Surg.* 2000;43(6):442–448.

40. Shafi S, Diaz-Arrastia R, Madden C, Gentilello L. Intracranial pressure monitoring in brain-injured patients is associated with worsening of survival. *J Trauma.* 2008;64(2):335–340.

41. Farahvar A, Gerber LM, Chiu YL, Carney N, Hartl R, Ghajar J. Increased mortality in patients with severe traumatic brain injury treated without intracranial pressure monitoring. *J Neurosurg.* 2012;117(4):729–734.

42. Stein SC, Georgoff P, Meghan S, Mirza KL, El Falaky OM. Relationship of aggressive monitoring and treatment to improved outcomes in severe traumatic brain injury. *J Neurosurg.* 2010;112(5):1105–1112.

43. Smith HP, Kelly Jr DL, McWhorter JM, et al. Comparison of mannitol regimens in patients with severe head injury undergoing intracranial monitoring. *J Neurosurg.* 1986;65(6):820–824.

44. Eisenberg HM, Frankowski RF, Contant CF, Marshall LF, Walker MD. High-dose barbiturate control of elevated intracranial pressure in patients with severe head injury. *J Neurosurg.* 1988;69(1):15–23.

45. Shiozaki T, Sugimoto H, Taneda M, et al. Effect of mild hypothermia on uncontrollable intracranial hypertension after severe head injury. *J Neurosurg.* 1993;79(3):363–368.

46. Ratanalert S, Phuenpathom N, Saeheng S, Oearsakul T, Sripairojkul B, Hirunpat S. ICP threshold in CPP management of severe head injury patients. *Surg Neurol.* 2004;61(5):429–434. discussion 434–425.

47. Marmarou A, Anderson RL, Ward JD, et al. Impact of ICP instability and hypotension on outcome in patients with severe head trauma. *J Neurosurg.* 1991;75(suppl 1):S159–S166.

48. Chambers IR, Treadwell L, Mendelow AD. Determination of threshold levels of cerebral perfusion pressure and intracranial pressure in severe head injury by using receiver-operating characteristic curves: an observational study in 291 patients. *J Neurosurg.* 2001;94(3):412–416.

49. Resnick DK, Marion DW, Carlier P. Outcome analysis of patients with severe head injuries and prolonged intracranial hypertension. *J Trauma.* 1997;42(6):1108–1111.

50. Young JS, Blow O, Turrentine F, Claridge JA, Schulman A. Is there an upper limit of intracranial pressure in patients with severe head injury if cerebral perfusion pressure is maintained? *Neurosurg Focus.* 2003;15(6):E2.

51. Kahraman S, Dutton RP, Hu P, et al. Heart rate and pulse pressure variability are associated with intractable intracranial hypertension after severe traumatic brain injury. *J Neurosurg Anesthesiol.* 2010;22(4):296–302.

52. Venkatesh B, Garrett P, Fraenkel DJ, Purdie D. Indices to quantify changes in intracranial and cerebral perfusion pressure by assessing agreement between hourly and semi-continuous recordings. *Intensive Care Med.* 2004;30(3):510–513.

53. Zanier ER, Ortolano F, Ghisoni L, Colombo A, Losappio S, Stocchetti N. Intracranial pressure monitoring in intensive care: clinical advantages of a computerized system over manual recording. *Crit Care*. 2007;11(1):R7.

54. Vik A, Nag T, Fredriksli OA, et al. Relationship of "dose" of intracranial hypertension to outcome in severe traumatic brain injury. *J Neurosurg*. 2008;109(4):678–684.

55. Lazaridis C, Desantis SM, Smielewski P, et al. Patient-specific thresholds of intracranial pressure in severe traumatic brain injury. *J Neurosurg*. 2014;120(4):893–900.

56. Czosnyka M, Smielewski P, Kirkpatrick P, Laing RJ, Menon D, Pickard JD. Continuous assessment of the cerebral vasomotor reactivity in head injury. *Neurosurgery*. 1997;41(1):11–17, discussion 17–19.

62 How Should Traumatic Brain Injury Be Managed?

Danielle K. Sandsmark, Larami MacKenzie, W. Andrew Kofke

The morbidity and mortality resulting from traumatic brain injury (TBI) stem not only from the primary brain damage caused by the initial impact but also from the secondary insults that follow. Although the primary injury occurs nearly immediately and is largely irreversible, secondary insults include a variety of ischemic, metabolic, and inflammatory disturbances that occur in the vulnerable brain tissue. These insults develop over hours to days after injury. Given the delayed presentation, these secondary insults represent an opportunity for clinical intervention. Recognition and treatment of these evolving processes are critical to ensuring optimal outcome following serious brain injury.

In the following discussion, we outline the evidence supporting various intensive care unit (ICU) practices in the management of the severely brain injured to prevent secondary brain damage. We follow and summarize the general format of the Brain Trauma Foundation (BTF) management guidelines.[1] The specific studies that are included were evaluated with GRADE (Grading of Recommendations Assessment, Development and Evaluation) criteria, as detailed in Table 62-1.

SYSTEMIC BLOOD PRESSURE AND OXYGENATION

Background

Both hypotension and hypoxemia contribute to secondary brain injury and influence outcomes after trauma.[2] Because of ethical constraints, it is not possible to perform randomized studies to establish absolute thresholds for oxygenation and blood pressure support. In the following section, we discuss the available evidence that can provide some guidance to these thresholds.

Evidence

Hypoxemia

Analysis of the prospectively collected Traumatic Coma Data Bank showed that episodes of hypoxemia (partial pressure of oxygen in arterial blood [Pao_2] <60 mm Hg or apnea/cyanosis in the field) in the acute period after injury were associated with increased mortality.[2] Studying prehospital trauma patients, Stocchetti et al.[3] found that hypoxemia (defined as a peripheral oxygen saturation <60%) at the accident scene was associated with a universally poor prognosis (death or severe disability), as was severe hypotension (defined as systolic blood pressure <60 mm Hg). In 3240 patients included in the San Diego County trauma registry, both hypoxemia (Pao_2 <110 mm Hg) and extreme hyperoxemia were associated with increased mortality and poorer clinical outcomes in survivors of TBI.[4] Hypoxemia in head-injured patients cared for in the ICU also increases mortality.[5]

Hypotension

Similar results have been reported with prehospital and in-hospital hypotension.[6] A single episode of hypotension with a systolic blood pressure lower than 90 mm Hg was associated with increased morbidity and doubled mortality.[2] Similarly, Marmarou and colleagues[7] used the Traumatic Coma Data Bank to study 428 patients with severe TBI and found that as the proportion of systolic blood pressure measurements <80 mm Hg or intracranial pressure (ICP) >20 mm Hg increased, patient outcome worsened. A series of prospective studies by Vassar and colleagues[8] evaluating resuscitative fluids given before hospital admission in hypotensive trauma patients demonstrated that hyperosmolar fluid resuscitation (7.5% hypertonic saline [HTS] ± dextran) more effectively raised blood pressure than isotonic solutions, and patients who received hyperosmolar resuscitation had better outcomes than predicted. In the subset of trauma patients with a Glasgow Coma Scale (GCS) score of 8 or less, the hyperosmolar treatment group fared significantly better than the isotonic group. A follow-up prospective study looking specifically at prehospital resuscitation of hypotensive patients with severe TBI showed no difference in neurologic outcome at 6 months in patients resuscitated with hypertonic fluids versus conventional fluid resuscitation.[9]

Recommendations

Hypoxemia and hypotension are associated with poor outcomes from TBI and should be avoided. GRADE B evidence supports a threshold value of 90 mm Hg systolic and Pao_2 mm Hg less than 60 with O_2 saturation less than 90%, respectively.

441

Table 62-1 GRADE System: Determination of the Quality of Evidence

Underlying method
1. RCT
2. Downgraded RCT or upgraded observational studies
3. Well-done observational studies
4. Case series or expert opinion

Factors that may decrease the strength of evidence
1. Poor quality of planning and implementation of available RCTs, suggesting high likelihood of bias
2. Inconsistency of results (including problems with subgroup analyses)
3. Indirectness of evidence (differing population, intervention, control, outcomes, comparison)
4. Imprecision of results
5. High likelihood of reporting bias

Main factors that may increase the strength of evidence
1. Large magnitude of effect (direct evidence, RR≥2 with no plausible confounders)
2. Very large magnitude of effect with RR≥5 and no threats to validity (by two levels)
3. Dose-response gradient

RCT, randomized controlled trial; *RR,* relative risk.

CEREBRAL PERFUSION THRESHOLDS

Background

On the basis of Pouiselle's law describing laminar flow, cerebral blood flow (CBF) is directly related to the cerebral perfusion pressure (CPP), which is defined as mean arterial pressure (MAP) – ICP and is inversely related to the cerebral vascular resistance (CVR) (CBF = CPP/CVR). Under normal conditions, CBF remains constant despite changes in CPP by constriction and dilation of the cerebral blood vessels, termed *cerebral autoregulation.* After brain injury, cerebral autoregulation is often disrupted such that blood vessel radius either remains constant, despite changes in MAP and CPP, or varies directly (inversely) with CPP. In both cases, even small changes in CPP can trigger alterations in CBF, blood flow velocity, and ICP, which, in turn, compromises oxygen and glucose delivery to the brain tissue. Given the lack of tools to directly and continuously measure CBF, CPP has been used as a monitoring parameter reflective of cerebral perfusion.

Evidence

Low CPP (generally defined as less than 50 mm Hg), typically caused by systemic hypotension (low MAP) or intracranial hypertension (high ICP), is associated with poor clinical outcome as well as poor physiologic variables, including jugular venous oxygen saturation, brain oxygen saturation, and cerebral microdialysis parameters.[10-13]

Rosner and Daughton originally reported management on head-injured patients based on CPP thresholds.[14] They studied 34 patients and used a variety of interventions to achieve CPP greater than 70 mm Hg and concluded that this was associated with a decreased mortality and an improvement in functional outcome over prior cohorts, although it was unclear whether this was just due to a lower incidence of systemic hypotension.[15] Follow-up studies, however, suggested that there were risks of CPP augmentation. Robertson et al.[16] performed a randomized controlled trial (RCT) of CPP-guided versus ICP-guided management and found a fivefold increase in the development of acute respiratory distress syndrome (ARDS) in patients managed by CPP, presumably a consequence of overenthusiastic fluid resuscitation. Contant et al.[17] found a similar incidence of ARDS in their CPP-managed TBI patients. This complication was associated with an increased risk of mortality and poor neurologic outcome.

TBI is, by its very nature, a heterogeneous disease process with varying cerebral physiologies not only between patients but also between brain regions in a single patient. Thus, it is likely overly simplistic to believe that every individual (or, perhaps, every region of the brain) requires the same CPP to maintain adequate perfusion and avoid hyperperfusion or ICP changes. To this end, methods to measure individual cerebral autoregulation have been developed. Steiner et al.[18] retrospectively calculated a correlation coefficient defining the relationship between CPP and ICP to determine the CPP at which autoregulation was best preserved. When the mean CPP was maintained near the level of autoregulation, there was an association with better outcomes; patients whose CPPs were either higher or lower than the optimal CPP faired more poorly. These data suggest that CPP can be optimized on an individual basis with adjunctive physiologic monitoring. However, the efficacy of this approach remains to be tested in large, prospective RCTs.

Another consideration in optimizing CPP is how the CPP is measured. Lassen originally defined CPP based on "arterial blood pressure measured at the level of the head," using the tragus of the ear as an external landmark.[19] However, there is much heterogeneity in current practice, and the MAP is often measured at the level of the right atrium.[20] When the head of the bed is elevated, as it should be for the management of head-injured patients, MAP measurements at the level of the right atrium may be higher than those measured at the tragus by up to 18 mm Hg, thereby overestimating CPP.[21] This variability in practice may contribute to difficulty in defining optimal CPP and MAP targets after head injury. In this regard, the Neuroanesthesia Society of Great Britain and Ireland and the Society of British Neurologic Surgeons recently issued a joint position statement advocating for measurement of CPP at the level of the tragus in patients with TBI (http://www.nasgbi.org.uk/media/uploads/NASGBI_and_SBNS_CPP_statement_final.pdf).

Recommendation

We recommend measuring CPP at the level of the tragus. Low CPP, generally defined as less than 50 mm Hg, should be prevented (GRADE B). Augmentation of CPP with fluids should be avoided because of the risk of iatrogenic complications based on GRADE B evidence. Adjunctive physiologic monitors to determine the CPP at which autoregulation is optimized may be helpful to individualize care, but there is currently no evidence to support a recommendation regarding their use.

INTRACRANIAL PRESSURE THRESHOLDS

Background

The bony, rigid skull and vertebral canal contain a fixed volume including the brain parenchyma, cerebrospinal fluid (CSF), and blood, creating a nearly incompressible system. Any increase in the volume of one of these compartments is met first with a compensatory shift in another compartment (e.g., CSF shifting down the less rigid spinal column). When compensatory changes are exhausted, however, the ICP increases dramatically and can cause secondary brain injury due to brain compression, herniation, and cerebral perfusion compromise. However, treatment of ICP must be balanced with the potential side effects of medical and pharmacologic ICP management.

Evidence

There are no prospective randomized studies designed to determine the threshold for initiation of ICP-reducing therapy. Several prospective observational studies reviewed suggest that outcomes improve when ICP is maintained at less than 20 to 25 mm Hg and that brain herniation is more likely above these thresholds.[7,22,23] However, in situations without intracranial mass lesions, ICP greater than 20 mm Hg may be tolerated.[24]

Chesnut et al.[25] performed the first study to compare outcomes in brain-injured patients who had their management guided by ICP monitoring with those who did not. In this study, the focus was on monitoring ICP, not its treatment. Thus, both arms underwent ICP-reducing therapy. In this population, there was no difference in ICU length of stay or 14-day or 6-month mortality in those who had aggressive management to maintain ICP less than 20 mm Hg compared with patients who were managed on the basis of clinical examination and radiographic imaging alone. The generalizability of these findings has been questioned,[26] but this study raises the important point that ICP monitoring in and of itself may not influence clinical outcomes.

Recommendations

Despite an absence of high-quality evidence, in most cases, an ICP higher than 20 to 25 mm Hg should be an indication to increase ICP-reducing therapy (GRADE C). This must be tempered with the iatrogenic risks of ICP-lowering therapy. When ICP monitoring is unavailable, management based on clinical examination and imaging is reasonable based on the available evidence.

SEIZURE PROPHYLAXIS

Background

Posttraumatic seizures (PTSs) are classified as early (<7 days after TBI) or late (>7 days after TBI). The incidence of PTS varies from 4% to 25% early and 9% to 42% late in untreated TBI patients.[27] Early PTS may contribute to secondary brain injury by inducing cerebral hypermetabolism, elevated ICP, and hypertension. It has been proposed that early PTSs beget late PTSs and epilepsy through neuronal kindling. Epilepsy can have a significant impact on quality of life in TBI survivors.[28]

Evidence

Temkin et al. performed a randomized, placebo-controlled trial in 404 patients with severe head trauma who received phenytoin or placebo for 1 year after head injury.[29] They found that patients receiving phenytoin had a decrease in the incidence of seizures in the acute period (<7 days) but no difference in late seizures. The same group found that both valproic acid and phenytoin also decreased seizures in the acute period.[30] The BTF meta-analysis concluded that anticonvulsant prophylaxis with phenytoin, carbamazapine, or valproic acid is indicated in the first 7 days after TBI but longer treatment is not warranted.[1] The Cochrane meta-analysis[31] of 11 RCTs and the American Academy of Neurology meta-analysis[32] of 8 RCTs arrived at similar conclusions.

Given the potential toxicities and need for drug level monitoring with both phenytoin and valproic acid, neurointensivists have begun to use levetiracetam for seizure prophylaxis after TBI.[33] In a retrospective review, Caballero et al. found that rates of seizure activity were not different between patients treated with levetiracetam and those treated with phenytoin.[34] Levetiracetam therapy was slightly cheaper. Larger, prospective studies are needed to determine if levetiracetam is efficacious and cost-effective in preventing acute seizures after TBI.

Recommendations

Seizure prophylaxis is indicated in the first 7 days after TBI for seizure prophylaxis (GRADE A). Phenytoin, valproic acid, and carbamazepine are all reasonable antiseizure medications for prophylaxis. In the absence of PTS, treatment should be stopped after 7 days. Levetiracetam may be a reasonable option for seizure prophylaxis in patients in whom phenytoin is contraindicated, but further studies are needed. There is no evidence to support antiepileptic administration for longer than 7 days after TBI in the absence of clinical or electrophysiologic seizure activity.

MANAGEMENT OF ELEVATED INTRACRANIAL PRESSURE: HYPERVENTILATION

Background

During hyperventilation, carbon dioxide concentrations fall, resulting in constriction of cerebral blood vessels. Vasoconstriction decreases CBF to reduce intravascular volume in the cranial cavity and lower ICP. In this regard, voluntary hyperventilation may be one of the first clinical signs of elevated ICP as consequent tissue acidosis from high ICP produces compensatory hyperventilation. Similarly, hyperventilation and maintenance of a modestly lower partial pressure of carbon dioxide in arterial blood ($Paco_2$) (30 to 35 mm Hg) are the first measures that can be used to lower ICP in the mechanically ventilated patient. Given that hypocarbia triggers intracranial vasoconstriction, the risk of decreased CBF and resultant cerebral ischemia as a consequence of hyperventilation must be considered, although hyperventilation has not been reported to cause brain injury in the absence of TBI.

Evidence

Several studies of CBF suggest that CBF is dangerously low in the acute period after TBI, leading the BTF to advise against aggressive hyperventilation (Paco$_2$ <25 mm Hg) after TBI.[1] Muizelaar et al.[35] performed a prospective, randomized study of hyperventilation in TBI and found a worse functional outcome, though no difference in mortality, at 3 and 6 months, but not at 12 months, in the hyperventilated patients.

Recommendations

Prolonged prophylactic hyperventilation to Paco$_2$ of 25 to 30 mm Hg should be avoided in TBI patients (GRADE B) because of risks of cerebral ischemia. It may be justified if accompanied by a monitoring of CBF adequacy. It also may be justified as a temporary intervention in emergency and temporary sudden increases in ICP such as with life-threatening herniation syndromes. Hypercarbia (Paco$_2$>45) should be avoided as this can trigger hyperemia, decreased CPP, and potentially trigger a sudden ICP elevation. There is insufficient evidence to determine the effect of hyperventilation on patient outcome after TBI.

MANAGEMENT OF ELEVATED INTRACRANIAL PRESSURE: HYPEROSMOLAR THERAPY

Background

Osmotic agents are thought to lower ICP primarily by drawing free water out of the brain parenchyma and into the systemic vasculature. The simplest way to maintain a modest osmotic gradient is to maintain the serum sodium on the upper range of normal (~145) in the euvolemic patient. When a stronger gradient is needed, mannitol and HTS are the two most commonly used agents.

Evidence

Although RCTs are lacking, mannitol and HTS are both effective agents for lowering ICP after TBI. Mannitol was superior to barbiturates in ICP control, maintenance of CPP, and mortality when given as a 20% bolus at 1 g/kg and repeated to maintain ICP greater than 20.[36]

Early studies focused on the use of HTS for resuscitation in trauma patients.[37,38] Shackford and colleagues were the first to specifically look at HTS infusion and ICP, finding that HTS significantly lowered ICP.[39] Several studies report efficacy of HTS in decreasing ICP, notably being effective in cases where ICP is refractory to mannitol therapy.[40,41] A trial evaluating equiosmolar doses of mannitol and 3% HTS in the operating room revealed an equivalent effect on "brain relaxation," suggesting equivalent ICP reduction with equiosmolar therapy.[42]

Another prospective, randomized study of 20 TBI patients looked at the effect of equivalent volumes of 7.5% HTS and 20% mannitol (2400 mOsm/kg HTS, 1160 mOsm/kg mannitol), showing a lower incidence of treatment failure with HTS.[38] A recent study using brain tissue oxygen monitoring in TBI found that, compared with 0.75 g/kg 20% mannitol, 7.5% HTS boluses were associated with lower ICP and higher CPP and cardiac output. They concluded that in patients with severe TBI and elevated ICP refractory to previous mannitol treatment, 7.5% HTS administered as second-tier therapy is associated with a significant increase of brain oxygenation and improved cerebral and systemic hemodynamics.[43]

Recommendations

Both mannitol and HTS are effective in the treatment of elevated ICP based on GRADE B evidence. Although small studies suggest that HTS may result in better ICP control in patients who no longer respond to mannitol therapy, no RCTs have directly compared the two treatments. As such, it is not possible to recommend one agent over the other agent. Other factors, such as volume status or kidney function, may favor use of one agent over another but should be assessed on a case-by-case basis.

MANAGEMENT OF ELEVATED INTRACRANIAL PRESSURE: SURGICAL DECOMPRESSIVE THERAPY

Background

When severe cerebral edema causes elevated ICP, decompressive craniectomy, a surgical procedure in which a portion of the skull is removed and the dura is opened, can provide definitive management. With the rigid cranium opened, brain swelling can occur outside of the cranial cavity without compromising surrounding structures. The surgical approach varies depending on the site and extent of injury. Hemispheric, bifrontal, or bihemispheric bone flaps may be removed. A durotomy is also performed to provide additional space into which the swelling brain can expand. The use of decompressive craniectomy to control elevated ICP has a long history dating to the early twentieth century. Only recently has the procedure started to undergo scrutiny for impact on outcome.

Evidence

In 26 patients who underwent bifrontal craniectomy for the treatment of refractory elevated ICP after severe TBI, surgical intervention was associated with significant reductions in ICP, and outcomes were favorable in 69% of patients, a significant improvement over similarly described cohorts.[44] In this regard, Aarabi et al.[45] found that decompressive craniectomy significantly lowered ICP in 85% of patients and was associated with a favorable outcome in 51% of patients at 3 months.

On the basis of these initial observations, 155 patients with severe, diffuse TBI who had elevations in ICP refractory to standard first-line therapies were enrolled in the first RCT of craniectomy after TBI.[46] Subjects were randomized to undergo bifrontotemporoparietal craniectomy or standard medical therapy. Although decompressive craniectomy did control ICP and result in fewer ICU days, surgical intervention was associated with more unfavorable outcomes (death, vegetative state, or severe disability) than standard medical therapy. There remain questions, though, regarding the generalizability of these data, particularly given that a large proportion (27%) of patients in the surgical arm had bilateral unreactive pupils at randomization (as compared with 12% in the medical management arm), a clinical finding historically associated with very poor outcomes.[47]

Recommendations

Surgical decompressive therapy is an effective measure for the management of persistently elevated ICP. However, there is no evidence that decompression improves clinical outcomes. We recommend that surgical decompressive therapy be considered as a lifesaving measure in patients in whom other measures to control ICP have failed and who may have a chance of functional outcome. It is important that families consenting for this procedure be counseled that the surgical procedure may be lifesaving but does not guarantee a satisfactory functional outcome.

ANESTHETICS, ANALGESICS, AND SEDATIVES

Background

Pain and agitation after TBI contribute to ICP elevations and increased cerebral metabolic demand. Thus, controlling anxiety, pain, and agitation is an important first step toward controlling ICP after TBI. High-dose barbiturates, benzodiazepines, and propofol decrease metabolic rate in intact brain areas, resulting in decreased CBF and ICP. The use of these medications must be balanced with the need for careful neurologic clinical examinations that may be limited in the presence of sedating medications. Although the use of sedation is generally easy for the neurointensivist to justify when ICP is an issue, pain can be difficult to quantify in these severely injured patients.

Evidence

There is no prospective randomized data supporting treatment of pain and agitation as a means for preventing elevated ICP. In a single, prospective randomized study comparing propofol to morphine for sedation in TBI patients, propofol use was associated with a trend toward lower ICP that did not reach statistical significance. Post hoc analysis of patients who received high-dose propofol suggested a better neurologic outcome despite the lack of a difference in ICP, suggesting a potential neuroprotective effect. Barbiturates have been shown to decrease ICP[22] but are so often complicated by severe hypotension that these risks seem to outweigh any benefits.[1,48]

More recently, dexmedetomidine, an alpha-2 agonist, has been used to effectively control agitation and allow for serial neurologic examinations[49] and has been shown to decrease CBF without affecting cerebral metabolic rate.[50] When directly compared with propofol, dexmedetomidine and propofol had similar cerebral physiologic effects with

multimodal monitoring.[51] The effect of dexmedetomidine on intracranial pressure has not been studied.

Recommendations

Propofol is recommended for sedation in severe TBI over morphine with GRADE C evidence. GRADE A evidence suggests that barbiturates should *not* be given prophylactically for TBI. Barbiturate use is supported in cases of severe refractory intracranial hypertension with GRADE C evidence.

PROPHYLACTIC HYPOTHERMIA AND THERAPEUTIC NORMOTHERMIA

Background

Fever is common in patients with severe brain injuries and has been associated with poor outcome.[52-54] The mechanisms by which fever worsens outcomes are unclear but likely include potentiation of inflammatory cascades, increased tissue metabolic demand, and excitotoxicity. As such, fever control (induced normothermia) is frequently employed early in the care of brain-injured neurocritical care patients.

Hypothermia (generally defined as cooling to 32 to 33° C, though protocols vary) appears to be neuroprotective in preclinical[55] and single institution human studies and improves neurologic outcomes after cardiac arrest.[56,57] These data suggest that it may be useful in the care of TBI patients.

Evidence

Studies have been conflicting regarding the efficacy of prophylactic hypothermia in TBI. Most consistent have been studies demonstrating the beneficial impact of hypothermia on ICP control.[58] Although hypothermia can aid in ICP control, the influence on patient outcome has been less obvious. Despite the preclinical evidence of neuroprotection associated with hypothermia, a randomized, prospective multicenter trial failed to show improvement when TBI patients were treated with induced hypothermia.[59] This study was limited by significant heterogeneity in therapeutic protocols between centers. A follow-up analysis suggested that better outcomes were achieved in high-volume centers.[60] Several meta-analyses concluded that evidence was insufficient to confidently recommend the use of prophylactic hypothermia in TBI.[61-64] In the BTF analysis, although a mortality effect favoring hypothermia was not significant, there was a statistically significant 46% increased chance of a good outcome in the hypothermic patients.[1] Further analysis indicated that a minimum duration of 48 hours of induced hypothermia was needed to see a protective effect but was associated with an increased risk for pneumonia. The BTF and American Association of Neurological Surgeons thus issued a level III recommendation for cautious and selective use of moderate hypothermia for TBI.

Since those recommendations, several additional studies have been reported. One proposed limitation of the earlier studies was a relatively late induction of hypothermia. Clifton et al.[65] conducted a prospective, multicenter,

RCT of hypothermia versus normothermia induced 2 to 5 hours after injury. The study was terminated early because of futility, showing no benefit of hypothermia despite a relatively fast time to cooling. Recently Maekawa et al.[66] reported a prospective, multicenter, RCT of prolonged hypothermia (32 to 34°C for > 72 hours) versus monitored temperature management (35 to 37°C) after TBI but found no improvement in neurologic outcome. Similarly, in children with severe TBI, hypothermia did not reduce mortality or improve functional outcome over fever control.[67]

It is possible that hypothermia may cause additional physiologic effects (immunosuppression, bleeding diathesis, and cardiac arrhythmias, among others) and complications due to related therapies (for example, induced paralysis, shivering control) that may negate the positive effects of cooler temperature. In this regard, a case series comparing prophylactic hypothermia at 33°C versus 35°C after severe TBI found equivalent ICP control at the milder hypothermia target with fewer complications, including hypokalemia, infection, ventricular tachycardias, pulmonary embolus, renal failure, and tendency to lower mortality.[68] Fever control (induced normothermia), rather than true hypothermia, with an intravascular cooling catheter similarly controlled ICP in 21 patients with severe TBI.[69] Although the effect of induced normothermia after TBI has not been prospectively studied, studies of other serious brain injuries, including stroke[70] and subarachnoid hemorrhage,[71,72] have been mixed.

Recommendations

In severe TBI, there is GRADE C evidence for selective and cautious application of prophylactic moderate hypothermia from 32 to 35°C for 48 hours. The higher temperature may provide equivalent ICP control with fewer adverse effects. Rewarming should be done slowly to minimize the possibility of a rebound increase in ICP. Therapeutic normothermia (monitored temperature management) using endovascular cooling is supported by GRADE D evidence. Hyperthermia should be avoided.

BRAIN OXYGEN MONITORING

Background

CBF ensures delivery of glucose and oxygen to the brain parenchyma and should be proportional to the metabolic demands of the tissue. Brain oxygen monitors have been used as indirect indicators of adequate CBF.

Oxygen delivery to the brain can be measured both globally (whole brain) and regionally. Jugular bulb catheters use a fiberoptic oximeter to measure the content of oxygen in the jugular veins to measure global brain oxygenation. The jugular venous oxygen concentration is compared with the oxygen content in the arterial system; the difference between the two ($SvjO_2$) serves as a surrogate measure of the balance between CBF and metabolic demand (normal values: 55% to 69%). Regional oxygenation can be measured using a Clarke-type electrode. Oxygen molecules diffuse from the brain parenchyma into the probe through a diffusible membrane and are reduced at the cathode,

creating an electrical current that is proportional to the partial pressure of oxygen in brain tissue ($PbtO_2$) in the sampled region (normal values $Pbto_2$>20 mm Hg).

Evidence

In the BTF meta-analysis,[1] numerous studies of jugular bulb oxygen monitoring in TBI were reviewed. Worse outcomes were seen in patients who had episodes of $SvjO_2$ of less than 50%, as may occur in tissue ischemia or states of high metabolic demand such as status epilepticus. Episodes of $SvjO_2$ higher than 75%, which may be associated with hyperemia or infarcted, metabolically inactive tissue, were also associated with poor outcomes. These studies suggest that $SvjO_2$ be kept between 50% and 75%. However, there are no randomized prospective studies that test this hypothesis.

Using a regional brain oxygen monitor, Meixensberger et al.[73] compared 53 patients who had brain oxygen–directed therapy with 40 historic controls who had ICP/CPP–directed therapy. They found that, over the whole monitoring period, the partial pressure of brain oxygen was higher in the group who received brain oxygen–directed therapy; this was not statistically significant. Spiotta et al.[74] prospectively compared 70 patients with severe TBI who received brain oxygen–directed therapy with 53 patients receiving ICP/CPP–directed therapy and found that patients who had brain oxygen–directed therapy had improved survival and clinical outcomes at 3 months. In patients who had brain oxygen monitoring and later died, there was a longer mean duration of compromised brain oxygen and a lower rate of response to efforts to increase brain oxygen. Using historic controls, Stiefel and colleagues[75] compared the impact of a change in local practice to use $PbtO_2$ to guide therapy and reported a significant improvement in outcome. This report was neither prospective nor randomized, and the historic controls had a higher mortality than would otherwise have been expected.

However, not all studies have found an improvement in patient outcome with brain oxygen–directed therapy. Adamides et al.[76] studied 30 patients who had brain oxygen monitoring. Twenty patients in whom treatment was aimed at targeting a predefined goal brain oxygenation value (>15 mm Hg) had less cerebral hypoxia during the duration of monitoring, but neurologic outcome at 6 months was not different between groups. Martini et al.[77] studied 123 patients who underwent brain tissue oxygen monitoring compared with 506 patients who had ICP-directed therapy. The study found that patients treated on the basis of brain oxygen thresholds had longer lengths of stay in the ICU and a greater use of clinical resources without any improvement in survival or neurologic outcome at hospital discharge. Notably, patients who received brain oxygen–directed therapy had more severe injury at the time of enrollment as measured by admission GCS and injury severity scores.

Although the effect of brain oxygen–guided management on patient outcomes (and whether that is even the best endpoint to measure) remains to be determined, $PbtO_2$ or $SvjO_2$ monitoring does provide unique insight into aspects of brain physiology not provided by other monitors. For example, Eriksson et al.[78] found that survivors of severe head injury had significantly higher brain oxygen values than nonsurvivors, though there was no difference in ICP and CPP values for the two groups. Thus brain oxygen monitoring may provide unique physiologic information that can be used in conjunction with other physiologic monitors in the management of these complex patients to optimize their clinical outcomes.

Recommendations

GRADE C evidence supports the use of $SvjO_2$ and $PbtO_2$ monitoring as supplements to ICP monitoring in TBI. $SvjO_2$ of less than 50% and $PbtO_2$ less than 15 mm Hg should be avoided. The extent of time and the depth of the drop in brain oxygen values below these thresholds likely also affect outcome. Clinicians are cautioned regarding the lack of prospective randomized studies documenting an impact of the use of these modalities on outcome after severe TBI. Toxicity from the therapy recommended to achieve these goals (e.g., prolonged 100% oxygen) must be weighed against the lack of more robust evidence supporting their use.

STEROIDS

Background

Corticosteroids have been used extensively to decrease brain edema from brain tumors and inflammatory processes. Therefore corticosteroids have been examined for their effects on secondary injury due to brain swelling following TBI.

Evidence

Saul et al. first explored the use of high-dose methylprednisolone (5 mg/kg/day) in patients with severe TBI but found no difference in outcomes at 6 months.[79] Braakman et al. similarly found no benefit from high-dose dexamethasone given within 6 hours of injury.[80] In 2005, a meta-analysis of 20 studies including more than 12,000 patients concluded that there was an increased risk of death associated with the use of corticosteroids,[81] and thus their use is not recommended by the Brain Trauma Foundation.[1]

Recommendations

Corticosteroids should not be given after TBI (Grade A).

NUTRITION

Background

Hypermetabolism and nitrogen wasting have long been reported in patients after head injury, resulting in an increase of approximately 140% of the expected metabolic expenditure.[82-84]

Evidence

Among 797 severe TBI patients treated at 22 trauma centers, patients who were not fed within 5 days after TBI had a twofold increase in mortality.[85] Results were even worse when feeding was delayed for 7 days; mortality in that cohort was increased fourfold. The researchers found that the amount of nutrition during the first 5 days inversely correlated with mortality even after correcting for other factors known to affect mortality after TBI. They were able to calculate a 30% to 40% increase in mortality for every 10 kcal/kg decrease in caloric intake.

A few small studies have compared enteral with parenteral nutrition after TBI and have found no substantial differences between methods of feeding.[86,87]

AUTHORS' RECOMMENDATIONS

There is GRADE B evidence that full enteral or parenteral nutritional support should be implemented at least by day 5 after injury in patients without evidence of previous malnutrition.

REFERENCES

1. Brain Trauma Foundation. *Guidelines for the Management of Severe Traumatic Brain Injury*; 2007. 1–116.
2. Chesnut RM, Marshall SB, Piek J, Blunt BA, Klauber MR, Marshall LF. Early and late systemic hypotension as a frequent and fundamental source of cerebral ischemia following severe brain injury in the Traumatic Coma Data Bank. *Acta Neurochir Suppl (Wien)*. 1993;59:121–125.
3. Stocchetti N, Furlan A, Volta F. Hypoxemia and arterial hypotension at the accident scene in head injury. *J Trauma*. 1996;40(5):764–767.
4. Davis DP, Meade W, Sise MJ, et al. Both hypoxemia and extreme hyperoxemia may be detrimental in patients with severe traumatic brain injury. *J Neurotrauma*. 2009;26(12):2217–2223.
5. Jones PA, Andrews PJ, Midgley S, et al. Measuring the burden of secondary insults in head-injured patients during intensive care. *J Neurosurg Anesthesiol*. 1994;6(1):4–14.
6. Manley G, Knudson MM, Morabito D, Damron S, Erickson V, Pitts L. Hypotension, hypoxia, and head injury: frequency, duration, and consequences. *Arch Surg*. 2001;136(10):1118–1123.
7. Marmarou A, Anderson RL, Ward JD, Choi SC, Young HF. Impact of ICP instability and hypotension on outcome in patients with severe head trauma. *J Neurosurg*. 1991;75:S59–S66.
8. Vassar MJ, Fischer RP, O'Brien PE, et al. A multicenter trial for resuscitation of injured patients with 7.5% sodium chloride. The effect of added dextran 70. The Multicenter Group for the Study of Hypertonic Saline in Trauma Patients. *Arch Surg*. 1993;128(9):1003–1011. discussion1011–3.
9. Cooper DJ, Myles PS, McDermott FT, et al. Prehospital hypertonic saline resuscitation of patients with hypotension and severe traumatic brain injury: a randomized controlled trial. *JAMA*. 2004;291(11):1350–1357.
10. Chan KH, Miller JD, Dearden NM, Andrews PJ, Midgley S. The effect of changes in cerebral perfusion pressure upon middle cerebral artery blood flow velocity and jugular bulb venous oxygen saturation after severe brain injury. *J Neurosurg*. 1992;77(1):55–61.
11. Andrews PJD, Sleeman DH, Statham PFX, et al. Predicting recovery in patients suffering from traumatic brain injury by using admission variables and physiologic data: a comparison between decision tree analysis and logistic regression. *J Neurosurg*. 2002;97(2):326–336.
12. Clifton GL, Miller ER, Choi SC, Levin HS. Fluid thresholds and outcome from severe brain injury. *Crit Care Med*. 2002;30(4):739–745.
13. Nelson DW, Thornquist B, MacCallum RM, et al. Analyses of cerebral microdialysis in patients with traumatic brain injury: relations to intracranial pressure, cerebral perfusion pressure and catheter placement. *BMC Med*. 2011;9(1):21.
14. Rosner MJ, Daughton S. Cerebral perfusion pressure management in head injury. *J Trauma*. 1990;30(8):933–940. discussion940–1.

15. Chesnut RM. Avoidance of hypotension: conditio sine qua non of successful severe head-injury management. *J Trauma.* 1997; 42(suppl 5):S4–S9.

16. Robertson CS, Valadka AB, Hannay HJ, et al. Prevention of secondary ischemic insults after severe head injury. *Crit Care Med.* 1999;27(10):2086–2095.

17. Contant CF, Valadka AB, Gopinath SP, Hannay HJ, Robertson CS. Adult respiratory distress syndrome: a complication of induced hypertension after severe head injury. *J Neurosurg.* 2001;95(4): 560–568.

18. Steiner LA, Czosnyka M, Piechnik SK, et al. Continuous monitoring of cerebrovascular pressure reactivity allows determination of optimal cerebral perfusion pressure in patients with traumatic brain injury. *Crit Care Med.* 2002;30(4):733–738.

19. Lassen NA. Cerebral blood flow and oxygen consumption in man. *Physiol Rev.* 1959;39(2):183–238.

20. Kosty JA, LeRoux PD, Levine J, et al. Brief report: a comparison of clinical and research practices in measuring cerebral perfusion pressure: a literature review and practitioner survey. *Anesth Analg.* 2013;117(3):694–698.

21. Rosner MJ, Coley IB. Cerebral perfusion pressure, intracranial pressure, and head elevation. *J Neurosurg.* 1986;65(5):636–641.

22. Eisenberg HM, Frankowski RF, Contant CF, Marshall LF, Walker MD. High-dose barbiturate control of elevated intracranial pressure in patients with severe head injury. *J Neurosurg.* 1988;69(1):15–23.

23. Ratanalert S, Phuenpathom N, Saeheng S, Oearsakul T, Sripairojkul B, Hirunpat S. ICP threshold in CPP management of severe head injury patients. *Surg Neurol.* 2004;61(5):429–434. discussion434–5.

24. Chambers IR, Treadwell L, Mendelow AD. Determination of threshold levels of cerebral perfusion pressure and intracranial pressure in severe head injury by using receiver-operating characteristic curves: an observational study in 291 patients. *J Neurosurg.* 2001;94(3):412–416.

25. Chesnut RM, Temkin N, Carney N, et al. A trial of intracranial-pressure monitoring in traumatic brain injury. *N Engl J Med.* 2012;367(26):2471–2481.

26. Ropper AH. Brain in a box. *N Engl J Med.* 2012;367(26):2539–2541.

27. Teasell R, Bayona N, Lippert C, Villamere J, Hellings C. Post-traumatic seizure disorder following acquired brain injury. *Brain Inj.* 2007; 21(2):201–214.

28. Kolakowsky-Hayner SA, Wright J, Englander J, Duong T, Ladley-O'Brien S. Impact of late post-traumatic seizures on physical health and functioning for individuals with brain injury within the community. *Brain Inj.* 2013;27(5):578–586.

29. Temkin NR, Dikmen SS, Wilensky AJ, Keihm J, Chabal S, Winn HR. A randomized, double-blind study of phenytoin for the prevention of post-traumatic seizures. *N Engl J Med.* 1990;323(8):497–502.

30. Temkin NR, Dikmen SS, Anderson GD, et al. Valproate therapy for prevention of posttraumatic seizures: a randomized trial. *J Neurosurg.* 1999;91(4):593–600.

31. Schierhout G, Roberts I. WITHDRAWN: Antiepileptic drugs for preventing seizures following acute traumatic brain injury. *Cochrane Database Syst Rev.* 2012;6:CD000173.

32. Chang BS, Lowenstein DH, Quality Standards Subcommittee of the American Academy of Neurology. Practice parameter: antiepileptic drug prophylaxis in severe traumatic brain injury: report of the Quality Standards Subcommittee of the American Academy of Neurology. *Neurology.* 2003;60(1):10–16.

33. Kruer RM, Harris LH, Goodwin H, et al. Changing trends in the use of seizure prophylaxis after traumatic brain injury: a shift from phenytoin to levetiracetam. *J Crit Care.* 2013;28(5):883.e9–883.e13.

34. Caballero GC, Hughes DW, Maxwell PR, Green K, Gamboa CD, Barthol CA. Retrospective analysis of levetiracetam compared to phenytoin for seizure prophylaxis in adults with traumatic brain injury. *Hosp Pharm.* 2013;48(9):757–761.

35. Muizelaar JP, Marmarou A, Ward JD, et al. Adverse effects of prolonged hyperventilation in patients with severe head injury: a randomized clinical trial. *J Neurosurg.* 1991;75(5):731–739.

36. Schwartz ML, Tator CH, Rowed DW, Reid SR, Meguro K, Andrews DF. The University of Toronto head injury treatment study: a prospective, randomized comparison of pentobarbital and mannitol. *Can J Neurol Sci.* 1984;11(4):434–440.

37. Vassar MJ, Perry CA, Gannaway WL, Holcroft JW. 7.5% sodium chloride/dextran for resuscitation of trauma patients undergoing helicopter transport. *Arch Surg.* 1991;126(9):1065–1072.

38. Vialet R, Albanèse J, Thomachot L, et al. Isovolume hypertonic solutes (sodium chloride or mannitol) in the treatment of refractory posttraumatic intracranial hypertension: 2 mL/kg 7.5% saline is more effective than 2 mL/kg 20% mannitol. *Crit Care Med.* 2003;31(6):1683–1687.

39. Shackford SR, Bourguignon PR, Wald SL, Rogers FB, Osler TM, Clark DE. Hypertonic saline resuscitation of patients with head injury: a prospective, randomized clinical trial. *J Trauma.* 1998;44(1):50–58.

40. Horn P, Münch E, Vajkoczy P, et al. Hypertonic saline solution for control of elevated intracranial pressure in patients with exhausted response to mannitol and barbiturates. *Neurol Res.* 1999;21(8):758–764.

41. Suarez JI, Qureshi AI, Bhardwaj A, et al. Treatment of refractory intracranial hypertension with 23.4% saline. *Crit Care Med.* 1998;26(6):1118–1122.

42. Rozet I, Tontisirin N, Muangman S, et al. Effect of equiosmolar solutions of mannitol versus hypertonic saline on intraoperative brain relaxation and electrolyte balance. *Anesthesiology.* 2007;107(5):697–704.

43. Oddo M, Levine JM, Frangos S, et al. Effect of mannitol and hypertonic saline on cerebral oxygenation in patients with severe traumatic brain injury and refractory intracranial hypertension. *J Neurol Neurosurg Psychiatr.* 2009;80(8):916–920.

44. Whitfield PC, Patel H, Hutchinson PJ, et al. Bifrontal decompressive craniectomy in the management of posttraumatic intracranial hypertension. *Br J Neurosurg.* 2001;15(6):500–507.

45. Aarabi B, Hesdorffer DC, Ahn ES, Aresco C, Scalea TM, Eisenberg HM. Outcome following decompressive craniectomy for malignant swelling due to severe head injury. *J Neurosurg.* 2006;104(4):469–479.

46. Cooper DJ, Rosenfeld JV, Murray L, et al. Decompressive craniectomy in diffuse traumatic brain injury. *N Engl J Med.* 2011;364(16): 1493–1502.

47. Attia J, Cook DJ. Prognosis in anoxic and traumatic coma. *Crit Care Clin.* 1998;14(3):497–511.

48. Roberts I, Sydenham E. Barbiturates for acute traumatic brain injury. *Cochrane Database Syst Rev.* 2012;12:CD000033.

49. Tang JF, Chen P-L, Tang EJ, May TA, Stiver SI. Dexmedetomidine controls agitation and facilitates reliable, serial neurological examinations in a non-intubated patient with traumatic brain injury. *Neurocrit Care.* 2011;15(1):175–181.

50. Wang X, Ji J, Fen L, Wang A. Effects of dexmedetomidine on cerebral blood flow in critically ill patients with or without traumatic brain injury: a prospective controlled trial. *Brain Inj.* 2013;27(13–14): 1617–1622.

51. James ML, Olson DM, Graffagnino C. A pilot study of cerebral and haemodynamic physiological changes during sedation with dexmedetomidine or propofol in patients with acute brain injury. *Anaesth Intensive Care.* 2012;40(6):949–957.

52. Saxena M, Andrews PJD, Cheng A, Deol K, Hammond N. Modest cooling therapies (35°C to 37.5°C) for traumatic brain injury. *Cochrane Database Syst Rev.* 2014;8:CD006811.

53. Bohman L-E, Levine JM. Fever and therapeutic normothermia in severe brain injury: an update. *Curr Opin Crit Care.* 2014;20(2):182–188.

54. Commichau C, Scarmeas N, Mayer SA. Risk factors for fever in the neurologic intensive care unit. *Neurology.* 2003;60(5):837–841.

55. Dietrich WD, Atkins CM, Bramlett HM. Protection in animal models of brain and spinal cord injury with mild to moderate hypothermia. *J Neurotrauma.* 2009;26(3):301–312.

56. Bernard SA, Gray TW, Buist MD, et al. Treatment of comatose survivors of out-of-hospital cardiac arrest with induced hypothermia. *N Engl J Med.* 2002;346(8):557–563.

57. Hypothermia after Cardiac Arrest Study Group. Mild therapeutic hypothermia to improve the neurologic outcome after cardiac arrest. *N Engl J Med.* 2002;346(8):549–556.

58. Jiang J, Yu M, Zhu C. Effect of long-term mild hypothermia therapy in patients with severe traumatic brain injury: 1-year follow-up review of 87 cases. *J Neurosurg.* 2000;93(4):546–549.

59. Clifton GL, Miller ER, Choi SC, et al. Lack of effect of induction of hypothermia after acute brain injury. *N Engl J Med.* 2001;344(8):556–563.

60. Clifton GL, Choi SC, Miller ER, et al. Intercenter variance in clinical trials of head trauma–experience of the National Acute Brain Injury Study: Hypothermia. *J Neurosurg.* 2001;95(5):751–755.

61. Sydenham E, Roberts I, Alderson P. Hypothermia for traumatic head injury. *Cochrane Database Syst Rev.* 2009;2:CD001048.

62. Alderson P, Gadkary C, Signorini DF. Therapeutic hypothermia for head injury. *Cochrane Database Syst Rev.* 2004;4:CD001048.

63. Harris OA, Colford JM, Good MC, Matz PG. The role of hypothermia in the management of severe brain injury: a meta-analysis. *Arch Neurol.* 2002;59(7):1077–1083.

64. McIntyre LA, Fergusson DA, Hébert PC, Moher D, Hutchison JS. Prolonged therapeutic hypothermia after traumatic brain injury in adults: a systematic review. *JAMA.* 2003;289(22):2992–2999.

65. Clifton GL, Valadka A, Zygun D, et al. Very early hypothermia induction in patients with severe brain injury (the National Acute Brain Injury Study: Hypothermia II): a randomised trial. *Lancet Neurol.* 2011;10(2):131–139.

66. Maekawa T, Yamashita S, Nagao S, Hayashi N, Ohashi Y. Prolonged mild therapeutic hypothermia versus fever control with tight hemodynamic monitoring and slow rewarming in patients with severe traumatic brain injury: a randomized controlled trial. *J Neurotrauma.* 2015;(32):422–429.

67. Adelson PD, Wisniewski SR, Beca J, et al. Comparison of hypothermia and normothermia after severe traumatic brain injury in children (Cool Kids): a phase 3, randomised controlled trial. *Lancet Neurol.* 2013;12(6):546–553.

68. Tokutomi T, Miyagi T, Takeuchi Y, Karukaya T, Katsuki H, Shigemori M. Effect of 35 degrees C hypothermia on intracranial pressure and clinical outcome in patients with severe traumatic brain injury. *J Trauma.* 2009;66(1):166–173.

69. Puccio AM, Fischer MR, Jankowitz BT, Yonas H, Darby JM, Okonkwo DO. Induced normothermia attenuates intracranial hypertension and reduces fever burden after severe traumatic brain injury. *Neurocrit Care.* 2009;11(1):82–87.

70. Hertog den HM, van der Worp HB, van Gemert HMA, et al. The Paracetamol (Acetaminophen) In Stroke (PAIS) trial: a multicentre, randomised, placebo-controlled, phase III trial. *Lancet Neurol.* 2009;8(5):434–440.

71. Badjatia N, Fernandez L, Schmidt JM, et al. Impact of induced normothermia on outcome after subarachnoid hemorrhage: a case-control study. *Neurosurgery.* 2010;66(4):696–700. discussion700–1.

72. Douds GL, Tadzong B, Agarwal AD, Krishnamurthy S, Lehman EB, Cockroft KM. Influence of Fever and hospital-acquired infection on the incidence of delayed neurological deficit and poor outcome after aneurysmal subarachnoid hemorrhage. *Neurol Res Int.* 2012;2012:479865.

73. Meixensberger J, Jaeger M, Väth A, Dings J, Kunze E, Roosen K. Brain tissue oxygen guided treatment supplementing ICP/CPP therapy after traumatic brain injury. *J Neurol Neurosurg Psychiatr.* 2003;74(6):760–764.

74. Spiotta AM, Stiefel MF, Gracias VH, et al. Brain tissue oxygen-directed management and outcome in patients with severe traumatic brain injury. *J Neurosurg.* 2010;113(3):571–580.

75. Bohman L-E, Heuer GG, Macyszyn L, et al. Medical management of compromised brain oxygen in patients with severe traumatic brain injury. *Neurocrit Care.* 2011;14(3):361–369.

76. Adamides AA, Rosenfeldt FL, Winter CD, et al. Brain tissue lactate elevations predict episodes of intracranial hypertension in patients with traumatic brain injury. *J Am Coll Surg.* 2009;209(4):531–539.

77. Martini RP, Deem S, Yanez ND, et al. Management guided by brain tissue oxygen monitoring and outcome following severe traumatic brain injury. *J Neurosurg.* 2009;111(4):644–649.

78. Eriksson EA, Barletta JF, Figueroa BE, et al. Cerebral perfusion pressure and intracranial pressure are not surrogates for brain tissue oxygenation in traumatic brain injury. *Clin Neurophysiol.* 2012;123(6):1255–1260.

79. Saul TG, Ducker TB, Salcman M, Carro E. Steroids in severe head injury: a prospective randomized clinical trial. *J Neurosurg.* 1981;54(5):596–600.

80. Braakman R, Schouten HJ, Blaauw-van Dishoeck M, Minderhoud JM. Megadose steroids in severe head injury. Results of a prospective double-blind clinical trial. *J Neurosurg.* 1983;58(3):326–330.

81. Alderson P, Roberts I. Corticosteroids for acute traumatic brain injury. *Cochrane Database Syst Rev.* 2005;1:CD000196.

82. Clifton GL, Robertson CS, Grossman RG, Hodge S, Foltz R, Garza C. The metabolic response to severe head injury. *J Neurosurg.* 1984;60(4):687–696.

83. Young B, Ott L, Norton J, et al. Metabolic and nutritional sequelae in the non-steroid treated head injury patient. *Neurosurgery.* 1985;17(5):784–791.

84. Deutschman CS, Konstantinides FN, Raup S, Thienprasit P, Cerra FB. Physiological and metabolic response to isolated closed-head injury. Part 1: Basal metabolic state: correlations of metabolic and physiological parameters with fasting and stressed controls. *J Neurosurg.* 1986;64(1):89–98.

85. Hartl R, Gerber LM, Ni Q, Ghajar J. Effect of early nutrition on deaths due to severe traumatic brain injury. *J Neurosurg.* 2008;109(1):50–56.

86. Borzotta AP, Pennings J, Papasadero B, et al. Enteral versus parenteral nutrition after severe closed head injury. *J Trauma.* 1994;37(3):459–468.

87. Justo Meirelles CM, de Aguilar-Nascimento JE. Enteral or parenteral nutrition in traumatic brain injury: a prospective randomised trial. *Nutr Hosp.* 2011;26(5):1120–1124.

63 How Should Aneurysmal Subarachnoid Hemorrhage Be Managed?

Paulomi K. Bhalla, Ting Zhou, Joshua M. Levine

Aneurysmal subarachnoid hemorrhage (SAH), a type of hemorrhagic stroke due to rupture of an intracranial aneurysm, affects approximately 30,000 Americans each year and has a mortality rate of nearly 45%.[1] At least 15% of people with SAH die before reaching the hospital. Of those who survive, a substantial proportion is left with significant disability.[2] Prompt diagnosis, treatment, and anticipation of complications may improve outcome. Case fatality rates have been declining and functional outcomes have been improving.[3] These changes in the natural history of SAH may be attributable to early aneurysm repair and aggressive management of medical complications. This chapter reviews major clinical management points and discusses the relevant literature.

EMERGENCY SETTING

In the emergency setting, once the diagnosis of SAH has been established, initial goals are to stabilize the patient's airway, breathing, and circulation. Early referral to a large-volume center with experienced vascular neurosurgeons, neuroendovascular specialists, and dedicated neurointensivists should be considered. Four studies have demonstrated that hospital volume of SAH patients and procedural experience correlate with improved mortality.[4-7]

SAH-RELATED COMPLICATIONS

Rebleeding

Aneurysmal rebleeding is one of the most serious initial threats to the patient. The incidence may be as high as 30%,[8] with the greatest risk (roughly 4%) during the first 24 hours.[9] Temporizing medical measures are used to reduce the risk of rebleeding until the culprit aneurysm is excluded from the circulation through surgical or endovascular means.

Medical Measures

Bed rest does not alter the incidence of rebleeding,[10] but it has become a standard practice. Blood pressure control is widely recommended to reduce the risk of aneurysmal rebleeding. The benefit of blood pressure reduction must be weighed against the risk of precipitating cerebral ischemia.[11] Although there are no prospective studies that demonstrate the efficacy of antihypertensive therapy, retrospective data suggest an association between hypertension and aneurysmal rebleeding.[12,13] Ohkuma et al. found a statistically significant increase in the incidence of prehospitalization rebleeding in patients whose systolic blood pressure was greater than 160 mm Hg.[13] Interpretation of these data is confounded by variable times at which rebleeding was observed and variations in antihypertensive therapies. Because rebleeding may be related to aneurysm expansion, which is largely dictated by changes in transmural pressure, surges in blood pressure may be more important than absolute levels of blood pressure.[13,14] Therefore, it is reasonable to treat extreme hypertension and to minimize blood pressure lability with a short-acting, intravenous agent that has a predictable dose–response relationship. Premorbid baseline blood pressure should be taken into consideration for setting blood pressure goals, and hypotension should be avoided.

Antifibrinolytics

Antifibrinolytic agents such as tranexamic acid and epsilon-aminocaproic acid have been well studied. Ten prospective randomized studies (1904 participants) have been performed (Table 63-1) and were included in a 2013 Cochrane Review.[15] In sum, death and poor outcome (death, vegetative state, or severe disability) were not influenced by treatment.[15-25] It appears that, although antifibrinolytic medications reduce the risk of rebleeding, their benefit is offset by an increased risk of cerebral infarction.[16,23,24] In several of these studies, patients received antifibrinolytic therapy for weeks, well after the risk for rebleeding had declined and the risk of delayed cerebral ischemia (DCI) increased. Two recent case-control studies have shown that an early and short course of epsilon-aminocaproic acid before exclusion of the aneurysm from the circulation might reduce the risk of rebleeding without significantly increasing complications.[26,27] In one study, patients treated

Table 63-1 **Summary of Randomized Controlled Trials Evaluating Antifibrinolytic Therapy in SAH**

Study, Year*	Number of Subjects (Intervention/No Intervention)	Study Design	Intervention	Control	Outcomes
Girvin, 1973	66 (39/27)		Episilon-aminocaproic acid	Standard treatment	No effect on rebleeding, ischemia, or mortality
van Rossum, 1977	51 (26/25)	DB, P	Tranexamic acid	Placebo	No effect on rebleeding or mortality
Chandra, 1978	39 (20/19)	DB, P	Tranexamic acid	Placebo	No effect on rebleeding or mortality
Maurice, 1978	79 (38/41)		Tranexamic acid	Standard treatment	No effect on rebleeding or mortality
Kaste, 1979	64 (32/32)	DB, P	Tranexamic acid	Placebo	No effect on rebleeding or mortality
Fodstad, 1981	59 (30/29)		Tranexamic acid	Standard treatment	No effect on rebleeding, cerebral ischemia, or mortality
Vermeulen, 1984	479 (241/238)	DB, P	Tranexamic acid	Placebo	Decreased rebleeding, increased cerebral ischemia; no effect on outcome or mortality
Tsementzis, 1990	100 (50/50)	DB, P	Tranexamic acid	Placebo	Increased cerebral ischemia; no effect on rebleeding, outcome, or mortality
Roos, 2000	452 (229/223)	DB, P	Tranexamic acid	Placebo	Decreased rebleeding; no effect on ischemia, outcome, or mortality
Hillman, 2002	505 (254/251)		Tranexamic acid	Standard treatment	Decreased rebleeding; no effect on cerebral ischemia, outcome, or mortality
ULTRA	940 (470/470)		*Tranexamic acid*	*Standard treatment*	*Primary endpoint: functional outcome; secondary endpoints: case fatality, rebleeding rate, complication rates*

*Items in italics indicate ongoing studies.
DB, double blind; *P*, placebo; *SAH*, subarachnoid hemorrhage.

with epsilon-aminocaproic acid had an eightfold increase in deep venous thrombosis without an increase in pulmonary embolism.[26] This nonrandomized study was not adequately powered to determine the effect of antifibrinolytic therapy on overall patient outcome. A Dutch multicenter, randomized, open-label study, Ultra-Early Tranexamic Acid after Subarachnoid Hemorrhage (ULTRA), began enrolling patients in 2013.[28] It is designed to study the effect on functional outcome (blinded endpoint) of early administration of tranexamic acid in patients with moderate to high-grade aneurysmal SAH for a duration of up to 24 hours. The results of this study might inform whether an early and short course of antifibrinolytic therapy is clinically warranted. The Neurocritical Care Society Consensus Guidelines advise that an early and short course of antifibrinolytic therapy should be considered for patients who are at high risk of rebleeding (such as those with high clinical grade) and in whom definitive aneurysm treatment will be delayed.[29] However, antifibrinolytic agents should be avoided in patients who are at high risk of thromboembolic complications and in whom the risk of rebleeding

is reduced. Patients treated with antifibrinolytic therapy should be monitored for systemic and cerebral thrombotic complications.

Surgical and Endovascular Measures

There are two primary methods for excluding aneurysms from the circulation: (1) surgical, in which a craniotomy is performed and a clip is placed across the aneurysm neck and (2) endovascular, in which detachable coils are placed into the aneurysm by means of catheter-based techniques. On occasion, an endovascular technique known as flow diversion may be used, in which a stent is placed into the parent vessel across the neck of the aneurysm, allowing blood flow to bypass the aneurysm. The International Subarachnoid Aneurysm Trial (ISAT) is the only large prospective trial comparing the two primary methods.[30] In this trial, 2143 of 9559 patients were deemed good candidates for either therapy and were randomized to surgical or endovascular aneurysm treatment. In the short term, endovascular therapy was associated with less disability (15.6% vs. 21.6%) but lower rates of complete aneurysm obliteration

(58% vs. 81%) and higher recurrent SAH rates (2.9% per year vs. 0.9% per year). At 1 year, there was no difference in mortality. Long-term follow-up of these patients found low rates of rebleeding from the treated aneurysm in both groups (10 in the coiling group, 3 in the clipped group), which was insignificant by intention-to-treat analysis. At 5 years, the risk of death was significantly lower in the endovascular arm compared with the surgical arm (11% vs. 14%), but in patients who survived there was no difference in good outcome (modified Rankin Scale [mRS] >2).[31]

Although endovascular therapy has proven to be effective in the short term, aneurysm re-canalization remains a significant limitation. In a retrospective analysis, aneurysm recurrence was found in 33.6% of coiled aneurysms within 1 month and up to 2 years at 0.5 to 24 (mean±SD) after treatment.[32] Another retrospective review suggested that the use of a high-porosity stent (to retain coils within the aneurysm) was associated with a higher rate of complete aneurysm obliteration but also with increased morbidity and mortality, likely due to the need for dual-antiplatelet therapy.[33] Therefore the use of stents should be avoided if safer alternatives exist.

Whether to clip or to coil an aneurysm is a complex decision that depends on patient factors (age, comorbidities), aneurysm factors (size, shape, location), and availability of local resources and expertise. On the basis of several single-institution retrospective case series and nonrandomized prospective studies, there is evidence that patients with middle cerebral artery (MCA) aneurysms and large (> 50 mL) hematomas might benefit from microsurgical clipping,[34-36] whereas patients who are older, are seen during the vasospasm period, have poor clinical grade, or have a basilar apex aneurysm might be considered for endovascular therapy.[35,37-39] Ideally, experienced neurosurgeons and interventional neuroradiologists collaboratively make the decision.[30]

Timing

In recent years, there has been a trend toward early aneurysm treatment. Multiple retrospective and prospective studies have established an association between a longer interval to treatment and increased risk of pretreatment hemorrhage. The International Cooperative study on the Timing of Aneurysm Surgery explored early versus late surgical intervention based on the neurosurgeons' intention to treat.[40] Patients whose surgery was planned for within the first 3 days had an overall mortality rate equal to the patients whose surgery was planned for between days 11 and 32. However, patients in the early surgical group had a significantly better clinical recovery than those whose surgery was delayed (P<.01). The patients with the highest mortality were those whose surgery was planned for days 7 to 10 after ictus, a time when risk of vasospasm and delayed cerebral injury is greatest. On the basis of this study, early surgery/endovascular therapy is recommended.

Hydrocephalus

Acute hydrocephalus (enlargement of the ventricles) occurs in 15% to 30% of SAH patients.[41-45] The presence of hydrocephalus correlates with worse radiographic and clinical grades and with an unfavorable prognosis.[41-44] The symptoms associated with hydrocephalus range from no symptoms to signs of intracranial hypertension, such as impairment of upward gaze, sixth nerve palsy, and headache. Hydrocephalus may be "noncommunicating" because of obstruction (by blood) within the ventricular system or "communicating" because of obstruction of cerebrospinal fluid (CSF) reabsorption into the venous system.

If severe, hydrocephalus may impair the level of consciousness and should be treated immediately with CSF diversion. Ventriculostomy is the most common method of treatment; however, in a select group of patients with communicating hydrocephalus, who are not at risk for central or tonsillar herniation, lumbar drainage may be reasonable. Two small, single-institution studies suggested that in appropriately selected patients, lumbar CSF drainage is associated with a reduction in "clinical vasospasm" (i.e., neurological deficits not attributable to other structural or metabolic causes).[46,47] The EARLYDRAIN (Outcome After Early Lumbar CSF-drainage in Aneurysmal SAH) trial is an ongoing two-arm randomized controlled study comparing the effect of early continuous lumbar CSF drainage and standard neurointensive care with standard neurointensive care alone on functional outcome (disability at 6 months).[48] CSF drainage usually leads to an improvement in symptoms.[45,49,50]

Hydrocephalus and the need for CSF diversion are typically temporary. In some patients, hydrocephalus does not resolve, and ongoing CSF diversion with a permanent indwelling shunt is necessary.[51] In a single-center, prospective, randomized controlled trial, extending the duration of weaning external ventricular drainage for more than 24 hours did not affect the need for permanent shunting and was associated with increased length of both intensive care unit (ICU) and hospital stay.[52] There is no role for routine fenestration of the lamina terminalis to decrease the rate of permanent shunting.[53] Data regarding treatment of hydrocephalus in SAH are largely retrospective; optimal management of patients with mild symptoms is unknown.

Seizures

The evidence regarding the incidence, prophylaxis, and treatment of seizures is mostly retrospective. The reported incidence of seizures after SAH varies from 8% to 35%.[54-60] In one retrospective cohort study, most seizures after SAH occurred before hospitalization, and the incidence of in-hospital seizures was 4.1%. These seizures occurred despite prophylaxis with an antiepileptic drug (AED) and occurred at least 1 week after aneurysmal rupture.[54] Risk factors associated with the development of seizures include ruptured MCA aneurysm, intracerebral hemorrhage, thicker cisternal clot, rebleeding, ischemic infarct, and a history of hypertension.[54-57] Two studies demonstrated no difference in outcome between patients who had seizures and those who did not.[54,58] However, a third study found that seizures at the time of hemorrhage were associated with poor outcome.[61]

The incidence of generalized convulsive status epilepticus (GCSE) is 0.2%, but the incidence of nonconvulsive status epilepticus (NSE) is much higher.[62,63] A prospective study found that 31% of stuporous or comatose SAH patients had NSE when monitored with continuous electroencephalography (cEEG). The mean onset of NSE was 18 days after hemorrhage.[63] GCSE and NSE are associated with worse outcome.[62-64] Therefore it is reasonable to use periodic or cEEG to assess unconscious patients and those who have a change in neurologic examination for seizures.

The benefit of prophylactic AEDs has not been definitively established.[65-67] It is reasonable to use AEDs before aneurysm treatment because of the risk of seizure-related rebleeding (due to a surge in blood pressure). However, there is no evidence to support the long-term use of AEDs in patients without a history of seizure. In fact, cumulative phenytoin exposure is associated with a worse cognitive outcome at 3 months.[68]

Delayed Cerebral Ischemia

DCI (also referred to as *delayed ischemic neurologic deficits* [DINDs]) is defined as neurologic deterioration presumed to be ischemic that lasts for more than an hour and that cannot be attributed to another cause.[69] DCI accounts for most morbidity and mortality from SAH; therefore its detection and treatment are the major foci of intensive care. Although historically attributed exclusively to cerebral vasospasm (narrowing of the large caliber arteries at the base of the brain), DCI likely has protean causes, including a local inflammatory and hypercoagulable state that result in formation of microthrombi and microembolism.[70] Consequently, consensus statements recommend that the term *vasospasm* be reserved to describe only radiologic findings of vessel narrowing and not clinical deterioration.[29,69] DCI may present with agitation followed by an indolent decrease in level of consciousness or focal neurologic deficits that vary depending on the affected arterial distribution.[71] Vasospasm and DCI usually begin at day 3 after bleed, peak at days 6 to 8, and resolve over 2 to 4 weeks.[71,72] Thickness of cisternal clot has been associated with the development of vasospasm.[73] Almost one third of patients who survive the initial SAH have DCI,[40,74] and approximately half of these patients die.[75]

The diagnosis of and the decision to treat DINDs due to vasospasm are made with an observed clinical deterioration along with the radiographic finding of vasospasm. For SAH patients who have impaired consciousness and in whom subtle clinical deteriorations are not easily seen, bedside monitoring modalities such as cEEG, transcranial Doppler ultrasound (TCD), and invasive physiologic monitors might serve as surrogates for clinical changes.

Detection: Monitoring for ischemia includes clinical, radiologic, and physiologic assessments. Although by definition, DCI is detected by serial neurologic examination, not all ischemic insults are clinically apparent, especially in comatose patients.

Radiologic monitoring includes methods to assess for cerebral vasospasm and methods that assess cerebral blood flow (CBF) (perfusion). The gold standard for vasospasm detection is invasive digital subtraction angiography (DSA). Risks associated with DSA include hematoma, infection, peripheral thromboembolic events, and stroke. The rate of neurologic complications in SAH patients is 1.8%.[76] Noninvasive angiography with computed tomography (CT) or magnetic resonance imaging (MRI) is less sensitive for detecting vasospasm.[77-80] CT angiography (CTA) has a sensitivity of 86% to 91.6%[77-79] and is better suited to detect vasospasm of proximal arterial segments. CTA has a high negative predictive value (95% to 99%); therefore it may be used as a screening tool to limit the use of DSA. Magnetic resonance angiography (MRA) has a sensitivity for vasospasm detection of 45.6% compared with conventional angiography.[80]

TCD detects increased cerebral blood flow velocity (CBFV) associated with vasospasm. This noninvasive study may be performed daily at the bedside and is less expensive than many other monitoring tests.[81] TCD is most useful in detecting evidence of vasospasm in the middle cerebral and basilar arteries.[81,82] Compared with DSA, TCD has a relatively high specificity for, but poor sensitivity (42% to 67%) for, vasospasm detection.[82,83] Several conditions other than cerebral vasospasm increase CBFV, such as increased blood pressure and hyperemia.[84,85] The Lindegaard ratio (hemispheric index), the ratio between the blood flow velocities in the MCA and the ipsilateral extracranial internal carotid artery, may be used to distinguish increased CBFV due to vasospasm from other causes. Lindegaard ratios between 3 and 6 correlate with mild and moderate vasospasm, whereas indices greater than 6 suggest severe vasospasm.[85] Importantly, elevated TCD velocities do not correlate with the development of DIND.[86] No study has shown that TCD monitoring affects outcome after SAH.

Although imaging blood flow may be a more direct way to assess for ischemia than imaging of blood vessels (for vasospasm), it has been less well studied. Methods for blood flow imaging include CT perfusion (CTP), xenon CT (Xe-CT), MR perfusion, and single-photon emission CT. In the ICU, CT-based imaging studies (CTP, Xe-CT) are typically more practical because they involve less time than MRI and nuclear imaging studies and may be done at the bedside with a portable CT scanner. Although Xe-CT is a well-established tool that provides quantitative blood flow information, xenon gas is no longer approved by the U.S. Food and Drug Administration for this use. Therefore Xe-CT blood flow imaging is currently not in clinical use. The literature regarding the utility of CTP consists of multiple small studies, and there are considerably fewer studies on the utility of MR perfusion. Neither CT nor MR perfusion imaging is widely used for detection of DCI, and further study of these modalities is required.

Physiologic monitoring for DCI includes invasive techniques, such as regional brain tissue oxygen monitoring, regional CBF monitoring, and regional biochemical monitoring, and noninvasive techniques, such as quantitative cEEG and near-infrared spectroscopy. Although there is much enthusiasm for regional brain tissue oxygen monitoring and cerebral microdialysis, there is little supportive evidence in this setting.[29] Although traditionally used to detect seizures, cEEG is also becoming a tool for detection of ischemia. Ischemia produces characteristic changes on EEG, namely loss of fast-frequency waves followed by an increase in slow-frequency waves and ultimately suppression of brain waves. Various software analytic tools are available that provide some measure of the relative proportion of fast waves to slow waves; therefore, they might allow cEEG to serve as a continuous, noninvasive ischemia detector. The optimal EEG parameters for DCI detection and the effect on outcome of therapy based on cEEG ischemia monitoring are unknown. The literature consists exclusively of small prospective and retrospective single-center observational studies that used varying definitions of DCI and that included patients with varying severities of SAH. These studies suggest that it might be possible to detect ischemia by cEEG 1 to 3 days before changes in clinical examination. As with other physiologic monitors, quantitative cEEG is not widely used and its utility requires further study.

Prevention and Treatment: Table 63-2 summarizes the randomized trials that have been performed on therapies to treat vasospasm and DCI. Therapy consists of medical and endovascular measures.

Hemodynamic Augmentation Strategies: Although induced hypertension, hypervolemia, and hemodilution ("Triple-H therapy") have historically been the mainstay of medical treatment for vasospasm and DIND, this strategy is at best supported by moderate quality evidence. Hypovolemia is associated with worsening vasospasm, and DCI and should be avoided[87-89]; however, volume loading is associated with harm. Two randomized controlled trials (RCTs) evaluated the effect of prophylactic hypervolemia on CBF and the incidence of vasospasm.[90,91] Neither study found a significant improvement in CBF, incidence of symptomatic vasospasm, or functional outcome in patients receiving hypervolemic therapy compared with those receiving normovolemic therapy.[90,91] Patients receiving hypervolemic therapy had more complications, including bleeding, congestive heart failure, and infection.[91] On the basis of these studies, prophylactic hypervolemia is not recommended, and patients should be maintained in a euvolemic state.

Induced hypertension is widely used and supported only by case series. The HIMALAIA (Hypertension Induction in the Management of AneurysmaL subArachnoid haemorrhage with secondary IschaemiA) trial is a Dutch multicenter, randomized, controlled, single-blinded study on the effect of induced hypertension on functional outcome and CBF in patients with DCI after SAH. This study began enrolling patients in 2014, and it is projected to be completed by July 2017.[92]

Endovascular Treatments: When neurologic deterioration due to vasospasm is refractory to maximal medical therapy, endovascular treatment should be considered. Transluminal balloon angioplasty mechanically dilates the vasospastic vessels to improve CBF. Although the effect is durable, balloon angioplasty is associated with a higher rate of vessel rupture beyond the level of the carotid and M1 segments and does not affect long-term outcome.[93,94] Disruption of aneurysm clips and thrombus formation are other recognized complications of balloon angioplasty.[95-97] Catheter-based intra-arterial delivery of vasodilators, including papaverine, verapamil, nicardipine, nimodipine, and milrinone, may be more effective in the treatment of vasospasm in the distal vessels.[98-102] Patients should be monitored for increased ICP and systemic hypotension during intra-arterial vasodilator therapy. RCTs to establish the efficacy of these agents are lacking.

Magnesium: Magnesium is a physiologic antagonist of calcium and has neuroprotective properties. Magnesium modulates calcium channels and relaxes vascular smooth muscles. Hypomagnesemia is associated with vasospasm and should be corrected.[103] Pilot data supporting an association between intravenous magnesium

therapy and improved clinical outcomes[104-108] were not corroborated in two multicenter, randomized, placebo-control trials. Both the IMASH (Intravenous Magnesium Sulphate for Aneurysmal Subarachnoid Hemorrhage)[109] and MASH-2 (Magnesium for Aneurysmal Subarachnoid Hemorrhage)[110] studies were unable to detect a functional outcome benefit at 6 months and 3 months, respectively, in patients treated with intravenous magnesium infusion compared with the placebo group. Although hypomagnesemia should be avoided, magnesium administration to achieve supranormal levels is not recommended.

Calcium Channel Blockers: Calcium channel blockers may improve outcome after SAH. Five double-blinded, placebo-controlled trials of oral nimodipine demonstrated improved functional outcomes despite no effect on the incidence or severity of vasospasm.[111-115] Two RCTs of intravenous nicardipine demonstrated no effect on 3-month outcome despite a reduction in the incidence of symptomatic vasospasm.[116,117] A Cochrane Review of 16 trials, involving 3361 patients, found that oral nimodipine alone reduced the risk of poor outcome by 33%. For intravenous nimodipine and other calcium channel blockers, the results were not statistically significant.[118] Patients with SAH should receive oral nimodipine 60 mg every 4 hours for 21 days.[119]

Statins: Statins have pleotropic vascular and neuroprotective effects, which created interest in their use for the treatment of SAH. Several small studies suggested that pravastatin and simvastatin administration was associated with a decreased incidence of vasospasm and DCI and a shorter duration of vasospasm.[120,121] In addition, mortality due to vasospasm and clinical outcomes at 6 months were improved.[122] However, in a well-designed multicenter RCT, 40 mg simvastatin instituted within 96 hours of SAH for up to 21 days was not associated with improved 6-month functional outcome (modified Rankin scale score).[123] Therefore de novo initiation of statin therapy is not recommended; however, continuation of statin therapy in patients with premorbid statin use is reasonable. An ongoing trial comparing the effects of 80 with 40 mg of simvastatin on outcome after SAH is currently underway.[124]

Hyponatremia

Approximately one third of SAH patients have hyponatremia.[89,125-127] Hyponatremia is associated with an increased incidence of DCI and is more common in patients with anterior communicating artery aneurysms, higher grade of SAH, and hydrocephalus.[89,125,126] Although hyponatremia may be due to the syndrome of inappropriate secretion of antidiuretic hormone (SIADH), treatment with fluid restriction is detrimental and leads to increased mortality from DCI.[89] Alternatively, hyponatremia may be due to cerebral salt wasting, a form of hypovolemic hyponatremia that is treated with volume replacement and salt.[128] Irrespective of the cause of hyponatremia, oral or intravenous sodium chloride is usually sufficient to correct mild hyponatremia. In patients with symptomatic vasospasm or severe hyponatremia, hypertonic saline may be given.[129] Two small prospective, randomized trials found that fludrocortisone may reduce natriuresis and prevent hyponatremia.[130,131] In patients with SIADH, a prospective trial found that conivaptan, an oral vasopressin receptor agonist, effectively corrects hyponatremia.[132]

Table 63-2 Summary of Randomized Controlled Trials Evaluating the Prevention of Vasospasm and DINDs in SAH

Study, Year*	Number of Subjects (Intervention/No Intervention)	Study Design	Intervention	Control	Outcomes
HEMODYNAMIC AUGMENTATION					
Lennihan, 2000	82 (41/41)		Hypervolemic therapy	Normovolemic therapy	No difference in symptomatic vasospasm
Egge, 2001	32 (16/16)		Hypervolemic hypertensive hemodilution therapy	Normovolemic therapy	No difference in DIND or TCD vasospasm
HIMALAIA	*240 (120/120)*		*Induced hypertension*	*Standard therapy without induced hypertension*	*Primary endpoint: functional outcome Secondary endpoints: adverse effects, CBF measured by perfusion CT*
MAGNESIUM THERAPY					
van den Bergh, 2005	283 (139/144)	DB, P	Magnesium IV	Placebo	Decreased incidence of DINDs; improved clinical outcome at 3 months
Veyna, 2002	40 (20/20)		Magnesium IV	Standard therapy	Trend toward improved clinical outcome
Wong, 2006	60 (?/?)	DB	Magnesium IV	Saline	Trend toward decrease in symptomatic vasospasm; decrease TCD vasospasm timeframe; no difference in clinical outcome
Schmid-Eisaeser, 2006	104 (53/51)		Magnesium IV	Nimodipine IV	Incidence of vasospasm and clinical outcome comparable
Muroi, 2008	58 (31/27)	P	Magnesium IV	Placebo	No difference in DINDs; improved clinical outcome at 3 months
IMASH, 2010	328 (169/159)	DB, P	Magnesium IV	Saline	No difference in clinical outcome at 6 months
MASH-2, 2012	1203 (606/597)	DB, P	Magnesium IV	Saline	No difference in clinical outcome at 3 months
CALCIUM CHANNEL BLOCKERS					
Allen, 1983	116 (56/60)	DB, P	Nimodipine PO	Placebo	Decreased incidence of DINDs
Philippon, 1986	70 (?/?)	DB, P	Nimodipine PO	Placebo	No difference in vasospasm; decreased incidence of DINDs; improved mortality
Neil-Dwyer, 1987	75 (?/?)	DB, P	Nimodipine PO	Placebo	Improved clinical outcome at 3 months
Petruk, 1988	154 (72/82)	DB, P	Nimodipine PO	Placebo	Decreased incidence of DINDs; improved clinical outcome at 3 months
Pickard, 1989	554 (278/276)	DB, P	Nimodipine PO	Placebo	Decreased incidence of DINDs; improved clinical outcome at 3 months
Haley, 1993	906 (449/457)	DB, P	Nicardipine IV	Placebo	Decreased incidence of vasospasm; no difference in clinical outcome
Haley, 1994	365 (184/181)	DB	High-dose nicardipine IV	Low-dose nicardipine IV	Incidence of vasospasm and clinical outcome comparable
STATIN THERAPY					
Lynch, 2005	39 (19/20)	DB, P	Simvastatin	Placebo	Decreased incidence of vasospasm
Tseng, 2005	80 (40/40)	DB, P	Pravastatin	Placebo	Decreased incidence of vasospasm and DINDs; improved mortality
Tseng, 2006	80 (40/40)	DB, P	Pravastatin	Placebo	Improved clinical outcome at 6 months
Chou, 2008	39 (19/20)	DB, P	Simvastatin	Placebo	No difference in vasospasm or DINDs; trend toward decreased mortality
STASH, 2014	812 (391/421)	DB, P	Simvastatin	Placebo	No difference in short- and long-term outcome
Wong	*240 (120/120)*	*DB*	*Simvastatin 80 mg*	*Simvastatin 40 mg*	*Presence of DIND at 1 month*
OTHER APPROACH					
Bulters, 2013	71 (35/36)		Intra-aortic balloon pump	Hypervolemic therapy	No difference in clinical outcome, mean cardiac output, or CBF

*Items in italics indicate ongoing studies.

CBF, cerebral blood flow; *CT,* computed tomography; *DB,* double blind; *DIND,* delayed ischemic neurologic deficit; *IV,* intravenously; *P,* placebo; *PO,* by mouth; *SAH,* subarachnoid haemorrhage; *TCD,* transcranial Doppler ultrasound.

Cardiac Dysfunction

Electrocardiographic Abnormalities: Ninety percent of patients with SAH experience cardiac arrhythmias, including supraventricular and ventricular premature complexes, supraventricular and ventricular tachyarrhythmias, and sinoatrial and atrioventricular block. Life-threatening arrhythmias—usually torsade de pointes or ventricular flutter/fibrillation—are seen in 3% to 4% of patients. They occur most commonly in the first 48 hours and are associated with QT prolongation and with hypokalemia. The clinical and radiographic findings of SAH do not correlate with the presence of arrhythmias.[133,134] Patients with QT prolongation are more likely to have increased serum cardiac troponin I.[135] A total of 6% to 12% of patients have ST-segment elevations or, more commonly, depressions.[134,135] These abnormalities are associated with neurogenic stunned myocardium (see later) and are not usually due to coronary artery disease or to coronary vasospasm.[136]

Cardiomyopathy: SAH patients are susceptible to a reversible cardiomyopathy known as neurogenic stunned myocardium. One purported mechanism is activation of the sympathetic nervous system with consequent catecholamine toxicity.[137] Fifteen percent of patients have global left ventricular dysfunction, and another 13% to 18% have regional wall motion abnormalities (RWMAs). The RWMAs do not respect coronary arterial vascular distributions but may occur in the distribution of myocardial sympathetic nerve terminals.[138-140] Predictors of neurogenic stunned myocardium include poor clinical grade, temporal proximity to aneurysm rupture, female gender, larger body surface area, larger left ventricular mass index, elevated serum cardiac troponin I, tachycardia, lower systolic blood pressure, higher doses of phenylephrine, and previous cocaine or amphetamine use.[140,141] RWMA most commonly affect the mid regions of the anteroseptal, anterior, inferoseptal, and anterolateral left ventricular walls (apical-sparing pattern) or the left ventricular base ("inverted Takotsubo" pattern). The apex occasionally is disproportionately involved ("Takotsubo" pattern). RWMAs are independent risk factors for DCI, death, and poor functional outcome.[142] Patients may have a range of symptoms from mild heart failure to cardiogenic shock. Treatment is supportive and prognosis is excellent.[140]

Fever

The incidence of fever in patients with SAH is 23% to 70%.[143-147] Risk factors for developing fever include the presence of intraventricular blood, older age, and poor clinical grade.[143,145,147] Pyrexia has been associated with poor clinical outcome in multiple studies.[145,147,148] In one prospective study, fever was associated with poor outcome independent of the presence of DCI, infection, or disease severity.[148] It remains unclear whether fever is merely a marker of disease severity or is causally related to poor outcome. In one case control study, compared with conventional fever management (with acetaminophen and water-cooled blankets), aggressive temperature control (with a modern servo-controlled temperature-management device) was associated with improved outcomes at 12 months, increased ICU length of stay, increased use of sedatives, and higher rates of tracheostomy.[149] Despite a paucity of evidence, fever control has become a standard of care.

Anemia

Anemia, defined as a hemoglobin level less than 10 g/dL, is common in patients with aneurysmal SAH and develops in 39% to 57% of patients.[150-152] Higher hemoglobin levels have been associated with improved outcomes in two retrospective studies,[153,154] and another study that incorporated positron-emission tomography (PET) studies found improved oxygen delivery without reduction in global CBF.[155] These benefits must be weighed against the increased rates of medical complications and infections associated with blood transfusion in this population.[151,156] A recent prospective, single-institution RCT trial compared hemoglobin transfusion thresholds of 10 and 11.5 g/dL and found no significant difference in rates of fever or ventilator days but less cortical infarction in the higher hemoglobin threshold group.[157] Further study is required to define the optimal triggers for red blood cell transfusion in patients with aneurysmal SAH.

CONCLUSION

The goal of critical care management of patients with SAH is to limit further neurologic injury. Prompt diagnosis and treatment of SAH are crucial. Anticipating complications from rebleeding, hydrocephalus, seizures, and DCI is imperative. Further prospective randomized trials are needed to establish the efficacy of new and existing therapies.

AUTHORS' RECOMMENDATIONS

- Rebleeding is the most serious initial threat to the patient with SAH. Aneurysms should be promptly clipped or coiled. Blood pressure should be controlled until the aneurysm is secured. An early and brief course of antifibrinolytic therapy until aneurysm treatment may be considered for patients who are at low risk of thromboembolic events.
- Prophylactic AEDs are reasonable in the acute setting, but there is no evidence supporting their long-term use.
- The maximal risk for DCI occurs between postbleed days 3 and 14. Vasospasm is one cause of DCI. The gold standard for vasospasm detection is conventional cerebral angiography; however, TCD may be used to monitor for vasospasm. The utility of monitoring for DCI with quantitative cEEG, near-infrared spectroscopy, and invasive physiologic probes requires further study.
- Treatment of DCI includes maintenance of euvolemia and induced hypertension. In patients with vasospasm and symptomatic ischemia refractory to medical measures, balloon angioplasty and intra-arterial vasodilator administration should be considered.
- Oral nimodipine improves outcome in SAH and should be given to all patients unless contraindicated.
- Hypomagnesemia should be corrected. Supplemental magnesium administration to achieve supranormal levels is not recommended.
- De novo initiation of statin therapy in the setting of acute SAH is not recommended.
- Hyponatremia, anemia, fever, and cardiac dysfunction are common medical complications of SAH.

REFERENCES

1. King Jr JT. Epidemiology of aneurysmal subarachnoid hemorrhage. *Neuroimaging Clin N Am.* 1997;7(4):659–668.
2. Johnston SC, Selvin S, Gress DR. The burden, trends, and demographics of mortality from subarachnoid hemorrhage. *Neurology.* 1998;50(5):1413–1418.
3. Nieuwkamp DJ, Setz LE, Algra A, Linn FH, de Rooij NK, Rinkel GJ. Changes in case fatality of aneurysmal subarachnoid haemorrhage over time, according to age, sex, and region: a meta-analysis. *Lancet Neurol.* 2009;8(7):635–642.
4. Johnston SC. Effect of endovascular services and hospital volume on cerebral aneurysm treatment outcomes. *Stroke.* 2000;31(1):111–117.
5. Bardach NS, Zhao S, Gress DR, et al. Association between subarachnoid hemorrhage outcomes and number of cases treated at California hospitals. *Stroke.* 2002;33(7):1851–1856.
6. Cross 3rd DT, Tirschwell DL, Clark MA, et al. Mortality rates after subarachnoid hemorrhage: variations according to hospital case volume in 18 states. *J Neurosurg.* 2003;99(5):810–817.
7. Berman MF, Solomon RA, Mayer SA, Johnston SC, Yung PP. . Impact of hospital-related factors on outcome after treatment of cerebral aneurysms. *Stroke.* 2003;34(9):2200–2207. 2004.
8. Winn HR, Richardson AE, Jane JA. The long-term prognosis in untreated cerebral aneurysms: I. the incidence of late hemorrhage in cerebral aneurysm: a 10-year evaluation of 364 patients. *Ann Neurol.* 1977;1(4):358–370.
9. Sundt Jr TM, Whisnant JP. Subarachnoid hemorrhage from intracranial aneurysms. Surgical management and natural history of disease. *N Engl J Med.* 1978;299(3):116–122.
10. Nibbelink DW, Torner JC, Henderson WG. Intracranial aneurysms and subarachnoid hemorrhage – report on a randomized treatment study. IV-A. Regulated bed rest. *Stroke.* 1977;8(2):202–218.
11. Wijdicks EF, Vermeulen M, Murray GD, Hijdra A, van Gijn J. The effects of treating hypertension following aneurysmal subarachnoid hemorrhage. *Clin Neurol Neurosurg.* 1990;92(2):111–117.
12. Fuji Y, Takeuchi S, Sasaki O, Minakawa T, Koike T, Tanaka R. Ultra-early rebleeding in spontaneous subarachnoid hemorrhage. *J Neurosurg.* 1996;84(1):35–42.
13. Ohkuma H, Tsurutani H, Suzuki S. Incidence and significance of early aneurysmal rebleeding before neurosurgical or neurological management. *Stroke.* 2001;32(5):1176–1180.
14. Stornelli SA, French J. Subarachnoid hemorrhage—factors in prognosis and management. *J Neurosurg.* 1964;21:769–780.
15. Baharoglu M, Germans M, Rinkel G, et al. *Antifibrinolytic therapy for aneurysmal subarachnoid haemorrhage (Cochrane Review). The Cochrane Collaboration.* John Wiley & Sons; 2013.
16. Hillman J, Fridriksson S, Nilsson O, Zhengquan Y, Säveland H, Jakobsson KE. Immediate administration of tranexamic acid and reduced incidence of early rebleeding after aneurysmal subarachnoid hemorrhage: a prospective randomized study. *J Neurosurg.* 2002;97(4):771–778.
17. Girvin JP. The use of antifibrinolytic agents in the preoperative treatment of ruptured intracranial aneurysms. *Trans Am Neurol Assoc.* 1973;98:150–152.
18. Van Rossum J, Wintzen AR, Endtz LJ, Schoen JHR, de Jonge H. Effect of tranexamic acid on rebleeding after subarachnoid hemorrhage: a double-blind controlled clinical trial. *Ann Neurol.* 1977;2:238–242.
19. Chandra B. Treatment of subarachnoid hemorrhage from ruptured intracranial aneurysm with tranexamic acid: a double-blind clinical trial. *Ann Neurol.* 1978;3:502–504.
20. Maurice-Williams RS. Prolonged antifibrinolysis: an effective nonsurgical treatment for ruptured intracranial aneurysms? *Brit Med J.* 1978;1:945–947.
21. Kaste M, Ramsay M. Tranexamic acid in subarachnoid hemorrhage. A double-blind study. *Stroke.* 1979;10:519–522.
22. Fodstad H, Forssell A, Liliequist B, Schannong M. Antifibrinolysis with tranexamic acid in aneurysmal subarachnoid hemorrhage: a consecutive controlled clinical trial. *Neurosurgery.* 1981;8:158–165.
23. Vermeulen M, Lindsay KW, Murray GD, et al. Antifibrinolytic treatment in subarachnoid hemorrhage. *N Engl J Med.* 1984;311:432–437.
24. Tsementzis SA, Hitchcock ER, Meyer CH. Benefits and risks of antifibrinolytic therapy in the management of ruptured intracranial aneurysms. A double-blind placebo-controlled study. *Acta Neurochirurgica.* 1990;102:1–10.
25. Roos Y, for the STAR-study group. Antifibrinolytic Treatment in Aneurysmal Subarachnoid Haemorrhage: a randomized placebo-controlled trial. *Neurology.* 2000;54:77–82.
26. Starke R, Kim G, Fernandez A, et al. Impact of a protocol for acute antifibrinolytic therapy on aneurysm rebleeding after subarachnoid hemorrhage. *Stroke.* 2008;39(9):2617–2621.
27. Harrigan M, Rajneesh K, Ardelt A, Fisher W. Short-term antifibrinolytic therapy before early aneurysm treatment in subarachnoid hemorrhage: effects on rehemorrhage, cerebral ischemia, and hydrocephalus. *Neurosurgery.* 2010;67(4):935–939.
28. Germans M, Post R, Coert B, Rinkel G, Vandertop W, Verbaan D. Ultra-early tranexamic acid after subarachnoid hemorrhage (ULTRA): study protocol for a randomized controlled trial. *Trials.* 2013;14:143.
29. Diringer MN, Cleck TP, Hemphill 3rd J, et al. Critical care management of patients following aneurysmal subarachnoid hemorrhage: recommendations from the Neurocritical Care Society's Multidisciplinary Consensus Conference. *Neurocrit Care.* 2011;15:211–240.
30. Molyneux AJ, Kerr RSC, Yu LM, et al. International subarachnoid aneurysm trial (ISAT) of neurosurgical clipping versus endovascular coiling in 2143 patients with ruptured intracranial aneurysms: a randomised comparison of effects on survival, dependency, seizures, rebleeding, subgroups, and aneurysm occlusion. *Lancet.* 2005;366(9488):809–817.
31. Molyneux AJ, Kerr RS, Birks J, ISAT Collaborators, et al. Risk of recurrent subarachnoid haemorrhage, death, or dependence and standardised mortality ratios after clipping or coiling of an intracranial aneurysm in the International Subarachnoid Aneurysm Trial (ISAT): long-term follow-up. *Lancet Neurol.* May 2009;8(5):427–433.
32. Raymond J, Guilbert F, Weill A, et al. Long-term angiographic recurrences after selective endovascular treatment of aneurysms with detachable coils. *Stroke.* 2003;34:1398–1403.
33. Piotin M, Blanc R, Spelle L, et al. Stent-assisted coiling of intracranial aneurysms: clinical and angiographic results in 216 consecutive aneurysms. *Stroke.* 2010;41(1):110–115.
34. Regli L, Dehdashti AR, Uske A, de Tribolet N. Endovascular coiling compared with surgical clipping for the treatment of unruptured middle cerebral artery aneurysms: an update. *Acta Neurochir Suppl.* 2002;82:41–46.
35. Bracard S, Lebedinsky A, Anxionnat R, et al. Endovascular treatment of Hunt and Hess grade IV and V aneurysms. *Am J Neuroradiol.* 2002;23:953–957.
36. Rinne J, Hernesniemi J, Niskanen M, Vapalahti M. Analysis of 561 patients with 690 middle cerebral artery aneurysms: anatomic and clinical features as correlated to management outcome. *Neurosurgery.* 1996;38:2–11.
37. Proust F, Gérardin E, Derrey S, et al. Interdisciplinary treatment of ruptured cerebral aneurysms in elderly patients. *J Neurosurg.* 2010;112:1200–1207.
38. Brilstra EH, Rinkel GJ, van der Graaf Y, van Rooij WJ, Algra A. Treatment of intracranial aneurysms by embolization with coils: a systematic review. *Stroke.* 1999;30:470–476.
39. Lusseveld E, Brilstra EH, Nijssen PC, et al. Endovascular coiling versus neurosurgical clipping in patients with a ruptured basilar tip aneurysm. *Neurol Neurosurg Psychiatry.* 2002;73:591–593.
40. Haley Jr EC, Kassell NF, Torner JC. The International Cooperative Study on the Timing of Aneurysm Surgery. The North American experience. *Stroke.* 1992;23(2):205–214.
41. Mehta V, Holness RO, Connolly K, et al. Acute hydrocephalus following aneurysmal subarachnoid hemorrhage. *Can J Neurol Sci.* 1996;23:40–45.
42. Suarez-Rivera O. Acute hydrocephalus after subarachnoid hemorrhage. *Surg Neurol.* 1998;49:563–565.
43. Lin CL, Kwan AL, Howng SL. Acute hydrocephalus and chronic hydrocephalus with the need of postoperative shunting after aneurysmal subarachnoid hemorrhage. *Kaohsiung J Med Sci.* 1999;15:137–145.
44. Sheehan JP, Polin RS, Sheehan JM, et al. Factors associated with hydrocephalus after aneurysmal subarachnoid hemorrhage. *Neurosurgery.* 1999;45:1120–1127. discussion 1127–1128.

45. Hasan D, Vermeulen M, Wijdicks EF, et al. Management problems in acute hydrocephalus after subarachnoid hemorrhage. *Stroke*. 1989;20:747–753.

46. Klimo Jr P, Kestle JR, MacDonald JD, Schmidt RH. Marked reduction of cerebral vasospasm with lumbar drainage of cerebrospinal fluid after subarachnoid hemorrhage. *J Neurosurg*. 2004;100:215–224.

47. Kwon OY, Kim YJ, Cho CS, Lee SK, Cho MK. The utility and benefits of external lumbar CSF drainage after endovascular coiling on aneurysmal/subarachnoid hemorrhage. *J Kor Neurosurg Soc*. 2008;43:281–287.

48. Bardutzky J, Witsch J, Jüttler E, Schwab S, Vajkoczy P, Wolf S. EARLYDRAIN- outcome after early lumbar CSF-drainage in aneurysmal subarachnoid hemorrhage: study protocol for a randomized controlled trial. *Trials*. September 14, 2011;12:203.

49. Rajshekhar V, Harbaugh RE. Results of routine ventriculostomy with external ventricular drainage for acute hydrocephalus following subarachnoid haemorrhage. *Acta Neurochir*. 1992;115:8–14.

50. Milhorat TH. Acute hydrocephalus after aneurysmal subarachnoid hemorrhage. *Neurosurgery*. 1987;20:15–20.

51. Gruber A, Reinprecht A, Bavinzski G, Czech T, Richling B. Chronic shunt-dependent hydrocephalus after early surgical and early endovascular treatment of ruptured intracranial aneurysm. *Neurosurgery*. 1999;44(3):503–509.

52. Klopfenstein JD, Kim LJ, Feiz-Erfan I, et al. Comparison of rapid and gradual weaning from external ventricular drainage in patients with aneurysmal subarachnoid hemorrhage: a prospective randomized trial. *J Neurosurg*. 2004;100:225–229.

53. Komotar RJ, Hahn DK, Kim GH, et al. Efficacy of lamina terminalis fenestration in reducing shunt-dependent hydrocephalus following aneurysmalaneurysmal subarachnoid hemorrhage: a systematic review: clinical article. *J Neurosurg*. 2009;111:147–154.

54. Rhoney DH, Tipps LB, Murry KR, et al. Anticonvulsant prophylaxis and timing of seizures after aneurysmal subarachnoid hemorrhage. *Neurology*. 2000;55:258–265.

55. Ohman J. Hypertension as a risk factor for epilepsy after aneurysmal subarachnoid hemorrhage and surgery. *Neurosurgery*. 1990;27:578–581.

56. Ukkola V, Heikkinen ER. Epilepsy after operative treatment of ruptured cerebral aneurysms. *Acta Neurochir*. 1990;106:115–118.

57. Hasan D, Schnonck RS, Avezaat CJ, Tanghe HL, van Gijn J, van der Lugt PJ. Epileptic seizures after subarachnoid hemorrhage. *Ann Neurol*. 1993;33(3):286–291.

58. Lin CL, Dumont AS, Lieu AS, et al. Characterization of perioperative seizures and epilepsy following aneurysmal subarachnoid hemorrhage. *J Neurosurg*. 2003;99(6):978–985.

59. Cabral RJ, King TT, Scott DF. Epilepsy after two different neurosurgical approaches to the treatment of ruptured intracranial aneurysm. *J Neurol Neurosurg Psychiatry*. 1976;39:1052–1056.

60. Kotila M, Waltimo O. Epilepsy after stroke. *Epilepsia*. 1992;33: 495–498.

61. Butzkueven H, Evans AH, Pitman A, et al. Onset seizures independently predict poor outcome after subarachnoid hemorrhage. *Neurology*. 2000;55(9):1315–1320.

62. Claassen J, Bateman BT, Willey JZ, et al. Generalized convulsive status epilepticus after nontraumatic subarachnoid hemorrhage: the nationwide inpatient sample. *Neurosurgery*. 2007;61(1):60–64. discussion 64–65.

63. Dennis LJ, Claassen J, Hirsch LJ, Emerson RG, Connolly ES, Mayer SA. Nonconvulsive status epilepticus after subarachnoid hemorrhage. *Neurosurgery*. 2002;51(5):1136–1143. discussion 1144.

64. Claassen J, Hirsch LJ, Frontera JA, et al. Prognostic significance of continuous EEG monitoring in patients with poor-grade subarachnoid hemorrhage. *Neurocrit Care*. 2006;4(2):103–112.

65. Sbeih I, Tamas LB, O'Laoire SA. Epilepsy after operation for aneurysms. *Neurosurgery*. 1986;19(5):784–788.

66. O'Laoire SA. Epilepsy following neurosurgical intervention. *Acta Neurochir Suppl*. 1990;50:52–54.

67. Shaw MD. Post-operative epilepsy and the efficacy of anticonvulsant therapy. *Acta Neurochir Suppl*. 1990;50:55–57.

68. Naidech AM, Kreiter KT, Janjua N, et al. Phenytoin exposure is associated with functional and cognitive disability after subarachnoid hemorrhage. *Stroke*. 2005;36(3):583–587.

69. Vergouwen M, Vermeulen M, van Gijn J, et al. Definition of delayed cerebral ischemia after aneurysmal subarachnoid hemorrhage as an outcome event in clinical trials and observational studies: proposal of a multidisciplinary research group. *Stroke*. 2010;41(10):2391–2395.

70. Stein SC, Levine JM, Nagpal S, et al. Vasospasm as the sole cause of cerebral ischemia: how strong is the evidence? *Neurosurg Focus*. 2006;21(3):E2.

71. Heros RC, Zervas NT, Varsos V. Cerebral vasospasm after subarachnoid hemorrhage: an update. *Ann Neurol*. 1983;14:599–608.

72. Fisher CM, Roberson GH, Ojemann RG. Cerebral vasospasm with ruptured saccular aneurysm—the clinical manifestations. *Neurosurgery*. 1977;1:245–248.

73. Fisher CM, Kistler JP, Davis JM. Relation of cerebral vasospasm to subarachnoid hemorrhage visualized by computerized tomographic scanning. *Neurosurgery*. 1980;6:1–9.

74. Haley Jr EC, Kassell NF, Apperson-Hansen C, Maile M, Alves W, and the Participants. A randomized, double-blind, vehicle-controlled trial of tierilazad mesylate in patients with aneurysmal subarachnoid hemorrhage: a cooperative study in North America. *J Neurosurg*. 1997;86:467–474.

75. Kassell NF, Boarini DJ, Adams Jr HP, et al. Overall management of ruptured aneurysm: comparison of early and late operation. *Neurosurgery*. 1981;9:120–128.

76. Cloft HJ, Joseph GJ, Dion JE. Risk of cerebral angiography in patients with subarachnoid hemorrhage, cerebral aneurysm, and arteriovenous malformation: a meta-analysis. *Stroke*. 1999;30(2):317–320.

77. Otawara Y, Ogasawara K, Ogawa A, Sasaki M, Takahashi K. Evaluation of vasospasm after subarachnoid hemorrhage by use of multi slice computed tomographic angiography. *Neurosurgery*. 2002;51(4):939–942.

78. Anderson GB, Ashforth R, Steinke DE, Findlay JM. CT angiography for the detection of cerebral vasospasm in patients with acute subarachnoid hemorrhage. *Am J Neuroradiol*. 2000;21(6):1011–1015.

79. Chaudhary SR, Ko N, Dillon WP, et al. Prospective evaluation of multidetector-row CT angiography for the diagnosis of vasospasm following subarachnoid hemorrhage: a comparison with digital subtraction angiography. *Cerebrovasc Dis*. 2008;25 (1–2):144–150.

80. Tamatani S, Sasaki O, Takeuchi S, Fujii Y, Koike T, Tanaka R. Detection of delayed cerebral vasospasm, after rupture of intracranial aneurysms, by magnetic resonance, angiography. *Neurosurgery*. 1997;40(4):748–753.

81. Sloan MA, Alexandrov AV, Tegeler CH, et al. Assessment: Transcranial Doppler ultrasonography: Report of the Therapeutics and Technology Assessment Subcommittee of the American Academy of Neurology. *Neurology*. 2004;62:1468–1481.

82. Sloan MA, Haley Jr EC, Kassell NF, et al. Sensitivity and specificity of transcranial Doppler ultrasonography in the diagnosis of vasospasm following subarachnoid hemorrhage. *Neurology*. 1989;39:1514–1518.

83. Lysakowski C, Walder B, Costanza M, Ramer M. Transcranial Doppler versus angiography in patients with vasospasm due to a ruptured cerebral aneurysm. *Stroke*. 2001;32:2292–2298.

84. Manno EM, Gress DR, Schwamm LH, et al. Effects of induced hypertension on transcranial Doppler ultrasound velocities in patients after subarachnoid hemorrhage. *Stroke*. 1998;29:422–428.

85. Lindegaard KF, Nornes H, Bakke SJ, Sorteberg W, Natstad P. Cerebral vasospasm diagnosis by means of angiography and blood velocity measurements. *Acta Neurochir*. 1989;100(1–2):12–24.

86. Ekelund A, Saveland H, Romner B, Brandt L. Is transcranial Doppler sonography useful in detecting late cerebral ischaemia after aneurysmal subarachnoid haemorrhage? *Br J Neurosurg*. 1996;10(1):19–25.

87. Maroon JC, Nelson PB. Hypovolemia in patients with subarachnoid hemorrhage: therapeutic implications. *Neurosurgery*. 1979;4:223–226.

88. Solomon RA, Post KD, McMurtry JG. Depression of circulating blood volume after subarachnoid hemorrhage: Implications for treatment of symptomatic vasospasm. *Neurosurgery*. 1984;15:354–361.

89. Wijdicks EF, Vermeulen M, Hijdra A, van Gijn J. Hyponatremia and cerebral infarction in patients with ruptured intracranial aneurysms: Is fluid restriction harmful? *Ann Neurol*. 1985;17:137–140.

90. Lennihan L, Mayer SA, Matthew EF, et al. Effect of hypervolemic therapy on cerebral blood flow after subarachnoid hemorrhage: a randomized control trial. *Stroke.* 2000;31:383–391.

91. Egge A, Waterloo K, Sjoholm H, Solberg T, Ingebrigtsen T, Romner B. Prophylactic hyperdynamic postoperative fluid therapy after aneurysmal subarachnoid hemorrhage: a clinical, prospective, randomized, controlled study. *Neurosurgery.* 2001;49:593–606.

92. Gathier CS, van den Bergh WM, Slooter AJ, HIMALAIA-Study Group. HIMALAIA (Hypertension Induction in the Management of AneurysmaL subArachnoid haemorrhage with secondary IschaemiA): a randomized single-blind controlled trial of induced hypertension vs. no induced hypertension in the treatment of delayed cerebral ischemia after subarachnoid hemorrhage. *Int J Stroke.* 2014;9(3):375–380.

93. Polin RS, Coenen VA, Hansen CA, et al. Efficacy of transluminal angioplasty for the management of symptomatic cerebral vasospasm following aneurysmal subarachnoid hemorrhage. *Neurosurg.* 2000;92:284–290.

94. Zwienenberg-Lee M, Hartman J, Rudisill N, Madden L. Effect of prophylactic transluminal balloon angioplasty on cerebral vasospasm and outcome in patients with Fisher grade III subarachnoid hemorrhage: results of a phase II multicenter, randomized, clinical trial. *Stroke.* 2008;39(6):1759–1765.

95. Higashida RT, Halbach VV, Cahan LD, et al. Transluminal angioplasty for treatment of intracranial arterial vasospasm. *J Neurosurg.* 1989;71(5 Pt 1):648–653.

96. Higashida RT, Halbach VV, Dormandy B, et al. Endovascular treatment of intracranial aneurysms with a new silicone microballoon device: technical considerations and indications for therapy. *Radiology.* 1990;174(3 Pt 1):687–691.

97. Higashida RT, Halbach VV, Dowd CF, et al. Intravascular balloon dilatation therapy for intracranial arterial vasospasm: patient selection, technique, and clinical results. *Neurosurg Rev.* 1992;15:89–95.

98. Kassell NF, Helm G, Simmons N, Phillips CD, Cail WS. Treatment of cerebral vasospasm with intra-arterial papaverine. *J Neurosurg.* 1992;77(6):848–852.

99. Feng L, Fitzsimmons BF, Young WL, et al. Intraarterially administered verapamil as adjunct therapy for cerebral vasospasm: safety and 2-year experience. *Am J Neuroradiol.* 2002;23(8):1284–1290.

100. Badjatia N, Topcuoglu MA, Pryor JC, et al. Preliminary experience with intra-arterial nicardipine as a treatment for cerebral vasospasm. *Am J Neuroradiol.* 2004;25(5):819–826.

101. Biondi A, Ricciardi GK, Puybasset L, et al. Intra-arterial nimodipine for the treatment of symptomatic cerebral vasospasm after aneurismal subarachnoid hemorrhage: preliminary results. *Am J Neuroradiol.* 2004;25(6):1067–1076.

102. Fraticelli AT, Cholley BP, Losser MR, Saint Maurice JP, Payen D. Milrinone for the treatment of cerebral vasospasm after aneurismal subarachnoid hemorrhage. *Stroke.* 2008;39(3):893–898.

103. van den Bergh WM, Algra A, van der Sprenkel JW, Tulleken CA, Rinkel GJ. Hypomagnesemia after aneurysmal subarachnoid hemorrhage. *Neurosurgery.* 2003;52(2):276–281. discussion 281–2.

104. van den Berg WM, Algra A, van Kooten F, et al. Magnesium sulfate in aneurysmal subarachnoid hemorrhage: a randomized controlled trial. *Stroke.* 2005;36(5):1011–1015.

105. Veyna RS, Seyfried D, Burke, et al. Magnesium sulfate therapy after aneurysmal subarachnoid hemorrhage. *J Neurosurg.* 2002;96(3):510–514.

106. Wong GK, Chan MT, Boet R, Poon WS, Gin T. Intravenous magnesium sulfate after aneurysmal subarachnoid hemorrhage: a prospective randomized pilot study. *J Neurosurg Anesthesiol.* 2006;18(2):142–148.

107. Schmid-Elsaesser R, Kunz M, Zausinger S, Prueckner S, Briegel J, Steiger HJ. Intravenous magnesium versus nimodipine in the treatment of patients with aneurysmal subarachnoid hemorrhage: a randomized study. *Neurosurgery.* 2006;58(6):1054–1065. discussion 1054–1065.

108. Muroi C, Terzic A, Fortunati M, Yonekawa Y, Keller E. Magnesium sulfate in the management of patients with aneurysmal subarachnoid hemorrhage: a randomized, placebo-controlled, dose-adapted trial. *Surg Neurol.* 2008;69(1):33–39. discussion 39.

109. Wong GK, Poon WS, Chan MT, et al. IMASH Investigators. Intravenous magnesium sulphate for aneurysmal subarachnoid hemorrhage (IMASH): a randomized, double-blinded, placebo-controlled, multicenter phase III trial. *Stroke.* 2010;41(5):921–926.

110. Dorhout Mees SM, Algra A, Vandertop WP, et al. MASH-2 Study Group. Magnesium for aneurysmal subarachnoid hemorrhage (MASH-2): a randomized placebo-controlled trial. *Lancet.* 2012;380(9836):44–49.

111. Allen GS, Ahn HS, Preziosi TJ, et al. Cerebral arterial spasm—a controlled trial of nimodipine in patients with subarachnoid hemorrhage. *N Eng J Med.* 1983;308(11):619–624.

112. Phillippon J, Grob R, Dagreou F, Guggiari M, Rivierez M, Viars P. Prevention of vasospasm in subarachnoid haemorrhage. A controlled study with nimodipine. *Acta Neurochir (Wien).* 1986;82(3–4):110–114.

113. Neil-Dwyer G, Mee E, Dorrance D, Lowe D. Early intervention with nimodipine in subarachnoid hemorrhage. *Eur Heart J.* 1987;8(Suppl K):41–47.

114. Petruck KC, West M, Mohr G, et al. Nimodipine treatment in poor-grade aneurysm patients. Results of a multicenter double-blind placebo-controlled trial. *J Neurosurg.* 1988;68(4):505–517.

115. Pickard JD, Murray GD, Illingworth R, et al. Effect of oral nimodipine on cerebral infarction and outcome after subarachnoid haemorrhage: British aneurysm nimodipine trial. *Br Med J.* 1989;298(6674):636–642.

116. Haley Jr EC, Kassell NF, Torner JC. A randomized controlled trial of high-dose intravenous nicardipine in aneurysmal subarachnoid hemorrhage. A report of the Cooperative Aneurysm Study. *J Neurosurg.* 1993;78(4):537–547.

117. Haley Jr EC, Kassell NF, Torner JC, Truskowski LL, Germanson TP. A randomized trial of two doses of nicardipine in aneurysmal subarachnoid hemorrhage. A report of the Cooperative Aneurysm Study. *J Neurosurg.* 1994;80(5):788–796.

118. Dorhout Mees SM, Rinkel GJ, Feigin VL, et al. Calcium antagonists for aneurysmal subarachnoid hemorrhage. *Cochrane Database Syst Rev.* 2007;3:CD000277.

119. Mayberg MR, Batjer HH, Dacey R, et al. Guidelines for the management of aneurysmal subarachnoid hemorrhage. A statement for healthcare professionals from a special writing group of the Stroke Council, American Heart Association. *Circulation.* 1994;90(5):2592–2605.

120. Tseng MY, Czosnyka M, Richards H, Pickard JD, Kirkpatrick PJ. Effects of acute treatment with pravastatin on cerebral vasospasm, autoregulation, and delayed ischemic deficits after aneurysmal subarachnoid hemorrhage: a phase II randomized placebo-controlled trial. *Stroke.* 2005;36(8):1627–1632.

121. Lynch JR, Wang H, McGirt MJ, et al. Simvastatin reduces vasospasm after aneurysmal subarachnoid hemorrhage: results of a pilot randomized clinical trial. *Stroke.* 2005;36(9):2024–2026.

122. Tseng MY, Hutchinson PJ, Czosnyka M, Richards H, Pickard JD, Kirkpatrick PJ. Effects of acute pravastatin treatment on intensity of rescue therapy, length of inpatient stay, and 6-month outcome in patients after aneurysmal subarachnoid hemorrhage. *Stroke.* 2007;38(5):1545–1550.

123. Kirkpatrick PJ, Turner CL, Smith C, Hutchinson PJ, Murray GD, STASH Collaborators. Simvastatin in aneurysmal subarachnoid hemorrhage (STASH): a multicenter randomized phase III trial. *Lancet Neurol.* 2014;13(7):666–675.

124. Wong GK, Liang M, Lee MW, Po YC, Chan KY, Poon WS. High-dose simvastatin for aneurysmal subarachnoid hemorrhage: a multicenter, randomized, controlled, double-blind clinical trial protocol. *Neurosurgery.* 2013;72(5):840–844.

125. Hasan D, Wijdicks EF, Vermeulen M. Hyponatremia is associated with cerebral ischemia in patients with aneurysmal subarachnoid hemorrhage. *Ann Neurol.* 1990;27(1):106–108.

126. Sayama T, Inamura T, Matsushima T, Inoha S, Inoue T, Fukui M. High incidence of hyponatremia in patients with ruptured anterior communicating artery aneurysms. *Neurol Res.* 2000;22(2):151–155.

127. Qureshi AI, Suri MF, Sung GY, et al. Prognostic significance of hypernatremia and hyponatremia among patients with aneurysmal subarachnoid hemorrhage. *Neurosurgery.* 2002;50(4):749–755.

128. Wijdicks EF, Vermeulen M, ten Haaf JA, Hijdra A, Bakker WH, van Gijn J. Volume depletion and natriuresis in patients with a ruptured intracranial aneurysm. *Ann Neurol.* 1985;18(2):211–216.

129. Suarez JI, Qureshi AI, Parekh PD, et al. Administration of hypertonic (3%) sodium chloride/acetate in hyponatremic patients with symptomatic vasospasm following subarachnoid hemorrhage. *J Neurosurg Anesthesiol.* 1999;11(3):178–184.

130. Hasan d, Lindsay KW, Wijdicks EF, et al. Effect of fludrocortisone acetate in patients with subarachnoid hemorrhage. *Stroke.* 1989;20(9):1156–1161.

131. Mori T, Katayama Y, Kawamata T, Hirayama T. Improved efficiency of hypervolemic therapy with inhibition of natriuresis by fludrocortisone in patients with aneurysmal subarachnoid hemorrhage. *J Neurosurg.* 1999;91(6):947–952.

132. Ghali JK, Koren MJ, Taylor JR, et al. Efficacy and safety of oral conivaptan: a V1A/V2 vasopressin receptor antagonist, assessed in a randomized, placebo-controlled trial in patients with euvolemic or hypervolemic hyponatremia. *J Clin Endocrinol Metab.* 2006;91(6):2142–2152.

133. Andreoli A, di Pasquale G, Pinelli G, Grazi P, Tognetti F, Testa C. Subarachnoid hemorrhage: frequency and severity of cardiac arrhythmias. A survey of 70 cases studied in the acute phase. *Stroke.* 1987;18(3):558–564.

134. Di Pasquale G, Pinelli G, Andreoli A, Manini G, Grazi P, Tognetti F. Holter detection of cardiac arrhythmias in intracranial subarachnoid hemorrhage. *Am J Cardiol.* 1987;59(6):596–600.

135. Sommargren CE, Zaroff JG, Banki N, Drew BJ. Electrocardiographic repolarization abnormalities in subarachnoid hemorrhage. *J Electrocardiol.* 2002;35(Suppl):257–262.

136. Kono T, Morita H, Kuroiwa T, Onaka H, Takatsuka H, Fujiwara A. Left ventricular wall motion abnormalities in patients with subarachnoid hemorrhage: neurogenic stunned myocardium. *J Am Coll Cardiol.* 1994;24(3):636–640.

137. Lambert G, Naredi S, Eden E, Rydenhag B, Friberg P. Monoamine metabolism and sympathetic nervous activation following subarachnoid haemorrhage: influence of gender and hydrocephalus. *Brain Res Bull.* 2002;58(1):77–82.

138. Zaroff JG, Rordorf GA, Ogilvy CS, Picard MH. Regional patterns of left ventricular systolic dysfunction after subarachnoid hemorrhage: evidence for neurally mediated cardiac injury. *J Am Soc Echocardiogr.* 2000;13(8):774–779.

139. Kothavale A, Banki NM, Kopelnik A, et al. Predictors of left ventricular regional wall motion abnormalities after subarachnoid hemorrhage. *Neurocrit Care.* 2006;4(3):199–205.

140. Banki N, Kopelnik A, Tung P, et al. Prospective analysis of prevalence, distribution, and rate of recovery of left ventricular systolic dysfunction in patients with subarachnoid hemorrhage. *J Neurosurg.* 2006;105(1):15–20.

141. Tung P, Kopelnik A, Banki N, et al. Predictors of neurocardiogenic injury after subarachnoid hemorrhage. *Stroke.* 2004;35(2):548–551.

142. Van der Bilt I, Hasan D, van den Brink R, SEASAH Investigators, et al. Cardiac dysfunction after aneurysmal subarachnoid hemorrhage: relationship with outcome. *Neurology.* 2014;82(4):351–358.

143. Fernandez A, Schmidt JM, Claassen J, et al. Fever after subarachnoid hemorrhage: risk factors and impact on outcome. *Neurology.* 2007;68:1013–1019.

144. Dorhout Mees SM, Luitse MJ, van den Bergh WM, Rinkel GJ. Fever after aneurysmal subarachnoid hemorrhage: relation with extent of hydrocephalus and amount of extravasated blood. *Stroke.* 2008;39:2141–2143.

145. Kilpatrick MM, Lowry DW, Firlik AD, Yonas H, Marion DW. Hyperthermia in the neurosurgical intensive care unit. *Neurosurgery.* 2000;47:850–855.

146. Badjatia N. Fever control in the neuro-ICU: why, who and when? *Curr Opin Crit Care.* 2009;15(2):79–82.

147. Zhang G, Zhang JH, Qin X. Fever increased in-hospital mortality after subarachnoid hemorrhage. *Acta Neurochir Suppl.* 2011;110(Pt 1):239–243.

148. Oliveira–Filho J, Ezzeddine MA, Segal AZ, et al. Fever in subarachnoid hemorrhage: relationship to vasospasm and outcome. *Neurology.* 2001;56(10):1299–1304.

149. Badjatia N, Fernandez L, Schmidt JM, et al. Impact of induced normothermia on outcome after subarachnoid hemorrhage: a case-control study. *Neurosurgery.* 2010;66(4):696–700.

150. Sampson TR, Dhar R, Diringer MN. Factors associated with the development of anemia after subarachnoid hemorrhage. *Neurocrit Care.* 2010;12(1):4–9.

151. Kramer AH, Gurka MJ, Nathan B, Dumont AS, Kassell NF, Bleck TP. Complications associated with anemia and blood transfusion in patients with aneurysmal subarachnoid hemorrhage. *Crit Care Med.* 2008;36(7):2070–2075.

152. Giller CA, Wills MJ, Giller AM, Samson D. Distribution of hematocrit values after aneurysmal subarachnoid hemorrhage. *J Neuroimaging.* 1998;8(3):169–170.

153. Naidech AM, Drescher J, Ault ML, Shaibani A, Batjer HH, Alberts MJ. Higher hemoglobin is associated with less cerebral infarction, poor outcome, and death after subarachnoid hemorrhage. *Neurosurgery.* 2006;59(4):775–779.

154. Naidech AM, Jovanovic B, Wartenberg KE, et al. Higher hemoglobin is associated with improved outcome after subarachnoid hemorrhage. *Crit Care Med.* 2007;35(10):2383–2389.

155. Dhar R, Zazulia AR, Videen TO, Zipfel GJ, Derdeyn CP, Diringer MN. Red blood cell transfusion increases cerebral oxygen delivery in anemic patients with subarachnoid hemorrhage. *Stroke.* 2009;40(9):3039–3044.

156. Levine J, Kofke A, Cen L, et al. Red blood cell transfusion is associated with infection and extracerebral complications after subarachnoid hemorrhage. *Neurosurgery.* 2010;66(2):312–318.

157. Naidech AM, Shaibani A, Garg RK, et al. Prospective, randomized trial of higher goal hemoglobin after subarachnoid hemorrhage. *Neurocrit Care.* 2010;13(3):313–320.

64 How Should Acute Ischemic Stroke Be Managed in the Intensive Care Unit?

Allie M. Massaro, Scott E. Kasner, Joshua M. Levine

Stroke is the fourth leading cause of death in the United States and is a leading cause of long-term disability for adults.[1,2] The health-care cost of stroke patients in 2010 was estimated at $37 billion. Acute ischemic stroke (AIS) accounts for almost 90% of all stroke subtypes.[1] Comprehensive stroke centers have been shown to reduce mortality and morbidity.[3,4] Neurointensive intensive care units (NICUs) play an integral role in comprehensive stroke centers and have been associated with reduced in-hospital mortality and length of hospitalization.[5,6] The cornerstone of therapy in the NICU is to minimize secondary brain injury.

Roughly 15% to 20% of ischemic stroke patients require intensive care.[7] There are no universally agreed on intensive care unit (ICU) admission criteria for patients with AIS; however, common indications include the presence of hemorrhagic transformation, the presence or risk of significant cerebral edema and herniation, intubation due to brainstem compression, hemodynamic instability, and postprocedural or postsurgical care.[8]

EMERGENCY SETTING

Stroke remains a clinical diagnosis; therefore history and physical examination are critical. Given the narrow therapeutic window for acute treatment, timely diagnosis and identification of symptom onset are essential. Approximately 1 to 2 million neurons are lost per minute of delay.[9] Intravenous (IV) recombinant tissue plasminogen activator (rt-PA) (alteplase [Activase]) is the only medication approved by the U.S. Food and Drug Administration for the treatment of AIS.[10] The randomized multicenter National Institute of Neurological Disorders and Strokes (NINDS) rt-PA study demonstrated roughly double the odds of a very favorable outcome in patients who were treated with rt-PA within 3 hours of symptom onset compared with placebo.[10] This benefit was observed at 3 months in the primary outcome of a composite of the National Institutes of Health (NIH) Stroke Scale (NIHSS), modified Rankin Scale (mRS), Barthel Index, and Glasgow Outcome Scale.[10] Subsequent randomized trials, including Alteplase Thrombolysis for Acute Noninterventional Therapy in Ischemic

Stroke (ATLANTIS),[11] European Cooperative Acute Stroke Study (ECASS),[12] and ECASSII,[13] failed to show benefit for thrombolysis in the 3- to 6-hour time window. ESCASS III, however, identified a significant but slightly smaller benefit in patients treated with rt-PA between 3 and 4.5 hours of symptom onset (mRS 0 to 1 in 52.4% treatment arm vs. placebo 45.2%).[14] A recent meta-analysis of 27 randomized trials (n = 10,187) reviewing thrombolysis in AIS showed that thrombolysis (IV and intraarterial) up to 6 hours after AIS significantly reduced morbidity and mortality at 3 to 6 months (odds ratio [OR] 0.85; confidence interval [CI], 0.78 to 0.93)[15] and that treatment within 3 hours was associated with more benefit (OR, 0.66; 95% CI, 0.56 to 0.79).[15]

The major contraindications to IV rt-PA include major surgery within the past 14 days, international normalized ratio (INR) greater than 1.7, platelet count less than 100,000, history of intracerebral hemorrhage, and sustained blood pressure greater than 185/110 mm Hg.[10] The American Heart Association/American Stroke Association (AHA/ASA) recommends administration of IV rt-PA (0.9 mg/kg with 10% given as a bolus and the remainder as an infusion over 1 hour) to eligible patients within 4.5 hours of stroke symptom onset and a door-to-needle time of less than 60 minutes.[8] Many centers have adopted an approach that was developed in Helsinki, Finland, in which suspected acute stroke patients are taken directly from the door to the computed tomography (CT) scanner and, if eligible, are given IV rt-PA immediately after the CT scan, reducing door-to-needle time to about 20 minutes.[16]

Given worse outcomes in patients ineligible for IV rt-PA, especially for those with middle cerebral artery (MCA) occlusions, intra-arterial rt-PA has been evaluated for safety and efficacy. The Prolyse in Acute Cerebral Thromboembolism (PROACT) study randomized 40 patients to intra-arterial infusion of prourokinase or placebo. The treatment arm was associated with a significant increase in vessel recanalization; however, there was a concomitant increase in symptomatic intracerebral hemorrhage (sICH) (15.4% vs. 7.1%).[17] PROACT II, a multicenter single blind trial in which 180 patients were randomized to treatment with intra-arterial prourokinase plus heparin or heparin alone demonstrated improved outcome at 90 days for patients with stroke due to MCA occlusion who were treated with prourokinase within 6 hours of symptom onset.[18] The primary endpoint of mRS 0 to 2 was achieved in 40% of the treatment arm and 25% in the control group, with a 66% recanalization rate in the treatment group versus 18% in the control group. There was an increase in early sICH in the treatment arm (10% vs. 2%).[18] This study opened the window for intervention for AIS to up to 6 hours with intra-arterial thrombolysis.

Nonpharmacologic approaches to thrombolytic therapy have also been developed. Four devices are available in the United States: the MERCI retriever,[19] the Penumbra suction catheter,[20] the Solitaire stentriever,[21] and the Trevo retrieval system.[22] Each has been shown to successfully open thrombosed arteries, but none has been subjected to a randomized comparison to placebo or IV tissue plasminogen activator (tPA). The one randomized clinical trial (RCT) in this arena compared the MERCI with Solitaire devices and found improved recanalization rates and clinical outcomes with the Solitaire stentriever.[21]

The combination of IV and endovascular thrombolytic therapy has also been studied. The Interventional Management of Acute Stroke (IMS) series of trials evaluated the feasibility and safety of combining IV rt-PA and intra-arterial thrombolysis.[23,24] Ultimately the IMS III randomized trial of standard IV rt-PA versus IV rt-PA followed by intra-arterial thrombolysis was stopped early because of futility after more than 650 patients were randomized.[24] There was no significant difference in functional outcome (mRS of 2 or less) at 90 days (40.8% with endovascular therapy, 38.7% with IV rt-PA). On the basis of these data, the AHA/ASA suggested that it is reasonable to consider endovascular thrombolytic therapy in patients who are not candidates for IV rt-PA or for patients with a proximal MCA occlusion who are at an experienced stroke center with qualified interventionalists.[8] Evidence does not support substitution of intra-arterial thrombolysis for IV rt-PA.

There is emerging evidence to support the use of therapeutic protocols that combine rt-PA and intra-arterial stenting. The EXTEND-IA (Extending the Time for Thrombolysis in Emergency Neurological Deficits–Intra-arterial) study,[25] based in Australia and New Zealand, randomized patients already receiving rt-PA (0.9 mg/kg) for AIS, within 4.5 hours of onset, to endovascular thrombectomy with the Solitaire FR (Flow Restoration) stent retriever or to continue receiving IV rt-PA alone. The study was limited to patients with strokes in specified locations (internal carotid and middle cerebral arteries) and who had clearly salvageable brain tissue: the ischemic core had to be less than 70 mL on CT perfusion imaging.

Only 70 patients were enrolled in the trial before it was stopped because of significant outcome benefits in the intervention (stent) group. There were two observable benefits. First, the proportion of ischemic tissue that was reperfused was significantly greater in the endovascular-therapy group than in the rt-PA–only group (median, 100% vs. 37%; $P < .001$). In addition, there were significant neurologic improvements at 3 and 90 days. There were no significant differences in death or intracranial hemorrhage. Endovascular therapy was initiated at a median of 210 minutes after the onset of stroke symptoms.

A Dutch multicenter study, MR CLEAN (Multicenter Randomized Clinical trial of Endovascular treatment for Acute ischemic stroke in the Netherlands),[26] randomized patients with proximal arterial occlusion (distal intracranial carotid artery, middle cerebral artery [M1 or M2], or anterior cerebral artery [A1 or A2]), in the anterior cerebral circulation, within 6 hours of symptom onset, 89% of whom were receiving rt-PA, to intra-arterial therapy—intra-arterial rt-PA or endovascular stenting, or standard therapy—the majority of whom received continued IV thrombolysis. Five hundred patients were enrolled at 16 centers, and 190 of 223 patients randomized to the "intra-arterial" group received endovascular stents. There was significant improvement in functional outcome at 90 days in the intervention group, as measured by the modified Rankin Score (0 to 2) (32.6% vs. 19.1%; OR, 1.67; CI, 1.21 to 2.30; absolute risk reduction [ARR], 13.5%; number needed to treat [NNT], 8). There were no significant differences in mortality or intracranial hemorrhage.

The ESCAPE (Endovascular Treatment for Small Core and Proximal Occlusion Ischemic Stroke) trial[27] was a large, international, 22-center trial that randomized a similar cohort of patients with proximal intracranial occlusion in the anterior circulation but stretched the time limit to 12 hours after symptoms had become apparent. Of the 316 participants enrolled, 238 received IV alteplase, and of those, 120 received endovascular stenting. Again, the study was stopped early for efficacy; mortality was significantly reduced in the group who received endovascular stents (10.4% vs. 19.0% in the control group; $P = .04$; ARR, 8.6%; NNT, 12). The intervention group also had significantly better functional outcomes at 90 days (53.0% vs. 29.3% in the control group; $P < .001$; ARR, 23.7%; NNT, <5). There was no difference in the development of intracranial hemorrhage (3.6% vs. 2.7%, control group; $P = .75$).

In summary, endovascular stenting appears to be a highly effective therapy for patients suitable for thrombolysis who have proximal anterior circulation or middle cerebral strokes, small infarct cores, reasonably good collateral circulation, and rapid access to an interventional neuroradiology unit.

CRITICAL CARE MANAGEMENT

Airway, Ventilation, and Oxygenation

As in all medical emergencies, airway management is paramount. In AIS, common reasons for intubation include depressed level of consciousness, hypoventilation, and oropharyngeal dysfunction that may increase the risk of aspiration. In patients with brainstem infarction, and less commonly with hemispheric infarction, protective swallow and cough reflexes may be diminished, leading to airway compromise. A major therapeutic goal is prevention of further tissue hypoxia and worsening of brain injury. The need for intubation portends a poor prognosis, with 50% mortality in 30 days.[28] Tracheostomy is recommended for patients with brainstem dysfunction that compromises central respiratory drive or that results in bulbar palsies and in patients with prolonged mechanical ventilation. Tracheostomy allows for less sedation, increased patient comfort, less airway dead space, and decreased work of breathing. A prospective randomized trial, Stroke-related Early Tracheostomy versus Prolonged Orotracheal Intubation in Neurocritical Care Trial (SETPOINT), evaluated the optimal timing of tracheostomy in ventilated patients with severe stroke.[29] Early tracheostomy (within 1 to 3 days of intubation) was safe, did not increase length of stay in the ICU, and decreased the need for sedation; however, its effect on mortality and outcome is unknown.[29] It is reasonable to discuss tracheostomy with the AIS patient or family members on a case-by-case basis and when the patient is expected to be intubated for more than 7 to 10 days.

Studies in nonintubated patients with AIS do not support the use of supplemental oxygenation unless oxygen saturation falls below 94%.[8] Hypoxia should be evaluated and treated similar to that for any critically ill patient. In practice, most nonintubated stroke patients do not require supplemental oxygen.

BLOOD PRESSURE CONTROL AND CARDIAC CARE

High blood pressure after AIS occurs in up to 80% of patients.[8,30] The ideal blood pressure after AIS is unknown; however, both high and low blood pressures are associated with poor outcome.[31,32] Ideally, blood pressure should be monitored continuously by an intra-arterial catheter to detect rapid fluctuations. High blood pressure is associated with an increased risk of recurrent AIS within 14 days; patients in whom systolic blood pressure (SBP) is more than 200 mm Hg have a 50% or more greater risk of recurrence compared with patients in whom SBP is 130 mm Hg.[31] There is a U-shaped relationship between blood pressure and mortality.[31,32] A post hoc analysis of data from the International Stroke Trial (IST) suggests that for every 10 mm Hg below 150 mm Hg the risk of early death increases by nearly 18%, and for every 10 mm Hg above 150 mm Hg early death increases by 3.8%.[31] A smaller observational study suggested that for every 10 mm Hg below 180 mm Hg of SBP, the risk of early poor outcome increased by 25%, whereas for every 10 mm Hg above 180 mm Hg, the risk of poor outcome increased by 23%.[32] It is presumed that hypertension is associated with poor outcome because of increased risk of recurrent stroke, hemorrhagic conversion of ischemic infarct, continued vascular damage, and worsening of cerebral edema.

Although hypertension is associated with poorer outcome, the impact of lowering blood pressure is unclear. The angiotensin-receptor blocker candesartan for treatment of acute stroke trial (SCAST) randomized more than 2000 patients to an angiotensin-receptor blocker (candesartan) or a placebo for 1 week after stroke. At 6 months the treatment group had a significantly lower blood pressure but also a higher risk of poor functional outcome as measured by the mRS (OR, 1.17).[33] Current recommendations from the AHA/ASA include permissive hypertension for patients who did not receive thrombolytic therapy (SBP <220 mm Hg; diastolic blood pressure [DBP], < 120 mm Hg). For patients who are to be treated with rt-PA, blood pressure should be maintained below 185/110 mm Hg before drug administration and below 180/105 mm Hg for the first 24 hours after treatment.[8] In most patients, blood

pressure declines without any medical intervention.[34] If antihypertensive therapy is needed, then the drug of choice should be short acting and have a reliable dose-response curve. Although labetalol and nicardipine are commonly used in the ICU, there are no data to guide choice of optimal antihypertensive agents.

Frank hypotension is relatively uncommon in stroke patients and should be avoided. Patients who have hypotension should be evaluated for myocardial ischemia and for aortic dissection, which may be causally related to the stroke. Neurogenic myocardial stunning may result from the stroke and may result in cardiogenic shock. Between 10% and 18% of patients with AIS have an elevated serum troponin level.[35,36] Patients who become hypotensive after thrombolytic therapy should be promptly evaluated for extracranial hemorrhage and for cardiac tamponade from hemopericardium.

Pharmacologic augmentation of blood pressure in patients who are normotensive (induced hypertension) is not routinely recommended. Theoretically, induced hypertension might increase cerebral blood flow to ischemic regions of brain. Small pilot studies suggest that raising blood pressure with vasopressors might be safe, but its impact on outcome is not known.[37,38]

FLUID MANAGEMENT

Stroke patients can become volume depleted from insensible losses and decreased oral intake from dysphagia and altered mental status. Euvolemia should be maintained in all patients. IV fluids should be dosed and adjusted daily based on clinical determination of volume status. There is no evidence to support routine placement of a central venous catheter to guide volume administration by measurement of central venous pressure. Isotonic crystalloid IV fluid solutions, such as 0.9% saline, Normosol-R, or Plasma Lyte 148, are preferred. Hypotonic solutions increase cerebral edema and exacerbate brain injury.[8] Hypertonic solutions have not been proven to be beneficial. A large randomized double-blinded trial found no benefit to administration of 25% albumin compared with normal saline with respect to 90-day outcome.[39]

GLUCOSE CONTROL

Hyperglycemia is present in up to one third of AIS patients and in observational studies is independently associated with poor outcomes.[40-42] Whether hyperglycemia is a marker of injury severity or is causally related to brain injury, or both, remains unclear. Deleterious effects of hyperglycemia might include increased brain tissue acidosis, increased blood–brain barrier permeability, and increased odds of hemorrhagic transformation.[41,43] Persistent hyperglycemia (>200 mg/dL) within the first 24 hours after stroke correlates with expansion of stroke volume and poor neurologic outcome.[42] The optimal blood glucose level is unknown, and treatment targets vary across guidelines. In the Intensive Insulin Therapy Trial (ITT), AIS patients were randomized to receive intensive insulin infusion (<126 mg/dL) versus standard subcutaneous insulin treatment for 24 hours. Intensive insulin therapy was associated with better glucose control over the first 24 hours but also with increased infarct size on magnetic resonance imaging.[44] A 2014 Cochrane review analyzed 1583 patients from 11 RCTs and suggested that intensive insulin therapy was associated with an increased risk of symptomatic hypoglycemia and did not affect functional outcome or mortality.[45] The Stroke Hyperglycemia Insulin Network Effort (SHINE) trial is an ongoing multicentered, randomized double-blinded trial that aims to compare aggressive glycemic control with IV insulin to maintain blood glucose in the range of 80 to 130 mg/dL versus "routine" glycemic control with subcutaneous insulin to a target of below 180 mg/dL.[46] Current AHA/ASA guidelines recommend maintenance of glucose between 140 and 180 mg/dL (7 to 10 mmol/L) and use of an insulin infusion if needed.[8] Frequent monitoring of blood glucose levels should be performed, and hyperglycemia should be minimized.

Hypoglycemia is a potential mimic of AIS, and serum glucose levels should be checked in the emergency setting. Hypoglycemia after AIS is uncommon and is typically related to diabetic medications.[8] Hypoglycemia (glucose level <60 mg/dL [3.3 mmol/L]) should be identified and treated rapidly.

TEMPERATURE

Fever occurs in 25% to 50% of patients with AIS and is consistently and independently associated with increased morbidity and mortality in cohort studies.[47-49] Fever on admission and within the first 24 hours after stroke onset is associated with worse outcome.[50,51] For each 1°C increase in admission body temperature, the relative risk of poor outcome increases by 2.2.[52] Fever may be due to a systemic inflammatory response, but an infectious cause should be sought.

Although fever control is recommended as standard of care, there have been no randomized trials of fever control. Trials have, however, examined fever prevention. In the Paracetamol (Acetaminophen) in Stroke (PAIS) trial, patients with admission temperature (36°C to 39°C) were randomized to paracetamol (6 g) or placebo within 12 hours of stroke onset. There was no difference between groups in outcome (mRS) at 3 months.[53] A post hoc analysis identified a modest increase in functional improvement in patients with baseline temperature higher than 37°C. To corroborate these results, a PAIS II trial is currently ongoing.[54]

Patients who have hypothermia may have reduced mortality and better long-term outcomes.[52,55] The impact of therapeutic hypothermia on outcome is unknown. Two clinical trials have shown feasibility of both surface and endovascular cooling methods in patients with AIS.[56,57] The Intravascular Cooling in the Treatment of Stroke (ICTuS-L) trial suggested that the combination of hypothermia (induced by an endovascular cooling catheter) and thrombolysis is feasible. Hypothermia was not associated with an increased risk of bleeding; however, there was an association with pneumonia.[58] The ongoing ICTuS 2/3 study aims to further test the safety of hypothermia and the difference in outcome between patients treated with hypothermia plus thrombolysis and patients treated with thrombolysis alone.[59] An international multicenter phase III clinical trial is also underway to determine whether hypothermia improves functional outcome after AIS.[60]

HEMOGLOBIN MANAGEMENT

Both anemia and polycythemia may be deleterious in patients with AIS. A prospective cohort study of more than 800 AIS patients showed an association between anemia and increased mortality, and the worst outcomes present in those with both low and high hemoglobin levels (i.e., a "U-shaped" relationship between hemoglobin and outcome).[61] A retrospective analysis of 109 patients with AIS showed that low hemoglobin count and red blood cell transfusion was associated with prolonged NICU stay and duration of mechanical ventilation but was not associated with mortality or 3-month functional outcome.[62] In this study nearly all patients (97.2%) had anemia, and one third received blood transfusions (at the discretion of the physician), which did not confer an advantage in long-term outcome.[62]

The impact of red blood cell transfusion on outcome is unclear, and no prospective randomized trials have addressed the optimal transfusion threshold in patients with AIS. In the general critical care population, a meta-analysis demonstrated an increased risk of health-care–associated infections, such as pneumonia and sepsis, with a liberal transfusion policy (hemoglobin count <10 g/dL) compared with a restrictive policy (hemoglobin count <7 g/dL).[63] A second meta-analysis showed that restrictive blood transfusion (hemoglobin count <7 g/dL) was associated with a decreased incidence of coronary events, bacterial infections, and mortality.[64]

In patients with AIS, the risks associated with both anemia and red blood cell transfusion should be weighed on an individual basis. It is recommended that both anemia and aggressive transfusion practice be avoided.

ANTITHROMBOTIC MEDICATIONS

For patients who are not candidates for reperfusion therapy, antithrombotic therapy is the mainstay of treatment. The Chinese Acute Stroke Trial (CAST), a randomized placebo-controlled trial of more than 20,000 patients, and the International Stroke Trial (IST), a randomized trial of almost 20,000 patients, demonstrated a decrease in ischemic stroke recurrence rate when aspirin was given within 48 hours of symptom onset (1.6% vs. 2.1%; P=.01; and 2.8% vs. 3.9%; P<.001, respectively), with no significant increase in hemorrhagic conversion.[65,66] In the CAST study, there was also a small but significant decrease in mortality in aspirin-treated patients (3.3% vs. 3.9%).[65] Treatment effect was independent of age, stroke severity, and stroke subtype.

More recent studies corroborate the benefit of early antithrombotic drug administration in patients with AIS. In the Fast Assessment of Stroke and Transient Ischemic Attack to Prevent Early Recurrence (FASTER) trial, almost 400 patients with transient ischemic attack (TIA) or stroke

(NIHSS <4) were randomized to treatment with clopidogrel or placebo and simvastatin or placebo. All patients also received aspirin. The clopidogrel arm had a 7.1% stroke risk within 90 days compared with 10.8% in the placebo arm (risk ratio, 0.7 [95% CI, 0.3 to 1.2]; ARR, 3.8% [95% CI, 9.4 to 1.9]; P = .19).[67] In the randomized, double-blinded placebo controlled Clopidogrel with Aspirin in Acute Minor Stroke or Transient Ischemic Attack (CHANCE) trial, 5170 Chinese patients were assigned to clopidogrel and aspirin or to placebo plus aspirin within 24 hours of minor stroke or TIA.[68] The primary endpoint, stroke at 90 days, occurred in 8.2% of patients in the clopidogrel-aspirin group and in 11.7% of the aspirin-alone group (hazard ratio, 0.68; 95% CI, 0.57 to 0.81; P <.001). There was no difference in hemorrhage rate (0.3%). An ongoing randomized, double-blinded, placebo-controlled study in the United States, the Platelet-Oriented Inhibition in New TIA and Minor Ischemic Stroke (POINT) trial, is assessing the impact on outcome (ischemic vascular event at 90 days) of clopidogrel and aspirin initiated within 12 hours of symptom onset. Additional antiplatelet agents are also being studied. The Acute Stroke of Transient Ischemic Attack Treated with Aspirin or Ticagrelor and Patient Outcomes (SOCRATES) trial is an ongoing double-blinded RCT that aims to compare the effect on outcome of ticagrelor versus aspirin.

Currently, most patients with AIS should be treated with aspirin 325 mg within 24 to 48 hours after stroke symptom onset.[8] The primary effect of aspirin is a reduction in early recurrent stroke.[8] Aspirin is not recommended as a substitute for rt-PA. For patients who receive thrombolysis, antithrombotic agents must be avoided for the first 24 hours. Aspirin is usually initiated after a head CT obtained 24 hours after rt-PA administration demonstrates absence of intracerebral hemorrhage. There is no convincing evidence to support the use of other oral antiplatelet agents such as clopidogrel, dipyridamole, ticagrelor, and ticlopidine. Administration of IV antiplatelet agents, such as the glycoprotein IIb/IIIa inhibitor (abcixamab), is largely ineffective.[69]

Data do not support the routine use of systemic anticoagulation with heparin in AIS.[8] Therapeutic heparin may be considered in select patients with carotid artery dissection, although there are no randomized clinical trials to support this practice.[70] The decision about whether to use systemic anticoagulation in the acute to subacute period should be made on a case-by-case basis. A detailed discussion is beyond the scope of this chapter.

MALIGNANT INFARCTION

Malignant infarction refers to life-threatening cerebral edema from AIS. It is observed in 1% to 10% of patients with supratentorial infarction[71-73] and typically in patients with occlusion of the internal carotid artery or proximal MCA (Fig. 64-1).[71] Peak swelling usually occurs 2 to 5 days after stroke onset, but up to one third of patients may have neurologic deterioration in the first 24 hours.[74,75] Clinical features of malignant infarction include headache, declining level of consciousness, nausea/vomiting, paralysis ipsilateral to the hemispheric infarction, and signs of brainstem dysfunction. The prognosis of malignant infarctions

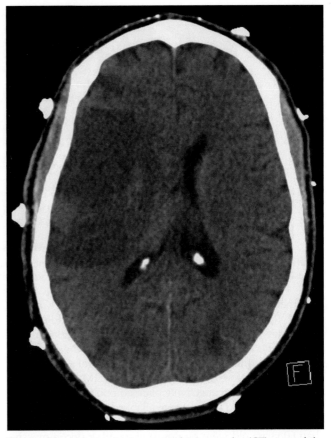

Figure 64-1. Noncontrast computed tomography (CT) scan of the head showing a right malignant middle cerebral artery (MCA) ischemic stroke with surrounding edema and midline shift.

is poor, with mortality of up to 80% in malignant MCA infarction.[76,77] In a retrospective case-controlled study, predictors of malignant infarction included early hypodensity involving more than 50% of the MCA territory, a history of hypertension or heart failure, increased baseline white blood cell count, and involvement of additional vascular territories.[78] An autopsy series of 192 patients identified 45 patients with nonlacunar malignant MCA territory strokes, and predictors of malignant edema included younger age, no history of stroke, carotid occlusion, higher heart weight, and abnormal ipsilateral circle of Willis, with a slight predominance of female sex.[79]

Medical therapy has limited success in patients with malignant infarction. Measures to decrease intracranial pressure (ICP) such as hyperventilation, osmotic therapy, steroids, and barbiturates are not effective long-term therapies.[80-82] ICP monitors are not routinely used because of the focal nature of the compressive lesion, which may cause herniation without a global rise in ICP.

In contrast to medical therapy, surgical intervention has been shown to decrease both mortality and functional disability. Surgery provides an immediate reduction in ICP and improvement in blood flow and allows the brain to herniate out of the craniectomy defect instead of toward the brainstem. There have been four randomized clinical trials looking at functional outcome after decompressive surgery: Decompressive Craniectomy in Malignant Middle Cerebral Artery Infarcts (DECIMAL), Decompressive Surgery for the

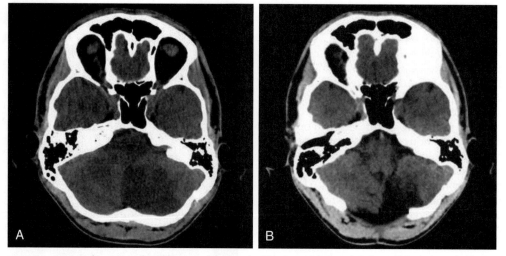

Figure 64-2. Noncontrast computed tomography (CT) scan of the head with an acute ischemic infarct of the left cerebellar hemisphere. **A,** There is mass effect and effacement of the fourth ventricle. **B,** After suboccipital decompressive hemicraniectomy.

Treatment of Malignant Infarction of the Middle Cerebral Artery (DESTINY), Hemicraniectomy after Middle Cerebral Artery Infarction with Life-threatening Edema trial (HAMLET), and Decompressive Surgery for the Treatment of Malignant Infarction of the Middle Cerebral Artery (DESTINY II).[83-86] Before the completion of DECIMAL, DESTINY, and HAMLET, a prospectively planned pooled meta-analysis was undertaken to hasten the available data and reliably estimate treatment effect.[75] In total, 93 patients who were no more than 60 years old were randomized to either decompressive surgery within 48 hours of AIS or conservative management. Surgery was associated with improved functional outcome and reduced mortality (28% vs. 78% in the medical arm). The probability of having an mRS of less than 3 (moderate disability but able to walk unassisted) nearly doubled; however, the probability of having an mRS of 4 (severe disability, unable to attend to bodily needs, cannot walk without assistance) increased more than 10 times.[75] The NNT was 2 to prevent one death, 2 to prevent mRS of 5 or death, and 4 to prevent mRs of 4 or death.[75]

DESTINY II evaluated the role of decompressive hemicraniectomy versus conservative management in older patients (>60 years) with MCA stroke.[86] Hemicraniectomy improved the primary outcome of survival without severe disability (defined as mRS 0 to 4) at 6 months (38% vs. 18%). However, most survivors required assistance with most bodily needs, and no patients had an mRS of 0 to 2 (survival with no disability or minor disability).[86]

Although hemicraniectomy improves mortality, functional outcomes are improved to some extent and only in patients younger than 60 years. The decision to pursue decompressive hemicraniectomy should be made on an individual basis.

CEREBELLAR INFARCTION

Cerebellar infarction often presents with minor, seemingly benign symptoms such as ataxia and dysarthria; however, patients may experience precipitous fatal deterioration. Cerebellar infarctions are life threatening because the posterior fossa is a relatively small and rigid compartment. Edema from cerebellar infarction may therefore result in direct compression of the brainstem, compression of the fourth

ventricle and acute noncommunicating hydrocephalus, and upward or downward cerebellar herniation (Fig. 64-2).[87-89] In patients who have acute hydrocephalus, an external ventricular drain may be placed to rapidly drain cerebral spinal fluid and lower ICP; however, there remains a risk of upward herniation.[87,88,90,91] Suboccipital decompressive craniectomy (SDC) is a lifesaving intervention that is less controversial than decompressive hemicraniectomy.[92,93] There are no RCTs guiding timing or patient selection for SDC; however, its benefit is considered self-evident, and it is recommended as the therapy of choice by the ASA to relieve both hydrocephalus and acute brainstem compression.[8]

COMPLICATIONS OF ISCHEMIC STROKE

Hemorrhagic Transformation and Complications of Thrombolytic Therapy

The risk of spontaneous hemorrhagic transformation of AIS is generally low (0.6%) but increases with the use of IV rt-PA or intra-arterial thrombolytic therapy.[10,66] The risk of symptomatic intracerebral hemorrhage after IV rt-PA is about 5%, and after intra-arterial pharmacologic or mechanical thrombolysis is 10%.[10,94] Predictors of hemorrhagic transformation include age, high NIHSS, elevated serum glucose level, and early mass effect.[95,96]

Treatment of spontaneous hemorrhagic conversion is generally supportive. With any decline in neurologic status during thrombolysis the infusion should be immediately stopped, and emergent noncontrast head CT should be obtained, along with complete blood count and coagulation profile. No therapy has been proven successful in reversing the effects of rt-PA; reasonable options include fibrinogen, cryoprecipitate, fresh frozen or thawed plasma (FFP or TP), and platelets. Neurosurgical consultation may be helpful in select cases where there is concern for increased ICP and mass effect.

A rare complication of rt-PA is angioedema, which occurs in 1% to 3% of patients. It typically manifests 30 to 120 minutes after the initial infusion and classically occurs contralateral to the ischemic lesion.[97] Activation of the complement and kinin cascades due to the presence of increased plasmin has been implicated. This risk is increased in patients taking angiotensin-converting enzyme inhibitors, which act along a similar pathway.[98] Management for mild angioedema includes administration of 50 mg IV diphenhydramine followed by 100 mg of IV methylprednisolone or nebulized epinephrine.[99] In cases where there is airway compromise, urgent intubation or establishment of an emergency surgical airway may be required.

Additional complications associated with intra-arterial therapy include arterial perforation, intracranial arterial embolization, subarachnoid hemorrhage, groin site pseudoaneurysm, and retroperitoneal hematoma. These complications occur infrequently (<5%).[100] In a retrospective case series, postoperative patients treated with intra-arterial therapy for AIS had a higher risk of systemic bleeding (25%), usually at the surgical site.[101]

Seizures

The incidence of seizure after stroke has a reported range of 2% to 33%, depending on the study design;[102-104] however, prospective studies suggest a lower frequency of 2% to 8%.[105-110] Although clinical seizures in the acute setting are relatively uncommon, prolonged electroencephalography reveals nonconvulsive seizures in up to one third of patients with an abnormal level of consciousness.[111,112] Risk factors for seizure include greater stroke severity, cortical infarction, a cardioembolic cause of AIS, and hemorrhagic conversion.[106,110] In theory, seizures may worsen stroke outcome by increasing the risk of aspiration, causing blood pressure and vital sign fluctuations, and increasing ICP. However, mounting evidence suggests an association between burden of antiepileptic drug exposure and worse cognitive outcomes.[105,113,114] It is recommended to treat seizures aggressively if they occur but not to administer prophylactic anticonvulsants. Electroencephalogram monitoring should be considered in AIS patients with depressed levels of consciousness, although data are lacking regarding the impact on the outcome of treating nonconvulsive seizures.

AUTHORS' RECOMMENDATIONS

- Patients with AIS should be cared for at a comprehensive stroke center with the availability of a NICU.
- IV rt-PA is recommended within 4.5 hours of symptom onset for eligible patients.
- Patients with proximal anterior circulation lesions who are suitable for rt-PA, with moderate-sized stroke area and good collateral circulation, appear to be ideal candidates for endovascular stent placement. Endovascular therapy in this setting significantly reduces mortality and improves 90-day functional outcome.
- Oral administration of aspirin (initial dose, 325 mg) within 24 to 48 hours is indicated for most patients.
- Permissive hypertension is acceptable in the acute setting with goal SBP below 220 mm Hg and DBP below 120 mm Hg or, in a patient treated with rt-PA, below 180/105 mm Hg.
- Decompressive craniectomy for malignant supratentorial cerebral infarction is lifesaving; however, advanced patient age increases the risk of severe disability and should be discussed on a case-by-case basis.
- Suboccipital decompressive crainiectomy for space-occupying cerebellar infarction is recommended to treat hydrocephalus and reduce brainstem compression.

REFERENCES

1. Go AS, Mozaffarian D, Roger VL, et al. Heart disease and stroke statistics–2014 update: a report from the American Heart Association. *Circulation.* 2014;129(3):e28–e292.
2. Prevalence and most common causes of disability among adults–United States, 2005. *MMWR Morb Mortal Wkly Rep.* 2009;58(16):421–426.
3. Stroke Unit Trialists' Collaboration. Collaborative systematic review of the randomised trials of organised inpatient (stroke unit) care after stroke. *BMJ.* 1997;314:1151–1159.
4. Govan L, Weir CJ, Langhorne P. Organized inpatient (stroke unit) care for stroke. *Stroke.* 2008;39:2402–2403.
5. Suarez JI. Outcome in neurocritical care: advances in monitoring and treatment and effect of a specialized neurocritical care team. *Crit Care Med.* 2006;34(suppl 9):S232–S238.
6. Suarez JI, Zaidat OO, Suri MF, et al. Length of stay and mortality in neurocritically ill patients: impact of a specialized neurocritical care team. *Crit Care Med.* 2004;32(11):2311–2317.
7. Zazulia AR. Critical care management of acute ischemic stroke. *Continuum Lifelong Learn Neurol.* 2009;15(3):68–82.
8. Jauch EC, Saver JL, Adams Jr HP, et al. Guidelines for the early management of patients with acute ischemic stroke: a guideline for healthcare professionals from the American Heart Association/American Stroke Association. *Stroke.* 2013;44(3):870–947.
9. Saver JL, Fonarow GC, Smith EE, et al. Time to treatment with intravenous tissue plasminogen activator and outcome from acute ischemic stroke. *JAMA.* 2013;309(23):2480–2488.
10. NINDS rt-PA Stroke Study Group. Tissue plasminogen activator for acute ischemic stroke. *N Engl J Med.* 1995;333:1581–1588.
11. Clark WM, Wissman S, Albers GW, Jhamandas JH, Madden KP, Hamilton S. Recombinant tissue-type plasminogen activator (Alteplase) for ischemic stroke 3 to 5 hours after symptom onset. The ATLANTIS Study: a randomized controlled trial. Alteplase Thrombolysis for Acute Noninterventional Therapy in Ischemic Stroke. *JAMA.* 1999;282(21):2019–2026.
12. Hacke W, Kaste M, Fieschi C, et al. Intravenous thrombolysis with recombinant tissue plasminogen activator for acute hemispheric stroke. The European Cooperative Acute Stroke Study (ECASS). *JAMA.* 1995;274(13):1017–1025.
13. Hacke W, Kaste M, Fieschi C, et al. Randomised double-blind placebo-controlled trial of thrombolytic therapy with intravenous alteplase in acute ischaemic stroke (ECASS II). Second European-Australasian Acute Stroke Study Investigators. *Lancet.* 1998;352(9136):1245–1251.
14. Hacke W, Kaste M, Bluhmki E, et al. Thrombolysis with alteplase 3 to 4.5 hours after acute ischemic stroke. *N Engl J Med.* 2008;359(13):1317–1329.
15. Wardlaw JM, Murray V, Berge E, del Zoppo GJ. Thrombolysis for acute ischaemic stroke. *Cochrane Database Syst Rev.* 2014;7:CD000213.
16. Meretoja A, Strbian D, Mustanoja S, Tatlisumak T, Lindsberg PJ, Kaste M. Reducing in-hospital delay to 20 minutes in stroke thrombolysis. *Neurology.* 2012;79(4):306–313.
17. del Zoppo GJ, Higashida RT, Furlan AJ, Pessin MS, Rowley HA, Gent M. PROACT: a phase II randomized trial of recombinant pro-urokinase by direct arterial delivery in acute middle cerebral artery stroke. PROACT Investigators. Prolyse in Acute Cerebral Thromboembolism. *Stroke.* 1998;29(1):4–11.
18. Furlan A, Higashida R, Wechsler L, et al. Intra-arterial prourokinase for acute ischemic stroke. The PROACT II study: a randomized controlled trial. Prolyse in Acute Cerebral Thromboembolism. *JAMA.* 1999;282(21):2003–2011.
19. Smith WS, Sung G, Starkman S, et al. Safety and efficacy of mechanical embolectomy in acute ischemic stroke: results of the MERCI trial. *Stroke.* 2005;36(7):1432–1438.
20. The penumbra pivotal stroke trial: safety and effectiveness of a new generation of mechanical devices for clot removal in intracranial large vessel occlusive disease. *Stroke.* 2009;40(8):2761–2768.
21. Saver JL, Jahan R, Levy EI, et al. Solitaire flow restoration device versus the Merci Retriever in patients with acute ischaemic stroke (SWIFT): a randomised, parallel-group, non-inferiority trial. *Lancet.* 2012;380(9849):1241–1249.
22. Nogueira RG, Lutsep HL, Gupta R, et al. Trevo versus Merci retrievers for thrombectomy revascularisation of large vessel occlusions in acute ischaemic stroke (TREVO 2): a randomised trial. *Lancet.* 2012;380(9849):1231–1240.

23. The Interventional Management of Stroke (IMS) II Study. *Stroke*. 2007;38(7):2127–2135.
24. Broderick JP, Palesch YY, Demchuk AM, et al. Endovascular therapy after intravenous t-PA versus t-PA alone for stroke. *N Engl J Med*. 2013;368(10):893–903.
25. Campbell BC, EXTEND-IA Investigators, et al. Endovascular therapy for ischemic stroke with perfusion-imaging selection. *N Engl J Med*. March 12, 2015;372(11):1009–1018.
26. Berkhemer OA, MR CLEAN Investigators, et al. A randomized trial of intraarterial treatment for acute ischemic stroke. *N Engl J Med*. January 1, 2015;372(1):11–20.
27. Goyal M, ESCAPE Trial Investigators, et al. Randomized assessment of rapid endovascular treatment of ischemic stroke. *N Engl J Med*. March 12, 2015;372(11):1019–1030.
28. Bushnell CD, Phillips-Bute BG, Laskowitz DT, Lynch JR, Chilukuri V, Borel CO. Survival and outcome after endotracheal intubation for acute stroke. *Neurology*. 1999;52(7):1374–1381.
29. Bosel J, Schiller P, Hook Y, et al. Stroke-related Early Tracheostomy versus Prolonged Orotracheal Intubation in Neurocritical Care Trial (SETPOINT): a randomized pilot trial. *Stroke*. 2013;44(1):21.
30. Qureshi AI, Ezzeddine MA, Nasar A, et al. Prevalence of elevated blood pressure in 563,704 adult patients with stroke presenting to the ED in the United States. *Am J Emerg Med*. 2007;25(1):32–38.
31. Leonardi-Bee J, Bath PM, Phillips SJ, Sandercock PA. Blood pressure and clinical outcomes in the International Stroke Trial. *Stroke*. 2002;33(5):1315–1320.
32. Castillo J, Leira R, Garcia MM, Serena J, Blanco M, Davalos A. Blood pressure decrease during the acute phase of ischemic stroke is associated with brain injury and poor stroke outcome. *Stroke*. 2004;35(2):520–526.
33. Sandset EC, Bath PM, Boysen G, et al. The angiotensin-receptor blocker candesartan for treatment of acute stroke (SCAST): a randomised, placebo-controlled, double-blind trial. *Lancet*. 2011;377(9767):741–750.
34. Phillips SJ. Pathophysiology and management of hypertension in acute ischemic stroke. *Hypertension*. 1994;23(1):131–136.
35. Jensen JK, Kristensen SR, Bak S, Atar D, Hoilund-Carlsen PF, Mickley H. Frequency and significance of troponin T elevation in acute ischemic stroke. *Am J Cardiol*. 2007;99(1):108–112.
36. Kerr G, Ray G, Wu O, Stott DJ, Langhorne P. Elevated troponin after stroke: a systematic review. *Cerebrovasc Dis*. 2009;28(3):220–226.
37. Marzan AS, Hungerbuhler HJ, Studer A, Baumgartner RW, Georgiadis D. Feasibility and safety of norepinephrine-induced arterial hypertension in acute ischemic stroke. *Neurology*. 2004;62(7):1193–1195.
38. Hillis AE, Ulatowski JA, Barker PB, et al. A pilot randomized trial of induced blood pressure elevation: effects on function and focal perfusion in acute and subacute stroke. *Cerebrovasc Dis*. 2003;16(3):236–246.
39. Ginsberg MD, Palesch YY, Hill MD, et al. High-dose albumin treatment for acute ischaemic stroke (ALIAS) Part 2: a randomised, double-blind, phase 3, placebo-controlled trial. *Lancet Neurol*. 2013;12(11):1049–1058.
40. Weir CJ, Murray GD, Dyker AG, Lees KR. Is hyperglycaemia an independent predictor of poor outcome after acute stroke? Results of a long-term follow up study. *BMJ*. 1997;314(7090):1303–1306.
41. Williams LS, Rotich J, Qi R, et al. Effects of admission hyperglycemia on mortality and costs in acute ischemic stroke. *Neurology*. 2002;59(1):67–71.
42. Baird TA, Parsons MW, Phanh T, et al. Persistent poststroke hyperglycemia is independently associated with infarct expansion and worse clinical outcome. *Stroke*. 2003;34(9):2208–2214.
43. Lindsberg PJ, Roine RO. Hyperglycemia in acute stroke. *Stroke*. 2004;35(2):363–364.
44. Rosso C, Corvol JC, Pires C, et al. Intensive versus subcutaneous insulin in patients with hyperacute stroke: results from the randomized INSULINFARCT trial. *Stroke*. 2012;43(9):2343–2349.
45. Bellolio MF, Gilmore RM, Ganti L. Insulin for glycaemic control in acute ischaemic stroke. *Cochrane Database Syst Rev*. 2014;1:CD005346.
46. Bruno A, Durkalski VL, Hall CE, et al. The Stroke Hyperglycemia Insulin Network Effort (SHINE) trial protocol: a randomized, blinded, efficacy trial of standard vs. intensive hyperglycemia management in acute stroke. *Int J Stroke*. 2014;9(2):246–251.
47. Azzimondi G, Bassein L, Nonino F, et al. Fever in acute stroke worsens prognosis: a prospective study. *Stroke*. 1995;26:2040–2043.
48. Grau AJ, Buggle F, Schnitzler P, Spiel M, Lichy C, Hacke W. Fever and infection early after ischemic stroke. *J Neurol Sci*. 1999;171(2):115–120.
49. Wrotek SE, Kozak WE, Hess DC, Fagan SC. Treatment of fever after stroke: conflicting evidence. *Pharmacotherapy*. 2011;31(11):1085–1091.
50. Castillo J, Davalos A, Marrugat J, Noya M. Timing for fever-related brain damage in acute ischemic stroke. *Stroke*. 1998;29(12):2455–2460.
51. Wang Y, Lim LL, Levi C, Heller RF, Fisher J. Influence of admission body temperature on stroke mortality. *Stroke*. 2000;31(2):404–409.
52. Reith J, Jorgensen HS, Pedersen PM, et al. Body temperature in acute stroke: relation to stroke severity, infarct size, mortality, and outcome. *Lancet*. 1996;347(8999):422–425.
53. den Hertog HM, van der Worp HB, van Gemert HM, et al. The Paracetamol (Acetaminophen) In Stroke (PAIS) trial: a multicentre, randomised, placebo-controlled, phase III trial. *Lancet Neurol*. 2009;8(5):434–440.
54. de Ridder IR, de Jong FJ, den Hertog HM, et al. Paracetamol (Acetaminophen) in stroke 2 (PAIS 2): Protocol for a randomized, placebo-controlled, double-blind clinical trial to assess the effect of high-dose paracetamol on functional outcome in patients with acute stroke and a body temperature of 36.5°C or above. *Int J Stroke*. 2015;10(3):457–462.
55. Kammersgaard LP, Jorgensen HS, Rungby JA, et al. Admission body temperature predicts long-term mortality after acute stroke: the Copenhagen Stroke Study. *Stroke*. 2002;33(7):1759–1762.
56. De Georgia MA, Krieger DW, Abou-Chebl A, et al. Cooling for Acute Ischemic Brain Damage (COOL AID): a feasibility trial of endovascular cooling. *Neurology*. 2004;63(2):312–317.
57. Krieger DW, De Georgia MA, Abou-Chebl A, et al. Cooling for acute ischemic brain damage (cool aid): an open pilot study of induced hypothermia in acute ischemic stroke. *Stroke*. 2001;32(8):1847–1854.
58. Hemmen TM, Raman R, Guluma KZ, et al. Intravenous thrombolysis plus hypothermia for acute treatment of ischemic stroke (ICTuS-L): final results. *Stroke*. 2010;41(10):2265–2270.
59. Lyden PD, Hemmen TM, Grotta J, Rapp K, Raman R. Endovascular therapeutic hypothermia for acute ischemic stroke: ICTuS 2/3 protocol. *Int J Stroke*. 2014;9(1):117–125.
60. van der Worp HB, Macleod MR, Bath PM, et al. EuroHYP-1: European multicenter, randomized, phase III clinical trial of therapeutic hypothermia plus best medical treatment vs. best medical treatment alone for acute ischemic stroke. *Int J Stroke*. 2014;9(5):642–645.
61. Tanne D, Molshatzki N, Merzeliak O, Tsabari R, Toashi M, Schwammenthal Y. Anemia status, hemoglobin concentration and outcome after acute stroke: a cohort study. *BMC Neurol*. 2010;10:22.
62. Kellert L, Schrader F, Ringleb P, Steiner T, Bosel J. The impact of low hemoglobin levels and transfusion on critical care patients with severe ischemic stroke: STroke: RelevAnt Impact of HemoGlobin, Hematocrit and Transfusion (STRAIGHT)—an observational study. *J Crit Care*. 2014;29(2):236–240.
63. Rohde JM, Dimcheff DE, Blumberg N, et al. Health care-associated infection after red blood cell transfusion: a systematic review and meta-analysis. *JAMA*. 2014;311(13):1317–1326.
64. Salpeter SR, Buckley JS, Chatterjee S. Impact of more restrictive blood transfusion strategies on clinical outcomes: a meta-analysis and systematic review. *Am J Med*. 2014;127(2):124–131. e123.
65. CAST (Chinese Acute Stroke Trial) Collaborative Group. CAST: randomised placebo-controlled trial of early aspirin use in 20,000 patients with acute ischemic stroke. *Lancet*. 1997;349:1641–1649.
66. International Stroke Trial Collaborative Group. The International Stroke Trial (IST): a randomised trial of aspirin, heparin, both, or neither among 19435 patients with acute ischaemic stroke. *Lancet*. 1997;349:1569–1581.
67. Kennedy J, Hill MD, Ryckborst KJ, Eliasziw M, Demchuk AM, Buchan AM. Fast assessment of stroke and transient ischaemic attack to prevent early recurrence (FASTER): a randomised controlled pilot trial. *Lancet Neurol*. 2007;6(11):961–969.
68. Wang Y, Wang Y, Zhao X, et al. Clopidogrel with aspirin in acute minor stroke or transient ischemic attack. *N Engl J Med*. 2013;369(1):11–19.

69. Adams Jr HP, Effron MB, Torner J, et al. Emergency administration of abciximab for treatment of patients with acute ischemic stroke: results of an international phase III trial: Abciximab in Emergency Treatment of Stroke Trial (AbESTT-II). *Stroke.* 2008;39(1):87–99.

70. Lyrer P, Engelter S. Antithrombotic drugs for carotid artery dissection. *Cochrane Database Syst Rev.* 2003;3:CD000255.

71. Flechsenhar J, Woitzik J, Zweckberger K, Amiri H, Hacke W, Juttler E. Hemicraniectomy in the management of space-occupying ischemic stroke. *J Clin Neurosci.* 2013;20(1):6–12.

72. Shaw CM, Alvord Jr EC, Berry RG. Swelling of the brain following ischemic infarction with arterial occlusion. *Arch Neurol.* 1959;1:161–177.

73. Frank JI. Large hemispheric infarction, deterioration, and intracranial pressure. *Neurology.* 1995;45:1286–1290.

74. Qureshi AI, Suarez JI, Yahia AM, et al. Timing of neurologic deterioration in massive middle cerebral artery infarction: a multicenter review. *Crit Care Med.* 2003;31(1):272–277.

75. Vahedi K, Hofmeijer J, Juettler E, et al. Early decompressive surgery in malignant infarction of the middle cerebral artery: a pooled analysis of three randomised controlled trials. *Lancet Neurol.* 2007;6(3):215–222.

76. Hacke W, Schwab S, Horn M, Spranger M, DeGeorgia M, von Kummer R. The 'malignant' middle cerebral artery territory infarction: clinical course and prognostic signs. *Arch Neurol.* 1996;53:309–315.

77. Berrouschot J, Sterker M, Bettin S, Koster J, Schneider D. Mortality of space-occupying ('malignant') middle cerebral artery infarction under conservative intensive care. *Intensive Care Med.* 1998;24(6):620–623.

78. Kasner SE, Demchuk AM, Berrouschot J, et al. Predictors of fatal brain edema in massive hemispheric ischemic stroke. *Stroke.* 2001;32(9):2117–2123.

79. Jaramillo A, Gongora-Rivera F, Labreuche J, Hauw JJ, Amarenco P. Predictors for malignant middle cerebral artery infarctions: a postmortem analysis. *Neurology.* 2006;66(6):815–820.

80. Hofmeijer J, van der Worp HB, Kappelle LJ. Treatment of space-occupying cerebral infarction. *Crit Care Med.* 2003;31(2):617–625.

81. Righetti E, Celani MG, Cantisani T, Sterzi R, Boysen G, Ricci S. Glycerol for acute stroke. *Cochrane Database Syst Rev.* 2000;4:CD000096.

82. Schwab S, Spranger M, Schwarz S, Hacke W. Barbiturate coma in severe hemispheric stroke: useful or obsolete? *Neurology.* 1997;48(6):1608–1613.

83. Vahedi K, Vicaut E, Mateo J, et al. Sequential-design, multicenter, randomized, controlled trial of early decompressive craniectomy in malignant middle cerebral artery infarction (DECIMAL Trial). *Stroke.* 2007;38(9):2506–2517.

84. Juttler E, Schwab S, Schmiedek P, et al. Decompressive Surgery for the Treatment of Malignant Infarction of the Middle Cerebral Artery (DESTINY): a randomized, controlled trial. *Stroke.* 2007;38(9):2518–2525.

85. Hofmeijer J, Kappelle LJ, Algra A, Amelink GJ, van Gijn J, van der Worp HB. Surgical decompression for space-occupying cerebral infarction (the Hemicraniectomy After Middle Cerebral Artery infarction with Life-threatening Edema Trial [HAMLET]): a multicentre, open, randomised trial. *Lancet Neurol.* 2009;8(4):326–333.

86. Juttler E, Unterberg A, Woitzik J, et al. Hemicraniectomy in older patients with extensive middle-cerebral-artery stroke. *N Engl J Med.* 2014;370(12):1091–1100.

87. Greenberg J, Skubick D, Shenkin H. Acute hydrocephalus in cerebellar infarct and hemorrhage. *Neurology.* 1979;29(3):409–413.

88. Horwitz NH, Ludolph C. Acute obstructive hydrocephalus caused by cerebellar infarction. Treatment alternatives. *Surg Neurol.* 1983;20(1):13–19.

89. Jensen MB, St Louis EK. Management of acute cerebellar stroke. *Arch Neurol.* 2005;62(4):537–544.

90. Hornig CR, Rust DS, Busse O, Jauss M, Laun A. Space-occupying cerebellar infarction. Clinical course and prognosis. *Stroke.* 1994;25(2):372–374.

91. Mathew P, Teasdale G, Bannan A, Oluoch-Olunya D. Neurosurgical management of cerebellar haematoma and infarct. *J Neurol Neurosurg Psychiatry.* 1995;59(3):287–292.

92. Pfefferkorn T, Eppinger U, Linn J, et al. Long-term outcome after suboccipital decompressive craniectomy for malignant cerebellar infarction. *Stroke.* 2009;40(9):3045–3050.

93. Chen HJ, Lee TC, Wei CP. Treatment of cerebellar infarction by decompressive suboccipital craniectomy. *Stroke.* 1992;23(7):957–961.

94. Furlan A, Higashida R, Wechsler L, et al. Intra-arterial prourokinase for acute ischemic stroke. The PROACT II study: a randomized controlled trial. *JAMA.* 1999;282:2003–2011.

95. The NINDS rt-PA Stroke Study Group. Intracerebral hemorrhage after intravenous t-PA therapy for ischemic stroke. *Stroke.* 1997;28:2109–2118.

96. Heuschmann PU, Kolominsky-Rabas PL, Roether J, et al. Predictors of in-hospital mortality in patients with acute ischemic stroke treated with thrombolytic therapy. *JAMA.* 2004;292(15):1831–1838.

97. Ottomeyer C, Hennerici MG, Szabo K. Raising awareness of orolingual angioedema as a complication of thrombolysis in acute stroke patients. *Cerebrovasc Dis.* 2009;27(3):307–308.

98. Hill MD, Barber PA, Takahashi J, Demchuk AM, Feasby TE, Buchan AM. Anaphylactoid reactions and angioedema during alteplase treatment of acute ischemic stroke. *CMAJ.* 2000;162(9):1281–1284.

99. Lee K. *The NeuroICU Book.* The McGraw Hill Companies; 2012.

100. Schellinger PD, Fiebach JB, Mohr A, Ringleb PA, Jansen O, Hacke W. Thrombolytic therapy for ischemic stroke–a review. Part II–Intra-arterial thrombolysis, vertebrobasilar stroke, phase IV trials, and stroke imaging. *Crit Care Med.* 2001;29(9):1819–1825.

101. Chalela JA, Katzan I, Liebeskind DS, et al. Safety of intra-arterial thrombolysis in the postoperative period. *Stroke.* 2001;32(6):1365–1369.

102. Burn J, Dennis M, Bamford J, Sandercock P, Wade D, Warlow C. Epileptic seizures after a first stroke: the Oxfordshire Community Stroke Project. *BMJ.* 1997;315(7122):1582–1587.

103. Bladin CF, Alexandrov AV, Bellavance A, for the Seizures After Stroke Study Group, et al. Seizures after stroke: a prospective multicenter study. *Arch Neurol.* 2000;57(11):1617–1622.

104. Camilo O, Goldstein LB. Seizures and epilepsy after ischemic stroke. *Stroke.* 2004;35(7):1769–1775.

105. Ryvlin P, Montavont A, Nighoghossian N. Optimizing therapy of seizures in stroke patients. *Neurology.* 2006;67(12 suppl 4):S3–S9.

106. Bladin CF, Alexandrov AV, Bellavance A, et al. Seizures after stroke: a prospective multicenter study. *Arch Neurol.* 2000;57(11):1617–1622.

107. Lamy C, Domigo V, Semah F, et al. Early and late seizures after cryptogenic ischemic stroke in young adults. *Neurology.* 2003;60(3):400–404.

108. Giroud M, Gras P, Fayolle H, Andre N, Soichot P, Dumas R. Early seizures after acute stroke: a study of 1,640 cases. *Epilepsia.* 1994;35(5):959–964.

109. Kilpatrick CJ, Davis SM, Tress BM, Rossiter SC, Hopper JL, Vandendriesen ML. Epileptic seizures in acute stroke. *Arch Neurol.* 1990;47(2):157–160.

110. Beghi E, D'Alessandro R, Beretta S, et al. Incidence and predictors of acute symptomatic seizures after stroke. *Neurology.* 2011;77(20):1785–1793.

111. Jordan KG. Nonconvulsive status epilepticus in acute brain injury. *J Clin Neurophysiol.* 1999;16(4):332–340. discussion 353.

112. Drislane FW. Presentation, evaluation, and treatment of nonconvulsive status epilepticus. *Epilepsy Behav.* 2000;1(5):301–314.

113. Goldstein LB, Matchar DB, Morgenlander JC, Davis JN. Influence of drugs on the recovery of sensorimotor function after stroke. *J Neuro Rehab.* 1990;4:137–144.

114. Goldstein LB. Common drugs may influence motor recovery after stroke. The Sygen In Acute Stroke Study Investigators. *Neurology.* 1995;45(5):865–871.

How Should Status Epilepticus Be Managed?

Debbie H. Yi, Kathryn A. Davis, Joshua M. Levine

Status epilepticus (SE) may be defined as continuous clinical and/or electrographic seizures lasting at least 5 minutes or recurrent discrete seizures without interictal recovery of consciousness.[1] It is a medical emergency and requires prompt recognition and treatment to limit morbidity and mortality. Few randomized controlled trials exist to inform treatment, and practice algorithms vary. In response to the heterogeneity of practice, in 2012, the Neurocritical Care Society published authoritative evidence-based expert consensus guidelines for the evaluation and management of status epilepticus.[2] This chapter provides background on the epidemiology, classification, pathophysiology, and causes of SE and focuses on evidence-based clinical management.

EPIDEMIOLOGY

Studies pertaining to the epidemiology of SE are limited by the changing definitions of SE over time and underreporting. For more than 50% of cases, SE is the result of a patient's first seizure.[1] The incidence is thought to be grossly underestimated but has been cited as 65,000 to 150,000 in the United States per year.[3] In a prospective population analysis of SE in Richmond, Virginia, patients were followed for 30 days after seizures were controlled or to the time of death. The incidence was found to be 41 per 100,000 per year, and there was a bimodal age distribution with clustering in the first year of life and in people older than 60 years. Those older than age 60 had the highest incidence and the highest rate of recurrence. Overall mortality was 22% despite a pediatric mortality of approximately 3%.[4]

CLASSIFICATION

A common way to categorize SE is based on whether seizures are focal or generalized and whether consciousness is impaired. In simple partial SE (also termed *epilepsia partialis continua* when there is motor involvement), seizures emanate from a focal brain region and produce focal symptoms (e.g., unilateral twitching of a limb, aphasia) without impairment of consciousness. In complex partial SE, seizures emanate from a focal brain region, produce focal symptoms, and are associated with impaired consciousness. In generalized SE, seizures involve the entire brain, and consciousness is always impaired. Generalized and complex partial SE is considered more threatening than simple partial SE. The latter typically does not require treatment in an intensive care unit (ICU) and will not be addressed in this chapter. In the ICU, SE often occurs in patients who have preexisting altered mental status from other causes (e.g., cardiac arrest, traumatic brain injury). Therefore, for practical purposes in the ICU, seizures may be classified as (1) convulsive or nonconvulsive and (2) responsive to therapy or refractory. Convulsive SE consists of tonic-clonic movements (rhythmic jerking) and altered mental status (either as coma, lethargy, or confusion). On electroencephalogram (EEG), there are bilateral, symmetric discharges.[1] More than half of patients with generalized convulsive SE respond to a single antiepileptic drug (AED).[5] Development of generalized convulsive SE during hospitalization, older age, and longer duration and severity of impaired consciousness are associated with a poor outcome.[2] Nonconvulsive SE (NCSE) is defined as seizure activity without convulsions (shaking) and is only reliably diagnosed with an EEG. In the ICU, NCSE might be included on the differential diagnosis of any patient with altered mental status. Patients with NCSE may have alterations in behavior, including agitation; aggression; alterations in thought, including confusion and psychosis; and alterations in level of arousal, ranging from lethargy to coma. There may be subtle motor signs, such as muscle twitching, nystagmus, or eye deviation, or none at all.[6] Factors associated with a poor outcome include more serious illness as the cause of seizures, severely altered mental status, and longer seizure duration.[2] Refractory SE may be defined as SE that does not abate after standard initial treatments, typically a benzodiazepine and a bolus of an AED.[5] Refractory SE may be convulsive ("clinical") or nonconvulsive ("subclinical" or "electrographic"). This diagnosis can be subjective because it is sometimes difficult to ascertain whether "adequate" therapy was administered (e.g., in the prehospital or emergency department setting). Patients with a more severe cause, advanced age, longer seizure duration, and high APACHE-2 (Acute Physiology and Chronic Health Evaluation II) scores have worse outcomes.[2]

PATHOPHYSIOLOGY

Seizures have an immediate and often dramatic direct effect on systemic and cerebral physiology at the organ, cellular, and molecular level. SE may result in secondary systemic complications that contribute to morbidity and mortality.

Widespread neuronal depolarization during SE results in a significant increase in the cerebral metabolic rate for oxygen. Because of metabolic autoregulation, this leads to increased systemic blood pressure and cardiac output and results in an increase in cerebral blood flow. In turn, this causes an increase in cerebral blood volume, which causes increased intracranial pressure. This can be especially problematic in patients with low intracranial compliance and can result in catastrophic intracranial hypertension and death. Systemic complications of SE include hypoxia, hypotension, metabolic acidosis, hyperthermia, rhabdomyolysis, and hypoglycemia. Hyperthermia is a result of the increased motor activity seen in seizures. For this reason, patients can also manifest secondary rhabdomyolysis and metabolic acidosis. Initial acute hypertension may give way to normotension or even hypotension. Low blood pressure potentiates brain damage because of inadequate cerebral perfusion. Hypoglycemia can be seen in late SE.[1] Prolonged seizures cause a massive release of glutamate that initiates a cascade of processes, including mitochondrial dysfunction, oxidative stress, inflammatory reactions, and immunosuppression.[7] This eventually leads to neuronal excitotoxicity and injury as well as cellular ischemia and, inevitably, cell death. Animal studies suggest deleterious effects on neurons when there is more than 30 minutes of seizure activity.[1]

ETIOLOGIES

Virtually any insult to the brain may cause seizures and SE. SE may be due to acute insults, such as metabolic abnormalities (e.g., hypoglycemia, hyponatremia); hypoxia; global brain ischemia (e.g., cardiac arrest); medications; toxic ingestions; withdrawal from alcohol, benzodiazepines, and other toxins; infectious or autoimmune encephalitis; sepsis; cerebral vascular insults (bleeding more often than ischemia); acute traumatic brain injury; hypertensive encephalopathy; eclampsia; and neurosurgery. SE may also result from remote structural injury to the brain, including prior head injury, meningitis, stroke, or hypoxic-ischemic encephalopathy. It is frequently observed in patients with epilepsy because of their underlying seizure disorder, because of subtherapeutic AED levels, or because of a superimposed insult (e.g., infection). However, up to 50% of patients who have SE have no prior history of seizures.[8]

MANAGEMENT

SE is a medical emergency. Time is of the essence to prevent permanent brain injury and to limit systemic complications. The longer SE lasts, the less likely it will respond to therapy.[9] Treatment of seizures and diagnostic efforts typically proceed in parallel. Initial measures involve stabilization of the airway, breathing, and circulation coupled with emergent efforts to terminate seizures. Seizure termination occurs in successive stages, which are described in detail in the following sections. Definitive seizure control should be obtained within 60 minutes of onset if possible. There is a scarcity of randomized controlled studies to inform the optimal bundle of therapies (preferred drugs, dosages, sequence of administration) for SE, and the treatment approach outlined is largely the product of observational data and expert opinion (Figs. 65-1 and 65-2).

FIRST-TIER (EMERGENCY) THERAPIES

A short-acting benzodiazepine is the initial drug of choice for seizure termination. Intravenous (IV) access should be

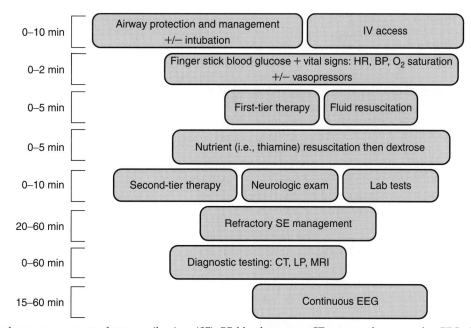

Figure 65-1. Critical care management of status epilepticus (*SE*). *BP*, blood pressure; *CT*, computed tomography; *EEG*, electroencephalogram; *HR*, heart rate; *IV*, intravenous; *LP*, lumbar puncture; *MRI*, magnetic resonance imaging; *O₂*, oxygen. (*Adapted from the Neurocritical Care Society's Guidelines for the Evaluation and Management of Status Epilepticus [Neurocrit Care. 2012;17:3–23.]*)

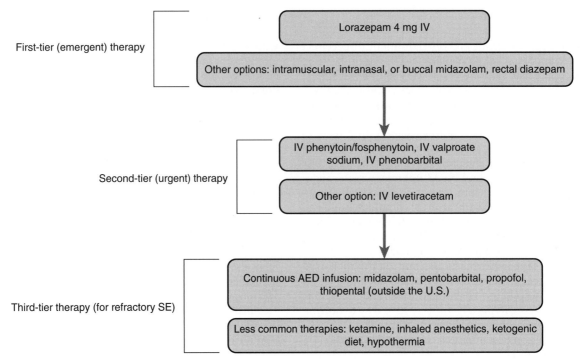

First-tier (emergent) therapy

Lorazepam 4 mg IV

Other options: intramuscular, intranasal, or buccal midazolam, rectal diazepam

Second-tier (urgent) therapy

IV phenytoin/fosphenytoin, IV valproate sodium, IV phenobarbital

Other option: IV levetiracetam

Third-tier therapy (for refractory SE)

Continuous AED infusion: midazolam, pentobarbital, propofol, thiopental (outside the U.S.)

Less common therapies: ketamine, inhaled anesthetics, ketogenic diet, hypothermia

Figure 65-2. Treatment algorithm for status epilepticus (*SE*). *AED*, antiepileptic drug; *IV*, intravenous.

obtained immediately, and therapy typically begins with administration of lorazepam (4 mg IV). This decision is guided by the double-blind multicenter Veterans Administration cooperative trial, in which 384 patients with generalized convulsive SE were randomized to one of four initial IV treatments: (1) diazepam (0.15 mg/kg) followed by phenytoin (18 mg/kg), (2) lorazepam (0.1 mg/kg), (3) phenobarbital (15 mg/kg), or (4) phenytoin (18 mg/kg). The study endpoint ("success") was defined as cessation of motor and electrographic seizures within 20 minutes of the start of drug infusion and no seizure recurrence within 40 minutes. Treatments ordered by success were as follows: lorazepam (64.9%), phenobarbital (55.8%), diazepam and phenytoin (55.8%), and phenytoin (43.6%; *P* = .02 for overall comparison among the four groups). In an intention-to-treat analysis, the difference between groups was no longer significant. The authors concluded that lorazepam is more effective than phenytoin (*P* = .002 for pairwise comparison), and although it is no more effective than phenobarbital or diazepam plus phenytoin, it is easier to use.[3] If the first dose of IV lorazepam fails to terminate seizures, then a second dose should be administered within 5 to 10 minutes in conjunction with a second-line AED. If IV access has not been established, then intraosseous access should be considered. Alternatively, IV, intramuscular (IM), intranasal, or buccal midazolam, or rectal diazepam, may be administered. Midazolam is likely as effective as lorazepam and has more predictable pharmacokinetics. A double-blind, randomized, noninferiority trial of 448 subjects with SE suggested that in the prehospital setting, IM midazolam was safe and at least as effective as IV lorazepam for seizure termination.[10] In parallel with efforts to abort seizures, the cause of SE is sought, and select life-threatening causes (e.g., bacterial meningitis, viral encephalitis, hypoxia) are empirically

treated. IV access must be expeditiously obtained. If oxygenation or ventilation is compromised, then intubation is performed. It is imperative to understand that neuromuscular blocking (NMB) agents will stop tonic-clonic activity but will have no impact on seizures. Once NMBs are administered, it must be assumed that SE is still present until proven otherwise (with EEG). For patients who have SE and fever or in whom there is history or examination findings suggestive of meningoencephalitis, empiric antibiotics and acyclovir are administered, and unless contraindicated, a lumbar puncture should be performed. Routine laboratory testing includes measurement of serum glucose and electrolytes, blood urea nitrogen, creatinine, liver function tests, and AED levels. When there is a suspicion for a toxic cause or there is no clear cause of seizures, a urine toxicology screen and measurement of the levels of alcohol, salicylates, acetaminophen, and tricyclics may be helpful. Metabolic abnormalities, such as hypoglycemia or hyponatremia, should be treated immediately if they are considered causative. If SE is due to hypoglycemia or hyponatremia, then correction of the underlying abnormality usually obviates the need for AED therapy.

SECOND-TIER (CONTROL) THERAPIES

The vast majority of patients with SE will require second-tier AED therapy. If first-tier therapies were successful in aborting seizures, then the goal of second-tier therapies is to prevent recurrence. If first-tier therapies were unsuccessful, then the goal of second-tier therapies is to terminate SE. The aim of second-tier therapy is to rapidly achieve a therapeutic AED level and to sustain it with scheduled maintenance doses. The optimal second-tier AED is unknown, and both data and expert opinion are conflicting. Available options include IV phenytoin, fosphenytoin, sodium valproate, levetiracetam, and phenobarbital (phenobarbitone). Given the lack of data, no strong recommendations may be made for one particular AED over another; selection of an agent is typically based on local protocol or based on individual patient and drug characteristics. A thorough knowledge of AED side effects is crucial to anticipate and rapidly respond to complications. IV phenytoin is diluted in propylene glycol, resulting in a highly basic solution. Infiltration into soft tissue may result in severe injury ("purple glove syndrome") that, in extreme cases, may result in limb amputation. Phenytoin is associated with significant hypotension, particularly at rapid infusion rates, and may cause arrhythmias. Fosphenytoin is a prodrug developed as an alternative to phenytoin.[11] It is not diluted in propylene glycol; therefore it likely does not carry the same risk of soft tissue injury. As with phenytoin, fosphenytoin administration may be complicated by hypotension and arrhythmias. Monitoring of cardiac rhythm and blood pressure is mandatory for safe administration. Sodium valproate is associated with hyperammonemia, thrombocytopenia, hepatotoxicity, and pancreatitis. Levetiracetam is relatively well tolerated; however, there exists only level IIb evidence for its efficacy as a second-line agent. Phenobarbital and midazolam are associated with respiratory depression, hypotension, and deep sedation.

THIRD-TIER THERAPIES (FOR REFRACTORY SE)

SE that does not respond to first- and second-tier therapy may be considered refractory. There are no data to guide the optimal waiting period for initiation of third-tier therapies. Current recommendations based on expert opinion suggest immediate initiation of treatment.[2] Treatment options include (1) repeating bolus administration of a second-tier AED, and if seizures persist, then initiation of a continuous infusion of an AED at anesthetic doses or (2) directly resorting to a continuous AED infusion. Options for continuous AED infusions include midazolam, pentobarbital, propofol, and thiopental (thiopentone). Lack of sufficient comparative data regarding relative safety and effectiveness preclude a recommendation of one AED over the other; the choice of agent is dictated by local protocol or by consideration of patient and drug characteristics. Less common therapies include ketamine, volatile inhaled anesthetics, a ketogenic diet, and mild to moderate hypothermia. These are supported only by case reports and are not recommended as routine therapies.[12-15] The dose of medication (infusion rate) should be titrated to the lowest dose necessary to achieve an EEG endpoint—either seizure cessation or burst suppression (alternating high-amplitude electrical activity [bursts] and periods of no apparent brain activity [suppression]).[16] There are no data to suggest that one approach is better than the other; however, consideration should be given to the side effect profile of individual agents and context-sensitive half-life.

From this perspective, propofol causes significantly more hypotension than benzodiazepines, but it is more titratable with a shorter duration of action. Barbiturates have a large volume of distribution and undergo zero-order kinetics, resulting in prolonged duration of action. Continuous electroencephalography is widely used to guide therapy in refractory SE, although there is a lack of data to guide duration of use. Data are lacking to guide duration of pharmacologic coma.[17] Customarily, burst suppression is achieved for 24 to 48 hours followed by gradual weaning of the anesthetic while monitoring for recurrent seizures with continuous EEG. Should SE recur during weaning of an AED infusion, then the dose is increased to achieve seizure suppression, and an additional AED may be necessary. If a continuous infusion of one AED fails to suppress seizures, then adding a second agent or switching therapy should be considered.

NATURAL HISTORY AND PROGNOSIS

The longer SE persists, the more difficult it becomes to terminate the seizures. With the progression of SE, there are changes to the GABA (γ-aminobutyric acid)–receptor action, NMDA (*N*-methyl-D-aspartate) receptor–mediated transmission, receptor trafficking, and mitochondrial function. These changes are thought to contribute to refractoriness. (The North London Convulsive Status Epilepticus in Childhood Surveillance Study [NLSTEPSS] found that when prehospital treatment was not administered, there was an association with episodes of SE longer than 60 minutes).[8] Patients treated within an hour had 80% success rate at terminating seizure activity. If 2 or more hours elapsed, then 40% to 50% were successfully terminated. If SE lasts longer than 60 minutes, then there is 30% mortality.[3] Functional outcome is affected by the duration of refractory SE. There is a 21% likelihood of a return to baseline function after refractory SE as compared with 63% for nonrefractory SE.[18,19] However, there are case reports of patients being treated for weeks to months and still making an excellent functional recovery.[19]

AUTHORS' RECOMMENDATIONS

- SE is defined as continuous clinical and/or electrographic seizures lasting at least 5 minutes or recurrent discrete seizures without interictal recovery of consciousness.
- SE may occur in any ICU, consequent of a medley of clinical conditions.
- Morbidity and mortality directly correlate with the duration of seizures.
- Therapy is directed at terminating, as quickly as possible, the seizures by using an escalating therapeutic protocol, and at detecting and treating the underlying cause (if any).
- Initial therapy usually involves administration of a rapidly acting benzodiazepine (lorazepam or midazolam), followed by AEDs, such as phenytoin or valproate.
- For refractory cases, general anesthetic agents are administered, usually titrated, to specified EEG endpoints.
- Functional outcome appears to be dependent on the duration of seizure activity.

REFERENCES

1. Working Group on Status Epilepticus. Treatment of convulsive status epilepticus. *JAMA*. 1993;270(7):854–859.
2. Neurocritical Care Society Status Epilepticus Guideline Writing Committee, Brophy GM, Bell R, et al. Guidelines for the evaluation and management of status epilepticus. *Neurocrit Care*. 2012;17(1):3–23.
3. Treiman DM, Meyers PD, Walton NY, et al. A comparison of four treatments for generalized convulsive status epilepticus. *N Engl J Med*. 1998;339(12):792–798.
4. DeLorenzo RJ, Hauser WA, Towne AR, et al. A prospective, population-based epidemiologic study of status epilepticus in Richmond. *Virginia*. 1996;46(4):1029–1035.
5. Mayer SA, Claassen J, Lokin J, Mendelsohn F, Dennis LJ, Fitzsimmons B-F. Refractory status epilepticus. *Arch Neurol*. 2002;59:205–210.
6. Walker M. Status epilepticus: an evidence based guide. *BMJ*. 2005;331(673):673–677.
7. Löscher W, Brandt C. Prevention or modification of epileptogenesis after brain insults: experimental approaches and translational research. *Pharmacol Rev*. 2010;62(4):668–700.
8. Shearer P, Riviello J. Generalized convulsive status epilepticus in adults and children: treatment guidelines and protocols. *Emerg Med Clin NA*. 2011;29(1):51–64.
9. Neligan A, Shorvon SD. Prognostic factors, morbidity and mortality in tonic clonic status epilepticus: a review. *Epilepsy Res*. 2011;93(1):1–10.
10. Silbergleit R, Durkalski V, Lowenstein D, et al. Intramuscular versus intravenous therapy for prehospital status epilepticus. *N Engl J Med*. 2012;366(7):591–600.
11. Fischer JH, Patel TV, Fischer PA. Fosphenytoin. *Clin Pharmacokinet*. 2003;42(1):33–58.
12. Mewasingh LD, Sekhara T, Aeby A, Christiaens FJC, Dan B. Oral ketamine in paediatric non-convulsive status epilepticus. *Seizure*. 2003;12(7):483–489.
13. *Treatment of Refractory Status Epilepticus with Inhalational Anesthetic Agents Isoflurane and Desflurane*. 2004:1–6.
14. Nam SH, Lee BL, Lee CG, et al. The role of ketogenic diet in the treatment of refractory status epilepticus. *Epilepsia*. 2011;52(11):e181–e184.
15. Corry JJ, Dhar R, Murphy T, Diringer MN. Hypothermia for refractory status epilepticus. *Neurocrit Care*. 2008;9(2):189–197.
16. Amzica F. Basic physiology of burst-suppression. *Epilepsia*. 2009;50(s12):38–39.
17. Sutter R, Marsch S, Fuhr P, Kaplan PW, Rüegg S. Anesthetic drugs in status epilepticus: risk or rescue? A 6-year cohort study. *Neurology*. 2014;82(8):656–664.
18. Novy J, Logroscino G, Rossetti AO. Refractory status epilepticus: a prospective observational study. *Epilepsia*. 2010;51(2):251–256.
19. Legriel S, Azoulay E, Resche-Rigon M, et al. Functional outcome after convulsive status epilepticus. *Crit Care Med*. 2010;38(12):2295–2303.

66 How Should Guillain-Barré Syndrome Be Managed in the ICU?

Joy Vijayan, Nobuhiro Yuki

Guillain-Barré syndrome (GBS) is a rapidly progressive motor, sensory, and autonomic neuropathic disorder that may present to critical care with acute respiratory failure or bulbar palsy. Correct diagnosis and implementation of therapy usually results in favorable outcomes. This chapter considers management of GBS in the intensive care unit (ICU).

PATHOGENESIS

GBS is a prototype of a postinfectious autoimmune disease. Most patients develop GBS 1 to 3 weeks after a microbial infection.[1] Histopathologically, GBS can be divided into acute inflammatory demyelinating polyneuropathy and acute motor axonal neuropathy based on the site of involvement of the inflammatory process within the peripheral nerve (Fig. 66-1). Infections such as *Campylobacter jejuni* or cytomegalovirus induce the development of antibodies that subsequently bind to target antigens on the peripheral nerves as a result of molecular mimicry. These autoantibodies attach to the outer surface of Schwann cells or axonal membranes at the nodes of Ranvier, resulting in activation of the compliment system. This subsequently leads to the detachment of the paranodal myelin, resulting in motor conduction failure and muscle weakness.

DIAGNOSIS

The presentation of GBS and related conditions can be heterogeneous, making the clinical diagnosis at times challenging. Classically, GBS presents with a rapidly progressive weakness of the extremities with variable involvement of the bulbar and respiratory muscles. There are localized subtypes of GBS that tend to involve only a specific group of muscles (Table 66-1).[2] These include (1) the pharyngeal-cervical-brachial subtype with involvement of the bulbar and proximal upper limb muscles; (2) the paraparetic subtype; and (3) the bifacial variant, which presents with isolated facial weakness. Miller Fisher syndrome (MFS), which presents with ophthalmoplegia, ataxia, and areflexia, is a variant of GBS. MFS may present in incomplete form as acute ophthalmoplegia or acute ataxic neuropathy. Bickerstaff brainstem encephalitis, which presents with hypersomnolence, ophthalmoplegia, and ataxia, is a central nervous system subtype of MFS. Some of these patients go on to have involvement of other groups of muscles and thus phenotypically resemble the classical type of GBS. Pharyngeal-cervical-brachial weakness, MFS, and Bickerstaff encephalitis are often misdiagnosed as having brainstem stroke, myasthenia gravis, botulism, or Wernicke encephalopathy (Table 66-2).

Nerve conduction studies and cerebrospinal fluid (CSF) analysis are not always conclusive, especially at admission, and the diagnosis should be based on clinical grounds (Table 66-3). A lumbar puncture is performed primarily to rule out infectious processes, such as Lyme disease, or malignancies, such as lymphoma. Albuminocytologic dissociation (elevation in CSF protein [>0.55 g/L] without an elevation in white blood cells) is present in approximately 50% of patients with GBS during the first week of illness. Brain and spinal imaging studies are unhelpful. A history of antecedent infectious symptoms such as sore throat, cough, or diarrhea is useful for the clinical diagnosis as well as the presence of distal paraesthesias immediately before, and at the onset of, weakness or ataxia.

PREDICTORS

Need for Mechanical Ventilation

The development of respiratory compromise requiring mechanical ventilation is the most common fatal complication of GBS and occurs in up to 30% of patients. Early identification of respiratory deterioration and transfer to critical care usually leads to a positive outcome. There are several prediction tools that are used to recognize the development of respiratory dysfunction. The Erasmus GBS Respiratory Insufficiency Score (EGRIS) is a point-based tool (Table 66-4) that can accurately predict the probability of development of respiratory failure in 90% of patients. Figure 66-2 shows the clinical variables used in this tool, including the days between onset of weakness and admission, the presence of facial and bulbar weakness, and the Medical Research Council (MRC) sum score (a sum of the MRC scores of six different muscles measured bilaterally, ranging from 0 [tetraplegic] to 60 [normal]).[3]

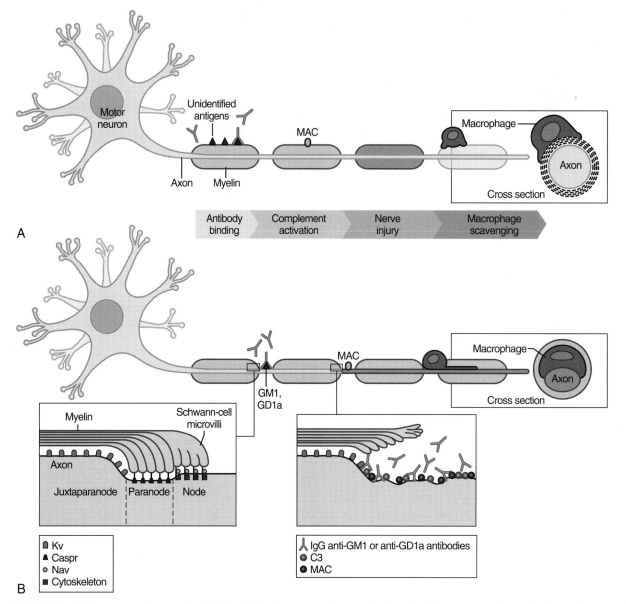

Figure 66-1. Possible immunopathogenesis of GBS. **A,** The immunopathogenesis of acute inflammatory demyelinating polyneuropathy. Although autoantigens have yet to be unequivocally identified, autoantibodies may bind to myelin antigens and activate complement. This is followed by the formation of membrane attack complex (*MAC*) on the outer surface of Schwann cells and the initiation of vesicular degeneration. Macrophages subsequently invade myelin and act as scavengers to remove myelin debris. **B,** The immunopathogenesis of acute motor axonal neuropathy. Myelinated axons are divided into four functional regions: the nodes of Ranvier, paranodes, juxtanodes, and internodes. Gangliosides GM1 and GD1a are strongly expressed at the nodes of Ranvier, where the voltage-gated sodium (Nav) channels are localized. Contactin-associated protein (*Caspr*) and voltage-gated potassium (*Kv*) channels are respectively present at the paranodes and juxtanodes. Immunoglobulin G (*IgG*) anti-GM1 or anti-GD1a autoantibodies bind to the nodal axolemma, leading to MAC formation. This results in the disappearance of Nav clusters and the detachment of paranodal myelin, which can lead to nerve-conduction failure and muscle weakness. Axonal degeneration may follow at a later stage. Macrophages subsequently invade from the nodes into the periaxonal space, scavenging the injured axons. (*Adapted from Yuki N, Hartung HP. Guillain-Barré syndrome.* N Engl J Med *2012;336:2294–2304. With permission from Massachusetts Medical Society.*)

The French Cooperative study prospectively analyzed a group of 722 patients to identify possible predictors of need for mechanical ventilation. The six predictors included time from onset to admission of less than 7 days, inability to cough, inability to stand, inability to lift the elbows or head, and elevated liver enzymes. Mechanical ventilation was required in more than 85% of patients with at least four predictors. The authors also recommended monitoring patients in the ICU if they have one of these predictors.[4] A second French study looking at objective parameters noted that a reduction in vital capacity by 20% and peroneal nerve conduction block was associated with an increased risk of need for mechanical ventilation.[5]

There have been several studies that have used serial assessment of spirometric parameters to indicate the need for mechanical ventilation. Factors associated with progression to respiratory failure included vital capacity of less than 20 mL/kg, maximal inspiratory pressure of less than 30 cm H_2O, maximal expiratory pressure of less than 40 cm H_2O, or a reduction of more than 30% in any of the above parameters from baseline at admission.[6,7]

Table 66-1 **Clinical Features of Guillain-Barré Syndrome, Miller Fisher Syndrome, and Their Subtypes**			
	Pattern of Weakness	**Ataxia**	**Hypersomnolence**
Guillain-Barré syndrome	**Four limbs**	**Yes**	
• Pharyngeal-cervical-brachial weakness	Bulbar/cervical/upper limbs		
Incomplete form			
• Acute pharyngeal weakness	Bulbar		
• Bifacial weakness with paraesthesias	Facial		
• Paraparetic Guillain-Barré syndrome	Lower limbs		
Miller Fisher syndrome	**Ophthalmoplegia**	**Yes**	
Incomplete forms			
• Acute ophthalmoparesis	Ophthalmoplegia		
• Acute ataxic neuropathy	No weakness	Yes	
• Acute ptosis	Ptosis		
• Acute mydriasis	Paralytic mydriasis		
Central nervous system subtype			
• Bickerstaff brainstem encephalitis	Ophthalmoplegia		Yes
Incomplete form			
• Acute ataxic hypersomnolence	No weakness		Yes

Mortality

The reported mortality rate in GBS ranges from 3% to 11%.[8,9] Factors associated with increased mortality included advanced age, antecedent gastroenteritis, grade of disability on the Hughes disability scale, an axonal type of neuropathy, a shorter latency from onset to nadir of illness, and longer disease duration. Pneumonia and cardiac dysrhythmias were the main cause death. Of importance, mortality occurred with almost equal frequency during the progressive, plateau, and recovery phase of the illness. The presence of concomitant medical comorbidities has been shown to increase the overall mortality in certain GBS study groups in comparison with cohorts with isolated GBS.

Poor Long-Term Outcome

There are several prognostic factors and scoring scales used to predict the long-term outcome of patients with GBS.[10] The factors that have been used commonly are the Erasmus GBS Outcome Score (EGOS; Table 66-5)[11] and the modified EGOS (mEGOS) score (Table 66-6).[12] The former scoring scale takes into consideration the age, presence of diarrhea, and the disability functional score at admission and is used to predict the patients' probability of ambulating independently at 6 months after the hospital admission (Fig. 66-3). The newer version, or mEGOS (Fig. 66-4), relies on the same variables except that the MRC sum score replaces the disability functional score (i.e., the sum of scores ranges from 0 [tetraplegic] to 60 [normal] and is a measure of six different muscle groups from both sides). The outcome measures include the functional disability at 4 weeks, 3 months, and 6 months after hospital admission.

Table 66-2 **Differential Diagnosis of Guillain-Barré Syndrome, Miller Fisher Syndrome, and Their Subtypes**
Guillain-Barré Syndrome
• Acute spinal cord disease
• Carcinomatous or lymphomatous meningitis
• Myasthenia gravis
• Critical illness neuropathy
• Thiamine deficiency
• Corticosteroid-induced myopathy
• Toxins (e.g., neurotoxic shellfish poisoning)
• Acute hypophosphatemia
• Prolonged use of neuromuscular blocking drugs
• Tick paralysis
• West Nile poliomyelitis
• Acute intermittent porphyria
Miller Fisher Syndrome, Bickerstaff Brainstem Encephalitis, and Pharyngeal-Cervical-Brachial Weakness
• Basilar artery occlusion
• Myasthenia gravis
• Wernicke encephalopathy
• Botulism
• Brainstem encephalitis
• Diphtheria
• Tick paralysis
Paraparetic Variant
• Lumbosacral plexopathy
• Diabetic
• Neoplastic
• Inflammatory (e.g., sarcoidosis)
• Infective (e.g., cytomegalovirus, Lyme disease)
• Lesions of cauda equine
Bifacial weakness with paraesthesias
• Lyme disease
• Sarcoidosis

Table 66-3 Diagnostic Criteria for Guillain-Barré Syndrome, Miller Fisher Syndrome and Their Subtypes

Core Clinical Features	Supportive Features
• Relatively symmetric pattern of limb *and/or* motor cranial nerve weakness[a,b] • Monophasic illness pattern *and* interval between onset and nadir of weakness between 12 hours and 28 days *and* subsequent plateau • Absence of identifies alternative diagnosis	• Antecedent infectious symptoms[c] • Presence of distal paraesthesias before or at the onset of weakness • Cerebrospinal fluid albuminocytologic dissociation[d]
1. Guillain-Barré syndrome	
• Weakness in all four limbs[a,e,f] *and* areflexia/hyporeflexia[g]	• Neurophysiologic evidence of neuropathy
1.1 Pharyngeal-cervical-brachial weakness	
• Oropharyngeal weakness *and* neck weakness *and* arm weakness *and* arm areflexia/hyporeflexia[a,b,h] • Absence of leg weakness *and* ataxia[i,j]	• Neurophysiologic evidence of neuropathy • Presence of anti-GT 1a or anti-GQ1b
1.2 Paraparetic Guillain-Barré syndrome	
• Leg weakness *and* areflexia/hyporeflexia[a] • Absence of arm weakness	• Neurophysiologic evidence of neuropathy
1.3 Bifacial weakness with paraesthesias	
• Facial weakness *and* areflexia/hyporeflexia[a] • Absence of ophthalmoplegia *and* limb weakness	
2. Miller Fisher syndrome	
• Ophthalmoparesis *and* ataxia *and* areflexia/hyporeflexia[a,b,k,l] • Absence of limb weakness[m] *and* hypersomnolence	• Presence of anti-GQ1b antibodies
2.1 Bickerstaff brainstem encephalitis	
• Hypersomnolence *and* ophthalmoparesis *and* ataxia[a,b,n] • Absence of limb weakness[m]	• Presence of anti-GQ1b antibodies

[a]Weakness may be asymmetric or unilateral.
[b]In Miller Fisher syndrome, Bickerstaff brainstem encephalitis, and pharyngeal-cervical-brachial weakness, the clinical severity of each component may vary from partial to complete. In acute ataxic neuropathy and acute ataxic hypersomnolence, there is no weakness.
[c]The presence of upper respiratory infectious symptoms or diarrhea 3 days to 6 weeks before the onset of neurologic symptoms.
[d]Cerebrospinal fluid with total white cell count <50 cells/μL and protein above the normal laboratory range.
[e]Weakness usually starts in the legs and ascends but may start in the arms. Weakness may be mild, moderate, or complete paralysis.
[f]Cranial nerve-innervated muscles or respiratory muscles may be involved.
[g]Muscle stretch reflexes may be normal or exaggerated in 10% of cases.
[h]The absence of certain features indicated incomplete pharyngeal-cervical-brachial weakness as follows: absence of upper limb weakness with and without neck weakness.
[i]Leg weakness may vary considerably, but oropharyngeal, neck, and arm weakness should be more prominent.
[j]The presence of additional features indicates overlap with other Guillain-Barré syndrome variants as follows: ataxia *and* ophthalmoplegia, "overlap with Miller Miller Fisher syndrome; ataxia *without* ophthalmoplegia, overlap with acute ataxic neuropathy": ataxia *and* ophthalmoplegia *and* disturbed consciousness, "overlap with Bickerstaff brainstem encephalitis."
[k]The absence of certain features indicates incomplete Miller Fisher syndrome as follows: absence of ataxia, acute ophthalmoparesis; absence of ophthalmoparesis, acute ataxic neuropathy.
[l]The presence of a single feature indicates incomplete Miller Fisher syndrome as follows: ptosis, acute ptosis; mydriasis, acute mydriasis.
[m]The presence of limb weakness indicates overlap by GBS.
[n]The absence of certain features indicates incomplete Bickerstaff brainstem encephalitis as follows: ophthalmoplegia, acute ataxic hypersomnolence.

MANAGEMENT

Monitoring

The development of respiratory and cardiac dysfunction usually runs in tandem with the progression of the active disease phase. Prompt recognition of the evolution of the neurologic deficits and recognition of worsening respiratory and cardiac function with timely intervention can lead to satisfactory outcomes in most GBS patients. It is imperative that these patients are closely monitored for worsening pharyngeal weakness with incipient development of a compromised airway and frequently assessed for respiratory muscle weakness through bedside clinical examination or lung function studies.

The initial clinical course of patients with GBS is characterized by a rapidly evolving weakness of the extremities. The subsequent evolution and severity of disease is varied. Respiratory failure and the need for mechanical ventilation is one of the most serious short-term complications of GBS, and early triaging to critical care can be of paramount importance. Historic clues that would suggest the need for early intubation include a hyperacute presentation with a very short latent period from onset to nadir, involvement of bulbar muscles, inability to converse in full sentences, complaints of shortness of breath, and difficulty in generating a good cough. Clinical signs that can suggest impending respiratory compromise include weak neck muscles, a poor cough, reduced chest expansion, paradoxical abdominal

Table 66-4 Erasmus GBS Respiratory Insufficiency Score

Measure	Categories	Score
Days between onset of weakness and hospital admission	>7 days	0
	4-7days	1
	≤3 days	2
Facial and/or bulbar weakness at hospital admission	Absence	0
	Presence	1
Medical Research Council sum score at hospital admission	60-51	0
	50-41	1
	40-31	2
	30-21	3
	≤20	4
Erasmus GBS	Respiratory Insuffciency Score	0-7

GBS, Guillain-Barré syndrome.

Table 66-5 Erasmus GBS Outcome Score

	Categories	Score
Age at onset (years)	≥60	1
	41-60	0.5
	≤40	0
Diarrhea (≤4 weeks)	Absence	0
	Presence	1
GBS disability score (at 2 weeks after entry)	0 or 1	1
	2	2
	3	3
	4	4
	5	5
Erasmus GBS	Outcome Score	1-7

GBS, Guillain-Barré syndrome.

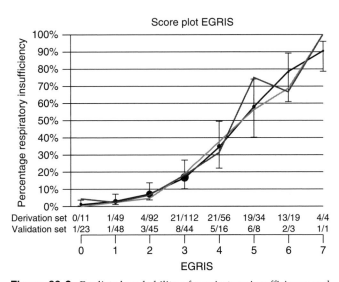

Figure 66-2. Predicted probability of respiratory insufficiency and observed percentage of mechanical ventilation (MV) in derivation and validation cohorts according to the Erasmus GBS Respiratory Insufficiency Score (*EGRIS*). The black line reflects the predicted probability of respiratory insufficiency derived from the combined cohorts. The size of bullets in the graph reflects the size of the patient group with a corresponding EGRIS score in the combined cohorts (n=565). The dark gray line reflects the observed percentage of MV in the derivation cohort (n=377), and the light gray line reflects this percentage in the validation cohort (n=188). Above the line are the number of patients requiring MV with a defined EGRIS in the derivation and validation cohorts. *(Adapted from Walgaard C, Lingsma HF, Ruts L, et al. Prediction of respiratory insufficiency in Guillain-Barré syndrome.* Ann Neurol. *2010; 67:781–787. With permission from John Wiley & Sons.)*

Table 66-6 Modified Erasmus GBS Outcome Scores

Prognostic Factors	Score	Prognostic Factors	Score
Age at onset (years)		Age at onset (years)	
≤40	0	≤40	0
41-60	1	41-60	1
>60	2	>60	2
Preceding diarrhea*		Preceding diarrhea	
Absent	0	Absent	0
Present	1	Present	1
MRC sum score (at hospital admission)		MRC sum score (at day 7 of admission)	
51-60	0	51-60	0
41-50	2	41-50	3
31-40	4	31-40	6
0-30	6	0-30	9
mEGOS	0-9	mEGOS	0-12

*Diarrhea in the 4 weeks preceding the onset of weakness.
GBS, Guillain-Barré syndrome; *mEGOS*, Modified Erasmus GBS Outcome Score; *MRC*, Medical Research Council.

movements, and a single breath count less than 20.[13-15] Weakness of the axial muscles including the neck flexors and the truncal muscles run in parallel with diaphragmatic weakness and other respiratory muscles. A normal person with good ventilatory reserve would be able to count up to 50 in a single breath after a deep inspiration. Inability to count beyond 25 and 10 roughly correlates with a vital capacity not greater than 2 L and 1 L, respectively. Counts less than 15 are associated with substantial respiratory compromise. Prediction models or clinical tools such as the ones mentioned above can be of assistance in triaging patients to the ICU.

The recommended monitoring for worsening respiratory functions includes clinical assessment done every

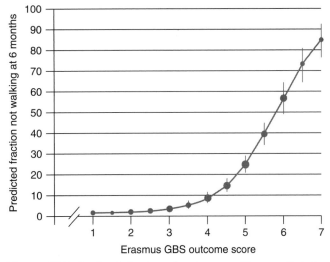

Figure 66-3. Predicted fraction of patients unable to walk independently at 6 months after randomization on the basis of the Erasmus Guillain-Barré syndrome (*GBS*) outcome score (n = 762). Vertical bars indicate 95% confidence intervals. Point sizes are proportionate to the number of patients with a specific score. The probability of not walking independently at 6 months is given by the equation $1/(1 + \exp[8.2 - 1.4 \times EGOS])$. (*Adapted from van Koningsveld R, Steyerberg EW, Hughes RAC, et al. A clinical prognostic scoring system for Guillain-Barré syndrome. Lancet Neurol. 2007;6:589–594. With permission from Elsevier Limited.*)

weak cough and a subjective sense of dyspnea, one less than 25 mL/kg is associated with a weak inspiratory sigh with development of peripheral microatelectasis and increasing pulmonary vascular shunt, and a value less than 15 mL/kg or 1 L (<30% to 35% of predicted) is considered an indication for elective intubation and ventilation. Thus serial monitoring of the vital capacity, negative inspiratory force (NIF), and the maximum expiratory pressure are useful parameters for predicting worsening respiratory functions. The "20/30/40" rule is often used as a parameter to estimate need for intubation and mechanical ventilation. Any drop in vital capacity below 20 mL/kg, a NIF less than −30 cm H_2O, and a maximum expiratory pressure less than 40 cm H_2O indicates impending respiratory compromise and the need for intubation and mechanical ventilation. There is likely no benefit in using noninvasive ventilation as a bridge or alternative to intubation. Elective intubation and ventilation has been found to be associated with a reduced incidence of pneumonia and shorter duration of mechanical ventilation.[17,18]

Ventilatory Management

Intubation and Mechanical Ventilation

There are several precautions that should to be taken once the decision has been made to intubate and mechan-

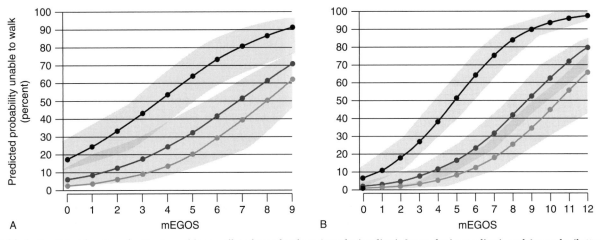

Figure 66-4. Predicted fraction of patients unable to walk independently at 4 weeks (*top lines*), 3 months (*center lines*), and 6 months (*bottom lines*) on the basis of modified Erasmus GBS Outcome Score (*mEGOS*) at hospital admission (**A**) and at day 7 of admission (**B**). The gray areas around the bottom two lines represent 90% confidence intervals. (*Adapted from Walgaard C, Lingsma HF, Ruts L, et al. Early recognition of poor prognosis in Guillain-Barré syndrome. Neurology 2011;76:968–975. With permission from Lippincott Williams and Wilkins.*)

2 to 4 hours and periodic spirometric assessment.[16] The possibility of deteriorating respiratory function at night, when ventilation is solely dependent on the diaphragmatic muscles during the rapid eye movement stage of sleep, should be a period of concern, and close observation is required. There is also a drop of approximately 10% in the forced vital capacity when assuming the recumbent position in comparison to the upright position. Normal forced vital capacity is approximately 60 to 70 mL/kg and is expressed as a percentage of a predicted value based on the age, ethnicity, and anthropological features of the subject. A vital capacity of less than 30 mL/kg is associated with a

ically ventilate the GBS patient. Autonomic dysfunction is a common complication. Patients are at elevated risk of hemodynamic instability at the time of intubation associated with the vasodilatory effects of anesthetic agents and reduced venous return associated with positive pressure ventilation.[19,20] Severe hyperkalemia may be associated with the use of succinylcholine in patients with GBS, and alternative neuromuscular blocking agents should be used, if necessary.

No randomized controlled trials of mechanical ventilation strategy in GBS have been performed. The approach will clearly be determined by the degree of respiratory muscle weakness and the capacity to trigger the ventilator. Patients with GBS usually have normal lungs; therefore meticulous attention should be paid to avoidance of ventilator-induced lung injury (VILI) and ventilator-associated pneumonia. A sensible approach would be to use volume assist-control ventilation, with tidal volume limited to 6 mL/kg or less (predicted body weight) initially with minute ventilation set to maintain partial pressure of carbon dioxide in arterial blood ($Paco_2$) within normal limits, and fraction of inspired oxygen targeted as close as possible to room air (0.21%). Positive end-expiratory pressure should be administered to prevent atelectasis and atelectrauma.[21] The patient may subsequently transition to pressure support, proportional assisted, or neutrally assisted ventilation, but to date, few data beyond case reports support one approach over another.

Weaning and Ventilator Liberation

Weaning and ventilator liberation in GBS is a major challenge for the intensivist.[22,23] Prolonged and careless mechanical ventilation may lead to complications that include ventilator-associated pneumonia, development of tracheal injury, VILI, laryngotracheal stenosis, and diaphragmatic atrophy. Premature extubation may result in respiratory distress, myocardial ischemia, and gastropulmonary aspiration.

Tracheostomy

Tracheostomy improves patient comfort, resulting in minimal sedation; it reduces the risk of laryngeal and vocal cord damage; it enhances airway toilet; and it facilitates liberation from mechanical ventilation. The timing of tracheostomy is unclear and depends on local culture, physician preference, and disease trajectory. If mechanical ventilation is likely to exceed 2 weeks, then tracheostomy at that stage would appear appropriate.[23] Clinical clues that would suggest the need for tracheostomy include persisting neck and proximal arm weakness, severe autonomic instability, development of ventilator-associated pneumonia, or advanced age. The integrated pulmonary function ratio based on the summed vital capacity and the inspiratory and expiratory pressure can be used to predict the need for a tracheostomy.[24] A pulmonary function ratio is obtained at day 12 after intubation and is calculated by dividing the pulmonary function score at day 12 with that obtained at day 1. A ratio of less than 1 is highly unlikely to be associated with a successful liberation and is an indicator for early tracheostomy. The sensitivity of a pulmonary function ratio of less than 1 for predicting that the duration of ventilation would be more than 3 weeks was 70%, and the specificity and positive predictive value was 100%. If pulmonary function tests are improving, then tracheostomy can be deferred for an additional week. Percutaneous dilatational tracheostomy, which is cosmetically more acceptable and associated with a lower risk of decannulation, is preferred over the conventional surgical approach.

Indication for Temporary Pacing

Autonomic dysfunction consequent of GBS may result in cardiovascular instability. This involves dysfunction or hyperactivity of the sympathetic and parasympathetic arm of the autonomic nervous system.[26] Dysautonomia is more likely to occur in patients who are mechanically ventilated. Common abnormalities vary from relatively innocuous sinus tachycardia to the more serious and life-threatening arrhythmias as a result of vagally mediated bradycardia and cardiac asystole. This may necessitate the need for atropine and temporary pacing. Monitoring for dysautonomia includes frequent electrocardiographic recording and measurement of supine and standing blood pressure. Those with significant sinus tachycardia, episodic arrhythmias, or blood pressure fluctuation should be transferred to the ICU for telemetry and continuous blood pressure measurement. Persistent bradyarrhythmia is an indication for temporary pacemaker insertion. A fluctuating blood pressure level ("roller coaster") is a well-described complication in GBS, and this can be clinically challenging. In general, if vasopressors or antihypertensives are to be administered, short-acting agents (e.g., esmolol, nicardipine) are preferable. Care should be taken with dosage because patients with GBS can be extremely sensitive to even small doses of vasoactive agents because of possible denervation supersensitivity. Autonomic and motor dysfunction generally simultaneously resolve.

Immunotherapy

Treatment specifically targeted at the primary pathophysiologic process of GBS is initiated once the patient's life-threatening hemodynamic and respiratory problems have been addressed.[27] The principal intervention is immunotherapy. Plasma exchange and intravenous immunoglobulin (IVIG) have been shown to be effective in hastening the recovery of patients with GBS. The greatest benefit is in patients with profound motor weakness and ventilator failure. Patients with associated autonomic instability, or pressor-dependent septic shock, are administered IVIG rather than plasma exchange. Due consideration should be given to the associated underlying medical comorbidities while these specific treatment modalities are initiated.

Intravenous Immunoglobulin

IVIG acts by neutralizing pathogenic antibodies and inhibiting autoantibody-mediated complement activation, resulting in reduced nerve injury and faster clinical improvement, as compared with no treatment. IVIG has replaced plasma exchange as the treatment of choice because of its greater convenience and availability. The standard treatment regimen involves administering 2 g/kg immunoglobulin over a period of 5 days.[28] The pharmacokinetics of immunoglobulin vary among patients, and some patients have a smaller increase in serum immunoglobulin G (IgG) after administration of immunoglobulin. These patients are likely to have a poorer outcome, with fewer able to walk unaided at 6 months. A second course of immunoglobulin in severely unresponsive patients was reported to be beneficial in one study.[29,30]

Plasma Exchange

Plasma exchange is most effective when it is started within the first 2 weeks after disease onset.[31] Plasma exchange nonspecifically removes antibodies and complement and appears to be associated with reduced nerve damage and more rapid clinical improvement as compared with supportive treatment alone. The usual regimen is five exchanges over a period of 2 weeks, with a total exchange of five plasma volumes.

The combination of plasma exchange followed by a course of IVIG is not significantly better than plasma exchange or IVIG alone. Neither prednisolone nor methylprednisolone can significantly accelerate recovery or improve long-term outcome in patients with GBS. One study showed that combined administration of IVIG and methylprednisolone was not more effective than IVIG alone, although an analysis corrected for known prognostic factors suggested a short-term effect.[32]

Supportive Treatment

The management of GBS also involves several other supportive measures. These include addressing the standard medical comorbidities seen in ICU patients as well as dealing with conditions that are unique to GBS.[33]

Deep Vein Thrombosis

GBS patients are at high risk for the development of deep vein thrombosis (DVT) as a result of prolonged immobilization due to weakness of all four extremities. There have been no clinical trials that have addressed pharmacologic or mechanical approaches to prophylaxis against DVT in GBS. The duration of prophylaxis is unclear as is whether to actively screen patients for thrombosis. Prophylactic treatment with subcutaneous heparin or low-molecular-weight heparinoids (LMWHs) likely reduces the incidence of DVT. In the perioperative literature, elasticated support stockings (TED [thromboembolism-deterrent hose]) and sequential compression devices (SCDs) have been shown to reduce the incidence of DVT by as much as 70%. We recommend the use of LMWHs, SCDs, and TED. Aggressive prophylaxis should continue until there is significant recovery of motor function and the patient is able to ambulate.

Adynamic Ileus

Constipation in GBS is a commonly encountered clinical symptom and can result from multiple factors, including immobilization, opioids, electrolyte imbalance, and dehydration. Moreover, GBS patients are at increased risk of having adynamic ileus, either independently or in conjunction with other features of autonomic involvement. Frequent monitoring of the abdominal girth and bowel sounds are essential components of daily care. Recommendations are made on the basis of anecdotal reports. Patients should be administered stool softeners because voiding may be compromised. Erythromycin and neostigmine have been used in the treatment of patients with adynamic ileus. Although bladder function is frequently compromised, GBS patients are routinely catheterized as part of standard nursing care.

Syndrome of Inappropriate ADH Secretion of Antidiuretic Hormone

The syndrome of inappropriate secretion of antidiuretic hormone (SIADH) is seen in up to 50% of patient with GBS.[34] SIADH is also considered to be a prognostic indicator, with lower sodium levels associated with a poor outcome. The exact mechanism of hyponatremia in SIADH is not understood. Downward osmotic resetting and enhanced tubular sensitivity to ADH are some of the proposed mechanisms. Prompt recognition of this clinical entity is an essential aspect of ICU management to prevent complications such as disorientation and seizures.

Neuropathic Pain

Neuropathic pain is a frequently reported symptom in most patients with GBS. These symptoms involve the distal extremities and occur over the shoulder and lower back in those with radicular involvement. In one study, pain was reported by 89% of the patients and was severe in half. Seventy-five percent of these patients required opioid analgesia in addition to acetaminophen (paracetamol) and nonsteroidal inflammatory agents.[35] Opioids are problematic in that they may induce bowel and bladder dysfunction. In 10% of patients, nonopioid analgesics such as gabapentin and carbamazepine were required.[35] Both gabapentin[36] and carbamazepine[37] have been shown to significantly reduce pain symptoms, compared with placebo, in GBS.

Patients with GBS may also suffer in the ICU as a consequence of anxiety, insomnia, and delirium. Carefully titrated anxiolytics and night sedatives are recommended, particularly in the early progressive stage of the disease.

AUTHORS' RECOMMENDATIONS

- GBS is an acute-onset motor, sensory, and autonomic neuropathy that likely results after infection and may manifest as demyelination or axonal degeneration.
- GBS patients usually present to the ICU in respiratory failure for mechanical ventilation after progressive loss of respiratory reserve.
- Morphologically, the lungs are normal; mechanical ventilation is required for failure of the thoracic pump, particularly during sleep. Ventilation strategy should include meticulous attention to lung stretch and the fraction of inspired oxygen. Early tracheostomy should be considered.
- IVIG is the current standard medical therapy, and plasma exchange, which is more complex and expensive, is reserved for severe cases.
- Autonomic dysfunction may manifest as tachyarrhythmias or bradyarrhythmias, hypertension or hypotension, or all of these. Care must be taken to avoid overtreatment and a prolonged rebound effect, particularly with antihypertensives.
- Bladder and bowel dysfunction are to be expected, as are fluid and electrolyte abnormalities. Patients are at high risk for DVT.
- Neuropathic pain, anxiety, and depression are major problems for patients with GBS in the ICU. Aside from empathy and reassurance, a multimodal anxiolytic and analgesic strategy may be required.

REFERENCES

1. Yuki N, Hartung HP. Guillain-Barré syndrome. *N Engl J Med.* 2012;336:2294–2304.
2. Wakerley BR, Uncini A, Yuki N, GBS Classification Group. Guillain-Barré and Miller Fisher syndromes—new diagnostic classification. *Nat Rev Neurol.* 2014;10:537–544.
3. Walgaard C, Lingsma HF, Ruts L, et al. Prediction of respiratory insufficiency in Guillain-Barré syndrome. *Ann Neurol.* 2010;67:781–787.

4. Sharshar T, Chevret S, Bourdain F, et al. Early predictors of mechanical ventilation in Guillain- Barré syndrome. *Crit Care Med.* 2003;31:278–283.
5. Durand MC, Porcher R, Orlikowski D, et al. Clinical and electrophysiological predictors of respiratory failure in Guillain-Barré syndrome: a prospective study. *Lancet Neurol.* 2006;5:1021–1028.
6. Lawn ND, Fletcher DD, Henderson RD, et al. Anticipating mechanical ventilation in Guillain-Barré syndrome. *Arch Neurol.* 2001;58:893–898.
7. Hughes RAC. Management of acute neuromuscular respiratory paralysis. *J R Coll Physicians Lond.* 1998;32:254–259.
8. Wong AH, Umapathi T, Shahrizaila N, et al. The value of comparing mortality of Guillain-Barré syndrome across different regions. *J Neurol Sci.* 2014;344:60–62.
9. van den Berg B, Bunschoten C, van Doorn PA. Mortality in Guillain-Barré syndrome. *Neurol.* 2013;80:1650–1654.
10. The Italian Guillain-Barré Study Group. The prognosis and main prognostic indicators of Guillain-Barré syndrome: a multicenter prospective study of 297 patients. *Brain.* 1996;119:2053–2061.
11. van Koningsveld R, Steyerberg EW, Hughes RAC, et al. A clinical prognostic scoring system for Guillain-Barré syndrome. *Lancet Neurol.* 2007;6:589–594.
12. Walgaard C, Lingsma HF, Ruts L, et al. Early recognition of poor prognosis in Guillain-Barré syndrome. *Neurol.* 2011;76:968–975.
13. Bella I, Chad DA. Neuromuscular disorders and acute respiratory failure. *Neurol Clin.* 1998;16:391–417.
14. Mehta S. Neuromuscular diseases causing acute respiratory failure. *Respir Care.* 2006;51:1016–1021.
15. Yavagal DR, Mayer SA. Respiratory complications of rapidly progressive neuromuscular syndromes: Guillain-Barré syndrome and myasthenia gravis. *Semin Respir Crit Care Med.* 2002;23:221–229.
16. Green DM. Weakness in the ICU: Guillain-Barré syndrome, myasthenia gravis, and critical illness polyneuropathy/myopathy. *Neurologist.* 2005;11:338–347.
17. Ropper AH, Gress DR, Diringer MN, et al. *Neurological and Neurosurgical Intensive Care.* 4th ed. Philadelphia: Lippincott Williams and Wilkins; 2004:279–294.
18. Orlikowski D, Prigent H, Sharshar T, et al. Respiratory dysfunction in Guillain-Barré syndrome. *Neurocrit Care.* 2004;1:415–422.
19. Dalos NP, Borel C, Hanley DF. Cardiovascular autonomic dysfunction in Guillain-Barré syndrome: therapeutic implications of Swan-Ganz monitoring. *Arch Neurol.* 1988;45:115–117.
20. Pfeiffer G, Schiller B, Kruse J, et al. Indicators of dysautonomia in severe Guillain-Barré syndrome. *J Neurol.* 1999;246:1015–1022.
21. Dhar R. Neuromuscular respiratory failure. *Continuum Lifelong Learning Neurol.* 2009;15:40–67.
22. MacIntyre NR. Evidence-based ventilator weaning and discontinuation. *Respir Care.* 2004;49:830–836.
23. Lawn ND, Wijdicks EF. Tracheostomy in Guillain-Barré syndrome. *Muscle Nerve.* 1999;22:1058–1062.
24. Lawn ND, Wijdicks EF. Post-intubation pulmonary function test in Guillain-Barré syndrome. *Muscle Nerve.* 2000;23:613–616.
25. Flachenecker P, Wermuth P, Hartung HP, et al. Quantitative assessment of Cardiovascular autonomic function in Guillain-Barré syndrome. *Ann Neurol.* 1997;42:171–179.
26. Zochodne DW. Autonomic involvement in Guillain-Barré syndrome: a review. *Muscle Nerve.* 1994;17:1145–1155.
27. van den Berg B, Walgaard C, Drenthen J, et al. Guillain-Barré syndrome: pathogenesis, diagnosis, treatment and prognosis. *Nat Rev Neurol.* 2014;10:469–482.
28. Patwa HS, Chaudhry V, Katzberg H, et al. Evidence-based guideline: intravenous immunoglobulin in the treatment of neuromuscular disorders: report of the Therapeutics and Technology Assessment Subcommittee of the American Academy of Neurology. *Neurology.* 2012;78:1009–1015.
29. van der Meché FGA, Schmitz PIM, Dutch Guillain-Barré Study Group. A randomized trial comparing intravenous immune globulin and plasma exchange in Guillain-Barré syndrome. *N Engl J Med.* 1992;336:1123–1129.
30. Kuitwaard K, de Gelder J, Tio-Gillen AP, et al. Pharmacokinetics of intravenous immunoglobulin and outcome in Guillain-Barré syndrome. *Ann Neurol.* 2009;66:597–603.
31. The Guillain-Barré syndrome Study Group. Plasmapheresis and acute Guillain-Barré syndrome. *Neurology.* 1985;35:1096–1104.
32. Hughes RAC, Swan AV, Raphael JC, et al. Immunotherapy for Guillain Barré syndrome: a systematic review. *Brain.* 2007;130:2245–2257.
33. Hughes RAC, Wijdicks FM, Benson E, et al. Supportive care for patients with Guillain-Barré syndrome. *Arch Neurol.* 2005;62:1194–1198.
34. Saifudheen K, Jose J, Gafoor VA, et al. Guillain-Barré syndrome and SIADH. *Neurology.* 2011;76:701–704.
35. Moulin DE, Hagen N, Feasby TE, Amireh R, Hahn A. Pain in Guillain-Barré syndrome. *Neurology.* 1997;48328–48331.
36. Pandey CK, Bose N, Garg G, et al. Gabapentin for the treatment of pain in Guillain-Barré syndrome: a double-blinded, placebo-controlled, crossover study. *Anesth Analg.* 2002:951719–951723.
37. Tripathi M, Kaushik S. Carbamazepine for pain management in Guillain-Barré syndrome patients in the intensive care unit. *Crit Care Med.* 2000:28655–28658.

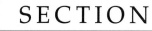

NUTRITION, GASTROINTESTINAL, AND HEPATIC CRITICAL CARE

67 Is It Appropriate to "Underfeed" the Critically Ill Patient?

Naomi E. Cahill, Daren K. Heyland

Critically ill patients are often hypermetabolic and can rapidly become nutritionally compromised.[1] Iatrogenic malnutrition is prevalent in these patients and has been associated with increased morbidity and mortality.[2] Consequently, the provision of nutrition therapy is an integral part of standard patient care. Current Clinical Practice Guidelines for feeding the critically ill patient recommend initiation of nutrition support within 24 to 48 hours of intensive care unit (ICU) admission. Furthermore, they recommend using enteral nutrition (EN) in preference to the parenteral route.[3-7]

Despite agreement across published guidelines on the route and timing of artificial nutrition, though, controversy exists over what the feeding target or optimal dose of calories should be. The Surviving Sepsis Campaign guidelines, updated in 2012, recommend avoiding "mandatory full caloric feeding in the first week but rather suggest low dose feeding (e.g., up to 500 calories per day), advancing as tolerated (Grade 2B [i.e., weak recommendation based on evidence of moderate quality])."[8] This concept of "low dose," "permissive underfeeding," or "hypocaloric" feeding was initially proposed more than a decade ago as a strategy to reduce the metabolic complications associated with the acute stress response.[9,10] In fact, unplanned hypocaloric feeding is common in clinical practice because of disruptions in delivery of EN as a result of gastrointestinal intolerance, fasting for procedures, and routine nursing practices.[11,12] Feedings provided to most critically ill patients do not meet nutritional requirements, and observational studies report that average energy intakes are approximately 60% of calculated requirements.[12,13]

In contrast to the updated Surviving Sepsis Campaign guidelines, the Canadian Critical Care Nutrition guidelines, updated in 2013, do not recommend this practice of underfeeding (whether intentional or not) and recommend "when starting EN in critically ill patients, [that] strategies to optimize delivery of nutrition (starting at target rate, higher thresholds of gastric residual volumes, use of prokinetics and small bowel feedings) should be considered, and in patients with Acute Lung Injury, an initial strategy of trophic feeds for 5 days should not be considered."[6] These disparate recommendations have led to confusion among critical care practitioners. This problem has important clinical and policy implications. On the one hand, it may result in the implementation of an inappropriate and potentially harmful therapy; on the other hand, it may stimulate a sense of complacency such that the importance of nutrition as a therapeutic modality may result in worse patient outcomes. Steps to facilitate the timely resolution of this controversy are warranted.

OBSERVATIONAL STUDIES ON HYPOCALORIC NUTRITION IN CRITICALLY ILL PATIENTS

Over the past decade, several observational studies have examined the association between energy intake and clinically important outcomes in critically ill patients. Nine observational studies have demonstrated that caloric debt or feeding less than goal calories is associated with worse clinical outcomes.[14-22] However, four additional studies found contrasting results, indicating that providing close to goal calories has adverse effects in critically ill patients.[23-26] Different methodological approaches may account for the inconsistent conclusions across these observational studies. Consequently, we conducted a large observational study to evaluate the association between caloric intake and clinical outcome. Our data, using a pooled dataset of 7872 mechanically ventilated critically ill patients from 352 ICUs from within 33 countries and including only those patients who remained in the ICU for at least 96 hours, showed that the result is highly dependent on the statistical methods used.[21] When the most robust statistical method (i.e., excluding patients who permanently progressed to oral feeding within 4 days and basing the 12-day average proportion of prescribed calories received only on ICU days before permanent progression to oral intake, in addition to adjusting for evaluable days and covariates) was applied, we observed that 60-day hospital mortality in patients receiving more than two thirds of their caloric prescription was significantly lower than patients receiving less than one-third of their caloric prescription (odds ratio [OR], 0.67, 95%; confidence interval [CI], 0.56 to 0.79; $P \le .0001$). Furthermore, these results indicated that providing approximately more than 80% of prescribed calories was associated with the optimal clinical outcome. Similar results were observed in a more recent analysis restricted to 2270 patients with an ICU admission diagnosis of sepsis.[22] Thus, on the basis of these large-scale "real world" observational studies, one would conclude that "underfeeding" the critically ill patient (including patients with sepsis) is not appropriate. As stated in our prior publication, though, "the causal association between nutritional intake and outcome cannot be definitively established by any observational study. No perfect adjustment is available despite our best efforts to account for the confounding effects of the duration of artificial nutrition."[27] To truly find the answer, we need to seek evidence from randomized controlled trials (RCTs).

RANDOMIZED CONTROLLED TRIALS OF INTENTIONAL UNDERFEEDING

Over the past four years, three RCTs comparing intentional hypocaloric and full feeding early in the course of ICU stay have been published.[28-30] The first of these, by Arabi et al., adopted a 2×2 factorial design to examine the effect of permissive underfeeding (i.e., 60% to 70% of calculated energy requirements) compared with feeding to goal calories (i.e., 90% to 100% of calculated energy requirements) and of intensive insulin therapy compared with conventional insulin therapy on the clinical outcomes of critically ill patients.[28] A total of 240 predominantly medical (83%) patients with the mean age of 51 years and body mass index (BMI) of 28.5 kg/m^2 were enrolled in this single-center study. Those allocated to the permissive underfeeding group received on average $59.0 \pm 16.1\%$ of their goal calories compared with $71.4 \pm 22.8\%$ in the target feeding group ($P < .0001$ although the target goal in the second group was not reached). The primary outcome of 28-day mortality was not significantly different between the two groups (18.3% vs. 23.3%, relative risk [RR] 0.79; 95% CI, 0.48 to 1.29; $P = .34$), but hospital mortality was significantly lower in the permissive underfeeding group compared with the target feeding group (30.0% vs. 42.5%: RR, 0.71; 95% CI, 0.50 to 0.99, $P = .04$). No other differences were observed. Arabi et al. are currently repeating this trial in multiple centers, the results of which are anticipated in the near future (Current Controlled Trials Register Number: ISRCTN68144998).

In the second single-center pilot RCT conducted by Petros et al., 100 critically ill patients who were predicted to require artificial nutrition for at least 3 days were randomized to receive either early (within 24 hours of ICU admission) full feeding or hypocaloric feeding (50% of their estimated caloric requirements based on 25 kcal/kg/day regimen).[29] Patients allocated to the hypocaloric feeding group received on average 42.6% of their caloric requirements whereas patients allocated to the full feeding group received on average 75.5% of goal calories ($P = .0001$). The primary endpoint was the rate of nosocomial infections during ICU stay. Significantly more infections were detected in patients in the hypocaloric group compared with the full feeding group (12 of 46 [26.1%] vs. 6 of 54 [11.1%], $P = .046$). No other differences were observed in clinical outcomes.

In another single-center pilot RCT,[30] 83 patients with a mean age of 52 years and a BMI of 30.5 kg/m^2, who were admitted to a surgical ICU and projected to require artificial nutrition for more than 48 hours, were randomized to hypocaloric (i.e., 50% of calculated caloric requirements) or full feeding (i.e., 100% of calculated caloric requirements). Patients randomized to the hypocaloric arm received significantly fewer calories compared with patients in the full feeding arm (983 [standard deviation [SD], 61] vs. 1338 [SD, 92] kcal; $P = .019$). The primary outcome was the proportion of patients acquiring infection. No significant differences were observed (RR, 70.7% [29 of 41] in the hypocaloric arm and 76.2% [32 of 42] in the full feeding arm; $P = .57$, adjusted OR, 0.82; 95% CI, 0.28 to 2.39). No differences were observed in other infectious or clinical outcomes.

Given the disparate and preliminary nature of the results of these three studies, it is prudent to wait for the results of the larger multicenter trials before making conclusions regarding early intentional underfeeding.

RANDOMIZED CONTROLLED TRIALS OF TROPHIC FEEDS

Two RCTs, conducted by the same research group aimed to test the hypothesis that initial trophic EN (i.e., provision of small volume of EN) would decrease gastrointestinal complications and improve outcomes.[31,32] In the first single-center study,[31] 200 patients (mean age, 54 years; BMI, 28.7 kg/m^2) with acute respiratory failure expected to require mechanical ventilation for at least 72 hours were enrolled and allocated to receive either full-energy EN (EN initiated at 25 mL/hr within 12 hours of randomization and advanced every 6 hours until goal rate achieved [within 1 to 2 days]) or trophic EN (EN initiated at 10 mL/hr and advancing to full-energy EN on study day 6). For study days 1 to 5, patients in the full-energy group received significantly more calories than patients in the trophic EN group (1418 ± 686 kcal/day vs. 300 ± 149 kcal/day, $P \leq .001$). Overall, there was a trend toward less gastrointestinal intolerance (26.5% vs. 39.2%; $P = .08$), less gastric residual volumes of more than 300 mL (2.1% vs. 7.5%; $P \leq .001$), and less diarrhea (19.1% vs. 24.1%; $P = .08$) in the trophic EN group. No differences were observed in clinical outcomes or infectious complications.

The second, more recent RCT was a large, multicenter study conducted in 44 ICUs in the United States.[32] The research team adopted a 2×2 factorial design with the intention of also evaluating the effectiveness of omega-3 fatty acid supplementation (the Early versus Delayed Enteral Nutrition [EDEN] study). A total of 1000 patients with a mean age of 52 years, a BMI of 30 kg/m^2, and a diagnosis of acute lung injury (ALI) were randomized to receive the same full-energy or trophic EN interventions as described for the previous single-center RCT. Patients randomized to the full-energy EN group received significantly more calories in the first 5 days than patients in the trophic EN group (1300 ± 82 vs. 400 ± 25 kcal/day, $P = .001$) and achieved the goal rate within 1.3 ± 1.2 days compared with 6.7 ± 1.8 days ($P = .001$). Overall, there was a significantly lower incidence of gastric residual volumes of greater than 300 mL (2.2% vs. 4.9%, $P \leq .001$) and a trend toward less diarrhea (16.5% vs. 18.7%, $P = .16$) and vomiting (1.7% vs. 2.2%, $P = .05$) in the trophic EN group. The authors reported no significant differences in ventilator-free days, infections, 60-day mortality, physical function, cognitive performance, and other outcomes at 6 and 12 months. There was a trend, though, toward improved 6-minute walk test scores with full feeding, and more patients who received trophic feeding were admitted to a physical rehabilitation facility (57 [23%] vs. 30 [14%]; *P* = .01).[33,34]

Therefore data from these two trials of trophic feeding do not indicate that it improved clinical outcomes, but it may reduce gastrointestinal complications. The absence of harm from trophic feeds in the initial 6 days of ICU stay may reflect the underpowered nature of these studies, and early trophic feeding may negatively affect long-term recovery and physical function.

RANDOMIZED CONTROLLED TRIALS OF EARLY ENHANCED ENTERAL NUTRITION

We identified seven trials designed to answer the questions "Is enterally providing more calories compared with fewer calories during this early phase beneficial?" Four RCTs that have linked increased energy intake from EN begun early in the course of critical illness with improved patient-centered outcomes,[35-38] one RCT evaluated a bundle comprising active supervision of nutrition provision together with delivery of near target energy requirements determined by repeated energy measurements,[39] and two cluster RCTs evaluated the effects of an enhanced feeding protocol intended to increase EN delivery.[40,41]

The first RCT by Taylor et al. investigated the effects of early enhanced EN on clinical outcomes in 82 mechanically ventilated patients with severe head injury randomized to receive either standard early EN or enhanced early EN.[35] Enteral feeding was started within 24 hours of the injury in both groups. In the control group, patients received EN starting at 15 mL/hr, which was increased incrementally as tolerated according to a predefined protocol. In the intervention group, patients received EN starting at the rate that would meet their full energy requirements. During the first week after head injury, patients in the enhanced EN group received significantly more calories than patients in the control group (59.2% vs. 36.8% of caloric goal, *P* ≤ .001). There was a trend toward improved neurologic outcome 3 months after injury in the intervention group (proportion with good neurologic recovery 25 of 41 [61%] vs. 35 of 41 [85%]; *P* = .08), but this difference was not apparent at 6 months, suggesting that the aggressively fed group had a faster time to recovery. Patients in the intervention group also had fewer overall complications, including infections, up to 6 months after the initial injury (37% vs. 61%; *P* = .046). There was no difference in mortality (12.2% in the intervention group and 14.6% in the control group), although the study was not adequately powered for this endpoint.

The second RCT comparing the use of early enhanced EN to standard early EN was conducted by Desachy et al.[36] One hundred patients admitted to two ICUs were enrolled and randomized to either initiate EN within 24 hours at goal rate (i.e., to achieve a caloric intake of 25 kcal/kg) or to initiate EN within 24 hours at 25 mL/hr with gradual increase to goal rate. Patients in the study group received significantly more calories than the control group (1715 ± 331 kcal/day vs. 1297 ± 331 kcal/day, *P* ≤ .001), achieving on average 95% of their energy needs compared with 76% in the control group. The incidence of high gastric residual volumes of more than 300 mL was greater in the early enhanced EN group (*P* = .04). There was no difference in the mortality, hospital, and ICU length of stay or incidence of adverse events necessitating withdrawal of EN.

The third single-center RCT, conducted by Braunshweig et al., aimed to evaluate the influence of intensive medical nutrition therapy in patients with ALI.[37] A total of 78 patients, the majority of whom were well nourished, were enrolled and randomized to receive either intensive administration of EN (>75% of goal calories) or standard care. Patients in the intervention group received 84.2% of goal calories compared with 55.4% in the control group (*P* ≤ .0001). The trial was stopped early because of safety concerns surrounding the significantly higher mortality rate in the intensive EN group (40% vs. 15.6%, *P* = .017).

The fourth, and most recent, trial, conducted in five ICUs in Australia, randomized 112 mechanically ventilated patients who were expected to require EN for more than 2 days to receive a concentrated 1.5-kcal/mL EN solution or a standard 1-kcal/mL EN solution.[38] Study EN was provided for the duration of the patients' ICU stay up to a maximum of 10 days. Patients allocated to the concentrated EN group received significantly more calories than patients in the standard EN group (2040 ± 578 vs. 1504 ± 573 kcal, *P* ≤ .001). The study was not powered to detect differences in adverse events or clinical outcomes. There was a trend, though, toward longer 90-day survival in the concentrated EN group (*P* = .057).

The fifth RCT evaluating the "dose" of nutritional support was a multicenter cluster-RCT of algorithms for critical care enteral and parenteral therapy in 14 Canadian ICUs (ACCEPT [algorithms for critical-care enteral and parenteral therapy]).[40] This trial evaluated the impact of evidence-based feeding algorithms on nutrition practices and patient outcomes. Four hundred and ninety-nine patients, ages 16 years or older, who were expected to stay in the ICU at least 48 hours were enrolled in the study. An intensive educational program was provided at the sites assigned to the intervention group. ICUs assigned to the control group did not receive any of the interventions. Patients at the intervention hospitals received significantly more days of EN per 10 days (6.7 vs. 5.4 days; *P* = .042), had a significantly shorter length of hospital stay (25 vs. 35 days; *P* = .003), and demonstrated a trend toward reduced mortality (27% vs. 37%; *P* = .058). Length of ICU stay was not different between the two groups, though (10.9 vs. 11.8 days; *P* = .7). Admittedly, it is difficult to understand how such a small difference in the dose of EN is associated with such large changes in clinical outcomes.

To confirm these observations, Doig and colleagues performed a complex, multifaceted intervention in 27 community and teaching hospitals in Australia and New Zealand. The trial involved 18 different strategies to change nutrition practice, including an evidence-based feeding algorithm.[41] ICUs randomized to receive the intervention participated in a 2-day guideline development conference that included an educational workshop on the use of the 18 interventions to be used to implement the new guidelines. The study found that EN was initiated earlier in patients from intervention ICUs (0.75 vs. 1.37 days; *P* < .001) and patients achieved the caloric goal more often

(6.10 vs. 5.02 days per 10 fed-patient days; $P = .03$). In addition, more patients were never fed in the control ICUs (28.2 vs. 5.7%; $P \le .001$). No significant differences were observed in any of the measured clinical outcomes, though.

Finally, a single-center pilot RCT conducted in Israel aimed to determine if tight caloric control improved hospital survival.[39] One hundred and thirty patients were randomized to have their nutritional requirements guided either by repeated resting energy expenditure (REE) measurements or by a single, initial weight-based measurement. Although the mean REE was not different between the study and control groups, the mean energy delivered was significantly higher in the study group (2086 ± 460 vs. 1480 ± 356 kcal/day; $P = .01$). An intention-to-treat analysis showed a trend toward improved mortality in the study group (32.3% vs. 47.7%; $P = .058$). However, the study group also had a longer duration of mechanical ventilation (16.1 ± 14.7 days vs. 10.5 ± 8.3 days; $P = .03$) and ICU stay (17.2 ± 14.6 days vs. 11.7 ± 8.4 days; $P = .04$) as well as more infectious complications (37 vs. 20; $P = .05$). These discrepant results need to be further explored.

META-ANALYSIS OF RANDOMIZED CONTROLLED TRIALS OF UNDERFEEDING FULL FEEDING

To illuminate our deliberation about the appropriateness of underfeeding in the critical care setting, we conducted a meta-analysis to aggregate the results of these recent RCTs of hypocaloric EN, trophic feeding, and enhanced early EN.[42] The studies by Martin et al. and Doig et al. were cluster RCTs; thus the unit of analysis was the ICU and not the individual patient. Therefore the results of these trials were not included. In addition, data from the study by Singer et al. were omitted because some patients received supplemental parenteral nutrition. Overall, there was no difference in ICU (RR, 1.01; 95% CI, 0.70 to 1.45; $P = .96$) or hospital mortality (RR, 1.14; 95% CI, 0.85 to 1.50; $P = .38$; Fig. 67-1), hospital length of stay (weighted mean difference [WMD] –0.16; 95% CI, –3.41, 3.72), or infectious complications (RR, 0.88; 95% CI, 0.70 to 1.59; $P = .25$; Fig. 67-2) in patients who received more EN compared with less EN.

WHERE DO WE GO FROM HERE?

In sum, the 13 observational studies and 12 RCTs detailed in this review do not appear to favor either feeding to goal or underfeeding. In fact, recent trials have, in some respects, muddied the water further and led to conflicting practice recommendations. These studies and discussions do not account for the heterogeneity of critically ill patients. Clearly, some subgroups of patients are at a greater nutritional risk and may therefore benefit from more aggressive nutrition therapy in the ICU, whereas "low-risk" patient populations would not be expected to derive benefit from increased caloric delivery. For example, review of the characteristics of patients enrolled in the EDEN trial of trophic versus full feeding reveals that, on average, they were young (52 years), well nourished (BMI 30 kg/m^2), and had a short ICU stay (requiring mechanical ventilation for 5 days).[32] The null results observed in this trial may be a function of the low nutrition risk nature of the population.

In lieu of a definitive answer, it may be reasonable to propose that nutritional requirements depend on nutrition risk. If a patient is well nourished and not expected to have a protracted clinical course, then underfeeding in the first week of ICU may be acceptable. Conversely, underfeeding a high-risk patient may have a detrimental effect on their clinical course and long-term outcomes. We would recommend that future research priorities in critical care nutrition include the following:

- Developing, validating, and applying nutrition risk assessment tools, such as the NUTrition Risk in the Critically ill Score (NUTRIC score)[43] to determine who might benefit the most from full feeding.
- Conducting high-quality, large-scale RCTs of nutrition interventions in the ICU targeting high-risk patients or patients stratified by nutritional risk.
- Considering long-term effects of nutrition interventions such as physical function, muscle mass, and quality of life together with the historically evaluated short-term outcomes of ICU and hospital mortality, length of stay, and infectious complications.
- Defining the optimal caloric prescription for critically ill patients to enable more accurate measurement of full feeding.
- Acquiring data on the nutritional status and nutritional intake of patients after ICU discharge because the benefits of optimizing nutrition within the ICU may be compromised if postdischarge provision is poor.

Until future trials elucidate the role of intentional underfeeding in ICU patients, critical care practitioners should continue to attempt to assess the nutritional risk of their patients and provide early and adequate EN using 80% goal calories as a quality benchmark.[27] This can be successfully operationalized at the bedside through innovative feeding protocols and monitoring tools such as the PEP uP protocol.[44] In high-risk patients in whom enteral delivery is proactive, strategies to optimize enteral nutrition delivery (prokinetics, postpyloric feeding) should be considered. In addition, recent data suggest that early supplemental parenteral nutrition may be warranted.[45] Conversely, if low-risk patients receive less than 80% goal calories, their intake should continue to be monitored, but no additional steps are required.

APPENDIX I: SUMMARY OF SEARCH STRATEGY

For the location of relevant articles, four bibliographic databases (Medline, Embase, CINAHL, and the Cochrane Library) were searched. Search terms included *nutritional support* or *enteral nutrition* or *energy intake* or *hypocaloric feeding* or *trophic feeding* or *energy debt* and *critical care* or *critical illness* or *intensive care units*. These searches spanned from 1996 to December 2014. In addition, personal files and relevant review articles were searched for additional studies. There were no language restrictions on included studies. Data only reported in abstract form were excluded.

Study or subgroup	High EN Events	Total	Less EN Events	Total	Weight	Risk ratio M-H, Random, 95% CI	Year	Risk ratio M-H, Random, 95% CI
1.2.1 Achieving target dose of EN								
Desachy 2008	14	50	11	50	12.7%	1.27 [0.64, 2.53]	2008	
Peake 2014	10	57	14	55	11.8%	0.69 [0.33, 1.42]	2014	
Braunschweig 2014	16	40	6	38	9.6%	2.53 [1.11, 5.79]	2014	
Subtotal (95% CI)		**147**		**143**	**34.2%**	**1.28 [0.63, 2.58]**		
Total events	40		31					
Heterogeneity: Tau^2 = 0.25; Chi^2 = 5.42, df = 2 (P = .07); I^2 = 63%								
Test for overall effect: Z = 0.68 (P = .50)								
1.2.2 Hypocaloric EN								
Arabi 2011	51	120	36	120	27.3%	1.42 [1.00, 2.00]	2011	
Petros 2013	17	54	17	46	17.3%	0.85 [0.49, 1.47]	2013	
Charles 2014	4	42	3	41	3.8%	1.30 [0.31, 5.46]	2014	
Subtotal (95% CI)		**216**		**207**	**48.3%**	**1.20 [0.85, 1.69]**		
Total events	72		56					
Heterogeneity: Tau^2 = 0.02; Chi^2 = 2.40, df = 2 (P = .30); I^2 = 17%								
Test for overall effect: Z = 1.03 (P = .30)								
1.2.3 Trophic vs. full feeds								
Rice 2011	20	102	22	98	17.5%	0.87 [0.51, 1.50]	2011	
Subtotal (95% CI)		**102**		**98**	**17.5%**	**0.87 [0.51, 1.50]**		
Total events	20		22					
Heterogeneity: Not applicable								
Test for overall effect: Z = 0.49 (P = .62)								
Total (95% CI)		**465**		**448**	**100.0%**	**1.14 [0.85, 1.52]**		
Total events	132		109					
Heterogeneity: Tau^2 = 0.05; Chi^2 = 9.12, df = 6 (P = .17); I^2 = 34%								
Test for overall effect: Z = 0.88 (P = .38)								
Test for subgroup differences: Chi^2 = 1.10, df = 2 (P = .58), I^2 = 0%								

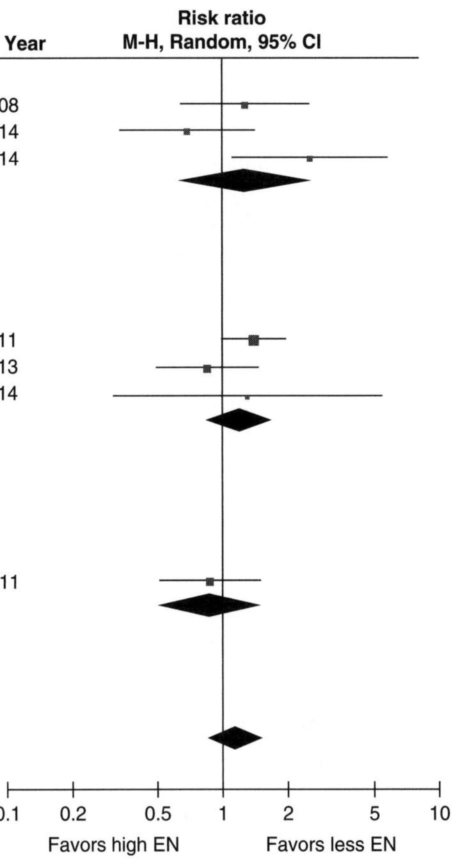

0.1 0.2 0.5 1 2 5 10
Favors high EN   Favors less EN

Figure 67-1. Meta-analysis of randomized controlled trials evaluating the effect of underfeeding versus full feeding on hospital mortality in critically ill patients. *CI*, confidence intervals; *EN*, enteral nutrition. (*Reproduced with permission from www.criticalcarenutrition.com.*)

Study or subgroup	High EN Events	Total	Less EN Events	Total	Weight	Risk ratio M-H, Random, 95% CI	Year	Risk ratio M-H, Random, 95% CI
1.3.1 Achieving Target Dose of EN								
Taylor 1999	25	41	35	41	26.6%	0.71 [0.54, 0.94]	1999	
Braunschweig 2014	5	40	8	38	4.2%	0.59 [0.21, 1.66]	2014	
Subtotal (95% CI)		**81**		**79**	**30.8%**	**0.71 [0.54, 0.92]**		
Total events	30		43					
Heterogeneity: Tau^2 = 0.00; Chi^2 = 0.14, df = 1 (P = .71); I^2 = 0%								
Test for overall effect: Z = 2.57 (P = .01)								
1.3.2 Hypocaloric EN								
Arabi 2011	56	120	53	120	26.5%	1.06 [0.80, 1.39]	2011	
Petros 2013	6	54	12	46	5.3%	0.43 [0.17, 1.05]	2013	
Charles 2014	24	42	23	41	19.6%	1.02 [0.70, 1.48]	2014	
Subtotal (95% CI)		**216**		**207**	**51.4%**	**0.93 [0.66, 1.31]**		
Total events	86		88					
Heterogeneity: Tau^2 = 0.04; Chi^2 = 3.73, df = 2 (P = .15); I^2 = 46%								
Test for overall effect: Z = 0.39 (P = .69)								
1.3.3 Trophic vs. full feeds								
Rice 2011	33	102	30	98	17.8%	1.06 [0.70, 1.59]	2011	
Subtotal (95% CI)		**102**		**98**	**17.8%**	**1.06 [0.70, 1.59]**		
Total events	33		30					
Heterogeneity: Not applicable								
Test for overall effect: Z = 0.26 (P = .79)								
Total (95% CI)		**399**		**384**	**100.0%**	**0.88 [0.70, 1.10]**		
Total events	149		161					
Heterogeneity: Tau^2 = 0.03; Chi^2 = 8.31, df = 5 (P = .14); I^2 = 40%								
Test for overall effect: Z = 1.15 (P = .25)								
Test for subgroup differences: Chi^2 = 3.23, df = 2 (P = .20), I^2 = 38.0%								

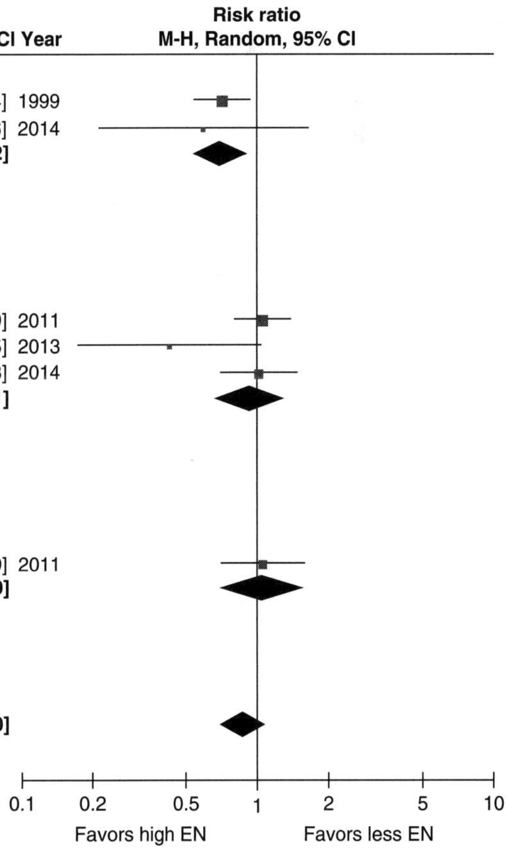

0.1 0.2 0.5 1 2 5 10
Favors high EN   Favors less EN

Figure 67-2. Meta-analysis of randomized controlled trials evaluating the effect of underfeeding versus full feeding on infections in critically ill patients. *CI*, confidence intervals; *EN*, enteral nutrition. (*Reproduced with permission from www.criticalcarenutrition.com.*)

Studies were included in the review process if they met the following criteria:

- *Study design:* RCT or meta-analysis
- *Population:* Mechanically ventilated, critically ill adult patients
- *Intervention (if applicable):* Intentional underfeeding, early aggressive versus early lower-dose EN
- *Outcomes:* At least one of the following: mortality (ICU, hospital, long-term), length of stay, infectious and noninfectious complication.

Because our goal was to determine the optimal amount of energy to feed the critically ill, we excluded studies that examined protein intake and outcomes. In contrast to the purported benefits of energy restriction, protein restriction is associated with worse clinical outcomes in animal models and clinical studies.[46] We also excluded studies that considered only obese patients because these studies apply to a minority of critically ill patients, limiting our ability to apply results to general clinical practice.

AUTHORS' RECOMMENDATIONS

- Most critically ill patients receive only 49% to 70% of their calculated energy requirements.
- The results of observational studies suggest that the optimal dose of enteral nutrition (EN) is greater than 25% but less than 82% goal calories.
- RCTs of studies of route of delivery and timing of feeding suggest that early aggressive EN is associated with improved clinical outcomes, but using PN in preference to EN or supplementing EN with PN does not confer any additional benefits.
- RCT level evidence on the optimal amount of energy to provide critically ill patients is lacking.
- Strategies to achieve 100% goal calories with EN should be pursued.

REFERENCES

1. Monk DN, Plank LD, Franch-Arcas G, et al. Sequential changes in the metabolic response in critically injured patients during the first 25 days after blunt trauma. *Ann Surg.* 1996;223:395–405.
2. Heyland DK, Dhaliwal R, Wang M, et al. The prevalence of iatrogenic underfeeding in the nutritionally 'at-risk' critically ill patient: Results of an international, multicenter, prospective study. *Clin Nutr.* 2015;34:659–666.
3. Heyland DK, Dhaliwal R, Drover JW, et al. Canadian clinical practice guidelines for nutrition support in mechanically ventilated, critically ill adult patients. *JPEN J Parenter Enteral Nutr.* 2003;27:355–373.
4. Doig GSS, Simpson F. *Evidence-Based Guidelines for Nutritional Support of the Critically Ill: Results of a Bi-National Guideline Development Conference.* Sydney: EvidenceBased.net; 2005.
5. Kreymann KG, Berger MM, Deutz NE, et al. ESPEN Guidelines on Enteral Nutrition: Intensive care. *Clin Nutr.* 2006;25:210–223.
6. McClave SA, Martindale RG, Vanek VW, et al. Guidelines for the Provision and Assessment of Nutrition Support Therapy in the Adult Critically Ill Patient: Society of Critical Care Medicine (SCCM) and American Society for Parenteral and Enteral Nutrition (A.S.P.E.N.). *JPEN J Parenter Enteral Nutr.* 2009;33:277–316.
7. Dhaliwal R, Cahill N, Lemieux M, et al. The Canadian critical care nutrition guidelines in 2013: an update on current recommendations and implementation strategies. *Nutr Clin Pract.* 2014;29:29–43.
8. Dellinger RP, Levy MM, Rhodes A, et al. Surviving Sepsis Campaign: international guidelines for management of severe sepsis and septic shock, 2012. *Intensive Care Med.* 2013;39:165–228.
9. Patino JF, de Pimiento SE, Vergara A, et al. Hypocaloric support in the critically ill. *World J Surg.* 1999;23:553–559.
10. Huang YC, Yen CE, Cheng CH, et al. Nutritional status of mechanically ventilated critically ill patients: comparison of different types of nutritional support. *Clin Nutr.* 2000;19:101–107.
11. Rice TW, Swope T, Bozeman S, et al. Variation in enteral nutrition delivery in mechanically ventilated patients. *Nutrition.* 2005;21:786–792.
12. Cahill NE, Dhaliwal R, Day AG, et al. Nutrition therapy in the critical care setting: what is "best achievable" practice? An international multicenter observational study. *Crit Care Med.* 2010;38:395–401.
13. Heyland DK, Heyland RD, Cahill NE, et al. Creating a culture of clinical excellence in critical care nutrition: the 2008 "Best of the Best" award. *JPEN J Parenter Enteral Nutr.* 2010;34:707–715.
14. Rubinson L, Diette GB, Song X, et al. Low caloric intake is associated with nosocomial bloodstream infections in patients in the medical intensive care unit. *Crit Care Med.* 2004;32:350–357.
15. Villet S, Chiolero RL, Bollmann MD, et al. Negative impact of hypocaloric feeding and energy balance on clinical outcome in ICU patients. *Clin Nutr.* 2005;24:502–509.
16. Dvir D, Cohen J, Singer P. Computerized energy balance and complications in critically ill patients: an observational study. *Clin Nutr.* 2006;25:37–44.
17. Petros S, Engelmann L. Enteral nutrition delivery and energy expenditure in medical intensive care patients. *Clin Nutr.* 2006;25:51–59.
18. Rimdeika R, Gudaviciene D, Adamonis K, et al. The effectiveness of caloric value of enteral nutrition in patients with major burns. *Burns.* 2006;32:83–86.
19. Faisy C, Lerolle N, Dachraoui F, et al. Impact of energy deficit calculated by a predictive method on outcome in medical patients requiring prolonged acute mechanical ventilation. *Br J Nutr.* 2009;101:1079–1087.
20. Alberda C, Gramlich L, Jones N, et al. The relationship between nutritional intake and clinical outcomes in critically ill patients: results of an international multicenter observational study. *Intensive Care Med.* 2009;35:1728–1737.
21. Heyland DK, Cahill N, Day AG. Optimal amount of calories for critically ill patients: depends on how you slice the cake!. *Crit Care Med.* 2011;39:2619–2626.
22. Elke G, Wang M, Weiler N, et al. Close to recommended caloric and protein intake by enteral nutrition is associated with better clinical outcome of critically ill septic patients: secondary analysis of a large international nutrition database. *Crit Care.* 2014;18:R29.
23. Krishnan JA, Parce PB, Martinez A, et al. Caloric intake in medical ICU patients: consistency of care with guidelines and relationship to clinical outcomes. *Chest.* 2003;124:297–305.
24. Hise ME, Halterman K, Gajewski BJ, et al. Feeding practices of severely ill intensive care unit patients: an evaluation of energy sources and clinical outcomes. *J Am Diet Assoc.* 2007;107:458–465.
25. Ibrahim EH, Mehringer L, Prentice D, et al. Early versus late enteral feeding of mechanically ventilated patients: results of a clinical trial. *JPEN J Parenteral Enteral Nutr.* 2002;26:174–181.
26. Arabi YM, Haddad SH, Tamim HM, et al. Near-target caloric intake in critically ill medical-surgical patients is associated with adverse outcomes. *JPEN J Parenteral Enteral Nutr.* 2010;34:280–288.
27. Heyland DK, Cahill N, Day AG. Optimal amount of calories for critically ill patients: Depends on how you slice the cake! *Crit Care Med.* 2011;39:2691–2699.
28. Arabi YM, Tamim HM, Dhar GS, et al. Permissive underfeeding and intensive insulin therapy in critically ill patients: a randomized controlled trial. *Am J Clin Nutr.* 2011;93:569–577.
29. Petros S, Horbach M, Seidel F, et al. Hypocaloric vs Normocaloric Nutrition in Critically Ill Patients: A Prospective Randomized Pilot Trial. *JPEN J Parenter Enteral Nutr.* April 3, 2014. [Epub ahead of print].
30. Charles EJ, Petroze RT, Metzger R, et al. Hypocaloric compared with eucaloric nutritional support and its effect on infection rates in a surgical intensive care unit: a randomized controlled trial. *Am J Clin Nutr.* 2014;100:1337–1343.
31. Rice TW, Mogan S, Hays MA, et al. Randomized trial of initial trophic versus full-energy enteral nutrition in mechanically ventilated patients with acute respiratory failure. *Crit Care Med.* 2011;39:967–974.
32. Rice TW, Wheeler AP, Thompson BT, et al. Initial trophic vs full enteral feeding in patients with acute lung injury: the EDEN randomized trial. *JAMA.* 2012;307:795–803.
33. Needham DM, Dinglas VD, Morris PE, et al. Physical and cognitive performance of patients with acute lung injury 1 year after initial trophic versus full enteral feeding. EDEN trial follow-up. *Am J Respir Crit Care Med.* 2013;188:567–576.

34. Needham DM, Dinglas VD, Bienvenu OJ, et al. One year outcomes in patients with acute lung injury randomised to initial trophic or full enteral feeding: prospective follow-up of EDEN randomised trial. *BMJ*. 2013;346:f1532.

35. Taylor SJ, Fettes SB, Jewkes C, et al. Prospective, randomized, controlled trial to determine the effect of early enhanced enteral nutrition on clinical outcome in mechanically ventilated patients suffering head injury. *Crit Care Med*. 1999;27:2525–2531.

36. Desachy A, Clavel M, Vuagnat A, et al. Initial efficacy and tolerability of early enteral nutrition with immediate or gradual introduction in intubated patients. *Intensive Care Med*. 2008;34:1054–1059.

37. Braunschweig CA, Sheean PM, Peterson SJ, et al. Intensive nutrition in acute lung injury: a clinical trial (INTACT). *JPEN J Parenter Enteral Nutr*. 2015;39:13–20.

38. Peake SL, Davies AR, Deane AM, et al. Use of a concentrated enteral nutrition solution to increase calorie delivery to critically ill patients: a randomized, double-blind, clinical trial. *Am J Clin Nutr*. 2014;100:616–625.

39. Singer P, Anbar R, Cohen J, et al. The tight calorie control study (TICACOS): a prospective, randomized, controlled pilot study of nutritional support in critically ill patients. *Intensive Care Med*. 2011;37:601–609.

40. Martin CM, Doig GS, Heyland DK, et al. Multicentre, cluster-randomized clinical trial of algorithms for critical-care enteral and parenteral therapy (ACCEPT). *CMAJ*. 2004;170:197–204.

41. Doig GS, Simpson F, Finfer S, et al. Effect of evidence-based feeding guidelines on mortality of critically ill adults: a cluster randomized controlled trial. *JAMA*. 2008;300:2731–2741.

42. Critical Care Nutrition. *Practice Guidelines 2013*; 2014.

43. Heyland DK, Dhaliwal R, Jiang X, et al. Identifying critically ill patients who benefit the most from nutrition therapy: the development and initial validation of a novel risk assessment tool. *Crit Care*. 2011;15:R268.

44. Heyland DK, Murch L, Cahill N, et al. Enhanced protein-energy provision via the enteral route feeding protocol in critically ill patients: results of a cluster randomized trial. *Crit Care Med*. 2013;41:2743–2753.

45. Doig GS, Simpson F, Sweetman EA, et al. Early parenteral nutrition in critically ill patients with short-term relative contraindications to early enteral nutrition: a randomized controlled trial. *JAMA*. 2013;309:2130–2138.

46. Weijs PJ. Fundamental determinants of protein requirements in the ICU. *Curr Opin Clin Nutr Metab Care*. 2014;17:183–189.

68 How Does Critical Illness Alter the Liver?

Michael Bauer, Andreas Kortgen

Liver alterations are common in critical illness. These changes can be attributed to diverse factors, including systemic inflammation and poor perfusion but also to drugs and parenteral nutrition.[1-4] Damage ranges from self-limited abnormalities in liver chemistry to fulminant organ failure. In addition, critical illness elicits profound changes in the concentrations of acute-phase proteins, plasma peptides synthesized by the liver as part of the response to a "danger" signal. Although some of these proteins help to control damage, the functions of others are obscure. Critical illness also induced a reprogramming of metabolic function. Finally, there is a severity-dependent disruption of phase I and II biotransformation and bile transport (i.e., excretory failure with important implications for pharmacotherapy in the intensive care unit [ICU]). The hepatobiliary excretory machinery appears exceptionally sensitive to inflammation.[5,6] As a result, impaired excretion occurs in the absence of traditional markers of (ischemic) liver cell death, such as serum transaminases.[3] Importantly, these changes—acute-phase protein elaboration, altered metabolism, and disrupted biotransformation—occur in parallel. With increasing severity of liver impairment, other functions, most notably synthesis of coagulatory proteins and glucose homeostasis, fail and impaired clearance of toxic compounds affects other organs, as in the case of hepatic encephalopathy. Although fulminant liver failure in previously healthy patients is rare, a deterioration of a preexisting liver disease is more common. The extent of the dysfunction is often underestimated, especially in surgical patients, and is associated with substantial morbidity and mortality. Episodes of decompensated cirrhosis are manifested as variceal bleeding, renal insufficiency, and encephalopathy.

MECHANISMS AND MANIFESTATION OF LIVER DYSFUNCTION

The liver is a highly perfused organ, and there are complex mechanisms to regulate liver microcirculatory blood flow. Under pathophysiologic conditions, these regulatory mechanisms can become ineffective and impaired. Together with macrocirculatory changes, an altered microcirculation may lead to profound changes in critically ill patients and may even reduce effective sinusoidal blood flow. Globally reduced (e.g., in hemorrhagic shock, right heart failure, mechanical ventilation) or redistributed (i.e., sepsis, anaphylaxis, endocrinopathies) blood flow with shunting are mechanisms for ischemic damage. Shunts can be intrahepatic or extrahepatic. In patients with chronic liver disease and portal hypertension, an especially large amount of portal blood can be redirected via extrahepatic shunts. Conversely, increased liver blood flow in acute hepatitis has also been described.

Ischemic damage to the liver may accompany low flow states (i.e., shock) or reflect congestion as a consequence of right heart failure. When severe, ischemia characteristically leads to cell death in the pericentral region of the hepatic acinus, which is reflected in an increase in serum levels of glutamate dehydrogenase. Hypoxic hepatitis leading to centrolobular hepatocellular necrosis is associated with a rapid increase in serum aminotransferases (aspartate and alanine aminotransferase) with levels up to 20 times the upper limit of normal.[1]

Impaired excretory function is a frequent manifestation of critical illness. Development of jaundice as a complication of severe trauma or life-threatening disease was only observed with the widespread establishment of ICUs in the 1960s. This finding may well be related to prototypical therapeutic ICU interventions such as multiple transfusions, parenteral nutrition, and potentially hepatotoxic medications.[7] In a large Austrian multicentric cohort, an early increase in plasma bilirubin (>2 mg/dL), noted in approximately 10% of critically ill intensive care patients, was a strong independent risk factor for subsequent mortality.[8]

Hepatocellular excretory dysfunction in the critically ill might result from altered blood flow or transmembrane transport. However, it is more frequently associated with systemic inflammation than with ischemic damage. Sepsis accounts for approximately 20% of jaundice cases. This number is surpassed as a cause only by malignant compression of the bile duct.[9] Many basolateral and canalicular transport proteins are downregulated in critically ill patients. This response most likely reflects sensitivity to inflammatory stimuli.[3,10] Alterations in hepatocellular enzyme expression and activity, including those modulating phase I and II metabolism, may lead to profound changes in endobiotic and xenobiotic detoxification.[4] Ductal cholestasis is another characteristic of hepatic dysfunction in the critically ill. This abnormality is most often seen in association with prolonged shock, in which impaired arterial perfusion may result in ischemic injury to the biliary system. Although hepatocellular impairment is most often fully reversible, ductular damage can lead to persistent alterations that may progress to secondary sclerosing cholangitis, an underappreciated long-term sequel of critical illness that carries a very poor prognosis.[11]

The incidence of excretory impairment is underestimated by traditional "static" measures, such as serum transaminases or bilirubin. In contrast, "dynamic" tests, such as solute clearance, are much more sensitive. Hepatobiliary transport systems are essential for the uptake and excretion of various compounds, including bile acids and xenobiotics, and this partial function is best monitored by a functional test such as dye excretion.

IMPACT OF LIVER DYSFUNCTION ON CRITICAL CARE PHARMACOLOGY

Liver disease induces complex changes in the handling of drugs. These alterations are often unpredictable and may affect pharmacokinetics and pharmacodynamics. Therefore administration of medications to these patients must be carefully evaluated and strictly controlled, a mandate that is especially important when dosing drugs with a narrow therapeutic index. The additional risk of (hepatotoxic) side effects must be taken into account, and extreme caution is recommended when such drugs are used. Whenever possible, therapeutic monitoring should be performed, and dosage should be adjusted based on measured pharmacokinetic and pharmacodynamics properties. For some drugs, such as sedatives or analgesics, titrating dosage according to clinical effect may be sufficient. However, in the critically ill, it is essential that initial underdosing be avoided. This issue is especially germane with respect to antibiotic therapy in septic patients, where early and effective drug levels are essential for patient survival. In general, the following recommendations for dosing of drugs eliminated by hepatic metabolism and excretion should be observed in critically ill patients:

1. In drugs with a high extraction ratio (>0.6), oral/enteral application leads to high first-pass metabolism and therefore low bioavailability. A reduction in hepatic blood flow due to shunting (intrahepatic, extrahepatic, or artificial following transjugular intrahepatic portosystemic shunt) or cirrhosis may substantially increase the bioavailability of such drugs. Thus, reducing initial doses and titrating maintenance doses should be considered for drugs with a high hepatic extraction ratio.
2. Intravenous administration of drugs is usually more reliable and predictable. If liver blood flow is reduced, then maintenance doses should be reduced. Conversely, administration of prodrugs that have to be metabolized to their active form in the liver can result in reduced availability of the active drug (e.g., clopidogrel, enalapril).[12]
3. For drugs with a low hepatic extraction ratio (<0.3), clearance is dependent on the intrinsic capacity of the elimination pathway and on the fraction of drug that is not protein bound. Impairment of specific elimination mechanisms must be taken into account. For drugs with protein binding less than 90%, maintenance, but not initial, doses should be reduced. The amount of reduction can be estimated based on the severity of liver dysfunction. For example, in patients with liver dysfunction consistent with Child-Turcotte-Pugh (CTP) Class A, doses should be dropped to 50% of normal. A decrease to 25% of the normal dose is recommended in Class B dysfunction, whereas the more severe impairment associated with Class C requires the use of drug monitoring.[12] These recommendations have limitations because the CTP score represents a rough approximation of impairment and each individual elimination mechanism may be differentially affected. Because phase II metabolism may be less severely impaired, drugs solely metabolized via this pathway should be preferentially used.
4. For drugs with a low hepatic extraction ratio and high protein binding, changes in pharmacokinetics are unpredictable. Therefore drug monitoring is recommended wherever possible, and the unbound fraction should be measured.
5. For hydrophilic substances, such as β-lactam antibiotics, an increased initial dosage should be considered in patients with ascites and edema because the volume of distribution may be substantially increased.[12] However, for maintenance dosage of these drugs, the potential for renal dysfunction must be considered.

Recent reports suggest that liver function tests can be used to predict the required drug dosages. For example, the disappearance rate of indocyanine green from the plasma may be used to determine the appropriate argatroban maintenance dose in critically ill patients with heparin-induced thrombocytopenia type II, whereas the methacetin breath test can predict the increase in tacrolimus trough levels after liver transplantation.[13-15] In the future, such testing might be used to govern therapy in which monitoring drug levels is not possible or where correct determination of the initial dose is crucial with respect to toxicity/side effects or therapeutic effect.

HEPATIC ADAPTATION TO CRITICAL ILLNESS: THE ACUTE-PHASE RESPONSE

Critical illness elicits profound changes in the plasma proteome. Many of the affected peptides are predominantly synthesized in the liver and are referred to as "acute-phase proteins." Proteins may be upregulated (as in the case of C-reactive protein) or downregulated (as in the case of albumin). The response is presumed to be adaptive, and, indeed, some acute-phase proteins have been shown to control damage and to participate in tissue repair. However, the role of many acute-phase reactants is unknown. In the clinical setting, measurements of acute-phase proteins have diagnostic or prognostic value. Reprogramming of metabolic function occurs in parallel with a severity-dependent disruption of phase I and II biotransformation and canalicular transport. Thus activation of the acute-phase response may not be entirely adaptive but may be associated with excretory impairment.

Overall, a deterioration of hepatobiliary excretion reflects an early and poor prognostic event in the critically ill. This change has important implications for monitoring and pharmacotherapy in the ICU. Early recognition, supportive care, and effective treatment of the underlying disease process as well as avoidance of hepatotoxic drugs are the cornerstones of management of liver dysfunction in the critical care setting.

AUTHORS' RECOMMENDATIONS

- Liver dysfunction in critical illness can be attributed to diverse factors, including systemic inflammation and poor perfusion but also to drugs and parenteral nutrition.
- The hepatobiliary excretory machinery appears exceptionally sensitive to inflammation; changes in acute phase protein elaboration, altered metabolism, and disrupted biotransformation may occur without changes in traditional liver function tests (e.g., transaminases).
- Hyperbilirubinemia or frank jaundice is a common complication of critical illness—and strongly predicts mortality. It results from downregulation of many basolateral and canalicular transport proteins.
- Liver disease induces complex changes in the handling of drugs. It is essential that initial underdosing be avoided—particularly with antibiotics. Drug dosing should be adjusted for hepatic extraction ratio, protein binding, and the type of metabolism (phase I versus phase II).
- Plasma protein levels may change in critical illness, specifically reprioritization of visceral proteins for acute phase compounds (such as CRP). It is unclear whether this is adaptive or pathologic.

REFERENCES

1. Fuhrmann V, Jäger B, Zubkova A, Drolz A. Hypoxic hepatitis – epidemiology, pathophysiology and clinical management. *Wien Klin Wochenschr*. 2010;122:129–139.
2. Vanwijngaerden YM, et al. Critical illness evokes elevated circulating bile acids related to altered hepatic transporter and nuclear receptor expression. *Hepatology*. 2011;54:1741–1752.
3. Kortgen A, Paxian M, Werth M, et al. Prospective assessment of hepatic function and mechanisms of dysfunction in the critically ill. *Shock*. 2009;32:358–365.
4. Recknagel P, Gonnert FA, Westermann M, et al. Liver dysfunction and phosphatidylinositol-3-kinase signalling in early sepsis: experimental studies in rodent models of peritonitis. *PLoS Med*. 2012;9:e1001338.
5. Geier A,P, Fickert M, Trauner. Mechanisms of disease: mechanisms and clinical implications of cholestasis in sepsis. *Nat Clin Pract Gastroenterol Hepatol*. 2006;3:574–585.
6. Gonnert FA, Recknagel P, Hilger I, Claus RA, Bauer M, Kortgen A. Hepatic excretory function in sepsis: implications from biophotonic analysis of transcellular xenobiotic transport in a rodent model. *Crit Care*. 2013;17:R67.
7. Marshall JC. New translational research provides insights into liver dysfunction in sepsis. *PLoS Med*. 2012;9:e1001341.
8. Kramer L, Jordan B, Druml W, et al. Incidence and prognosis of early hepatic dysfunction in critically ill patients-a prospective multicenter study. *Crit Care Med*. 2007;35:1099–1104.
9. Whitehead MW, Hainsworth I, Kingham JG. The causes of obvious jaundice in South West Wales: perceptions versus reality. *Gut*. 2001;48:409–413.
10. Andrejko KM, Raj NR, Kim PK, Cereda M, Deutschman CS. AL-6 modulates sepsis-induced decreases in transcription of hepatic organic anion and bile acid transporters. *Shock*. 2008;29:490–496.
11. Ruemmele P, Hofstaedter F, Gelbmann CM. Secondary sclerosing cholangitis. *Nat Rev Gastroenterol Hepatol*. 2009;6:287–295.
12. Delco F, Tchambaz L, Schlienger R, Drewe J, Krähenbühl S. Dose adjustments in patients with liver disease. *Drug Saf*. 2005;28:529–545.
13. Link A, Girndt M, Selejan S, Mathes A, Böhm M, Rensing H. Argatroban for anticoagulation in continuous renal replacement therapy. *Crit Care Med*. 2009;37:105–110.
14. Parker BM, Cywinski JB, Alster JM, et al. Predicting immunosuppressant dosing in the early postoperative period with noninvasive indocyanine green elimination following orthotopic liver transplantation. *Liver Transpl*. 2008;14:46–52.
15. Lock JF, Malinowski M, Schwabauer E, et al. Initial graft function is a reliable predictor of tacrolimus trough levels during the first post-transplant week. *Clin Transplant*. 2011;25:436–443.

69 How Is Acute Liver Failure Managed?

Mark T. Keegan

Acute liver failure (ALF) is a catastrophic condition that results in multiple organ failure. The severity of the illness and the rapidity of clinical deterioration in a previously healthy individual are alarming to patients, their families, and the health-care team. Support of the patient with ALF requires the full armamentarium of therapies available in the modern intensive care unit (ICU) and may require orthotopic liver transplantation (OLT).[1] Survival rates have increased significantly in recent years.[2,3]

Acute liver failure (the preferred term) is defined as the onset of hepatic encephalopathy (HE) and coagulopathy within 26 weeks of jaundice in a patient without preexisting liver disease. Terms that signify the duration of illness such as O'Grady's "hyperacute" (<7 days), "acute" (7 to 21 days), and "subacute" (21 days to 26 weeks); Bernuau's "fulminant" (<2 weeks) and "subfulminant" (2 to 12 weeks); and Mochida's fulminant (<8 weeks) and "late onset" (8 to 24 weeks) are popular but less useful because they do not have prognostic significance distinct from the etiology.[4-6]

In 2011, the American Association for the Study of Liver Diseases (AASLD) updated its position paper detailing the management of ALF.[7] Recommendations of the U.S. Acute Liver Failure Study Group for the ICU management of such patients were published in 2007.[8] The rarity, heterogeneity, severity, and speed of progression of ALF mean that there is a paucity of randomized controlled trials evaluating therapies, and many interventions are empiric or based on expert opinion.

EPIDEMIOLOGY

ALF is rare. In developed countries, an incidence of between 1 and 6 cases per million people per year has been reported.[9-11] Approximately 2000 cases of ALF occur per year in the United States.[12] Rates are probably higher in locations with high rates of infective hepatitis and/or lack of resources for treatment, but incidence data are sparse. The etiology of ALF differs depending on the geographic location. In the United States and Europe, medications are responsible for most cases.[1] Acetaminophen is the principal culprit and accounted for 46% of the 1696 cases of adult ALF in the U.S. Acute Liver Failure Registry.[3,13] As described by Larson in a prospective, multicenter study,

many acetaminophen-induced cases of ALF result from unintentional acetaminophen overdose.[14] Approximately three quarters of cases of ALF in this study were in women, and most patients were between 26 and 45 years of age. More recent estimates suggest that acetaminophen may account for up to 50% of cases of ALF.[15] In other parts of the world, viruses (especially hepatitis A, B, D, and E) are the principal causes. There are several other causes of ALF as detailed in Table 69-1.[16]

CLINICAL PRESENTATION

Although initially a liver insult, ALF quickly becomes a multisystem disease. Loss of hepatocyte function (including host defense functions) and release of cellular debris and inflammatory mediators lead to a generalized inflammatory process. The stigma of chronic liver disease is absent. HE and coagulopathy are the characteristic features of ALF, and both may progress rapidly over days or even hours. Diagnosis of ALF is made on clinical grounds, aided by laboratory analysis. Imaging studies (e.g., hepatic ultrasound to assess the patency of the liver's vascular supply) and liver biopsy may aid in the elucidation of the cause of ALF, but the latter is not usually performed.

INITIAL ASSESSMENT AND MANAGEMENT

Most patients are initially admitted to hospital under the care of a general medical, gastroenterology or liver service. When the diagnosis of ALF has been made, a referral center with a liver transplant program should be contacted for advice on management and consideration for transfer.[1,3,7] Some have suggested that waiting for the development of HE to diagnose ALF leads to crucial delays in treatment. When HE develops in a patient with ALF, ICU care is usually warranted because of the potential for further deterioration and the need for interventions such as intubation, mechanical ventilation, and hemodynamic support. Several institutions have developed formal protocols for management of patients with ALF.[17] Although the utility of such protocols has not been studied in a controlled trial, they may help to ensure that all relevant aspects of the patient's care are addressed.

Table 69-1 **Causes of Acute Liver Failure**
A. Viral Hepatitis A virus, hepatitis B virus ± hepatitis D virus, hepatitis E virus, herpes simplex virus, cytomegalovirus, Epstein–Barr virus, varicella zoster virus, adenovirus, hemorrhagic fever viruses
B. Drugs and toxins Dose dependent: Acetaminophen, carbon tetrachloride, yellow phosphorus, *Amanita phalloides, Bacillus cereus* toxin, sulfonamides, tetracycline, methyldioxymethamphetamine (ecstasy), herbal remedies Idiosyncratic: Volatile anesthetics (especially halothane), isoniazid, rifampicin, valproic acid, nonsteroidal anti-inflammatory drugs, disulfiram
C. Vascular Right heart failure, Budd-Chiari syndrome, veno-occlusive disease, shock liver (ischemic hepatitis), heat stroke
D. Metabolic Acute fatty liver of pregnancy, Wilson disease, Reye syndrome, galactosemia, hereditary fructose intolerance, tyrosinemia
E. Miscellaneous Malignant infiltration (liver metastases, lymphoma), autoimmune hepatitis, sepsis
F. Indeterminate Includes primary graft nonfunction in liver transplant recipients

Modified from Saas DA, Shakil AO. *Liver Transplant.* 2005;11:594–605.

PROGNOSIS

With supportive therapy, some patients with ALF will spontaneously recover hepatic function. However, in many other cases, the patient will die without OLT. Of 1696 patients with ALF in the U.S. Acute Liver Failure Study Group dataset, overall patient survival was 71%.[3] Although these survival figures are much better than in the pretransplantation era, ALF remains a life-threatening disease entity. The main causes of death are cerebral edema with subsequent herniation and multiple organ failure. In data reported by Lee, 660 (39%) of the 1696 patients were listed for transplantation; of these, 409 were transplanted with 371 survivors and 38 deaths. Eight hundred and twenty-six survived without transplantation, and 461 died without transplantation.[3] In a 2-year follow-up by Fontana et al., long-term survival was significantly higher in 262 transplant recipients compared with 506 patients who survived without the need for transplantation, perhaps because of underlying comorbidities.[18]

The timing of transplantation is crucial. Delay in listing for transplantation may result in the patient's demise before a donor organ is found or may result in perioperative mortality. Premature listing may result in OLT being performed in patients who might otherwise have spontaneously recovered liver function. Multiple prognostic scoring systems have been developed in an effort to identify those patients at high risk of mortality.[19,20] The most commonly used criteria are those developed by O'Grady and colleagues in the United Kingdom. These are commonly known as the King's College criteria.[21] They were developed in a cohort of 588 patients with ALF who were managed medically between 1973 and 1985. The criteria differentiate between acetaminophen-induced ALF and ALF

Table 69-2 **Potentially Helpful Indicators of Poor Prognosis* in Patients with ALF**
Etiology • Idiosyncratic drug reaction • Acute hepatitis B (and other non-hepatitis A viral infections) • Autoimmune hepatitis • Mushroom poisoning • Wilson disease • Budd-Chiari syndrome • Indeterminate cause
Coma grade on admission • III or IV

King's College criteria
• Acetaminophen-induced ALF
  • Strongly consider OLT listing if arterial lactate >3.5 mmol/L after early fluid resuscitation
  • List for OLT if pH <7.3 or arterial lactate >3.0 mmol/L after adequate fluid resuscitation
  • List for OLT if all three of the following occur within a 24-hour period: grade III or IV HE, INR >6.5, creatinine >3.4 mg/dL
• Non-acetaminophen–induced ALF
  • List for OLT if INR >6.5 and encephalopathy present (irrespective of grade)
  • List for OLT if encephalopathy present (irrespective of grade) and any three of the following are present:
    - Age <10 or >40 years[†]
    - Jaundice for >7 days before development of encephalopathy[†]
    - INR ≥3.5
    - Serum bilirubin ≥17 mg/dL
    - Unfavorable cause such as Wilson disease, idiosyncratic drug reaction, seronegative hepatitis

From Lee W, et al. Introduction to the Revised American Association for the Study of Liver Diseases Position Paper on Acute Liver Failure 2011. *Hepatology.* 2012; 55:965-967.

*Note that none of these factors, with the exception of Wilson disease and possibly mushroom poisoning, are either necessary or sufficient to indicate the need for immediate liver transplantation

[†]These criteria, in particular, have not been found to be predictive of outcome in recent analyses.

ALF, acute liver failure; *HE,* hepatic encephalopathy; *INR,* international normalized ratio; *OLT,* orthotopic liver transplantation

due to other causes. They use pH, the international normalized ratio (INR), creatinine, grade of encephalopathy, age, duration of jaundice, and bilirubin level for prognostication. These criteria have been determined to have clinically acceptable specificity but more limited sensitivity.[22] Other well-known prognostic systems include the Clichy criteria (which use encephalopathy grade, factor V concentration, and age) and the Japanese criteria (age, encephalopathy, bilirubin level, and coagulopathy).[5,6] The ALF Early Dynamic (ALFED) model of Kumar et al. is a prediction model that is based on the changes in INR, serum bilirubin, arterial ammonia, and HE.[23] A recent systematic review of prediction models noted that studies of new models were associated with methodological flaws and that the performance of any new model has yet to be evaluated prospectively in a large cohort of patients.[24] There are insufficient data to recommend a particular scheme because none have been found to discriminate well enough and some are methodologically flawed or biased or equate transplantation with death.[8] Table 69-2 identifies potentially helpful indicators of poor prognosis in patients with ALF.[25] The etiology of ALF appears to be the most important factor, albeit with imperfect sensitivity and specificity.

The United Network for Organ Sharing (UNOS), the donor organ allocation body in the United States, has criteria that must be satisfied before a patient may be listed as a Status IA candidate for liver transplantation (the highest priority for organ allocation). These include "acute liver failure with a life expectancy of less than seven days without a liver transplant" or "primary graft non-function, hepatic artery thrombosis and acute Wilson's disease."

THERAPY FOR SPECIFIC CAUSES

The cause of the ALF should be sought because it will have implications for both therapy and prognosis.[7] Diagnosis of the cause of ALF requires a detailed history, multiple serologic and imaging tests, and potentially liver biopsy.

On the basis of several studies, *N*-acetylcysteine (NAC) has been shown to be effective in the treatment of acetaminophen toxicity.[14,26,27] The availability of the antidote, coupled with the frequency with which ALF is caused by acetaminophen toxicity, mean that an acetaminophen level should be drawn in every patient with ALF.[20] Acetaminophen toxicity may be indicated by the presence of very high serum transaminases and low bilirubin levels and assays for toxicity-related serum acetaminophen-containing protein adducts. NAC should be administered even if there is doubt regarding the timing or dose of ingestion or of the plasma concentration of acetaminophen. Oral administration has largely been replaced by intravenous (IV) administration.[7] The duration of NAC administration is determined by clinical condition rather than by time or serum acetaminophen concentration. Dosing may need to be continued beyond 72 to 96 hours.[8] In addition to the administration of NAC, patients with known or suspected acetaminophen overdose within 4 hours of presentation should have activated charcoal administered just before starting NAC.[7]

Drug-induced hepatotoxicity (apart from that induced by acetaminophen) is usually idiosyncratic and typically occurs during the first 6 months of therapy. Antibiotics (especially antituberculous medications), nonsteroidal anti-inflammatories, and anticonvulsants are most commonly implicated.[3,28,29] There are no specific antidotes, but the offending agent should be identified and stopped. Herbal and nutritional supplements also may cause acute liver injury, and information regarding such supplements should be sought from the patient and family. If the cause of ALF remains indeterminate, even after liver biopsy, then further investigation of potential drug or toxin exposure should be made. In data from the U.S. Acute Liver Failure Study Group, 11% of patients with ALF were deemed to have (non-acetaminophen) drug-induced ALF, and the entity was especially common in women and minorities.[29] Transplant-free (3-week) survival was poor (27.1%), but with highly successful transplantation in 42.1%, overall survival was 66.2%.

Viral hepatitis has become a relatively infrequent cause of ALF in the United States but is more common elsewhere. Hepatitis A and B accounted for 4% and 8%, respectively, of cases of ALF in the U.S. multicenter cohort.[3,13] Acute hepatitis D may cause acute liver dysfunction in a patient with preexisting hepatitis B, and hepatitis E may cause ALF in endemic areas, especially in pregnancy.[30] Care of a patient with acute viral hepatitis is mainly supportive. Lamivudine, used in chronic hepatitis B infection, has been reported to be of use for the treatment of hepatitis B-associated ALF, although a clinical trial has not been performed.[7] Although ALF secondary to herpes simplex or varicella zoster virus infection is rare, treatment with acyclovir has been recommended for suspected or documented cases and transplantation considered.

ALF may develop as an acute presentation of autoimmune hepatitis. Corticosteroids (prednisolone starting at 40 to 60 mg/day) are often administered in this scenario, although this practice is based on theory and case series, and, in fact, is not supported by the large retrospective analysis of Karkhanis et al.[31] Transplantation may be required.

Acute fatty liver of pregnancy is a rare disease that may occur in the second half of pregnancy, most often in the third trimester. It resolves with delivery of the fetus. Liver transplantation has been performed for this condition but should not be necessary with early diagnosis and prompt delivery.[32]

Wilson disease is an uncommon cause of ALF (2% to 3% of cases in the U.S. Acute Liver Failure Group cohort) but carries a grim prognosis without transplantation. Features of Wilson disease include low serum ceruloplasmin, high serum and urinary copper, hemolysis, Kayser-Fleischer rings (seen on slit-lamp examination), very low serum alkaline phosphatase and uric acid, and a bilirubin (milligram per deciliter)/alkaline phosphatase (IU/L) ratio greater than 2.[33] Although penicillamine treatment may be used in Wilson disease, it is not recommended in the setting of ALF.[34] Rather, other measures to reduce serum copper and prevent further hemolysis (e.g., plasmapheresis) should be initiated while the patient is waiting for an emergent liver transplant.

Amanita phalloides (mushroom) poisoning has been treated with penicillin G, NAC, and silibinin although controlled trials have not been performed, and the latter is not available as a licensed drug in the United States.[35]

When ALF is due to an acute ischemic injury or severe congestive heart failure, treatment of the underlying cause is required, and the prognosis is related to the response to therapy of the inciting insult.

Abdominal pain, prominent hepatomegaly, and ascites may indicate acute hepatic vein thrombosis (Budd-Chiari syndrome), which may present as ALF.[36] Liver transplantation is indicated based on high survival rates in case series, provided underlying malignancy is excluded. Malignant infiltration of the liver sufficient to cause ALF is a contraindication to liver transplantation and indicates a very poor prognosis.

HEPATIC ENCEPHALOPATHY

HE is one of the hallmarks of ALF.[37] In contrast to patients with chronic liver disease, the development of HE in a patient with ALF often is associated with the development of cerebral edema and elevations in intracranial pressure

(ICP). Cerebral edema is especially likely to develop in those patients with a short interval between jaundice and development of HE. Cerebral edema with subsequent herniation is the leading cause of death in patients with grade IV encephalopathy (see later) and may occur in up to 80% of these patients.

There are two main theories regarding the development of cerebral edema in ALF. It is likely that both play a role.[38,39] Glutamine is the end product of brain ammonia metabolism and may accumulate in astrocytes, causing alterations in neurotransmitter synthesis, impairment of mitochondrial function, and changes in osmolality, which ultimately lead to cerebral edema. In addition, failure of cerebral autoregulation that develops as a result of ALF leads to cerebral vasodilatation with a subsequent increase in cerebral blood flow and cerebral edema. The increase in ICP leads to a decrease in cerebral perfusion pressure (CPP) and the development of cerebral ischemia. In accordance with the Monro-Kellie doctrine, cerebral edema in the fixed confines of the skull will ultimately lead to herniation and death. Hyponatremia, cytokine production, and the development of seizures each may contribute to the development of cerebral ischemia.

HE develops rapidly in patients with ALF. Alterations in mental status are initially subtle but may progress to coma. There are four grades of HE (Table 69-3), and the grade of encephalopathy correlates with the development of cerebral edema and with outcome. Cerebral edema is uncommon in grade I or II, but it occurs in 25% to 35% and 65% to 75% in patients with grades III and IV encephalopathy, respectively. The prognosis worsens when grade IV encephalopathy is complicated by cerebral edema and is further worsened if renal failure is present. Furthermore, the development of infection alters the progression of HE.[40] Although ammonia levels correlate poorly with the severity of HE, an arterial ammonia greater than 200 µg/dL within 24 hours of the development of grade III or IV HE is predictive of herniation.[41]

Treatment of Hepatic Encephalopathy and Elevated Intracranial Pressure

Grades I and II Hepatic Encephalopathy

The management of patients with HE depends on the grade. On the basis of the experience at the institution, patients with grade I HE may be managed on a general ward, with skilled nursing in a quiet environment, but in most institutions such patients should be managed in an ICU. If, and when, grade II HE develops, ICU care is indicated. A computed tomography (CT) scan of the head should be performed to exclude causes of mental status change other than HE (e.g., intracranial hemorrhage, space-occupying lesion), although transport to the CT scanner may be dangerous, especially if the patient's airway is not protected. Although CT scans may demonstrate cerebral edema in patients with advanced HE, intracranial hypertension may not be detected.[42]

Administration of sedatives to patients with grade I or II HE should be avoided if possible because they will confound the detection of signs that might indicate progression to the next stage of encephalopathy. Nonetheless, small doses of short-acting antipsychotics (e.g., haloperidol, benzodiazepines, or dexmedetomidine) may be required to control agitation.

On the basis of a belief that ammonia plays a role in the pathogenesis of cerebral edema in patients with ALF, lactulose has been administered to patients with HE. In a study by Alba, it was associated with a small increase in survival time but no difference in the severity of encephalopathy or overall outcome.[43] The AASLD position paper recommends that "in early stages of encephalopathy, lactulose may be used either orally or rectally to effect a bowel purge, but should not be administered to the point of diarrhea, and may interfere with the surgical field by increasing bowel distension during liver transplantation."[7] Nonabsorbable antibiotics (rifaximin neomycin) also are not proven to be of use in ALF, and neomycin carries a risk of nephrotoxicity.

Grades III and IV Hepatic Encephalopathy

A patient who progresses to Grade III HE requires endotracheal intubation for airway protection. The choice of sedative or induction agents to be administered before intubation is left to the discretion of the practitioner because there are no studies to demonstrate the advantage of one regimen over another in this circumstance. It is intuitive that a drug regimen that minimizes the risk of increasing ICP should be used. Therefore propofol is a reasonable choice in this situation. If a muscle relaxant is used, then a nondepolarizing neuromuscular blocker (e.g., cisatracurium) offers some advantages over succinylcholine in terms of its effect on ICP.

Grade	Mental Status	Tremor	EEG
I	Euphoria; occasionally depression; fluctuant mild confusion; slowness of mentation and affect; untidy, slurred speech; disorder in sleep rhythm	Slight	Usually normal
II	Accentuation of grade I; drowsiness; inappropriate behavior; able to maintain sphincter control	Present (easily elicited)	Abnormal; generalized slowing
III	Sleeps most of the time but arousable; incoherent speech; marked confusion	Usually present if patient can cooperate	Always abnormal
IV	Not arousable; may or may not respond to painful stimuli	Usually absent	Always abnormal

Table 69-3 Grades of Hepatic Encephalopathy

Modified from Sass DA, Shakil AO. *Gastroenterol Clin N Am.* 2003;32:1195–1211.
EEG, Electroencephalogram.

Intracranial Pressure Monitoring

The use of ICP monitoring devices in ALF is subject to ongoing debate.[7,44-46] Proponents of ICP monitoring argue that such monitoring will allow rational use of the therapies detailed below. Others suggest that the risks of monitoring outweigh its value. The U.S. Acute Liver Failure Study Group has provided data on ICP monitoring in patients with ALF.[47,48] In the most recent data evaluating 629 patients with ALF, ICP monitoring was used in 140 patients (22%). Compared with controls, patients with ICP monitoring were younger and more likely to be on renal replacement therapy (RRT). Hemorrhagic complications were rare. Half of those for whom ICP data were available had elevated ICP with associated increased mortality. Overall 21-day mortality was similar in patients with ICP monitors (33%) and controls (38%; *P* = .24). When stratifying by acetaminophen status and adjusting for confounders, however, CP monitor placement did not affect 21-day mortality in patients with acetaminophen-induced ALF but was associated with increased 21-day mortality in ALF of other cause.

The performance of a randomized clinical trial to answer the question of whether ICP monitoring should be used would require a relatively large number of patients and has not been performed thus far. The AASLD position paper recommends that "intracranial pressure monitoring is recommended in ALF patients with high grade hepatic encephalopathy, in centers with expertise in ICP monitoring, in patients awaiting and undergoing liver transplantation."[7]

The risks of ICP monitoring include bleeding and infection. The former is especially worrisome in these coagulopathic patients. The ICP monitoring device of choice has traditionally been an epidural catheter. These have relatively low associated risks for intracranial hemorrhage but may be less accurate than other devices. Subdural or intraparenchymal monitors provide improved reliability at the cost of increased bleeding risk. Coagulopathy needs to be treated before placement of an ICP monitor, and newer agents for the treatment of coagulopathy (see later) may alter the threshold for placement of such devices.[49] Definitive recommendations for INR or platelet count are not available.

There are insufficient data to recommend the use of transcranial Doppler or jugular venous bulb oximetry in patients with ALF.

Maintenance of Cerebral Perfusion Pressure

CPP is mean arterial pressure (MAP) minus ICP. The management goal for patients with cerebral edema is to limit ICP *and* to maintain CPP. Targets for CPP are subjects of debate, but a goal ICP less than 25 mm Hg and a CPP more than 60 mm Hg seem reasonable.[7,44,50] A CPP greater than 70 mm Hg may be of further advantage if that level can be achieved.[7,51] An ICP greater than 40 mm Hg and a prolonged period of time with a CPP less than 50 mm Hg are strongly associated with poor neurological recovery in patients with ALF, although the data are not sufficient to contraindicate OLT.[52] It may be necessary to augment MAP to attain and maintain a satisfactory CPP (see the later section on hemodynamic support). Systemic hypertension may be treated with conventional agents such as labetalol or hydralazine. Continuous infusions of nicardipine offer some theoretical advantage over the traditionally used sodium nitroprusside.

Control of Elevations of ICP in Patients with Grade III or IV HE

General Measures: Patients with elevated ICP (defined as an ICP >20 to 25 for more than 1 minute or a CPP <50) should be managed in a quiet environment. Head elevation to 20 to 30 degrees and avoidance of obstruction to venous return (e.g., head rotation, tight endotracheal tube ties) are recommended. Endotracheal tube suctioning should be kept to a minimum, and consideration should be given to administration of a bolus of a sedative agent such as propofol or lidocaine before suctioning. Hypoxemia and hypercapnia will increase ICP, and every effort should be made to avoid these.

Sedation and Analgesia: Patients in grade III or IV HE should be sedated as one measure to control ICP. Because of its rapid onset and offset (even in patients with liver disease), propofol seems an excellent choice for sedation to control ICP in patients with ALF. Wijdicks and Nyberg reported the use of propofol in seven patients with ALF who had ICP monitors in situ. At a median dose of 50 μg/kg/min, propofol alone appeared to control ICP, although the study was observational and there were several confounders.[53]

The induction of a "barbiturate coma" by administration of pentobarbital or sodium thiopental has been used to treat refractory intracranial hypertension in ALF, although studies are uncontrolled. Forbes and colleagues administered thiopental to patients with ALF, refractory intracranial hypertension, and poor prognosis and demonstrated reductions in ICP.[54] Side effects are numerous and include hemodynamic compromise and apnea.

Patients receiving infusions of propofol or barbiturates may require pressor support to maintain optimum hemodynamics.

Opiate infusions typically are used to treat discomfort and as adjunctive sedative agents. Fentanyl may be a better choice than morphine or meperidine because the last two are longer acting and have active metabolites that may accumulate in hepatic or renal dysfunction.

Mannitol: Mannitol is the only therapy proven in a controlled trial to reduce intracranial hypertension and improve survival in patients with ALF. Canalese and colleagues randomized 44 patients with ALF to receive mannitol (1 g/kg as required), dexamethasone (32 mg IV then 8 mg IV every 6 hours), both drugs, or neither drug for the treatment of elevated ICP.[55] Dexamethasone did not affect survival, but among patients who developed cerebral edema, those who received mannitol had significantly better survival than those who did not. The dose of mannitol has not been definitively established, and boluses of between 0.25 and 1 g/kg have been used, although doses on the lower end of this range are associated with fewer adverse effects. Limitations to the use of mannitol include the development of acute renal failure or hyperosmolality (serum osmolality >320 mOsm/L). The prophylactic administration of mannitol in ALF has not been studied.

Hypertonic Saline: Murphy et al. performed a randomized trial of the use of 30% (hypertonic) saline to maintain serum sodium concentrations between 145 and 155 mEq/L in patients with ALF and encephalopathy. They demonstrated that induction and maintenance of hypernatremia can reduce the incidence and severity of intracranial hypertension.[56] A survival benefit was not demonstrated, and the role of prophylactic hypertonic saline remains unproven, but its use is recommended by the AASLD "in patients at highest risk of developing cerebral edema."[7] Theoretically, and on the basis of literature in the neurosurgical population, hypotonic solutions and hyponatremia should be avoided because of the risk of worsening cerebral edema.

Treatment of Fever: Fever exacerbates intracranial hypertension in patients with ALF, and measures to maintain normothermia, including cooling blankets and fans, should be used in the febrile patient (see the later discussion on therapeutic hypothermia). Nonsteroidal antiinflammatory drugs and acetaminophen are relatively contraindicated because of the potential for nephrotoxicity and further hepatotoxicity, although their use has not been studied extensively in this population and they have been used to treat fever in patients with ALF.[1,37]

Hyperventilation: Hyperventilation to a partial pressure of carbon dioxide in arterial blood ($Paco_2$) of less than 30 mm Hg causes cerebral vasoconstriction and rapidly reduces ICP in patients with cerebral edema. Prophylactic hyperventilation, however, did not reduce the incidence of cerebral edema in a randomized controlled trial of 20 patients with ALF.[57] Furthermore, marked hypocapnia (to a $Paco_2 \leq 25$ mm Hg) or sustained hypocapnia may cause cerebral ischemia. Accordingly, the use of therapeutic hyperventilation is reserved for situations in which life-threatening cerebral edema is present and has proven refractory to other measures. Use of hyperventilation in this circumstance should be temporary—for at most a few hours.[7] Maintenance of a $Paco_2$ between 30 and 40 mm Hg is a reasonable goal.[8]

Seizure Prophylaxis: The development of seizures will markedly increase cerebral oxygen requirements, increase ICP, and may cause or worsen cerebral edema. Subclinical seizure activity was noted in 30% of patients with ALF studied by Ellis in a clinical trial.[58] The AASLD position paper recommends that phenytoin be given for control of seizures, although supporting data are scarce.[7] Benzodiazepines also may be administered, for both their antiseizure and sedative properties, but their metabolism and clearance are greatly decreased in liver failure. Prophylactic IV phenytoin was shown to reduce the incidence of seizures in this group of 42 patients, but the beneficial effects of phenytoin could not be documented in a confirmatory study.[59] The use of prophylactic phenytoin is not supported by current evidence. Electroencephalography should be performed in grade III or IV HE if myoclonus is present, if a sudden unexplained deterioration in neurologic status occurs, or when barbiturate coma is being used for management of cerebral edema.[8,59]

Indomethacin: Tofteng administered bolus doses of indomethacin to a series of 12 patients with ALF and cerebral edema and demonstrated a reduction in ICP and an increase in CPP.[60] Further data are awaited.

Nonabsorbable disaccharides, benzodiazepine receptor antagonists, or dopaminergic agonists have not been proven to be beneficial for the treatment of HE according to systematic reviews of the literature.[61-63]

A randomized placebo-controlled trial of L-ornithine L-aspartate (LOLA), a drug that facilitates the detoxification and excretion of ammonia, failed to demonstrate a decline in arterial ammonia or an improvement in survival.[64]

COAGULOPATHY

As is the case with cerebral edema, the development of a coagulopathy is a hallmark of ALF. Coagulopathy has multiple causes. These include platelet dysfunction (quantitative and qualitative), hypofibrinogenemia, and inadequate coagulation factor synthesis.[65] However, despite markedly elevated INR, overall hemostasis may be preserved by compensatory mechanisms.[66] The thromboelastogram (TEG) is commonly used to aid in the management of coagulopathy in patients with liver disease, especially in patients undergoing liver transplantation, but TEG use has not been studied in a randomized controlled trial. In the absence of bleeding, correction of coagulopathy by administration of fresh frozen plasma (FFP) is not required and may confound assessment of progression of the disease.[20] When invasive procedures are planned or when the patient is bleeding, it is appropriate to treat coagulopathy.[7,8] Almost 40 years ago, Gazzard showed that FFP administration did not reduce morbidity or mortality in ALF.[67] Vitamin K is typically given to patients with ALF because some have subclinical vitamin K deficiency at the time of presentation. There is some debate regarding the threshold for administration of platelets, although in the absence of bleeding or plans for invasive procedures a value of greater than 10 to 20×10^9/L seems acceptable. If invasive procedures are planned, then a platelet count of at least 50×10^9/L should be attained. Cryoprecipitate should be administered when the fibrinogen level is less than 100 mg/dL. Recombinant factor VIIa (rVIIa; 40 µg/kg) was demonstrated to be of use to transiently correct the coagulopathy of ALF and allow performance of invasive procedures in two nonrandomized studies in (a total of) 26 patients who met King's College criteria for liver transplantation.[68] Thrombosis is a potential side effect. In patients with persistent coagulopathy despite FFP administration and in those who have contraindications to rVIIa, therapeutic plasmapheresis may be beneficial.[49,69] Many clinicians would advocate treatment of extreme coagulopathy (e.g., INR >7), even if invasive procedures are not planned.[20]

INFECTION

As documented by Rolando and colleagues in a study of 50 consecutive patients, individuals with ALF are at risk for bacterial and fungal infection.[70,71] Gram-positive cocci, enteric gram-negative bacilli, and *Candida* species are the most commonly isolated organisms. Disseminated infection may be a contraindication to transplantation. Although the use of prophylactic antimicrobial therapy may reduce the incidence of infection in certain patients with ALF, a survival benefit has not been demonstrated. Although recent evidence suggests that the presence of infection or the systemic inflammatory response syndrome influences the progression of encephalopathy in ALF, there is currently no evidence to show that administration of antimicrobials alters this relationship.[72] Surveillance for symptoms and signs of infection should be part of the management of a patient with ALF, although this recommendation is empiric.[7] Initiation of antibiotics is recommended when surveillance cultures reveal significant isolates, in grade III or IV HE, in the presence of refractory hypotension and if the systemic inflammatory response syndrome is present.[8] Broad-spectrum antibacterial agents are typically used and vancomycin added if intravascular catheter-related bloodstream infection or methicillin-resistant *Staphylococcus aureus* infection is suspected. Low-dose amphotericin is a part of ALF protocols at some institutions.

Rolando et al. studied 108 patients with ALF in a prospective randomized fashion to compare the incidence of infection in patients given IV antimicrobials with and without enteral antimicrobials.[73] The addition of enteral antimicrobials did not decrease the incidence of infection.

ACUTE KIDNEY INJURY

A retrospective analysis of data from 1604 patients in the U.S. Acute Liver Failure Study Group demonstrated that 70% of patients with ALF developed acute kidney injury (AKI), and 30% underwent RRT.[74] AKI is associated with increased mortality and may be caused by various mechanisms. These include hypovolemia and hypoperfusion, nephrotoxins, or hepatorenal syndrome.[75] In the cohort reported by Tujios, AKI was more common in those with more severe liver dysfunction, in advanced encephalopathy, in the elderly, and in those with acetaminophen-induced ALF. AKI affected short- and long-term outcomes, but it rarely resulted in chronic kidney disease (only 4% of survivors were dialysis dependent), and patients with acetaminophen-induced ALF/AKI had better outcomes than those with other causes. Davenport performed a prospective, randomized controlled trial in patients with combined acute liver and renal failure to compare the effect of various modes of dialysis on hemodynamics.[76] Continuous modes of dialysis were associated with less hemodynamic compromise. Furthermore, continuous RRT is less likely to provoke an elevation in ICP or pulmonary pressures than is intermittent dialysis.[77] Continuous RRT may be continued in the operating room during liver transplantation.[78]

HEMODYNAMIC SUPPORT

Distributive shock often develops in patients with ALF and may lead to multiple organ failure. Hypovolemia occurs secondary to transudation of fluid into the extravascular space and decreased oral intake. A central venous catheter should be placed to facilitate infusion of vasoactive medications and to monitor filling pressures. A pulmonary artery catheter may be used to guide hemodynamic therapy, and although there is debate regarding the appropriateness of the use of pulmonary artery catheters, there are no studies specific for patients with ALF. The initial treatment of hypotension should be with IV normal saline. Despite adequate

fluid resuscitation, a low systemic vascular resistance in ALF often results in persistent hypotension. Hemodynamic derangements may compromise cerebral, renal, and hepatic perfusion with subsequent worsening of organ dysfunction. The recommended goal MAP is 75 mm Hg, although this is not supported by data.[7,79] When ICP is elevated, the MAP goal may need to be altered upward to maintain a CPP between 60 and 80 mm Hg.[79] The optimal choice of pressor is unknown because, despite some limited studies, there are no definitive trials to identify the best vasoactive agent. Norepinephrine, dopamine, and epinephrine are reasonable choices to achieve hemodynamic goals. Most centers use norepinephrine, which may best augment peripheral organ perfusion while minimizing tachycardia and preserving splanchnic (thereby hepatic) blood flow.[7,79] Norepinephrine may offer some advantages over dopamine in patients with cerebral injury and may be a better choice than epinephrine for splanchnic perfusion in patients with distributive shock. Vasopressin may be added, but its use is controversial, and a small study of terlipressin in ALF (six patients with ALF and HE) at a dose that did not alter systemic hemodynamics demonstrated worsening of cerebral hyperemia and intracranial hypertension.[80]

Adrenal insufficiency may be present in patients with liver failure and administration of corticosteroids (e.g., hydrocortisone 200 mg/day) should be considered when refractory hypotension is present. Although there are some data to support this practice, most are from patients with chronic liver failure rather than ALF, and significant controversy exists regarding steroid supplementation in critically ill patients.[81]

MECHANICAL VENTILATION

Patients with ALF need airway protection when grade III encephalopathy develops and will need mechanical ventilation if respiratory failure or severe metabolic acidosis occurs. Acute respiratory distress syndrome (ARDS) may develop, and a low tidal volume strategy is indicated. Because of the presence of cerebral edema, the respiratory rate should be increased to maintain satisfactory minute ventilation and permissive hypercapnia should not be used. It is unclear whether prophylactic use of low tidal volume in patients with ALF will delay or avoid the development of ARDS, although some evidence exists in non-ALF patients.[82] It is unknown whether higher levels of applied positive end-expiratory pressure (PEEP) cause ischemic hepatic damage. When PEEP is required to achieve acceptable oxygenation in patients with ALF and ARDS, it should be applied, recognizing that adequate systemic oxygenation is essential for optimum hepatic function. In addition, lungs that have been injured demonstrate a reduction in compliance, which will offset transmission of pressure to the liver.[83]

GASTROINTESTINAL BLEEDING

Gastrointestinal bleeding is a risk with all critically ill patients, especially if they require mechanical ventilation. Accordingly, there is a significant risk of gastrointestinal bleeding in individuals with ALF, although this risk is presumably less than in patients with cirrhosis, portal hypertension, and esophageal or gastric varices. In two controlled trials involving 75 patients, H2 blockers, but not antacids, were associated with a decreased incidence of bleeding in patients with ALF. Accordingly, H2 blockers or, by extension, proton pump inhibitors should be administered to patients with ALF.[7,84]

METABOLIC CONCERNS

Metabolic derangements—often severe—occur in ALF, and frequent monitoring of acid-base status and metabolic parameters is required. Alkalosis and acidosis may occur, and the latter may be especially refractory when ALF is accompanied by acute renal failure. Infusions of sodium bicarbonate or a nonsodium buffer such as tris(hydroxymethyl) aminomethane or initiation of continuous RRT with a bicarbonate-rich infusate are often required. Impaired hepatic gluconeogenesis in ALF patients makes use of "tight" glycemic control potentially problematic. Hyperglycemia may worsen cerebral edema in patients with ALF, but hypoglycemia must be avoided. Hypoglycemia may be profound and occult because of encephalopathy or sedation. Boluses of 50% dextrose solutions and continuous dextrose infusions are often required to maintain normoglycemia. Phosphate and magnesium may be low and require repeated supplementation.

NUTRITION

Patients with ALF manifest a catabolic state and increased energy expenditure.[85] Nutritional support is recommended, although studies on which to base therapy are limited. Enteral feeding should be initiated early in the course of ALF, usually by nasogastric or nasojejunal tube. Severe protein restriction should be avoided. The AASLD position paper recommends 60 g of protein per day, although 1 to 1.2 g of protein per kilogram of estimated dry weight may be more appropriate.[7] A Cochrane Database review of the use of branched-chain amino acids in ALF and HE did not find convincing evidence of a beneficial effect, although the trials performed in this field were mostly of poor methodological quality.[86] Parenteral nutrition should be used if enteral nutrition is contraindicated or not tolerated. Both enteral and parenteral nutrition reduce the incidence of stress ulceration. Lipid emulsions appear to be safe in patients with ALF.[87]

TRANSPLANTATION

Although ALF may resolve with only supportive interventions, especially in patients with acetaminophen-induced ALF, OLT is the only definitive therapy for the condition. The therapy has not been evaluated in a prospective clinical trial for patients with ALF, but there is little doubt as to its effectiveness. Overall survival for patients with ALF has increased from 15% in the pretransplant era to 60% or better in the posttransplant era.[13] Some of the improved survival rates (which are as high as 80% to 90% in some series) are

due to improvements in ICU management that also have resulted in an increase in spontaneous survival rates. ALF is the only condition designated as UNOS Status I (highest priority for donor liver allocation). OLT is not universally available, and only 10% of liver transplantations are performed in patients with ALF.[88,89] In the U.S. Acute Liver Failure Study Group series, 29% of patients underwent OLT and 25% of patients listed for transplantation died on the waiting list.[13] In the Nordic countries' experience, 73% of 315 patients listed received a transplant, and 16% died without transplant.[10] Mortality after OLT in the first year is higher for patients with ALF than for patients transplanted for other reasons (1-year survival rate 79% for OLT in setting of ALF vs. approximately 90% for other causes), and most deaths occur from infection within the first 3 months.[89] Outcome is worse for older recipients, those who receive older or partial grafts, and those receiving non-ABO identical grafts.[89,90] Longer term survival, though, is better than in those transplanted for chronic liver disease.

MANAGEMENT DURING AND AFTER LIVER TRANSPLANTATION

Although there are insufficient data to recommend any specific management of patients with ALF during OLT, guidelines based on expert opinion have been published.[8,79] If an ICP monitor has been placed before OLT, then it should be continuously monitored intraoperatively because ICP may increase, especially at the time of reperfusion. Intraoperative management should follow the MAP, ICP, and CPP goals used preoperatively. Whether to perform the technique of venovenous bypass is a matter of surgeon preference because no definitive data on its role in minimizing swings in cerebral perfusion exist.

AREAS OF CONTROVERSY

Therapeutic Hypothermia

In experimental animal models, mild-moderate hypothermia has been demonstrated to prevent development of brain edema in ALF, possibly by altering brain ammonia or glucose metabolism or preventing hyperemia. On the basis of these theoretical benefits, reports of the use of therapeutic hypothermia in patients with ALF have demonstrated promise.[91,92] Hypothermia (cooling to core temperature of 33 to 34° C) has been used as a "bridge to transplant" or to control ICP during transplant surgery. Such therapy may be associated with infections, coagulopathy, and arrhythmias, and therapeutic hypothermia in ALF has not been subjected to rigorous scrutiny. Multicenter, randomized, controlled clinical trials are needed to confirm that hypothermia in ALF secures brain viability and improves survival without causing harm.

N-acetylcysteine for Non-Acetaminophen–Induced ALF

NAC may have a role in non-acetaminophen-induced ALF[93]; however, studies have been inconclusive thus far.

In a randomized, double-blind, multicenter placebo controlled trial, IV NAC improved transplant-free survival in patients with early-stage non-acetaminophen–related ALF. Patients with advanced coma grades did not benefit from NAC.[94]

Hepatectomy and Auxiliary Transplantation

Some investigators have proposed that liver-derived pro-inflammatory cytokines may be important in producing intracranial hypertension in ALF.[95] The use of hepatectomy has been advocated in patients with ALF, refractory circulatory dysfunction, and intracranial hypertension, assuming that OLT will be performed thereafter. Data to support such a practice, however, are sparse and consist of case reports and uncontrolled case series.[96-98] Hepatectomy cannot be recommended at this time. Auxiliary liver transplantation is a technique in which a partial liver graft is placed either heterotopically or orthotopically while leaving part of the native liver in situ in the hope that the native liver will regenerate. A European multicenter study demonstrated the feasibility and potential utility of this technique.[99] Recently, Lodge and colleagues have performed emergency subtotal hepatectomy and auxiliary OLT for acetaminophen-induced ALF with encouraging early results in a nonrandomized case series.[100] At this time, though, no clear indications for auxiliary liver transplantation exist, and a randomized clinical trial has not taken place.

Living-Donor Liver Transplantation for ALF

The advent of living-donor liver transplantation adds a further option to the management of ALF.[101] Its use in children is well established.[102] Case series in adults report 5-year survival rates of up to 80%.[103-105] The ethical difficulties already associated with this procedure in patients with cirrhosis, though, are greatly increased in the scenario of ALF when the acuity of the situation has the potential to lead to rushed or incompletely informed decision-making.[106]

Liver Support Systems

The "holy grail" for the treatment of ALF is a liver support device to replace the detoxification, metabolic, and synthetic functions of the liver.[107] Such a system could be used as a bridge to liver transplantation, or preferably to complete recovery of the patient's native liver. Trials for the assessment of liver support devices are complicated by the fact that many patients are diverted to liver transplantation before the response to therapy with the device can be established. Furthermore, ALF is a "catch-all" phrase for a heterogenous group of disorders with different etiologies and rates of progression. There have been several approaches to the development of an "artificial liver." The first systems removed toxins through hemodialysis, hemofiltration, or hemoperfusion. Newer systems combine hemodialysis with adsorption to albumin or charcoal. Living hepatocytes (porcine or derived from human hepatocellular cancer cells) are the basis of

"bioartificial liver" devices. Demetriou and colleagues published the results of a randomized, clinical trial evaluating a porcine bioartificial liver in 171 patients with ALF.[108] Overall, survival was no different between the intervention (71% survival) and control (62%) groups. The survival gap widened when the 27 patients who had primary graft nonfunction were excluded, but it did not reach statistical significance. Meta-analyses (based on few subjects) evaluating the utility of artificial liver support systems in ALF have provided conflicting results.[109,110] The use of commercially available artificial systems based on albumin dialysis (Molecular Adsorbent Recirculating System [MARS]) and fractionated plasma separation and adsorption (Prometheus) has not been demonstrated to improve survival, although most studies have been in patients with acute or chronic liver failure. Saliba and colleagues, though, in a randomized controlled trial involving 102 patients with ALF, were unable to show a benefit with MARS, although the trial was confounded by the fact that many of the patients in the study were quickly transplanted.[111]

SUMMARY

ALF is a complex, multisystem illness that develops after a catastrophic hepatic insult. It is characterized by coagulopathy and HE accompanied by cerebral edema and elevated ICP. The etiology is dependent on geographic location, with drugs and toxins causing more than half of the cases in developed countries. Care of the patient requires a multidisciplinary approach and the full armamentarium of ICU support (Tables 69-4 and 69-5). The rarity of the condition and the rapidity of its development mean that there is a paucity of randomized clinical trials evaluating therapies for ALF. The U.S. Acute Liver Failure Study Group has published a consensus document with recommendations for specific aspects of ICU care of these patients. Although some patients will recover spontaneously, for patients with poor prognosis liver transplantation is the only definitive treatment. Survival rates after liver transplantation are approximately 75% to 90%. The efficacy of artificial liver support devices in ALF remains unproven.

Table 69-4 Important Summary Documents and Guidelines for the Management of Acute Liver Failure

Authors	Year	Organization	Type of Document
Lee et al. 2012	2012	American Association for the Study of Liver Diseases	Position paper on the management of acute liver failure: Update
Stravitz et al. 2007	2007	United States Acute Liver Failure Study Group	Recommendations for intensive care of patients with acute liver failure

Table 69-5 Selected Randomized Studies in the Management of Acute Liver Failure

Study, Year	Number of Subjects (Intervention, No Intervention)	Study Design	Intervention	Control	Outcomes
Canalese et al. 1982	44 patients with ALF (4 groups)	Prospective, randomized, controlled trial	Dexamethasone alone, mannitol alone, both dexamethasone and mannitol	Neither	Dexamethasone did not affect survival among patients who developed cerebral edema, survival was better in mannitol group
Bhatia et al. 2004	42 patients with ALF (22 patients given prophylactic phenytoin, 22 controls)	Prospective, randomized, controlled trial	Prophylactic phenytoin administration	Usual therapy	Similar rates of cerebral edema, need for mechanical ventilation, incidence of seizures, mortality
Gazzard et al. 1975	20 patients with acetaminophen-induced ALF (10 intervention, 10 controls)	Prospective, randomized, controlled trial	FFP 300 mL every 6 hours	Usual therapy	No difference in morbidity or mortality between intervention and control groups
Davenport et al. 1993	32 patients (12 intermittent RRT, 20 continuous RRT)	Prospective, randomized, controlled trial of patients with ALF and acute renal failure	Continuous RRT	Intermittent RRT	Patients in intermittent RRT had significantly lower cardiac indices and MAP
Demetriou et al. 2004	171 patients (85 bioartificial liver, 86 control)	Prospective, randomized, controlled, multicenter trial in patients with severe ALF	HepatAssist bioartificial liver (patients were allowed to undergo liver transplantation)	Usual therapy (including potential liver transplantation)	30-day survival 71% for bioartificial liver vs 62% for control ($P = .26$).
Acharya et al. 2009	201 patients	Prospective, randomized, placebo-controlled, trial in patients with ALF	LOLA infusions (30 g daily over 3 days) HepatAssist bioartificial liver (patients were allowed to undergo liver transplantation)	Placebo	No improvement in encephalopathy grade or survival with LOLA administration

ALF, acute liver failure; *FFP,* fresh frozen plasma; *LOLA,* L-ornithine L-aspartate; *RRT,* renal replacement therapy.

AUTHOR'S RECOMMENDATIONS

- The diagnosis of ALF should prompt discussion with a referral center for consideration of transfer and potential liver transplantation.
- The U.S. Acute Liver Failure Study Group has published recommendations for the ICU management of patients with ALF.
- The cause of ALF should be determined because specific therapies exist for certain conditions. Acetaminophen overdose is a common cause of ALF and should be treated with NAC. The utility of NAC in non-acetaminophen ALF remains controversial
- Assessment of prognosis is important, and the King's College criteria are often used, although they are not absolutely predictive.
- Patients with grade III HE should be intubated for airway protection.
- Although monitoring of ICP has not been demonstrated to improve mortality in patients with ALF, the practice is common.

An ICP of less than 25 mm Hg and a CPP greater than 60 mm Hg should be targeted.
- Treatment for elevations of ICP includes general supportive measures, sedation, and osmotherapy with mannitol or hypertonic saline. Therapeutic hypothermia and hyperventilation are controversial.
- Coagulopathy should be treated only if invasive procedures are planned, if the patient is actively bleeding, or if the coagulopathy is extreme.
- Metabolic derangements should be treated aggressively and nutrition should be initiated.
- Transplantation is the only definitive treatment for ALF, and, provided there are no contraindications, the patient should receive a highest priority listing for liver transplantation.
- The performance of hepatectomy and auxiliary transplantation and the use of liver support devices remain unproven.

REFERENCES

1. Bernal W, Wendon J. Acute liver failure. *N Engl J Med.* 2013;369:2525–2534.
2. Bernal W, Hyyrylainen A, Gera A, et al. Lessons from look-back in acute liver failure? A single centre experience of 3300 patients. *J Hepatol.* 2013;59:74–80.
3. Lee WM. Acute liver failure. *Semin Respir Crit Care Med.* 2012;33:36–45.
4. O'Grady JG, Schalm SW, Williams R. Acute liver failure: redefining the syndromes. *Lancet.* 1993;342:273–275.
5. Bernuau J, Rueff B, Benhamou J. Fulminant and subfulminant liver failure: definitions and causes. *Semin Liver Dis.* 1986;6:97–106.
6. Mochida S, Nakayama N, Matsui A, Nagoshi S, Fujiwara K. Re-evaluation of the Guideline published by the Acute Liver Failure Study Group of Japan in 1996 to determine the indications of liver transplantation in patients with fulminant hepatitis. *Hepatol Res.* 2008;38:970–979.
7. Lee W, Stravitz R, Larson A. Introduction to the revised American Association for the Study of Liver Diseases position paper on acute liver failure 2011. *Hepatology.* 2012;55:965–967.
8. Stravitz RT, Kramer AH, Davern T, et al. Intensive care of patients with acute liver failure: recommendations of the U.S. Acute Liver Failure Study Group. *Crit Care Med.* 2007;35:2498–2508.
9. Bower WA, Johns M, Margolis HS, Williams IT, Bell BP. Population-based surveillance for acute liver failure. *Am J Gastroenterol.* 2007;102:2459–2463.
10. Brandsaeter B, Hockerstedt K, Friman S, et al. Fulminant hepatic failure: outcome after listing for highly urgent liver transplantation-12 years experience in the nordic countries. *Liver Transpl.* 2002;8:1055–1062.
11. Escorsell A, Mas A, de la Mata M. Acute liver failure in Spain: analysis of 267 cases. *Liver Transpl.* 2007;13:1389–1395.
12. Hoofnagle JHCR, Shapiro C, et al. Fulminant hepatic failure: summary of a workshop. *Hepatology.* 1995;21:240–252.
13. Ostapowicz G, Fontana RJ, Schiodt FV, et al. Results of a prospective study of acute liver failure at 17 tertiary care centers in the United States. *Ann Intern Med.* 2002;137:947–954.
14. Larson AM, Polson J, Fontana RJ, et al. Acetaminophen-induced acute liver failure: results of a United States multicenter, prospective study. *Hepatology.* 2005;42:1364–1372.
15. Nourjah P, Ahmad SR, Karwoski C, Willy M. Estimates of acetaminophen (Paracetomal)-associated overdoses in the United States. *Pharmacoepidemiol Drug Saf.* 2006;15:398–405.
16. Sass DA, Shakil AO. Fulminant hepatic failure. *Liver Transpl.* 2005;11:594–605.
17. Daas M, Plevak DJ, Wijdicks EF, et al. Acute liver failure: results of a 5-year clinical protocol. *Liver Transpl Surg.* 1995;1:210–219.
18. Fontana RJ, Ellerbe C, Durkalski VE, et al. Two-year outcomes in initial survivors with acute liver failure: results from a prospective, multicentre study. *Liver Int.* 2015;35:370–380.
19. Shakil AO, Kramer D, Mazariegos GV, Fung JJ, Rakela J. Acute liver failure: clinical features, outcome analysis, and applicability of prognostic criteria. *Liver Transpl.* 2000;6:163–169.
20. Lee WM, Stravitz RT, Larson AM. Introduction to the revised American Association for the Study of Liver Diseases position paper on acute liver failure 2011. *Hepatology.* 2012;55:965–967.
21. O'Grady JGAG, Hayllar KM, et al. Early indicators of prognosis in fulminant hepatic failure. *Gastroenterology.* 1989;97:439–445.
22. McPhail MJ, Wendon JA, Bernal W. Meta-analysis of performance of Kings's College Hospital Criteria in prediction of outcome in non-paracetamol-induced acute liver failure. *J Hepatol.* 2010;53:492–499.
23. Kumar R, Shalimar SH, et al. Prospective derivation and validation of early dynamic model for predicting outcome in patients with acute liver failure. *Gut.* 2012;61:1068–1075.
24. Wlodzimirow KA, Eslami S, Chamuleau RA, Nieuwoudt M, Abu-Hanna A. Prediction of poor outcome in patients with acute liver failure-systematic review of prediction models. *PLoS One.* 2012;7:e50952.
25. Bernal W, Auzinger G, Dhawan A, Wendon J. Acute liver failure. *Lancet.* 2010;376:190–201.
26. Smilkstein MJ, Knapp GL, Kulig KW, Rumack BH. Efficacy of oral *N*-acetylcysteine in the treatment of acetaminophen overdose. Analysis of the national multicenter study (1976 to 1985). *N Engl J Med.* 1988;319:1557–1562.
27. Keays R, Harrison PM, Wendon JA, et al. Intravenous acetylcysteine in paracetamol induced fulminant hepatic failure: a prospective controlled trial. *BMJ.* 1991;303:1026–1029.
28. Leise MD, Poterucha JJ, Talwalkar JA. Drug-induced liver injury. *Mayo Clin Proc.* 2014;89:95–106.
29. Reuben A, Koch DG, Lee WM. Drug-induced acute liver failure: results of a U.S. multicenter, prospective study. *Hepatology.* 2010;52:2065–2076.
30. Schiodt FV, Davern TJ, Shakil AO, McGuire B, Samuel G, Lee WM. Viral hepatitis-related acute liver failure. *Am J Gastroenterol.* 2003;98:448–453.
31. Karkhanis J, Verna EC, Chang MS, et al. Steroid use in acute liver failure. *Hepatology.* 2014;59:612–621.
32. Hay JE. Liver disease in pregnancy. *Hepatology.* 2008;47:1067–1076.
33. Korman JD, Volenberg I, Balko J, et al. Screening for Wilson disease in acute liver failure: a comparison of currently available diagnostic tests. *Hepatology.* 2008;48:1167–1174.
34. Roberts EA, Schilsky ML. A practice guideline on Wilson disease. *Hepatology.* 2003;37:1475–1492.
35. Broussard CN, Aggarwal A, Lacey SR, et al. Mushroom poisoning–from diarrhea to liver transplantation. *Am J Gastroenterol.* 2001;96:3195–3198.
36. Menon KV, Shah V, Kamath PS. The Budd-Chiari syndrome. *N Engl J Med.* 2004;350:578–585.
37. Wendon J, Lee W. Encephalopathy and cerebral edema in the setting of acute liver failure: pathogenesis and management. *Neurocrit Care.* 2008;9:97–102.
38. Blei AT. Brain edema in acute liver failure: can it be prevented? Can it be treated? *J Hepatol.* 2007;46:564–569.
39. Bjerring PN, Eefsen M, Hansen BA, Larsen FS. The brain in acute liver failure. A tortuous path from hyperammonemia to cerebral edema. *Metabol Brain Dis.* 2009;24:5–14.
40. Vaquero J, Polson J, Chung C, et al. Infection and the progression of hepatic encephalopathy in acute liver failure. *Gastroenterology.* 2003;125:755–764.
41. Clemmesen JO, Larsen FS, Kondrup J, Hansen BA, Ott P. Cerebral herniation in patients with acute liver failure is correlated with arterial ammonia concentration. *Hepatology.* 1999;29:648–653.
42. Wijdicks EFM PD, Rakela J, et al. Clinical and radiologic features of cerebral edema in fulminant hepatic failure. *Mayo Clin Proc.* 1995;70:119–124.
43. Alba L, Hay JE, Angulo P. Lactulose therapy in acute liver failure. *J Hepatol.* 2002;36:33A.
44. Raghavan M, Marik PE. Therapy of intracranial hypertension in patients with fulminant hepatic failure. *Neurocrit Care.* 2006;4:179–189.
45. Wendon JA, Larsen FS. Intracranial pressure monitoring in acute liver failure. A procedure with clear indications. *Hepatology.* 2006;44:504–506.
46. Bernuau J, Durand F. Intracranial pressure monitoring in patients with acute liver failure: a questionable invasive surveillance. *Hepatology.* 2006;44:502–504.
47. Vaquero J, Fontana RJ, Larson AM, et al. Complications and use of intracranial pressure monitoring in patients with acute liver failure and severe encephalopathy. *Liver Transpl.* 2005;11:1581–1589.
48. Karvellas CJ, Fix OK, Battenhouse H, Durkalski V, Sanders C, Lee WM. Outcomes and complications of intracranial pressure monitoring in acute liver failure: a retrospective cohort study. *Crit Care Med.* 2014;42:1157–1167.
49. Le TV, Rumbak MJ, Liu SS, Alsina AE, van Loveren H, Agazzi S. Insertion of intracranial pressure monitors in fulminant hepatic failure patients: early experience using recombinant factor VII. *Neurosurgery.* 2010;66:455–458.
50. Lidofsky SD, Bass NM, Prager MC, et al. Intracranial pressure monitoring and liver transplantation for fulminant hepatic failure. *Hepatology.* 1992;16:1–7.
51. Rosner MJ, Rosner SD, Johnson AH. Cerebral perfusion pressure: management protocol and clinical results. *J Neurosurg.* 1995;83:949–962.
52. McCashland TM, Shaw Jr BW, Tape E. The American experience with transplantation for acute liver failure. *Semin Liver Dis.* 1996;16:427–433.
53. Wijdicks EF, Nyberg SL. Propofol to control intracranial pressure in fulminant hepatic failure. *Transplant Proc.* 2002;34:1220–1222.
54. Forbes A, Alexander GJ, O'Grady JG, et al. Thiopental infusion in the treatment of intracranial hypertension complicating fulminant hepatic failure. *Hepatology.* 1989;10:306–310.

55. Canalese J, Gimson AE, Davis C, Mellon PJ, Davis M, Williams R. Controlled trial of dexamethasone and mannitol for the cerebral oedema of fulminant hepatic failure. *Gut.* 1982;23:625–629.

56. Murphy N, Auzinger G, Bernel W, Wendon J. The effect of hypertonic sodium chloride on intracranial pressure in patients with acute liver failure. *Hepatology.* 2004;39:464–470.

57. Ede RJ, Gimson AE, Bihari D, Williams R. Controlled hyperventilation in the prevention of cerebral oedema in fulminant hepatic failure. *J Hepatol.* 1986;2:43–51.

58. Ellis AJ, Wendon JA, Williams R. Subclinical seizure activity and prophylactic phenytoin infusion in acute liver failure: a controlled clinical trial. *Hepatology.* 2000;32:536–541.

59. Bhatia V, Batra Y, Acharya SK. Prophylactic phenytoin does not improve cerebral edema or survival in acute liver failure–a controlled clinical trial. *J Hepatol.* 2004;41:89–96.

60. Tofteng F, Larsen FS. The effect of indomethacin on intracranial pressure, cerebral perfusion and extracellular lactate and glutamate concentrations in patients with fulminant hepatic failure. *J Cereb Blood Flow Metab.* 2004;24:798–804.

61. Als-Nielsen B, Gluud LL, Gluud C. Non-absorbable disaccharides for hepatic encephalopathy: systematic review of randomised trials. *BMJ.* 2004;328:1046.

62. Als-Nielsen B, Gluud LL, Gluud C. Dopaminergic agonists for hepatic encephalopathy. *Cochrane Database Syst Rev.* 2004:CD003047.

63. Als-Nielsen B, Gluud LL, Gluud C. Benzodiazepine receptor antagonists for hepatic encephalopathy. *Cochrane Database Syst Rev.* 2004:CD002798.

64. Acharya SK, Bhatia V, Sreenivas V, Khanal S, Panda SK. Efficacy of L-ornithine L-aspartate in acute liver failure: a double-blind, randomized, placebo-controlled study. *Gastroenterology.* 2009;136:2159–2168.

65. Lisman T, Leebeek FW. Hemostatic alterations in liver disease: a review on pathophysiology, clinical consequences, and treatment. *Dig Surg.* 2007;24:250–258.

66. Stravitz RT, Lisman T, Luketic VA, et al. Minimal effects of acute liver injury/acute liver failure on hemostasis as assessed by thromboelastography. *J Hepatol.* 2012;56:129–136.

67. Gazzard BG, Henderson JM, Williams R. Early changes in coagulation following a paracetamol overdose and a controlled trial of fresh frozen plasma therapy. *Gut.* 1975;16:617–620.

68. Shami VM, Caldwell SH, Hespenheide EE, Arseneau KO, Bickston SJ, Macik BG. Recombinant activated factor VII for coagulopathy in fulminant hepatic failure compared with conventional therapy. *Liver Transpl.* 2003;9:138–143.

69. Munoz SJ, Ballas SK, Moritz MJ, et al. Perioperative management of fulminant and subfulminant hepatic failure with therapeutic plasmapheresis. *Transplant Proc.* 1989;21:3535–3536.

70. Rolando N, Harvey F, Brahm J, et al. Fungal infection: a common, unrecognised complication of acute liver failure. *J Hepatol.* 1991;12:1–9.

71. Rolando N, Harvey F, Brahm J, et al. Prospective study of bacterial infection in acute liver failure: an analysis of fifty patients. *Hepatology.* 1990;11:49–53.

72. Rolando N, Wade J, Davalos M, Wendon J, Philpott-Howard J, Williams R. The systemic inflammatory response syndrome in acute liver failure. *Hepatology.* 2000;32:734–739.

73. Rolando N, Wade JJ, Stangou A, et al. Prospective study comparing the efficacy of prophylactic parenteral antimicrobials, with or without enteral decontamination, in patients with acute liver failure. *Liver Transpl Surg.* 1996;2:8–13.

74. Tujios SR, Hynan LS, Vazquez MA, et al. Risk factors and outcomes of acute kidney injury in patients with acute liver failure. *Clin Gastroenterol Hepatol.* 2015;13:352–359.

75. Gines P, Guevara M, Arroyo V, Rodes J. Hepatorenal syndrome. *Lancet.* 2003;362:1819–1827.

76. Davenport A, Will EJ, Davidson AM. Improved cardiovascular stability during continuous modes of renal replacement therapy in critically ill patients with acute hepatic and renal failure. *Crit Care Med.* 1993;21:328–338.

77. Davenport A. Renal replacement therapy in the patient with acute brain injury. *Am J Kidney Dis.* 2001;37:457–466.

78. Nadim MK, Annanthapanyasut W, Matsuoka L, et al. Intraoperative hemodialysis during liver transplantation: a decade of experience. *Liver Transpl.* 2014;20:756–764.

79. Stravitz RT, Kramer DJ. Management of acute liver failure. *Nat Rev Gastroenterol Hepatol.* 2009;6:542–553.

80. Shawcross DL, Davies NA, Mookerjee RP, et al. Worsening of cerebral hyperemia by the administration of terlipressin in acute liver failure with severe encephalopathy. *Hepatology.* 2004;39:471–475.

81. Marik PE. Adrenal-exhaustion syndrome in patients with liver disease. *Intensive Care Med.* 2006;32:275–280.

82. Gajic O, Dara SI, Mendez JL, et al. Ventilator-associated lung injury in patients without acute lung injury at the onset of mechanical ventilation. *Crit Care Med.* 2004;32:1817–1824.

83. Saner FH, Olde Damink SW, Pavlakovic G, et al. Positive end-expiratory pressure induces liver congestion in living donor liver transplant patients: myth or fact. *Transplantation.* 2008;85:1863–1866.

84. Macdougall BR, Bailey RJ, Williams R. H2-receptor antagonists and antacids in the prevention of acute gastrointestinal haemorrhage in fulminant hepatic failure. Two controlled trials. *Lancet.* 1977;1:617–619.

85. Walsh TS, Wigmore SJ, Hopton P, Richardson R, Lee A. Energy expenditure in acetaminophen-induced fulminant hepatic failure. *Crit Care Med.* 2000;28:649–654.

86. Als-Nielsen B, Koretz RL, Kjaergard LL, Gluud C. Branched-chain amino acids for hepatic encephalopathy. *Cochrane Database Syst Rev.* 2003:CD001939.

87. Munoz SJ. Nutritional therapies in liver disease. *Semin Liver Dis.* 1991;11:278–291.

88. Simpson KJ, Bates CM, Henderson NC, et al. The utilization of liver transplantation in the management of acute liver failure: comparison between acetaminophen and non-acetaminophen etiologies. *Liver Transpl.* 2009;15:600–609.

89. Germani G, Theocharidou E, Adam R, et al. Liver transplantation for acute liver failure in Europe: outcomes over 20 years from the ELTR database. *J Hepatol.* 2012;57:288–296.

90. Bernal W, Cross TJ, Auzinger G, et al. Outcome after wait-listing for emergency liver transplantation in acute liver failure: a single centre experience. *J Hepatol.* 2009;50:306–313.

91. Vaquero J. Therapeutic hypothermia in the management of acute liver failure. *Neurochem Int.* 2012;60:723–735.

92. Jalan R, OD SW, Deutz NE, Lee A, Hayes PC. Moderate hypothermia for uncontrolled intracranial hypertension in acute liver failure. *Lancet.* 1999;354:1164–1168.

93. Sklar GE, Subramaniam M. Acetylcysteine treatment for non-acetaminophen-induced acute liver failure. *Ann Pharmacother.* 2004;38:498–500.

94. Lee WM, Hynan LS, Rossaro L, et al. Intravenous *N*-Acetylcysteine improves transplant-free survival in early stage non-acetaminophen acute liver failure. *Gastroenterology.* 2009;137:856–864.

95. Jalan R, Pollok A, Shah SH, Madhavan K, Simpson KJ. Liver derived pro-inflammatory cytokines may be important in producing intracranial hypertension in acute liver failure. *J Hepatol.* 2002;37:536–538.

96. So SK, Barteau JA, Perdrizet GA, Marsh JW. Successful retransplantation after a 48-hour anhepatic state. *Transplant Proc.* 1993;25:1962–1963.

97. Guirl MJ, Weinstein JS, Goldstein RM, Levy MF, Klintmalm GB. Two-stage total hepatectomy and liver transplantation for acute deterioration of chronic liver disease: a new bridge to transplantation. *Liver Transpl.* 2004;10:564–570.

98. Ringe B, Lubbe N, Kuse E, Frei U, Pichlmayr R. Management of emergencies before and after liver transplantation by early total hepatectomy. *Transplant Proc.* 1993;25:1090.

99. Chenard-Neu MP, Boudjema K, Bernuau J, et al. Auxiliary liver transplantation: regeneration of the native liver and outcome in 30 patients with fulminant hepatic failure—a multicenter European study. *Hepatology.* 1996;23:1119–1127.

100. Lodge JP, Dasgupta D, Prasad KR, et al. Emergency subtotal hepatectomy: a new concept for acetaminophen-induced acute liver failure. *Ann Surg.* 2008;247:238–249.

101. Trotter JF, Wachs M, Everson GT, Kam I. Adult-to-adult transplantation of the right hepatic lobe from a living donor. *N Engl J Med.* 2002;346:1074–1082.

102. Liu CL, Fan ST, Lo CM, et al. Live donor liver transplantation for fulminant hepatic failure in children. *Liver Transpl.* 2003;9:1185–1190.

103. Campsen J, Blei AT, Emond JC, et al. Outcomes of living donor liver transplantation for acute liver failure: the adult-to-adult living donor liver transplantation cohort study. *Liver Transpl.* 2008;14:1273–1280.

104. Ikegami T, Taketomi A, Soejima Y, et al. Living donor liver transplantation for acute liver failure: a 10-year experience in a single center. *J Am Coll Surg.* 2008;206:412–418.

105. Kilic M, Aydin U, Noyan A, et al. Live donor liver transplantation for acute liver failure. *Transplantation.* 2007;84:475–479.

106. Abouna GJ. Emergency adult to adult living donor liver transplantation for fulminant hepatic failure—is it justifiable? *Transplantation.* 2001;71:1498–1500.

107. Williams R. The elusive goal of liver support–quest for the Holy Grail. *Clin Med.* 2006;6:482–487.

108. Demetriou AA, Brown Jr RS, Busuttil RW, et al. Prospective, randomized, multicenter, controlled trial of a bioartificial liver in treating acute liver failure. *Ann Surg.* 2004;239:660–667.

109. Stutchfield BM, Simpson K, Wigmore SJ. Systematic review and meta-analysis of survival following extracorporeal liver support. *Br J Surg.* 2011;98:623–631.

110. Zheng Z, Li X, Li Z, Ma X. Artificial and bioartificial liver support systems for acute and acute-on-chronic hepatic failure: a meta-analysis and meta-regression. *Exp Ther Med.* 2013;6:929–936.

111. Saliba F, Camus C, Durand F, et al. Albumin dialysis with a noncell artificial liver support device in patients with acute liver failure: a randomized, controlled trial. *Ann Intern Med.* 2013;159:522–531.

70 How Does Critical Illness Alter the Gut? How Does One Manage These Alterations?

Rohit Mittal, Mara Serbanescu, Kevin W. McConnell

Alterations in the gut and immune function are proposed to play an important role in the pathophysiology and progression of critical illness, especially in sepsis.[1-6] Because the treatment of most aspects of critical illness is supportive, significant research efforts are focused on targeting and preventing the changes that occur in these two complex systems in efforts to devise new therapeutic options. This review focuses on the changes that take place in the gut and therapeutic interventions that may be available in the future.

DEFINING THE GUT

The gut is a complex ecosystem with multiple components that are altered in critical illness. Globally, the gut can be divided into two components: (1) the commensal bacterial microbiome and (2) the structures that provide intestinal integrity or barrier function. The two components are separated by a layer of mucus, which serves as the first barrier separating intraluminal contents and commensal bacteria from the epithelium (Fig. 70-1).[7] We analyze each in more detail to determine how therapeutic modulation of the intestinal microflora or gut integrity may be used to treat septic patients (Fig. 70-2).

UNDERSTANDING AND ALTERING THE MICROBIOME FOR THERAPEUTIC BENEFIT

Perhaps the most striking aspect of the gut is that it plays host to nearly 100 trillion bacteria, which serve an important symbiotic function for the host.[8,9] The multitude of organisms within the gut exist in differing populations over the life of the host and can be altered by diet, stress, disease, and iatrogenic methods.[8,10] It is increasingly recognized that these bacterial populations play a key role in the pathogenesis and pathophysiology of critical illness, and they have become a target for therapeutic interventions. To understand how altering the gut bacteria can be beneficial,

one must first understand how the microbiome is affected during critical illness and how it may contribute to propagating the disease.

Isolation of enteric bacteria from blood cultures suggests that bacteria are able to translocate across the intestinal barrier into the bloodstream via the portal circulation.[11] However, this process has not been definitively confirmed because portal vein blood samples from trauma patients have failed to isolate enteric bacteria.[12] Rather, bacteria have been isolated from mesenteric lymph nodes in cirrhosis, in portal hypertension, and after hepatectomy.[13-15] These findings suggest that translocation may occur under specific disease states, but hematogenous spread of bacteria is unlikely.

In studying the intestinal microbial environment, a growing body of evidence suggests that changes in bacterial populations, gene expression, and microenvironment are able to potentiate illness. In mice, intestinal *Pseudomonas* alters its own gene expression and transforms into a more virulent form after hepatectomy,[16,17] an effect that is directly potentiated by the administration of morphine.[18] This virulent transformation can be halted by phosphate supplementation or by the prevention of hypophosphatemia,[19] highlighting the importance of maintaining a "healthy" intestinal microbiome.[20] Intestinal microbes constantly survey the surrounding bacterial populations and the microenvironment. Changes in either that may indicate "stress" will lead bacteria to alter their numbers and gene expression, a concept referred to as "quorum sensing."[21] During health, normal host bacteria produce bacteriocins that inhibit growth of other bacteria, particularly pathogenic ones.[21,22] This response suggests that virulent transformation might be prevented by therapeutically altering the microbiome. Changes of this nature can be accomplished through supplementation of healthy bacteria, destruction/elimination of pathogenic organisms, or replacement of the entire microbiologic population.

The demonstration of changes in the microbiome led to the development of probiotics and synbiotics that supplement the gut with live bacteria and nutrients to support their growth. Prophylactic probiotic/synbiotic administration reduces the incidence of ventilator-associated pneumonias and infectious complications in trauma patients and those undergoing major abdominal surgery.[23,24] In the setting of pediatric necrotizing enterocolitis, probiotics may also reduce the associated mortality.[25] However, because probiotic/synbiotic administration has not been shown to significantly alter mortality and in rare instances has resulted in bacteremia, the therapeutic benefit of these agents remains to be determined.[26]

In efforts to attack the problem from a different point of view, ongoing research has examined selective decontamination of the digestive tract (SDD) for critically ill patients. In SDD, broad-spectrum antibiotics are administered prophylactically to prevent bacterial overgrowth.[27-29] Although SDD may reduce the incidence of ventilator-associated pneumonias, concerns over the development of bacterial resistance have limited its use.[30-32] A detailed analysis of the risks, benefits, and application of SDD can be found in Chapter 46.

Restoration of the distal gut microbiome to that of a healthy host via fecal transplantation has emerged as a novel and promising therapeutic option for critically ill patients with several disorders.[33] Perturbations in the intestinal microbiome are inciting factors for several gastrointestinal diseases, of which *Clostridium difficile* infection is a prime example, and fecal transplantation seeks to target these disease processes.[34-37] There is also growing evidence that fecal transplantation can correct alterations in the microbiome that play an important role in inflammatory bowel disease, with a reduction in symptoms and even disease remission in a select group of these patients.[38] Although fecal transplantation may benefit select groups of patients,[39,40] its role as a first-line therapy in critically ill patients remains unclear.

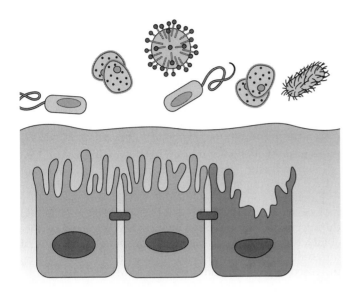

Figure 70-1. The intestinal microbiome is made of up interactions between various populations of commensal bacterial. These bacteria are contained within the gut through components of intestinal integrity, which include the mucous layer and intercellular junctional complex (IJC). Epithelial cell apoptosis or alterations in the mucous layer or IJC impair intestinal integrity.

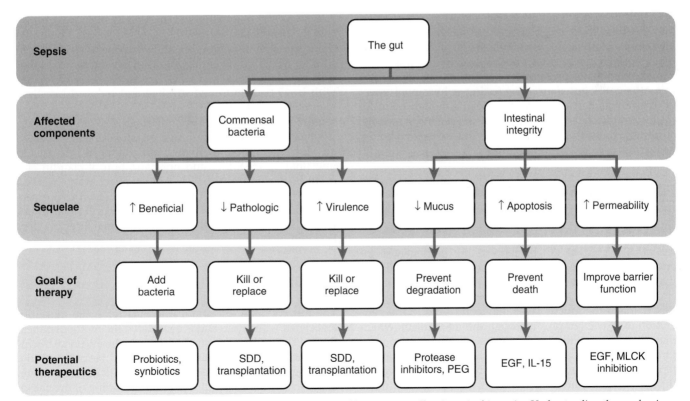

Figure 70-2. Sepsis alters the behavior and populations of commensal bacteria as well as intestinal integrity. Understanding the mechanisms by which sepsis alters the gut is vital to creating targeted therapies for critically ill patients. *EGF*, epidermal growth factor; *IL*, interleukin; *MLCK*, myosin light chain kinase; *PEG*, polyethylene glycol; *SDD*, selective decontamination of the digestive tract.

CRITICAL ILLNESS AND ALTERATIONS IN INTESTINAL INTEGRITY

The intestinal epithelium is made up of a single layer of columnar cells that are produced in the crypts of Lieberkühn and migrate upward toward the villous tip, where they are exfoliated into the intestinal lumen.[6] These cells are responsible for nutrient absorption, they provide a barrier against intraluminal contents and bacteria, and they communicate with the immune system. Epithelial cells are held together by an intercellular junctional complex, forming a selective barrier allowing for paracellular transport of ions and solutes.[41] Alterations in the mucus layer and the intercellular junctional complexes impair gut barrier function, whereas epithelial cell apoptosis impairs intestinal integrity (Fig. 70-1).

Mucus-producing epithelial cells secrete a layer of glycosylated proteins that lines the gut and forms a hydrophobic barrier. This protective layer can be altered during states of stress.[7] In critical illness, the mucous layer becomes thinner and loses its hydrophobicity, potentially increasing gut injury. The degree of intestinal injury directly correlates with the extent of mucous layer loss.[42] This effect appears to result, in part, from mucous degradation by pancreatic proteases and digestive enzymes.[43,44] The proteolytic effects of these compounds can then cause autodigestion (i.e., direct injury to intestinal epithelium).[45] Although isolated loss of the mucous layer is not sufficient to cause systemic organ dysfunction, it does appear to play a synergistic role in the process.

In animal models, treatment with the protease inhibitors 6-amidino-2-naphtyl *p*-guanidinobenzoate di-methanesulfate, transexamic acid, or aprotinin-attenuated autodigestion and thus intestinal and systemic injury, a benefit that may be related to reduced reactive oxygen species.[46,47] High molecular weight polyethylene glycol also preserved mucus-producing cells and maintained hydrophobicity.[48] Female rates have preservation of the mucus layer, and this attenuates gut injury, suggesting a hormonal effect on the mucus barrier.[49] Unfortunately, although many of these therapies have shown promise in preclinical models, additional translational and clinical data are needed before being implemented in clinical practice.

ROLE OF INTESTINAL LYMPH IN CRITICAL ILLNESS

Although evidence has not supported a role for the hematogenous spread of gut bacteria in the pathogenesis of critical illness, data generated in the last decade indicate that mesenteric lymph may activate neutrophils and cause endothelial cell injury.[50] In particular, pancreatic enzymes that damage the mucus layer may contribute to the generation of "toxic lymph," although the mechanism, which may involve reactive oxygen species, remains poorly understood.[51,52] In animal models, ligation of the mesenteric lymph duct prevents critical illness–induced myocardial dysfunction and lung injury.[53-57] A practical treatment option would need to focus on preventing generation of toxic lymph, perhaps by minimized reactive oxygen species or inhibiting pancreatic proteases.

GUT EPITHELIAL LAYER AND INTESTINAL INTEGRITY

The gut and spleen are the only systems in which apoptosis is significantly increased in sepsis and critical illness.[58,59] Toll-like receptor 4 expression by intestinal epithelial cells mediates proliferation and apoptosis.[60] The relationship between gut epithelial apoptosis and survival from experimental sepsis is multifactorial, reflecting the model of sepsis, timing, and degree of cell death.[61] In one animal model, gut epithelial apoptosis can be prevented through overexpression of the antiapoptotic protein Bcl-2.[62,63]

The connection between intestinal epithelial cells includes a tight junction complex containing multiple proteins, including occludins, claudins, and junctional adherens molecules. Activation of myosin light chain kinase (MLCK) (an intracellular protein kinase) results in activation of intracellular zonula occludens (ZO) proteins, which leads to junctional complex contraction and allows paracellular molecular transport.[7,64] This gut barrier function is altered during critical illness, leading to increased intestinal permeability. Proposed mechanisms include altered expression of intracellular ZO and intercellular proteins.[7,65,66] In addition, increased expression and activation of MLCK during critical illness may lead to increased contraction of the junctional complex and increased intestinal permeability.[67,68]

Although there are no clinically available agents that prevent gut epithelial apoptosis, two options have shown promise. Epidermal growth factor (EGF) is a cytoprotective peptide that improves intestinal integrity. In septic animals, EGF treatment normalized gut epithelial proliferation and apoptosis and provided a significant survival advantage.[69,70] This protective benefit persists when EGF is selectively overexpressed in enterocytes, suggesting that the benefits arise from these cells.[71] Another potential therapeutic option involves the cytokine interleukin 15 (IL-15), which exerts antiapoptotic effects on natural killer cells, dendritic cells, and CD8 T cells. Septic mice treated with IL-15 had improved survival and reduced intestinal apoptosis.[72] Although EGF and IL-15 show promise, they require further study before clinical use. Preventing hyperpermeability may also improve intestinal integrity. ML-9, an MLCK inhibitor, attenuated burn-induced increases in intestinal permeability and normalization of claudin and occludin levels in mice.[68] A similar effect was observed with PIK (membrane permeant inhibitor of MLCK), a second MLCK inhibitor.[73] Therefore targeting the machinery responsible for the maintenance of intestinal integrity may be a potential therapy in critically ill patients.

CONCLUSIONS

The gut plays an important role in driving the mortality associated with sepsis and is considered the motor of critical illness. The process reflects alterations in the intestinal microbiome and loss of intestinal integrity and barrier function. Although the therapeutic options for critically ill patients are currently limited, improved understanding of the pathophysiology of critical illness has identified new potential targets for pharmacologic intervention. Additional translational and clinical research is needed to demonstrate clinical utility.

AUTHORS' RECOMMENDATIONS

- The gut plays an important role in driving the mortality associated with sepsis and is considered the motor of critical illness.
- The gut plays host to nearly 100 trillion bacteria. These bacterial populations play a key role in the pathogenesis and pathophysiology of critical illness.
- The process reflects alterations in the intestinal microbiome and loss of intestinal integrity and barrier function.
- Although the therapeutic options for critically ill patients are currently limited (e.g., selective gut or oral decontamination), improved understanding of the pathophysiology of critical illness has identified new potential targets for pharmacologic intervention.
- Epidermal growth factor (EGF) and IL-15 are promising treatments, in preclinical testing, for maintaining gut barrier function.
- Additional translational and clinical research is needed to demonstrate clinical utility.

REFERENCES

1. Angus DC, Linde-Zwirble WT, Lidicker J, Clermont G, Carcillo J, Pinsky MR. Epidemiology of severe sepsis in the United States: analysis of incidence, outcome, and associated costs of care. *Crit Care Med.* 2001;29(7):1303–1310.
2. Martin GS, Mannino DM, Eaton S, Moss M. The epidemiology of sepsis in the United States from 1979 through 2000. *N Engl J Med.* 2003;348(16):1546–1554.
3. Gaieski DF, Edwards JM, Kallan MJ, Carr BG. Benchmarking the incidence and mortality of severe sepsis in the United States. *Crit Care Med.* 2013;41(5):1167–1174.
4. Carrico CJ, Meakins JL, Marshall JC, Fry D, Maier RV. Multiple-organ-failure syndrome. *Arch Surg.* 1986;121(2):196–208.
5. Hotchkiss RS, Karl IE. The pathophysiology and treatment of sepsis. *N Engl J Med.* 2003;348(2):138–150.
6. Clark JA, Coopersmith CM. Intestinal crosstalk: a new paradigm for understanding the gut as the "motor" of critical illness. *Shock.* 2007;28(4):384–393.
7. Turner JR. Intestinal mucosal barrier function in health and disease. *Nat Rev Immunol.* 2009;9(11):799–809.
8. Cho I, Blaser MJ. The human microbiome: at the interface of health and disease. *Nat Rev Genet.* 2012;13(4):260–270.
9. Eckburg PB, Bik EM, Bernstein CN, et al. Diversity of the human intestinal microbial flora. *Science.* 2005;308(5728):1635–1638.
10. Arumugam M, Raes J, Pelletier E, et al. Enterotypes of the human gut microbiome. *Nature.* 2011;473(7346):174–180.
11. Quigley EM. Passing the bug–translocation, bacteremia, and sepsis in the intensive care unit patient: is intestinal decontamination the answer? *Crit Care Med.* 2011;39(5):1202–1203.
12. Moore FA, Moore EE, Poggetti R, et al. Gut bacterial translocation via the portal vein: a clinical perspective with major torso trauma. *J Trauma.* 1991;31(5):629–636. discussion 636–628.
13. Liu X, Li H, Lu A, et al. Reduction of intestinal mucosal immune function in heat-stressed rats and bacterial translocation. *Int J Hyperthermia.* 2012;28(8):756–765. North American Hyperthermia Group.
14. Nishigaki E, Abe T, Yokoyama Y, et al. The detection of intraoperative bacterial translocation in the mesenteric lymph nodes is useful in predicting patients at high risk for postoperative infectious complications after esophagectomy. *Ann Surg.* 2014;259(3):477–484.
15. Mizuno T, Yokoyama Y, Nishio H, et al. Intraoperative bacterial translocation detected by bacterium-specific ribosomal rna-targeted reverse-transcriptase polymerase chain reaction for the mesenteric lymph node strongly predicts postoperative infectious complications after major hepatectomy for biliary malignancies. *Ann Surg.* 2010;252(6):1013–1019.
16. Babrowski T, Romanowski K, Fink D, et al. The intestinal environment of surgical injury transforms *Pseudomonas aeruginosa* into a discrete hypervirulent morphotype capable of causing lethal peritonitis. *Surgery.* 2013;153(1):36–43.
17. Seal JB, Alverdy JC, Zaborina O, An G. Agent-based dynamic knowledge representation of *Pseudomonas aeruginosa* virulence activation in the stressed gut: Towards characterizing host-pathogen interactions in gut-derived sepsis. *Theor Biol Med Model.* 2011;8:33.
18. Babrowski T, Holbrook C, Moss J, et al. *Pseudomonas aeruginosa* virulence expression is directly activated by morphine and is capable of causing lethal gut-derived sepsis in mice during chronic morphine administration. *Ann Surg.* 2012;255(2):386–393.
19. Zaborin A, Gerdes S, Holbrook C, Liu DC, Zaborina OY, Alverdy JC. *Pseudomonas aeruginosa* overrides the virulence inducing effect of opioids when it senses an abundance of phosphate. *PLoS One.* 2012;7(4):e34883.
20. Carlisle EM, Poroyko V, Caplan MS, Alverdy J, Morowitz MJ, Liu D. Murine gut microbiota and transcriptome are diet dependent. *Ann Surg.* 2013;257(2):287–294.
21. Schuijt TJ, van der Poll T, de Vos WM, Wiersinga WJ. The intestinal microbiota and host immune interactions in the critically ill. *Trends Microbiol.* 2013;21(5):221–229.
22. Gillor O, Etzion A, Riley MA. The dual role of bacteriocins as anti- and probiotics. *Appl Microbiol Biotechnol.* 2008;81(4):591–606.
23. Morrow LE, Kollef MH, Casale TB. Probiotic prophylaxis of ventilator-associated pneumonia: a blinded, randomized, controlled trial. *Am J Respir Crit Care Med.* 2010;182(8):1058–1064.
24. Shimizu K, Ogura H, Asahara T, et al. Probiotic/synbiotic therapy for treating critically ill patients from a gut microbiota perspective. *Dig Dis Sci.* 2013;58(1):23–32.
25. AlFaleh K, Anabrees J. Probiotics for prevention of necrotizing enterocolitis in preterm infants. *Cochrane Database Syst Rev.* 2014;4. CD005496.
26. Theodorakopoulou M, Perros E, Giamarellos-Bourboulis EJ, Dimopoulos G. Controversies in the management of the critically ill: the role of probiotics. *Int J Antimicrob Agents.* 2013;(suppl 42):S41–S44.
27. Silvestri L, de la Cal MA, van Saene HK. Selective decontamination of the digestive tract: the mechanism of action is control of gut overgrowth. *Intensive Care Med.* 2012;38(11):1738–1750.
28. Silvestri L, van Saene HK, Petros AJ. Selective digestive tract decontamination in critically ill patients. *Expert Opin Pharmacother.* 2012;13(8):1113–1129.
29. Oudemans-van Straaten HM, Endeman H, Bosman RJ, et al. Presence of tobramycin in blood and urine during selective decontamination of the digestive tract in critically ill patients, a prospective cohort study. *Crit Care.* 2011;15(5):R240.
30. Walden AP, Bonten MJ, Wise MP. Should selective digestive decontamination be used in critically ill patients? *BMJ.* 2012;345:e6697.
31. van der Meer JW, Vandenbroucke-Grauls CM. Resistance to selective decontamination: the jury is still out. *Lancet Infect Dis.* 2013;13(4):282–283.
32. Daneman N, Sarwar S, Fowler RA, Cuthbertson BH. Effect of selective decontamination on antimicrobial resistance in intensive care units: a systematic review and meta-analysis. *Lancet Infect Dis.* 2013;13(4):328–341.
33. Brandt LJ, Reddy SS. Fecal microbiota transplantation for recurrent clostridium difficile infection. *J Clin Gastroenterol.* 2011;(suppl 45):S159–S167.
34. Brandt LJ. American Journal of Gastroenterology Lecture: intestinal microbiota and the role of fecal microbiota transplant (FMT) in treatment of *C. difficile* infection. *Am J Gastroenterol.* 2013;108(2):177–185.
35. Borody TJ, Khoruts A. Fecal microbiota transplantation and emerging applications. *Nat Rev Gastroenterol Hepatol.* 2012;9(2):88–96.
36. Borody TJ, Campbell J. Fecal microbiota transplantation: techniques, applications, and issues. *Gastroenterol Clin North Am.* 2012;41(4):781–803.
37. Khoruts A, Sadowsky MJ. Therapeutic transplantation of the distal gut microbiota. *Mucosal Immunol.* 2011;4(1):4–7.
38. Colman RJ, Rubin DT. Fecal microbiota transplantation as therapy for inflammatory bowel disease: a systematic review and meta-analysis. *J Crohns Colitis.* 2014;8(12):1569–1581.
39. Khoruts A, Weingarden AR. Emergence of fecal microbiota transplantation as an approach to repair disrupted microbial gut ecology. *Immunol Lett.* 2014;162(2 Pt A):77–81.
40. Sha S, Liang J, Chen M, et al. Systematic review: faecal microbiota transplantation therapy for digestive and nondigestive disorders in adults and children. *Aliment Pharmacol Ther.* 2014;39(10):1003–1032.
41. McConnell KW, Coopersmith CM. Epithelial cells. *Crit Care Med.* 2005;33(suppl 12):S520–S522.

42. Lu Q, Xu DZ, Sharpe S, et al. The anatomic sites of disruption of the mucus layer directly correlate with areas of trauma/hemorrhagic shock-induced gut injury. *J Trauma.* 2011;70(3):630–635.

43. Sharpe SM, Qin X, Lu Q, et al. Loss of the intestinal mucus layer in the normal rat causes gut injury but not toxic mesenteric lymph nor lung injury. *Shock.* 2010;34(5):475–481.

44. Chang M, Alsaigh T, Kistler EB, Schmid-Schonbein GW. Breakdown of mucin as barrier to digestive enzymes in the ischemic rat small intestine. *PLoS One.* 2012;7(6):e40087.

45. Chang M, Kistler EB, Schmid-Schonbein GW. Disruption of the mucosal barrier during gut ischemia allows entry of digestive enzymes into the intestinal wall. *Shock.* 2012;37(3):297–305.

46. Mittal R, Coopersmith CM. Redefining the gut as the motor of critical illness. *Trends Mol Med.* 2014;20(4):214–223.

47. Fishman JE, Levy G, Alli V, Sheth S, Lu Q, Deitch EA. Oxidative modification of the intestinal mucus layer is a critical but unrecognized component of trauma hemorrhagic shock-induced gut barrier failure. *Am J Physiol Gastrointest Liver Physiol.* 2013;304(1):G57–G63.

48. Valuckaite V, Seal J, Zaborina O, Tretiakova M, Testa G, Alverdy JC. High molecular weight polyethylene glycol (PEG 15-20) maintains mucosal microbial barrier function during intestinal graft preservation. *J Surg Res.* 2013;183(2):869–875.

49. Sheth SU, Lu Q, Twelker K, et al. Intestinal mucus layer preservation in female rats attenuates gut injury after trauma-hemorrhagic shock. *J Trauma.* 2010;68(2):279–288.

50. Senthil M, Brown M, Xu DZ, Lu Q, Feketeova E, Deitch EA. Gut-lymph hypothesis of systemic inflammatory response syndrome/multiple-organ dysfunction syndrome: validating studies in a porcine model. *J Trauma.* 2006;60(5):958–965. discussion 965–957.

51. Caputo FJ, Rupani B, Watkins AC, et al. Pancreatic duct ligation abrogates the trauma hemorrhage-induced gut barrier failure and the subsequent production of biologically active intestinal lymph. *Shock.* 2007;28(4):441–446.

52. Senthil M, Watkins A, Barlos D, et al. Intravenous injection of trauma-hemorrhagic shock mesenteric lymph causes lung injury that is dependent upon activation of the inducible nitric oxide synthase pathway. *Ann Surg.* 2007;246(5):822–830.

53. Badami CD, Senthil M, Caputo FJ, et al. Mesenteric lymph duct ligation improves survival in a lethal shock model. *Shock.* 2008;30(6):680–685.

54. Lee MA, Yatani A, Sambol JT, Deitch EA. Role of gut-lymph factors in the induction of burn-induced and trauma-shock-induced acute heart failure. *Int J Clin Exp Med.* 2008;1(2):171–180.

55. Watkins AC, Caputo FJ, Badami C, et al. Mesenteric lymph duct ligation attenuates lung injury and neutrophil activation after intraperitoneal injection of endotoxin in rats. *J Trauma.* 2008;64(1):126–130.

56. Sambol JT, Lee MA, Caputo FJ, et al. Mesenteric lymph duct ligation prevents trauma/hemorrhage shock-induced cardiac contractile dysfunction. *J Appl Physiol.* 2009;106(1):57–65.

57. Deitch EA. Gut lymph and lymphatics: a source of factors leading to organ injury and dysfunction. *Ann N Y Acad Sci.* 2010;1207(suppl 1):E103–E111.

58. Takasu O, Gaut JP, Watanabe E, et al. Mechanisms of cardiac and renal dysfunction in patients dying of sepsis. *Am J Respir Crit Care Med.* 2013;187(5):509–517.

59. Hotchkiss RS, Swanson PE, Freeman BD, et al. Apoptotic cell death in patients with sepsis, shock, and multiple organ dysfunction. *Crit Care Med.* 1999;27(7):1230–1251.

60. Neal MD, Sodhi CP, Dyer M, et al. A critical role for TLR4 induction of autophagy in the regulation of enterocyte migration and the pathogenesis of necrotizing enterocolitis. *J Immunol.* 2013;190(7):3541–3551.

61. Vyas D, Robertson CM, Stromberg PE, et al. Epithelial apoptosis in mechanistically distinct methods of injury in the murine small intestine. *Histol Histopathol.* 2007;22(6):623–630.

62. Coopersmith CM, Chang KC, Swanson PE, et al. Overexpression of Bcl-2 in the intestinal epithelium improves survival in septic mice. *Crit Care Med.* 2002;30(1):195–201.

63. Coopersmith CM, Stromberg PE, Dunne WM, et al. Inhibition of intestinal epithelial apoptosis and survival in a murine model of pneumonia-induced sepsis. *JAMA.* 2002;287(13):1716–1721.

64. Suzuki T. Regulation of intestinal epithelial permeability by tight junctions. *Cell Mol Life Sci.* 2013;70(4):631–659.

65. Epstein MD, Tchervenkov JI, Alexander JW, Johnson JR, Vester JW. Increased gut permeability following burn trauma. *Arch Surg.* 1991;126(2):198–200.

66. Rupani B, Caputo FJ, Watkins AC, et al. Relationship between disruption of the unstirred mucus layer and intestinal restitution in loss of gut barrier function after trauma hemorrhagic shock. *Surgery.* 2007;141(4):481–489.

67. Cunningham KE, Turner JR. Myosin light chain kinase: pulling the strings of epithelial tight junction function. *Ann N Y Acad Sci.* 2012;1258:34–42.

68. Chen C, Wang P, Su Q, Wang S, Wang F. Myosin light chain kinase mediates intestinal barrier disruption following burn injury. *PLoS One.* 2012;7(4):e34946.

69. Clark JA, Clark AT, Hotchkiss RS, Buchman TG, Coopersmith CM. Epidermal growth factor treatment decreases mortality and is associated with improved gut integrity in sepsis. *Shock.* 2008;30(1):36–42.

70. Geng Y, Li J, Wang F, et al. Epidermal growth factor promotes proliferation and improves restoration after intestinal ischemia-reperfusion injury in rats. *Inflammation.* 2013;36(3):670–679.

71. Clark JA, Gan H, Samocha AJ, et al. Enterocyte-specific epidermal growth factor prevents barrier dysfunction and improves mortality in murine peritonitis. *Am J Physiol Gastrointest Liver Physiol.* 2009;297(3):G471–G479.

72. Inoue S, Unsinger J, Davis CG, et al. IL-15 prevents apoptosis, reverses innate and adaptive immune dysfunction, and improves survival in sepsis. *J Immunol.* 2010;184(3):1401–1409.

73. Zahs A, Bird MD, Ramirez L, Turner JR, Choudhry MA, Kovacs EJ. Inhibition of long myosin light-chain kinase activation alleviates intestinal damage after binge ethanol exposure and burn injury. *Am J Physiol Gastrointest Liver Physiol.* 2012;303(6):G705–G712.

ENDOCRINE CRITICAL CARE

71 Is There a Place for Anabolic Hormones in Critical Care?

Nicholas Heming, Virginie Maxime, Djillali Annane

Anabolism is the enzymatic process by which nutrients and energy are used to synthesize molecules in living cells. In contrast, catabolism involves chemical reactions that lead to the degradation of molecules. During growth, anabolic processes dominate, either through increased biosynthesis or decreased molecular degradation. In healthy subjects, energy is produced through the catabolism of carbohydrates and fat, whereas proteins and amino acids are used to generate new structures (i.e., for anabolism). When patients become acutely ill, amino acids from muscle are used to synthesize acute-phase proteins and to generate glucose de novo (i.e., for gluconeogenesis), but this process is limited and adaptive. However, in critical illness, two distinct phases have been described.[1] The first is similar to what is seen in acute illness and is similarly characterized by the diversion of energy and anabolism toward vital organs and the immune system. This response is partially mediated by the endocrine system. Protracted critical illness constitutes the second phase. It is often maladaptive, with uncompensated catabolism leading to major nitrogen loss and muscle wasting, and is characterized by a globally decreased endocrine response.[2] Increased catabolism may be responsible for insufficient wound healing, prolonged mechanical ventilation, and extended hospital lengths of stay. Aggressive nutritional support during this second phase has failed to prevent muscle wasting.[3,4] It has been hypothesized that hormone supplementation during the protracted phase of critical illness may favor anabolism. Four hormones having anabolic properties may be of interest in the critical care setting: androgens, insulin, growth hormone, and thyroid hormone. The following chapter reviews the evidence regarding the safety and efficacy of anabolic hormone supplementation in critically ill adults.

ANDROGENS

Androgens, or male sex hormones, are synthesized by a series of enzymatic reactions initiated using cholesterol. Cholesterol is first converted into pregnenolone and its metabolite progesterone. These two hormones are converted into 17-hydroxypregnenolone (17-OH-pregnenolone) and 17-hydroxyprogesterone (17-OH-progesterone), respectively, and then into dehydroepiandrosterone (DHEA) and androstenedione. Of note, 17-OH-pregnenolone and 17-OH-progesterone are also precursors of cortisol. DHEA (as well as DHEA-S, the sulfated form of DHEA that predominates in the circulation) and androstenedione, although adrenal androgens, are considered to be largely inactive.[5,6] Serum DHEA levels are increased during septic shock, whereas those of DHEA-S are decreased. The increase in DHEA concentration may follow the increase in cortisol levels seen during septic shock.[7] DHEA is converted to androstenedione via 3-β-hydroxysteroid dehydrogenase, which is then converted to testosterone by 17-β-hydroxysteroid dehydrogenase. Testosterone can also be converted to estradiol by the aromatase enzyme (Fig. 71-1).

Testosterone is the most abundantly produced and the most clinically relevant androgen. It is secreted by the interstitial cells of Leydig in the testes and by the adrenal glands in males and females.[5,8] Testosterone secretion is regulated by luteinizing hormone (LH) produced in the anterior pituitary. LH secretion is stimulated by gonadotropin-releasing hormone (GnRH), which is produced by the hypothalamus. Circulating testosterone is bound to albumin or to the sex hormone-binding globulin.[9] Serum concentrations of testosterone are 12 to 31 nmol/L in healthy males and 0.52 to 2.6 nmol/L in healthy females. Testosterone remains in the circulation for no more than a few hours, after which it has either been transported to its target tissues or degraded. At a cellular level, testosterone or its intracellular metabolite, dihydrotestosterone, binds to a nuclear receptor protein complex. This complex migrates to the cell nucleus and induces DNA transcription. Testosterone has well-documented anabolic properties.[10] It induces hypertrophy of type I and II muscle fibers and increases the number of skeletal muscle satellite cells.[11,12] Testosterone also promotes the differentiation of multipotent mesenchymal cells into myocytes and inhibits their differentiation into adipocytes.[13,14] Finally, androgens may alter other physiologic parameters via nongenomic signaling pathways that involve lipid and protein metabolism.[15]

Studies in animal models of trauma hemorrhage and sepsis have demonstrated that females have stronger immune responses and better survival rates than males.[16,17] In the critically ill, though, clinical evidence of an association between female gender and improved outcome is weak and relies on an inconclusive or contradictory literature.[18,19]

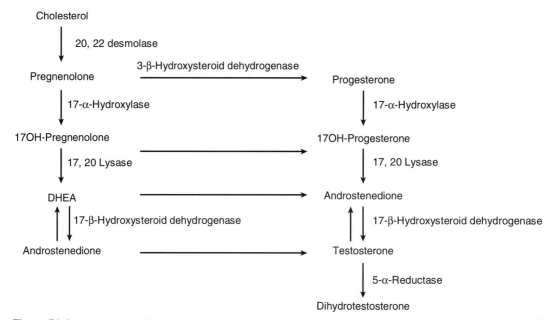

Figure 71-1. Biosynthesis of androgens. *DHEA,* dehydroepiandrosterone. *(Adapted from Miller and Auchus [2011].[86])*

During acute illness, testosterone concentrations are low, whereas LH levels are increased.[20] In patients with prolonged critical illness, serum testosterone, LH, and GnRH concentrations are low.[21,22] For example, in some patients with chronic obstructive pulmonary disease or human immunodeficiency virus–associated wasting syndromes, administration of synthetic androgens induced a gain in muscle mass and strength and improved respiratory function.[23,24] In men with severe burn injuries, testosterone reduced protein catabolism.[25] The synthetic androgen oxandrolone, which has been approved by the U.S. Food and Drug Administration as an adjunctive therapy after surgery or trauma, may reduce weight loss, improve functional status, and increase wound healing.[26,27] However, a large trial involving oxandrolone administration to trauma patients failed to demonstrate any significant benefit.[28] Another trial, performed in ventilator-dependent surgical patients, found that oxandrolone prolonged the duration of mechanical ventilation.[29] Data from trials assessing the effect of testosterone supplementation in critically ill patients on patient-centered outcomes are scarce. Although data are limited, the safety profile of androgens may be favorable. Likewise, data on testosterone precursor (such as DHEA) supplementation in the critically ill are also lacking.

Overall, in the critically ill, androgen supplementation may have some benefits on nutritional endpoints in select subgroups of patients. Additional trials are still needed before the routine use of such a therapeutic approach could be suggested for caring for the critically ill.

INSULIN

Insulin is formed by two peptide chains—a 21-amino acid A chain and a 30-amino acid B chain—that are linked by disulfide bonds.[30] The hormone regulates carbohydrate metabolism by promoting glucose entry into cells.

Insulin is produced by the beta cells of the islets of Langerhans of the pancreas.[5] The gene for insulin is highly conserved and encodes a single chain precursor. Various factors, including glucose, glucagon, cholecystokinin, and gastric inhibitory polypeptide, induce insulin secretion. Insulin secretion is inhibited by catecholamines and somatostatin. Monomers of insulin, the active form of the hormone, are mostly unbound in the circulation. The half-life of circulating insulin is extremely short, approximately 6 minutes, ensuring that carbohydrate homeostasis occurs almost instantaneously. The fasting serum concentration of insulin ranges from 28 to 108 pmol/L in healthy individuals.

The insulin receptor has strong analogies with the insulin-like growth factor-1 (IGF-1) receptor. Both belong to the receptor tyrosine kinase family.[31] On ligand binding, intracellular portions of the receptor are activated. Activation is followed by the recruitment of adaptor proteins and downstream signaling proteins.[32] One of the downstream signals involves the mitogen-activated protein kinase cascade, which plays a role in modulating cellular proliferation, differentiation, and survival. Insulin receptors can also recruit the insulin receptor substrate adaptor, inducing the activation of phosphoinositide 3-kinase. This enzyme indirectly increases the amount of glucose that is captured by the organism.[33] In addition to its effect on carbohydrate metabolism, insulin also plays a role in protein metabolism and storage, but the mechanics leading to the modification of protein metabolism are still unknown.

Insulin increases the translation of mRNA as well as the rate of transcription of selected DNA genetic sequences. Insulin inhibits the catabolism of proteins, decreases the rate of amino acid release by muscle cells, and stimulates the transport of amino acids into the cells. Insulin inhibits the activity of enzymes promoting gluconeogenesis. Because gluconeogenesis relies on amino acids, insulin indirectly conserves protein and amino acid stores.[34] Insulin promotes protein synthesis in cultured cells, in isolated muscles, and in vivo in animals.[35,36] A trial conducted in healthy human volunteers, using isotopic tracers, showed that insulin promotes muscle anabolism by stimulating protein synthesis.[37] Reports from trials conducted in burned patients indicate that infusion of insulin improved protein synthesis.[38,39]

Numerous trials assessing the administration of insulin to general populations of critically ill patients have been conducted in recent years. The aim of these trials was to assess the effect of glucose control on mortality; thus they did not focus on the anabolic effects. A large monocentric trial found that surgical intensive care unit (ICU) patients treated with intensive insulin therapy (target blood glucose levels between 80 and 110 mg/dL) had lower ICU mortality than patients managed with conventional treatment (blood glucose between 180 and 200 mg/dL).[40] A second monocentric trial did not find significant differences in survival rates in medical ICU patients with or without intensive insulin therapy.[41] Subgroup analyses revealed that intensive insulin therapy reduced the mortality rate in patients hospitalized in the ICU for more than 3 days.[41] The Glucontrol multicenter trial compared intensive insulin therapy (target blood glucose between 4.4 and 6.1 mmol/L) with conventional treatment (target blood glucose between 7.8 and 10.0 mmol/L) in the critically ill.[42] In this trial, which was prematurely stopped because of a high number of protocol violations, ICU mortality was similar in both groups. Intensive insulin therapy was associated with an increased incidence of hypoglycemia.[42] The Nice-Sugar trial, including more than 6000 patients, compared intensive insulin therapy (target blood glucose range of 81 to 108 mg/dL), to conventional treatment (target of ≤180 mg/dL).[43] Mortality at day 90 and the incidence of hypoglycemia were significantly higher in the intensive insulin therapy group.[43] The VISEP (Efficacy of Volume Substitution and Insulin Therapy in Severe Sepsis) trial included ICU patients with severe sepsis. In this trial, the mean score for organ failure and the number of deaths at 28 days were not significantly different between the intensive insulin therapy group (target blood glucose levels 80 to 110 mg/dL) and the conventional treatment group (target blood glucose levels 180 to 200 mg/dL). This trial was stopped prematurely because of a significant increase in the incidence of hypoglycemia with the experimental intervention.[44] Lastly, glucose variability might be an independent prognostic factor in critically ill patients.[45,46]

Current guidelines for the management of sepsis recommend administering insulin to control hyperglycemia.[47] As a general rule, physicians should target a blood glucose level of less than 180 mg/dL during ICU stay. There is no specific recommendation for the administration of insulin as an anabolic hormone.

GROWTH HORMONE

Growth hormone (GH) is structurally similar to prolactin and placental lactogen. Production of GH is positively controlled by the GH releasing hormone (GHRH) and ghrelin. Both are subjected to pulsatile release from the hypothalamus and act on the anterior pituitary to induce pulsatile release of GH. Ghrelin is also produced by the stomach and

pancreas.[48,49] Stress, physical exercise, hypoglycemia, and elevated concentrations of insulin induce the production of GHRH. By contrast, somatostatin, hyperglycemia, obesity, and hypercorticisolism inhibit GHRH production.[50,51] The serum half-life of GH is between 20 and 30 minutes. The fasting serum concentration of GH in healthy adults is less than 5 ng/mL. GH plays an anabolic role on protein and glucose metabolism, and it stimulates bone growth.[52] The hormone acts either directly through the GH receptors or via the effect of other GHs that have a structure similar to proinsulin and stimulate the uptake of amino acids and inhibit the degradation of muscle proteins.[53,54] The most important of these hormones is IGF-1, produced by hepatocytes under the influence of GH.[55] IGF-1 is a negative feedback regulator of GH and GHRH. IGF-1 stimulates protein synthesis and decreases the degradation of skeletal muscle proteins.[54] More than 90% of circulating IGF-1 is bound to the IGF binding proteins (IGFBPs).[50]

Critically ill patients have major nitrogen loss associated with muscle wasting. This state has some similarities to that of patients suffering from chronic GH deficiency.[56] The acute phase of a critical illness is characterized by an increased production of pituitary hormones, especially GH, and peripheral resistance to their effects. Overall production of GH is raised through an upsurge in the number and the intensity of pulses and is associated with heightened GH concentrations between pulses and attenuated oscillatory activity.[57] Underlying mechanisms may include increased levels of GHRH and decreased levels of somatostatin. Indeed, in the ICU, elevated GH concentrations seem to be associated with an increased risk of death.[58] In addition, IGF-1 levels are decreased because of the downregulated expression of liver GH receptors[59] or the decreased levels of the main carrier protein IGFBP-3, which is also regulated by GH. These changes are considered adaptive because they could direct the use of glucose, fatty acids, and amino acids toward the production of energy rather than anabolism.[60] During the chronic phase of critical illness, GH and IGF-1 levels decrease even further because of the dramatically reduced pulse amplitude only partially offset by the increased frequency of these same pulses. This neuroendocrine dysfunction seems to be secondary to decreased ghrelin levels. Indeed, high concentrations of ghrelin seem to be associated with a favorable outcome.[61]

IGF-I promotes proliferation and differentiation in muscle cell lines.[62] The administration of GH or of IGF-1 to healthy animals induces muscle hypertrophy.[63] Both GH and IGF-1 administration to animals suffering from burns or major surgery are associated with improved nitrogen balance and immune responsiveness.[64,65]

Exploratory trials in man show that GH supplementation is associated with a positive nitrogen balance both in patients with and without severe sepsis.[66,67] One trial reported that GH supplementation after major surgery was associated with a positive nitrogen balance and improved peripheral muscular testing.[68] However, two separate multicenter trials in general ICU populations showed that the administration of recombinant human GH was associated with an increased in-hospital mortality rate.[69] Current guidelines do not recommend the use of GH in the critically ill.[70] The administration of GH releasing peptide-2 (GHRP-2), which is an agonist of ghrelin, is more effective than GHRH for increasing circulating levels of GH, IGF-1, and IGFBP.[71] Additional studies are needed to confirm the efficacy and safety of this treatment. The administration of insulin to the critically ill increases circulating levels of GH and peripheral resistance to GH.[72] Peripheral resistance to GH during protracted illness could be protective.[50]

Opotherapy for GH deficiency is harmful during the acute phase of critical illness. Further studies are needed to examine the effects of GHRH on anabolism during protracted critical illness.

THYROID HORMONES

Thyroid hormones (THs) are synthesized in the thyroid gland. TH synthesis requires the prohormone thyroglobulin and iodine, obtained through normal dietary intake. Tyrosine residues on thyroglobulin can bind iodine once, forming monoiodotyrosine (MIT), or twice, forming diiodotyrosine (DIT). The combination of two DIT residues results in the formation of thyroxine (T_4). The combination of one MIT with one DIT residue results in the formation of triiodothyronine (T_3) or of the biologically inactive 3,3',5'-triiodothyronine (reverse T_3 or rT_3).[73] These hormones have the same thyronine structure but differ by the number and position of iodine atoms. T_4 is converted by type 1 deiodinase into the more active T_3. Type 2 deiodinase converts T_4 into T_3 and also converts rT_3 into T_2 (diiodothyronine). Type 3 deiodinase degrades THs, converting T_4 into rT_3 and T_3 into T_2. The hypothalamic thyroid-releasing hormone (TRH) controls the release of thyroid-stimulating hormone (TSH), which originates in the pituitary gland. In turn, TSH stimulates the production of T_3 and T_4. TSH has a basal level of constant secretion over which pulses are released. TSH is inhibited by somatostatin and dopamine as well as feedback from T_3 and T_4.[74] Approximately 80% of THs are transported bound to T_4-binding globulin, whereas 20% are bound to transthyretin or albumin. Serum concentration of free T_3 is between 4 and 9 pmol/L, whereas the concentration of free T_4 is between 9 and 25 pmol/L and that of TSH is between 0.1 and 4.5 µIU/mL. The half-life of T_4 is 6 to 7 days, whereas that of T_3 is 24 hours. THs enter the cell and bind to nuclear receptors, which mediate the activity of THs via modification of transcriptional activity. THs upregulate all cellular metabolic activities by increasing the number and the activity of mitochondria and accelerating the active transport of ions (potassium, sodium) and glucose across cell membranes. THs also upregulate metabolic activities via nongenomic pathways (i.e., through other means than TH nuclear receptor binding).[75] Physiologic amounts of THs have an anabolic effect and enhance protein synthesis.

In animal models, THs are necessary for anabolism,[76] but supraphysiologicl levels of THs are catabolic. In the ICU, up to 70% of patients have a "nonthyroidal illness syndrome" in which levels of T_3 are diminished and T_4 levels are normal or lowered in the absence of thyroidal disease. TSH is not increased.[77] These anomalies are caused by peripheral mechanisms. Type 1 deiodinase activity is decreased; thus less T_4 is deiodinated into T_3, whereas the activity of type 3 deiodinase is increased, inactivating THs.[78] The activity of type 2 deiodinase remains almost unchanged during the acute phase of critical illness. Patients also have reduced levels of TH-binding protein, causing lower levels of circulating T_4. Decreased levels of intracellular transport and of intranuclear receptor expression could be an adaptive mechanism, aimed at increasing tissue levels of the hormones, especially in the liver and the skeletal muscle.[79,80]

During protracted illness, hormonal disturbances are the consequence of hypothalamic–pituitary axis insufficiency: TRH and TSH levels are low.[81] Decreased TRH secretion could be induced by raised levels of T_3 at the hypothalamic level, either via upregulation of type 2 deiodinase or a downregulation of type 3 deiodinase activity.[82] Consequently, secretion of TSH is also modified. TSH pulsatility is lost, and the amplitude of each pulse is decreased. The pathophysiologic mechanisms explaining these modifications are incompletely understood but may include imbalance in proinflammatory and anti-inflammatory cytokines. However, their exact role remains controversial in animal and human studies.

Clinical trials of TH supplementation were undertaken in several small cohorts. T_4 supplementation increased mortality in patients with acute renal failure.[83] T_3 supplementation increased heart rate and vascular resistances without affecting mortality after major cardiac surgery.[84] The administration of TRH, associated with GHRH or GHRP-2, restored normal TSH and T_3 levels without increasing rT_3 levels.[85] None of these trials showed any clinically relevant beneficial effect of TH supplementation in adults previously devoid of thyroidal disease.

Overall, there is no evidence suggesting any significant benefit from the administration of THs or GHs to the critically ill. Anabolic steroid androgens might improve surrogate outcomes such as weight gain after major surgery or burns. Finally, insulin, which is now broadly given to ICU patients to control blood glucose, may also provide some anabolic effects.

AUTHORS' RECOMMENDATIONS

- Administration of TH or GH to the critically ill is not recommended.
- The synthetic androgen oxandrolone may be used as an adjunctive therapy to promote weight gain after surgery or trauma.
- Insulin, used as part of a blood glucose control strategy, may have some anabolic effects.

REFERENCES

1. Van den Berghe G, de Zegher F, Bouillon R. Clinical review 95: acute and prolonged critical illness as different neuroendocrine paradigms. *J Clin Endocrinol Metab.* 1998;83:1827–1834.
2. Puthucheary ZA, Rawal J, McPhail M, et al. Acute skeletal muscle wasting in critical illness. *JAMA.* 2013;310:1591–1600.
3. Streat SJ, Beddoe AH, Hill GL. Aggressive nutritional support does not prevent protein loss despite fat gain in septic intensive care patients. *J Trauma.* 1987;27:262–266.
4. Hart DW, Wolf SE, Herndon DN, et al. Energy expenditure and caloric balance after burn: increased feeding leads to fat rather than lean mass accretion. *Ann Surg.* 2002;235:152–161.
5. Guyton AC. *Textbook of Medical Physiology.* 11th ed. Saunders Co.; 2005.

6. Shea JL, Wongt P-Y, Chen Y. Free testosterone: clinical utility and important analytical aspects of measurement. *Adv Clin Chem.* 2014;63:59–84.

7. Arlt W, Hammer F, Sanning P, et al. Dissociation of serum dehydroepiandrosterone and dehydroepiandrosterone sulfate in septic shock. *J Clin Endocrinol Metab.* 2006;91:2548–2554.

8. Federman DD. The biology of human sex differences. *N Engl J Med.* 2006;354:1507–1514.

9. Fortunati N. Sex hormone-binding globulin: not only a transport protein. What news is around the corner? *J Endocrinol Invest.* 1999;22:223–234.

10. Bhasin S, Storer TW, Berman N, et al. The effects of supraphysiologic doses of testosterone on muscle size and strength in normal men. *N Engl J Med.* 1996;335:1–7.

11. Sinha-Hikim I, Artaza J, Woodhouse L, et al. Testosterone-induced increase in muscle size in healthy young men is associated with muscle fiber hypertrophy. *Am J Physiol Endocrinol Metab.* 2002;283:E154–E164.

12. Sinha-Hikim I, Roth SM, Lee MI, Bhasin S. Testosterone-induced muscle hypertrophy is associated with an increase in satellite cell number in healthy, young men. *Am J Physiol Endocrinol Metab.* 2003;285:E197–E205.

13. Singh R, Artaza JN, Taylor WE, Gonzalez-Cadavid NF, Bhasin S. Androgens stimulate myogenic differentiation and inhibit adipogenesis in C3H 10T1/2 pluripotent cells through an androgen receptor-mediated pathway. *Endocrinology.* 2003;144:5081–5088.

14. Bhasin S, Taylor WE, Singh R, et al. The mechanisms of androgen effects on body composition: mesenchymal pluripotent cell as the target of androgen action. *J Gerontol A Biol Sci Med Sci.* 2003;58:M1103–M1110.

15. Mauras N, Hayes V, Welch S, et al. Testosterone deficiency in young men: marked alterations in whole body protein kinetics, strength, and adiposity. *J Clin Endocrinol Metab.* 1998;83:1886–1892.

16. Wichmann MW, Ayala A, Chaudry IH. Male sex steroids are responsible for depressing macrophage immune function after trauma-hemorrhage. *Am J Physiol.* 1997;273:C1335–C1340.

17. Zellweger R, Wichmann MW, Ayala A, Stein S, DeMaso CM, Chaudry IH. Females in proestrus state maintain splenic immune functions and tolerate sepsis better than males. *Crit Care Med.* 1997;25:106–110.

18. Croce MA, Fabian TC, Malhotra AK, Bee TK, Miller PR. Does gender difference influence outcome? *J Trauma.* 2002;53:889–894.

19. Valentin A, Jordan B, Lang T, Hiesmayr M, Metnitz PGH. Gender-related differences in intensive care: a multiple-center cohort study of therapeutic interventions and outcome in critically ill patients. *Crit Care Med.* 2003;31:1901–1907.

20. Lephart ED, Baxter CR, Parker CR. Effect of burn trauma on adrenal and testicular steroid hormone production. *J Clin Endocrinol Metab.* 1987;64:842–848.

21. Sharshar T, Bastuji-Garin S, De Jonghe B, et al. Hormonal status and ICU-acquired paresis in critically ill patients. *Intensive Care Med.* 2010;36:1318–1326.

22. Van den Berghe G, Weekers F, Baxter RC, et al. Five-day pulsatile gonadotropin-releasing hormone administration unveils combined hypothalamic-pituitary-gonadal defects underlying profound hypoandrogenism in men with prolonged critical illness. *J Clin Endocrinol Metab.* 2001;86:3217–3226.

23. Schols AM, Soeters PB, Mostert R, Pluymers RJ, Wouters EF. Physiologic effects of nutritional support and anabolic steroids in patients with chronic obstructive pulmonary disease. A placebo-controlled randomized trial. *Am J Respir Crit Care Med.* 1995;152:1268–1274.

24. Strawford A, Barbieri T, Van Loan M, et al. Resistance exercise and supraphysiologic androgen therapy in eugonadal men with HIV-related weight loss: a randomized controlled trial. *JAMA.* 1999;281:1282–1290.

25. Ferrando AA, Sheffield-Moore M, Wolf SE, Herndon DN, Wolfe RR. Testosterone administration in severe burns ameliorates muscle catabolism. *Crit Care Med.* 2001;29:1936–1942.

26. Demling RH, Orgill DP. The anticatabolic and wound healing effects of the testosterone analog oxandrolone after severe burn injury. *J Crit Care.* 2000;15:12–17.

27. Jeschke MG, Finnerty CC, Suman OE, Kulp G, Mlcak RP, Herndon DN. The effect of oxandrolone on the endocrinologic, inflammatory, and hypermetabolic responses during the acute phase postburn. *Ann Surg.* 2007;246:351–360.

28. Gervasio JM, Dickerson RN, Swearingen J, et al. Oxandrolone in trauma patients. *Pharmacotherapy.* 2000;20:1328–1334.

29. Bulger EM, Jurkovich GJ, Farver CL, Klotz P, Maier RV. Oxandrolone does not improve outcome of ventilator dependent surgical patients. *Ann Surg.* 2004;240:472–478.

30. Adams MJ, Blundell TL, Dodson EJ, et al. Structure of rhombohedral 2 zinc insulin crystals. *Nature.* 1969;224:491–495.

31. Hubbard SR, Till JH. Protein tyrosine kinase structure and function. *Annu Rev Biochem.* 2000;69:373–398.

32. De Meyts P, Whittaker J. Structural biology of insulin and IGF1 receptors: implications for drug design. *Nat Rev Drug Discov.* 2002;1:769–783.

33. Pessin JE, Saltiel AR. Signaling pathways in insulin action: molecular targets of insulin resistance. *J Clin Invest.* 2000;106:165–169.

34. Barthel A, Schmoll D. Novel concepts in insulin regulation of hepatic gluconeogenesis. *Am J Physiol Endocrinol Metab.* 2003;285:E685–E692.

35. Manchester KL, Young FG. The effect of insulin on incorporation of amino acids into protein of normal rat diaphragm in vitro. *Biochem J.* 1958;70:353.

36. Airhart J, Arnold JA, Stirewalt WS, Low RB. Insulin stimulation of protein synthesis in cultured skeletal and cardiac muscle cells. *Am J Physiol.* 1982;243:C81–C86.

37. Biolo G, Declan Fleming RY, Wolfe RR. Physiologic hyperinsulinemia stimulates protein synthesis and enhances transport of selected amino acids in human skeletal muscle. *J Clin Invest.* 1995;95:811–819.

38. Sakurai Y, Aarsland A, Herndon DN, et al. Stimulation of muscle protein synthesis by long-term insulin infusion in severely burned patients. *Ann Surg.* 1995;222:283–294, 294–297.

39. Ferrando AA, Chinkes DL, Wolf SE, Matin S, Herndon DN, Wolfe RR. A submaximal dose of insulin promotes net skeletal muscle protein synthesis in patients with severe burns. *Ann Surg.* 1999;229:11–18.

40. Van den Berghe G, Wouters P, Weekers F, et al. Intensive insulin therapy in critically ill patients. *N Engl J Med.* 2001;345:1359–1367.

41. Van den Berghe G, Wilmer A, Hermans G, et al. Intensive insulin therapy in the medical ICU. *N Engl J Med.* 2006;354:449–461.

42. Preiser J-C, Devos P, Ruiz-Santana S, et al. A prospective randomised multi-centre controlled trial on tight glucose control by intensive insulin therapy in adult intensive care units: the Glucontrol study. *Intensive Care Med.* 2009;35:1738–1748.

43. NICE-SUGAR Study Investigators, Finfer S, Chittock DR, et al. Intensive versus conventional glucose control in critically ill patients. *N Engl J Med.* 2009;360:1283–1297.

44. Brunkhorst FM, Engel C, Bloos F, et al. Intensive insulin therapy and pentastarch resuscitation in severe sepsis. *N Engl J Med.* 2008;358:125–139.

45. Hermanides J, Vriesendorp TM, Bosman RJ, Zandstra DF, Hoekstra JB, Devries JH. Glucose variability is associated with intensive care unit mortality. *Crit Care Med.* 2010;38:838–842.

46. Meyfroidt G, Keenan DM, Wang X, Wouters PJ, Veldhuis JD, Van den Berghe G. Dynamic characteristics of blood glucose time series during the course of critical illness: effects of intensive insulin therapy and relative association with mortality. *Crit Care Med.* 2010;38:1021–1029.

47. Dellinger RP, Levy MM, Rhodes A, et al. Surviving sepsis campaign: international guidelines for management of severe sepsis and septic shock: 2012. *Crit Care Med.* 2013;41:580–637.

48. Kojima M, Hosoda H, Date Y, Nakazato M, Matsuo H, Kangawa K. Ghrelin is a growth-hormone-releasing acylated peptide from stomach. *Nature.* 1999;402:656–660.

49. Nass R, Gaylinn BD, Thorner MO. The ghrelin axis in disease: potential therapeutic indications. *Mol Cell Endocrinol.* 2011;340:106–110.

50. Mesotten D, Van den Berghe G. Changes within the GH/IGF-I/IGFBP axis in critical illness. *Crit Care Clin.* 2006;22:17–28.

51. Giustina A, Veldhuis JD. Pathophysiology of the neuroregulation of growth hormone secretion in experimental animals and the human. *Endocr Rev.* 1998;19:717–797.

52. Berneis K, Keller U. Metabolic actions of growth hormone: direct and indirect. *Baillières Clin Endocrinol Metab.* 1996;10:337–352.

53. Humbel RE. Insulin-like growth factors I and II. *Eur J Biochem.* 1990;190:445–462.

54. Froesch ER, Schmid C, Schwander J, Zapf J. Actions of insulin-like growth factors. *Annu Rev Physiol.* 1985;47:443–467.

55. Brown GM, Kirpalani SH. A critical review of the clinical relevance of growth hormone and its measurement in the nuclear medicine laboratory. *Semin Nucl Med.* 1975;5:273–285.
56. Ruokonen E, Takala J. Dangers of growth hormone therapy in critically ill patients. *Curr Opin Clin Nutr Metab Care.* 2002;5:199–209.
57. Ross R, Miell J, Freeman E, et al. Critically ill patients have high basal growth hormone levels with attenuated oscillatory activity associated with low levels of insulin-like growth factor-I. *Clin Endocrinol (Oxf).* 1991;35:47–54.
58. Schuetz P, Müller B, Nusbaumer C, Wieland M, Christ-Crain M. Circulating levels of GH predict mortality and complement prognostic scores in critically ill medical patients. *Eur J Endocrinol.* 2009;160:157–163.
59. Dahn MS, Lange MP, Jacobs LA. Insulinlike growth factor 1 production is inhibited in human sepsis. *Arch Surg.* 1988;123:1409–1414.
60. Van den Berghe G. Dynamic neuroendocrine responses to critical illness. *Front Neuroendocrinol.* 2002;23:370–391.
61. Koch A, Sanson E, Helm A, Voigt S, Trautwein C, Tacke F. Regulation and prognostic relevance of serum ghrelin concentrations in critical illness and sepsis. *Crit Care.* 2010;14:R94.
62. Florini JR, Ewton DZ, Coolican SA. Growth hormone and the insulin-like growth factor system in myogenesis. *Endocr Rev.* 1996;17:481–517.
63. Adams GR, McCue SA. Localized infusion of IGF-I results in skeletal muscle hypertrophy in rats. *J Appl Physiol Bethesda Md 1985.* 1998;84:1716–1722.
64. Inaba T, Saito H, Fukushima R, et al. Effects of growth hormone and insulin-like growth factor 1 (IGF-1) treatments on the nitrogen metabolism and hepatic IGF-1-messenger RNA expression in postoperative parenterally fed rats. *JPEN.* 1996;20:325–331.
65. Shimoda N, Tashiro T, Yamamori H, Takagi K, Nakajima N. Effects of growth hormone and insulin-like growth factor-1 on protein metabolism, gut morphology, and cell-mediated immunity in burned rats. *Nutrition.* 1997;13:540–546.
66. Voerman BJ, Strack van Schijndel RJ, Groeneveld AB, de Boer H, Nauta JP, Thijs LG. Effects of human growth hormone in critically ill nonseptic patients: results from a prospective, randomized, placebo-controlled trial. *Crit Care Med.* 1995;23:665–673.
67. Voerman HJ, van Schijndel RJ, Groeneveld AB, et al. Effects of recombinant human growth hormone in patients with severe sepsis. *Ann Surg.* 1992;216:648–655.
68. Jiang ZM, He GZ, Zhang SY, et al. Low-dose growth hormone and hypocaloric nutrition attenuate the protein-catabolic response after major operation. *Ann Surg.* 1989;210:513–524.
69. Takala J, Ruokonen E, Webster NR, et al. Increased mortality associated with growth hormone treatment in critically ill adults. *N Engl J Med.* 1999;341:785–792.
70. Critical evaluation of the safety of recombinant human growth hormone administration: statement from the growth hormone research society. *J Clin Endocrinol Metab.* 2001;86:1868–1870.
71. Van den Berghe G, Wouters P, Weekers F, et al. Reactivation of pituitary hormone release and metabolic improvement by infusion of growth hormone-releasing peptide and thyrotropin-releasing hormone in patients with protracted critical illness. *J Clin Endocrinol Metab.* 1999;84:1311–1323.
72. Mesotten D, Wouters PJ, Peeters RP, et al. Regulation of the somatotropic axis by intensive insulin therapy during protracted critical illness. *J Clin Endocrinol Metab.* 2004;89:3105–3113.
73. Bianco AC, Salvatore D, Gereben B, Berry MJ, Larsen PR. Biochemistry, cellular and molecular biology, and physiological roles of the iodothyronine selenodeiodinases. *Endocr Rev.* 2002;23:38–89.
74. Yen PM. Physiological and molecular basis of thyroid hormone action. *Physiol Rev.* 2001;81:1097–1142.
75. Davis PJ, Davis FB. Nongenomic actions of thyroid hormone. *Thyroid.* 1996;6:497–504.
76. Flaim KE, Li JB, Jefferson LS. Effects of thyroxine on protein turnover in rat skeletal muscle. *Am J Physiol.* 1978;235:E231–E236.
77. Farwell AP. Nonthyroidal illness syndrome. *Curr Opin Endocrinol Diabetes Obes.* 2013;20:478–484.
78. Peeters RP, Wouters PJ, Kaptein E, van Toor H, Visser TJ, Van den Berghe G. Reduced activation and increased inactivation of thyroid hormone in tissues of critically ill patients. *J Clin Endocrinol Metab.* 2003;88:3202–3211.
79. Thijssen-Timmer DC, Peeters RP, Wouters P, et al. Thyroid hormone receptor isoform expression in livers of critically ill patients. *Thyroid.* 2007;17:105–112.
80. Chopra IJ, Huang TS, Beredo A, Solomon DH, Chua Teco GN, Mead JF. Evidence for an inhibitor of extrathyroidal conversion of thyroxine to 3,5,3'-triiodothyronine in sera of patients with nonthyroidal illnesses. *J Clin Endocrinol Metab.* 1985;60:666–672.
81. Fliers E, Noppen NW, Wiersinga WM, Visser TJ, Swaab DF. Distribution of thyrotropin-releasing hormone (TRH)-containing cells and fibers in the human hypothalamus. *J Comp Neurol.* 1994;350:311–323.
82. Arem R, Wiener GJ, Kaplan SG, Kim HS, Reichlin S, Kaplan MM. Reduced tissue thyroid hormone levels in fatal illness. *Metabolism.* 1993;42:1102–1108.
83. Acker CG, Singh AR, Flick RP, Bernardini J, Greenberg A, Johnson JP. A trial of thyroxine in acute renal failure. *Kidney Int.* 2000;57:293–298.
84. Klemperer JD, Klein I, Gomez M, et al. Thyroid hormone treatment after coronary-artery bypass surgery. *N Engl J Med.* 1995;333:1522–1527.
85. Van den Berghe G, Wouters P, Carlsson L, Baxter RC, Bouillon R, Bowers CY. Leptin levels in protracted critical illness: effects of growth hormone-secretagogues and thyrotropin-releasing hormone. *J Clin Endocrinol Metab.* 1998;83:3062–3070.
86. Miller WL, Auchus RJ. The molecular biology, biochemistry, and physiology of human steroidogenesis and its disorders. *Endocr Rev.* 2011;32:81–151.

72 How Do I Diagnose and Manage Acute Endocrine Emergencies in the ICU?

Noelle N. Saillant, Carrie A. Sims

Endocrine emergencies are frequently encountered in the intensive care unit (ICU). This chapter will focus on several of the more common disorders, including diabetic hyperglycemia, thyroid storm, myxedema coma, and adrenal insufficiency. Understanding the pathophysiology of these different disease states will enable the intensivist to make a rapid diagnosis, initiate proper therapy, and avoid major pitfalls.

DIABETIC KETOACIDOSIS

Diabetic ketoacidosis (DKA) is a life-threatening hyperglycemic condition that accounts for over 140,000 annual hospital admissions.[1] With improved therapy, the age-adjusted mortality rate has fallen dramatically and is currently less than 5%.[2,3] Although DKA is considered a pathognomonic complication of insulin-dependent diabetes (type 1), 5% to 30% of people with type 2 diabetes may have this condition. The defining features of DKA include metabolic acidosis (arterial pH <7.35 with bicarbonate <16 mEq/L), hyperglycemia (>250 mg/dL), and ketonemia. The severity of DKA can be graded as mild, moderate, or severe according to the degree of metabolic acidosis and the presence of an altered mental status (Table 72-1).[4,5]

Pathophysiology

DKA is a dysregulated catabolic state that occurs in the setting of insulin deficiency coupled with high levels of counter-regulatory hormones such as glucagon, cortisol, catecholamines, and growth hormone.[6] This hormonal imbalance inhibits carbohydrate metabolism with a preferential shift toward fat metabolism. Impaired glucose uptake, increased gluconeogenesis, and enhanced lipolysis all contribute to a marked increase in serum glucose.[7] To compensate for the increase in osmolarity, water is shifted from the intracellular to the extracellular compartment. Because the kidney cannot effectively reabsorb glucose in the presence of marked hyperglycemia, an osmotic diuresis ensues. Hypovolemia and profound electrolyte depletion soon follow.

DKA is defined by the development of acidosis. As the liver oxidizes free fatty acids, ketones (acetone, beta-hydroxybutyrate, and acetoacetate) are generated. These ketones are relatively strong acids and deplete the body's buffering capacity.[8]

Clinical Presentation

The symptoms of DKA are directly related to hyperglycemia and acidosis. Hyperglycemia leads to polyuria, polydipsia, and dehydration. The generation of ketoacids results in nausea, vomiting, and abdominal pain.[9] The metabolic acidosis also triggers compensatory hyperventilation with acetone excretion leading to a classic fruity odor on the patient's breath. Although an increased white blood cell count is common even in the absence of an infection, a fever is rare and should prompt an aggressive search for a concomitant infection. Likewise, an altered mental status is not typical and warrants further investigation.

Therapy

In 2009, the American Diabetes Association published an updated consensus statement regarding the management of DKA in terms of fluids, electrolytes, and insulin therapy.[4]

Fluid and Electrolyte Replacement

Volume replacement is the initial therapy, and isotonic saline (0.9% NaCl) should be infused rapidly (1 to 2 L/h), even if the serum sodium is elevated. After intravascular volume repletion, fluids can be changed to 0.45% NaCl if the serum sodium is 140 mEq/L or greater.

Almost all patients with DKA will have an overall potassium deficit, primarily reflecting urinary losses; however, serum potassium is often initially elevated because potassium is shifted out of cells in response to the insulin deficiency and hyperosmolality. With insulin therapy, potassium is returned to the intracellular space. Profound hypokalemia can result and may lead to life-threatening cardiac arrhythmias and respiratory muscle weakness. Potassium replacement should be initiated when the serum potassium concentration falls below 5.0 to 5.2 mEq/L.

Table 72-1 Diagnostic Criteria for DKA and HHS

Criteria	DKA			HHS
	Mild	Moderate	Severe	
Plasma glucose (mg/dL)	>250	>250	>250	>600
Arterial pH	7.25-7.30	7.00-7.24	<7.00	>7.30
Serum bicarbonate (mEq/L)	15-18	10 to <15	<10	>18
Urine ketones*	Positive	Positive	Positive	Small
Serum ketones*	Positive	Positive	Positive	Small
Effective serum osmolality†	Variable	Variable	Variable	>320
Anion gap‡	>10	>12	>12	Variable
Alteration in mental state	Alert	Alert/drowsy	Stupor/coma	Stupor/coma

*Nitroprusside reaction method.
†Effective serum osmolality = 2[measured Na^+] + glucose/18.
‡Anion gap = [Na^+] − ([Cl^-] + [HCO_3^-]).
DKA, diabetic ketoacidosis; *HHS*, hyperglycemic state.
Adapted from the 2009 American Diabetes Association consensus statement.[4]

If there urine output is adequate (>50 mL/h), potassium should be included in each liter of intravenous (IV) fluid (20 to 30 mEq) with the goal of maintaining the potassium in the range of 4.0 to 5.0 mEq/L.[6]

Likewise, phosphate levels in DKA are often deceptively elevated on presentation despite total body phosphate depletion. Although phosphate replacement has not been associated with improved clinical outcomes, supplementation is prudent when the serum phosphate concentration is less than 1.0 mg/dL to avoid cardiopulmonary muscle weakness.[4,9]

Despite significant acidosis (pH >7.0), supplemental bicarbonate is rarely needed and may contribute to worsening intracellular acidosis and may increase the risk of hypokalemia and cerebral edema.[10-12] Bicarbonate supplementation should only be considered when the arterial pH is less than 6.9 and should be terminated once a pH greater than 7.0 is achieved.[4]

Insulin Therapy

Insulin therapy should only be initiated *after* adequate volume replacement and once the serum potassium is 3.3 mEq/L or greater. Once these goals have been achieved, a continuous infusion of regular insulin is recommended.[4,13] Although a bolus of insulin has been traditionally used, a randomized trial has recently demonstrated this "priming" bolus is unnecessary, and effective glycemic control can be achieved by starting the insulin drip at 0.14 U/kg/h.[4] Glucose levels should decrease by 50 to 70 mg/dL/h. The insulin infusion rate should be doubled until there is a steady rate of decline in the serum glucose concentration. Glucose should be hourly monitored by finger stick and confirmed by frequent serum glucose measurements. It is important to note, however, that the serum glucose will normalize before ketoacid production stops.

Insulin therapy should be continued along with supplemental glucose until the anion gap normalizes. An abrupt discontinuation of insulin can lead to a recurrence of hyperglycemia and ketoacidosis. Conversely, to prevent hypoglycemia, it is recommended that glucose be added to IV fluids and the insulin infusion adjusted once the serum glucose falls to 250 mg/dL or less. Normalization of glucose levels and reversal of the metabolic acidosis and anion gap should prompt a switch to subcutaneous (SQ) insulin, although the IV and SQ should overlap for several hours.[6]

Precipitating Factors

In most cases, a precipitating cause of DKA can be identified. Although noncompliance or inadequate insulin therapy (i.e., insulin pump failure) can initiate a hyperglycemic crisis, DKA is frequently associated with infection. Myocardial ischemia, stroke, or other acute medical illness can also precipitate a diabetic crisis and should be carefully investigated. Finally, DKA has been associated with the use of glucocorticoids, thiazides, pentamidine, second-generation antipsychotics, and sympathomimetic agents including cocaine.[4,5,14,15]

Complications

Major complications are rare and frequently attributable to underlying medical conditions; however, several DKA-specific complications warrant mention. Cerebral edema is an uncommon complication that primarily develops in children.[18,19] Clinical symptoms include headache and behavioral and mental status changes that may rapidly progress to seizures, coma, and death. If neurologic findings progress beyond lethargy and behavioral changes, then the mortality rate is over 70%, with only 7% to 14% of patients recovering without permanent disability. Treatment is primarily supportive. Mannitol, hypertonic saline, and dexamethasone have been used, but their role has not been subjected to study.[20] This devastating complication can be minimized by gradually correcting the sodium, water, and glucose abnormalities. Pulmonary edema can occur on occasion as the result of overzealous fluid replacement, poor cardiac function, or reduced osmotic pressure.

HYPEROSMOLAR HYPERGLYCEMIC STATE

Although various terms have been used in the past, the syndrome of hyperglycemia-induced volume depletion without acidosis is now referred to as a "hyperglycemic hyperosmolar state" (HHS) to capture the range of clinical variability involved.[21] Although most patients with HHS have type 2 diabetes, 20% of patients will have no previous history of diabetes.[22] In contrast to DKA, HHS occurs infrequently but carries a much higher mortality rate.[23,24] Importantly, patients usually do not die because of the severe hypertonicity associated with HHS, but rather as the result of the comorbidities that precipitated or developed during the treatment of HHS.[25]

The hallmark features of HHS are hyperglycemia (glucose >600 mg/dL), hyperosmolality (>320 mOsm/kg), and volume depletion with an average total body water deficit of 9 L.[26] Unlike DKA, HHS is not associated with a significant acidosis. Mild ketonemia, however, does not preclude the diagnosis (Table 72-1).

Pathophysiology

The pathogenesis of HHS is similar to DKA. Traditionally, in HHS, serum insulin levels were thought to be sufficient to prevent the severe ketogenesis, but not high enough to prevent hyperglycemia.[7] This theory, though, is not supported by measurements of serum insulin. More likely, the lack of ketogenesis in HHS is related to lower levels of counter-regulatory hormones (e.g., glucagon, catecholamines).[27]

As with DKA, insulin deficiency coupled with an altered counter-regulatory hormone profile leads to increased gluconeogenesis and impaired glucose use. Large amounts of glucose saturate the urine and impair the concentrating capacity of the kidney. If adequate fluid intake is preserved and renal perfusion is maintained, then major hyperglycemia will not develop. If renal function deteriorates because of underlying kidney disease or intravascular volume depletion, though, plasma glucose levels will increase, and hyperosmolality will develop. Profound hyperglycemia (glucose >600 mg/dL) and hyperosmolality (>320 mOsm/kg) lead to an exuberant osmotic diuresis and severe dehydration.

Clinical Presentation

Although HHS typically occurs in the elderly, it may occur at any age. Symptoms are primarily related to hyperglycemia (e.g., polydipsia, polyuria, fatigue, and visual disturbances) and profound dehydration (e.g., weakness, anorexia, weight loss, dizziness, confusion, and lethargy). The most common clinical presentation is altered mental status and neurologic symptoms.[21] Central nervous symptoms typically occur when the osmolality reaches 230 to 330 mOsm/kg and range from headache to seizures to coma.

Therapy

Although there are some important differences, the treatment of DKA and HHS are very similar.

Fluid and Electrolyte Replacement

Fluid and electrolyte deficits are often more profound than those seen with DKA, but they may not be appreciated on the initial chemistry values. Volume resuscitation is the mainstay of therapy and can lower serum glucose by as much as 50%. This is primarily due to improved renal perfusion and subsequent excretion of glucose. After the initial resuscitation, corrected serum sodium should be calculated with the following equation:

$$\text{Corrected Na}^+ = 1.6\,(\text{glucose} - 100)/100.$$

Replacement of one half of the fluid deficit within the initial 12 hours followed by the remainder over the next 12 to 24 hours is recommended. More gradual administration may be needed in patients younger than 20 years to avoid cerebral edema.[28]

The free water deficit can be estimated with the following formula:

$$\text{Free water deficit} = \text{TBW} \times (([\text{Na}^+]_{\text{calc}}/[\text{Na}^+]_{\text{normal}}) - 1)$$

where

TBW (total body water) = body weight (kg) × 0.6 for males (or 0.5 for females).

Although the initial potassium levels may be normal or elevated, patients with HHS have a significant potassium deficit. Replacement should be initiated when serum values are between 3.3 and 5.3 mEq/L if urine output is sufficient. Phosphate and magnesium replacement are only needed when levels are extremely low.[4]

Insulin Therapy

Adequate intravascular volume resuscitation should precede instituting insulin therapy to prevent vascular collapse. As with DKA, a potassium level of 3.3 mEq/L or less should be treated before initiating insulin therapy. The rate of decrease of glucose tends to be more precipitous in HHS than in DKA because these patients tend to be more volume depleted. The serum glucose should be maintained between 250 and 300 mg/dL until the plasma osmolality is

315 mOsm/kg or less and the patient is mentally alert.[4] The use of a SQ insulin protocol to initially treat HHS has not been investigated.

Precipitating Factors

The two most common precipitating factors in the development of HSS are inadequate insulin therapy and infection.[29] Because infection precipitates 60% of HHS cases, cultures should be taken and antibiotics should be instituted early.[23] Myocardial infarction or stroke also may provoke the release of counter-regulatory hormones and promote gluconeogenesis. Medications that affect carbohydrate metabolism (e.g., glucocorticoids, thiazide diuretics, phenytoin, beta blockers) may also play a contributing role, and an association with alcohol and cocaine use has been observed.[29,30]

Complications

Although serious complications are frequently the result of underlying comorbidities, subclinical rhabdomyolysis is common in HHS and may contribute to acute renal failure. Cerebral edema has also been described but is thankfully rare.

AUTHORS' RECOMMENDATIONS

- Normal saline should be administered slowly so that the estimated water and sodium deficits can be corrected over the first 24 hours. For the risk of cerebral edema to be minimized, plasma osmolality should not be reduced by more than 3 mosmol/kg/h.
- IV insulin therapy—a bolus followed by an infusion—is recommended.
- Dextrose should be added to the IV fluids once serum glucose levels reach 300 mg/dL. Serum glucose levels should be maintained between 250 and 300 mg/dL until the osmolality is 315 mOsm/kg or less and the patient is mentally alert.
- Supplemental potassium chloride should be given when the serum potassium concentration is 5.3 mEq/L or less. Potassium replacement should be given before starting insulin therapy if the serum concentration is less than 3.3 mEq/L.

THYROTOXIC CRISIS

Thyrotoxic crisis, or thyroid storm, is an acute, potentially life-threatening state that occurs in patients with untreated or incompletely treated hypothyroidism. Although the incidence of hyperthyroidism ranges between 0.02% and 1.3%, only 1% to 2% of patients with thyrotoxicosis will develop thyroid storm.[31-35] If untreated, the mortality from thyroid storm can be extremely high (90%). With early management, mortality is 10% to 20%.[31,34,35]

Pathophysiology

Thyroid hormone secretion is tightly regulated by the hypothalamic-pituitary-thyroid axis. Thyrotropin-releasing hormone (TRH) is released from the hypothalamus and stimulates the synthesis and secretion of thyroid-stimulating hormone (TSH). In turn, TSH controls the synthesis and secretion of the thyroid hormones, thyroxine (T_4) and triiodothyronine (T_3). Over 99.5% of serum T_4 and T_3 are protein bound and metabolically inactive. The small percentage of free T_4 and T_3 influence metabolic function and modulate the release of TRH and TSH via negative feedback.[36]

Interestingly, T_4 has limited activity and must be converted to the more active hormone T_3 by deiodinases. More than 80% of the available T_3 is synthesized in peripheral tissues such as the kidney and liver. T_3 directly binds to cytoplasmic thyroid hormone receptor complexes and migrates with additional regulatory elements to the nucleus to directly activate or inhibit expression of genes encoding proteins that modulate cellular metabolism, adrenergic responsiveness, and thermoregulation.[37] Hyperthyroidism typically results from an overactive thyroid nodule or gland. Less commonly, excessive pituitary secretion of TSH or the overingestion of thyroid hormone can result in hyperthyroidism.[38] The pathologic transition from hyperthyroidism to thyroid storm is not fully understood, but it usually occurs in the setting of surgery, sepsis, injury, or other acute medical illness. Although total thyroid hormone levels may not be significantly higher than those observed in uncomplicated thyrotoxicosis, higher levels of free thyroid hormone and lower levels of binding proteins have been demonstrated.[39] Elevated catecholamines in acute illness or trauma may further stimulate the synthesis and release of thyroid hormone.

Clinical Presentation

Thyroid storm can occur in the setting of hyperthyroidism from any cause, but it most frequently occurs as a complication of Graves disease. Thyroid storm classically presents with fever (>38.5° C) and profound tachycardia. Other cardiac findings may include atrial fibrillation, congestive heart failure, hypotension, and shock.[40] Gastrointestinal symptoms include nausea, vomiting, diarrhea, abdominal pain, and occasionally liver failure.[41] Gastrointestinal fluid losses may be profound, and dehydration may contribute to multiorgan failure. Central nervous system symptoms are common and range from confusion to psychosis to coma.[37]

Serum T_4 or T_3 values cannot be used to differentiate thyrotoxicosis from thyroid storm—the diagnosis must be made on clinical grounds. Burch and Wartofsky developed a clinical scoring system to standardize the diagnosis (Table 72-2). A score of 45 or more is highly suggestive of thyroid storm, a score of 25 to 44 is concerning for impending thyroid storm, and a score less than 25 makes thyroid storm unlikely.[36]

In addition to altered thyroid parameters, elevated blood urea nitrogen and creatinine, hypercalcemia, anemia, thrombocytopenia, leukocytosis or leukopenia, and hyperglycemia may be present. Liver function tests are frequently elevated. Concomitant adrenal insufficiency, especially in the setting of Graves disease, should be ruled out.[42]

Treatment

The therapeutic goals of treating thyroid storm are to (1) decrease hormone production and secretion, (2) block the conversion of T_4 to T_3, and (3) antagonize the

Table 72-2 **Diagnostic Scoring System for Thyroid Storm**	
Physiologic Parameters	**Points**
THERMOREGULATORY DYSFUNCTION	
Temperature (°F)	
99-99.9	5
100-100.9	10
101-101.9	15
102-102.9	20
103-103.9	25
≥104.0	30
CENTRAL NERVOUS SYSTEM DYSFUNCTION	
Absent	0
Mild (agitation)	10
Moderate (delirium, psychosis, extreme lethargy)	20
Severe (seizures, coma)	30
GASTROINTESTINAL-HEPATIC DYSFUNCTION	
Absent	0
Moderate (nausea, vomiting, diarrhea, abdominal pain)	10
Severe (unexplained jaundice)	20
CARDIOVASCULAR DYSFUNCTION	
Tachycardia (beats/min)	
90-109	5
110-119	10
120-129	15
≥140	25
Congestive Heart Failure	
Absent	0
Mild (pedal edema)	5
Moderate (bibasilar rales)	10
Severe (pulmonary edema)	15
Atrial Fibrillation	
Absent	0
Present	10
PRECIPITATING EVENT	
Absent	0
Present	10

Adopted from Burch HB, Wartofsky L. Life-threatening thyrotoxicosis. Thyroid storm. *Endocrinol Metab Clin N Am* 1993:22:263–277.[36]

catecholaminergic effects of thyroid hormone (Table 72-3 and Figure 72-1).

Decrease Hormone Production and Secretion

Thionamides such as propylthiouracil and methimazole will effectively block new thyroid hormone synthesis, but they do not prevent the release of stored hormone.[43,44]

Thionamides also have immunosuppressive properties that decrease expression of antithyroptropin-receptor antibodies.[37] Propylthiouracil also inhibits the peripheral conversion of T_4 to T_3.

High-dose iodine administration can acutely block the release of T_4 and T_3. Iodine products, though, should only be given after thyroid synthesis has been blocked for several hours. If synthetic function is not adequately inhibited, then the iodine bolus will enhance thyroid hormone synthesis and can exacerbate the thyrotoxicosis.[45] Iodine enrichment will also complicate postcrisis treatment options.

Iopanoic acid and other iodinated oral radiographic contrast agents have extremely high iodine concentrations and can be used, off-label, in lieu of iodine solutions. In addition to decreasing thyroid hormone release, these agents attenuate the effects of thyroid hormone by decreasing the hepatic uptake of T_4, inhibiting the peripheral conversion of T_4 to T_3 and blocking the cellular binding of T_4 and T_3.[38,46] Thyroid synthesis should be blocked before use to prevent enriched thyroid hormone production.

Lithium carbonate also can block the formation and release of thyroid hormone and is an option for patients who are allergic to iodine.[37] Because of a narrow therapeutic window, lithium is not considered a first-line therapy.[47] Lastly, ʟ-carnitine blocks the nuclear uptake of thyroid hormone and has been suggested as a treatment of thyrotoxicosis in combination with methimazole.[48]

Decrease Peripheral Conversion of T_4 to T_3

Glucocorticoids can effectively reduce the peripheral deiodination of T_4 to T_3 and may be helpful in modulating the autoimmune disorder of Graves disease. Glucocorticoids are used even with "normal" cortisol levels because steroid therapy may improve survival.[49-51]

As previously mentioned, propylthiouracil and iopanoic acid also decrease the peripheral deiodination of T_4 to T_3. In contrast, cholestyramine reduces circulating thyroid hormone by inhibiting enterohepatic recirculation.[51] Finally, there are case reports describing the use of plasmaphoresis, hemoperfusion, and plasma exchange as methods for reducing autoimmune antibodies, immune complexes, and thyroid levels in critically ill patients refractory to conventional therapies.[52-56]

Antagonize Adrenergic Effects of Thyroid Hormone

β-Adrenergic blockade remains a mainstay of therapy but should be used cautiously in patients with congestive heart failure. In addition to their antiadrenergic effects, beta blockers also inhibit the peripheral conversion of T_4 to T_3. In addition to the expected cardiac effects, these agents markedly improve agitation, confusion, psychosis, diaphoresis, diarrhea, and fever.[33] Diltiazem, a calcium channel antagonist, may provide an alternative method of controlling adrenergic symptoms.[57,58]

Supportive Care

Supportive care is essential and should be provided in an ICU environment. Atrial fibrillation is observed in up to 40% of patients with thyroid storm. Many patients will require vigorous fluid resuscitation. If hypotension persists despite adequate volume resuscitation, then vasopressors

Table 72-3 Pharmacologic Management of Thyroid Storm

Medication	Mechanism of Action	Dosage
Propylthiouracil	Inhibits new hormone synthesis; decreases T_4 to T_3 conversion	200-400 mg po q 6-8 hr
Methimazole	Inhibits new hormone synthesis	20-25 mg po q 6 hr
Lugol solution	Blocks release of hormone from gland	4-8 drops po q 6-8 hr
Saturated solution of potassium iodide (SSKI)	Blocks release of hormone from gland	5 drops po q 6 hr
Iopanoic acid	Blocks release of hormone from gland; inhibits T_4 to T_3 conversion	1 g po q 8 hr for 24 hr then 500 mg po q 12 hr
Lithium carbonate	Blocks release of hormone from gland; inhibits new hormone synthesis	300 mg po q 8 hr
Cholestyramine	Decreases enterohepatic resorption of thyroid hormone	4 g po qid
Propranolol	β-Adrenergic blockade; decreases T_4 to T_3 conversion	1-2 mg IV q 10-15 min 20-120 mg po q 4-6 hr
Esmolol	β-Adrenergic blockade	50-100 µg/kg/min
Diltiazem	Decreases adrenergic symptoms	5-10 mg/hr IV 60-120 mg po q 6-8 hr
Reserpine	Decreases secretion of catecholamines	2.5-5 mg IM q 4-6 hr
Guanethidine	Decreases secretion of catecholamines	30-40 mg po q 6 hr
Hydrocortisone	Decreases T_4 to T_3 conversion; vasomotor stability	100 g IV q 8 hr

IM, intramuscular; *IV,* intravenous; T_3, triiodothyronine; T_4, thyroxine.

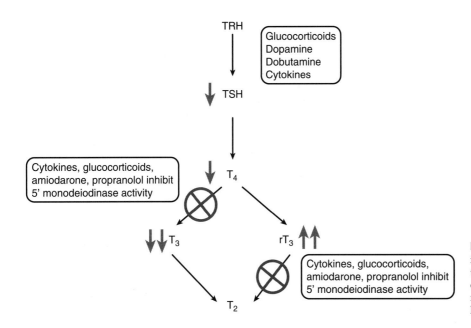

Figure 72-1. Changes in hypothalamic-pituitary-thyroid axis in critical illness. rT_3, reverse triiodothyronine; T_2, diiodothyronine; T_3, triiodothyronine T_4, thryroxine; *TRH,* thyrotropin-releasing hormone; *TSH,* thyroid-stimulating hormone.

may be needed and hydrocortisone supplementation should be considered.

Hyperpyrexia should be treated with external cooling methods and acetaminophen. Salicylates, such as aspirin, should be avoided because they can inhibit hormone-protein binding and increase free hormone levels.[48]

Precipitating Factors

An infection, acute medical illness, or sympathomimetic agents may precipitate the development of thyroid storm

by increasing circulating catecholamines.[59] Amiodarone and other iodinated medications may also precipitate thyrotoxicosis and subsequent thyroid crisis in those with underlying thyroid disease. Finally, withdrawal or noncompliance with antithyroid medications may contribute to thyrotoxicosis.[47]

Definitive Treatment

Patients with a history of thyroid storm should undergo definitive treatment with either radioactive iodine ablation or surgical thyroidectomy. If iodine was used in management of the acute crisis, then radioactive ablation should be postponed several months until the iodine stores are depleted. Surgical resection can be performed after treatment with iodine, although there is an increased risk of perioperative thyroid storm. This risk is substantially decreased if thyroid hormone levels are carefully monitored and normalized before surgery.

AUTHORS' RECOMMENDATIONS

- Thyroid storm is a rare condition that presents with exaggerated features of hyperthyroidism.
- Thyroid function tests cannot be used that differentiate thyrotoxicosis from thyroid storm.
- Pharmacologic treatment of thyroid storm includes thionamides to decrease hormone synthesis, a beta blocker to antagonize the adrenergic effects, a steroid to decrease peripheral hormone conversion, and occasionally iodine to prevent hormone release.
- Hydrocortisone is given for the increased risk of concomitant adrenal insufficiency and to inhibit the peripheral conversion of T_4 to T_3.
- After resolution of the crisis, patients should be evaluated for definitive management (e.g., radioiodine ablation or surgical thyroidectomy).

MYXEDEMA COMA

Myxedema coma is the result of severe, decompensated hypothyroidism leading to a depressed mental status, hypotension, and hypothermia. It is a serious, but rare, medical emergency that carries a high mortality rate (20% to 50%) even with early diagnosis and appropriate therapy.[61-63]

Pathophysiology

Decreased thyroid function results in a depressed basal metabolic rate, decreased oxygen consumption, and impaired energy production. The cardiovascular system is particularly susceptible. Decreased β-adrenergic responsiveness and diminished thermogenesis lead to increased systemic vascular resistance, diastolic hypertension, and decreased blood volume.[64,65] In addition, depressed myocardial contractility and bradycardia result in low cardiac output, profound hypotension, and diminished cerebral perfusion.[66]

Primary hypothyroidism occurs when there is permanent loss or atrophy of thyroid tissue and accounts for 90% to 95% of cases of myxedema coma. Most patients will have an elevated serum TSH level and low free T_4 values. Although myxedema coma can occur in patients with hypothalamic or pituitary dysfunction (central hypothyroidism), this is extremely rare (<5% of cases).[64] These patients will have a normal or low TSH value in the setting of a low free T_4 concentration.

Clinical Presentation

Patients with hypothyroidism are frequently elderly women. Physical findings include dry skin, thin hair, a hoarse voice, and delayed deep tendon reflexes. Classically, mucin deposition (myxedema) may cause nonpitting edema of the hands and feet, periorbital swelling, and macroglossia.

Progression to myxedema coma is characterized by mental status changes and hypothermia. In a retrospective review of 24 patients, 88% presented with a temperature less than 94° F (34° C).[67] Importantly, the mortality of myxedema correlates directly with the degree of hypothermia, and a core temperature less than 90° F (32° C) is associated with a worse prognosis.[64]

Myxedema coma is associated with derangements of every organ system. Cardiovascular findings include bradycardia, prolongation of the QT interval, heart block, depressed cardiac contractility, and hypotension.[68] Without the administration of thyroid hormone, hypotension may become refractory to vasopressor support. Central depression and respiratory muscle weakness also frequently result in hypoventilation, respiratory acidosis, and hypoxemia.[69,70] As such, most patients require mechanical ventilation.[64,70] Finally, gastrointestinal complaints are common and decreased gastrointestinal motility limits the use of oral medications and enteral nutrition. Therefore thyroid hormone treatment should be intravenously given.

Laboratory values are notable for hyponatremia and hypoglycemia.[71-73] Although infection is frequently a precipitating cause of myxedema coma, an elevated white blood cell count is frequently absent.

Therapy

Given the lethality of untreated myxedema coma, therapy should be instituted without waiting for laboratory confirmation. Before therapy is initiated, though, thyroid function tests should be drawn. In addition to measuring serum TSH and free T_4, a cortisol level should also be obtained. Appropriate hormonal supplementation will normalize the basal metabolic rate and reverse all symptoms and signs of hypothyroidism.[74] Some neuromuscular and psychiatric symptoms, however, may take months to disappear.[75]

Hormonal Replacement Therapy

Given the rarity of myxedema coma, there are no randomized clinical trials comparing treatment regimens. Thyroid hormone therapy is critical, but it may precipitate cardiac arrhythmias or ischemia. In addition, thyroid replacement may unmask coexisting adrenal insufficiency and precipitate an adrenal crisis.[76] Hydrocortisone should be given in conjunction with thyroid replacement.[64]

Because the conversion of T_4 to T_3 is impaired in severe hypothyroidism, IV T_3 may be preferable given its greater biologic availability. T_3 rapidly achieves effective tissue levels and may positively affect survival.[77] Moreover, T_3 crosses the blood-brain barrier more readily than T_4 and may hasten the improvement of neurologic symptoms.[78] Treatment with IV T_4 can also be used. Because the patient's inherent tissue deiodinase activity is required to convert T_4 to T_3, significant clinical improvement may take 1 to 3 days. This slower onset of action, though, theoretically decreases the likelihood of cardiac complications.[79]

A third treatment option is to supplement both T_4 and T_3. In theory, this provides T_3 at a subtherapeutic dose for immediate action as well as a loading dose of T_4. Although there are no clinical studies validating this approach, this regimen attempts to provide physiologic balance between efficacy and safety.[64]

Precipitating Factors

The presence of a precipitating infection or concurrent acute illness should be investigated. Typical signs of infection (e.g., fever, tachycardia) may not be present in the patient with myxedema coma, and patients who die frequently have unrecognized infection and sepsis. Empiric antibiotics are warranted until cultures are proven negative.

Monitoring Therapy

Patients should be carefully monitored for the development of tachyarrhythmias or myocardial ischemia during IV thyroid administration. Initially, TSH and free T_4 levels should be closely followed to prevent overtreatment. In patients with central hypothyroidism, TSH levels will not reflect the adequacy of treatment, and free T_4 levels should be monitored and maintained in the upper-normal range.

AUTHORS' RECOMMENDATIONS

- Treatment of myxedema coma should be initiated without waiting for the results of thyroid function tests.
- The optimal strategy for thyroid hormone replacement remains controversial. Regimens include IV T_3, T_4, or a combination of both hormones.
- IV hydrocortisone should be given in conjunction with thyroid hormone replacement.
- Empiric antibiotics should be initiated until cultures are proven negative.

REFERENCES

1. Centers for Disease Control and Prevention. *Diabetes Surveillance System, National Hospital Discharge Survey, National Center for Health Statistics.* Atlanta: U.S. Department of Health and Human Services; 2012. Retrieved May 28, 2014, from: http://www.cdc.gov/diabetes/statistics/dkafirst/fig1.htm.
2. Lin SF, Lin JD, Huang YY. Diabetic ketoacidosis: comparisons of patient characteristics, clinical presentations and outcomes today and 20 years ago. *Chang Gung Med J.* 2005;28(1):24–30.
3. Fishbein HA, Palumbo PJ. Acute metabolic complications in diabetes. In: *Diabetes in America. National Diabetes Data Group.* National Institutes of Health; 1995:283–291.
4. Kitabchi AE, Miles JM, Umpierrez GE, Fisher JN. Hyperglycemic crises in adult patients with diabetes. *Diabetes Care.* 2009;32:1335–1343.
5. Kitabachi AE, Umpierrez GE, Murphy MB, Krieshberg RA. Hyperglycemic crisis in adult patients with diabetes: a consensus statement from the American Diabetes Association. *Diabetes Care.* 2006;29:2739–2748.
6. Kitabachi AE, Umpierrez GE, Murphy MB, et al. Management of hyperglycemic crisis in patients with diabetes. *Diabetes Care.* 2001;24:131–153.
7. Corwell B, Knieght B, Oliveri L, Willis GC. Current diagnosis and treatment of hyperglycemic emergencies. *Emerg Med Clin North Am.* 2014;32(2):437–452.
8. Delaney MF, Zisman A, Kettyle WM. Diabetic ketoacidosis and hyperglycemic hyperosmolar nonketotic syndrome. *Endorinol Metab Clin North Am.* 2000;29:683–705.
9. Umpierrez G, Freire AX. Abdominal pain in patients with hyperglycemic crisis. *J Crit Care.* 2002;17:63–67.
10. Barsotti MM. Potassium phosphate and potassium chloride in the treatment of diabetic ketoacidosis. *Diabetes care.* 1980;3:569.
11. Viallon A, Zeni F, Lafond P, et al. Does bicarbonate therapy improve the management of severe diabetic ketoacidosis. *Crit Care Med.* 1999;27:2690–2693.
12. Glaser NS, Wooten-Gorges SL, Buonocore MH, et al. Frequency of subclinical cerebral edema in children with diabetic ketoacidosis. *Pediatr Diabetes.* 2006;7:75–80.
13. Barski L, Kezerle L, Zeller L, Zektser M, Jotkowitz. New approaches to the use of insulin in patients with diabetic ketoacidosis. *Eur J Intern Med.* 2013;24:213–216.
14. Umpierrez GE, Cuervo R, Karabell A, et al. Treatment of diabetic ketoacidosis with subcutaneous insulin aspart. *Diabets Care.* 2005;28:1856–1861.
15. Morris LR, Murphy MB, Kiabchi AE. Bicarbonate therapy in severe diabetic ketoacidosis. *Ann Intern Med.* 1986;105:836–840.
16. Newcomer JW. Second generation (atypical) antipsycotics and metabolic effects: a comprehensive literature review. *CNS Drugs.* 2005;19(suppl 1):1–93.
17. Nyenwe EA, Longanthan RS, Blum S, et al. Active use of cocaine: an independent risk factor for recurrent diabetic ketoacidosis in a city hospital. *Endocrine Practice.* 2007;13:22–29.
18. Cameron FJ, Scratch SE, Nadebaum C, et al. Neurological consequences of diabetic ketoacidosis at the initial presentation of type 1 diabetes in a prospective cohort study of children. *Diabetes Care.* 2014;37(6):1554–1562.
19. Wiggam MI, O'Kane MJ, Harper R, et al. Treatment of diabetic ketoacidosis using normalization of blood 3-hydroxybutrate concentration as the endpoint of emergency management. A randomized controlled study. *Diabetes Care.* 1997;20:1347–1352.
20. Glaser N, Barnett P, McCaslin I, et al. Risk factors for cerebral edema in children with diabetic ketoacidosis. *N Eng J Med.* 2001;344:264–269.
21. Wachtel TJ. The diabetic hyperosmolar state. *Clin Geriatr Med.* 1990;6:797–806.
22. Wolfsdorf J, Glaser N, Sperling MA. Diabetic ketoacidosis in infants, children, and adolescents: a consensus statement from the American Diabetes Association. *Diabetes Care.* 2006;29:1150–1159.
23. Ennis ED, Stahl EJVB, Kreisberg RA. The hyperosmolar hyperglycaemic syndrome. *Diabetes Rev.* 1994;2:115–126.
24. Wachtel TJ, Silliman RA, Lamberton P. Prognositc factors in the diabetic hyperosmolar state. *J Am Geriatr Soc.* 1978;35:737–741.
25. Pinies JA, Cairo G, Gaztambide S, et al. Course and prognosis of 132 patients with diabetic nonketotic hyperosmolar state. *Diabetes Metab.* 1994;20:43–48.
26. Delaney MF, Zisman A, Kettyle WM. Diabetic ketoacidosis and hyperglycemic hyperosmolar nonketotic syndrome. *Endocrinol Metab Clin North Am.* 2000;29:683–705.
27. Siperstein M. Diabetic ketoacidosis and hyperosmolar coma. *Endocrinol Metab Clin North Am.* 1992;21:415–432.
28. Yared Z, Chiasson JL. Ketoacidosis and the hypersomolar hyperglycemic state in adult diabetic patients: diagnosis and treatment. *Minerva Med.* 2003;94:409–418.
29. Nugent BW. Hyperosmolar hyperglycemic state. *Emerg Med Clin N Am.* 2005;23:629–648.
30. Magee MF, Bhatt BA. Management of decompensated diabetes: diabetic ketoacidosis and hyperglycemic hyperosmolar syndrome. *Crit Care Clin.* 2001;17:75–106.
31. Akamizu T, Satoh T, Isozaki O, et al. Diagnostic criteria, clinical features, and incidence of thyroid storm based on nationwide surveys. *Thyroid.* 2012;22(7):661.
32. Morales AE, Rosenbloom AL. Death caused by hyperglycemic hyperosmolar state at the onset of type 2 diabetes. *J Pediatr.* 2004;144:270–273.
33. Stathatos N, Wartofsky L. Thyrotoxic storm. *J Int Care Med.* 2002;17:1–7.
34. Canaris GJ, Manowitz NR, Mayor G, Ridgway EC. The Colorado thyroid disease prevalence study. *Arch Intern Med.* 2000;160:263–277.
35. Aoki Y, Belin RM, Clickner R, et al. Serum TSH and total T4 in the United States population and their association with participant characteristics: National Health and Nutrition Examination Survey (NHANES 1999-2002). *Thyroid.* 2007;17:1211–1223.
36. Burch HB, Wartofsky L. Life-threatening thyrotoxicosis. Thyroid storm. *Endocrinol Metab Clin N Am.* 1993;22:263–277.
37. Nayuk B, Burman K. Thyrotoxicosis and thyroid storm. *Endocrinol Metab Clin N Am.* 2006:663–686.

38. Tsai MJ, O'Malley BW. Molecular mechanisms of action of steroid/thyroid receptor superfamily members. *Ann Rev Biochem.* 1994;63:451.

39. Goldberg PA, Inzucchi SE. Critical issues in endocrinology. *Clin Chest Med.* 2003;24:583–606.

40. Sarlis NJ, Gourgiotis L. Thyroid emergencies. *Rev Endocr Metab Disord.* 2003;4:129–136.

41. Dabon-Almirante CL, Surks M. Clinical and laboratory diagnosis of thyrotoxicosis. *Endocrinol Metab Clin N Am.* 1998;27:25–35.

42. Stathatos N, Wartofsky L. Thyrotoxic storm. *J Intensive Care Med.* 2002;17:1–7.

43. Glauser J, Strange GR. Hypothyroidism and hyperthyroidism in the elderly. *Emerg Med Rep.* 2002;1:1–12.

44. Nabil N, Miner DJ, Amatruda JM. Methimazole: an alternative route of administration. *J Clin Endocrinol Metab.* 1982;54:180–181.

45. Walter RM, Bartle WR. Rectal administration of propylthiouracil in the treatment of Graves' disease. *Am J Med.* 1990;88:69.

46. Tyer N, Kim TY, Martinez DS. Review on oral cholcystographic agents for the management of hyperthyroidism. *Endocr Pract.* August 2014:1–6.

47. Papi G, Corsello SM, Pontecorvi A. Clinical concepts on thyroid emergencies. *Front Endocrinol.* 2014;5(102):1–11.

48. Benvenga S, Ruggeri RM, Russo A, et al. Usefulness of L-carnitine, a naturally occurring inhibitor of thyroid hormone action, in iatrogenic hyperthyroidism: a randomized, double-blind, placebo-controlled clinical trial. *J Clin Endocrinol Metab.* 2001;86:3579–3594.

49. Wartofsky L, Ransil BJ, Ingbar SH. Inhibition by iodine of the release of thyroxine from the thyroid glands of patients with thyrotoxicosis. *J Clin Invest.* 1970;49:78–86.

50. Dluhy RG. The adrenal cortex in thyrotoxicosis. In: Braverman LE, Utiger RD, eds. *Werner's and Ingbar's the Thyroid.* 9th ed. Philadelphia: Lipincott, Williams and Wilkins; 2005:660–664.

51. Mazzaferri EL, Skillman TG. Thyroid storm. A review of 22 episodes with special emphasis on the use of guanethidine. *Arch Intern Med.* 1969;124:684–690.

52. Solomon BL, Wartofsky L, Burman KD. Adjunctive cholestyramine therapy for thyrotoxicosis. *Clin Endocrinol.* 1993;38:39–43.

53. Ashkar FS, Katims RB, Smoak III WM, Gilson AJ. Thyroid storm treatment with blood exchange and plasmapheresis. *JAMA.* 1970;214:1275–1279.

54. Burman KD, Yeager HC, Briggs WA, et al. Resin hemoperfusion: a method of removing circulating thyroid hormones. *J Clin Endocrinol Metab.* 1976;42:70–78.

55. Pons-Estel GJ, Salemi GE, Serrano RM, et al. Therapeutic plasma exchange for the management of refractory systemic autoimmune diseases: report of 31 cases and review of the literature. *Autoimmun Rev.* 2011;10(11):679–684.

56. Muller C, Perrin P, Faller B, et al. The role of plasma Echange in the thyroid storm. *Ther Apher Dial.* 2011;15(6):522–531.

57. Duggal J, Singh S, Kuchinic P, et al. Utility of esmolol in thyroid crisis. *Can J Clin Pharm.* 2006;13:292–295.

58. Kelestimur F, Aksu A. The effect of diltiazem on the manifestations of hyperthyroidism and thyroid function tests. *Exp Clin Endocrinol Diabetes.* 1996;104:38–42.

59. Milner MR, Gelman KM, Phillips RA, et al. Double-blind crossover trial of diltiazem versus propranolol in the management of thyrotoxic symptoms. *Pharmacotherapy.* 1990;10:100–106.

60. Goldberg PA, Inzucchi SE. Critical issues in endocrinology. *Clin Chest Med.* 2003;24:583–606.

61. Sherman SI, Simonson L, Ladenson PW. Clinical and socioeconomic predispositions to complicated thyrotoxicosis: a predictable and preventable syndrome? *Am J Med.* 1996;101:192–198.

62. Sarlis NJ, Gourgiotis L. Thyroid emergencies. *Rev Endocr Metab Disord.* 2003;4:129–136.

63. Hylander B, Rosenqvist U. Treatment of myxoedema coma – factors associated with fatal outcome. *Acta Endocrinol.* 1985;108:65–71.

64. Wartofsky L. Myxedema coma. *Endocrinol Metab Clin N Am.* 2006;35:687–698.

65. Wall CR. Myxedema coma: diagnosis and treatment. *Am Fam Physician.* 2000;62:2485–2490.

66. Kwaku MP, Burman KD. Myxedema coma. *J Intensive Care Med.* 2007;22:224–231.

67. Sanders V. Neurologic manifestations of myxedema coma. *N Eng J Med.* 1962;266:547–551.

68. Matthew V, Misgar RA, Ghosh S, et al. Myxedema coma: a new look into an old crisis. *J Thyroid Res.* 2011:1–7.

69. Reinhardt W, Mann K. Incidence, clinical picture and treatment of hypothyroid coma: results of a survey. *Med Klin.* 1997;92:521–524.

70. Zwillich CW, Pierson DJ, Hofeldt FD, et al. Ventilatory control in myxedema and hypothyroidism. *N Eng J Med.* 1975;292:662–665.

71. Marinez FJ, Bermudez-Gomez M, Celli BR. Hypothyroidism: a reversible cause of diaphragmatic dysfunction. *Chest.* 1989;96:1059–1063.

72. Iwasaki Y, Oisa Y, Yamauchi K, et al. Osmoregulation of plasma vasopressin in myxedema. *J Clin Endocrinol Metab.* 1990;70:534–539.

73. Skowsky RW, Kiuchi TA. The role of vasopressin in the impaired water excretion of myxedema. *Am J Med.* 1971;51:41–53.

74. Fliers E, Wiersinga WM. Myxedema coma. *Rev Endocr Metabol Disord.* 2003;4:137–141.

75. Zulewski H, Muller B, Exer P, et al. Estimation of tissue hypothyroidism by a new clinical score: evaluation of patients with various grades of hypothyroidism and controls. *J Clin Endocrinol Metab.* 1997;82:771.

76. Al-Adsani H, Hoffer LJ, Silva JE. Resting energy is sensitive to small dose changes in patients on chronic thyroid hormone replacement. *J Clin Endocrinol Metab.* 1997;82:1118–1125.

77. Bigos ST, Rigway EC, Kouridas IA, et al. Spectrum of pituitary alterations with mild and severe thyroid impairment. *J Clin Endocrinol Metab.* 1978;36:317–325.

78. Pereira VG, Haron ES, Lima-Neto N, et al. Management of myxedema coma: report on three successfully treated cases with nasogastric or intravenous administration of triiodothyronine. *J Endocrinol Invest.* 1982;5:331–334.

79. Hylander B, Rosenqvist U. Treatment of myxoedema coma: factors associated with fatal outcomes. *Acta Endocrin.* 1985;108:65–71.

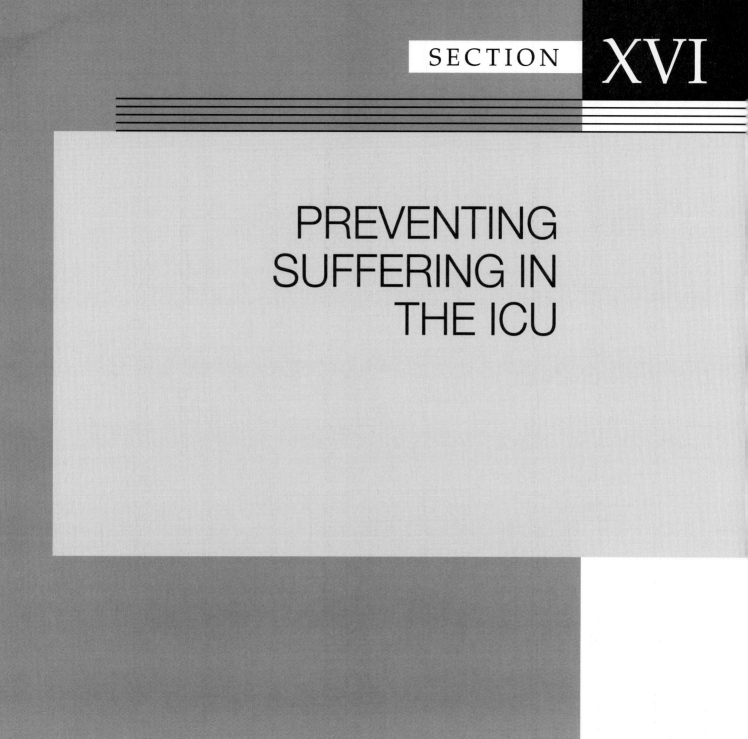

SECTION XVI

PREVENTING SUFFERING IN THE ICU

73 How Does One Diagnose, Treat, and Reduce Delirium in the Intensive Care Unit?

E. Wesley Ely, Arna Banerjee, Pratik P. Pandharipande

Delirium, a disturbance of consciousness and cognition, may occur in up to 80% of intensive care unit (ICU) patients and is frequently underdiagnosed.[1-3] Delirium is associated with longer durations of mechanical ventilation and ICU length of stay as well as an increased risk of death, disability, and long-term cognitive dysfunction.[4-8]

This chapter aims to broadly define delirium, discuss the associated subtypes and risk factors, and provide the basis for clinicians to develop strategies aimed at preventing and treating delirium in their practice settings.

DEFINITION

The *Diagnostic and Statistical Manual of Mental Disorders* (*DSM-5*)[9] defines delirium as (1) disturbance of consciousness (i.e., reduced clarity of awareness of the environment) with reduced ability to focus, sustain, or shift attention. (2) A change in cognition (e.g., memory deficit, disorientation, language disturbance) or development of a perceptual disturbance that is not better accounted for by a preexisting, established, or evolving dementia. (3) The disturbance develops over a short period (usually hours to days) and tends to fluctuate during the course of the day. (4) There is evidence from the history, physical examination, or laboratory findings that the disturbance is caused by a direct physiologic consequence of a general medical condition, an intoxicating substance, medication use, or more than one cause.

Delirium has been further differentiated according to the level of alertness; the motoric subtypes consist of hyperactive, hypoactive, and mixed subtypes.[10] Distribution of delirium in medical and surgical patients suggests that the hypoactive subtype, characterized by a flat affect, withdrawal, apathy, or lethargy, is the most prevalent. The hyperactive delirious patient is described as agitated, restless, violent, or emotionally labile. Although challenging to manage clinically, the weight of evidence suggests a better overall prognosis for the hyperactive patient compared with the hypoactive delirious patient.[11] Nevertheless, two published studies contradict these findings, suggesting either that the hyperactive subtype carries a poorer

prognosis[12] or that there is no difference in outcomes by subtype.[13] The rates of prevalence of the subtypes of delirium in the ICU are 1.6% for the hyperactive subtype, 43.5% for the hypoactive subtype, and 54.1% for the mixed subtype.[10] The Delirium Motor Subtype Scale may aid in making this diagnosis.[14]

RISK FACTORS

The causes of delirium are multifactorial. The risk factors can be divided into predisposing factors (i.e., host factors) and precipitating factors (Table 73-1). Patients in the hospital at a higher risk for having delirium include patients with dementia, chronic illness, advanced age, existing infection, and depression. Modifiable risk factors such as hypertension, poor nutrition, substance withdrawal, and tobacco use have also been shown to be associated with development of delirium in the hospital. Iatrogenic or potentially modifiable factors include hypoxia, metabolic and electrolyte disturbances, infection, dehydration, hyperthermia, sepsis, psychoactive medications, and sleep deprivation.[15-17] There has been much research on postoperative delirium, especially in those undergoing cardiopulmonary bypass, with a retrospective study showing a decreased incidence of delirium in patients pretreated with statins.[18] ICU statin use has been associated with reduced delirium, especially early during sepsis, whereas the discontinuation of a previously used statin was associated with increased delirium.[19,20] Benzodiazepine use has also been associated with an increased incidence of delirium.[21-23] In addition, heart surgery without cardiopulmonary bypass appears to confer an advantage in decreasing delirium, suggesting that electrolyte or metabolic disturbances play a role in the development of delirium.[24]

PATHOGENESIS

The pathogenesis of delirium is complex and still poorly understood. Maldonado has postulated that the different mechanisms that may play a role in delirium are all

Table 73-1 **Risk Factors for Delirium**

Host Factors	Acute Illness	Iatrogenic and Environmental Factors
Age 65 years or older	Acidosis	Immobilization
Male sex	Anemia	Medications (e.g., opioids, benzodiazepines)
Alcoholism	Fever, infection, sepsis	Anticholinergic drugs
Apolipoprotein E4 polymorphism	Hypotension	Alcohol or drug withdrawal
Cognitive impairment	Metabolic disturbances (e.g., sodium, calcium, blood urea nitrogen, bilirubin)	Sleep disturbances
Dementia	Respiratory disease	—
History of delirium	—	—
Depression	—	—
Hypertension	—	—
Smoking	—	—
Vision or hearing impairment	—	—

"complementary, rather than competing." Imbalance or derangement of multiple neurotransmitter systems has been implicated in the pathophysiology of delirium.

NEUROINFLAMMATORY RESPONSE HYPOTHESIS

Inflammatory mediators such as cytokines and chemokines are readily expressed in critical illness, trauma, sepsis, and after surgical interventions. Animal studies have demonstrated that the release of endogenous inflammatory mediators correlates with exacerbated cognitive and motor symptoms[25] and increased vascular permeability in the brain.[26] Studies have shown that sepsis, severe sepsis, and septic shock are characterized by significantly elevated C-reactive protein (CRP), S-100β, and cortisol in those patients with delirium compared with those without delirium.[27-29] Cerebral autoregulation is disturbed and inflammation may impede endothelial function of the cerebral vasculature, thus making the blood–brain barrier more permeable to inflammatory insults. In support of this theory, a recent study in ICU patients has shown that endothelial dysfunction is associated with greater duration of delirium.[30] In another study, higher levels of procalcitonin at ICU admission were associated with prolonged duration of brain dysfunction, and higher levels of CRP showed trends toward an association.[31] In addition, inflammation upregulates γ-aminobutryic acid (GABA)$_A$ receptors in the brain, contributing to the inhibitory tone within the

brain and reducing brain synaptic connectivity.[32] Thus, the iatrogenic administration of GABA-ergic medications such as benzodiazapines probably further contributes to the inhibition of neural pathways and increases the risk of delirium.

CHOLINERGIC DEFICIENCY HYPOTHESIS

Impaired oxidative metabolism in the brain results in a cholinergic deficiency. The finding that hypoxia impairs acetylcholine synthesis supports this hypothesis. The reduction in cholinergic function results in an increase in the levels of glutamate, dopamine, and norepinephrine in the brain. Serotonin and GABA are also reduced, possibly contributing to delirium.[33,34]

MONOAMINE AXIS HYPOTHESIS

Dopamine, norepinephrine, and serotonin have been implicated in acute brain dysfunction in the ICU. Dopamine is thought to increase the excitability of neurons, and acetylcholine and GABA decrease neuronal excitability.[35] Norepinephrine activity has been associated with hyperactive delirium,[33] and the elevated norepinephrine levels seen after traumatic brain injury have been associated with poor neurologic status, decreased survival, and longer hospital length of stay.[36]

Serotonin

Elevated serotonin levels have been associated with impaired learning and memory and may be indirectly involved in the pathogenesis of acute brain dysfunction.[33]

AMINO ACID HYPOTHESIS

Amino acid entry into the brain is regulated by a sodium-independent large neutral amino acid transporter type-1. Increased cerebral uptake of tryptophan and phenylalanine, compared with that of other large neutral amino acids, can lead to elevated levels of dopamine and norepinephrine, two neurotransmitters that have been implicated in the pathogenesis of delirium.[37-39] Although tryptophan has been postulated to play a role in delirium, a major pathway for its metabolism also exists via the kynurenine pathway. Activation of this pathway in the presence of inflammation may produce neurotoxic metabolites, which may predispose patients to delirium.[40]

IMPAIRED OXIDATIVE METABOLISM

Oxygen deprivation in the brain through either hypoxia or hypoperfusion has been implicated in delirium. Engel and Romano discussed delirium as a state of "cerebral insufficiency" as early as 1959, when they showed that delirium was accompanied by diffuse slowing on electroencephalogram, suggesting a reduction in brain metabolism.[41] This may be further accentuated in the patient

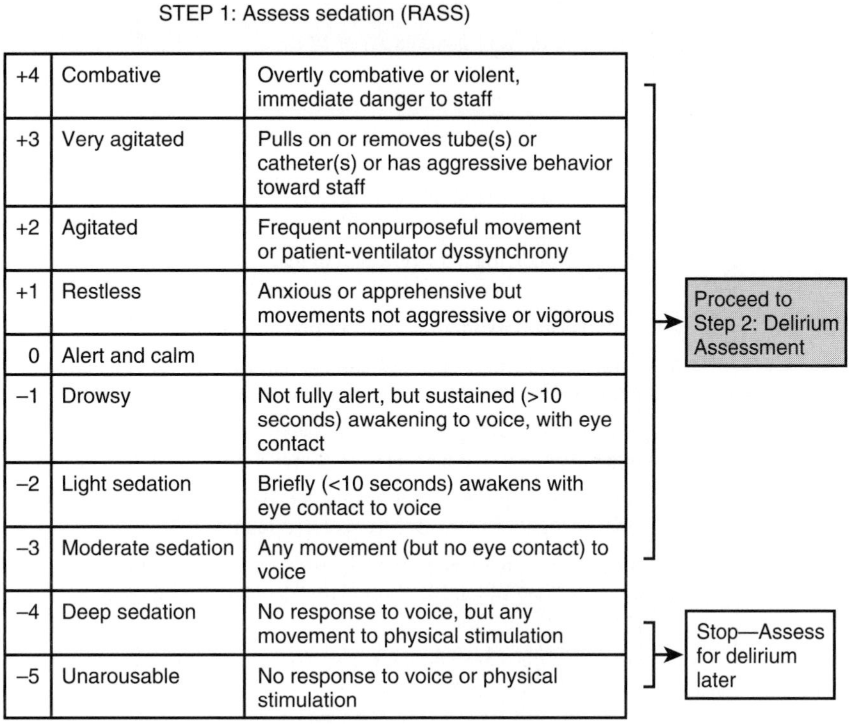

STEP 1: Assess sedation (RASS)
+4 Combative Overtly combative or violent, immediate danger to staff
+3 Very agitated Pulls on or removes tube(s) or catheter(s) or has aggressive behavior toward staff
+2 Agitated Frequent nonpurposeful movement or patient-ventilator dyssynchrony
+1 Restless Anxious or apprehensive but movements not aggressive or vigorous
0 Alert and calm
–1 Drowsy Not fully alert, but sustained (>10 seconds) awakening to voice, with eye contact
–2 Light sedation Briefly (<10 seconds) awakens with eye contact to voice
–3 Moderate sedation Any movement (but no eye contact) to voice
–4 Deep sedation No response to voice, but any movement to physical stimulation
–5 Unarousable No response to voice or physical stimulation
Proceed to Step 2: Delirium Assessment
Stop—Assess for delirium later

Figure 73-1. Richmond Agitation-Sedation Scale (*RASS*),[36,37] used to determine the level of sedation.

who already has compromised blood flow secondary to vascular dementia. Decreases in oxidative metabolism, as well as acetylcholine release, have been demonstrated in the aging brain,[42] and preexisting cognitive dysfunction in the elderly patient, suggestive of chronic changes from vascular insufficiency, has been shown to be the most significant predictor of the development of delirium in the postoperative period.[43]

RECOGNITION OF DELIRIUM

Early recognition of delirium is important, if only to avoid lengthening its course through exacerbation by iatrogenic factors. Therefore clinicians must use assessment tools that allow for timely, accurate assessment by a broad range of practitioners in various settings. Recognition becomes additionally difficult in the ICU setting because patients may have a purposefully altered sensorium secondary to sedation administered for procedures, pain, or mechanical ventilation. Therefore, assessment of a patient for delirium becomes a two-step process because it is important for the clinician first to establish the current level of sedation before assessing the patient for delirium. Examples of scales that can be used to assess sedation include the Ramsay Sedation Scale,[44] the Riker Sedation-Agitation Scale,[45] and the Richmond Agitation-Sedation Scale (RASS).[46,47]

Once the level of sedation has been established and the patient is responsive to verbal stimulus, it is then appropriate for the clinician to assess for the presence of delirium. Although there have been multiple instruments validated for use in non-ICU patients, only two are validated for diagnosing delirium in mechanically ventilated patients: the Intensive Care Delirium Screening Checklist (ICDSC)[48] and the Confusion Assessment Method for the

1: Acute onset of mental status changes or a fluctuating course?
Yes
No
2: Inattention?
No
Not delirium (CAM-ICU negative)
Yes
No
3: Disorganized thinking?
No
4: Altered level of consciousness?
Yes
Yes
Delirium present (CAM-ICU positive)

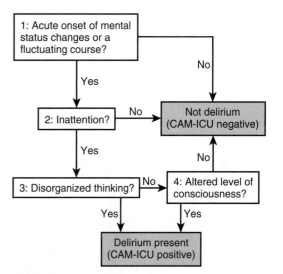

Figure 73-2. Confusion Assessment Method for the Intensive Care Unit (*CAM-ICU*), used to determine the presence or absence of delirium after the level of sedation has been assessed. *(From Ely EW, Inouye SK, Bernard GR, et al. Delirium in mechanically ventilated patients: Validity and reliability of the confusion assessment method for the intensive care unit [CAM-ICU].* JAMA. *2001;286:2703–2710.)*

ICU (CAM-ICU). The CAM-ICU is a scale that is based on the Confusion Assessment Method[49,50] but is amended to increase its applicability in the ICU setting. It takes a trained ICU nurse approximately 2 minutes to complete the CAM-ICU, and accuracy over a set of 471 paired observations in the ICU setting resulted in an accuracy rate of 98.4% with excellent inter-rater reliability.[49] It has been validated in multiple ICU settings.[51,52]

A combination of the RASS for assessment of sedation (Fig. 73-1) followed by the CAM-ICU (Fig. 73-2) or

Table 73-2 **Intensive Care Delirium Screening Checklist**

Patient Evaluation

Altered level of consciousness (A-E)	Deep sedation/coma over entire shift [SAS= 1, 2; RASS = -4,-5] = Not assessable Agitation [SAS = 5, 6, or 7; RASS= 1-4] at any point = 1 point Normal wakefulness [SAS = 4; RASS = 0] over the entire shift = 0 points Light sedation [SAS = 3; RASS= -1, -2, -3]: = 1 point (if no recent sedatives) = 0 points (if recent sedatives)
Inattention	Difficulty in following a conversation or instructions. Easily distracted by external stimuli. Difficulty in shifting focuses. Any of these scores 1 point.
Disorientation	Any obvious mistake in time, place, or person scores 1 point.
Hallucinations-delusion-psychosis	The unequivocal clinical manifestation of hallucination or of behavior probably due to hallucination or delusion. Gross impairment in reality testing. Any of these scores 1 point.
Psychomotor agitation or retardation	Hyperactivity requiring the use of additional sedative drugs or restraints to control potential danger to oneself or others. Hypoactivity or clinically noticeable psychomotor slowing.
Inappropriate speech or mood	Inappropriate, disorganized, or incoherent speech. Inappropriate display of emotion related to events or situation. Any of these scores 1 point.
Sleep/wake cycle disturbance	Sleeping less than 4 hours or waking frequently at night (do not consider wakefulness initiated by medical staff or loud environment). Sleeping during most of the day. Any of these scores 1 point.
Symptom fluctuation	Fluctuation of the manifestation of any item or symptom over 24 hours scores 1 point.
Total score (0-8)	

the ICDSC (Table 73-2) can be used for the establishment of delirium in ICU patients. The diagnosis of delirium using the CAM-ICU (after establishing a RASS score of −3 or less) requires (1) acute change or fluctuation in mental status (feature 1), *and* (2) inattention (feature 2), *and* (3) one of the following: (a) disorganized thinking (feature 3) *or* (b) altered level of consciousness (feature 4). Only those patients with a RASS score of −3 and higher are alert enough to respond to the test and thus can be assessed for delirium. For diagnosis of delirium with the ICDSC, patients who score at least 4 points are considered to have delirium.

Some recent studies have questioned whether delirium evaluations should be done while on sedation.[53,54] It is important to note that a small subset of patients (~10%) may have rapidly reversible sedation-related delirium[53]; that is, their delirium resolves when sedation is turned off. Unfortunately, in the study evaluating rapidly reversible delirium, most patients continued to have persistent delirium even after sedation was interrupted. Thus, when feasible, delirium evaluation should also be done after interruption of sedation; however, delirium evaluations should not be forgone just because a patient is on sedation because the omission would be far worse than overdiagnosing delirium in a handful of patients.

PRIMARY PREVENTION

The prevention of delirium in the ICU requires constant reassessment of patients' clinical courses and treatments. Several potential pathophysiologic contributors to delirium have been previously outlined. All have endpoints associated with cellular mechanisms, suggesting that avoiding metabolic derangements, including electrolyte abnormalities, hypoglycemia, hypoxia, dehydration, and hyperthermia, are paramount in the prevention of delirium.

Medications have long been implicated in the development of delirium, either because of their side effects or their direct effects on the central nervous system. The number of medications administered[15] and their psychoactive effects[55] are suggestive of precipitating delirium.

Another potential risk factor for delirium is alteration of the sleep cycle. Disruption of the sleep–wake cycle in the ICU may be necessary to continuously monitor and manage the critically ill patient. However, the toll on the patient may be high because multiple studies have shown that sleep disruption has detrimental effects on cognition and memory even in the healthy, non-ICU patient.[56] Maintaining a sleep–wake cycle whenever possible through nonpharmacologic or pharmacologic means may help prevent delirium.[57]

There has been some debate about whether the "protocolization" of patient care may reduce the incidence of delirium. In a study that included 852 general medical patients older than 70 years, standardized geriatrician-led protocols were developed for six risk factors of delirium: cognitive impairment, sleep deprivation, immobility, visual impairment, hearing impairment, and dehydration. Using these protocols resulted in a 40% reduction in the initial development of delirium in the intervention patients (95 vs. 16%).[58] When these patients were assessed after 6 months for 10 outcomes, including items such as functional status, cognitive status, delirium, and rehospitalization, only incontinence was slightly less common in the intervention group.[59]

Patients in the ICU frequently receive continuous intravenous analgesics and sedatives. Accumulation in individual patients can predispose to a withdrawal syndrome on discontinuation. Because substance-induced delirium is one of the etiologies recognized by the *DSM-5*, it is no surprise that analgesic and sedative polypharmacy contribute significantly; hence, strategies to reduce exposure to psychoactive medications need to be implemented.[60]

For the improvement of patient outcome and recovery, a liberation strategy focusing on the ABCDEs (Awakening and Breathing Trials, Choice of appropriate sedation, Delirium monitoring and management, and Early mobility and Exercise) has been proposed and shown to decrease the incidence of delirium and coma and improve other patient outcomes.[61,62]

Awaken the Patient Daily

Benzodiazepines are known to increase the risk of delirium in a dose-dependent manner.[22,23] Many studies have shown that protocolized target-based sedation and daily spontaneous awakening trials reduce the number of days on mechanical ventilation. This also exposes the patient to lower cumulative doses of sedatives.[63,64]

Spontaneous Breathing Trials

Studies have shown that daily interruption of mechanical ventilation is superior to other varied approaches to ventilator weaning.[65] Thus incorporation of spontaneous breathing trials into practice reduced the total time on mechanical ventilation.

Coordination of Daily Awakening and Daily Breathing

The Awakening and Breathing controlled trial[66] combined the spontaneous awakening trial with the spontaneous breathing trial. This combination was associated with shorter duration of mechanical ventilation, a 4-day reduction in hospital length of stay, a remarkable 32% decrease in risk of dying at 1 year, and no long-term neuropsychological consequences of waking patients during critical illness.[67] Although delirium duration was not decreased, coma duration was reduced. Thus more patients in the intervention group qualified for delirium evaluation as compared with the control group, where they were more likely to be in a state of coma so ineligible for delirium evaluation.

Choosing the Right Sedative Regimen in Critically Ill Patients

Numerous studies have confirmed that benzodiazepines are associated with poor clinical outcomes.[1,23,68] Two studies comparing dexmedetomidine (alpha-2 agonist) to benzodiazepine infusions showed that the former reduced the burden of brain dysfunction.[71-73]

Delirium Management

The Society of Critical Care Medicine (SCCM) has published guidelines recommending routine monitoring for delirium in all ICU patients.[60] Pharmacologic therapy for delirium should only be attempted after correcting any contributing factors or underlying physiologic abnormalities.

Exercise and Early Mobility

Morris et al.[74] showed that early initiation of physical therapy in ICU patients was associated with decreased length of ICU and hospital polypharmacy. Schweikert et al.[75] looked at the efficacy of combining daily interruption of sedation with physical and occupational therapy on patient outcomes. Patients in the intervention arm had better functional outcomes at discharge, and early physical therapy was also associated with a 50% decrease in the duration of delirium in ICU and hospital stay. Needham et al.[76] conducted a quality improvement project with the use of a multidisciplinary team that focused on reducing sedation use. The authors reported that benzodiazepine use decreased and the patients had improved sedation and delirium status. A decrease in ICU and hospital length of stay was also noted.

We have included an empirical protocol (Fig. 73-3) that we use to treat delirium in ICU settings that is based on the current SCCM Clinical Practice Guidelines. It is merely an example of such a protocol, and the use of a similar protocol should be updated with current data and designed to be implemented specifically at an individual institution. The choice of particular antipsychotics is not described because there are limited data guiding such recommendations.

PHARMACOLOGIC INTERVENTION

Although antidelirium medications in either the preventive or treatment stage are appealing, there are currently none available that have the ability to alter the outcome of delirium. Before administering new psychotropic medications to the delirious patient, one must rule out all reversible causes that may be either the underlying etiology of the delirium or that may be exacerbating the current situation. Reversible causes that could precipitate or exacerbate delirium include hypoxia, hypercarbia, hypoglycemia, metabolic derangements, infection, or shock. Once a decision is made to use antipsychotic medications (typical or atypical), these medications should be individualized (and minimized) to avoid associated adverse events.

Recommendations for delirium treatment strategies suggest that dexmedetomidine may be a better treatment strategy than one that is benzodiazepine based. There is no evidence for routine use of antipsychotic therapy for the treatment of delirium. Cholinesterase inhibitors should not be used to prevent or treat delirium.[77]

Haloperidol is a medication frequently used in the ICU for delirium. It may be given at an initial intravenous dose of 2 to 5 mg (0.5 to 2 mg in the elderly) and then repeated every 6 hours. Guidelines suggest a maximum dose of 20 mg/day. The recent HOPE-ICU (HalOPeridol Effectiveness in ICU delirium) trial unfortunately showed no benefit of treatment with haloperidol, but it still may be considered for acute agitation (hyperactive delirium). However, haloperidol must be used with caution because it has various adverse effects, including dystonias, neuroleptic malignant syndrome, extrapyramidal effects, and, the most worrisome, torsades de pointes. It should not be given to patients with electrocardiographic evidence of prolonged QT interval. QT interval daily measurements are recommended when haloperidol is initiated.

Any of the atypical antipsychotic medications (olanzapine, risperidone, quetiapine, ziprasidone) may be considered, although data on their efficacy in treating delirium are sparse. In a small, 36-patient randomized

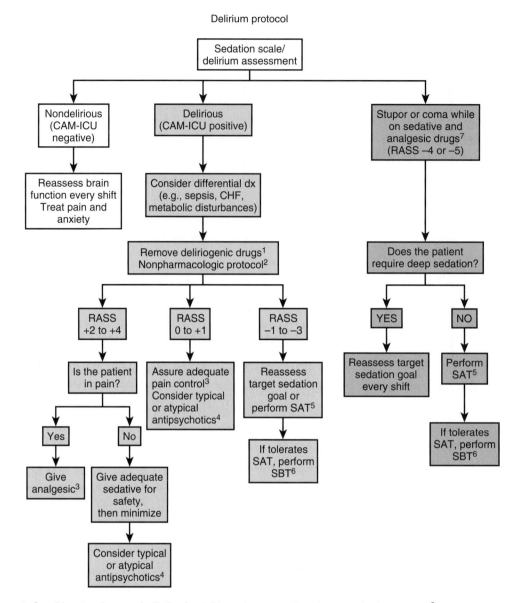

1. Consider stopping or substituting for deliriogenic medications such as benzodiazepines, anticholinergic medications (metochlorpromide, H2 blockers, promethazine, diphenhydramine), steroids, etc.
2. See nonpharmacologic protocol at right
3. Analgesia – Adequate pain control may decrease delirium. Consider intermittent narcotics if feasible. Asses with objective tool.
4. Typical or atypical antipsychotics – While tapering or discontinuing sedatives, consider haloperidol 2 to 5 mg IV initially (0.5–2 mg in elderly) and then q 6 hours. Guideline for max haloperidol dose is 20 mg/day due to ~60% D_2-receptor saturation. May also consider using any of the atypicals (e.g., olanzapine, quetiapine, risperidone, ziprasidone, or abilifide). Discontinue if high fever, QTc prolongation, or drug-induced rigidity.
5. Spontaneous Awakening Trial (SAT) – Stop sedation or decrease infusion (especially benzodiazepines) to awaken patient as tolerated.
6. Spontaneous Breathing Trial (SBT) – CPAP trial if on ≤50% and ≤8 PEEP and SpO_2 >90%
7. Sedatives and analgesics may include benzodiazepines, propofol, dexmedetomidine, fentanyl, or morphine

Nonpharmacologic protocol[2]
Orientation
Provide visual and hearing aids
Encourage communication and reorient patient repetitively
Have familiar objects from patient's home in the room
Attempt consistency in nursing staff
Allow television during day with daily news
Nonverbal music
Environment
Sleep hygiene: Lights off at night, on during day.
Sleep aids (zolpidem, mirtazapine)
Control excess noise (staff, equipment, visitors) at night
Ambulate or mobilize patient early and often
Clinical parameters
Maintain systolic blood pressure >90 mm Hg
Maintain oxygen saturation >90%
Treat underlying metabolic derangements and infections

Figure 73-3. An example of an empirical protocol used for the treatment of delirium in an intensive care unit setting. *CAM-ICU,* Confusion Assessment Method for the Intensive Care Unit; *CHF,* congestive heart failure; *CPAP,* continuous positive airway pressure; *dx,* diagnosis; *PEEP,* positive end-expiratory pressure; *RASS,* Richmond Agitation-Sedation Scale. *(Courtesy Dr. E. W. Ely, http://www.icudelirium.org.)*

controlled trial, quetiapine was shown to be more efficacious in resolution of the first episode of delirium compared with placebo. Likewise, single-dose riperidone has been shown to reduce delirium in cardiac ICU patients. These drugs also need to be used with caution and discontinued if high fever, QT prolongation, or drug-induced rigidity occurs.

AUTHORS' RECOMMENDATIONS

- Delirium is a disturbance of consciousness and cognition occurring over a short period. It is associated with significantly increased morbidity and mortality in critically ill patients.
- Subtypes of delirium include hyperactive, hypoactive, and mixed. The subtype may carry a prognostic implication, with hyperactive having a better prognosis.
- Many risk factors are associated with delirium, and some of these are modifiable or preventable by the clinician, such as hypoxia, metabolic and electrolyte disturbances, infection, dehydration, hyperthermia, sepsis, psychoactive medications, and sleep deprivation.
- Various cellular and metabolic processes are proposed causes for delirium, all of which are likely interrelated.
- There are multiple validated assessment tools for delirium. Patients in the ICU must first be assessed for their level of sedation (with a scale such as the RASS) and then for the presence of delirium (with a scale such as the CAM-ICU or the ICDSC).
- Minimizing sedation by using tactics such as daily interruptions for sedation helps reduce the exposure to deliriogenic psychoactive medications.
- Benzodiazepines should be avoided in the ICU, except for the treatment of specific conditions. Alternatives for sedation include haloperidol, atypical antipsychotics, dexmedetomidine, and remifentanil, although additional studies are required to determine the role of these medications in preventing and treating delirium.

REFERENCES

1. Dubois MJ, Bergeron N, Dumont M, Dial S, Skrobik Y. Delirium in an intensive care unit: a study of risk factors. *Intensive Care Med.* 2001;27(8):1297–1304.
2. Ely EW, Gautam S, Margolin R, et al. The impact of delirium in the intensive care unit on hospital length of stay. *Intensive Care Med.* 2001;27(12):1892–1900.
3. Pisani MA, Murphy TE, Van Ness PH, Araujo KL, Inouye SK. Characteristics associated with delirium in older patients in a medical intensive care unit. *Arch Intern Med.* 2007;167(15):1629–1634.
4. Pandharipande P, Girard T, Jackson J, et al. Long-term cognitive impairment after critical illness. *N Engl J Med.* 2013;369(14):1306–1316.
5. Girard TD, Jackson JC, Pandharipande PP, et al. Delirium as a predictor of long-term cognitive impairment in survivors of critical illness. *Crit Care Med.* 2010;38(7):1513–1520.
6. Ely E, Shintani A, Truman B, Speroff T, Gordon S, Harrell F. Delirium as a predictor of mortality in mechanically ventilated patients in the intensive care unit.[see comment]. *JAMA.* 2004;291:1753–1762.
7. Pisani M, Kong S, Kasl S, Murphy T, Araujo K, Van Ness P. Days of delirium are associated with 1-year mortality in an older intensive care unit population. *Am J Respir Crit Care Med.* 2009:200904.
8. Shehabi Y, Riker R, Bokesch P, Wisemandle W. Delirium duration and mortality in lightly sedated, mechanically ventilated intensive care unit patients. *Crit Care Med.* 2010;38(12):2311–2318.
9. American Psychiatric Association. *The Diagnostic and Statistical Manual of Mental Disorders: DSM 5.* bookpointUS; 2013.
10. Pandharipande P, Cotton BA, Shintani A, et al. Motoric subtypes of delirium in mechanically ventilated surgical and trauma intensive care unit patients. *Intensive Care Med.* 2007;33(10):1726–1731.
11. Kiely DK, Jones RN, Bergmann MA, Marcantonio ER. Association between psychomotor activity delirium subtypes and mortality among newly admitted postacute facility patients. *J Gerontol A Biol Sci Med Sci.* 2007;62(2):174–179.
12. Marcantonio ER, Ta T, Duthrie E, Resnick NM. Delirium severity and psychomotor types: their relationship with outcomes after hip fracture repair. *J Am Geriatr Soc.* 2002;50:850–857.
13. Camus V, Gonthier R, Dubos G, Schwed P, Simeone I. Etiologic and outcome profiles in hypoactive and hyperactive subtypes of delirium. *J Geriatr Psychiatry Neurol.* 2001;13:38–42.
14. Meagher D, Adamis D, Leonard M, et al. Development of an abbreviated version of the Delirium Motor Subtyping Scale (DMSS-4). *Int Psychogeriatr.* 2014;26(04):693–702.
15. Inouye SK, Charpentier PA. Precipitating factors for delirium in hospitalized elderly persons. Predictive model and interrelationship with baseline vulnerability. *JAMA.* 1996;275(11):852–857.
16. McNicoll L, Pisani MA, Zhang Y, Ely EW, Siegel MD, Inouye SK. Delirium in the intensive care unit: occurrence and clinical course in older patients. *J Am Geriatr Soc.* 2003;51(5):591–598.
17. Lin S-M, Huang C-D, Liu C-Y, et al. Risk factors for the development of early-onset delirium and the subsequent clinical outcome in mechanically ventilated patients. *J Crit Care.* 2008;23(3):372–379.
18. Katznelson R, Djaiani GN, Borger MA, et al. Preoperative use of statins is associated with reduced early delirium rates after cardiac surgery. *Anesthesiology.* 2009;110(1):67–73.
19. Pandharipande P, Shintani A, Hughes C, et al. Statin use and the daily risk of delirium in a prospective cohort of critically ill patients. *Am J Respir Crit Care Med.* 2012;185:A3646.
20. Morandi A, Hughes CG, Thompson JL, et al. Statins and delirium during critical illness: a multicenter, prospective cohort study. *Crit Care Med.* 2014;42(8):1899–1909.
21. McPherson JA, Wagner CE, Boehm LM, et al. Delirium in the Cardiovascular Intensive Care Unit: exploring modifiable risk factors. *Crit Care Med.* 2013;41(2):405.
22. Pandharipande P, Cotton B, Shintani A, et al. Prevalence and risk factors for development of delirium in surgical and trauma intensive care unit patients. *J Trauma.* 2008;65(1):34–41.
23. Pandharipande P, Shintani A, Peterson J, et al. Lorazepam is an independent risk factor for transitioning to delirium in intensive care unit patients. *Anesthesiology.* 2006;104(1):21–26.
24. Bucerius J, Gummert JF, Borger MA, et al. Predictors of delirium after cardiac surgery delirium: effect of beating-heart (off-pump) surgery. *J Thoracic Cardiovasc Surg.* 2004;127(1):57–64.
25. Maldonado JR. Pathoetiological model of delirium: a comprehensive understanding of the neurobiology of delirium and an evidence-based approach to prevention and treatment. *Crit Care Clin.* 2008;24(4):789–856.
26. Cunningham C, Campion S, Lunnon K, et al. Systemic inflammation induces acute behavioral and cognitive changes and accelerates neurodegenerative disease. *Biol Psychiatry.* 2009;65(4):304–312.
27. van Munster BC, Bisschop PH, Zwinderman AH, et al. Cortisol, interleukins and S100B in delirium in the elderly. *Brain Cognition.* 2010;74(1):18–23.
28. Pfister D, Siegemund M, ll-Kuster S, et al. Cerebral perfusion in sepsis-associated delirium. *Crit Care.* 2008;12(3):R63.
29. MacDonald A, Adamis D, Treloar A, Martin F. C-reactive protein levels predict the incidence of delirium and recovery from it. *Age Ageing.* 2007;36. [Epub ahead of print].
30. Hughes CG, Morandi A, Girard TD, et al. Association between endothelial dysfunction and acute brain dysfunction during critical illness. *Anesthesiology.* 2013;118(3):631.
31. McGrane S, Girard TD, Thompson JL, et al. Procalcitonin and C-reactive protein levels at admission as predictors of duration of acute brain dysfunction in critically ill patients. *Crit Care.* 2011;15(2):R78.
32. Sanders RD. Hypothesis for the pathophysiology of delirium: Role of baseline brain network connectivity and changes in inhibitory tone. *Med hypotheses.* 2011;77(1):140–143.
33. Hshieh TT, Fong TG, Marcantonio ER, Inouye SK. Cholinergic deficiency hypothesis in delirium: a synthesis of current evidence. *J Gerontol Series A: Biol Sci Med Sci.* 2008;63(7):764–772.
34. Plaschke K, Hill H, Engelhardt R, et al. EEG changes and serum anticholinergic activity measured in patients with delirium in the intensive care unit. *Anaesthesia.* 2007;62(12):1217–1223.

35. Trzepacz PT. Is there a final common neural pathway in delirium? Focus on acetylcholine and dopamine. *Semin Clin Neuropsychiatry.* 2000;5:132–148.

36. Tran TY, Dunne IE, German JW. Beta blockers exposure and traumatic brain injury: a literature review. *Neurosurg Focus.* 2008;25(4):E8.

37. Van Der Mast RC, Fekkes D, Moleman P, Pepplinkhuizen L. Is postoperative delirium related to reduced plasma tryptophan? *Lancet.* 1991;338(8771):851–852.

38. Wurtman RJ, Hefti F, Melamed E. Precursor control of neurotransmitter synthesis. *Pharmacol Rev.* 1980;32(4):315–335.

39. Pandharipande P, Morandi A, Adams J, et al. Plasma tryptophan and tyrosine levels are independent risk factors for delirium in critically ill patients. *Intensive Care Med.* 2009;35(11):1886–1892.

40. Wilson JRA, Morandi A, Girard TD, et al. The association of the kynurenine pathway of tryptophan metabolism with acute brain dysfunction during critical illness. *Crit Care Med.* 2012;40(3):835.

41. Engel GL, Romano J. Delirium, a syndrome of cerebral insufficiency. *J Chronic Dis.* 1959;9(3):260–277.

42. Gibson GE, Peterson C. Aging decreases oxidative metabolism and the release and synthesis of acetylcholine. *J Neurochem.* 1981;37(4):978–984.

43. Robinson TN, Raeburn CD, Tran ZV, Angles EM, Brenner LA, Moss M. Postoperative delirium in the elderly: risk factors and outcomes. *Ann Surg.* 2009;249(1):173–178.

44. Ramsay MA, Keenan SP. Measuring level of sedation in the intensive care unit. *JAMA.* 2000;284:441–442.

45. Riker R, Picard J, Fraser G. Prospective evaluation of the Sedation-Agitation Scale for adult critically ill patients. [see comment] *Crit Care Med.* 1999;27:1325–1329.

46. Sessler C, Gosnell M, Grap M, Brophy G, O'Neal P, Keane K. The Richmond Agitation-Sedation Scale: validity and reliability in adult intensive care unit patients. *Am J Respir Crit Care Med.* 2002;166:1338–1344.

47. Ely EW, Truman B, Shintani A, et al. Monitoring sedation status over time in ICU patients: reliability and validity of the Richmond Agitation-Sedation Scale (RASS). *JAMA.* 2003;289(22):2983–2991.

48. Bergeron N, Dubois MJ, Dumont M, Dial S, Skrobik Y. Intensive Care Delirium Screening Checklist: evaluation of a new screening tool. *Intensive Care Med.* 2001;27(5):859–864.

49. Ely E, Inouye S, Bernard G, et al. Delirium in mechanically ventilated patients: validity and reliability of the confusion assessment method for the intensive care unit (CAM-ICU). *JAMA.* 2001;286:2703–2710.

50. Inouye S, van Dyck C, Alessi C, Balkin S, Siegal A, Horwitz R. Clarifying confusion: the confusion assessment method. *Ann Intern Med.* 1990;113(12):941–948.

51. Pun B, Gordon S, Peterson J, et al. Large-scale implementation of sedation and delirium monitoring in the intensive care unit: a report from two medical centers. *Crit Care Med.* 2005;33(6):1199.

52. Soja S, Pandharipande P, Fleming S, et al. Implementation, reliability testing, and compliance monitoring of the Confusion Assessment Method for the Intensive Care Unit in trauma patients. *Intensive Care Med.* 2008;34(7):1263–1268.

53. Patel SB, Poston JT, Pohlman A, Hall JB, Kress JP. Rapidly reversible, sedation-related delirium versus persistent delirium in the intensive care unit. *Am J Respir Crit Care Med.* 2014;189(6):658–665.

54. Haenggi M, Blum S, Brechbuehl R, Brunello A, Jakob SM, Takala J. Effect of sedation level on the prevalence of delirium when assessed with CAM-ICU and ICDSC. *Intensive Care Med.* 2013;39(12):2171–2179.

55. Marcantonio ER, Juarez G, Goldman L, et al. The relationship of postoperative delirium with psychoactive medications. *JAMA.* 1994;272(19):1518–1522.

56. Yoo S-S, Hu PT, Gujar N, Jolesz FA, Walker MP. A deficit in the ability to form new human memories without sleep. *Nature Neurosci.* 2007;10(3):385–392.

57. Kamdar BB, King LM, Collop NA, et al. The effect of a quality improvement intervention on perceived sleep quality and cognition in a medical ICU. *Critical Care Med.* 2013;41(3):800.

58. Inouye SK, Bogardus Jr ST, Charpentier PA, et al. A multicomponent intervention to prevent delirium in hospitalized older patients. *N Engl J Med.* 1999;340(9):669–676.

59. Bogardus Jr ST, Desai MM, Williams CS, Leo-Summers L, Acampora D, Inouye SK. The effects of a targeted multicomponent delirium intervention on postdischarge outcomes for hospitalized older adults. *Am J Med.* 2003;114(5):383–390.

60. Barr J, Fraser GL, Puntillo K, et al. Clinical practice guidelines for the management of pain, agitation, and delirium in adult patients in the intensive care unit. *Crit Care Med.* 2013;41(1):263–306.

61. Balas MC, Vasilevskis EE, Burke WJ, et al. Critical care nurses' role in implementing the "ABCDE bundle" into practice. *Crit Care Nurse.* 2012;32(2):35–47.

62. Vasilevskis EE, Pandharipande PP, Girard TD, Ely EW. A screening, prevention, and restoration model for saving the injured brain. *Crit Care Med.* 2010;38(10 0):S683.

63. Kollef MH, Levy NT, Ahrens TS, Schaiff R, Prentice D, Sherman G. The use of continuous i.v. sedation is associated with prolongation of mechanical ventilation. *Chest.* 1998;114(2):541–548.

64. Kress J, Pohlman A, O'Connor M, Hall J. Daily interruption of sedative infusions in critically ill patients undergoing mechanical ventilation. *N Engl J Med.* 2000;342:1471–1477.

65. Ely E, Baker A, Dunagan D, et al. Effect on the duration of mechanical ventilation of identifying patients capable of breathing spontaneously. *N Engl J Med.* 1996;335:1864–1869.

66. Girard T, Kress J, Fuchs B, et al. Efficacy and safety of a paired sedation and ventilator weaning protocol for mechanically ventilated patients in intensive care (Awakening and Breathing Controlled trial): a randomised controlled trial. *Lancet.* 2008;371:126–134.

67. Jackson J, Girard T, Gordon S, et al. Long-term cognitive and psychological outcomes in the Awakening and Breathing Controlled trial. *Am JRespir Crit Care Med.* 2010:200903.

68. Marcantonio ER, Goldman L, Orav EJ, Cook EF, Lee TH. The association of intraoperative factors with the development of postoperative delirium. *Am J Med.* 1998;105(5):380–384.

69. Carson SS, Kress JP, Rodgers JE, et al. A randomized trial of intermittent lorazepam versus propofol with daily interruption in mechanically ventilated patients. *Crit Care Med.* 2006;34(5):1326–1332.

70. Breen D, Karabinis A, Malbrain M, et al. Decreased duration of mechanical ventilation when comparing analgesia-based sedation using remifentanil with standard hypnotic-based sedation for up to 10 days in intensive care unit patients: a randomised trial [IS-RCTN47583497]. *Crit Care.* 2005;9(3):R200–R210.

71. Pandharipande PP, Pun BT, Herr DL, et al. Effect of sedation with dexmedetomidine vs lorazepam on acute brain dysfunction in mechanically ventilated patients: the MENDS randomized controlled trial. *JAMA.* 2007;298(22):2644–2653.

72. Pandharipande P, Sanders R, Girard T, et al. Effect of dexmedetomidine versus lorazepam on outcome in patients with sepsis: an a priori-designed analysis of the MENDS randomized controlled trial. *Crit Care.* 2010;14:R38.

73. Riker R, Shehabi Y, Bokesch P, Ceraso D, Wisemandle W, Koura F. Dexmedetomidine vs midazolam for sedation of critically ill patients. *JAMA.* 2009;301:489–499.

74. Morris PE, Goad A, Thompson C, et al. Early intensive care unit mobility therapy in the treatment of acute respiratory failure. *Crit Care Med.* 2008;36(8):2238–2243.

75. Schweickert W, Pohlman M, Pohlman A, et al. Early physical and occupational therapy in mechanically ventilated, critically ill patients: a randomised controlled trial. *Lancet.* 2009;373:1874–1882.

76. Needham DM, Korupolu R, Zanni JM, et al. Early physical medicine and rehabilitation for patients with acute respiratory failure: a quality improvement project. *Arch Phys MedRehabil.* 2010;91(4):536–542.

77. Devlin JW, Fraser GL, Ely EW, Kress JP, Skrobik Y, Dasta JF. Pharmacological management of sedation and delirium in mechanically ventilated ICU patients: remaining evidence gaps and controversies. *Semin Respir Crit Care Med.* 2013;34(2):201–215.

TRAUMA, OBSTETRICS, AND ENVIRONMENTAL INJURIES

74 How Should Trauma Patients Be Managed in the Intensive Care Unit?

Brian P. Smith, Patrick M. Reilly

Each year, in the United States, more than 2.5 million people are killed or hospitalized as a result of traumatic injuries.[1] Over one quarter of these patients are treated in an intensive care unit (ICU) at some point during their hospital stays.[2] With mortality rates exceeding 20% for the most severely injured patients (injury severity score [ISS] > 25),[3] it stands to reason that the delivery of high-quality health care to trauma patients in an ICU setting plays a paramount role in their resuscitation and recovery.

INFRASTRUCTURE

The first step in the provision of high-quality trauma ICU care is delivery of the trauma patient to an ICU capable of rendering that care. In this regard, trauma patients should be cared for at hospitals with specialty trauma services. Population-based estimates have demonstrated a relative risk (RR) for mortality of 0.80 (95% confidence interval [CI], 0.66 to 0.98) for trauma patients treated at trauma centers compared with case mix-matched patients treated at nontrauma centers.[4] Multiple studies have confirmed this model of care as successful and cost effective.[4-6] There remains debate regarding the source of this outcome advantage. Specifically, it is unclear whether the advantage derives from the absolute volume of the trauma center or the level of trauma center designation (and the resources associated with that designation).[7-10]

There is much less uncertainty about the role of intensivists in caring for these patients. In 2006, Nathens and colleagues demonstrated that, when compared with "open" ICUs, the intensivist model was associated with an RR of death of 0.78 among trauma patients in a large multicenter prospective cohort study.[11] This effect was more pronounced among elderly patients (RR of death, 0.55), in ICUs in trauma centers (RR of death, 0.64), and in units directed by surgically trained intensivists (RR of death, 0.67). Similar data have shown not only improved mortality but also lower ICU mortality, lower ventilator-associated pneumonia rates, and increased ventilator-free days among ICUs that actively engage intensivists in the care of trauma patients.[12-14] This model has been expanded to trauma care in the combat zone, with favorable effects on

morbidity and mortality among combat-injured patients cared for by intensivists.[15]

Finally, perhaps the most important factor contributing to the better care afforded by trauma centers and staffed with specifically trained personnel is the availability of ICU beds themselves. Emergency department lengths of stay continue to increase, and much of the early part of resuscitation occurs within the confines of the emergency department or the trauma bay.[16,17] Providing ICU-level care within the trauma bay can be a challenging task. Evidence suggests that emergency department length of stay is directly linked to increased rates of pneumonia and death.[18,19] One response to this problem is implementation of an "open trauma bed" protocol to improve throughput from the trauma bay. In this study sample, the emergency department length of stay was decreased by nearly 1 hour after the protocol was instituted.[20] Other investigators have demonstrated similar results, supported by cost-effectiveness data, by staffing an open ICU bed with an otherwise unassigned charge nurse.[21] However, it remains unclear how these protocols affect patients who are displaced from the ICU to generate bed availability.

RESUSCITATION

The primary goal of the intensivist caring for a trauma patient should be the recognition of shock and the implementation of resuscitation strategies to capture and reverse the associated abnormal physiology. The diagnosis of shock must be made with a high clinical index of suspicion because ongoing occult hypoperfusion (which occurs in up to 85% of severely injured trauma patients) has been associated with increased morbidity and mortality.[22-24] Several modalities of quantifying resuscitative efforts beyond standard vital signs have been proposed. They can be classified broadly into invasive monitors (such as pulmonary artery [PA] catheters, peripheral arterial catheters, and gastric tonometers), noninvasive monitors (such as bedside ultrasonography and bioreactance monitoring), and biomarkers (such as arterial or venous lactate, base deficit, and arterial or mixed venous oxygen saturation).

Invasive Hemodynamic Monitoring

Optimal oxygen (O_2) delivery relies heavily on adequate cardiac performance. Therefore, optimization of cardiac output (CO) is a key feature of any resuscitative effort. Historically, PA catheterization was the mainstay of invasive hemodynamic monitoring. However, routine use of these devices has become less common,[24a] and they seem most efficacious among older trauma patients and those who arrive in severe shock.[25]

Several commercially available products are available to estimate CO with less intrusion than PA catheterization. For instance, the lithium indicator dilution technique utilizes central venous catheterization and cannulation of the femoral or axillary artery to measure heart function. Similarly, there exist proprietary algorithms capable of estimating CO via transpulmonary thermodilution methods. Finally, volume responsiveness based on stroke volume variation transduced by a peripherally inserted arterial catheter can be calculated by several devices. Although all of these systems show promise in regards to their low complication rates, their efficacy in guiding fluid resuscitation of trauma patients remains unknown. Animal hemorrhagic shock models suggest that these devices might be unreliable, most commonly underestimating CO.[26-28] It is conceivable that as these technologies evolve, they will be capable of estimating cardiac function similar to pulmonary arterial cannulation without the need to traverse the right side of the heart and dwell within the pulmonary arterial system.

Noninvasive Hemodynamic Monitoring

Impedance cardiography and bioreactance are two methods of quantifying cardiac function without invasive monitoring. Both methods use electrophysiology to measure how changes in aortic blood volume and flow influence transmission of a known electrical current across the thorax. These technologies have been studied in multiple ICU settings and show modest correlation with traditional PA catheter thermodilution.[29,30] To date, there is one prospective observational study of this technology in trauma patients, demonstrating an association of bioreactance monitoring and shortened hospital length of stay.[31] However, it should be noted that the comparison groups were historic controls, and changes in hospital admission and discharge practices might have confounded the analysis.

Ultrasonography has been used as a triage tool in the trauma bay for many years and has recently become an important test for the intensivist who cares for trauma patients. Several investigators have shown that bedside ultrasonography of the cava and heart can demonstrate hypovolemic shock and the response to plasma expansion.[32-35] Most of these studies are limited by their retrospective nature; however, a recent randomized trial indicated that use of limited transthoracic echocardiograms during trauma resuscitation was associated with decreased intravenous fluid administration and improved survival.[36] Confirmatory studies are required. However, the repeatability, relatively low cost, and noninvasiveness of this diagnostic tool seem promising.

Biomarkers

The mainstay of trauma resuscitation has been biochemical endpoints of resuscitation. Although many have been investigated, the two that have been most useful in caring for trauma patients are serum lactate and base deficit. Both of these tests are sensitive measures of hypoperfusion[37,38]; however, the interpretation of these tests can be clouded by hepatic and/or renal dysfunction. Abnormal lactate and base deficit have been associated with morbidity and mortality.[39,40] Measurement of lactate and base deficit might be useful guides for resuscitative progress because mortality has been associated with increased time to normalization of serum lactate.[41] Likewise, in one study of trauma patients with increasing base deficit despite resuscitation, 65% were found to have ongoing hemorrhage, suggesting the potential utility of this test as an adjunct to the resuscitative efforts.[42] The most recent recommendation on the topic developed by the Eastern Association for the Surgery of Trauma suggests using at least one of these measures to quantify the need for ongoing resuscitation.[22]

There is mounting evidence that these studies, performed as point of care (POC) tests, decrease the time to diagnosis and intervention, reduce the total volume of blood draws, and shorten ICU lengths of stay.[43-45] POC thromboelastography can also be considered to help guide blood product administration during resuscitation in the trauma bay as well as the ICU.[46,47]

Special Considerations of Shock

Hypovolemic Shock

Hypovolemic shock from uncontrolled hemorrhage is the quintessential form of shock among trauma patients. Much work has been done to advance the care of trauma patients, both in control of hemorrhage (permissive hypotension, fluid restrictive resuscitation, damage control surgery, applications of tourniquets, topical hemostatic agents, endovascular occlusion, etc.) as well as replacement of intravascular volume (colloid, isotonic and hypertonic crystalloid, balanced salt solutions, blood products, massive transfusion protocols, etc.). Details of these techniques can be found elsewhere in this text. Suffice it to say that mastery of hemorrhage control and fluid resuscitation is critical to the cessation and reversal of hemorrhagic shock.

Septic Shock

Trauma patients with septic shock should be cared for according to the Surviving Sepsis Guidelines.[48] Although no studies, to date, have demonstrated any outcome advantage in particular to trauma patients, this body of work remains the most comprehensive summary of sepsis management in most patients. Particular mention should be made of two details. First, source control can be particularly challenging in trauma patients with multiple injured systems. Practitioners must rely heavily on physical examination, coupled with various methods of diagnostic imaging to guide interventions. This is particularly true in hostile abdomens and thoraces, in which some patients will undoubtedly benefit from percutaneous drainage rather than more traditional surgical exposures. Second, antibiotic stewardship is fundamental to trauma ICUs. The data supporting de-escalation of antibacterial therapy as a means of quelling antibiotic resistance are lacking. However, the recent emergence of increasingly resistant organisms coincident with the common practice of empiric broad-spectrum antibiotic therapy lends strong credence to a linkage between these phenomena. Consequentially, strong consideration should be given to narrowing antibacterial coverage when culture data are available in appropriate patient groups.[49-51] There is no evidence that trauma patients (even those with much "spillage" or "contamination") benefit from extended empiric coverage. Likewise, the "open abdomen" strategy of patient care does not necessarily mandate use of antibiotics in the absence of other indicators of infection.[52]

In addition, those practitioners who care for trauma patients must remain vigilant for signs of severe sepsis or septic shock through the duration of each patient's encounter. Either might very well be the inciting event that leads to a patient's trauma and admission, or it might very well bring a trauma patient back to the hospital from inpatient physical therapy, skilled nursing, or even home. And patients remain susceptible to the diagnosis at every point in between.

Neurogenic Shock

The incidence of neurogenic shock in patients with cervical spinal cord injuries is 20%.[53] The optimal treatment of the bradycardia and hypotension that define this pathophysiology remains unknown, but treatment with intravascular volume expansion as well as pharmacologic management with vasoactive, chronotropic, and inotropic medications might be indicated.[53-55] On occasion, the use of electrical cardiac stimulation, by way of percutaneous or intravascular pacers, might be valuable.[56] Therefore, the ICU should be capable of managing these various modes of hemodynamic support for patients with this injury complex.

Cardiogenic Shock

The combination of increasing age among trauma patients and higher numbers of high-speed motor vehicle accidents has contributed to increasing numbers of clinically significant cardiac injuries. It is estimated that up to 20% of road traffic deaths are associated with blunt injuries to the heart.[57] Recognition of cardiac compromise can be challenging because many of these patients suffer concomitant injuries resulting in mixed shock physiology.[58,59] Signs of systemic hypotension in the face of elevated central venous pressure should raise concern for cardiogenic shock. Otherwise, clinicians must maintain a high index of suspicion based on the mechanism of injury despite potentially silent clinical signs. Patients with suspected blunt cardiac injury should be screened with electrocardiogram and troponin I. The negative predictive value of these combined tests approaches 100%.[59] The care of patients with cardiogenic shock is detailed elsewhere in this text. The care of trauma patients, in particular, must be guided by experienced traumatologists, in consultation with cardiologists, weighing the risks and benefits of interventions in the setting of potentially competing priorities.

Special Considerations of Trauma Patients

The Open Cavity

The use of damage control surgery and resuscitation has resulted in many critically ill trauma patients presenting to the ICU with open body cavities.[60,61] It is not unusual for patients to spend days recovering from the initial physiologic insult before these cavities can be closed. In this regard, it is paramount that ICUs specializing in the care of trauma patients be familiar with management of severe biomechanical and physiologic derangements that occur as chest and abdominal wall geometry are altered. Advanced modes of mechanical ventilation might be necessary for patients with packed thoraces. Likewise, the open abdomen might require skilled nursing wound care with negative pressure dressings and supplemented nutritional strategies for gastrointestinal drainage and discontinuity.

Traction/Immobility

Damage control orthopedic surgery (early external fixation followed by definitive treatment) has become increasingly common among polytrauma patients.[62-65] Therefore, the number of patients with large external fixation devices in the ICU has increased. Likewise, ICU patients might be cared for with pelvic stabilization devices (sheets and commercially available pelvic binders) and/or spinal column stabilizing devices (cervical spine bracing devices such as cervical collars or Halo systems, thoracolumbosacral orthosis braces). Although these techniques are helpful to the recovery of various injuries, they oftentimes limit mobility and access to soft tissue care. Therefore, particular attention must be paid to these trauma patients to ensure adequate wound care and prevention of the secondary complications of immobility.

Venous Thromboembolism Prophylaxis

Venous thromboembolism (VTE) is a common complication in patients with major trauma.[66] The risk is compounded by various factors, such as the systemic inflammatory response to major trauma, immobility, and the hypercoagulable state associated with major surgery, bone fractures, and the use of invasive vascular devices. It is important for the ICU to practice aggressive evaluation for VTE with protocolized care to help prevent the (potentially fatal) sequelae of VTE.[67,68] Implementation of VTE prevention strategies in the form of "smart order sets" or risk assessment models has been associated with decreased rates of radiographically documented VTE (2.5% vs. 0.7%) and a 39% RR reduction of hospital-acquired VTE in some patient groups.[69,70] Clinicians must also be familiar with evidence-based best practice guidelines to help reduce VTE risk, particularly for trauma patients.[71,72]

INTENSIVE CARE UNIT PROTOCOLS

Guideline-based care (in the form of agreed-upon practice patterns, guidelines, or protocols) plays an important role in the delivery of high-quality intensive care therapies to patients with traumatic injuries. Studies have demonstrated that implementation of trauma systems, including things such as early management guidelines and consensus-developed clinical practice guidelines and protocols, are associated with decreasing odds of death (odds ratio [OR] 0.45; 95% CI, 0.27 to 0.76), standardized care, and improved resource utilization.[73,74] They are natural extensions of the algorithmic approach to the triage of life-threatening injuries suggested by the Advanced Trauma Life Support (ATLS) curriculum.[75] It is impossible to list every ICU trauma guideline within the context of this chapter, but consideration should be given to several management strategies. Indeed, this approach has been advocated for management of, among others, elevated intracranial pressure, spinal cord injury and rehabilitation, sedation and delirium, pain control, mechanical ventilation and weaning, use of enteral and parenteral nutrition, glucose control, utilization of bladder catheters, blood transfusions, antibiotic stewardship, prophylaxis of stress ulcers and venous thromboembolic disease, early mobilization and physical therapy, and use of various ICU devices (such as central and peripherally inserted catheters, arterial lines, and ICU specialty beds). Importantly, virtually none of these interventions is based on high-level evidence. However, the central theme of the guidelines (i.e., that improved outcomes for injured patients) can be obtained through better organization, and planning of trauma care should be maintained.[76] Some researchers have found that major deviations from clinical management guidelines are associated with a 3-fold increase in mortality among trauma patients (adjusted OR 3.28; 95% CI, 1.53 to 7.03).[77] Similarly, an intervention as simple as strict adherence to a daily rounding checklist has been linked to improved outcomes, such as decreased ventilator-associated pneumonia rates, relative to partial compliance with the same checklist (3.5% vs. 13.4%, $P = .04$).[78]

TERTIARY EXAMINATION

A common pitfall of caring for trauma patients (particularly those who are critically ill) is failure to recognize missed injuries.[79] This results from many variables, including severe physiologic derangements, inability of the patient to participate in the history and physical examination, handoffs of care, and multiple service lines assuming care of different injury complexes. So-called "missed injuries" can result in significant morbidity and even death.[80,81] Several mechanisms have been proposed to help decrease the rate of missed injuries. Most are extensions of the tertiary survey proposed by Enderson in 1990.[82] Technologic advances should also help to reduce missed injury rates as faster and more detailed medical imaging becomes increasingly affordable and mobile. Access to electronic medical records and the use of handheld communication devices and electronic checklists should also help expedite recognition and communication of previously undocumented injuries.

THE EXTENDED INTENSIVE CARE UNIT TEAM

Physical Therapy

More than 25% of patients with multiple injuries and extended ICU lengths of stay develop long-term limitations of range of motion unrelated to their injuries, 30% are unable to return to work, and nearly 50% suffer permanent sensory deficits.[83,84] Early mobilization plays a fundamental role in the battle against ICU-acquired weakness. Therefore, integration of an aggressive physical and occupational therapy service into the daily care of these patients is paramount in their recovery.[85-88] This seems particularly true among patients requiring blood transfusions during the ICU stay.[89]

Pharmacy

There is increasing evidence that the presence of a clinical pharmacist at ICU rounds improves outcomes of ICU patients.[90-93] Clinical pharmacists serve as a direct link to the main hospital pharmacies. They are often well versed in hospital antibiograms, they have critical training in drug–drug interactions, and they provide continuity of care among the prehospital setting, the ICU stay, and the transition to other levels of care. There is good evidence demonstrating an association with engaged clinical pharmacists and decreased adverse drug events, as well as cost savings in trauma centers.[94]

SUMMARY

Traumatic injuries account for many ICU admissions each year. These patients are best served at dedicated trauma centers with access to multimodality diagnostic and treatment options. Care teams should be led by intensive trained physicians with knowledge and experience in various resuscitative techniques, and team members should represent various disciplines including nursing, pharmacy, and physical therapy. The ICU should be capable of and familiar with POC testing, invasive and noninvasive monitoring, and appropriate triage of critically ill patients. Most importantly, the care of the trauma patient in the ICU should integrate algorithmic approaches to diagnosis and treatment incorporating resources from evidence-based guidelines and expert-level opinions.

AUTHORS' RECOMMENDATIONS

- Critically ill trauma patients should be cared for by a team of trained intensivists in a designated trauma center ICU.
- Intensivists should be well trained in the recognition and treatment of shock, and they should maintain a high index of suspicion for various shock states based on history, physical examination, and mechanism of injury.
- Trauma ICUs should be familiar with and capable of monitoring patients with invasive, noninvasive, and POC testing based on patient needs and severity of illness.
- ICU protocols should be used to guide trauma care, with particular attention paid to VTE prophylaxis. ICU care should also account for the management of open body cavities and trauma variables such as skeletal traction.

REFERENCES

1. Centers for Disease Control and Prevention. Web-based Injury Statistics Query and Reporting System (WISQARS). http://www.cdc.gov/injury/WISQARS/; Accessed 18.08.14.
2. Nathens AB, Maier RV, Jurkovich GJ, et al. The delivery of critical care services in US trauma centers: is the standard being met? *J Trauma*. 2006;60:773–784.

3. Dutton RP, Stansbury LG, Leone S, et al. Trauma mortality in mature trauma systems: are we doing better? An analysis of trauma mortality patterns, 1997-2008. *J Trauma.* 2010;69:620–626.

4. MakKenzie EJ, Rivara FP, Jurkavich GJ, et al. A national evaluation of the effect of trauma-center care on mortality. *N Engl J Med.* 2006;354:366–378.

5. Sampalis JS, Denis R, Lavoie A, et al. Trauma care regionalization: a process-outcome evaluation. *J Trauma.* 1999;46:565–579.

6. MacKenzie EJ, Weir S, Rivara FP, et al. The value of trauma center care. *J Trauma.* 2010;69:1–10.

7. Nathens AB, Jurkovich GJ, Maier RV, et al. Relationship between trauma center volume and outcomes. *JAMA.* 2001;285:1164–1171.

8. Demetriades D, Martin M, Salim A, et al. The effect of trauma center designation and trauma volume on outcomes in specific severe injuries. *J Trauma.* 2005;242:512–517.

9. Bennett KM, Vaslef S, Pappas TN, et al. The volume-outcomes relationship for United States level I trauma centers. *J Surg Res.* 2011;167:19–23.

10. Minei JP, Fabian TC, Guffey DM, et al. Incerased trauma center volume is associated with improved survival after severe injury. *Ann Surg.* 2014;260:456–465.

11. Nathens AB, Rivara FP, MacKenzie EJ, et al. The impact of an intensivist-model ICU on trauma-related mortality. *Ann Surg.* 2006;244:545–552.

12. Multz AS, Chalfin DB, Samson IM, et al. A "closed" medical intensive care unit (MICU) improves resource utilization when compared with an "open" MICU. *Am J Med Respir Crit Care Med.* 1998;157:1468–1473.

13. Ghorra S, Reinert SE, Cioffi W, et al. Analysis of the effect of conversion from open to closed surgical intensive care unit. *Ann Surg.* 1999;229:163–171.

14. Pronovost PJ, Jenckes MW, Dorman T, et al. Organizational characteristics of intensive care units related to outcomes of abdominal aortic surgery. *JAMA.* 1999;281:1310–1317.

15. Lettieri CJ, Shah AA, Greenburg DL. An intensivist-directed intensive care unit improves clinical outcomes in a combat zone. *Crit Care Med.* 2009;37:1256–1260.

16. Fromm Jr RE, Gibbs LR, McCallum WG, et al. Critical care in the emergency department: a time based study. *Crit Care Med.* 1993;21:970–976.

17. Derlet RW, Richards JR. Overcrowding in the nation's emergency departments: complex causes and disturbing effects. *Ann Emerg Med.* 2000;35:63–68.

18. Carr BG, Kaye AJ, Wiebe DJ, et al. Emergency department length of stay: a major risk factor for pneumonia in intubated blunt trauma patients. *J Trauma.* 2007;63:9–12.

19. Mowery NT, Dougherty SD, Hildreth AN, et al. Emergency department length of stay is an independent predictor of hospital mortality in trauma activation patients. *J Trauma.* 2011;70:1317–1325.

20. Bhakta A, Bloom M, Warren H, et al. The impact of implementing a 24/7 open trauma bed protocol in the surgical intensive care unit on throughput and outcomes. *J Trauma Acute Care Surg.* 2013;75:97–101.

21. Fryman L, Talley C, Kearney P, Bernard A, Davenport D. Maintaining an open trauma intensive care unit bed for rapid admission can be cost-effective. *J Trauma Acute Care Surg.* 2015;79:98–103.

22. Tisherman SA, Barie P, Bokhari F, et al. Clinical practice guideline: endpoints of resuscitation. *J Trauma.* 2004;57:898–912.

23. Scalea TM, Maltz S, Yelon J, et al. Resuscitation of multiple trauma and head injury: role of crystalloid fluids and inotropes. *Crit Care Med.* 1994;20:1610–1615.

24. Abou-Khalil B, Scalea TM, Trooskin SZ, et al. Hemodynamic responses to shock in young trauma patients: need for invasive monitoring. *Crit Care Med.* 1994;22:633–639.

24a. Rajaram SS, Desai NK, Kalra A, et al. Pulmonary artery catheters for adult patients in intensive care. *Cochrane Database Syst Rev.* 2013;2:CD003408. doi: 10.1002/14651858.CD003408.pub3. 10.1002/14651858.CD003408.

25. Friese RS, Shafi S, Gentilello LM. Pulmonary artery catheter use is associated with reduced mortality in severely injured patients: a National Trauma Data Bank analysis of 53,312 patients. *Crit Care Med.* 2006;34:1597–1601.

26. Lee CH, Wang JY, Huang KL, et al. Unreliability of pulse contour-derived cardiac output in piglets simulating acute hemorrhagic shock and rapid volume expansion. *J Trauma.* 2010;68:1357–1361.

27. Piehl MD, Manning JE, McCurdy SL, et al. Pulse contour cardiac output analysis in a piglet model of severe hemorrhagic shock. *Crit Care Med.* 2008;36:1189–1195.

28. Cooper ES, Muir WW. Continuous cardiac output monitoring via arterial pressure waveform analysis following severe hemorrhagic shock in dogs. *Crit Care Med.* 2007;37:1724–1729.

29. Kamath SA, Dranzer MH, Tassisa G, et al. Correlation of impedance cardiography with invasive hemodynamic measurements in patients with advanced heart failure: the BioImpedance CardioGraphy (BIG) substudy of the Evaluation Study of Congestive Heart Failure and Pulmonary Artery Catheterization Effectiveness (ESCAPE) Trial. *Am Heart J.* 2009;158:217–223.

30. Kieback AG, Borges AC, Schink T, et al. Impedance cardiography versus invasive measurements of stroke volume index in patients with chronic heart failure. *Int J Cardiol.* 2010;143:211–213.

31. Dunham CM, Chirichella TJ, Gruber BS, et al. Emergency department noninvasive (NICOM) cardiac outputs are associated with trauma activation, patient injury severity and host conditions and mortality. *J Trauma Acute Care Surg.* 2012;73:479–485.

32. Ferrada P, Vanguri P, Anand RJ, et al. A, B, C, D, echo: limited transthoracic echocardiogram is a useful tool to guide therapy for hypotension in the trauma bay–a pilot study. *J Trauma Acute Care Surg.* 2013;74:220–223.

33. Yanagawa Y, Sakamoto T, Okada Y. Hypovolemic shock evaluated by sonographic measurement of the inferior vena cava during resuscitation in trauma patients. *J Trauma.* 2007;63:1245–1248.

34. Carr BG, Dean AJ, Everett WW, et al. Intensivist bedside ultrasound (INBU) for volume assessment in the intensive care unit: a pilot study. *J Trauma.* 2007;63:495–500.

35. Nguyen A, Plurad DS, Bricker S, et al. Flat or fat? Inferior vena cava ratio is a marker for occult shock in trauma patients. *J Surg Res.* 2014;192:263–267.

36. Ferrada P, Evans D, Wolfe L, et al. Findings of a randomized controlled trial using limited transthoracic echocardiogram (LTTE) as a hemodynamic monitoring tool in the trauma bay. *J Trauma Acute Care Surg.* 2014;76:31–37.

37. Rutherford EJ, Morris Jr JA, Reed GW, et al. Base deficit stratifies mortality and determines therapy. *J Trauma.* 1992;33:417–423.

38. Manikis P, Jankowski S, Zhang H, et al. Correlation of serial blood lactate levels to organ failure and mortality after trauma. *Am J Emerg Med.* 1995;13:619–622.

39. McNelis J, Marini CP, Jurkiewicz A, et al. Prolonged lactate clearance is associated with increased mortality in the surgical intensive care unit. *Am J Surg.* 2001;182:481–485.

40. Davis JW, Kaups KL. Base deficit in the elderly: a marker of severe injury and death. *J Trauma.* 1998;45:873–877.

41. Abramson D, Salea TM, Hitchcock R, et al. Lactate clearance and survival following injury. *J Trauma.* 1993;35:584–588.

42. Davis JW, Shackford SR, Mackersie SC, et al. Base deficit as a guide to volume resuscitation. *J Trauma.* 1988;28:1464–1467.

43. Weber CF, Görlinger K, Meininger G, et al. Point-of-care testing: a prospective, randomized clinical trial of efficacy in coagulopathic cardiac surgery patients. *Anesthesiology.* 2012;117:531–547.

44. Rossi AF, Khan DM, Hannan R, et al. Goal-directed medical therapy and point-of-care testing improve outcomes after congenital heart surgery. *Intensive Care Med.* 2005;31:98–104.

45. Meybohm P, Zacharowski K, Weber CF. Point-of-care coagulation management in intensive care medicine. *Crit Care.* 2013;17:218–227.

46. Feinman M, Cotton BA, Haut ER. Optimal fluid resuscitation in trauma: type, timing and total. *Curr Opin Crit Care.* 2014;20:366–372.

47. Tapia NM, Chang A, Norman M. TEG-guided resuscitation is superior to standardized MTP resuscitation in massively transfused penetrating trauma patients. *J Trauma Acute Care Surg.* 2013;74:378–385.

48. Dellinger RP, Levy MM, Rhodes A, et al. Surviving sepsis campaign: international guidelines for management of severe sepsis and septic shock: 2012. *Crit Care Med.* 2013;41:580–637.

49. Eachempati SR, Hydo LJ, Shou J, et al. Does de-escalation of antibiotic therapy for ventilator-associated pneumonia affect the likelihood of recurrent pneumonia or mortality in critically ill surgical patients? *J Trauma.* 2009;66:1343–1348.

50. Rello J, Vidaur L, Sandiumenge A, et al. De-escalation therapy in ventilator-associated pneumonia. *Crit Care Med.* 2004;32:2183–2190.

51. Masterton R. Antibiotic de-escalation. *Crit Care Clin.* 2011;27:149–162.

52. Dutton WD, Diaz Jr JJ, Miller RS, et al. Critical care issues in managing complex open abdominal wound. *J Intensive Care Med.* 2012;27:167–171.

53. Guly HR, Bouamra O, Lecky FE, et al. The incidence of neurogenic shock in patients with isolated spinal cord injury in the emergency department. *Resuscitation.* 2008;76:57–62.

54. Zipnick RI, Scalea TM, Trooskin SZ, et al. Hemodynamic responses to penetrating spinal cord injuries. *J Trauma.* 1993;35:578–582.

55. Dumont RJ, Verma S, Okonkwo DO, et al. Acute spinal cord injury, part II: contemporary pharmacotherapy. *Clin Neuropharmacol.* 2001;24:265–279.

56. Bilello JF, Davis JW, Cunningham MA, et al. Cervical spinal cord injury and the need for cardiovascular intervention. *Arch Surg.* 2003;138:1127–1129.

57. Parmly LF, Manion WC, Mattingly TW. Non penetrating traumatic injury of the heart. *Circulation.* 1958;18:371–396.

58. Pretre R, Chilcott M. Blunt trauma to the heart and great vessels. *N Engl J Med.* 1997;336:626–632.

59. Clancy K, Velopulos C, Bilaniuk JW, et al. Screening for blunt cardiac injury: an Eastern Association for the Surgery of Trauma practice management guideline. *J Trauma Acute Care Surg.* 2012;73:s301–s306.

60. Rotondo MF, Schwab CW, McGonigal MD, et al. 'Damage control': an approach for improved survival in exsanguinating penetrating abdominal injury. *J Trauma.* 1993;35:375–382.

61. Burch JM, Ortiz VB, Richardson RJ, et al. Abbreviated laparotomy and planned reoperation for critically injured patients. *Ann Surg.* 1992;215:476–484.

62. Hoey BA, Schwab CW. Damage control surgery. *Scand J Surg.* 2009;91:92–103.

63. Nowotarski PJ, Turen CH, Brumback RJ, et al. Conversion of external fixation to intramedullary nailing for fractures of the shaft of the femur in multiply injured patients. *J Bone Joint Surg Am.* 2000;82:781–788.

64. Pape HC, Hildebrand F, Pertschy S, et al. Changes in the management of femoral shaft fractures in polytrauma patients: from early total care to damage control orthopedic surgery. *J Trauma.* 2002;53:452–461.

65. Taeger G, Ruchholtz S, Waydhas C, et al. Damage control orthopedics in patients with multiple injuries is effective, time saving, and safe. *J Trauma.* 2005;59:409–416.

66. Geerts WH, Code KI, Jay RM, et al. A prospective study of venous thromboembolism after major trauma. *N Engl J Med.* 1994;331:1601–1606.

67. Tooher R, Middleton P, Pham C, et al. A systematic review of strategies to improve prophylaxis for venous thromboembolism in hospitals. *Ann Surg.* 2005;241:397–415.

68. Maynard G, Stein J. Designing and implementing effective venous thromboembolism prevention protocols: lessons from collaborative efforts. *J Thromb Thrombolysis.* 2010;29:159–166.

69. Zeidan AM, Streiff MB, Lau BD, et al. Impact of a venous thromboembolism prophylaxis "smart order set": improved compliance, fewer events. *Am J Heme.* 2013;88:545–549.

70. Maynard GA, Morris TA, Jenkins IH, et al. Optimizing prevention of hospital-acquired venous thromboembolism (VTE): prospective validation of a VTE risk assessment model. *J Hosp Med.* 2010;5:10–18.

71. Rogers FB, Cipolle MD, Velmahos G, et al. Practice management guidelines for the prevention of venous thromboembolism in trauma patients: the EAST Practice Management Guidelines Workgroup. *J Trauma.* 2002;53:142–164.

72. Guyatt GH, Akl EA, Crowther M, et al. Executive summary: antithrombotic therapy and prevention of thrombosis, 9th ed: American College of Chest Physicians Evidence-Based Clinical Practice Guidelines. *Chest.* 2012;141:s7–s47.

73. Brennan PW, Everest ER, Griggs WM, et al. Risk of death among cases attending South Australian Major Trauma Services after severe trauma: the first 4 years of operation of a state trauma system. *J Trauma.* 2002;53:333–339.

74. Simons R, Eliopoulos V, Laflamme D, et al. Impact on process of trauma care delivery 1 year after the introduction of a trauma program in a provincial trauma center. *J Trauma.* 1999;46:811–816.

75. American College of Surgeons Committee on Trauma. *Advanced Trauma Life Support Program for Doctors.* 9th ed. Chicago: American College of Surgeons; 2013.

76. Mock C, Lormond JD, Goosen J, et al. *Guidelines for Essential Trauma Care.* Geneva: World Health Organization; 2004.

77. Rice TW, Morris S, Tortella BJ, et al. Deviations from evidence-based clinical management guidelines increase mortality in critically injured trauma patients. *Crit Care Med.* 2012;40:778–786.

78. Dubose J, Teixeira PGR, Inaba K, et al. Measureable outcomes of quality improvement using a daily quality rounds checklist: one-year analysis in a trauma intensive care unit with sustained ventilator associated pneumonia reduction. *J Trauma.* 2010;69:855–860.

79. Angle N, Coimbra R, Hoyt DB. Pitfalls in the management of the trauma patient in the intensive care unit. *Trauma.* 1999;1:301–305.

80. Janjua KJ, Sugrue M, Deane SA. Prospective evaluation of early missed injuries and the role of tertiary trauma survey. *J Trauma.* 1998;44:1000–1006.

81. Buduhan G, McRitchie DI. Missed injuries in patients with multiple trauma. *J Trauma.* 2000;49:600–605.

82. Enderson BL, Reath DB, Meadors J, et al. The tertiary trauma survey: a prospective study of missed injury. *J Trauma.* 1990;30:666–669.

83. Grotz M, Hohensee A, Remmers D, et al. Rehabilitation results of patients with multiple injuries and multiple organ failure and long-term intensive care. *J Trauma.* 1997;42:919–926.

84. Baldry Currens JA. Evaluation of disability and handicap following injury. *Injury.* 2000;31:99–106.

85. De Jonghe B, Lacherade J-C, Sharshar T, et al. Intensive care unit-acquired weakness: risk factors and prevention. *Crit Care Med.* 2009;37:s309–s315.

86. Griffiths RD, Hall JB. Intensive care unit-acquired weakness. *Crit Care Med.* 2010;38:779–787.

87. Nordon-Craft A, Moss M, Quan D, et al. Document Intensive care unit-acquired weakness: implications for physical therapist management. *Phys Ther.* 2012;92:1494–1506.

88. Yosef-Brauner O, Adi N, Ben Shahar T, et al. Effect of physical therapy on muscle strength, respiratory muscles and functional parameters in patients with intensive care unit-acquired weakness. *Clin Respir J.* 2015;9:1–6.

89. Parsons EC, Kross EK, Ali NA, et al. Red blood cell transfusion is associated with decreased in-hospital muscle strength among critically ill patients requiring mechanical ventilation. *J Crit Care.* 2013;28:1079–1085.

90. Papadopoulos J, Rebuck JA, Lober C, et al. The critical care pharmacist: an essential intensive care practitioner. *Pharmacother.* 2002;22:1484–1488.

91. Kane SL, Weber RJ, Dasta JF. The impact of critical care pharmacists on enhancing patient outcomes. *Intensive Care Med.* 2003;29:691–698.

92. MacLaren R, Bond CA, Martin SJ, et al. Clinical and economic outcomes of involving pharmacists in the direct care of critically ill patients with infections. *Crit Care Med.* 2008;36:3184–3189.

93. Preslaski CR, Lat I, MacLaren R, et al. Pharmacist contributions as members of the multidisciplinary ICU team. *Chest.* 2013;144:1687–1695.

94. Hamblin S, Rumbaugh K, Miller R. Prevention of adverse drug events and cost savings associated with PharmD interventions in an academic Level I trauma center: an evidence-based approach. *J Trauma Acute Care Surg.* 2012;73:1484–1490

75 What Is Abdominal Compartment Syndrome and How Should It Be Managed?

Noelle N. Saillant, Lewis J. Kaplan

Abdominal compartment syndrome (ACS) is defined by the presence of organ dysfunction that can be attributed to elevated intra-abdominal pressure (IAP).[1] ACS is the end result of a cumulative increase in IAP above the upper limit of normal (normal 5 to 11 mm Hg) to values defining intra-abdominal hypertension (IAH). IAH is defined as the sustained or repetitive pathologic elevation of IAP to 12 mm Hg or more and is graded and classified according to a four-tiered continuum articulated by consensus by the World Society of Abdominal Compartment Syndrome (WSACS; www.wsacs.org; Table 75-1).[1-3] To understand how best to prevent, identify, and treat IAH and ACS, one needs to understand the pathophysiology, monitoring, categorization, and management techniques before and after ACS is diagnosed.

PATHOPHYSIOLOGY AND MECHANISM OF ACTION

The pathophysiology of ACS is complex. Rising IAP provides a clue that changes in arterial inflow, venous outflow, and the space occupied by viscera and intra-abdominal fluid have created disequilibrium in the normal pressure-volume relationship. Typical adult IAP ranges from 0 to 5 mm Hg; however, obesity, pregnancy, and advanced age may elevate the baseline. A recent study showed that IAP increased between 0.14 and 0.23 mm Hg for each increase in body mass index unit and 0.20 mm Hg/year for advancing age.[5] Open abdominal surgery also may elevate the measured IAP.[1]

ACS may be further classified as primary, secondary, or recurrent. Primary ACS develops as a direct result of an abdominal injury or other surgical abdominal emergency (i.e., intestinal perforation or ischemia). Secondary ACS reflects a response to a condition that is not of primary abdominal origin (e.g., visceral edema and/or the acute accumulation of ascites secondary to massive volume resuscitation). Lastly, recurrent ACS develops after successful medical or surgical therapy for primary or secondary ACS. The classic example is IAP secondary to application of a temporary closure device used to secure an open abdomen after initial successful surgical decompression. Blood, ascites, or visceral edema (or any

combination of the three) may increase the IAP and re-create the ACS. Likewise, external compression from an excessively tight binder may also dangerously elevate IAP. Regardless of cause, ACS affects every organ system in a deleterious fashion.[1,2,7] Risk factors for the development of ACS are detailed in Table 75-2.

DIAGNOSIS

Physical examination performs poorly as a diagnostic aid in IAH with a sensitivity of 60%.[8]

Pressure-Volume Metrics

Pressure-volume metrics that aid in monitoring abdominal pressure include the following:

1. Bladder pressures: IAP can be measured with an indwelling bladder catheter and the use of a protocolized transbladder technique that has been approved by the WSACS.[1,2] Problematic measurements may result when the patient is agitated or not supine and when the transducer is not zeroed at the mid-axillary line.
2. Abdominal perfusion pressure (APP), defined as

   $$APP = MAP \text{ (mean arterial pressure)} - IAP$$

   where a normal value is greater than 50 mm Hg.

   Trending the APP may be a useful parameter to follow progression of IAH, but the absolute number does not define ACS. At this time, the WSACS makes "no recommendation" regarding APP as an endpoint of resuscitation or management.[1,2]

Adjunctive Measurements

1. A decreased urine output (UOP) may identify incipient acute kidney injury (AKI) secondary to rising IAP but is equally likely to reflect other problems (e.g., septic AKI, chronic kidney disease [stage III or greater]). UOP is not useful in anuric or dialysis-dependent patients.[9]
2. Elevated airway pressure may aid in identification of dynamic changes in abdominal pressure–volume relationships. When on volume-cycled ventilation, where the tidal volume (V_T) is fixed, increased abdominal

Table 75-1 **IAH Grading Classification**	
Grade	**IAP (mm Hg)**
I	12-15
II	16-20
III	21-25
IV	>25

IAH, intra-abdominal hypertension; *IAP,* intra-abdominal pressure.
From Harman PK, Kron IL, McLaachlan HD, et al. Elevated intraabdominal
pressure and renal function. *Ann Surg.* 1982;196:594–597.

Table 75-2 **Risk Factors for the Development of ACS**
Acidosis (pH<7.2)
Hypothermia (core temperature<33° C)
Massive transfusion (>10 U of packed red blood cells) or resuscitation (>5 L of colloid or crystalloid per 24 hours)
Coagulopathy (platelets <55,000 or activated partial thromboplastin >2 times normal or international normalized ratio >1.5)
Severe sepsis/septic shock (AECC definitions) regardless of source
Bacteremia
Intra-abdominal infection and/or abscess
Hepatic dysfunction or cirrhosis with ascites
Mechanical ventilation
Elevated PEEP or the presence of auto-PEEP
Abdominal surgery (especially with tight fascial closures or massive incisional hernia repair)
Disordered intestinal motility
Intestinal volvulus or intestinal obstruction (mechanical or functional)
Peritoneal or retroperitoneal space occupying lesions
Major burn injury
Major traumatic injury
Body mass index >30 kg/m^2
Prone patient positioning
Acute pancreatitis
Damage control laparotomy
Laparoscopy with excessive inflation pressures
Peritoneal dialysis

Data from references 2 to 4.
ACS, abdominal compartment syndrome; *AECC,* American-European Consensus Conference; *PEEP,* positive end-expiratory pressure.

pressure will increase peak airway pressures. In pressure controlled ventilation, in which the peak pressure is fixed, rising IAP will lead to a decreased V_T. Escalating abdominal pressures will decrease the release volume on airway pressure release ventilation.[10]
3. Various other more sophisticated measures may track changes in pulmonary compliance, pulmonary elastance, and chest wall compliance but appear to provide less fidelity in presaging ACS than the measures noted above. Although ultrasound measurement of IVC diameter has proven useful in identifying hypovolemia, close correlation with IAP has not been noted.[11]

SYSTEMIC IMPACT OF ACS

Increased IAP results in dysfunction of the respiratory, cardiovascular, and renal systems.[12] Elevated ICP and depressed cerebral perfusion pressure (CPP) also may result from increased IAP and ACS.[13]

Cardiovascular System

Increases in IAP elevate intravascular and intrapleural pressures in a manner similar to progressively increased positive end-expiratory pressure (PEEP). Flow per unit time and the stroke volume per cardiac cycle are typically reduced, despite elevated intrathoracic pressures.[12-14]

Cardiac output (CO) decreases progressively as the IAP increases, principally as a result of decreased venous return (VR), diminished pulmonary flow, and impairment of left ventricular filling.[12] The magnitude of the decline in CO may depend on the patient's intravascular volume. One animal study demonstrated a 53% decrease in CO in hypovolemia but only a 17% decrease in euvolemia. CO increased in hypervolemic animals.[15] Thus hypovolemia exacerbates the cardiovascular effects of IAH and ACS.

Respiratory System

Progressive increases in IAP displace the hemidiaphragms cephalad, limiting alveolar filling and creating basilar and posterior alveolar collapse. As a result, adaptive hypoxic pulmonary vasoconstriction is activated and shunt increases. The decrease in pulmonary artery cross-sectional area creates a relative increase in pulmonary artery pressure, impairing right ventricular ejection. This sequence further decreases net pulmonary flow, exacerbating impaired oxygen (O_2) uptake and carbon dioxide (CO_2) off-loading. Complicating these untoward effects is progressive compression of the inferior vena cava (IVC), decreasing VR, further increasing IAP.[18] Increasing PEEP to improve oxygenation and compliance may further impede VR.[19-21] Plasma volume expansion may improve VR but can also increase extravascular lung water. It is clear that the management priority is to relieve the excessive IAH and to restore homeostasis. Alveolar recruitment should be an integral aspect of the management strategy and may help guide ventilation.

Renal System

The renal system is most readily evaluated by following UOP and laboratory data such as serum creatinine concentration. In patients with normal renal function, oliguria (UOP<0.5 mL/kg/hr) is the most commonly identified initial abnormality of IAH.[22] Although changes in creatinine as little as 0.3 mg/dL when accompanied by oliguria for 6 hours or more, meet criteria for AKI, an increase in the creatinine concentration is a late marker of impending AKI; thus, it is a poor index. Various more sensitive biomarkers (e.g., *N*-galactosamine) are gaining acceptance, but most have not been universally accepted.[23] It is important to recall that AKI may also reflect distorted flow or nephrotoxins and that septic AKI is the most common cause of AKI in the critically ill. In animal models of ACS, decompression failed to restore normal biochemistry despite clearly restoring a normal IAP.[24,25]

Although hypovolemic oliguria responds to volume expansion, the response in the presence of IAH and ACS is at best transient. Progressive compression of the IVC and renal veins is exacerbated by decreased flow secondary to compromised CO. These derangements compromise renal blood flow and glomerular filtration rate.[25] Consequently, an inadequate renal filtration gradient and renal perfusion pressure may importantly affect the development of IAH-induced AKI.[26] The filtration gradient is the pressure-driven mechanical force across the glomerulus and is determined by the difference between the glomerular filtration pressure (GFP) and the proximal tubular pressure (PTP). GFP is estimated by the difference between MAP and IAP, where $GFP = MAP - 2(IAP)$. In the presence of IAH or ACS, PTP is assumed to be equal to the IAP. Consequently, changes in IAP are more likely to exert a greater effect on renal function than changes in MAP.[27] Although IAP and renal vein compression recreate the findings of ACS in a laboratory model, extrinsic renal parenchymal compression does not. Interestingly, one model of Gerota fascia incision in the setting of visceral edema also helped reverse some abnormalities.[25,28,33]

Nonrenal Viscera

As IAH progresses to ACS, increasing IAP can compromise splanchnic blood flow. Animal studies indicate that ileal and gastric mucosal blood flow are specifically effected.[35] Hepatic arterial, portal venous, and hepatic microcirculatory blood flow decrease as IAH progresses and may impair hepatic energy production and small bowel tissue oxygen delivery and utilization.[36-41] Unrelieved IAH creates physiology similar to nonocclusive mesenteric ischemia and may lead to intestinal infarction and the need for resection.

Central Nervous System

Because central nervous system activity is dependent on cerebral blood flow, IAP increases that decrease CO and elevate central venous pressure (CVP) may compromise CPP (MAP—either CVP or intracranial pressure [ICP], whichever is higher). Although under normal conditions CVP exceeds ICP, the common association of abdominal injury and traumatic brain injury may make ICP clinically relevant. Indeed, animal studies indicate that elevated IAP increased ICP and decreased CPP, an effect reversed by decompression.[42-44]

Ocular System

The ACS has been associated with the rupture of retinal capillaries, resulting in the sudden onset of decreased central vision (Valsalva retinopathy). The mechanism behind this clinical entity is likely related to the venous hypertension stemming from increased intrathoracic pressure and impeded central VR. Retinal hemorrhage usually resolves within days to months, and no specific treatment is necessary.[45] This diagnosis should be considered in any patient with ACS who develops visual changes.

MANAGEMENT APPROACHES

The therapy for IAH and ACS is reduction in IAP. Achievement of this goal is determined by clinical circumstance and the etiology of the increased IAP. The WSACS has developed a process to address elements that contribute to IAH that includes positional changes, gastric or colonic decompression, temporary neuromuscular blockade, resuscitation with balanced component transfusion therapy, and limited intravenous crystalloid. The WSACS suggests a neutral fluid balance as a therapeutic goal when feasible. The role of albumin, diuretics, and renal support techniques is unclear. Secondary compartment syndrome from ascites may respond to percutaneous drainage.[48-51] A recent unrandomized study compared 31 cases of IAH/ACS managed with a 14FR pigtail catheter with 31 case controls: 81% (25 of 31) of the patients receiving a catheter avoided laparotomy, and 58% survived to discharge.[44] The article noted that evacuation of 1000 mL of volume or a decrease in abdominal pressure by 9 mm Hg was a predictor of successful percutaneous management of IAH. Importantly, the control cohort was surgically decompressed when ACS developed, whereas the treatment group was often decompressed before the development of ACS. Six of 31 patients managed with percutaneous methods developed a subsequent compartment syndrome and required laparotomy.[50] Because of these concerns, the WSASC assigned a grade of 1D (implementation strongly suggested despite very limited evidence) and has called for a randomized trial.[1] Catheter-based management is not recommended for management of visceral edema, retroperitoneal hematoma, or intraperitoneal hemorrhage.

The gold standard for the management of IAH that progresses to ACS is decompressive laparotomy. Although traditionally performed in the operating room (OR), a decompressive laparotomy may be safely undertaken in the intensive care unit (ICU) if mandated by the patient hemodynamic and respiratory instability. These procedures may be completed under deep sedation. Management with advanced ventilation appears to drive the need to operate in the ICU just as strongly as does hemodynamic instability that precludes safe transport as well as the time required for transport to the OR.[50] Repeat laparotomy, lavage, and temporary closure can also be safely achieved in the ICU setting.[51] The initial unpacking of a patient who has undergone a decompressive procedure may best be undertaken in the OR, but immediate relief of ACS can be emergently undertaken in the ICU.

Abdominal decompression is often associated with precipitous hemodynamic changes reflecting a sudden increase in VR. Heart rate often decreases, MAP increases, pulse pressure widens, and peak/mean/plateau pressures decrease with an increase in arterial oxygen saturation (Sao$_2$). The diaphragms are no longer displaced cephalad; thus, alveolar recruitment more readily occurs. Airway pressure release ventilation and pressure-based ventilation may then lead to substantial pulmonary distension in the increasingly compliant lungs.

On occasion, abdominal decompression may trigger unanticipated abrupt or worsened hypotension. Two possible etiologies have been proposed for this phenomenon: (1) an acute dilatation of the precapillary arteriolar sphincters[52] and (2) reperfusion of ischemic tissues, which releases vasoactive ischemic byproducts, including a large metabolic acid load.[53] Conflicting data regarding the use of bicarbonate-based solutions with regard to outcome have limited its use in the absence of a hyperchloremic acidosis.

Vacuum-based devices are currently recommended for the management of the open abdomen, although many temporary closure systems are available.[54,55] A systematic review of the available literature on open abdomen management highlighted a lack of prospective data on the effects of different approaches on outcome.[55]

Regardless of the technique selected, the many management priorities remain the same. The ability to easily gain access to the abdominal cavity for planned or unplanned reoperations is crucial during the early decompression period. The abdominal viscera must be protected from the exterior environment and from evaporative losses. Two issues merit special discussion: (1) protein loss and (2) creatinine clearance across the open abdomen. Aspirated fluid across the open abdomen contains approximately 2 g of protein per liter removed.[56] Accelerated protein loss is not routinely assessed, but it should be anticipated and addressed in the nutritional prescription. More importantly, reexploration and lavage with normotonic solution (commonly 0.9% normal saline solution [NSS] or lactated Ringer's solution) will mimic peritoneal dialysis. Although standard dialysis solutions have been evaluated as lavage solutions for the open abdomen, the focus has been on hemodynamic profile and visceral volume, not transperitoneal creatinine clearance. Understanding the contribution of the open abdomen to clearance may help inform pharmacologic dosing of therapeutic agents.

Finally, timing of definitive abdominal closure remains controversial after abdominal decompression. The open abdomen is associated with significant morbidity. Loss of abdominal domain and lateralization of the abdominal fascia may lead to large soft tissue deficits. Indeed, management with an open abdomen approach that leads to a giant ventral hernia is strongly associated with a reduced quality of life for up to 5 years after the index laparotomy.[57] Enterocutaneous or enteroatmospheric fistula are estimated to occur in 20% of patients managed with an open abdomen.[58,59] Evidence suggests that risk of complications, namely enteroatmospheric fistulization, increases if primary closure is delayed beyond 8 days.

The WSACS has endorsed protocolized efforts to obtain an early or at least same-hospital-stay abdominal fascial closure.[1] However, the best method of definitive closure remains controversial. Primary fascial closure is associated with a 30% hernia rate, and oftentimes it is not possible because of the large soft tissue defects and fascial retraction associated with open abdominal management. At this time, the role of component separation at index hospitalization is unclear. Functional closure utilizes a biologic mesh to bridge the resultant fascial defect. At best, there is an 80% hernia rate associated with this method of closure.[60-62]

Furthermore, avoidance of bioprosthetic mesh is suggested, according to WSACS guidelines. Finally, planned ventral hernia accepts the fascial defect with either a skin-only closure or split thickness skin grafting onto bowel. A time interval of 6 to 12 months allows dissolution of adhesion vascularity to minimize the risk of bowel injury at subsequent definitive closure.[61]

AUTHORS' RECOMMENDATIONS

- Early recognition and treatment are of prime importance when managing patients with IAH and ACS.
- Plasma volume expansion and relief of IAH or ACS may not reverse the untoward effect on end-organ function, especially within the renal system.
- ACS deleteriously affects blood flow and oxygen delivery in every organ system.
- Early intervention to manage IAH may retard progression to ACS and should be undertaken in a tiered fashion.
- It is important to measure bladder pressure in the correct fashion. Instilling too much irrigant may cause falsely elevated IAP readings and lead to overly aggressive treatment.
- ACS may occur even after decompressive laparotomy was performed, requiring loosening of the temporary abdominal dressings or unplanned laparotomy for management.

REFERENCES

1. Kirkpatrick AW, Roberts DJ, De Waele J, et al. Intra-abdominal hypertension and the abdominal compartment syndrome: updated concensus definitions and clinical practice guidelines from the World Society of Abdominal Compartment Syndrome. *Intensive Care Med*. 2013;39:1190–1206.
2. Malbrain NG, Cheatham ML, Kirkpatrick A, et al. Results from the international conference of experts on intra-abdominal hypertension and abdominal compartment syndrome. *Intensive Care Med*. 2006;32:1722–1732.
3. World Society of Abdominal Compartment Syndrome. 2013. Accessed 27.06.14, from https://www.wsacs.org.
4. Deleted in review.
5. Wilson A, Longhi J, Goldman C, Mcnatt S. Intra-abdominal pressure and the morbidly obese patient: the effect of body mass index. *J Trauma*. 2010;69(1):78–83.
6. Deleted in review.
7. Gracias VH, Braslow B, Johnson J, et al. Abdominal compartment syndrome in the open abdomen. *Arch Surg*. 2002;137:1298–1300.
8. Sugrue M, Bauman A, Jones F, et al. Clinical examination is an inaccurate predictor of intraabdominal pressure. *World J Surg*. 2002;26:1428–1431.
9. Mohmand H, Goldfarb S. Renal dysfunction associated with intra-abdominal hypertension and the abdominal compartment syndrome. *JASN*. 2011;22(4):615–621.
10. Pelosi P, Quintel M, Malbrain ML. Effect of intra-abdominal pressure on respiratory mechanics. *Acta Clin Belg Suppl*. 2007;62(1):78–88.
11. Wachsberg RH. Elevated intraabdominal pressure: sonographic observations. *J Ultrasound Med*. 2000;19:217–222.
12. Schein M, Wittmann DH, Aprahamian CC, et al. The abdominal compartment syndrome: the physiological and clinical consequences of elevated intra-abdominal pressure. *J Am Coll Surg*. 1995;180:745–753.
13. Cheatham M. Abdominal compartment syndrome. *Scand J Trauma Resusc Emerg Med*. 2009;17:10.
14. Cheatham M, Malbrain M. Abdominal perfusion pressure. In: Ivatury R, Cheatham M, Malbrain M, Sugrue M, eds. *Abdominal Compartment Syndrome*. Georgetown, TX: Landes Bioscience; 2006:69–81.
15. Wauters J, Claus P, Brosens N, et al. Relationship between abdominal pressure, pulmonary compliance, and cardiac preload in a porcine model. *Crit Care Res Pract*. 2012;2012:1–6.

16. Deleted in review.
17. Deleted in review.
18. Wittmann D. The compartment syndrome of the abdominal cavity. *J Intensive Care Med.* 2000;15:201–220.
19. Burchard KW, MCiombor D, McLeod MK, Slothman GJ, Gann DS. Positive end expiratory pressure with increased intra-abdominal pressure. *Surg Gynecol Obstet.* 1985;161:313–318.
20. Regli A, Mahendran R, Fysh ET, et al. Matching positive end-expiratory pressure to intra-abdominal pressure improves oxygenation in a porcine sick lung model of intra-abdominal hypertension. *Crit Care.* 2012;16(5):R208.
21. Krebs J, Pelosi P, Tsagogiorgas C, Alb M, Luecke T. Effects of positive end-expiratory pressure on respiratory function and hemodynamics in patients with acute respiratory failure with and without intra-abdominal hypertension: a pilot study. *Crit Care.* 2009;13(5):R160.
22. Dennen P, Douglas IS, Anderson R. Acute kidney injury in the intensive care unit: an update and primer for the intensivist. *Crit Care Med.* January 2010;38(1):261–275.
23. Ronco C. *N-GAL:* diagnosing AKI as soon as possible. *Crit Care.* 2007;11(6):173.
24. Mohmand H, Goldfarb S. Renal dysfunction associated with intra-abdominal hypertension and the abdominal compartment syndrome. *JASN.* 2011;22(4):615–621.
25. Doty JM, Saggi BH, Blocher CR, et al. Effects of increased renal parenchymal pressure on renal function. *J Trauma.* May 2000;48(5):874–877.
26. De Waele JJ, De Laet I. Intra-abdominal hypertension and the effect on renal function. *Acta Clin Belg Suppl.* 2007;2:371–374.
27. Sugrue M, Hallal A, D'Amours S. Intra-abdominal hypertension and the kidney. In: Ivatury RR, Cheatham ML, Malbrain MLNG, Sugrue M, eds. *Abdominal Compartment Syndrome.* Georgetown, Texas: Landes Biosciences; 2006:119–128.
28. Harman PK, Kron IL, McLaachlan HD, et al. Elevated intraabdominal pressure and renal function. *Ann Surg.* 1982;196:594–597.
29. Deleted in review.
30. Deleted in review.
31. Deleted in review.
32. Deleted in review.
33. Bloomfield GL, Blocher CR, Fakhry IF, et al. Elevated intra-abdominal pressure increases plasma renin activity and aldosterone levels. *J Trauma.* 1997;42:997–1005.
34. Deleted in review.
35. Diebel LN, Dulchavsky SA, Wilson RF. Effect of increased intra-abdominal pressure on mesenteric arterial and intestinal mucosal blood flow. *J Trauma.* 1992;33:45–49.
36. Caldwell CB, Ricotta JJ. Changes in visceral blood flow with elevated intraabdominal pressure. *J Surg Res.* 1987;43:14–20.
37. Nakatani T, Sakamoto Y, Kaneko I, et al. Effects of intraabdominal hypertension on hepatic energy metabolism in rabbits. *J Trauma.* 1997;43:192.
38. Pusajó JF, Bumaschny E, Agurrola A, et al. Postoperative intra-abdominal pressure: its relation to splanchnic perfusion, sepsis, multiple organ failure and surgical reintervention. *Intensive Crit Care Dig.* 1994;13:2–4.
39. Bongard F, Pianim N, Dubecz S, et al. Adverse consequences of increased intraabdominal pressure on bowel tissue oxygen. *J Trauma.* 1995;39:519–525.
40. Bloomfield GL, Ridings PC, Blocher CR, et al. Increased pleural pressure mediates the effects of elevated intra-abdominal pressure upon the central nervous and cardiovascular systems. *Surg Forum.* 1995;46:572–574.
41. Bloomfield GL, Ridings PC, Blocher CR, et al. Effects of increased intra-abdominal pressure upon intracranial and cerebral perfusion pressure before and after volume expansion. *J Trauma.* 1996;40:936–943.
42. Bloomfield GL, Ridings PC, Blocher CR, et al. A proposed relationship between increased intra-abdominal, intrathoracic, and intracranial pressure. *Crit Care Med.* 1997;25:496–503.
43. Priluck IA, Blodgett DW. The effects of increased intra-abdominal pressure on the eyes. *Nebr Med J.* 1996;81:8–9.
44. Reed SF, Britt RC, Collins J, et al. Aggressive surveillance and early catheter-directed therapy in the management of intra-abdominal hypertension. *J Trauma.* 2006;61:1359–1365.
45. Radenkovic DV, Bajec D, Ivancevic N, et al. Decompressive laparotomy with temporary abdominal closure versus percutaneous puncture with placement of abdominal catheter in patients with abdominal compartment syndrome during acute pancreatitis: background and design of multicenter, randomized, controlled study. *BMC Surg.* 2010;10:22.
46. Cheatham ML, Safcsak K. Percutaneous catheter decompression in the treatment of elevated intraabdominal pressure. *Chest.* 2011;140:1428–1435.
47. Latenser BA, Kowal-Vern A, Kimball D, et al. A pilot study comparing percutaneous decompression with decompressive laparotomy for acute abdominal compartment syndrome in thermal injury. *J Burn Care Rehabil.* 2002;23:190–195.
48. Piper G, Maerz LL, Schuster KM, et al. When the ICU is the operating room. *J Trauma Acute Care Surg.* 2013;74(3):871–875.
49. Diaz JJ, Mejia V, Subhawong AP, Subhawong T, Miller RS, O'Neill PJ. Protocol for bedside laparotomy in trauma and emergency general surgery: a low return to the operating room. *Am Surg.* 2005;1(11):986–991.
50. Shelly MP, Robinson AA, Hesford JW, et al. Haemodynamic effects following surgical release of increased intra-abdominal pressure. *Br J Anaesth.* 1987;59:800–805.
51. Morris JA, Eddy VA, Blinman TA, et al. The staged celiotomy for trauma: issues in unpacking and reconstruction. *Ann Surg.* 1993;217:576–586.
52. Perez D, Wildi S, Demartines N, et al. Prospective evaluation of vacuum-assisted closure in abdominal compartment syndrome and severe abdominal sepsis. *J Am Coll Surg.* 2007;205:586–592.
53. DJ1 R, Zygun DA, Grendar J, et al. Negative-pressure wound therapy for critically ill adults with open abdominal wounds: a systematic review. *J Trauma Acute Care Surg.* 2012;73(3):629–639.
54. Cheatham ML, Safcsak K, Brzezinski SJ, Lube MW. Nitrogen balance, protein loss, and the open abdomen. *Crit Care Med.* 2007;35:127.
55. Zarzaur BL, DiCocco JM, Fabian TC. Quality of life after abdominal reconstruction following open abdomen. *J Trauma.* 2011:285–291.
56. Miller RS, Morris Jr JA, Diaz Jr JJ, Herring MB, May AK. Complications after 344 damage-control open celiotomies. *J Trauma.* 2005;59(6):1365.
57. Rao M, Burke D, Finan PJ, Sagar PM. The use of vacuum-assisted closure of abdominal wounds: a word of caution. *Colorectal Dis.* 2007;9(3):266–268.
58. DiCocco JM, Magnotti LJ, Emmett KP, et al. Long-term follow-up of abdominal wall reconstruction after planned ventral hernia: a 15-year experience. *J Am Coll Surg.* 2010;210:686.
59. Diaz Jr JJ, Guy J, Berkes MB, et al. Acellular dermal allograft for ventral hernia repair in the compromised surgical field. *Am Surg.* 2006;72:1181.
60. Jin J, Rosen MJ, Blatnik J, et al. Use of acellular dermal matrix for complicated ventral hernia repair: does technique affect outcomes? *J Am Coll Surg.* 2007;205:654.
61. Jernigan TW, Fabian TC, Croce MA, et al. Staged management of giant abdominal wall defects: acute and long-term results. *Ann Surg.* 2003;238:349.
62. Diaz Jr JJ, Dutton WD, Ott MM, et al. Eastern Association for the Surgery of Trauma: a review of the management of the open abdomen–part 2 "Management of the open abdomen". *J Trauma.* 2011;71:502.

76 How Should Patients with Burns Be Managed in the Intensive Care Unit?

Marc G. Jeschke

More than 500,000 burn injuries occur annually in the United States.[1] Although most are minor, approximately 40,000 to 60,000 burn patients require admission to a hospital or major burn center for appropriate treatment every year.[2] The devastating consequences of burns have resulted in the allocation of significant clinical and research resources. This has led to improved care. Indeed, reports reveal a 50% decline in burn-related deaths and hospital admissions in the United States during the past 20 years. This reflects effective prevention strategies decreasing the number and severity of burns.[3,4] Advances in therapy strategies, based on implementation of critical care bundles, improved understanding of resuscitation, enhanced wound coverage, better support of the hypermetabolic response to injury, more appropriate infection control, and improved treatment of inhalation injury, improved the clinical outcome of this unique patient population. It is important to recognize that successful management of burn patients requires a diversified and multidisciplinary approach. This chapter gives an overview of the evidenced-based management of severely burned patients in the intensive care unit (ICU).

INITIAL ASSESSMENT AND EMERGENCY TREATMENT

All burned patients should initially be managed as trauma patients, following the guidelines of the American College of Surgeons Committee on Trauma and the Advanced Trauma Live Support Center.[5] The algorithms for trauma evaluation should be diligently applied to the burn patient. In particular, any wheezing, stridor, hoarseness, or tachypnea may be a sign of airway compromise. Tracheal tugging, carbonaceous sputum, soot around the patient's airway passages, and singed facial or nasal hair may suggest an airway burn or smoke inhalation. As in any trauma patient, progression to the next step in the primary survey is delayed until a proper airway is established and maintained.

Cardiac performance may be difficult to evaluate in the burn victim. In particular, burned extremities may impede the ability to obtain a blood pressure reading. In these situations, arterial lines, particularly femoral lines, are useful to monitor continuous blood pressure readings. Use of a pulmonary artery catheter (PAC) may be beneficial in the assessment of cardiovascular performance in certain situations (e.g., inadequate noninvasive monitoring, difficult-to-define end points of resuscitation),[6] but the general practicability, risk-to-benefit ratio, and lack of mortality reduction when the PAC is used have been widely criticized. Currently, there are no studies in burn patients that provide evidence-based recommendations. For disadvantages of the PAC to be overcome, less-invasive techniques have been developed.[7] None of these, though, is specific to burn patients. Several descriptive studies using PiCCO technology, in which cardiac performance is approximated with an arterial thermodilution catheter, have been conducted in burn patients.[8,9] Prospective trials are underway.

FLUID RESUSCITATION

Severe burns cause significant hemodynamic changes. These must be managed carefully to optimize intravascular volume, maintain end-organ tissue perfusion, and maximize oxygen delivery to the tissues.[10] Massive fluid shifts after severe burn injury result in the sequestration of fluid in burned and unburned tissue.[11] The result of this generalized edema may be burn shock, a leading cause of mortality in severely burned patients.[12-14] Therefore early and accurate fluid resuscitation of patients with major burns is critical for survival.[15] Calculations of fluid requirements are based on the amount of body surface involved in second- or third-degree burns (not first-degree burns). The "rule of nines" (Fig. 76-1, A) has been used to estimate the area of burned body surface, but this rule has limitations in children, in whom the head is proportionally larger than the body. A more accurate assessment can be made of burn injury, especially in children, by using the Lund and Browder chart, which takes into account changes associated with growth (Fig. 76-1, B). Various resuscitation formulas have been used. These differ in the amount of crystalloid and colloid to be given and in fluid tonicity (Table 76-1).[10,16] The modified Brooke and Parkland (Baxter) formulas are the most commonly used early resuscitation formulas,[17] but no formula will accurately predict the volume requirements of an individual patient.

556

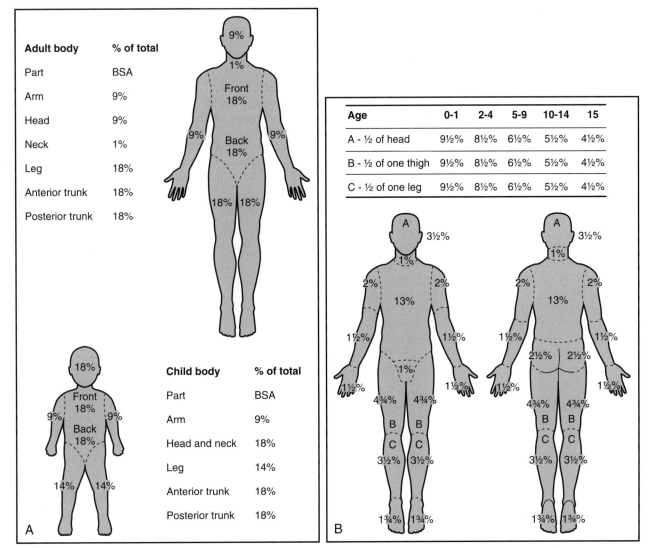

Figure 76-1. **A,** Estimation of burn size with the "rule of nines." **B,** Estimation of burn size with the Lund and Browder method. *BSA,* body surface area.

Table 76-1 Formulas for Estimating Adult Burn Patient Resuscitation Fluid Needs

Colloid Formula	Electrolyte	Colloid
Evans	Normal saline, 1.0 mL/kg/%burn	1.0 cc/kg/%burn
Brooke	Lactated Ringer's solution, 1.5 mL/kg/% burn	0.5 mL/kg
Slater	Lactated Ringer's solution, 2 L/24 hr	Fresh-frozen plasma, 75 mL/kg/24 hr
Crystalloid formulas Parkland Modified	Lactated Ringer's solution Lactated Ringer's solution	4 mL/kg/%burn 2 mL/kg/%burn
Hypertonic saline solutions Monafo Warden	Volume to maintain urine output at 30 mL/hr; fluid contains 250 mEq Na/L. Lactated Ringer's solution +50 mEq NaHCO₃ (180 mEq Na/L) for 8 hr to maintain urine output at 30-50 mL/hr. Lactated Ringer's solution to maintain urine output at 30-50 mL/hr beginning 8 hr postburn.	
Dextran formula (Demling)	Dextran 40 in saline, 2 mL/kg/hr for 8 hr. Lactated Ringer's solution, volume to maintain urine output at 30 mL/hr. Fresh-frozen plasma, 0.5 mL/kg/hr for 18 hr beginning 8 hr postburn.	

From Warden GD. Burn shock resuscitation. *World J Surg.* 1992; 16:16–23.
Na, sodium; *NaHCO₃,* sodium bicarbonate.

In children, maintenance requirements must be added to the resuscitation formula. The Galveston and Cincinnati Shriners Burns Hospitals have devised formulas (Table 76-2). Intravascular volume status must be reevaluated frequently during the acute phase. Fluid balance during burn shock resuscitation is typically measured by hourly urine output through an indwelling urethral catheter. It has been recommended to maintain a urine output of approximately 0.5 mL/kg per hour in adults[18] and 0.5 to 1.0 mL/kg per hour in patients weighing less than 30 kg.[19] No clinical studies, though, have identified the optimal hourly urine output to maintain vital organ perfusion during burn shock resuscitation. Because large volumes of fluid and electrolytes are administered initially and throughout the course of resuscitation, it is important to obtain baseline laboratory measurements.[20] Crystalloid, in particular lactated Ringer's solution, is the most popular resuscitation fluid currently used for burn patients.[21] Colloid and crystalloid solutions have been used. No outcome differences between the two have been identified despite extensive study.[22-25] Proponents of the use of crystalloid solutions alone report that other solutions, specifically colloids, are not better and are more expensive.[26] Nonetheless, most burn surgeons agree that patients with low serum albumin during burn shock may benefit from albumin supplementation to maintain oncotic pressure.[27]

INHALATION INJURY

Inhalation injury constitutes one of the most critical problems accompanying thermal insult, with mortality paralleling that for acute respiratory distress syndrome in patients requiring ventilator support for more than 1 week.[28,29] Early diagnosis of bronchopulmonary injury is initiated by a history of closed-space exposure; facial burns; or carbonaceous debris in the mouth, pharynx, or sputum.[30] There are few evidence-based data regarding inhalation injury, though. Therefore the standard diagnostic method is bronchoscopy. Endorf and Gamelli established a grading system for inhalation injury (0, 1, 2, 3, and 4) derived from findings at initial bronchoscopy and based on Abbreviated Injury Score criteria.[31] Bronchoscopic criteria that are consistent with inhalation injury included airway edema, inflammation, mucosal necrosis, presence of soot and charring in the airway, tissue sloughing, or carbonaceous material in the airway. At this time, though, there are neither uniform diagnosis criteria nor standardized treatment guidelines. Management of inhalation injury consists of ventilatory support, aggressive pulmonary

toilet, bronchoscopic removal of casts, and nebulization therapy.[10] According to the American Burn Association guidelines, prophylactic antibiotics are not indicated.

INFECTION/SEPSIS

Severely burned patients are susceptible to various infectious complications.[32] Because burns induce a systemic inflammatory response,[33] specific guidelines for the diagnosis and treatments of wound infection and sepsis in burns have been formulated (Table 76-3).

Table 76-3 Definition of Burn Sepsis

American Burn Association Consensus Definition on Burn Sepsis

- At least 3 of the following parameters:
  - T >38.5° C or <36.5° C
- Progressive tachycardia >90 beats/min in adults or >2 SD above age-specific norms in children
- Progressive tachypnea >30 beats/min in adults or >2 SD above age-specific norms in children
- WBC >12,000 or <4000 in adults or >2 SD above age-specific norms in children
- Refractory hypotension: SBP <90 mm Hg, MAP <70, or an SBP decrease >40 mm Hg in adults or < 2 SD below normal for age in children
- Thrombocytopenia: Platelet count <100,000/μL in adults, < 2 SD below norms in children
- Hyperglycemia: Plasma glucose >110 mg/dL or 7.7 mM/L in the absence of diabetes
- Enteral feeding intolerance (residual >150 mL/hr in children or 2 times feeding rate in adults; diarrhea >2500 mL/day for adults or >400 mL/day in children)

and

Pathologic tissue source identified: >105 bacteria on quantitative wound tissue biopsy or microbial invasion on biopsy

Bacteremia or fungemia

Documented infection as defined by Centers for Disease Control.

From Greenhalgh DG, Saffle JR, Holmes JH et al. American Burn Association consensus conference to define sepsis and infection in burns. *J Burn Care Res.* 2007; 28:776–790.
MAP, mean arterial pressure; *SBP,* systolic blood pressure; *SD,* standard deviation; *T,* temperature; *WBC,* white blood cell count.

Table 76.2 Formulas for Estimating Pediatric Resuscitation Needs

Cincinnati Shriners Burns Hospital	4 mL × kg × % total BSA burn + 1500 mL × m² BSA	1st 8 hr 2nd 8 hr 3rd 8 hr	Lactated Ringer's solution + 50 mg NaHCO₃ Lactated Ringer's solution Lactated Ringer's solution + 12.5 g albumin
Galveston Shriners Burns Hospital	5000 mL/m² BSA burn + 2000 mL/m² BSA	Lactated Ringer's solution + 12.5 g albumin	

BSA, body surface area; *NaHCO₃,* sodium bicarbonate.

BURN WOUND EXCISION

Methods for handling burn wounds have changed in recent decades. Increasingly, aggressive early tangential excision of the burn tissue and early wound closure primarily by skin grafts have led to significant improvement of mortality rates and substantially lower costs in this particular patient population.[10,34-37] Early wound closure also has been associated with decreased severity of hypertrophic scarring, joint contractures and stiffness, and quicker rehabilitation.[10,34] Techniques of burn wound excision have evolved substantially over the past decade. Published estimates of bleeding associated with these operations range between 3.5% and 5% of the blood volume for every 1% of the body surface excised.[38,39] Burn wound excision should occur in the operating room soon after the patient is admitted; however, sometimes excision may be necessary in the ICU.

METABOLIC RESPONSE AND NUTRITIONAL SUPPORT

The metabolic consequences of severe burn injury are profound, and their modulation constitutes an ongoing challenge for successful treatment. Metabolic rates of burn victims exceed those of most other critically ill patients and cause marked wasting of lean body mass within days of injury.[40] Failure to meet the subsequent energy and protein requirements may result in impaired wound healing, organ dysfunction, increased susceptibility to infection, and death.[41] Thus adequate nutrition is imperative. Because of the significant increase in postburn energy expenditure, high-calorie nutritional support was thought to decrease muscle metabolism,[42] but a randomized, double-blind, prospective study found that aggressive high-calorie feeding with a combination of enteral and parenteral nutrition was associated with increased mortality.[43] Therefore most authors recommend adequate calorie intake through early enteral feeding and avoidance of overfeeding.[10,40] Different formulas have been developed to address the specific energy requirements of burned adult and pediatric patients[44-46] (Tables 76-4 and 76-5). The caloric requirements in adult burn patients most often are calculated using the Curreri formula. This calls for 25 kcal/kg per day plus 40 kcal/%BSAB (percentage of total body surface area burned) per day.[47] Recommendations suggest administration of 1 to 2 g/kg per day of protein.[41] Because of glucose intolerance and futile cycling in critical illness, most ICUs provide a significant amount of caloric requirements as fat.[41,48] Burn patients exhibit lipid intolerance, though, that may result in hyperlipidemia and fatty liver infiltration that is associated with a higher incidence of infection and higher postoperative mortality rates.[49-51,52] Thus the extent to which exogenous lipid can be used as an energy source is limited.[48,53,54] Studies in a large cohort of severely burned children demonstrated that patients receiving a low-fat, high-carbohydrate diet had a significantly lower incidence of fatty liver on autopsy. Relative to historic controls, these patients had a significantly lower incidence of sepsis, prolonged

Table 76-4 Formulas for Estimating Caloric Requirements in Adult Burn Patients

Formula	Age/Sex	Equation
Harris-Benedict[84]	Men	$BEE\ (kcal/day) = 66.5 + (13.75 \times W) + (5.03 \times H) - (6.76 \times A)$
	Women	$BEE\ (kcal/day) = 655 + (9.56 \times W) + (1.85 \times H) - (4.68 \times A)$

Comment: Multiply BEE by stress factor of 1.2–2.0 (1.2–1.5 sufficient for most burns) to estimate caloric requirement.

Formula	Age/Sex	Equation
Curreri[44]	Age: 16-59 yr	$Calories\ (kcal/day) = (25 \times W) + (40 \times \%BSAB)$
	Age: >60 yr	$Calories = (20 \times W) + (65 \times \%BSAB)$

Comment: Specific for burns, may significantly overestimate energy requirements, maximum 50% BSAB.

A, age (yr); *BEE,* basal energy expenditure; *%BSAB,* percentage of total body surface area burned; *H,* height (cm); *W,* weight (kg).

Table 76-5 Formulas for Estimating Caloric Requirements in Pediatric Burn Patients

Formula	Sex/Age	Equation (daily requirement in kcal)
WHO[85]	Males	
	0-3 yr	$(60.9 \times W) - 54$
	3-10 yr	$(22.7 \times W) + 495$
	10-18 yr	$(17.5 \times W) + 651$
	Females	
	0-3 yr	$(61.0 \times W) - 51$
	3-10 yr	$(22.5 \times W) + 499$
	10-18 yr	$(12.2 \times W) + 746$
RDA[86]	0-6 mo	$108 \times W$
	6 mo to 1 yr	$98 \times W$
	1-3 yr	$102 \times W$
	4-10 yr	$90 \times W$
	11-14 yr	$55 \times W$
Curreri junior[87]	<1 yr	$RDA + (15 \times \%BSAB)$
	103 yr	$RDA + (25 \times \%BSAB)$
	4-15 yr	$RDA + (40 \times \%BSAB)$
Galveston infant[88]	0-1 yr	$2100\ kcal/m^2\ BSA + 1000\ kcal/m^2\ BSAB$
Galveston revised[46]	1-11 yr	$1800\ kcal/m^2\ BSA + 1300\ kcal/m^2\ BSAB$
Galveston adolescent[89]	12+	$1500\ kcal/m^2\ BSA + 1500\ kcal/m^2\ BSAB$

BSA, body surface area; *BSAB,* body surface area burned; *%BSAB,* percentage of total body surface area burned; *RDA,* Recommended Dietary Allowance (U.S.); *WHO,* World Health Organization.

survival, and significantly shorter stays in the ICU (grade C data). On the basis of these findings, I recommend that nutritional regimens for treatment of burn patients include a significantly reduced proportion of fat as the source of total caloric intake.

Diminished gastrointestinal absorption, increased urinary losses, altered distribution, and altered carrier protein concentrations after severe burns may lead to micronutrient deficiency. These deficiencies in trace elements and vitamins (Cu, Fe, Se, Zn, vitamins C and E) have been repeatedly described in major burns[55-57] and may lead to infectious complications, delayed wound healing, and stunting in children.[58] Thus supplementation would seem appropriate, but evidence-based practice guidelines are not currently available. Enhancing trace element status and antioxidant defenses by supplementing selenium, zinc, and copper was shown to decrease the incidence of nosocomial pneumonia in critically ill, severely burned patients in two consecutive, randomized double-blind trials.[59] Caution should be used to avoid toxic side effects.

MODULATION OF THE HORMONAL AND ENDOCRINE RESPONSE

Modification of adverse components of the hypermetabolic response to burn injury, particularly protein catabolism, would seem to be desirable. β-Adrenergic blockade, β-adrenergic supplementation, anabolic steroids, recombinant growth hormone, and insulin-like growth factor (IGF) are under active investigation. Various studies have demonstrated the potential beneficial effect of beta blockers in burn patients. In a single-center study, administration of propranolol in doses that decrease the heart rate by approximately 15% to 20% from baseline reduced the release of free fatty acids from adipose tissue, decreased hepatic triacylglycerol storage and fat accumulation, and reversed muscle protein catabolism.[60-62] In a retrospective study of adult burn patients, use of beta blockers was associated with decreased mortality, wound infection rate, and wound healing time.[63] Therefore beta blockers appear to have high potential as an anticatabolic treatment in severely burned patients.

Treatment with anabolic agents, such as oxandrolone, a testosterone analog, improved muscle protein catabolism through enhanced protein synthesis efficiency,[64] reduced weight loss, and increased donor site wound healing.[65] In a prospective randomized study, Wolf and colleagues demonstrated that administration of 10 mg of oxandrolone every 12 hours decreased hospital length of stay.[66] In a large prospective, double-blind, randomized single-center study, oxandrolone given at a dose of 0.1 mg/kg every 12 hours shortened acute hospital length of stay, maintained lean body mass, and improved body composition and hepatic protein synthesis.[67]

The use of recombinant human growth hormone in daily subcutaneous doses has been reported to accelerate donor site healing and restore earlier positive nitrogen balance.[68-70] Indeed, administration of 0.05 mg/kg of recombinant human growth hormone given over a 12-month period after burn injury significantly improved height, weight, lean body mass, bone mineral content, cardiac function, and muscle strength.[71] These findings are in contrast to those of Takala and colleagues[72] and with studies showing that growth hormone treatment induced hyperglycemia and insulin resistance.[70,73] It is likely that the prolonged catabolic nature of burn injury and perhaps the dose account for these discrepant results. IGF-1 has been shown to decrease the metabolic rate after burn injury and to increase whole-body anabolic activity without hyperglycemia or insulin resistance.[74] Studies by Van den Berghe and colleagues indicate that the use of IGF-1 alone is not effective in critically ill patients without burns.[74a] Again, the prolonged catabolic nature of burn injury may explain the difference.

GLUCOSE CONTROL

A prominent component of the hypermetabolic response after burn injury is hyperglycemia and insulin resistance.[75] These result from both an increase in hepatic gluconeogenesis and impaired insulin-mediated glucose transport into skeletal muscle cardiac muscle and adipose tissue.[76-79] Hyperglycemia and elevations in circulating insulin concentrations are of serious clinical concern. Hyperglycemia has been linked to impaired wound healing, increased infectious complications, and increased mortality.[80-83] A randomized controlled trial in severely burned pediatric patients indicated superiority for glucose control using insulin.[83a] Epub 2010 Apr 15.). Care providers need to be vigilant of an increased incidence of hypoglycemia that is associated with a 4- to 9-fold increase in morbidity and mortality.

CONCLUSION

Burn injuries alter several physiologic functions and are associated with substantial morbidity and mortality. Appropriate early and continued fluid resuscitation likely improves tissue perfusion and limits organ system failure. Likewise, early excision of burn wounds and topical antimicrobial agents may limit sepsis. Patients who have sustained an inhalation injury also may require additional support. Enteral tube feeding is useful to control stress ulceration, maintain intestinal mucosal integrity, and provide fuel for the resulting hypermetabolic state. β-Adrenergic blockade is recommended by many burn units as an anticatabolic treatment. Centralized care in burn units has promoted a concentrated team approach that has promoted clinical studies to examine such issues as fluid resuscitation, nutrition, wound excision, and temporary wound coverage. Further studies are required to address the primary determinants of death, inhalation injury complications, and pneumonia as well as to ameliorate pain and scar formation. Through the use of aggressive resuscitation, nutritional support, infection control, surgical therapy, and early rehabilitation, better psychological and physical results can be achieved for burn patients.

AUTHOR'S RECOMMENDATIONS

- Burn patients should be managed initially as trauma patients. Algorithms for trauma evaluation should be diligently applied to the burn patient.
- Early and accurate fluid resuscitation of patients with major burns is critical for survival, but overaggressive resuscitation should be avoided, particularly in small children younger than 4 years.
- Early diagnosis of bronchopulmonary injury is critical. Management of inhalation injury consists of ventilatory support, aggressive pulmonary toilet, bronchoscopic removal of casts, and nebulization therapy.
- Adequate nutritional intake through enteral tube feeding will aid in the control of stress ulceration, preserve intestinal mucosal integrity, and provide fuel for the resulting hypermetabolic state. Nutritional regimes for treatment of burn patients include a significantly reduced proportion of fat as the source of total caloric intake.
- Modulation of the hypermetabolic response improves outcomes.
- Hyperglycemia in burn patients is associated with increased complications and needs to be controlled to a target level of 130 mg/dL. Hypoglycemia needs to be avoided because it leads to increased mortality after burn.

REFERENCES

1. Guidelines for the operation of burn centers. *J Burn Care Res.* 2007;28:134–141.
2. Nguyen TT, Gilpin DA, Meyer NA, Herndon DN. Current treatment of severely burned patients. *Ann Surg.* 1996;223:14–25.
3. Brigham PA, McLoughlin E. Burn incidence and medical care use in the United States: estimates, trends, and data sources. *J Burn Care Rehabil.* 1996;17:95–107.
4. Wolf SE. Critical care in the severely burned: organ support and management of complications. In: Herndon DN, ed. *Total Burn Care.* 3rd ed. London: Saunders; 2007.
5. American College of Surgeons Committee on Trauma. *Resources of Optimal Care of the Injured Patient.* Chicago: American College of Surgeons; 1993.
6. Pulmonary Artery Catheter Consensus Conference. Consensus Statement. *Crit Care Med.* 1997;25:910–925.
7. Della Rocca G, Costas MG. Intrathoracic blood volume: Clinical Applications. In: Jean-Louis V, ed. *Yearbook of Intensive Care and Emergency Medicine.* Berlin: Springer; 2006:142–151.
8. Branski LK, Herndon DN, Byrd JF, et al. Transpulmonary thermodilution for hemodynamic measurements in severely burned children. *Crit Care.* 2011;15(2):R118. http://dx.doi.org/10.1186/cc10147. Epub 2011 Apr 21.
9. Kraft R, Herndon DN, Branski LK, Finnerty CC, Leonard KR, Jeschke MG. Optimized fluid management improves outcomes of pediatric burn patients. *J Surg Res.* May 1, 2013;181(1):121–128. http://dx.doi.org/10.1016/j.jss.2012.05.058. Epub 2012 Jun 6.
10. Ramzy PI, Barret JP, Herndon DN. Thermal injury. *Crit Care Clin.* 1999;15:333–352. ix.
11. Fodor L, Fodor A, Ramon Y, et al. Controversies in fluid resuscitation for burn management: literature review and our experience. *Injury.* 2006;37:374–379.
12. Carvajal HF. Fluid resuscitation of pediatric burn victims: a critical appraisal. *Pediatr Nephrol.* 1994;8:357–366.
13. Youn YK, LaLonde C, Demling R. The role of mediators in the response to thermal injury. *World J Surg.* 1992;16:30–36.
14. Warden GD. Burn shock resuscitation. *World J Surg.* 1992;16:16–23.
15. Wolf SE, Rose JK, Desai MH, et al. Mortality determinants in massive pediatric burns: an analysis of 103 children with > or = 80% TBSA burns (> or = 70% full-thickness). *Ann Surg.* 1997;225:554–565. discussion 565–569.
16. Pham TN, Cancio LC, Gibran NS. American Burn Association practice guidelines burn shock resuscitation. *J Burn Care Res.* 2008;29:257–266.
17. Holm C. Resuscitation in shock associated with burns: tradition or evidence-based medicine. *Resuscitation.* 2000;44:157–164.
18. Baxter CR, Shires T. Physiological response to crystalloid resuscitation of severe burns. *Ann N Y Acad Sci.* 1968;150:874–894.
19. Schwartz SI. Supportive therapy in burn care: consensus summary on fluid resuscitation. *J Trauma.* 1979;19(suppl 11):876–877.
20. Fabri PJ. Monitoring of the burn patient. *Clin Plast Surg.* 1986;13:21–27.
21. Greenhalgh DG. Burn resuscitation: the results of the ISBI/ABA survey. *Burns.* March 2010;36(2):176–182. http://dx.doi.org/10.1016/j.burns.2009.09.004. Epub 2009 Dec 16.
22. Perel P, Roberts I. Colloids versus crystalloids for fluid resuscitation in critically ill patients. *Cochrane Database Syst Rev.* 2007;4:CD000567.
23. Alderson P, Bunn F, Lefebvre C, et al. Human albumin solution for resuscitation and volume expansion in critically ill patients. *Cochrane Database Syst Rev.* 2004;4:CD001208.
24. Vincent JL, Sakr Y, Reinhart K, et al. Is albumin administration in the acutely ill associated with increased mortality? Results of the SOAP study. *Crit Care.* 2005;9:R745R754.
25. Cartotto R, Callum J. A review of the use of human albumin in burn patients. *J Burn Care Res.* November–December 2012;33(6):702–717. http://dx.doi.org/10.1097/BCR.0b013e31825b1cf6. Review.
26. Pruitt Jr BA, Mason Jr AD, Moncrief JA. Hemodynamic changes in the early postburn patient: the influence of fluid administration and of a vasodilator (hydralazine). *J Trauma.* 1971;11:36–46.
27. Warden GD. Fluid resuscitation and early management. In: Herndon DN, ed. *Total Burn Care.* 3rd ed. New York: Saunders; 2007:107–118.
28. Finnerty CC, Herndon DN, Jeschke MG. Inhalation injury in severely burned children does not augment the systemic inflammatory response. *Crit Care.* 2007;11:R22.
29. Thompson PB, Herndon DN, Traber DL, Abston S. Effect on mortality of inhalation injury. *J Trauma.* 1986;26:163–165.
30. Sheridan RL. Burns. *Crit Care Med.* 2002;30(suppl 11):S500S514.
31. Endorf FW, Gamelli RL. Inhalation injury, pulmonary perturbations, and fluid resuscitation. *J Burn Care Res.* 2007;28:80–83.
32. Pruitt Jr BA. Infection and the burn patient. *Br J Surg.* 1990;77:1081–1082.
33. Greenhalgh DG, Saffle JR, Holmes JH, et al. American Burn Association consensus conference to define sepsis and infection in burns. *J Burn Care Res.* 2007;28:776–790.
34. Atiyeh BS, Dham R, Kadry M, et al. Benefit-cost analysis of moist exposed burn ointment. *Burns.* 2002;28:659–663.
35. Lofts JA. Cost analysis of a major burn. *N Z Med J.* 1991;104:488–490.
36. Munster AM, Smith-Meek M, Sharkey P. The effect of early surgical intervention on mortality and cost-effectiveness in burn care, 1978–91. *Burns.* 1994;20:61–64.
37. Chan BP, Kochevar IE, Redmond RW. Enhancement of porcine skin graft adherence using a light-activated process. *J Surg Res.* 2002;108:77–84.
38. Budny PG, Regan PJ, Roberts AH. The estimation of blood loss during burns surgery. *Burns.* 1993;19:134–137.
39. Housinger TA, Lang D, Warden GD. A prospective study of blood loss with excisional therapy in pediatric burn patients. *J Trauma.* 1993;34:262–263.
40. Herndon DN, Tompkins RG. Support of the metabolic response to burn injury. *Lancet.* 2004;363:1895–1902.
41. Abdullahi A, Jeschke MG. Nutrition and Anabolic Pharmacotherapies in the Care of Burn Patients. *Nutr Clin Pract.* May 14, 2014. pii:0884533614533129. [Epub ahead of print] Review.
42. Hart DW, Wolf SE, Chinkes DL, et al. Effects of early excision and aggressive enteral feeding on hypermetabolism, catabolism, and sepsis after severe burn. *J Trauma.* 2003;54:755–761. discussion 761–754.
43. Herndon DN, Barrow RE, Stein M, et al. Increased mortality with intravenous supplemental feeding in severely burned patients. *J Burn Care Rehabil.* 1989;10:309–313.
44. Curreri PW, Richmond D, Marvin J, Baxter CR. Dietary requirements of patients with major burns. *J Am Diet Assoc.* 1974;65:415–417.

45. Allard JP, Pichard C, Hoshino E, et al. Validation of a new formula for calculating the energy requirements of burn patients. *JPEN J Parenter Enteral Nutr.* 1990;14:115–118.
46. Hildreth MA, Herndon DN, Desai MH, Broemeling LD. Current treatment reduces calories required to maintain weight in pediatric patients with burns. *J Burn Care Rehabil.* 1990;11:405–409.
47. Herndon DN, Curreri PW. Metabolic response to thermal injury and its nutritional support. *Cutis.* 1978;22:501–506. 514.
48. Demling RH, Seigne P. Metabolic management of patients with severe burns. *World J Surg.* 2000;24:673–680.
49. Garrel DR, Razi M, Lariviere F, et al. Improved clinical status and length of care with low-fat nutrition support in burn patients. *JPEN J Parenter Enteral Nutr.* 1995;19:482–491.
50. Mochizuki H, Trocki O, Dominioni L, et al. Optimal lipid content for enteral diets following thermal injury. *JPEN J Parenter Enteral Nutr.* 1984;8:638–646.
51. Barret JP, Jeschke MG, Herndon DN. Fatty infiltration of the liver in severely burned pediatric patients: autopsy findings and clinical implications. *J Trauma.* 2001;51:736–739.
52. Aarsland A, Chinkes D, Wolfe RR. Contributions of de novo synthesis of fatty acids to total VLDL-triglyceride secretion during prolonged hyperglycemia/hyperinsulinemia in normal man. *J Clin Invest.* 1996;98:2008–2017.
53. Jeschke MG, Herndon DN. Burns in children: standard and new treatments. *Lancet.* March 29, 2014;383(9923):1168–1178. http://dx.doi.org/10.1016/S0140-6736(13)61093-4. Epub 2013 Sep 11. Review.
54. Herndon DN, Nguyen TT, Wolfe RR, et al. Lipolysis in burned patients is stimulated by the beta 2-receptor for catecholamines. *Arch Surg.* 1994;129:1301–1304. discussion 1304–1305.
55. Cuthbertson DP, Fell GS, Smith CM, Tilstone WJ. Metabolism after injury. I. Effects of severity, nutrition, and environmental temperature on protein potassium, zinc, and creatine. *Br J Surg.* 1972;59:926–931.
56. Shakespeare PG. Studies on the serum levels of iron, copper and zinc and the urinary excretion of zinc after burn injury. *Burns Incl Therm Inj.* 1982;8:358–364.
57. Berger MM, Cavadini C, Bart A, et al. Cutaneous copper and zinc losses in burns. *Burns.* 1992;18:373–380.
58. Berger MM, Raffoul W, Shenkin A. Practical guidelines for nutritional management of burn injury and recovery: a guideline based on expert opinion but not including RCTs. *Burns.* 2008;34:141–143.
59. Berger MM, Eggimann P, Heyland DK, et al. Reduction of nosocomial pneumonia after major burns by trace element supplementation: aggregation of two randomised trials. *Crit Care.* 2006;10:R153.
60. Herndon DN, Hart DW, Wolf SE, et al. Reversal of catabolism by beta-blockade after severe burns. *N Engl J Med.* 2001;345:1223–1229.
61. Aarsland A, Chinkes D, Wolfe RR, et al. Beta-blockade lowers peripheral lipolysis in burn patients receiving growth hormone. Rate of hepatic very low density lipoprotein triglyceride secretion remains unchanged. *Ann Surg.* 1996;223:777–787. discussion 787–789.
62. Morio B, Irtun O, Herndon DN, Wolfe RR. Propranolol decreases splanchnic triacylglycerol storage in burn patients receiving a high-carbohydrate diet. *Ann Surg.* 2002;236:218–225.
63. Arbabi S, Ahrns KS, Wahl WL, et al. Beta-blocker use is associated with improved outcomes in adult burn patients. *J Trauma.* 2004;56:265–269. discussion 269–271.
64. Hart DW, Wolf SE, Ramzy PI, et al. Anabolic effects of oxandrolone after severe burn. *Ann Surg.* 2001;233:556–564.
65. Demling RH, Orgill DP. The anticatabolic and wound healing effects of the testosterone analog oxandrolone after severe burn injury. *J Crit Care.* 2000;15:12–17.
66. Wolf SE, Edelman LS, Kemalyan N, et al. Effects of oxandrolone on outcome measures in the severely burned: a multicenter prospective randomized double-blind trial. *J Burn Care Res.* 2006;27:131–139. discussion 140–141.
67. Jeschke MG, Finnerty CC, Suman OE, et al. The effect of oxandrolone on the endocrinologic, inflammatory, and hypermetabolic responses during the acute phase postburn. *Ann Surg.* 2007;246:351–360. discussion 360–362.
68. Gilpin DA, Barrow RE, Rutan RL, et al. Recombinant human growth hormone accelerates wound healing in children with large cutaneous burns. *Ann Surg.* 1994;220:19–24.
69. Meyer NA, Muller MJ, Herndon DN. Nutrient support of the healing wound. *New Horiz.* 1994;2:202–214.
70. Demling RH. Comparison of the anabolic effects and complications of human growth hormone and the testosterone analog, oxandrolone, after severe burn injury. *Burns.* 1999;25:215–221.
71. Przkora R, Herndon DN, Suman OE, et al. Beneficial effects of extended growth hormone treatment after hospital discharge in pediatric burn patients. *Ann Surg.* 2006;243:796–801. discussion 801–803.
72. Takala J, Ruokonen E, Webster NR, et al. Increased mortality associated with growth hormone treatment in critically ill adults. *N Engl J Med.* 1999;341:785–792.
73. Gore DC, Honeycutt D, Jahoor F, et al. Effect of exogenous growth hormone on glucose utilization in burn patients. *J Surg Res.* 1991;51:518–523.
74. Kupfer SR, Underwood LE, Baxter RC, Clemmons DR. Enhancement of the anabolic effects of growth hormone and insulin-like growth factor I by use of both agents simultaneously. *J Clin Invest.* 1993;91:391–396.
74a. Mesotten D, Van den Berghe. Changes within the growth hormone/insulin-like growth factor I/IGF binding protein axis during critical illness. *Endrocrinol Metab Clin North Am.* 2006;35:793–805.
75. Jeschke MG. Clinical review: Glucose control in severely burned patients - current best practice. *Crit Care.* July 25, 2013;17(4):232. http://dx.doi.org/10.1186/cc12678.
76. Jahoor F, Herndon DN, Wolfe RR. Role of insulin and glucagon in the response of glucose and alanine kinetics in burn-injured patients. *J Clin Invest.* 1986;78:807–814.
77. Gearhart MM, Parbhoo SK. Hyperglycemia in the critically ill patient. *AACN Clin Issues.* 2006;17:50–55.
78. Xin-Long C, Zhao-Fan X, Dao-Feng B, et al. Insulin resistance following thermal injury: An animal study. *Burns.* 2007;33:480–483.
79. Zauner A, Nimmerrichter P, Anderwald C, et al. Severity of insulin resistance in critically ill medical patients. *Metabolism.* 2007;56:1–5.
80. Guvener M, Pasaoglu I, Demircin M, Oc M. Perioperative hyperglycemia is a strong correlate of postoperative infection in type II diabetic patients after coronary artery bypass grafting. *Endocr J.* 2002;49:531–537.
81. McCowen KC, Malhotra A, Bistrian BR. Stress-induced hyperglycemia. *Crit Care Clin.* 2001;17:107–124.
82. Christiansen C, Toft P, Jorgensen HS, et al. Hyperglycaemia and mortality in critically ill patients: a prospective study. *Intensive Care Med.* 2004;30:1685–1688.
83. Jeschke MG, Pinto R, Kraft R, Finnerty CC, Kraft R. Hypoglycemia is associated with increased postburn morbidity and mortality in pediatric patients. *Crit Care Med.* May 2014;42(5):1221–1231.
83a. Jeschke MG, Kulp GA, Kraft R, Finnerty CC, Mlcak R, Lee JO, Herndon DN. Intensive insulin therapy in severely burned pediatric patients: a prospective randomized trial. *Am J Respir Crit Care Med.* 2010;182:351–359.
84. Harris JA, Benedict FG. A biometric study of human basal metabolism. *Proc Natl Acad Sci USA.* 1918;4:370–373.
85. Kleinman RE, Barness LA, Finberg L. History of pediatric nutrition and fluid therapy. *Pediatr Res.* 2003;54:762–772.
86. Food and Nutrition Board, Institute of Medicine. *Dietary Reference Intakes.* Washington, DC: National Academy Press; 2002.
87. Day T, Dean P, Adams M, et al. Nutritional requirements of the burned child: The Curreri Junior formula. *Proc Am Burn Assoc.* 1986;18(86).
88. Hildreth MA, Herndon DN, Desai MH, Broemeling LD. Caloric requirements of patients with burns under one year of age. *J Burn Care Rehabil.* 1993;14:108–112.
89. Hildreth M, Herndon D, Desai M, et al. Caloric needs of adolescent patients with burns. *J Burn Care Rehabil.* 1989;10:523–526.

77 What Is the Best Approach to Fluid Management, Transfusion Therapy, and the Endpoints of Resuscitation in Trauma?

Samuel A. Tisherman

Exsanguinating hemorrhage is a major cause of death from trauma. Rapid fluid resuscitation accompanied by aggressive efforts at hemostasis is required to save lives. Many questions regarding fluid resuscitation remain. These include the choice of fluid, indications for blood products, and the goals for fluid resuscitation before and after hemostasis is achieved.

Modern fluid resuscitation in trauma began in the early 1960s with the work of Shires and colleagues. During hemorrhage, fluid shifts from the interstitial space to the intravascular space because of changes in compartment pressures. Likewise, fluid initially shifts from cells into the interstitial space. As cells become ischemic during severe hemorrhagic shock (HS), however, failure of membrane ion pumps leads to a shift of fluids back into cells with resultant cellular swelling. Consequently, the interstitial space further loses fluid. Shires postulated that resuscitation with crystalloids, which fill the vascular and interstitial spaces, would be beneficial.[1] His animal studies demonstrated that survival improved with the addition of crystalloid (lactated Ringer's [LR] solution) to re-infusion of shed blood. Crystalloid resuscitation was quickly adopted in the military for resuscitation of trauma victims during the Vietnam conflict. Although this approach decreased the renal failure that had been seen in previous conflicts, it may have contributed to a new finding, "Da Nang lung" or "shock lung," which may have been acute respiratory distress syndrome (ARDS) or simply hydrostatic pulmonary edema from volume overload. Administration of LR solution quickly became a standard of the Advanced Trauma Life Support (ATLS) course and of care in prehospital and emergency department (ED) resuscitation of civilian trauma victims. Recent studies suggesting possible immunologic effects of LR solution have led to questions of this practice and a great interest in finding better alternatives as plasma substitutes.

Administration of blood to replace lost red blood cells has been another mainstay of resuscitation from HS. Although whole blood was initially used, blood banks have found that dividing the blood into packed red blood cells (PRBCs), fresh frozen plasma (FFP), and platelets is more efficient and economical. Recent studies have suggested that more rapid resuscitation with blood components that essentially reconstitute whole blood may be beneficial. Blood transfusions, however, have many potentially deleterious effects. Greater recognition of these effects has led to reconsideration of aggressive transfusion protocols once hemostasis has been achieved.

Endpoints for fluid resuscitation, similar to the fluids themselves, have undergone reconsideration in recent years. Although the trauma victim has ongoing hemorrhage (uncontrolled HS), normalization of blood pressure may increase bleeding and worsen outcome. Limited, or hypotensive, fluid resuscitation may be appropriate. Once hemostasis has been achieved, determining adequacy of resuscitation is critical. Standard parameters such as blood pressure, heart rate, and urine output are insufficient because many patients remain under-resuscitated, with "compensated hemorrhagic shock." Adjuvant tests are necessary to recognize this condition and ensure restoration of homeostasis.

PATHOPHYSIOLOGY OF HEMORRHAGIC SHOCK

HS is characterized by acute blood loss leading to decreased oxygen delivery to tissues. Although blood pressure and pulse are typically the clinical parameters used to determine the severity of shock, they lack sensitivity. In general, patients need to lose at least 30% to 40% of their blood volume to be hypotensive. An individual's response to hemorrhage may be affected by age, comorbid conditions, medications, and ingestion of drugs and alcohol. One of the most common mistakes of the novice clinician is to assume that the patient with a normal blood pressure is not in shock. Recognition and reversal of "compensated shock" is critical to achieve optimal outcomes.

Approximately 6% to 9% of trauma patients are in shock on admission. Of these, one third have exsanguinating hemorrhage, as evidenced by a lack of response to fluid resuscitation. These patients invariably require operative intervention and aggressive fluid resuscitation including blood products or they will die within minutes to hours. Another third of patients are classified as transient responders. They are initially hypotensive and improve with fluid resuscitation only to deteriorate again. They have less active bleeding than the first group, but their transient response can lull clinicians into a sense of complacency. Without ongoing resuscitation, operative intervention if necessary, and vigilance, they also have a high risk of dying or developing multiple organ dysfunction. The final third of these patients respond appropriately to fluid resuscitation and spontaneously achieve hemostasis. These patients are still at risk of hypoperfusion and organ dysfunction. In all trauma patients, early recognition of hypoperfusion, rapid restoration of homeostasis, and continued resuscitation to appropriate endpoints can reduce the risk of early cardiovascular collapse, development of organ system dysfunction, and death.

The inflammatory response to trauma may increase the risk of organ dysfunction and late death from trauma. Although laboratory studies have suggested therapies that could mitigate these deleterious cascades, none of these agents have made it to clinical use. Despite this, recent studies suggest that late deaths from multiple organ dysfunction and sepsis are actually rare.[2]

PRESENTATION OF AVAILABLE DATA BASED ON SYSTEMATIC REVIEW

Choice of Fluid. Although the use of crystalloids for resuscitation from traumatic HS has become standard, it seems that these solutions are not as innocuous as originally believed. Laboratory studies have demonstrated that crystalloids may exacerbate cellular injury. LR solution can cause an increase in oxidative burst and expression of adhesion molecules on neutrophils in human blood[3] and during HS in pigs.[4] No clinical studies have yet compared different crystalloids.

Modifications of LR solution (e.g., substituting the L-isomer of lactate or substitution of pyruvate or ketone bodies [β-hydroxybutyrate] for racemic lactate) can decrease the neutrophil activation and apoptosis.[5,6] In contrast, hypertonic saline (HTS) and fresh whole blood do not cause neutrophil activation.[7] HTS can attenuate immune-mediated cellular injury after trauma.[8]

Several small clinical trials have suggested a benefit of hypertonic solutions for resuscitation of trauma patients (Table 77-1). These studies explored the use of HTS alone or with a colloid added (e.g., hypertonic saline-dextan [HSD]) to prolong the intravascular volume expansion. Multiple studies[9-18] demonstrated that HTS or HSD increased blood pressure and volume expansion better than crystalloids but could not document improved survival. Mattox et al.[12] and Wade et al.[16] found that HSD improved survival in the subset of trauma patients who required operation, presumably more severely injured patients. Likewise, Bulger et al. found that HSD, compared with LR solution, improved ARDS-free survival only in patients who required more than 10 units of PRBCs.[19]

Regarding hypertonic fluids, Wade et al.[20] reviewed 14 trials of HTS or HSD and found that neither conferred a statistically significant survival benefit, but HSD seemed more promising. Given the potential physiologic benefit of HTS and the tactical advantage of small volume resuscitation for the military, the Resuscitation Outcomes Consortium (ROC) conducted a multicenter, prehospital, prospective, double-blind, randomized trial comparing normal saline, HTS, and HSD as the first resuscitation fluid in hypotensive trauma patients.[21] Survival to 28 days was not significantly different between groups.

The most recent Cochrane review of albumin administration found no benefit for patients with hypovolemia, burns, or hypoalbuminemia.[22] Increasing evidence suggests that starch solutions do not improve survival in the general intensive care unit (ICU) population and may increase the need for renal replacement therapy[23] or death.[24] These fluids currently have no role in trauma resuscitation.

The plasma substitutes discussed so far do not carry oxygen. Since the 1930s, there has been an interest in developing hemoglobin-based oxygen carriers (HBOCs) using hemoglobin (Hb) from red blood cells to provide oxygen-carrying capacity. Unconjugated Hb has severe renal and tissue toxicity. To decrease the nephrotoxicity and increase plasma half-life, researchers have developed various techniques to stabilize the Hb molecule. Some of these products may cause excessive vasoconstriction or oxidative damage. Diaspirin cross-linked Hb (HemAssist, Baxter Healthcare, Round Lake, Ill.) was the first product to undergo a randomized clinical trial in trauma patients. Unfortunately, the trial had to be discontinued early because of increased mortality in the subjects exposed to the product.[25] More recently, polymerized Hb derived from human blood (Poly-Heme, Northfield Laboratories, Evanston, Ill.) was compared with PRBCs in a small, randomized trial for trauma patients who required operations.[26] PolyHeme seemed safe and reduced the need for transfusion. A pivotal, randomized trial of PolyHeme compared with prehospital LR solution administration and early in-hospital blood transfusion demonstrated decreased allogeneic blood transfusion requirements, but no mortality benefit.[27] Other companies have been unable to conduct studies in trauma patients. Consequently, no HBOCs are currently available.

Transfusion. During the initial resuscitation of trauma victims, the ATLS course recommends that PRBCs be transfused after administering 1 to 2 L of crystalloid without an adequate hemodynamic response.[28] The goal is to acutely restore blood pressure and oxygen-carrying capacity.

Massive transfusions in trauma patients with HS lead to coagulopathy. The mechanisms involved in the development of the coagulopathy of trauma are complex.[29] Traditionally, management of the coagulopathy has been reactionary (i.e., administering FFP, cryoprecipitate, platelets, and calcium once the patient is coagulopathic). Military and civilian data suggest that a more proactive approach may be beneficial.[30-39] Administration of fresh whole blood, as available at times within the military, might be ideal,[40] but whole blood is not available from civilian blood banks. Consequently, a "hemostatic resuscitation" or "damage control resuscitation" approach involving the administration of FFP, platelets, and PRBCs in a 1:1:1 ratio has evolved. In addition to the ratio of the products, the

Table 77-1 **Summary of Clinical Trials**

Study, Year	Number of Subjects (Intervention/No Intervention)	Study Design	Intervention	Control	Outcomes
HYPERTONIC SALINE FOR HEMORRHAGIC SHOCK					
2011[21]	376 NS 256 HTS 220 HSD	DB	HTS/HSD	NS	No difference in 28-day survival.
2007[8]	36/26	DB	HSD	LR	Inhibit CD11b. Trend increase IL-1β, IL-10.
2007[19]	110/99	DB	HSD	LR	No difference ARDS-free survival. Improved ARDS-free survival if >10 U blood.
2006[89]	13/14	DB	HSD	NS	Promotes a more balanced inflammatory response.
2003[16]	120/110	DB	HSD	NS	Survival 83% vs. 76% overall (NS), 85% vs. 67% for patients requiring surgery ($P = .01$).
1993[14]	85 HTS 89 HS 84 NS	DB	HS or HSD	LR	HS improved survival compared with TRISS.
1992[18]	35/35/35	DB	HS or HSD	NS	No difference in survival. Better BP and volume expansion. Less fluid needed.
1991[9]	83/83	DB	HSD	LR	Improved BP. No change in survival.
1991[12]	211/211	DB	HSD	Crystalloid	No difference in survival, except patient who required operation. Improved BP, fewer complications.
1990[13]	32 HTS 23 HSD 51 LR	DB	HSD HS	LR	No safety issues except mild hyperchloremic acidosis.
1989[11]	48		HSD	PlasmaLyte A	Feasibility study.
1989[17]	32	DB	HSD	Crystalloid	No difference in survival.
TRANSFUSION					
2007[60]	240/439	Retrospective	Leukocyte-depleted PRBCs	Standard PRBCs	No difference in LOS or mortality.
2006[59]	286	Randomized	Leukocyte-depleted PRBCs	Standard PRBCs	No difference in infections, organ failures, mortality.
2006[55]	93/117	Prospective Operation Iraqi Freedom	Transfused	Not transfused	Higher ISS, HR, lower Hct, increased infection rate, ICU, and LOS.
2005[57]	102	Prospective, observational			The amount of transfused blood is independently associated with both the development of ARDS and hospital mortality.
2004[39]	954/8585	Prospective	Transfused	Not transfused	Older, higher ISS, lower GCS, more SIRS, higher mortality.
2004[38]	100/103 trauma patients	Prospective	Hb 7-9 g/dL	Hb 10-12 g/dL	No differences.
2003[41]	15,534	Prospective	Transfusion	Not transfused	Increase mortality (OR, 2.8), ICU, and LOS.
2002[43]	61	Prospective	Transfused		Older blood increased risk of infections.

Continued

Table 77-1 Summary of Clinical Trials—cont'd

Study, Year	Number of Subjects (Intervention/No Intervention)	Study Design	Intervention	Control	Outcomes
CLOTTING FACTOR REPLACEMENT					
2011[46]	DCR	Prospective and retrospective	Permissive hypotension, less crystalloid	Standard care, historical controls	DCR resulted in less crystalloid, more FFP, improved survival (OR, 0.4; CI, 0.18-0.9).
2011[45]	108/82	Prospective and retrospective	Permissive hypotension, less crystalloid	Standard care, historical controls	DCR was associated with increased survival (OR, 2.5; CI, 1.1-5.6).
2010[33]	214 patients receiving massive transfusion	Prospective and retrospective	Massive transfusion protocol	Standard care, historical controls	Factors that influenced survival were FFP/PRBC, platelets/PRBC, ISS, age, and total PRBCs.
2009[47]	442 patients receiving massive transfusion	Prospective and retrospective	Preemptive FFP and platelets	Standard care, historic controls	Mortality decreased from 31% to 20% long term. Thromboelastography was used to titrate.
2009[36]	37/40	Prospective and retrospective	1:1.5 FFP/PRBC, more rapid product availability	Standard care, historical controls	No difference in ratios, but more rapid administration was associated with improved mortality.
LIMITED FLUID RESUSCITATION FOR UNCONTROLLED HEMORRHAGE					
2011[69]	44/46	Prospective, randomized, intraoperative	MAP >50 mm Hg	MAP >65 mm Hg	Lower MAP group required fewer blood products, had less coagulopathy, and decreased early death.
2002[55]	55/55	Randomized	SBP >70 mm Hg	SBP >100 mm Hg	Survival 93% with no difference between groups.
1996[56]	527	Retrospective	Rapid infusion system used	Historical controls	Increased risk of dying 4.8×.
1994[54]	309/289	Randomized day of month	Delayed resuscitation	Immediate resuscitation	Improved survival: 70% vs. 62%. Decreased LOS.
1990[64]	6855	Retrospective	Prehospital fluid	No prehospital fluid	No difference in mortality.
ENDPOINTS OF RESUSCITATION FROM TRAUMA					
2002[62]	18/18	Prospective, nonrandomized	DO_2 500	DO_2 600	Less fluid and blood needed; similar outcome.
2000[61]	40/35	Prospective, randomized	Supranormal DO_2	Normal DO_2	Patients who achieve supranormal values increased survival, but no difference between groups in mortality, organ failure, or LOS.
1995[59]	50/75	Randomized	Supranormal DO_2	Normal DO_2	Improved survival (18% vs. 37%) and organ system failures.
1992[60]	33/34	Randomized	Supranormal DO_2	Normal DO_2	Decreased mortality, organ failure, LOS, ventilator days.
2006[60]	5995	Retrospective			Lactate did not correlate with mortality.
2003[67]	98	Prospective		Standard care	Admission lactate level correlates with ISS and 12-h lactate with survival.
1998[66]	100	Prospective	High BD	Low BD	Increase MOF and mortality, low oxygen use.
1998[65]	674	Observational			BD worse in nonsurvivors. No difference in pH.
1992[63]	3791	Retrospective			BD, age, injury mechanism, and head injury were associated with mortality using logistic regression.
1988[64]	209	Observational			Higher BD associated with lower BP and greater fluid resuscitation.

ARDS, acute respiratory distress syndrome; *BD,* base deficit; *BP,* blood pressure; *CI,* confidence interval; *DB,* double blind; *DCR,* damage control resuscitation; *DO₂,* oxygen delivery; *FFP,* fresh frozen plasma; *GCS,* Glasgow Coma Scale score; *Hb,* hemoglobin; *Hct,* hematocrit; *HR,* hazard ratio; *HSD,* hypertonic saline-dextran; *HTS,* hypertonic saline; *ICU,* intensive care unit; *IL,* interleukin; *ISS,* injury severity score; *LOS,* length of stay; *LR,* lactated Ringer's solution; *MAP,* mean arterial pressure; *MOF,* multiorgan failure; *NS,* normal saline; *OR,* odds ratio; *P,* placebo controlled; *PRBC,* packed red blood cell; *SBP,* systolic blood pressure; *SIRS,* systemic inflammatory response syndrome; *TRISS,* trauma and injury severity score.

rate of infusion may play a role because higher early infusion rates for FFP and platelets may be associated with improved survival.[41,42] It is not clear whether the absolute ratio or repletion of the "plasma deficit" (PRBC-FFP) is most important.[42] Not all studies have been as positive about the impact of early FFP administration.[43] These retrospective studies have been criticized for potential survival bias.[44] There have also been several studies of specific massive transfusion protocols that have suggested benefit compared with historic controls.[33,45-47] The Pragmatic, Randomized Optimal Platelets and Plasma Ratios study, designed to compare 1:1:1 resuscitation with 1:1:2, may provide more clarity to this issue.

For this hemostatic resuscitation strategy to be proactively applied, it is important to select patients who are at a high risk of requiring a massive transfusion. For example, the ABC score, which uses easily obtained clinical parameters in the ED (penetrating mechanism, systolic blood pressure of ≤90 mm Hg, heart rate of ≥120 beats/min, or positive focused assessment by sonography for trauma) may be very useful for predicting the need for massive transfusions with an area under the receiver operating characteristic curve of 0.84.[48]

Tranexamic acid (TxA) is an inhibitor of fibrinolysis that can decrease transfusion requirements during various elective surgical procedures. The Clinical Randomization of an Antifibrinolytic in Significant Hemorrhage 2 (CRASH-2) study compared, in a double-blind manner, TxA with placebo in 20,211 patients in 274 hospitals in 40 countries.[49] The investigators found that TxA significantly decreased mortality without increasing the risk of vascular occlusive events.

The precise role for other agents to reverse the complex coagulopathy of trauma, including activated factor VIIa,[50] fibrinogen concentrate, and prothrombin complex concentrates, remains unclear. Perhaps, titration of these agents with readily available, point-of-care tests, such as thromboelastometry, could prove useful.[51]

After the initial resuscitation and achievement of normovolemia, the indication for blood transfusion is based primarily upon Hb level. In the general ICU population, a restrictive transfusion threshold (Hb <7 g/dL) was as good, and possibly better, than a more liberal threshold (<10 g/dL).[52] A subset analysis of trauma patients found no differences in outcomes between the two transfusion thresholds, suggesting that the more restrictive strategy was safe.[53] Dunne et al.,[54,55] Malone et al.,[56] and Silverboard et al.[57] found strong associations between the amount of blood transfused in trauma patients and injury severity score (ISS), organ failure, length of stay (LOS), and mortality. Administration of blood stored for more prolonged periods of time may increase risk of infection.[58] Although some have postulated that complications of transfusions are related to leukocytes, leukocyte-depleted PRBCs seem to provide no benefit.[59,60] A more restrictive fluid resuscitation approach, along with a lung-protective strategy, may decrease the risk of the ARDS after trauma.[61]

Uncontrolled Hemorrhagic Shock. In most circumstances, the goal for fluid resuscitation is to restore normal blood pressure. For patients with active, uncontrolled hemorrhage, however, aggressive resuscitation may lead to increased bleeding and worse outcomes. This has been demonstrated in various animal models,[62] The optimal blood pressure goal during uncontrolled HS depends on the injury pattern as well as the type and rate of fluid resuscitation. How long this limited, hypotensive fluid resuscitation can be maintained is similarly unclear.[63]

In patients, Kaweski et al. retrospectively found that prehospital administration of fluids had no impact on mortality compared with no fluid administration.[64] Delayed resuscitation from HS was first tested in a randomized clinical trial by Bickell et al.[65] Patients with hypotension after penetrating torso trauma received either no fluid resuscitation or standard fluid resuscitation until undergoing operative intervention. Survival was slightly better in the delayed resuscitation group (70% vs. 62%).

In contrast, Turner et al. found no difference in outcome comparing standard prehospital fluid resuscitation and no fluid resuscitation strategies. There were no differences in outcomes between groups.

A trial by Dutton et al. that explored hypotensive resuscitation in the hospital in patients with both blunt and penetrating trauma victims did not demonstrate any difference in outcome, although survival was high in both groups.[66] In contrast, this group found that initial aggressive fluid resuscitation in severely injured trauma victims with the Rapid Infusion System increased the risk of dying almost fivefold.[67]

More recently, Duke et al. retrospectively examined the effect of "restrictive" fluid resuscitation in conjunction with a damage control resuscitation and damage control surgery strategy and found that the restrictive approach was associated with improved survival.[68] Morrison et al. demonstrated that hypotensive resuscitation of trauma patients in the operating room is associated with less coagulopathy and blood transfusion requirements and decreased early deaths from hemorrhage.[69]

In a recent meta-analysis, Wang et al. reviewed four randomized clinical trials and seven observational studies comparing a restrictive fluid resuscitation strategy and a more liberal strategy in trauma patients.[70] They found an increased risk of mortality with a liberal strategy in both randomized controlled trials and the observational studies.

Optimal management of the trauma patient with uncontrolled hemorrhage remains unclear. The ROC study group has completed a prehospital feasibility trial of a controlled (hypotensive) fluid resuscitation strategy compared with standard therapy in hypotensive trauma patients.[70a] The controlled strategy seemed safe and was associated with less early crystalloid administration and a suggestion of early mortality benefit, particularly with blunt trauma. A large-scale, randomized clinical trial is warranted.

Endpoints of Resuscitation. Once hemostasis is achieved, the first goal of fluid resuscitation in hypotensive trauma patients is to restore normal blood pressure, heart rate, and urine output. However, in many patients, vital signs alone may not identify "compensated shock," leaving some vascular beds inadequately perfused. Other clinical data are needed to identify this state and monitor further resuscitation.

Shoemaker and colleagues demonstrated that survivors of traumatic HS had higher levels of cardiac output, oxygen delivery, and oxygen consumption compared with nonsurvivors.[71,72] In small, randomized trials, they demonstrated that attempting to achieve these supranormal oxygen delivery values could improve survival.[73,74] Others have not been able to replicate these results.[75] Decreasing the oxygen delivery goals in the protocol produced similar outcomes with less fluid and blood product administration.[76]

Systemic evidence of inadequate tissue perfusion (i.e., compensated shock) can be identified by evidence of anaerobic metabolism. Lactate levels, base deficit, or serum bicarbonate correlate with survival.[77-83] Aggressive therapy to normalize these parameters may improve survival.[78,79]

Near-infrared spectroscopy and heart rate variability hold promise as noninvasive techniques that could be used in a continual fashion to optimize resuscitation.[84,85] The use of ultrasonographic estimation of volume status, expected volume responsiveness, and cardiac performance has become more standard in the ICU and early resuscitation of trauma patients.[86,87] Clear evidence of benefit from the use of these modalities is lacking. However, using ultrasound for monitoring and titrating fluid resuscitation would be a natural extension of its current use in the initial assessment of trauma patients. So far, none of these strategies has proved to be better than standard clinical parameters (blood pressure, heart rate, urine output) and acid–base parameters (base deficit, lactate).

INTERPRETATION OF DATA

Choice of Fluid. The standard initial fluid for resuscitation of trauma patients remains crystalloids, recognizing the potential deleterious effects and military strategic disadvantages of resuscitation with LR. There is no clear benefit of either HTS or HSD, neither of which is approved by the U.S. Food and Drug Administration for use in trauma resuscitation. On the basis of recent data, starch solutions have been removed from resuscitation algorithms. With this background and the potential benefit of the hemostatic resuscitation approach, many trauma centers have shifted in recent years toward almost exclusive early resuscitation with blood products for patients with severe HS.

Transfusion. There is no question that blood transfusions in patients with HS can be lifesaving, but it is also clear that they can also be detrimental. For patients in profound shock, initiation of PRBCs should begin as soon as possible. Early administration of plasma and platelets is associated with improved outcomes. The specific ratios of these products still need to be determined. Once hemostasis has been achieved and volume status is restored, however, administration of blood products should be minimized because the number of transfused units seems to be an independent risk factor for mortality.

Uncontrolled Hemorrhagic Shock. Although trauma victims have active hemorrhage, attempting to restore normal hemodynamics is likely to increase bleeding and worsen outcome. Hemostasis should be achieved as rapidly as possible. In the meantime, limited (hypotensive) fluid resuscitation should be considered. The specifics of optimal blood pressure level and safe duration of this approach are yet to be determined.

Endpoints of Resuscitation. A clinical practice guideline from the Eastern Association for the Surgery of Trauma recommended the use of lactate or base deficit as a readily measured and followed parameter to guide resuscitation.[88] If these values do not normalize rapidly, then the patient may still be under-resuscitated or may have ongoing bleeding. The optimal endpoint for resuscitation from HS is one that is easily measured, reproducible, and provides information to optimize resuscitation that is not available with standard clinical parameters. Although there are some promising new parameters to use as endpoints for resuscitation, more research is needed in this area.

SUMMARY

Optimal resuscitation of trauma victims with HS requires simultaneous efforts at hemostasis and fluid resuscitation. Crystalloids remain the initial plasma substitutes of choice. Early transfusions of PRBCs, FFP, and platelets are lifesaving, but they should be limited to the quantity that is absolutely necessary. While the patient is actively bleeding, fluid resuscitation should be limited to not aggravate bleeding, but still maintain a pulse. Once hemostasis has been achieved, fluid resuscitation should be aggressive to mitigate anaerobic metabolism as evidenced by improving lactate or base deficit.

AUTHOR'S RECOMMENDATIONS

- HS causes tissue ischemia that is followed by reperfusion injury and a systemic inflammatory response that can lead to multiple organ system dysfunction and death.
- Crystalloids remain the initial fluid of choice for resuscitation of patients with mild HS. Blood products should be administered early in patients with severe shock.
- During active hemorrhage, fluid resuscitation should be limited to avoid exacerbating hemorrhage. Once hemostasis has been achieved, fluid resuscitation should be aggressive to reverse tissue ischemia.
- After hemostasis, transfusions should be limited to maintain Hb above 7 g/dL. FFP and platelets should be administered to correct the coagulopathy of trauma.

REFERENCES

1. McClelland RN, Shires GT, Baxter CR, Coln CD, Carrico J. Balanced salt solution in the treatment of hemorrhagic shock. Studies in dogs. *JAMA*. March 13, 1967;199(11):830–834.
2. Tisherman SA, Schmicker RH, Brasel KJ, et al. detailed description of all deaths in both the shock and traumatic brain injury hypertonic saline trials of the resuscitation outcomes consortium. *Ann Surg*. 2015;261(3):586–590.
3. Stanton K, Alam HB, Rhee P, Llorente O, Kirkpatrick J, Koustova E. Human polymorphonuclear cell death after exposure to resuscitation fluids in vitro: apoptosis versus necrosis. *J Trauma*. June 2003;54(6):1065–1074.
4. Alam HB, Stanton K, Koustova E, Burris D, Rich N, Rhee P. Effect of different resuscitation strategies on neutrophil activation in a swine model of hemorrhagic shock. *Resuscitation*. January 2004;60(1):91–99.
5. Koustova E, Rhee P, Hancock T, et al. Ketone and pyruvate Ringer's solutions decrease pulmonary apoptosis in a rat model of severe hemorrhagic shock and resuscitation. *Surgery*. August 2003;134(2):267–274.

6. Koustova E, Stanton K, Gushchin V, Alam HB, Stegalkina S, Rhee PM. Effects of lactated Ringer's solutions on human leukocytes. *J Trauma*. May 2002;52(5):872–878.

7. Ayuste EC, Chen H, Koustova E, et al. Hepatic and pulmonary apoptosis after hemorrhagic shock in swine can be reduced through modifications of conventional Ringer's solution. *J Trauma*. January 2006;60(1):52–63.

8. Bulger EM, Cuschieri J, Warner K, Maier RV. Hypertonic resuscitation modulates the inflammatory response in patients with traumatic hemorrhagic shock. *Ann Surg*. April 2007;245(4):635–641.

9. Vassar MJ, Perry CA, Gannaway WL, Holcroft JW. 7.5% sodium chloride/dextran for resuscitation of trauma patients undergoing helicopter transport. *Arch Surg*. September 1991;126(9):1065–1072.

10. Holcroft JW, Vassar MJ, Turner JE, Derlet RW, Kramer GC. 3% NaCl and 7.5% NaCl/dextran 70 in the resuscitation of severely injured patients. *Ann Surg*. September 1987;206(3):279–288.

11. Maningas PA, Mattox KL, Pepe PE, Jones RL, Feliciano DV, Burch JM. Hypertonic saline-dextran solutions for the prehospital management of traumatic hypotension. *Am J Surg*. May 1989;157(5):528–533.

12. Mattox KL, Maningas PA, Moore EE, et al. Prehospital hypertonic saline/dextran infusion for post-traumatic hypotension. The U.S.A. Multicenter Trial. *Ann Surg*. May 1991;213(5):482–491.

13. Vassar MJ, Perry CA, Holcroft JW. Analysis of potential risks associated with 7.5% sodium chloride resuscitation of traumatic shock. [erratum appears in Arch Surg 1991 Jan;126(1):43] *Arch Surg*. October 1990;125(10):1309–1315.

14. Vassar MJ, Perry CA, Holcroft JW. Prehospital resuscitation of hypotensive trauma patients with 7.5% NaCl versus 7.5% NaCl with added dextran: a controlled trial. *J Trauma*. May 1993;34(5):622–632.

15. Mauritz W, Schimetta W, Oberreither S, Polz W. Are hypertonic hyperoncotic solutions safe for prehospital small-volume resuscitation? Results of a prospective observational study. *Euro J Emerg Med*. December 2002;9(4):315–319.

16. Wade CE, Grady JJ, Kramer GC. Efficacy of hypertonic saline dextran fluid resuscitation for patients with hypotension from penetrating trauma. *J Trauma*. May 2003;54(suppl 5):S144–S148.

17. Holcroft JW, Vassar MJ, Perry CA, Gannaway WL, Kramer GC. Use of a 7.5% NaCl/6% Dextran 70 solution in the resuscitation of injured patients in the emergency room. *Prog Clin Biol Res*. 1989;299:331–338.

18. Younes RN, Aun F, Accioly CQ, Casale LP, Szajnbok I, Birolini D. Hypertonic solutions in the treatment of hypovolemic shock: a prospective, randomized study in patients admitted to the emergency room. *Surgery*. April 1992;111(4):380–385.

19. Bulger EM, Jurkovich GJ, Nathens AB, et al. Hypertonic resuscitation of hypovolemic shock after blunt trauma. *Arch Surg*. 2007;143(2):139–148.

20. Wade CE, Kramer GC, Grady JJ, Fabian TC, Younes RN. Efficacy of hypertonic 7.5% saline and 6% dextran-70 in treating trauma: a meta-analysis of controlled clinical studies. *Surgery*. September 1997;122(3):609–616.

21. Bulger EM, May S, Kerby JD, et al. Out-of-hospital hypertonic resuscitation after traumatic hypovolemic shock: a randomized, placebo controlled trial. *Ann Surg*. March 2011;253(3):431–441.

22. Albumin Reviewers. Human albumin solution for resuscitation and volume expansion in critically ill patients. *Cochrane Database Syst Rev*. 2011;10:CD001208.

23. Myburgh JA, Finfer S, Bellomo R, et al. Hydroxyethyl starch or saline for fluid resuscitation in intensive care. *N Engl J Med*. 2012;367(20):1901–1911.

24. Zarychanski R, Abou-Setta AM, Turgeon AF, et al. Association of hydroxyethyl starch administration with mortality and acute kidney injury in critically ill patients requiring volume resuscitation: a systematic review and meta-analysis. *JAMA*. 2013;309(7):678–688.

25. Sloan EP, Koenigsberg M, Gens D, et al. Diaspirin cross-linked hemoglobin (DCLHb) in the treatment of severe traumatic hemorrhagic shock: a randomized controlled efficacy trial. *JAMA*. November 17, 1999;282(19):1857–1864.

26. Gould SA, Moore EE, Hoyt DB, et al. The first randomized trial of human polymerized hemoglobin as a blood substitute in acute trauma and emergent surgery. [see comment] *J Am Coll Surg*. August 1998;187(2):113–120.

27. Moore EE, Moore FA, Fabian TC, et al. Human polymerized hemoglobin for the treatment of hemorrhagic shock when blood is unavailable: the USA multicenter trial. *J Am Coll Surg*. January 2009;208(1):1–13.

28. *ATLS Student Manual*. 9th ed. Chicago, IL: American College of Surgeons; 2012.

29. Hess JR, Brohi K, Dutton RP, et al. The coagulopathy of trauma: a review of mechanisms. *J Trauma Acute Care Surg*. 2008;65(4):748–754.

30. Borgman MA, Spinella PC, Perkins JG, et al. The ratio of blood products transfused affects mortality in patients receiving massive transfusions at a combat support hospital. *J Trauma*. October 2007;63(4):805–813.

31. Holcomb JB, Fox EE, Wade CE. The PRospective Observational Multicenter Major Trauma Transfusion (PROMMTT) study. *J Trauma Acute Care Surg*. July 2013;75(1 suppl 1):S1–S2.

32. Holcomb JB, Zarzabal LA, Michalek JE, et al. Increased platelet:RBC ratios are associated with improved survival after massive transfusion. *J Trauma*. August 2011;71(2 suppl 3):S318–S328.

33. Shaz BH, Dente CJ, Nicholas J, et al. Increased number of coagulation products in relationship to red blood cell products transfused improves mortality in trauma patients. *Transfusion*. February 2010;50(2):493–500.

34. Zink KA, Sambasivan CN, Holcomb JB, Chisholm G, Schreiber MA. A high ratio of plasma and platelets to packed red blood cells in the first 6 hours of massive transfusion improves outcomes in a large multicenter study. *Am J Surg*. May 2009;197(5):565–570.

35. Teixeira PG, Inaba K, Shulman I, et al. Impact of plasma transfusion in massively transfused trauma patients. *J Trauma*. March 2009;66(3):693–697.

36. Riskin DJ, Tsai TC, Riskin L, et al. Massive transfusion protocols: the role of aggressive resuscitation versus product ratio in mortality reduction. *J Am Coll Surg*. August 2009;209(2):198–205.

37. Maegele M, Lefering R, Paffrath T, Tjardes T, Simanski C, Bouillon B. Red-blood-cell to plasma ratios transfused during massive transfusion are associated with mortality in severe multiple injury: a retrospective analysis from the Trauma Registry of the Deutsche Gesellschaft fur Unfallchirurgie. *Vox Sanguinis*. August 2008;95(2):112–119.

38. Holcomb JB, Wade CE, Michalek JE, et al. Increased plasma and platelet to red blood cell ratios improves outcome in 466 massively transfused civilian trauma patients. *Ann Surg*. September 2008;248(3):447–458.

39. Inaba K, Lustenberger T, Rhee P, et al. The impact of platelet transfusion in massively transfused trauma patients. *J Am Coll Surg*. November 2010;211(5):573–579.

40. Kauvar DS, Holcomb JB, Norris GC, Hess JR. Fresh whole blood transfusion: a controversial military practice. *J Trauma*. July 2006;61(1):181–184.

41. Simms ER, Hennings DL, Hauch A, et al. Impact of infusion rates of fresh frozen plasma and platelets during the first 180 minutes of resuscitation. *J Am Coll Surg*. August 2014;219(2):181–188.

42. de Biasi AR, Stansbury LG, Dutton RP, Stein DM, Scalea TM, Hess JR. Blood product use in trauma resuscitation: plasma deficit versus plasma ratio as predictors of mortality in trauma (CME). *Transfusion*. September 2011;51(9):1925–1932.

43. Scalea TM, Bochicchio KM, Lumpkins K, et al. Early aggressive use of fresh frozen plasma does not improve outcome in critically injured trauma patients. *Ann Surg*. October 2008;248(4):578–584.

44. Rajasekhar A, Gowing R, Zarychanski R, et al. Survival of trauma patients after massive red blood cell transfusion using a high or low red blood cell to plasma transfusion ratio. *Crit Care Med*. June 2011;39(6):1507–1513.

45. Cotton BA, Reddy N, Hatch QM, et al. Damage control resuscitation is associated with a reduction in resuscitation volumes and improvement in survival in 390 damage control laparotomy patients. *Ann Surg*. October 2011;254(4):598–605.

46. Duchesne JC, Barbeau JM, Islam TM, Wahl G, Greiffenstein P, McSwain Jr NE. Damage control resuscitation: from emergency department to the operating room. *Am Surg*. February 2011;77(2):201–206.

47. Johansson PI, Stensballe J. Effect of haemostatic control resuscitation on mortality in massively bleeding patients: a before and after study. *Vox Sanguinis*. February 2009;96(2):111–118.

48. Nunez TC, Voskresensky IV, Dossett LA, Shinall R, Dutton WD, Cotton BA. Early prediction of massive transfusion in trauma: simple as ABC (Assessment of Blood Consumption)? *J Trauma Acute Care Surg*. 2009;66(2):346–352.

49. CRASH-2 collaborators, Shakur H, Roberts I, et al. Effects of tranexamic acid on death, vascular occlusive events, and blood transfusion in trauma patients with significant haemorrhage (CRASH-2): a randomised, placebo-controlled trial. *Lancet*. July 3, 2010;376(9734):23–32.

50. Hauser CJ, Boffard K, Dutton R, et al. Results of the CONTROL trial: efficacy and safety of recombinant activated Factor VII in the management of refractory traumatic hemorrhage. *J Trauma*. September 2010;69(3):489–500.

51. Schochl H, Nienaber U, Hofer G, et al. Goal-directed coagulation management of major trauma patients using thromboelastometry (ROTEM)-guided administration of fibrinogen concentrate and prothrombin complex concentrate. *Crit Care*. 2010;14(2):R55.

52. Hebert PC, Wells G, Blajchman MA, et al. A multicenter, randomized, controlled clinical trial of transfusion requirements in critical care. *N Engl J Med*. February 11, 1999;340(6):409–417.

53. McIntyre L, Hebert PC, Wells G, et al. Is a restrictive transfusion strategy safe for resuscitated and critically ill trauma patients? *J Trauma*. September 2004;57(3):563–568.

54. Dunne JR, Malone DL, Tracy JK, Napolitano LM. Allogenic blood transfusion in the first 24 hours after trauma is associated with increased systemic inflammatory response syndrome (SIRS) and death. *Surg Infect*. 2004;5(4):395–404.

55. Dunne JR, Riddle MS, Danko J, Hayden R, Petersen K. Blood transfusion is associated with infection and increased resource utilization in combat casualties. *Am Surg*. July 2006;72(7):619–625.

56. Malone DL, Dunne J, Tracy JK, Putnam AT, Scalea TM, Napolitano LM. Blood transfusion, independent of shock severity, is associated with worse outcome in trauma. *J Trauma*. May 2003;54(5):898–905.

57. Silverboard H, Aisiku I, Martin GS, Adams M, Rozycki G, Moss M. The role of acute blood transfusion in the development of acute respiratory distress syndrome in patients with severe trauma. *J Trauma*. September 2005;59(3):717–723.

58. Offner PJ, Moore EE, Biffl WL, Johnson JL, Silliman CC. Increased rate of infection associated with transfusion of old blood after severe injury. *Arch Surg*. June 2002;137(6):711–716.

59. Nathens AB, Nester TA, Rubenfeld GD, Nirula R, Gernsheimer TB. The effects of leukoreduced blood transfusion on infection risk following injury: a randomized controlled trial. *Shock*. October 2006;26(4):342–347.

60. Phelan HA, Sperry JL, Friese RS. Leukoreduction before red blood cell transfusion has no impact on mortality in trauma patients. *J Surg Res*. March 2007;138(1):32–36.

61. Plurad D, Martin M, Green D, et al. The decreasing incidence of late posttraumatic acute respiratory distress syndrome: the potential role of lung protective ventilation and conservative transfusion practice. *J Trauma*. July 2007;63(1):1–7.

62. Mapstone J, Roberts I, Evans P. Fluid resuscitation strategies: a systematic review of animal trials. *J Trauma Acute Care Surg*. 2003;55(3):571–589.

63. Wu X, Stezoski J, Safar P, Tisherman SA. During prolonged (6 H) uncontrolled hemorrhagic shock (UHS) with hypotensive fluid resuscitation, mean arterial pressure (MAP) must be maintained above 60-70 mm Hg in rats. *Crit Care Med*. 2002;30(suppl):A40.

64. Kaweski SM, Sise MJ, Virgilio RW. The effect of prehospital fluids on survival in trauma patients. [see comment] *J Trauma*. October 1990;30(10):1215–1218.

65. Bickell WH, Wall Jr MJ, Pepe PE, et al. Immediate versus delayed fluid resuscitation for hypotensive patients with penetrating torso injuries. [see comment] *N Engl J Med*. October 27, 1994;331(17):1105–1109.

66. Dutton RP, Mackenzie CF, Scalea TM. Hypotensive resuscitation during active hemorrhage: impact on in-hospital mortality. [see comment] *J Trauma*. June 2002;52(6):1141–1146.

67. Hambly PR, Dutton RP. Excess mortality associated with the use of a rapid infusion system at a level 1 trauma center. [see comment] *Resuscitation*. April 1996;31(2):127–133.

68. Duke MD, Guidry C, Guice J, et al. Restrictive fluid resuscitation in combination with damage control resuscitation: time for adaptation. *J Trauma Acute Care Surg*. September 2012;73(3):674–678.

69. Morrison CA, Carrick MM, Norman MA, et al. Hypotensive resuscitation strategy reduces transfusion requirements and severe postoperative coagulopathy in trauma patients with hemorrhagic shock: preliminary results of a randomized controlled trial. *J Trauma*. March 2011;70(3):652–663.

70. Wang CH, Hsieh WH, Chou HC, et al. Liberal versus restricted fluid resuscitation strategies in trauma patients: a systematic review and meta-analysis of randomized controlled trials and observational studies. *Crit Care Med*. April 2014;42(4):954–961.

70a. Schreiber MA, Meier EN, et al. ROC investigators. A controlled resuscitation strategy is feasible and safe in hypotensive trauma patients: results of a prospective randomized pilot trial. *J Trauma Acute Care Surg*. 2015;78(4):687–695.

71. Shoemaker WC, Montgomery ES, Kaplan E, Elwyn DH. Physiologic patterns in surviving and nonsurviving shock patients. Use of sequential cardiorespiratory variables in defining criteria for therapeutic goals and early warning of death. *Arch Surg*. May 1973;106(5):630–636.

72. Bishop MH, Shoemaker WC, Appel PL, et al. Relationship between supranormal circulatory values, time delays, and outcome in severely traumatized patients. *Crit Care Med*. January 1993;21(1):56–63.

73. Bishop MH, Shoemaker WC, Appel PL, et al. Prospective, randomized trial of survivor values of cardiac index, oxygen delivery, and oxygen consumption as resuscitation endpoints in severe trauma. *J Trauma*. May 1995;38(5):780–787.

74. Fleming A, Bishop M, Shoemaker W, et al. Prospective trial of supranormal values as goals of resuscitation in severe trauma. *Arch Surg*. October 1992;127(10):1175–1179.

75. Velmahos GC, Demetriades D, Shoemaker WC, et al. Endpoints of resuscitation of critically injured patients: normal or supranormal? A prospective randomized trial. *Ann Surg*. September 2000;232(3):409–418.

76. McKinley BA, Kozar RA, Cocanour CS, et al. Normal versus supranormal oxygen delivery goals in shock resuscitation: the response is the same. *J Trauma*. November 2002;53(5):825–832.

77. Rutherford EJ, Morris Jr JA, Reed GW, Hall KS. Base deficit stratifies mortality and determines therapy. *J Trauma*. September 1992;33(3):417–423.

78. Davis JW, Shackford SR, Mackersie RC, Hoyt DB. Base deficit as a guide to volume resuscitation. *J Trauma*. October 1988;28(10):1464–1467.

79. Davis JW, Kaups KL, Parks SN. Base deficit is superior to pH in evaluating clearance of acidosis after traumatic shock. *J Trauma*. January 1998;44(1):114–118.

80. Kincaid EH, Miller PR, Meredith JW, Rahman N, Chang MC. Elevated arterial base deficit in trauma patients: a marker of impaired oxygen utilization. [see comment] *J Am Coll Surg*. October 1998;187(4):384–392.

81. Cerovic O, Golubovic V, Spec-Marn A, Kremzar B, Vidmar G. Relationship between injury severity and lactate levels in severely injured patients. *Intensive Care Med*. August 2003;29(8):1300–1305.

82. Fitzgibbons JP. Fluid, electrolyte, and acid-base management in the acutely traumatized patient. *Orthop Clin North Am*. July 1978;9(3):627–648.

83. Pal JD, Victorino GP, Twomey P, Liu TH, Bullard MK, Harken AH. Admission serum lactate levels do not predict mortality in the acutely injured patient. *J Trauma*. March 2006;60(3):583–587.

84. Cohn SM. Near-infrared spectroscopy: potential clinical benefits in surgery. *J Am Coll Surg*. August 2007;205(2):322–332.

85. Ryan ML, Ogilvie MP, Pereira BM, et al. Heart rate variability is an independent predictor of morbidity and mortality in hemodynamically stable trauma patients. *J Trauma*. June 2011;70(6):1371–1380.

86. Ferrada P, Murthi S, Anand RJ, Bochicchio GV, Scalea T. Transthoracic focused rapid echocardiographic examination: real-time evaluation of fluid status in critically ill trauma patients. *J Trauma*. January 2011;70(1):56–62.

87. Murthi SB, Hess JR, Hess A, Stansbury LG, Scalea TM. Focused rapid echocardiographic evaluation versus vascular cather-based assessment of cardiac output and function in critically ill trauma patients. *J Trauma Acute Care Surg*. May 2012;72(5):1158–1164.

88. Tisherman SA, Barie P, Bokhari F, et al. Clinical practice guideline: endpoints of resuscitation. *J Trauma*. October 2004;57(4):898–912.

89. Rizoli SB, Rhind SG, Shek PN, et al. The immunomodulatory effects of hypertonic saline resuscitation in patients sustaining traumatic hemorrhagic shock: a randomized, controlled, double-blinded trial. *Ann Surg*. January 2006;243(1):47–57.

78 How Should the Critically Ill Pregnant Patient Be Managed?

Lauren A. Plante

The critically ill pregnant woman presents many challenges to the intensivist, who must consider the needs of both mother and fetus in clinical decision-making.

Fortunately, the need for critical care services in the obstetric population is uncommon. Estimates from case series suggest that approximately 1 to 8 per 1000 obstetric admissions are admitted to an intensive care unit (ICU).[1,2] In addition, another 1% to 2% of critically ill women are treated in a labor and delivery unit or a specialized obstetric care unit.[3,4] These numbers may understate the scope of the problem because a large national population-based study of severe maternal morbidity has found that in 2008 to 2009, nearly 1.6% of delivery and postpartum hospitalizations in the United States were associated with severe maternal complications; purely antepartum admissions that did not result in delivery were not captured in this study.[5] Although the decision to admit or transfer an obstetric patient to the ICU varies with the range of services available at the institution and therefore not all women with severe maternal complications are counted in an ICU census, a recent state-level analysis calculated the ICU utilization rate as 419 per 100,000 deliveries.[6] Extrapolating to the nearly 4 million births in the United States during 2013,[7] nearly 17,000 pregnant or postpartum women in the United States would require ICU admission annually, at least 64,000 will sustain a major complication, and somewhere between 40,000 and 80,000 with a critical illness or potentially life-threatening complication will be treated within obstetric units, with or without the input of critical care specialists.

Special considerations in obstetrics include the "two-patient problem" (i.e., the balance of needs between mother and fetus) and the need for the clinician to factor in normal pregnancy physiology. Further complicating clinical decision making, a paucity of research has focused specifically on the critically ill pregnant patient. What follows is information, such as it exists, to assist the clinician caring for a pregnant or postpartum patient who has sepsis and one who needs ventilator support.

SEPSIS IN PREGNANCY

In most treatment trials, pregnant patients are explicitly barred from enrollment. Because severe sepsis and septic shock (aside from unsafe abortion) are not common in pregnancy, the epidemiology of sepsis in this population is not as well described as in a general medical-surgical population. The World Health Organization recently estimated 77,000 deaths worldwide per year from maternal sepsis, with 0.1% to 10% of all live births being complicated by some degree of maternal infection.[8] Criteria for sepsis or severe sepsis have been met in 3 to 9 per 10,000 deliveries in Europe[9,10]; Callaghan,[5] using data from the National Inpatient Sample, calculated 3 cases of sepsis per 10,000 delivery or postpartum hospitalizations in the United States, a figure that excludes antepartum hospitalizations not resulting in delivery.

The case-fatality rate for sepsis in the obstetric population is not known with any degree of certainty; however, the case-fatality rate for septic abortion specifically is as high as 20%.[11] Calculations based on birth statistics and the National Inpatient Sample,[5] although not provided in the original paper, would put the overall case-fatality rate for sepsis at delivery or postpartum at approximately 9%.

Sepsis may be obstetric or nonobstetric. Causes of obstetric sepsis include uterine infection (chorioamnionitis if undelivered, endomyometritis postpartum), septic abortion, and wound infection (cesarean or episiotomy wound); in addition, sepsis may follow invasive procedures such as amniocentesis, chorionic villus sampling, cervical cerclage, or percutaneous umbilical blood sampling. One of the few case series in the U.S. literature on septic shock in pregnancy[11a] reported half of the cases to have an obstetric cause whereas, of the 50% with nonobstetric causes, most were urinary in origin. However, more recent data from the U.K. Obstetric Surveillance System showed that 31% of severe sepsis cases in obstetric patients arose from the genital tract, another 20% were urinary in origin, and 26% had no identified source.[12]

WHAT CRITERIA SHOULD BE USED TO DIAGNOSE SEPSIS IN A PREGNANT OR POSTPARTUM PATIENT? ARE THESE DIFFERENT FROM THE GENERALLY ACCEPTED CRITERIA?

Criteria for the diagnosis of sepsis, originally promulgated in 1992, were reconfirmed in an international multispecialty

Table 78-1 Sepsis in Obstetrics Scoring System[14]

Variable	High Abnormal Range				Normal		Low Abnormal Range		
Score	+4	+3	+2	+1	0	−1	−2	−3	−4
Temperature (°C)	>40.9	39-40.9		38.5-38.9	36-38.4	34-35.9	32-33.9	30-31.9	<30
Systolic blood pressure (mm Hg)					>90		70-90		<70
Heart rate (beats/min)	>179	150-179	130-149	120-129	≤119				
Respiratory rate (breaths per minute)	>49	35-49		25-34	12-24	10-11	6-9		≤5
SpO₂ (%)					≥92%	90-91%		85-89%	<85%
WBC count (µ/L)	>39.9		25-39.9	17-24.9	5.7-16.9	3-5.6	1-2.9		<1
% Immature neutrophils			≥10%		<10%				
Lactic acid (mmol/L)			≥4		<4				

SpO₂, oxygen saturation by pulse oximetry; *WBC*, white blood cell.

conference in 2001. Their applicability in pregnancy, labor, or the immediate puerperium, however, is limited. There is considerable overlap between the normal physiologic parameters of pregnancy and the criteria used to make a diagnosis of systemic inflammatory response syndrome (SIRS) or sepsis. This may contribute both to a delayed recognition of sepsis among experienced obstetric care providers and to an overdiagnosis of sepsis in obstetric patients by critical care professionals. A recent systematic review of normal physiologic variables during pregnancy, labor, and the puerperium[13] demonstrated this dilemma in detail. In normal pregnancy, respiratory rates increase from the second to third trimester, with further increases in labor, and remain elevated postpartum. If the threshold for tachypnea is taken as a respiratory rate of 20 breaths per min, then the normal range in pregnancy includes this rate from the second trimester through the first few days postpartum. The normal range for maternal heart rate shows an overlap with the SIRS criterion for tachycardia (90 beats/min) in all stages of pregnancy. Normal white blood cell (WBC) count is also increased from the second trimester through the puerperium, again significantly overlapping the range identified as leukocytosis in the usual SIRS criteria. In fact, the mean WBC count in the first 2 days postpartum is 15×10^9/L, which would make it quite difficult to discriminate SIRS or sepsis by laboratory criteria in that period. Of the parameters analyzed, temperature alone is not affected by the fact of pregnancy (although the use of epidural analgesia in labor does increase the maternal temperature and could confound the diagnosis). In addition, both diastolic pressure and serum creatinine are known to decrease in pregnancy, which might call into question the threshold criteria commonly used for a diagnosis of severe sepsis.

A Sepsis in Obstetrics Score[14] was recently proposed as an indicator of maternal morbidity (Table 78-1). On the basis of the Rapid Emergency Medicine Score, itself a derivative of the APACHE (Acute Physiology and Chronic Health Evaluation) score, and the SIRS/sepsis criteria of the Surviving Sepsis Campaign (SSC), which were modified for pregnancy-specific parameters such as blood pressure, heart rate, and WBC count, the authors hoped to

refine a tool for predicting admission to the ICU within 48 hours after presentation to the emergency department in a group of pregnant and postpartum women in whom sepsis was suspected (Table 78-1). A cutoff score of 6 or more was found to have 89% sensitivity and 99% specificity for the outcome of interest, but the ICU admission rate of approximately 1% in the study population meant that the positive predictive value of the scoring system was only approximately 17%. This test performance was nevertheless better in predicting outcomes for obstetric patients with suspected sepsis than that of standard, nonmodified scoring systems such as the SIRS score alone or the Modified Early Warning System (MEWS).[15]

CAN THE SURVIVING SEPSIS CAMPAIGN GUIDELINES BE APPLIED IN CASES OF SEPSIS IN OBSTETRIC PATIENTS?

The SSC[16] is a multiorganizational effort to improve outcomes in sepsis and septic shock that is based on best available evidence. It recommends several goals, which are summarized in the following list, with commentary relating specifically to obstetric patients. There is no evidence base for these guidelines in a pregnant or postpartum patient, but there is no evidence against them either.

1. *Initial resuscitation for patients with sepsis-induced hypotension.* During the first 6 hours, target central venous pressure (CVP) 8 to 12 mm Hg, mean arterial pressure (MAP) greater than 65 mm Hg, urine output greater than 0.5 mL/kg/min, and mixed venous oxygen saturation 65%. Normalize lactate in patients with elevated lactate levels.

   MAP is commonly lower in pregnancy, which is a volume-loaded vasodilated state. MAP as low as 60 mm Hg may still be normal, and normal CVP is commonly lower than 8 mm Hg. Oncotic pressure is also lower in normal pregnancy; therefore, fluid loading with isotonic solution may predispose more easily to pulmonary edema. No pregnancy-specific guidelines or cutoffs have been proposed for these parameters.

2. *Blood cultures before antibiotic therapy, if this does not significantly delay starting antimicrobial therapy.*

   There is no reason this would not apply in pregnant/postpartum patients. One study in Finland reported on this specific policy for obstetric patients; 2% (of >40,000) were cultured for fever and had broad-spectrum antibiotics immediately administered. Bacteremia was confirmed in 5% of cases; only 1 of the 798 patients cultured had septic shock, for an incidence of 0.1%.[17]

3. *Imaging studies performed promptly to ascertain the source of infection.*

   Pregnant women can be imaged despite the fact of pregnancy, although there are some issues related to ionizing radiation. The American College of Obstetricians and Gynecologists recommends limiting the total radiation dose during pregnancy to 5 rad (5 cGy) because no fetal effects are known this low.[18] Substitute nonionizing modality if feasible (e.g., ultrasound, magnetic resonance imaging). If ionizing radiation is to be used, then shield the abdomen if possible. If ionizing radiation is required and the abdomen/pelvis is to be included in the field, then modify the technique to minimize the dose delivered to the fetus, and use dosimetry to tally the fetal dose.

4. *Initiation of broad-spectrum antibiotic therapy within 1 hour of diagnosis.*

   There is no reason this would not be feasible; however, the hemodynamic picture that characterizes normal pregnancy may result in overdiagnosing sepsis. The central hemodynamics of normal pregnancy include increased cardiac output, increased heart rate, decreased systemic vascular resistance, and a somewhat lower blood pressure.[19] Most but not all antibiotics can be used in pregnancy, although dose adjustments may be needed because of changes in pharmacokinetics (e.g., expanded plasma volume, increased glomerular filtration rate, increased protein binding).[20] Broad-spectrum coverage is reasonable in obstetrics patients. In a recent Finnish study of peripartum sepsis, more than 40 organisms were cultured, including aerobic gram-positive and gram-negative as well as anaerobic bacteria,[17] and extended-spectrum beta-lactamase–producing microbes should be considered in high-risk patients who do not respond to initial antibiotics.

5. *Reassessment of antibiotic therapy with clinical and microbiologic data to narrow antibiotic coverage when appropriate.*

   There are no data specific to pregnancy. When narrowing coverage, some consideration should be given to whether transplacental coverage is appropriate; some drugs do not cross the placenta well and may result in inadequate fetal treatment (e.g., erythromycin or azithromycin in the treatment of syphilis).[22]

6. *Seven to ten days of antibiotic therapy.*

   There is no evidence base specific to pregnancy, and no reason to recommend alteration in this goal.

7. *Source control.*

   There are no data specific to pregnancy. A significant proportion of cases of sepsis in pregnant/postpartum women localize to the uterus and would therefore require the uterus be emptied. This would generally equate to delivery. Fetuses less than 23 weeks gestational age are unlikely to survive outside of the uterus; at 23 and 24 weeks, survival rates of 26% and 55%, respectively, have been reported, at least at the highest-level neonatal intensive care facilities, although only 10% of those infants survive without major morbidity.[23] There are no data on antibiotics without delivery for women diagnosed with clinical sepsis attributed to intra-amniotic infection. Women with a diagnosis of subclinical intra-amniotic infection who were treated with antibiotics alone, in the hope of delaying delivery to a more favorable gestational age, have been observed to have a prolongation of pregnancy by days to weeks, with the only maternal morbidity recorded being a 3% rate of postpartum endometritis,[24] but with an infant death rate of 33% and major infant morbidity greater than 75%. It should be emphasized that patients with subclinical chorioamnionitis, who typically present only with preterm labor or membrane rupture, are unlikely to come to the ICU; if these patients cannot reasonably be managed without delivery, then there is no argument for managing clinical chorioamnionitis without it. There appears to be no place for deferring source control in pregnancy.

8. *Crystalloid as the fluid of choice for resuscitation.*

   There is no evidence to recommend one versus the other in pregnant patients with sepsis. Trials of crystalloid versus colloid have been performed to assess preloading before elective cesarean delivery with the patient under regional anesthesia, but extrapolation to sepsis would be inappropriate. Because the gradient between colloid oncotic pressure and pulmonary artery occlusion pressure is lower in pregnancy,[19] there may be more risk of pulmonary edema than in the nonobstetric patient.

9. *Norepinephrine as the first-choice vasopressor, to target initial MAP greater than 65 mm Hg.*

   No data exist to recommend a lower limit of MAP in pregnancy, but MAP is normally lower in pregnancy than in healthy nonpregnant controls.[25] Thus, a MAP of 65 mm Hg or greater may be too stringent. Although the MAP difference is 4 to 5 mm Hg lower in pregnancy, one cannot extrapolate to a recommendation to target 60 mm Hg instead. The uteroplacental circulation does not autoregulate, and compromised placental perfusion may be apparent by examination of the electronic fetal heart rate tracing: the tracing may allow individualization of the target MAP for the mother. Although norepinephrine, similar to epinephrine, vasopressin, and dopamine, has been used clinically in obstetric crises such as shock, there are limited data on safety or efficacy of any of these drugs in human pregnancy. During pregnancy, the response to vasoconstrictors, both endogenous and exogenous, is blunted; therefore, the usual therapeutic doses may not result in the expected effect.[26] No recommendation can be made. This decision must be individualized.

Space limits a discussion of the supportive therapies reviewed in SSC. Such therapies as transfusion of red cells and platelets, sedation, venous thrombosis prophylaxis, and stress ulcer prophylaxis are not proscribed during pregnancy. To avoid hyperinsulinemia in the fetus, one would generally target an upper maternal blood glucose level of 140 mg/dL or less rather than the SSC recommendation of 180 mg/dL or less.

ACUTE RESPIRATORY DISTRESS SYNDROME IN PREGNANCY

Acute respiratory distress syndrome (ARDS) is an uncommon disorder in pregnancy, with an incidence estimated at between 0.016% and 0.035% of deliveries, or roughly 1/3000 to 1/6000.[27,28] The incidence of acute lung injury (including ARDS) is estimated at roughly 80/100,000 patient-years in the general U.S. population.[29] The incidence of ARDS in pregnancy is calculated as 21 to 46 per 100,000 person-years[1] in the obstetric population, which is lower than the rate in the general population (although not, obviously, age-adjusted). The mortality rate for ARDS among obstetric patients was estimated as 24% to 44% among older case series,[27,28,30,31] and 33% in a more recent series,[32] neither of which is greatly different from the general population case-fatality rate of 38%.[29] A national review of Canadian hospital admissions between 1991 and 2002, however, found that the case-fatality rate among obstetric patients with ARDS in the absence of any major preexisting condition (e.g., diabetes, heart disease) was only 6%.[33]

WHAT IS THE OPTIMUM STRATEGY FOR MECHANICAL VENTILATION WHEN THE PATIENT IS PREGNANT?

There are no randomized controlled trials of ventilator strategies in the obstetric population. Many authorities recommend maintaining maternal oxygen saturation by pulse oximetry (SpO_2) greater than 95%, or partial pressure of oxygen in arterial blood (PaO_2) greater than 60 mm Hg "to preserve fetal wellbeing," but it is unclear what evidence supports this recommendation, at least in humans. Uteroplacental blood flow rather than maternal oxygenation per se is the major determinant of fetal oxygen delivery. The model for gas transport across the human placenta is thought to be that of a concurrent exchanger. The gradient between maternal and fetal oxygen content drives transfer. Because the oxygen content of fetal blood is low, the gradient is easily preserved: normal fetal umbilical venous partial pressure of oxygen (PO_2) (the most highly oxygenated blood in the system) is only 31 to 42 mm Hg.[34] The nature of a concurrent exchanger is such that oxygen saturation at the most highly oxygenated end of the fetal side is still lower than the least oxygenated end of the maternal circulation, represented by the uterine vein, or approximately the mixed venous saturation of oxygen (SvO_2). Only in the extreme case of a venous equilibrator could the two be equal, and under no circumstances can the fetal side be higher than the maternal venous side. Oxygen delivery to the fetus and to fetal organs, as to the adult, is represented by the product of blood flow and oxygen content.

Adaptive strategies in the fetus include higher affinity of fetal hemoglobin for oxygen and high cardiac output relative to size.

There is only one experimental trial of deliberate hypoxia in human pregnancy.[35] Ten women with normal pregnancies near term were exposed to a hypoxic gas mixture with a fraction of inspired oxygen (FIO_2) of approximately 0.1 (50% room air, 50% nitrogen) for 10 minutes, during which time SpO_2 decreased by 15%. Fetal parameters that are thought to represent fetal oxygenation (i.e., heart rate baseline and variability, fetal umbilical artery Doppler indices, and fetal middle cerebral artery Doppler indices) did not change during experimental maternal hypoxia. Direct sampling of fetal blood was not performed in this study.

In case series from the era preceding low-tidal-volume ventilation for ARDS, barotrauma rates were high in obstetric patients who underwent mechanical ventilation (i.e., 36% to 44%).[27,28] This compares unfavorably with the background rate of barotrauma of 11% among nonobstetric patients ventilated with "traditional" tidal volumes in ARDS.[36]

When undertaking a standard low-tidal-volume ventilation strategy for pregnant women with ARDS, the maternal partial pressure of carbon dioxide in arterial blood ($PaCO_2$) is probably of equal if not more importance than the PaO_2. CO_2 transfer across the placenta also requires a gradient; in this case the higher $PaCO_2$ of fetal blood diffuses across placental interface to the lower $PaCO_2$ of maternal blood. High maternal $PaCO_2$, as in permissive hypercapnia, would be expected to impede fetomaternal CO_2 transfer and promote fetal acidemia. In a small trial of CO_2 rebreathing in 35 healthy pregnant women, an increase in the maternal end-tidal CO_2 as high as 60 torr was associated with a loss of fetal heart rate variability in 57% of fetuses monitored, this being a proxy for fetal acidemia; 90% of fetuses thus affected normalized the tracing after test.[37]

Thus it would seem that a pregnant woman ventilated with the standard low-tidal-volume strategy could have the fetal heart rate tracing continuously monitored as a way of assessing fetal oxygenation and acid-base status. This would be irrelevant at very early gestational ages (e.g., before 24 weeks). If the tracing shows signs of fetal compromise, then interventions might include decreasing positive end-expiratory pressure (PEEP; to improve uterine blood flow by improving cardiac output) or increasing tidal volume so as to increase maternal pH and decrease maternal $PaCO_2$. Others have recommended focusing on attempts to increase maternal PaO_2, albeit without obvious evidence to support the intervention; this would require increasing FIO_2 rather than PEEP because of the effects of PEEP on cardiac output and therefore on uteroplacental perfusion.

Additional therapies that have been used for ARDS in the general population may be applied in the case of pregnancy, including inhaled nitric oxide and prone positioning, although creative use of buttresses or mattress cutouts may be required for proning, depending on the size of the gravid uterus. Fetal concerns should not be allowed to interfere with appropriate sedation of the mother. Neuromuscular blocking agents, if used, do not cross the placenta.

Delivery in itself does not seem to improve maternal survival in ARDS.[28,38,39] Fetal survival, however, is tightly linked to gestational age at delivery: this would imply a fetal benefit to continuing rather than interrupting pregnancy, assuming maternal and fetal condition permits.

WHAT IS THE ROLE OF EXTRACORPOREAL MEMBRANE OXYGENATION IN REFRACTORY ACUTE RESPIRATORY DISTRESS SYNDROME IN OBSTETERIC PATIENTS?

Extracorporeal membrane oxygenation (ECMO) is now more commonly applied and more generally available in adult patients with respiratory failure. The CESAR (Conventional Versus ECMO for Severe Adult Respiratory Failure) trial[40] showed a survival benefit of transfer to ECMO specialty centers for consideration of this intervention. Survival rates were 63% among patients who received ECMO compared with 47% of those not considered for ECMO. Although there were no obstetric patients enrolled in the CESAR trial, the year of the trial's publication also saw the worldwide pandemic of a novel influenza A virus, H1N1, which was significantly more severe among pregnant women than most other groups. A pragmatic approach to H1N1 respiratory failure, pioneered in Australia and New Zealand, meant that an unprecedented number of pregnant (and postpartum) patients were treated with ECMO.[41-43] This recent experience has led to an increasing willingness to consider ECMO for refractory respiratory failure among obstetric patients. A compilation of data from case reports and case series suggests that maternal survival on ECMO is approximately 80% and fetal survival is approximately 70%.[44] Because both antepartum and postpartum bleeding are of concern and may be catastrophic, it may be prudent to maintain a lower level of anticoagulation in these patients. Attention should also be paid to adequate venous drainage because the gravid uterus may compress the inferior vena cava when the patient is prone; thus, alterations in patient positioning or the addition of another venous outflow cannula may be required.

CONCLUSION

Care of the critically ill obstetric patient requires interpretation and adaptation of studies performed in the nonobstetric population. In most situations of critical illness in pregnancy, there are no randomized trials to guide the practitioner, and none are likely to be performed. Pregnancy physiology, uteroplacental perfusion, and fetal issues may require modifications in ICU management. A multidisciplinary approach, with careful assessment of treatment options, is expected to serve these patients best.

AUTHOR'S RECOMMENDATIONS

- Critical illness in pregnancy may result from diseases specific to pregnancy (pre-eclampsia, HELLP), diseases worsened by pregnancy (renal disease), and diseases unrelated to pregnancy (e.g., trauma).
- Most parturients are admitted to ICU after birth, most commonly as a result of hypertensive disease of pregnancy or postpartum hemorrhage.
- Pregnant patients have been specifically excluded from all major critical care trials.
- In general, what is good for the mother is good for the fetus. A multidisciplinary approach involving intensivists, obstetricians, and midwives/nurses with careful assessment of treatment options is expected to serve these patients best.
- Sepsis in pregnancy is either nonobstetric or obstetric—most commonly endometritis due to prolonged membrane rupture. The incidence is increasing and is principally associated with group A streptococcus.
- The diagnosis of sepsis is difficult because SIRS criteria are similar to the physiologic changes of pregnancy; raised inflammatory proteins and leukocytosis are normal during pregnancy.
- Resuscitation should be with balanced crystalloid; norepinephrine is the vasopressor of choice.
- ARDS in pregnancy is especially challenging; prone positioning is not advised. Consideration should be given to early delivery to optimize maternal welfare. ECMO has been used successfully.

REFERENCES

1. Keizer JL, Zwart JJ, Meerman RH, Harinck BIJ, Feuth HDM, van Roosmalen J. Obstetric intensive care admissions: a 12-year review in a tertiary care centre. *Eur J Obstet Gynecol Reprod Biol.* 2006;128:152–156.
2. Munnur U, Karnad DR, Bandi VDP, et al. Critically ill obstetric patients in an American and an Indian public hospital: comparison of case-mix, organ dysfunction, intensive care requirements, and outcomes. *Intensive Care Med.* 2005;31:1087–1094.
3. Ryan M, Hamilton V, Bowen M, McKenna P. The role of a high-dependency unit in a regional obstetric hospital. *Anaesthesia.* 2000;55:1155–1158.
4. Zeeman GG, Wendel GD, Cunningham FG. A blueprint for obstetric critical care. *Am J Obstet Gynecol.* 2003;188:532–536.
5. Callaghan WM, Creanga AA, Kuklina EV. Severe maternal morbidity among delivery and postpartum hospitalizations in the United States. *Obstet Gynecol.* 2012;120:1029–1036.
6. Wanderer JP, Leffert LR, Mhyre JM, Kuklina EV, Callaghan WM, Bateman BT. Epidemiology of obstetric-related intensive care unit admissions in Maryland, 1999-2008. *Crit Care Med.* 2013;41:1844–1852.
7. Hamilton BE, Martin JA, Osterman MJK, Curtin SC. Births: preliminary data for 2013. *Natl Vital Stat Rep.* May 29, 2014;63(2). Accessed online 20.09.14 at: http://www.cdc.gov/nchs/data/nvsr/nvsr63/nvsr63_02.pdf.
8. Dolea C, Stein C. *Global Burden of Maternal Sepsis in the Year 2000.* World Health Organization; 2003. Accessed online 02.03.09 at: http://www.who.int/healthinfo/statistics/bod_maternalsepsis.pdf.
9. Waterstone M, Bewley S, Wolfe C. Incidence and predictors of severe obstetric morbidity: case-control study. *BMJ.* 2001;322:1089–1094.
10. Zhang W-H, Alexander S, Bouvier-Colle M-H, Macfarlane A. Incidence of severe preeclampsia, postpartum haemorrhage and sepsis as a surrogate marker for severe maternal morbidity in a European population-based study: the MOMS-B survey. *BJOG.* 2005;112:89–96.
11. Finkeilman JD, De Feo FD, Heller PG, Afessa B. The clinical course of patients with septic abortion admitted to an intensive care unit. *Intensive Care Med.* 2004;30:1097–1102.
11a. Mabie WC, Barton JR, Sibai B. Septic shock in pregnancy. *Obstet Gynecol.* 1997;90:553–561.

12. Acosta CD, Kurinczuk JJ, Lucas DN, Tuffnell DJ, Sellers S, Knight M, on behalf of the United Kingdom Obstetric Surveillance System. Severe maternal sepsis in the UK, 2011-2012: A national case-control study. *PLoS Med*. 2014;11(7):e1001672.

13. Bauer ME, Bauer ST, Rajala B, et al. Maternal physiologic parameters in relationship to systemic inflammatory response syndrome criteria: a systematic review and meta-analysis. *Obstet Gynecol*. 2014;124:535–541.

14. Albright CM, Ali TN, Lopes V, Rouse DJ, Anderson BL. The sepsis in obstetrics score: a model to identify risk of morbidity from sepsis in pregnancy. *Am J Obstet Gynecol*. 2014;211:39. e1–8.

15. Lappen JR, Keene M, Lore M, Grobman WA, Gossett DR. Existing models fail to predict sepsis in an obstetric population with intrauterine infection. *Am J Obstet Gynecol*. 2010;203:573. e1–5.

16. Dellinger RP, Levy MM, Rhodes A, and the Surviving Sepsis Campaign Guidelines Committee, et al. Surviving Sepsis Campaign: international guidelines for management of severe sepsis and septic shock: 2012. *Crit Care Med*. 2013;41:580–637.

17. Kankuri E, Kurki T, Hiilesmaa V. Incidence, treatment and outcome of peripartum sepsis. *Acta Obstet Gynecol Scand*. 2003;82:730–735.

18. American College of Obstetricians and Gynecologists. Committee on Obstetric Practice. Committee Opinion no. 299, September 2004. Guidelines for diagnostic imaging during pregnancy. *Obstet Gynecol*. 2004;104:647–651.

19. Clark SL, Cotton DB, et al. Central hemodynamic assessment of normal term pregnancy. *Am J Obstet Gynecol*. 1989;161:1439–1444.

20. Nahum GG, Uhl K, Kennedy DL. Antibiotic use in pregnancy and lactation: what is known and not know about teratogenic and toxic risks. *Obstet Gynecol*. 2006;107:1120–1138.

21. Levy MM, Fink MP, Marshall JC, et al. 2001 SCCM/ESICM/ACCP/ATS/SIS International Sepsis Definitions Conference. *Crit Care Med*. 2003;31:1250–1256.

22. Zhou P, Qian Y, Xu J, Gu Z, Liao K. Occurrence of congenital syphilis after maternal treatment with azithromycin during pregnancy. *Sex Transm Dis*. 2007;34:472–474.

23. Stoll BJ, Hansen NI, Bell EF, et al. Neonatal outcomes of extremely preterm infants from the NICHD Neonatal Research Network. *Pediatrics*. 2010;126:443–456.

24. Miyazaki K, Furuhashi M, Matsuo K, et al. Impact of subclinical chorioamnionitis on maternal and neonatal outcomes. *Acta Obstet Gynecol*. 2007;86:191–197.

25. Macedo ML, Luminoso D, Savvidou MD, McEniery CM, Nicolaides KH. Maternal wave refections and arterial stiffness in normal pregnancy as assessed by applanation tonometry. *Hypertension*. 2008;51:1047–1051.

26. Magness RR, Rosenfeld CR. Systemic and uterine responses to alpha-adrenergic stimulation in pregnant and nonpregnant ewes. *Am J Obstet Gynecol*. 1986;155:897–904.

27. Mabie WC, Barton JR, Sibai BM. Adult respiratory distress syndrome in pregnancy. *Am J Obstet Gynecol*. 1992;167:950–957.

28. Catanzarite V, Willms D, Wong D, Landers C, Cousins L, Schrimmer D. Acute respiratory distress syndrome in pregnancy and the puerperium: causes, courses, and outcomes. *Obstet Gynecol*. 2001;97:760–764.

29. Rubenfeld GD, Caldwell E, Peabody E, et al. Incidence and outcomes of acute lung injury. *NEJM*. 2005;353:1685–1693.

30. Perry Jr KG, Martin RW, Blake PG, Roberts WE, Martin Jr JN. Maternal mortality associated with adult respiratory distress syndrome. *South Med J*. 1998;91:441–445.

31. Smith JL, Thomas F, Orme JF, Clemmer TP. Adult respiratory distress syndrome during pregnancy and the puerperium. *West Med J*. 1990;153:508–510.

32. Vasquez DN, Estenssoro E, Canales HS, et al. Clinical characteristics and outcomes of obstetric patients requiring ICU admission. *Chest*. 2007;131:718–724.

33. Wen SW, Huang L, Liston R, et al. Severe maternal morbidity in Canada, 1991-2001. *CMAJ*. 2005;173:759–764.

34. Nicolaides KH, Economides DL, Soothill PW. Blood gases, pH, and lactate in appropriate- and small-for-gestational-age fetuses. *Am J Obstet Gynecol*. 1989;161:996–1001.

35. Erkkola R, Pirhonen J, Polvi H. The fetal cardiovascular function in chronic placental insufficiency is different from experimental hypoxia. *Ann Chir Gynaecol*. 1994;83:76–79.

36. The Acute Respiratory Distress Syndrome Network. Ventilation with lower tidal volumes as compared with traditional tidal volumes for acute lung injury and the acute respiratory distress syndrome. *N Engl J Med*. 2000;342:1301–1308.

37. Fraser D, Jensen D, Wolfe LA, Hahn PM, Davies GAL. Fetal heart rate response to maternal hypocapnia and hypercapnia in late gestation. *J Obstet Gynaecol Can*. 2008;30(4):312–316.

38. Grisaru-Granovsky S, Ioscovich A, Hersch M, Schimmel M, Elstein D, Samueloff A. Temporizing treatment for the respiratory-compromised gravida: an observational study of maternal and neonatal outcome. *Int J Obstet Anesthesia*. 2007;16:261–264.

39. Tomlinson MW, Caruthers TJ, Whitty JE. Does delivery improve maternal condition in the respiratory-compromised gravida? *Obstet Gynecol*. 1998;91:108–111.

40. Peek GJ, Mugford M, Tiruvoipati R, for the CESAR trial collaboration, et al. Efficacy and economic assessment of conventional ventilator support versus extracorporeal membrane oxygenation for severe adult respiratory failure (CESAR): a multicentre randomised controlled trial. *Lancet*. 2009;374:1351–1363.

41. The ANZIC Influenza Investigators and Australasian Maternity Outcomes Surveillance System. Critical illness due to 2009 A/H1N1 influenza in pregnant and postpartum women: population based cohort study. *BMJ*. 2010;340:c1279.

42. Oloyumi-Obi T, Avery L, Schneider C, et al. Perinatal and maternal outcomes in critically ill obstetrics patients with pandemic H1N1 influenza A. *J Obstet Gynaecol Can*. 2010;32:443–447.

43. Dubar G, Azria E, Tesniere A, Dupont H, et al. French experience of 2009 A/H1N1v influenza in pregnant women. *PLoS ONE*. 2010;5(10):e13112.

44. Sharma NS, Wille KM, Bellot SC, Diaz-Guzman E. Modern use of extracorporeal life support in pregnancy and postpartum. *ASAIO J*. 2015;61(1):110–114.

79

How Do I Diagnose and Manage Patients Admitted to the ICU After Common Poisonings?

Jakub Furmaga, Kurt Kleinschmidt

Patients who are critically poisoned present significant diagnostic and therapeutic challenges to critical care staff. Unfortunately, there is no universally accepted management algorithm to aid in the evaluation despite the presence of so many harmful agents. The history is often unavailable, and providers must rely on physical examination, knowledge of toxidromes, and laboratory data to guide diagnosis and management.

In this chapter, we review diagnostic strategies using toxidromes and laboratory testing, describe acetaminophen (paracetamol, or N-acetyl-p-aminophenol [APAP]) and salicylate (acetylsalicylic acid [ASA]) toxicity in moderate detail, clarify the appropriate use of N-acetylcysteine (NAC) as an antidote for acetaminophen overdose, review the evidence behind urine alkalinization for salicylate overdose, and present the evidence behind various decontamination strategies.

DIAGNOSIS

Toxidromes

Toxidromes are constellations of signs and symptoms consistent with a specific group of xenobiotics and their unique effects on neuroreceptors (Table 79-1). The benefit of using toxidromes is that the correct management can be started without knowing the specific agent involved. For example, drugs that block acetylcholine at the muscarinic receptors can result in the anticholinergic toxidrome, which presents with tachycardia, dry skin, hypoactive bowel sounds, urinary retention, mydriasis, and in more severe cases, delirium. Regardless if it was caused by antihistamines, antipsychotics, or plants such as Jimsonweed, these symptoms should improve with the administration of physostigmine. The sympathomimetic toxidrome occurs after activation of norepinephrine and dopamine receptors by stimulants such as cocaine or amphetamine. These patients have tachycardia, diaphoresis, mydriasis, and delirium; regardless of the ingested agent, they will improve when treated with benzodiazepines (BZs). The anticholinergic and sympathomimetic toxidromes may initially appear similar; however, anticholinergic patients are "dry as a bone," whereas sympathomimetic patients are usually diaphoretic. The cholinergic toxidrome is the opposite of the anticholinergic and results from overstimulation of muscarinic and nicotinic receptors. It manifests as diaphoresis, salivation, lacrimation, urination, defecation, and miosis, with bradycardia, bronchospasm, and bronchorrhea being the life-threatening symptoms. Regardless of which organophosphate or carbamate caused these symptoms, atropine is the treatment. The opioid toxidrome results from overstimulation of the mu, kappa, and delta opiate receptors and presents with pinpoint pupils, respiratory depression, and decreased mental status. Antagonists of the opioid receptors, such as naloxone, reverse these symptoms. The sedative/hypnotics toxidrome is similar to that of opioids but has no pupillary changes and significantly less respiratory depression. There is no antidote for most of the causative agents except for flumazenil reversing BZ-related toxicity.

Correctly identified toxidromes can help guide antidote administration and improve the clinical picture without knowing the exact agent involved. However, poisoned patients often ingest many different agents that stimulate/block receptors that conflict with each other, thus clouding the presenting toxidrome.

Laboratory

Most hospitals offer urine drug screens; however, their routine use has not been shown to alter patient management or outcomes.[1] Interpretation can be difficult because different urine assays vary as to which agents, within a class, will be detected. Thus the false positives and false negatives from the assays will vary from institution to institution. Some general points can be made, though. A "positive" screen does not reflect current intoxication because clinical symptoms are generally gone long before the screen becomes "negative." For example, the tetrahydrocannabinol screen for marijuana can remain positive for weeks after an acute exposure and months after chronic exposure. BZ assays often yield false-negative results because not all of the BZs are biotransformed to the same detectable metabolite. Amphetamines are often

Table 79-1 Toxidromes: Clinical Presentations

Toxidrome	Vital Signs	Signs
Anticholinergic	HR ↑	Bowel sounds ↓ Delirium* Dry mouth Mydriasis or normal skin—dry, flushed
Sympathomimetic	HR ↑ BP ↑	Agitated Delirium* Mydriasis Skin—diaphoretic
Opioid	RR ↓ and/or shallow	Bowel sounds ↓ Mental status ↓ Miosis
Sedative-hypnotic	RR normal or ↓†	Mental status ↓
Cholinergic	HR ↓	Bronchoconstriction Bronchorrhea Diaphoresis Lacrimation Miosis Salivation Urination

BP, blood pressure; *HR*, heart rate; *RR*, respiratory rate; *↑*, increased; *↓*, decreased.
*If severe.
†If combined with other sedatives.

associated with false-positive results because of their structural similarity to many legal medications such as pseudoephedrine.

Quantitative serum levels are available for some medications. Measured levels that most commonly affect patient care in a setting of an ingestion are acetaminophen, salicylate, lithium, digoxin, methanol, and ethylene glycol. Phenytoin, valproic acid, and carbamazepine levels are often ordered to help with therapeutic dose monitoring. In an overdose, though, the presence of an elevated measurement is best used to confirm the drug's presence but rarely affects management because patients are observed until clinical improvement and not laboratory normalization.

DANGEROUS POISONINGS: TWO IMPORTANT AGENTS

Most toxic exposures in the United States are nonfatal. According to the 2012 report from the American Association of Poison Control Centers' National Poison Data System, only 0.1% of the reported exposures resulted in death.[2] However, acetaminophen and acetaminophen-containing products accounted for 8.0% of deaths (206 of the 2576 exposure related fatalities) and salicylates for 2.4% (61 of the 2576).[2] Errors occur in the evaluation and treatment of both of these common exposures. For example, a 2008 Maryland Poison Center study suggested that intravenous (IV) NAC administration errors for acetaminophen poisoning occur in approximately one third of cases and include incorrect doses, incorrect rate, interruption of therapy, and

unnecessary administration of NAC.[3] In addition, these agents are at times confused because they are commonly used over-the-counter analgesics. Thus the following section details the treatment of acetaminophen and salicylate overdose.

Acetaminophen

Most acetaminophen (APAP) is glucuronidated and sulfated to inactive, harmless metabolites in the liver (Fig. 79-1); however, approximately 5% to 10% is oxidized by the cytochrome P450 system into the hepatotoxic *N*-acetyl-*p*-benzoquinoneimine (NAPQI).[4] NAPQI is detoxified via conjugation with glutathione, which produces a nontoxic species that is renally eliminated.[5] After an APAP overdose, the glutathione supply is rapidly depleted, resulting in free NAPQI and subsequent hepatotoxicity. Hepatitis (as defined by aspartate aminotransferase [AST] > 1000 IU/L)[6] occurs after an ingestion of 150 mg/kg,[7] and higher doses can lead to acute liver failure (ALF).[8]

Because APAP toxicity has no early symptoms, a level is obtained in all cases of possible overdose. NAC is a partial antidote to APAP poisoning and acts to maintain or replenish depleted glutathione reserves in the liver. The Rumack-Matthew nomogram guides the use of NAC in acute (single-exposure) overdoses when the time of ingestion is known.[9] The treatment line is based on a 4-hour half-life starting with a toxic 4-hour serum concentration of 150 µg/mL. This screening tool has a sensitivity of almost 100% when strictly applied.[10] Levels before 4 hours after exposure generally do not guide therapy. Except in the setting of very large overdoses (>80 to 100 tablets) or co-ingestants that slow down gastrointestinal motility, serial APAP levels are unnecessary because of APAP's predictable absorption and elimination half-life. In cases of massive APAP ingestion, not only is complete absorption delayed but elimination half-life can also be prolonged to as much as 20.3 hours.[11]

A toxic level was traditionally treated with oral NAC for 72 hours (140 mg/kg followed by 70 mg/kg every 4 hours for 17 doses) in the United States. In Europe, Canada, and other territories, IV NAC has been used for decades. Acetadote, a pyrogen-free IV form of NAC, was approved in the United States in 2004. Acetadote is recommended for patients who were seen within 8 to 10 hours of acute ingestion and is administered with a 21-hour protocol: 150 mg/kg of NAC in 200 mL of 5% dextrose in water (D5W) over 1 hour, then 50 mg/kg in 500 mL of D5W over 4 hours, and then 100 mg/kg in 1000 mL of D5W over 16 hours. A recent cost analysis showed that an Acetadote regimen was less expensive than the generic oral NAC because of shortened hospital stay.[12] Both regimens are equally effective when started early[13]; however, one meta-analysis showed that for treatment started more than 18 hours after ingestion (late presenters), the 72-hour oral NAC formulation was more effective at preventing hepatotoxicity than the IV Acetadote. This difference was attributed to the oral NAC protocol's larger cumulative dose (1330 mg/kg vs. 300 mg/kg) and longer duration of treatment (72 hours vs. 21 hours).[14] Furthermore, late presenters who had already developed ALF had lower mortality and less progression to grade III/IV encephalopathy when given NAC compared with those

Acetaminophen metabolism diagram

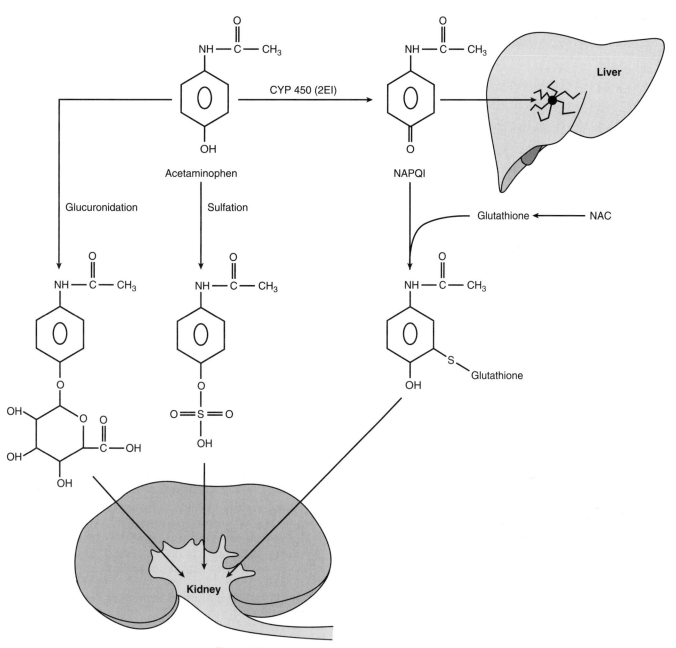

Figure 79-1. Acetaminophen metabolism diagram.

who had not.[15] On the basis of these data, many toxicologists advocate giving additional NAC (i.e., Acetadote bag #3: 100 mg/kg in 1000 mL of D5W over 16 hours) in addition to the 21-hour infusion for anyone who has continuously rising AST and for those with ongoing hepatitis (AST > 1000 IU/L). This is true even in situations when the APAP level becomes undetectable because it is its unmeasured metabolite, NAPQI, that is causing the liver injury.

Salicylates

Salicylate (ASA) poisoning is very common because of its availability in many stand-alone and combination products

for analgesia and fever and in liniments.[16] The salicylate toxidrome includes vomiting, hyperpnea, diaphoresis, dizziness, and hearing changes such as muffled hearing or tinnitus. Arterial blood gas shows mixed respiratory alkalosis and anion-gap metabolic acidosis. In chronic ingestion, patients often have an altered mental status and mimicking infection, and it is referred to as "pseudosepsis."[17]

Serum salicylate concentrations are most commonly reported in milligrams per deciliter. Therapeutic levels range from 10 to 30 mg/dL. Toxicity results from tissue distribution and not from the salicylate in the blood; thus serum levels and toxicity do not always correlate. For example, a serum salicylate level could be decreasing because

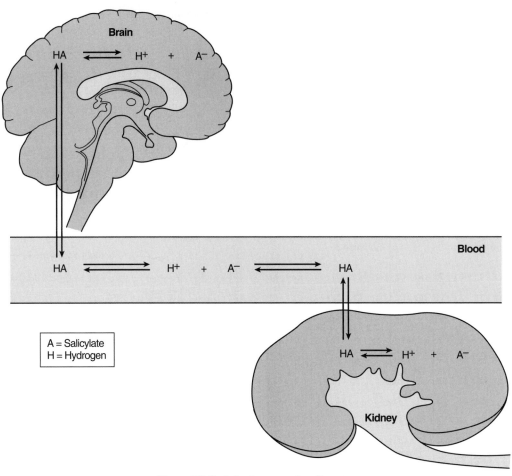

Figure 79-2. Salicylate excretion diagram.

salicylate is either being distributed into tissues (and the patient is becoming clinically sicker) or being eliminated by the kidneys (and the patient is clinically improving). Toxicity is considered to be resolving if (1) serial salicylate levels are no longer toxic (<30 mg/dL) and are decreasing and (2) the patient is clinically improving. It must be emphasized that salicylate evaluation is very different from that of APAP (in which treatment is primarily dictated by laboratory results) because ASA management depends on serial serum levels in conjunction with symptomatology.

Treatment of salicylate toxicity is focused on increased excretion (Fig. 79-2). Urine alkalinization enhances salicylate elimination by "trapping" the ASA ion in the renal tubules and improving its removal. In Prescott's study, urine alkalinization was achieved by adding three 50-mEq ampules of sodium bicarbonate into 1 L of D5W with 40 mEq of potassium chloride and infusing this mixture at 375 cc/hr (1.5 L total) for 4 hours (isotonic sodium bicarbonate preparations are commercially available in some territories).[18] The mean urine pH in these patients was 8.1 and resulted in a significant increase in urinary salicylate excretion. Forced diuresis was shown to be ineffective at improving elimination.[19] Hypokalemia must be avoided because intercalated cells in the distal tubules secrete hydrogen ions in exchange for potassium, thus preventing urine alkalinization and causing retention of salicylate.

In the more severe cases, hemodialysis should be considered. There are no definitive studies on the indications for hemodialysis; however, most toxicologists recommend it for the following scenarios:

- Level of 100 mg/dL or more in acute ingestion.
- Level of 60 mg/dL or more in chronic ingestion.
- In pregnant patients, a level of 60 mg/dL or more is very toxic to the fetus.
- Evidence of end-organ damage such as pulmonary or cerebral edema.
- Severe acid base disorder that is not resolving with resuscitation.
- Volume overload.

Another important clinical consideration is the endotracheal intubation of the salicylate-poisoned patient. Whether this is done for respiratory failure or airway protection, it is vital that the provider pays attention to the patient's acid base status. Massive overdose patients have severe metabolic acidosis for which their body compensates with hyperpnea. After intubation, providers must ensure the ventilator matches minute ventilation to the patient's initial compensation because failure to do so can lead to death from uncompensated metabolic acidosis.

MANAGEMENT PRINCIPLES

Before the 1960s, the standard treatment of poisoned patients was with medications that would have the opposite effect on neuroreceptors than the ingested substance (i.e., sedative ingestions would be treated with stimulants, stimulant exposures with sedatives). However, this approach caused many iatrogenic complications. In 1961, the "Scandinavian method" for treating patients after barbiturate poisoning was described. It used observation and respiratory support instead of the previously used gastric lavage and central analeptics. This new method decreased the mortality from barbiturate overdose from 20% to 1% to 2%.[20] This study caused a shift in the way poisoned patients were treated, with supportive care (i.e., respiratory and circulatory support) becoming the mainstay of treatment for most ingestions.

The approach to the undifferentiated comatose patient includes assessment for hypoglycemia and hypoxia and respiratory and circulatory stabilization. If there is suspicion for opiate overdose in a respiratory-depressed patient, then a trial of naloxone can be used before resorting to intubation. The competitive BZ antagonist flumazenil should not be used diagnostically in undifferentiated patients because it can precipitate intractable seizures in BZ-dependent patients.[21] However, the use of low-dose flumazenil has been safely used for treatment to improve respiratory status and prevent intubation. This risk and benefit analysis should be performed before every flumazenil administration.

DECONTAMINATION AND ENHANCED ELIMINATION

When all of the time-sensitive antidotes have been administered and the patient has been stabilized, the next step is to consider the use of decontamination to minimize patient's further exposure to the toxin. In theory, gastrointestinal decontamination decreases ongoing absorption of the remaining drug in the intestines. These strategies include gastric emptying (GE) through induction of emesis with ipecac or using gastric lavage, binding of unabsorbed toxins via single-dose activated charcoal (AC), and improved excretion with whole bowel irrigation (WBI). The effectiveness of these decontamination techniques is debatable; a few of the more influential clinical trials are discussed later.

GE eliminates substances still within the stomach. This was done either through induction of emesis with ipecac or lavage with a large-bore oral gastric tube. In a prospective study performed by Merigian et al., 808 poisoned patients were given AC with or without GE.[22] Not only was there no clinical benefit with GE, but those treated with GE were admitted to the intensive care unit twice as often and were intubated nearly 4 times more often than the control. These patients also experienced aspiration pneumonia at much higher rates (GE had 8 vs. 0 for no GE).[22]

WBI uses polyethylene glycol to mechanically flush out the bowel contents of the gastrointestinal tract. Volunteer studies have shown that WBI decreases the bioavailability of ingested drugs; however, no clinical improvement has been demonstrated. WBI is contraindicated in patients with bowel obstruction, perforation, ileus, hemodynamic instability, or compromised airways. WBI should be considered for sustained-release drugs, enteric coated medications, iron, and packets of illicit drugs.[23]

Multiple-dose activated charcoal (MDAC) is used to enhance elimination of already absorbed medications. MDAC involves repeated oral dosing of AC (first dose 50 g of AC with sorbitol and then 25 g of AC without sorbitol every 4 hours) to maintain the drug concentration gradient between the gut and the blood. This encourages migration of the drug from blood into the intestinal lumen ("gut dialysis"), where it binds to AC and is excreted. In addition, the persistent presence of AC disrupts the enterohepatic circulation of agents that undergo biliary elimination, thus enhancing their elimination. Certain toxins such as ASA are known to form bezoars, which MDAC is good at neutralizing. Although MDAC significantly increases drug elimination in animal and volunteer studies, it has not been shown to affect clinical outcomes.[24]

To summarize, there are several studies showing improved pharmacokinetic outcomes when decontamination/enhanced elimination techniques are used. However, there are no studies showing improvement in patient outcome. This does not mean that these techniques are not clinically beneficial; rather, because the incidence of serious ingestions in which they would help is so small, even the biggest studies were not powerful enough to detect this difference. Although there is lack of clinical benefit data, many toxicologists recommend AC for early ingestions of very toxic substances if patients are willing and able to drink it (low risk of aspiration). Likewise, for those who are critically ill and intubated (airway protected from possible aspiration), nasogastric administration of AC should also be considered.

AUTHORS' RECOMMENDATIONS

- The diagnosis of critically ill poisoned patients is facilitated by correct identification of toxidromes.
- A prolonged course of NAC should be administered to those with ongoing liver toxicity after acetaminophen overdose.
- Urine alkalinization enhances salicylate elimination.
- Good supportive care is the primary management for most poisoned patients; there are few true antidotes.
- GE with ipecac or gastric lavage has not been shown to benefit patients and may actually cause harm.
- AC may be considered in an awake and alert patient with a potentially fatal ingestion in whom aspiration is unlikely.
- WBI is useful in eliminating substances that are not affected by AC (such as iron or lithium).
- MDAC should be considered for patients poisoned with lethal amounts of salicylate, carbamazepine, dapsone, phenobarbital, quinine, or theophylline.

REFERENCES

1. Kellermann AL, et al. Impact of drug screening in suspected overdose. *Ann Emerg Med*. 1987;16(11):1206–1216.
2. Mowry JB, Spyker DA, Cantilena Jr LR, Bailey JE, Ford M. 2012 Annual Report of the American Association of Poison Control Centers' National Poison Data System (NPDS): 30th Annual Report. *Clin Toxicol*. 2013;51(10):949–1229.
3. Hayes BD, Klein-Schwartz W, Doyon S. Frequency of medication errors with intravenous acetylcysteine for acetaminophen overdose. *Ann Pharmacother*. 2008;42(6):766–770.
4. Corcoran GB, et al. Evidence that acetaminophen and N-hydroxyacetaminophen form a common arylating intermediate, N-acetyl-p-benzoquinoneimine. *Mol Pharmacol*. 1980;18(3):536–542.

5. Miller RP, Roberts RJ, Fischer LJ. Acetaminophen elimination kinetics in neonates, children, and adults. *Clin Pharmacol Ther.* 1976;19(3):284–294.

6. Smilkstein MJ, Knapp GL, Kulig KW, Rumack BH. Efficacy of oral N-acetylcysteine in the treatment of acetaminophen overdose. Analysis of the national multicenter study (1976 to 1985). *N Engl J Med.* 1988;319(24):1557–1562.

7. Prescott LF. Paracetamol overdosage. Pharmacological considerations and clinical management. *Drugs.* 1983;25(3):290–314.

8. Makin A, Williams R. The current management of paracetamol overdosage. *Br J Clin Pract.* 1994;48(3):144–148.

9. Rumack BH, Matthew H. Acetaminophen poisoning and toxicity. *Pediatr.* 1975;55(6):871–876.

10. Smilkstein MJ, Douglas DR, Daya MR. Acetaminophen poisoning and liver function. *N Engl J Med.* 1994;331(19):1310–1311. author reply 1311-2.

11. Gosselin S, Juurlink DN, Kielstein JT, et al. Extracorporeal treatment for acetaminophen poisoning: recommendations from the EXTRIP workgroup. *Clin Toxicol.* 2014:1–12.

12. Marchetti A, Rossiter R. Managing acute acetaminophen poisoning with oral versus intravenous N-acetylcysteine: a provider-perspective cost analysis. *J Med Econ.* 2009;12(4):384–391.

13. Green J, Heard K, Reynolds K, Albert D. Oral and intravenous acetylcysteine for treatment of acetaminophen toxicity: a systematic review and meta-analysis. *West J Emerg Med.* 2013;14(3):218–226.

14. Yarema MC, Johnson DW, Berlin RJ, et al. Comparison of the 20-hour intravenous and 72-hour oral acetylcysteine protocols for the treatment of acute acetaminophen poisoning. *YMEM.* 2009;54(4):606–614.

15. Harrison PM, Keays R, Bray GP, Alexander G. Improved outcome of paracetamol-induced fulminant hepatic failure by late administration of acetylcysteine. *Lancet.* 1990;335(8705):1572–1573.

16. Karsh J. Adverse reactions and interactions with aspirin. Considerations in the treatment of the elderly patient. *Drug Saf.* 1990;5(5):317–327.

17. Leatherman JW, Schmitz PG. Fever, hyperdynamic shock, and multiple-system organ failure. A pseudo-sepsis syndrome associated with chronic salicylate intoxication. *Chest.* 1991;100(5):1391–1396.

18. Prescott LF, Critchley J, Proudfoot AT. Diuresis or urinary alkalinisation for salicylate poisoning? *Br Med J (Clin Res Ed).* 1982;285(6352):1383–1386.

19. Prescott LF, et al. Diuresis or urinary alkalinisation for salicylate poisoning? *Br Med J (Clin Res Ed).* 1982;285(6352):1383–1386.

20. Clemmesen C, Nilsson E, Ruben H. Therapeutic trends in the treatment of barbiturate poisoning: The Scandinavian method. *Surv Anesthesiol KW.* 1962;6. N2 -(4).

21. Hojer J, Baehrendtz S. The effect of flumazenil (Ro 15-1788) in the management of self-induced benzodiazepine poisoning. A double-blind controlled study. *Acta Med Scand.* 1988;224(4):357–365.

22. Merigian KS, Woodard M, Hedges JR, Roberts JR, Stuebing R, Rashkin MC. Prospective evaluation of gastric emptying in the self-poisoned patient. *Am J Emerg Med.* 1990;8(6):479–483.

23. Position paper: whole bowel irrigation. *J Toxicol Clin Toxicol.* 2004;42(6):843–854.

24. Position statement and practice guidelines on the use of multi-dose activated charcoal in the treatment of acute poisoning. American Academy of Clinical Toxicology; European Association of Poisons Centres and Clinical Toxicologists. *J Toxicol Clin Toxicol.* 1999;37(6):731–751.

80 How Should Acute Spinal Cord Injury Be Managed in the ICU?

James Schuster, Matthew Piazza

Spinal cord injury (SCI) constitutes a major cause of morbidity in the trauma patient. The United States has the highest incidence of traumatic spinal cord injuries, with approximately 40 new cases per 1 million persons per year[1]; moreover, the economic burden of SCI exceeds $14 billion each year.[2] After prehospital stabilization and resuscitation, effective management of these patients relies on rapid, accurate clinical assessment and diagnosis of SCI and associated spine trauma, treatment tailored to the specific injury, prevention of complications, and early mobilization. The following chapter focuses on the evidence-based management of acute traumatic SCI in the intensive care unit (ICU).

PATHOPHYSIOLOGY OF SPINAL CORD INJURY

SCI occurs in two distinct phases. Primary injury is the immediate result of the initial traumatic insult—namely, sheer, compressive, or distractive forces that cause disruption of axons and blood vessels, leading to immediate neurologic dysfunction. Secondary injury evolves over the hours to days after the traumatic event and results from tissue hypoxia and ischemia—either at the cellular or systemic levels—inflammation, and neuronal hyperexcitability.

SCI is frequently observed in conjunction with trauma to the spinal column itself—bony fracture and/or dislocation, disc disruption, and ligamentous compromise—and may significantly contribute to neurologic dysfunction by exerting the aforementioned forces on the neural elements. Rapid diagnosis of spinal injuries is critical in the management of these patients. The absence of radiographic evidence of bony or ligamentous injury does not exclude spinal cord trauma, and the patient with unexplained poor findings from a neurologic examination may have underling cord injury. Furthermore, the same principle holds in patients who have abnormal results from a neurologic examination out of proportion to the degree of spinal column injury. Patients with severe cervical stenosis, diffuse idiopathic skeletal hyperostosis (DISH), rheumatoid arthritis, and baseline spinal instability are at the greatest risk.

CLINICAL ASSESSMENT

A detailed neurologic assessment is necessary to properly categorize the severity of the injury, guide management, and facilitate communication among practitioners. Although several neurologic assessment scales have been published in the literature, the American Spinal Injury Association (ASIA) Classifications Standards/International Standards for Neurological Classification of Spinal Cord Injury (ISNICSCI) is the most heavily validated clinical neurologic assessment scale and is considered the gold standard by many practitioners for the clinical evaluation of acute SCI patients.[3,4] There is currently class II evidence demonstrating significant interrater agreement, making this particular assessment scale appealing in terms of documenting and communicating serial examinations among practitioners.[5] The ASIA Impairment Scale (AIS) (Table 80-1) synthesizes the detailed neurologic assessment contained in the ASIA/ISNCSCI.

RADIOGRAPHIC ASSESSMENT AND COLLAR CLEARANCE IN THE CRITICALLY ILL TRAUMA PATIENT

Trauma patients with mechanisms of injury at risk for spine and SCI should be evaluated clinically before radiographic assessment. There is clear class I evidence regarding the initial radiographic assessment of such patients. Patients who are awake, alert, asymptomatic, and neurologically intact require neither radiographic imaging nor external cervical immobilization with collar.[6] Patients who have symptoms or whose mental status precludes clinical evaluation should be placed in a cervical collar and undergo high-quality computed tomography (CT) scanning or three-view plain radiographic imaging when CT scanning is unavailable.[6] CT scanning is superior to plain radiographs in the detection of cervical spine trauma.[7-11] The guidelines for further evaluation of these patients is less clear in the setting of normal CT or three-view radiographs, relying on class II and III evidence.

In the awake but symptomatic patient with normal CT or three-view radiographic imaging, some clinicians have advocated cervical spine clearance with normal dynamic flexion-extension films of the cervical spine or magnetic resonance imaging (MRI) to rule out ligamentous injury obtained within 48 hours of injury. The utility of either modality in identifying clinically significant cervical spine injury is controversial, though. A recent systematic review of the literature concluded that dynamic flexion-extension imaging is inferior to MRI at detecting ligamentous injury.[12] Moreover, flexion-extension films are largely dependent on patient cooperation. Duane et al. reported a relatively high rate of incomplete films (20.5%) and lower sensitivity compared with MRI, calling into question the clinical utility of this modality.[13] On the other hand, Schuster et al. found that in the setting of the neurologically intact patient with negative CT imaging, MRI did not detect clinically significant ligamentous injury.[14] Hence, given these limitations, either continuation of cervical collar until the patient is symptom free or cervical spine clearance at the discretion of the practitioner is a reasonable alternative in the symptomatic patient with negative CT imaging.

In the patient who is obtunded or comatose with negative CT imaging or three-view radiography, MRI or dynamic flexion-extension films are again available for further diagnostic evaluation and to assist in cervical spine clearance. As in awake, symptomatic patients, though, the marginal clinical value of these modalities is questionable. Prospective studies have demonstrated that flexion-extension adds little diagnostic value to CT imaging or plain radiographs in identifying clinically significant cervical spine injury.[15,16] Again, as in the awake patient, the high rate of inadequate films either due to poor imaging quality or incomplete motion may limit the interpretation of this study in the obtunded patient.[17] There are conflicting data within the literature regarding the utility of MRI in detecting clinically significant cervical spine injury. Multiple meta-analyses have demonstrated the merits of MRI

in detecting occult cervical spine injury with a normal CT scan, although each of these analyses included studies with heterogeneous cohorts, somewhat limiting their conclusions.[18,19] Panczykowksi et al. performed a meta-analysis comprising studies largely examining obtunded/intubated patients and showed that CT scanning alone could detect unstable cervical spine injury when compared with additional imaging modalities.[20] Interestingly, Stelfox et al. demonstrated that intubated trauma patients who had collar clearance by CT scan alone had fewer complications, were ventilator dependent for fewer days, and had shorter ICU and hospital lengths of stay.[21] Again, as in the case of the awake patient, cervical spine clearance in the setting of a normal CT may be deferred until the patient's mental status improves or may be cleared with physical examination on the basis of a normal CT alone. Halpern et al. showed that in patients who are likely to be cleared clinically in a relatively short period of time (2 weeks), it is safe and cost-effective to leave these patients in a cervical collar as opposed to obtaining an MRI.[22]

FREQUENTLY ENCOUNTERED INJURY PATTERNS

Although an extensive account of fracture/dislocation patterns and their management is beyond the scope of this text, we briefly review some of the more common fracture patterns of the spine.

Axial spine injuries extend from the occiput to C2. Occipital condyle fractures usually result from axial loading injuries (comminuted or linear type) and are usually stable; avulsion fractures of the condyle may result from distractive forces and should raise suspicion for atlanto-occipital dislocation (AOD) (see following discussion).

Primarily seen in high-velocity, high-impact trauma, AOD (Fig. 80-1) results from distraction injury, causing disruption of ligamentous structures that stabilize the

Table 80-1 **ASIA Impairment Scale**	
Grade	**Interpretation**
A-Complete injury	No motor or sensory function below the level of injury, including the sacral segments
B-Sensory incomplete injury	Preservation of sensory function, including sacral segments, below the level of injury, but no motor function
C-Motor incomplete injury	Preservation of motor function below the level of injury, including sacral segments, with more than half of muscle groups below the level of injury with muscle grades 0-2
D-Motor incomplete injury	Preservation of motor function below the level of injury, including sacral segments, with more than half of muscle groups below the level of injury with muscle grades 3-5
E-Normal	Normal neurological motor and sensory exam, including sacral segments

ASIA, American Spinal Injury Association.
Adapted from reference 77.

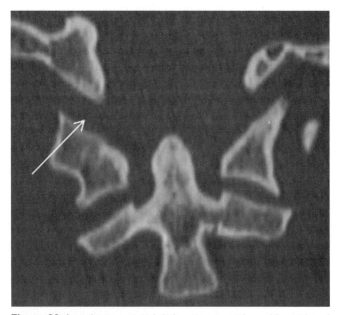

Figure 80-1. Atlanto-occipital dislocation as evidenced by widened C1-condyle interval on coronal computed tomography (*arrow*).

occipital-cervical junction. These patients may initially have normal results from a neurologic examination and progressive or fluctuating deficits, and this diagnosis can be easily missed. Moreover, concomitant traumatic brain injury is common among patients with AOD. Patients without a reliable examination or those with an unstable examination with a concerning mechanism should be evaluated for AOD. CT imaging, and in particular the condyle-C1 interval, is highly sensitive for the detection of AOD; other radiographic clues include prevertebral swelling; skull base or high cervical epidural, subdural, or subarachnoid hemorrhage; and occipital condyle avulsion fractures. MRI may be useful for direct visualization of the ligamentous structures and potential injury to the spinal cord. Ultimately, patients with AOD require surgical stabilization, usually with occipital-cervical fusion, frequently supplemented by external orthosis. Traction is not recommended in these patients and is associated with a tenfold increase in neurologic worsening compared with patients with subaxial cervical spine injuries.[23] Before the definitive surgical fixation, cervical spine immobilization must be ensured, particularly during transfers or turns.

C1 fractures involve two-point fractures in the anterior arch, the posterior arch, or a combination of both; four-point fractures give rise to the classic Jefferson fracture (Fig. 80-2). These fractures result from axial loading injuries, and stability depends on the integrity of the transverse ligament. If lateral displacement of the fracture fragments is significant, then these patients may require surgical fixation; otherwise, external immobilization is sufficient.

Bilateral C2 pars interarticularis fracture, or Hangman's fracture, usually result from axial loading and flexion injuries (Fig. 80-3). The stability of these fractures depends on the degree of C2-3 displacement or angulation. Fractures with minimal displacement generally heal well with external immobilization, whereas patients with significant displacement or angulation may signify disc disruption and may require reduction and surgical fixation.

Odontoid fractures are the most common C2 fracture with the pattern through the body of the dens the most frequent subtype (Fig. 80-4). Younger patients may heal

well with external orthosis with a halo vest. Significant displacement or angulation of the dens may require surgical stabilization. Elderly patients generally do not fair well either with external immobilization because of respiratory and swallowing issues or with surgical intervention because of higher risk profile, which poses a significant clinical dilemma. Surgical options include posterior C1-2 fusion or anterior odontoid screw placement.

Because of its mobility, the subaxial cervical spine (C3-T1) is prone to injury from various forces. Axial load forces can lead to compression deformities or more serious burst fractures. A combination of rotational, flexion, or distractive forces can lead to fracture-dislocation injuries with

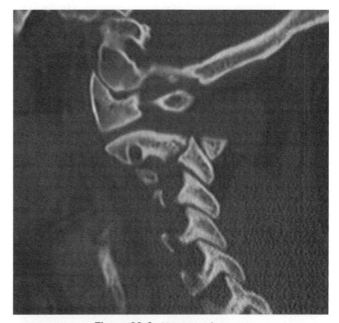

Figure 80-3. Hangman fracture.

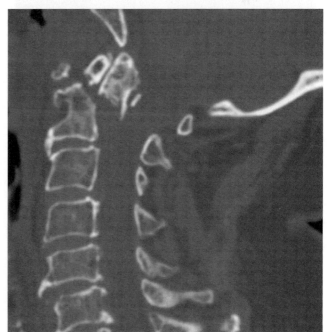

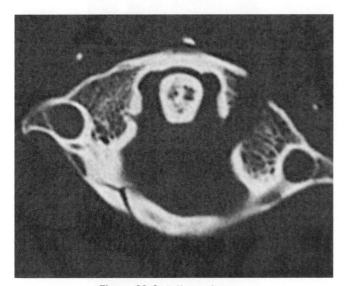

Figure 80-2. Jefferson fracture.

Figure 80-4. Type II odontoid fracture.

resultant SCI (Fig. 80-5); these injuries require emergency evaluation by a trained specialist.

The thoracic spine is structurally well reinforced by the rib cage; hence, significant forces are required to produce injuries. As such, when these injuries occur, they can be devastating (Fig. 80-6). The thoracolumbar junction is particularly prone to injury because it is the transition point between the thoracic spine and the relatively more mobile lumbar spine (Fig. 80-7). In general, the lower lumbar vertebrae are less mobile and less prone to injury.

SURGICAL DECISION MAKING

Surgical decision making and management rely on classification of injury, determination of an injury's stability and degree of compression of neural elements, and the accurate assessment of neurologic function. The goals of neurosurgical management of SCI consist of decompression of neural elements and stabilization of the spine, the timing of which depends on the patient's neurologic function.

Early decompression and stabilization in patients with incomplete injuries has become the prevailing trend.[24] Even with complete injuries, early surgical intervention results in earlier mobilization, reduced pulmonary complications, fewer days for patients to undergo mechanical ventilation, and shorter length of stay.[24-26] Rapid decompression of neural elements can be achieved with certain cervical spine fractures before definitive surgical

treatment with closed reduction with cervical traction using Gardner-Wells tongs performed under fluoroscopy; this procedure should be performed only by a skilled specialist. An exhaustive account of the various surgical approaches is beyond the scope of this text, and we refer

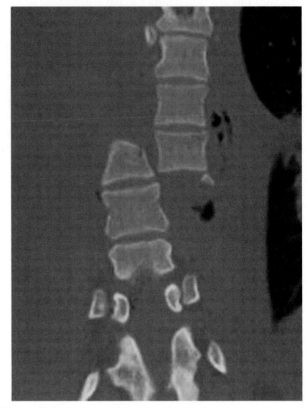

Figure 80-6. Fracture dislocation injury of thoracic spine causing cord transection.

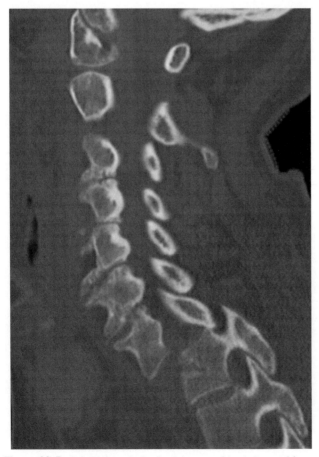

Figure 80-5. Subaxial cervical spine injury resulting in jumped facets.

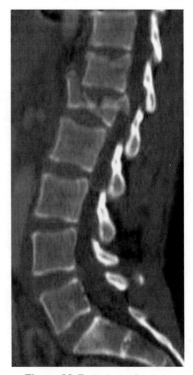

Figure 80-7. L1 burst fracture.

readers to references dedicated to the surgical treatment of spinal trauma.[27]

Several grading scales have been proposed to classify spinal injury and guide in surgical decision making. The Subaxial Cervical Spine Injury Classification (SCLICS)[28] and the Thoracolumbar Injury Classification and Severity Scale (TLICS)[29] are commonly used and ideal in that they include metrics for ligamentous integrity and neurologic function. Of note, greater emphasis is placed on incomplete neurologic injury, suspected spinal cord over nerve root injury, and injury patterns that suggest a high degree of instability (e.g., distraction, subluxation). Both the TLICS and SCLICS have shown to be safe and effective guides for surgical intervention in prospective studies.[30,31] Interestingly, the introduction of the TLICS score led to greater adoption of nonsurgical intervention.[32] The TLICS score has been validated and is reliable[33,34] whereas the SCLICS has been performed less well with regards to interrater variability.[35]

ACUTE TRAUMATIC CENTRAL CORD SYNDROME

Acute traumatic central cord syndrome (ATCCS) is a heterogenous clinical diagnosis that usually results from a hyperextension injury in which there is preferential damage to the medial anterior and posterior columns of the spinal cord (Fig. 80-8). Because of the somatotopic organization of corticospinal tracts, this typically leads to weakness in the upper extremities with relative

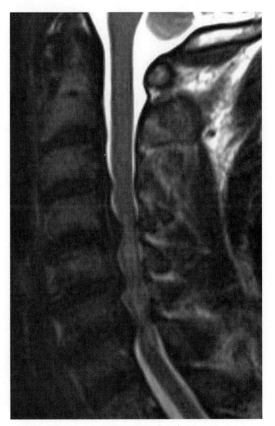

Figure 80-8. Acute central cord in patient with severe cervical stenosis.

sparing of the lower extremities, although this clinical presentation can be varied. In general, for the diagnosis of ACTSS to be made, the ASIA motor score in the upper extremities must be 10 points less than the corresponding score in the lower extremities.[36] This injury pattern may or may not be associated with bony or ligamentous disruption.

Patients with ATCCS are especially prone to further SCI secondary to hypotension; as a result, maintaining adequate perfusion pressure is imperative in the acute postinjury and perioperative periods. Because ATCCS frequently occurs in elderly patients, baseline pressures may be elevated relative to younger patients with SCI, and as a result, these patients may require higher mean arterial pressure (MAP) to maintain adequate spinal cord perfusion.

The timing of surgical intervention for ATCCS is somewhat controversial, although recent studies have demonstrated that surgery can be safely performed within 24 hours after injury and may lead to improved outcomes compared with delayed intervention. The surgical approach is variable and, in addition to surgeon preference, is guided by spinal alignment, the number of levels involved, the location of pathology, and the presence of other bony or ligamentous injuries.[25,37,38]

CORTICOSTEROID THERAPY

Several multicenter, prospective, randomized trials have been conducted to determine the efficacy of high-dose corticosteroid administration in patients with acute SCI. The National Acute Spinal Cord Injury Study (NASCIS) I compared high-dose with low-dose methylprednisolone (MP) and found no difference in neurologic function at 6 weeks, 6 months, and 1 year, although wound infection and death were more frequent in the high-dose group.[39,40] The NASCIS II trial published in 1990 was a multicenter, randomized, double-blinded trial comparing MP with naloxone or placebo in patient acute SCI; the authors found no significant difference in primary outcome measures, although a post hoc analysis revealed improvement in neurologic function at 6 months and 1 year in patients who received MP within 8 hours of injury.[41,42] A third trial, NASCIS III, was conducted that compared 24-hour MP with 48-hour MP administration and again found no significant difference in predetermined outcome measures, although a post hoc analysis revealed improved ASIA motor scores at 6 weeks and 6 months in the 48-hour MP group.[43] In the NASCIS II and NASCIS III studies, the post hoc analysis is considered class III evidence. Another multicenter, randomized, prospective trial was conducted to examine complication rates and found that patients who received MP had greater rates of respiratory complications and gastrointestinal bleeding.[44]

In summary, no class I or class II medical evidence exists supporting the clinical benefit of MP in the treatment of acute SCI. The class III evidence that has been published claims inconsistent effects likely related to random chance or selection bias. However, class I, II, and III evidence demonstrates that high-dose MP for the treatment of acute SCI is associated with numerous complications including death.[45]

HYPOTHERMIA AFTER SPINAL CORD INJURY

The application of hypothermia as a neuroprotective strategy in the setting of acute SCI has garnered significant interest. Animal data and small case series with both systemic hypothermia and regional/local hypothermia at the time of surgical decompression have demonstrated the potential for improved outcomes after SCI.[46-48] The current guidelines from the AANS/CNS (American Association of Neurological Surgeons/Congress of Neurological Surgeons) joint section on the spine provide a grade C (level 4 evidence) for the use of modest systemic hypothermia for SCI.[49] Large multicenter randomized trials are needed to explore the clinical utility of hypothermia after SCI.

DIAGNOSIS AND MANAGEMENT OF VERTEBRAL ARTERY INJURY

Patients who sustain SCI may have injury mechanisms that place them at risk for cervical artery injury. Rates of vertebral injury between 17% and 27.5% have been quoted in screened patients with highly suspicious injures[50-52] and an overall rate of 1.4% has been quoted among patients with any blunt cervical trauma.[53] Patients with fractures into the transverse foramen, occipital-cervical dislocation, associated skull base fractures, and subluxation/dislocation injuries may be at greatest risk.[50] Approximately 12% to 14% of patients will have a stroke attributable to cerebrovascular injury, and nearly half of these occur at the time of presentation.[53,54]

The Modified Denver Screening Criteria (Table 80-2) were designed to identify those patients at greatest risk for cerebrovascular injury after blunt trauma and guide the decision to obtain angiographic imaging.[55] Although the gold standard for diagnosis of cerebrovascular injury is conventional angiogram, CT angiography is an excellent, noninvasive alternative. Eastman et al. demonstrated class I evidence for the utility of CT angiography, quoting sensitivity and specificity of 97.7% and 100%, respectively.[56] Conventional angiography should still be considered, though, if endovascular intervention is a possibility.

Table 80-2 **Modified Denver Screening Criteria**
Arterial hemorrhage
Cervical bruit/thrill
Expanding cervical hematoma
Focal neurologic deficit
Neurologic examination inconsistent with head CT
Ischemic stroke on secondary head CT
Cervical spine, basilar skull, or severe facial (LeForte II/III) fracture
Diffuse axonal injury with GCS <6
Near hanging with anoxic brain injury

Adapted from reference 78.
CT, computed tomography; *GCS*, Glasgow Coma Scale score.

Only class III evidence exists for the treatment of blunt cerebrovascular injury. Several large retrospective studies have demonstrated that patients without any intervention have higher rates of stroke,[53,54] but there is no clear consensus regarding the utility of antiplatelet therapy, anticoagulation, or endovascular intervention. Potential endovascular treatment options include vessel/pseudoaneurysm embolization and stenting of the dissected vessel. The treatment decision should be tailored to the individual patient. Of note, patients who undergo endovascular stenting may require dual antiplatelet therapy, which may be relatively contraindicated in the complex trauma patient.

PENETRATING SPINAL CORD INJURY

Penetrating SCI (i.e., from bullets, shrapnel, knives) is a distinct clinical entity from blunt SCI and may be a frequent occurrence at urban and military trauma centers (Fig. 80-9). SCI in this setting can occur directly from the penetrating object itself and can occur indirectly from the blast effect of the penetrating object (e.g., as in the case of bullets, shrapnel). Hence, patients may have complete cord injuries without evidence of canal involvement of the penetrating object on imaging.[57] Management of these patients is largely supportive, and the role of surgery is poorly defined. Few studies have been published examining outcomes after

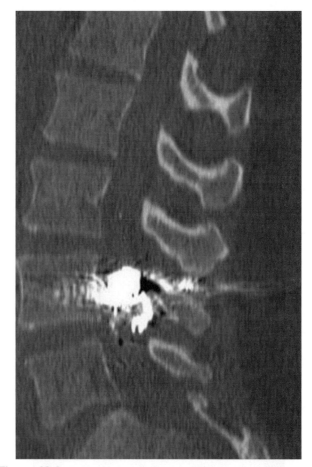

Figure 80-9. Penetrating gunshot to lumbar spine with bullet fragment in spinal canal.

surgery for decompression; these patients usually do not have improvement after surgery and run the risk of further injury or exacerbating cerebrospinal fluid leakage with operative exploration. Thoracolumbar injuries are rarely unstable (<1%) whereas reported rates of instability requiring surgery in the cervical spine reach 30%.[58,59] Patients with gunshot wound trajectories through hollow viscus organs may be at increased risk for neurologic and spinal infections.[60] A short course of antibiotics in this setting (<48 hours) may be sufficient for prophylaxis.[61,62]

HEMODYNAMIC SUPPORT

Patients who have sustained cervical or high thoracic cord injuries are at risk of abnormal systemic sympathetic tone resulting in bradycardia and hypotension. Hypotension in the setting of SCI can lead to ischemic insults to the cord itself, worsen neurologic dysfunction, and may result in multiorgan hypoperfusion injury. Class III evidence exists in support of maintaining MAP between 85 and 90 mm Hg for 7 days.[63-65] The data in support of this protocol used an arbitrary MAP threshold and duration of maintenance and was uncontrolled. Nevertheless, the improvement in outcome observed in these patients was considerable compared with outcomes in SCI patients before implementation of this protocol. Moreover, the decision to maintain MAPs should be specific to the patient, and one should consider the potential deleterious effects and prolonged immobilization required for vasopressor use.

Hemodynamic support should be administered with a combination of fluids and vasopressors. Patients with neurogenic shock often respond poorly to fluids because of peripheral vasodilation; over-resuscitation and aggressive use of fluids in these patients can lead to pulmonary and peripheral edema and abdominal compartment syndrome. Vasopressor choice largely depends on the level of the injury. Patients with cervical and high thoracic cord injury respond well to agents with inotropic, chronotropic, and vasoconstrictive agents, such as dopamine, epinephrine, and norepinephrine. Purely vasoconstrictive agents such as phenylephrine can worsen underlying bradycardia and should probably be avoided. Conversely, norepinephrine or phenylephrine may be an appropriate choice in SCI patients with low thoracic injury in whom systemic vasodilation is the primary cause of hypotension. Complications of prolonged vasopressor use are common among SCI patients, with approximately 74% of SCI patients experiencing an arrhythmia, ST segment changes, or troponin elevations.[66] In particular, complications are more frequent in older patients and those who are receiving inotropic/chronotropic agents.

AUTONOMIC DYSFUNCTION AND ORTHOSTATIC HYPOTENSION AFTER SPINAL CORD INJURY

After the acute phase of SCI in which hemodynamic support is targeted at maintaining cord perfusion, patients, especially those with high cord injuries, are at risk of symptomatic bradycardia and orthostatic hypotension,

which can lead to impaired mobilization. Numerous pharmacologic and nonpharmacologic methods are available to prevent orthostatic hypotension, although few data exist to support these interventions. Class II evidence exists for use of midodrine after SCI to reduce symptomatic orthostatic hypotension from a small, double-blinded, randomized clinical trial demonstrating improved exercise tolerance.[67] Other measures include increased salt intake, assistive compressive devices, and functional electrical stimulation. The latter involves stimulation of muscles around lower extremity veins, leading to increased return of blood flow to the heart and hence left ventricular preload; class II data from multiple randomized clinical trials provide evidence for its use in SCI patients with autonomic dysfunction.[68]

AIRWAY AND PULMONARY MANAGEMENT AFTER ACUTE SPINAL CORD INJURY

Patients with SCI, and in particular high cervical cord injury, are at significant risk for pulmonary complications. Impairment in accessory respiratory muscle and even diaphragmatic function leads to poor secretion clearance and low tidal volumes, placing these patients at risk for respiratory failure, ventilator dependence, atelectasis, and pneumonia. Patients with acute SCI, especially cervical cord injury, should have their airway secured soon after injury.[69] If endotracheal intubation is undertaken, then great care must be taken to ensure spinal alignment. The basic principles of mechanical ventilation in patients with SCI include adequate ventilator support while the risk of diaphragmatic atrophy is reduced.[70] Diaphragmatic atrophy can begin as soon as 18 hours after intubation, is related to the length of time on the ventilator, and is especially relevant in the SCI patient because these patients almost exclusively rely on the diaphragm for respiratory function. While mechanically ventilated, patients should have aggressive respiratory therapy to ensure adequate secretion clearance.

Most patients with complete cervical cord injury will require tracheostomy.[71] The most appropriate timing of tracheostomy in patients with respiratory failure after SCI is a subject of much debate in the literature. No randomized clinical trials have compared early with late tracheostomy. Retrospective data support early tracheostomy (within 7 to 10 days after injury). Previous studies have demonstrated a shorter ICU length of stay and reduction in time to ventilator wean.[72,73] Moreover, early tracheostomy appears safe after anterior cervical fusion without a significant increase in infection risk.[74]

VENOUS THROMBOEMBOLISM PROPHYLAXIS

Patients with SCI are high risk for the development of venous thromboembolism (VTE) secondary to prolonged immobility. VTE prophylaxis for SCI has been extensively studied. There exists class I evidence for the use of VTE prophylaxis for SCI.[75] In particular, low-dose heparin in combination with electrical stimulation is superior to low-dose heparin alone or placebo, and adjusted-dose heparin (1.5 times normal partial thromboplastin time) resulted in a lower incidence of VTE in SCI patients compared with low-dose heparin. Therapy should ideally be initiated within 72 hours.[75] VTE prophylaxis for 3 months after the initial injury is recommended on the basis of class II evidence; in patients who have significant improvement in neurologic function and mobilization and who can participate in aggressive physical therapy, the duration of VTE prophylaxis may be shortened.[75] With regard to the choice of anticoagulant, low-molecular-weight heparinoids are associated with lower rates of VTE and bleeding-related complications.[76] In patients who have a contraindication to anticoagulation, inferior vena cava filter placement should be considered.

CONCLUSION

Patients with suspected SCI require rapid clinical assessment, diagnosis, and management targeted at their disease. Although clear guidelines exist for clinical and radiographic evaluation, future prospective, randomized studies should focus on identifying optimal timing of surgery for patients with ACTSS, clarifying the role and duration of blood pressure augmentation during the acute period after injury. Furthermore, efforts aimed at the creation and implementation of neuroprotective strategies to improve outcomes after SCI are needed.

AUTHORS' RECOMMENDATIONS

- The initial assessment of the spine in trauma is clinically augmented by radiographic examinations determined by clinical suspicion, symptoms, and level of consciousness.
- CT assessment of the cervical spine is superior to plain radiographs. The role of MRI in this setting is unclear.
- Early surgical intervention is associated with more rapid mobilization and fewer medical complications.
- Corticosteroids are unlikely to be of benefit in acute SCI and are associated with a significant number of complications.
- Monitored temperature control may be of benefit, but it is currently unsupported by the clinical literature.
- Hypotension may be associated with absolute or relative hypovolemia in the setting of neurogenic shock. In general, vasopressor/inotropic therapy is more effective and associated with fewer complications than large-volume fluid administration.
- Respiratory failure associated with diaphragmatic and intercostal muscle weakness usually requires mechanical ventilation. Diaphragmatic atrophy is a common complication.
- Early tracheostomy results in more rapid liberation for mechanical ventilation and shorter ICU stay.
- Supportive measures in ICU include VTE prophylaxis, nutrition, psychological welfare, and aggressive monitoring for pressure sores.

REFERENCES

1. Devivo MJ. Epidemiology of traumatic spinal cord injury: trends and future implications. *Spinal Cord.* 2012;50(5):365–372.
2. Ma VY, Chan L, Carruthers KJ. Incidence, prevalence, costs, and impact on disability of common conditions requiring rehabilitation in the United States: stroke, spinal cord injury, traumatic brain injury, multiple sclerosis, osteoarthritis, rheumatoid arthritis, limb loss, and back pain. *Arch Phys Med Rehabil.* 2014;95(5):986e1–995e1.
3. Marino RJ, et al. International standards for neurological classification of spinal cord injury. *J Spinal Cord Med.* 2003;26(suppl 1): S50–S56.
4. Hadley MN, et al. Clinical assessment following acute cervical spinal cord injury. *Neurosurgery.* 2013;72(suppl 2):40–53.
5. Savic G, et al. Inter-rater reliability of motor and sensory examinations performed according to American Spinal Injury Association standards. *Spinal Cord.* 2007;45:444–451.
6. Ryken TC, et al. Radiographic assessment. *Neurosurgery.* 2013;72 (suppl 2):54–72.
7. Bailitz J, et al. CT should replace three-view radiographs as the initial screening test in patients at high, moderate, and low risk for blunt cervical spine injury: a prospective comparison. *J Trauma.* 2009;66:1605–1609.
8. Diaz JJ, et al. Are five-view plain films of the cervical spine unreliable? A prospective evaluation in blunt trauma patients with altered mental status. *J Trauma.* 2003;55:658–663. discussion 663-664.
9. Griffen MM, et al. Radiographic clearance of blunt cervical spine injury: plain radiograph or computed tomography scan?. *J Trauma.* 2003;55:222–226. discussion 226-227.
10. Mathen R, et al. Prospective evaluation of multislice computed tomography versus plain radiographic cervical spine clearance in trauma patients. *J Trauma.* 2007;62:1427–1431.
11. Schenarts PJ, et al. Prospective comparison of admission computed tomographic scan and plain films of the upper cervical spine in trauma patients with altered mental status. *J Trauma.* 2001;51:663–668. discussion 668-669.
12. Sierink JC, et al. Systematic review of flexion/extension radiography of the cervical spine in trauma patients. *Eur J Radiol.* 2013;82:974–981.
13. Duane TM, et al. Flexion-extension cervical spine plain films compared with MRI in the diagnosis of ligamentous injury. *Am Surg.* 2010;76:595–598.
14. Schuster R, et al. Magnetic resonance imaging is not needed to clear cervical spines in blunt trauma patients with normal computed tomographic results and no motor deficits. *Arch Surg.* 2005;140:762–766 (Chicago, Ill. : 1960).
15. Hennessy D, et al. Cervical spine clearance in obtunded blunt trauma patients: a prospective study. *J Trauma.* 2010;68:576–582.
16. Padayachee L, et al. Cervical spine clearance in unconscious traumatic brain injury patients: dynamic flexion-extension fluoroscopy versus computed tomography with three-dimensional reconstruction. *J Trauma.* 2006;60:341–345.
17. Griffiths HJ, et al. The use of forced flexion/extension views in the obtunded trauma patient. *Skeletal Radiol.* 2002;31:587–591.
18. Muchow RD, et al. Magnetic resonance imaging (MRI) in the clearance of the cervical spine in blunt trauma: a meta-analysis. *J Trauma.* 2008;64:179–189.
19. Schoenfeld AJ, et al. Computed tomography alone versus computed tomography and magnetic resonance imaging in the identification of occult injuries to the cervical spine: a meta-analysis. *J Trauma.* 2010;68:109–113. discussion 113-114.
20. Panczykowski DM, Tomycz ND, Okonkwo DO. Comparative effectiveness of using computed tomography alone to exclude cervical spine injuries in obtunded or intubated patients: meta-analysis of 14,327 patients with blunt trauma. *J Neurosurg.* 2011;115:541–549.
21. Stelfox HT, et al. Computed tomography for early and safe discontinuation of cervical spine immobilization in obtunded multiply injured patients. *J Trauma.* 2007;63:630–636.
22. Halpern CH, et al. Clearance of the cervical spine in clinically unevaluable trauma patients. *Spine (Phila Pa 1976).* 2010;35(18):1721–1728.
23. Theodore N, et al. The diagnosis and management of traumatic atlanto-occipital dislocation injuries. *Neurosurgery.* 2013;72(suppl 2):114–126.
24. Bellabarba C, et al. Does early fracture fixation of thoracolumbar spine fractures decrease morbidity or mortality? *Spine (Phila Pa 1976).* 2010;35(suppl 9):S138–S145.
25. Fehlings MG, et al. Early versus delayed decompression for traumatic cervical spinal cord injury: results of the Surgical Timing in Acute Spinal Cord Injury Study (STASCIS). *PLoS One.* 2012;7(2):e32037.
26. Schinkel C, Anastasiadis AP. The timing of spinal stabilization in polytrauma and in patients with spinal cord injury. *Curr Opin Crit Care.* 2008;14:685–689.
27. Fessler RG, Sekhar LN. *Atlas of Neurosurgical Techniques: Spine and Peripheral Nerves.* New York, NY: Thieme Medical Publishers; 2006.

28. Vaccaro AR, et al. The subaxial cervical spine injury classification system: a novel approach to recognize the importance of morphology, neurology, and integrity of the disco-ligamentous complex. *Spine (Phila Pa 1976)*. 2007;32(21):2365–2374.

29. Vaccaro AR, et al. A new classification of thoracolumbar injuries: the importance of injury morphology, the integrity of the posterior ligamentous complex, and neurologic status. *Spine (Phila Pa 1976)*. 2005;30(20):2325–2333.

30. Joaquim AF, et al. Clinical results of patients with thoracolumbar spine trauma treated according to the Thoracolumbar Injury Classification and Severity Score. *J Neurosurg Spine*. 2014;20:562–567.

31. Joaquim AF, et al. Clinical results of patients with subaxial cervical spine trauma treated according to the SLIC score. *J Spinal Cord Med*. 2014;37:420–424.

32. Joaquim AF, et al. Measuring the impact of the Thoracolumbar Injury Classification and Severity Score among 458 consecutively treated patients. *J Spinal Cord Med*. 2014;37:101–106.

33. Lewkonia P, Paolucci EO, Thomas K. Reliability of the thoracolumbar injury classification and severity score and comparison with the denis classification for injury to the thoracic and lumbar spine. *Spine*. 2012;37:2161–2167.

34. Rihn JA, et al. A review of the TLICS system: a novel, user-friendly thoracolumbar trauma classification system. *Acta Orthop*. 2008;79:461–466.

35. van Middendorp JJ, et al. The Subaxial Cervical Spine Injury Classification System: an external agreement validation study. *Spine J*. 2013;13:1055–1063.

36. Pouw MH, et al. Diagnostic criteria of traumatic central cord syndrome. Part 1: a systematic review of clinical descriptors and scores. *Spinal Cord*. 2010;48:652–656.

37. Aarabi B, et al. Management of acute traumatic central cord syndrome (ATCCS). *Neurosurgery*. 2013;72(suppl 2):195–204.

38. Fehlings MG, et al. Perioperative and delayed complications associated with the surgical treatment of cervical spondylotic myelopathy based on 302 patients from the AOSpine North America Cervical Spondylotic Myelopathy Study. *J Neurosurg Spine*. 2012;16(5):425–432.

39. Bracken MB, et al. Efficacy of methylprednisolone in acute spinal cord injury. *JAMA*. 1984;251(1):45–52.

40. Bracken MB, et al. Methylprednisolone and neurological function 1 year after spinal cord injury. Results of the National Acute Spinal Cord Injury Study. *J Neurosurg*. 1985;63(5):704–713.

41. Bracken MB, et al. A randomized, controlled trial of methylprednisolone or naloxone in the treatment of acute spinal-cord injury. Results of the Second National Acute Spinal Cord Injury Study. *N Engl J Med*. 1990;322(20):1405–1411.

42. Bracken MB, et al. Methylprednisolone or naloxone treatment after acute spinal cord injury: 1-year follow-up data. Results of the second National Acute Spinal Cord Injury Study. *J Neurosurg*. 1992;76(1):23–31.

43. Bracken MB, et al. Administration of methylprednisolone for 24 or 48 hours or tirilazad mesylate for 48 hours in the treatment of acute spinal cord injury. Results of the Third National Acute Spinal Cord Injury Randomized Controlled Trial. National Acute Spinal Cord Injury Study. *JAMA*. 1997;277(20):1597–1604.

44. Matsumoto T, et al. Early complications of high-dose methylprednisolone sodium succinate treatment in the follow-up of acute cervical spinal cord injury. *Spine*. 2001;26:426–430.

45. Hurlbert RJ, et al. Pharmacological therapy for acute spinal cord injury. *Neurosurgery*. 2013;72(suppl 2):93–105.

46. Hansebout RR, Hansebout CR. Local cooling for traumatic spinal cord injury: outcomes in 20 patients and review of the literature. *J Neurosurg Spine*. 2014;20(5):550–561.

47. Dididze M, et al. Systemic hypothermia in acute cervical spinal cord injury: a case-controlled study. *Spinal Cord*. 2013;51(5):395–400.

48. Levi AD, et al. Clinical application of modest hypothermia after spinal cord injury. *J Neurotrauma*. 2009;26(3):407–415.

49. Ahmad FU, Wang MY, Levi AD. Hypothermia for acute spinal cord injury–a review. *World Neurosurg*. 2014;82(1–2):207–214.

50. Lebl DR, et al. Vertebral artery injury associated with blunt cervical spine trauma: a multivariate regression analysis. *Spine*. 2013;38:1352–1361.

51. Mitha AP, et al. Clinical outcome after vertebral artery injury following blunt cervical spine trauma. *World Neurosurg*. 2013;80:399–404.

52. Mueller C-A, et al. Vertebral artery injuries following cervical spine trauma: a prospective observational study. *Eur Spine J*. 2011;20:2202–2209.

53. Stein DM, et al. Blunt cerebrovascular injuries: does treatment always matter? *J Trauma*. 2009;66:132–143. discussion 143-144.

54. Cothren CC, et al. Treatment for blunt cerebrovascular injuries: equivalence of anticoagulation and antiplatelet agents. *Arch Surg*. 2009;144:685–690 (Chicago, Ill. : 1960).

55. Biffl WL, et al. Optimizing screening for blunt cerebrovascular injuries. *Am J Surg*. 1999;178:517–522.

56. Eastman AL, et al. Computed tomographic angiography for the diagnosis of blunt cervical vascular injury: is it ready for prime-time?. *J Trauma*. 2006;60:925–929. discussion 929.

57. Mirovsky Y, et al. Complete paraplegia following gunshot injury without direct trauma to the cord. *Spine (Phila Pa 1976)*. 2005;30(21):2436–2438.

58. Cornwell 3rd EE, et al. Thoracolumbar immobilization for trauma patients with torso gunshot wounds: is it necessary? *Arch Surg*. 2001;136(3):324–327.

59. Beaty N, et al. Cervical spine injury from gunshot wounds. *J Neurosurg Spine*. 2014;21(3):442–449.

60. Schwed AC, et al. Abdominal hollow viscus injuries are associated with spine and neurologic infections after penetrating spinal cord injuries. *Am Surg*. 2014;80(10):966–969.

61. Pasupuleti LV, Sifri ZC, Mohr AM. Is extended antibiotic prophylaxis necessary after penetrating trauma to the thoracolumbar spine with concomitant intraperitoneal injuries? *Surg Infect (Larchmt)*. 2014;15(1):8–13.

62. Rabinowitz RP, et al. Infectious complications in GSW's through the gastrointestinal tract into the spine. *Injury*. 2012;43(7):1058–1060.

63. Ryken TC, et al. The acute cardiopulmonary management of patients with cervical spinal cord injuries. *Neurosurgery*. 2013;72(suppl 2):84–92.

64. Casha S, Christie S. A systematic review of intensive cardiopulmonary management after spinal cord injury. *J Neurotrauma*. 2011;28:1479–1495.

65. Vale FL, et al. Combined medical and surgical treatment after acute spinal cord injury: results of a prospective pilot study to assess the merits of aggressive medical resuscitation and blood pressure management. *J Neurosurg*. 1997;87(2):239–246.

66. Inoue T, et al. Medical and surgical management after spinal cord injury: vasopressor usage, early surgerys, and complications. *J Neurotrauma*. 2014;31:284–291.

67. Nieshoff EC, et al. Double-blinded, placebo-controlled trial of midodrine for exercise performance enhancement in tetraplegia: a pilot study. *J Spinal Cord Med*. 2004;27:219–225.

68. Krassioukov A, et al. A systematic review of the management of orthostatic hypotension after spinal cord injury. *Arch Phys Med Rehabil*. 2009;90:876–885.

69. Hassid VJ, et al. Definitive establishment of airway control is critical for optimal outcome in lower cervical spinal cord injury. *J Trauma*. 2008;65:1328–1332.

70. Galeiras Vázquez R, et al. Respiratory management in the patient with spinal cord injury. *BioMed Res Int*. 2013;2013:168757.

71. Menaker J, et al. Admission ASIA motor score predicting the need for tracheostomy after cervical spinal cord injury. *J Trauma Acute Care Surg*. 2013;75:629–634.

72. Choi HJ, et al. The effectiveness of early tracheostomy (within at least 10 days) in cervical spinal cord injury patients. *J Korean Neurosurg Soc*. 2013;54:220–224.

73. Romero J, et al. Tracheostomy timing in traumatic spinal cord injury. *Eur Spine J*. 2009;18:1452–1457.

74. Babu R, et al. Timing of tracheostomy after anterior cervical spine fixation. *J Trauma Acute Care Surg*. 2013;74:961–966.

75. Dhall SS, et al. Deep venous thrombosis and thromboembolism in patients with cervical spinal cord injuries. *Neurosurgery*. 2013;72(suppl 2):244–254.

76. Ploumis A, et al. Thromboprophylaxis in patients with acute spinal injuries: an evidence-based analysis. *J Bone Joint Surg Am*. 2009;91:2568–2576.

77. American Spinal Injury Association. *International Standards for Neurological Classification of Spinal Cord Injury*. Chicago, Il: American Spinal Injury Association; 2002.

78. Cothren CC, et al. Anticoagulation is the gold standard therapy for blunt carotid injuries to reduce stroke rate. *Arch Surg*. 2004;139(5):540–545. discussion 545-546.

HEMATOLOGY
CRITICAL CARE

81 When Is Transfusion Therapy Indicated in Critical Illness and When Is It Not?

Carrie Valdez, Babak Sarani

Transfusion of blood products is one of the most common therapies ordered in the intensive care unit (ICU). It is estimated that 4 million patients are transfused a total of 8 to 12 million units of packed red blood cells (PRBCs) each year in the United States alone and that most transfusions occur in either surgical or critically ill patients. Several studies in various countries have documented that the incidence of PRBC transfusion in the ICU varies between 20% and 50%.[1-5] In addition to anemia, approximately 40% of critically ill patients will have a low platelet count or elevation in their coagulation parameters at some point during their ICU stay. Most of these hematologic derangements, though, are asymptomatic, and numerous studies in the last decade have shown that outcome is either not changed or worsened after transfusion to normalize these values. Although there are some well-designed trials that can be used to formulate guidelines regarding transfusion of PRBCs in critically ill patients, there are no good studies that can be used to determine which patients benefit and which do not from platelet or plasma transfusion in the ICU. This chapter reviews the available evidence on best transfusion practices in the ICU, including a review of the use of recombinant factor VIIa and four-factor prothrombin complex concentrate (PCC).

BASIS FOR TRANSFUSION OF BLOOD PRODUCTS: BENEFITS AND RISKS

Outcomes related to transfusion practices are only now being studied in well-designed prospective trials. Although there are many trials related to transfusion of PRBCs, there is a dearth of information related to practice patterns and outcomes from use of non–red blood cell products in patients who are not actively hemorrhaging.

Packed Red Blood Cell Transfusion

The normal blood volume is 7 to 8% of ideal body weight. This corresponds to a hemoglobin (Hb) level of 14 to 16 g/dL and a hematocrit of 40 to 45%. Transfusion of red blood cells (RBCs) can restore circulating blood volume and oxygen-carrying capacity as described by the formula

$$Vo_2 = CO \times C_aO_2$$

where

$$C_aO_2 = \text{arterial oxygen content (mg\%/L)}$$
$$= [1.39*(Sao_2)* (Hb) + 0.003 \times Pao_2]$$

and

$$Vo_2 = \text{oxygen delivery (g\%/min)}$$
$$Hb = \text{hemoglobin level (g/dL)}$$
$$CO = \text{cardiac output (L/min)}$$
$$Sao_2 = \text{arterial oxygen saturation (\%)}$$
$$Pao_2 = \text{arterial oxygen tension (mm Hg)}$$

The body has many adaptive responses to increase oxygen delivery in the face of anemia (Table 81-1). It may be advantageous to increase oxygen (O_2) delivery by increasing the oxygen saturation or Hb concentration because increasing cardiac output can increase myocardial oxygen demand and may precipitate ischemia in patients with coronary artery disease.[6]

Anecdote and historical practices have dictated that the ideal Hb/hematocrit value in hospitalized patients is 10 g/dL or 30%. The basis for this claim lies in part on rheologic calculations suggesting that it is associated with an optimal balance between oxygen-carrying capacity (where high is better) and viscosity (where low is better). Such a balance would minimize cardiac work and maintain peripheral oxygen delivery. As recently as the 1990s, this recommendation was supported, in part, by two large retrospective studies in Jehovah's Witness populations that showed a significant increase in perioperative mortality if the preoperative Hb was 6 g/dL as opposed to 12 g/dL (odds ratio of 2.5 for each gram that the postoperative Hb was less than 8 g/dL; Table 81-2).[7,8] The risk of death was highest in patients with known cardiovascular disease.

A series of trials in postoperative patients have called into question the validity of these retrospective studies and suggested that the transfusion threshold should be individualized based on documentation of end-organ hypoxia. Two randomized studies of postcardiac surgery patients found no difference in morbidity in those randomized to a liberal versus restrictive transfusion strategy.[9,10] Although

Table 81-1 Physiologic Mechanisms to Increase Oxygen Delivery in Anemia

MECHANISMS THAT INCREASE ARTERIAL OXYGEN CONTENT

Increased production of erythropoietin, leading to increased Hb synthesis and Hb concentration

Rightward shift of Hb saturation curve due to increased 2,3-DPG permitting increased oxygen "off-loading" at capillary PO_2

MECHANISMS THAT INCREASE CARDIAC OUTPUT

Increased heart rate

Increased myocardial contractility

Decreased blood viscosity leading to decreased peripheral vascular resistance (afterload)

2,3-DPG, 2,3-diphosphoglycerate; *Hb,* hemoglobin; Po_2, partial pressure of oxygen.

Table 81-2 Postoperative Outcomes of Anemic Jehovah's Witnesses

Preoperative Hb Level (g/dL)	Mortality (%)
< 6	61.5
6.1–8	33
8.1–10	0
> 10	7.1

Hb, hemoglobin.
From Carson JL, Poses RM, Spence RK et al. Severity of anemia and operative mortality and morbidity. *Lancet* 1998;1:727–729.

Table 81-3 Thresholds for Transfusion in Stable Anemic Patients Without Risk for Potential Acute Blood Loss or Acute Surgical Stress

Hb < 8-10 g/dL
Acute myocardial infarction or ACS

Hb ≤ 7 g/dL
All other patients

ACS, acute coronary syndrome; *Hb,* hemoglobin.

Table 81-4 Thresholds for Transfusion in Stable Patients at High Risk for Acute Blood Loss

Hb ≤ 10 g/dL
Known disorders of hemostasis or RBC dyscrasia (e.g., sickle cell anemia)
All with anticipated estimated blood loss ≥ 1000 mL

Hb ≤ 7 g/dL
All other patients

Hb, hemoglobin; *RBC,* red blood cell.

the study by Hajjar et al. found a dose-dependent increase in morbidity after transfusion, the study by Murphy et al. found an increase in mortality but no change in morbidity in those randomized to the restrictive transfusion arm of the study. Reasons for this finding are uncertain considering that the mean difference in Hb level between the two arms was only 1 g/dL. Thus, although a restrictive strategy for blood transfusion after cardiac surgery may be desirable, the actual Hb trigger has yet to be determined. Another randomized study of elderly patients undergoing total hip arthroplasty similarly found no difference in morbidity or mortality in those randomized to an Hb transfusion threshold of 10 g/dL versus 8 g/dL,[11] whereas a retrospective study in a similar patient population found a significant increase in perioperative morbidity and no change in mortality.[12]

In a single prospective, randomized, blinded study, blood transfusion, used as part of a "sepsis bundle," was found to improve survival in patients with septic shock whose hemodynamic parameters did not correct with intravenous fluids.[13] Because the interventions in this study were delivered as a bundle, though, it is not possible to determine the relative impact of transfusion alone on outcome. More recently, an adequately powered, randomized, prospective study of critically ill patients with septic shock found no difference in mortality or need for ongoing critical care interventions, such as mechanical ventilation,

vasopressor use, or renal replacement therapy, between patients assigned to transfusion at an Hb trigger of 7 g/dL versus 9 g/dL.[14] Moreover, there was no change in the results in the subgroups of patients older than 70 years or those with known cardiovascular disease, although those with acute coronary syndrome (ACS) were excluded from this study. Reasons to account for this may be explained by the findings of three smaller randomized studies that found that PRBC transfusion does not improve oxygen delivery or uptake in septic patients in the ICU.[15-17]

Many recent studies have addressed the role of PRBC transfusion in asymptomatic, hemodynamically stable, nonbleeding, anemic critically ill patients. A single randomized, blinded, prospective study in 1999 and several subsequent observational studies found that patients who are transfused above an Hb value of 7 g/dL have either the same or better outcomes than those who are transfused to an Hb value of 10 g/dL.[3-5] These findings are consistent with many other studies and one meta-analysis that also documented an increased risk of infection after PRBC transfusion.[3,5,19-26] Other studies have documented an increased risk of death after RBC transfusion.[3,5] On the basis of these studies, current guidelines regarding PRBC transfusion in critically ill but asymptomatic and resuscitated (i.e., hemodynamically normal) patients call for an Hb transfusion trigger of 7 g/dL (Tables 81-3 and 81-4).[27]

There are no randomized studies evaluating a threshold for PRBC transfusion in patients with unstable angina or ACS, but a large post hoc analysis from the combined patient pool of three studies that were originally designed to evaluate efficacy of antiplatelet agents in those with myocardial ischemia found a significant increase in the hazard ratio in patients who were transfused to a hematocrit greater than 25%.[28] This finding has been corroborated in multiple other retrospective studies.[29-31] Conversely, a recent retrospective study of a highly select cohort of patients with ACS suggested a decrease in mortality for those transfused for an Hb trigger of 9 g/dL.[32] The authors caution, though, that the cohort enrolled in the study was not representative of typical patients with ACS; therefore the results of the trial may not be generalizable to the overall population of patients with ACS. Thus, although there are insufficient data upon which to firmly recommend a transfusion threshold below an Hb level of 10 g/dL in this cohort, transfusion to an Hb level between 8 and 10 g/dL may be reasonable in most patients, and the need for transfusion to a higher Hb level may be better reserved for patients with evidence of ongoing end-organ ischemia.

Transfusion of blood products carries many risks. These include transmission of blood-borne pathogens, transfusion-associated circulatory overload (TACO), transfusion-related acute lung injury (TRALI), and transfusion-related immunomodulation (TRIM). Clinically significant transfusion reaction is rare under current guidelines and is most commonly due to clerical error. Interestingly, this adverse event is rarely seen in exsanguinating patients. Although the reason for this is uncertain, it is likely due to alterations in the immune system resulting from severe injury massive transfusion.[33] TRALI and TRIM are most likely variants of the same disorder—an exaggerated inflammatory response and an altered or deranged immune system due to transfusion of foreign protein—and may explain the increased risk for infection.[34] TRALI may result from local (pulmonary) inflammation whereas TRIM may represent systemic immune derangement. Both entities are likely underreported because of a lack of unique diagnostic criteria and adequately designed studies aimed to address their incidence.

TRALI is defined as noncardiogenic pulmonary edema that occurs within 4 to 6 hours of transfusion. It has a reported incidence of 1:5000 to 1:10,000 transfusions[35] and is most common after transfusion of plasma. TRIM is best exemplified by reports showing the association between PRBC transfusion and infection* and reports documenting a chimeric state in which donor epitopes can be expressed by cells of transfused trauma patients years after the transfusion itself.[38-40] Mechanisms underlying TRIM are only now being elucidated. Co-transfusion of soluble proteins, such as human leukocyte antigen or fibrinogen/fibrin degradation products, and co-transfusion of disrupted white blood cell products have been proposed as possible explanations.[34]

Plasma Transfusion

The plasma portion of donated whole blood contains most of the necessary clotting factors of the coagulation cascade. Although there are decreased concentrations of factors V, VII, and VIII because of degradation and fibrinogen (factor I) because of dilution, spontaneous hemorrhage rarely occurs with factor concentrations greater than 25%.[41,42] Higher levels are needed, however, to arrest hemorrhage. Plasma is dosed as 10 to 15 mL/kg (ideal body weight), and generally 4 units will result in 40% to 60% factor recovery.[42] It should be noted that transfusion

of 5 units of random-donor platelets or 1 unit of single-donor platelets also results in the transfusion of 1 unit equivalent of plasma because platelets are suspended in plasma.[41] Plasma is commonly used in the ICU to rapidly treat coagulopathy with concomitant hemorrhage or in anticipation of an invasive procedure in a patient with coagulopathy.

Warfarin is an oral anticoagulant that is very commonly used to prevent thromboembolic disease from various causes. A retrospective study found that each 30-min delay in administration of the first unit of plasma decreases the odds of correction of warfarin-induced coagulopathy by 20% in patients with intracerebral bleeding, underscoring the need for rapid and accurate reversal of the drug in hemorrhaging patients.[44] Because the speed with which plasma can be administered is limited by its supply and the time required to thaw and prepare the product, use of PCCs to quickly restore clotting ability is becoming increasingly common. PCC provides a concentrated source of three or four vitamin-K-dependent coagulation factors. PCCs are stored in a lyophilized state and only require reconstitution. A type/screen is not needed, the product does not need to be thawed, and total volume of drug to be administered is less than 100 mL, thereby making administration significantly faster and with no risk of TACO. Multiple international organizations, including the American College of Chest Physicians, recommend a combination of PCC and vitamin K for emergency anticoagulation reversal.[45] A 2013 study by Sarode evaluated the efficacy and safety of PCC compared with plasma in patients on vitamin K antagonists presenting with major bleeding. Rapid international normalized ratio reduction was achieved in 62% of patients receiving PCC versus 10% of patients receiving plasma, demonstrating PCC superiority. The safety profile was similar between groups.[46]

There is wide variability in the manner in which physicians utilize plasma (fresh frozen plasma [FFP]) in non-bleeding patients with coagulopathy.[47] Many physicians use FFP prophylactically to reverse coagulopathy in nonbleeding patients despite published guidelines recommending against this and an unknown risk-benefit ratio.[48,49] Others cite mild coagulopathy as a reason to use FFP as a volume expander in nonbleeding volume-depleted patients.[50] To date, there are no universally agreed-upon guidelines for use of FFP in nonbleeding patients. Suggested indications and dosing are shown in Table 81-5.

Transfusion of plasma has the same risks as transfusion of RBCs, but the incidence of adverse events is higher for all possible complications. The most frequent adverse event associated with plasma transfusion is TRALI. Recent theory postulates that this reflects variability in plasma protein (and presumably antibody) content in the fluid being transfused.[35] This proposed mechanism is supported by a randomized, blinded, crossover study that found that this risk is higher after transfusion of plasma obtained from multiparous women.[51] A retrospective study found a 3-fold higher relative risk of infection in critically ill surgical patients who received FFP, a finding that is consistent with the risk of infection after PRBC transfusion.[52] Hemolytic transfusion reactions also are possible after transfusion of plasma because plasma contains variable titers of anti-A and anti-B antibody.

---

*References 20, 21, 23, 24, 36, 37.

Table 81-5 Indications for Transfusion of Plasma
Emergency reversal of warfarin-induced coagulopathy
Replacement of isolated coagulation protein deficiency
Massive transfusion
DIC with serious active bleeding
Liver disease with clinical bleeding and evidence of coagulation defect
Thrombotic thrombocytopenic purpura (TTP)
Replacement of clotting factors after apheresis therapy

DIC, disseminated intravascular coagulation.

Table 81-6 Indications for Transfusion of Cryoprecipitate
Hemophilia A (factor VIII deficiency)
von Willebrand disease
Fibrinogen deficiency
Dysfibrinogenemia
Factor XIII deficiency
Uremic platelet dysfunction

Cryoprecipitate Transfusion

Cryoprecipitate is the precipitated fraction obtained from thawing FFP at 4°C. This method of isolation means that cryoprecipitate is pooled from the FFP obtained from multiple donors. Cryoprecipitate is rich in factor VIII, von Willebrand factor, factor XIII, and fibronectin. Most importantly, it is the only blood component that contains concentrated fibrinogen; thus the main indication for its use is treatment of coagulopathy due to hypofibrinogenemia.[49] Therefore it may be useful in the management of disseminated intravascular coagulation (DIC) with hemorrhage and in reversal of thrombolytic agents (Table 81-6). Although an adequate dose of plasma can replete fibrinogen, hypofibrinogenemia can be reversed more quickly using cryoprecipitate. Cryoprecipitate is dosed as a 10-pack transfusion, in which each 10-pack raises the fibrinogen level 75%.[42] Bleeding patients with known von Willebrand deficiency should also receive cryoprecipitate to optimize platelet function whereas nonbleeding patients with this disorder can be treated with DDAVP.

Risks associated with transfusion of cryoprecipitate are the same as those reported for the other blood components. However, the incidence of TRALI and TRIM is probably lower than that associated with transfusion of plasma because the total volume of cryoprecipitate transfused is much less than plasma, minimizing the recipient's exposure to foreign protein antigen. The risk of transmission of blood-borne pathogens, though, may be higher because of the pooled nature of this product. There are no well-designed studies assessing outcomes or adverse events related to transfusion of cryoprecipitate.

Platelet Transfusion

Platelet transfusion is less common than RBC or plasma transfusion. The most common indication for platelet transfusion is decreased production followed by increased destruction of cells.[41] In the critically ill population, in which DIC is more prevalent, increased utilization of platelets can also lead to thrombocytopenia. Although the absolute platelet count may not correlate with function or ability to form a stable clot, it is generally agreed that spontaneous bleeding can occur with platelet counts less than 10,000 cells/μL.[53] Although not validated in studies, many clinicians recommend that a minimum platelet count of 50,000 cells/μL should be maintained, if possible, for patients at significant risk of bleeding (e.g., trauma, postoperative patients, or those about to undergo an invasive procedure associated with a significant risk of hemorrhage), and a target of 80,000 to 100,000 cells/μL is recommended for patients who are actively bleeding or at risk for intracranial hemorrhage.[41,54]

Although the platelet count can be determined easily and quickly, there is no reliable method to test platelet function. A possible exception is thromboelastography (TEG), one of two available viscoelastographic means of assessing clot formation and lysis. Limited evidence from observational data suggests that TEG is able to diagnose platelet dysfunction after trauma.[55] Unfortunately, effects on blood product transfusion, mortality, and other outcomes remain unproven in randomized trials.[56]

There are no studies that can be used to recommend timing and volume of platelet transfusion in nonbleeding critically ill patients. Furthermore, although there are no good studies to determine the effect that use of aspirin or nonsteroidal anti-inflammatory agents has on hemorrhage after injury, a review of the literature suggests that use of aspirin may worsen intracranial hemorrhage after traumatic brain injury.[57] An open-label, ex vivo study in volunteers showed that platelet transfusion can reverse the platelet dysfunction caused by clopidrogel,[58] and platelet transfusion may be prudent in patients with traumatic brain injury who were prescribed antiplatelet medications, including nonsteroidal anti-inflammatory agents. The efficacy of platelet transfusion to reverse the effects of antiplatelet medications for other causes of hemorrhage remains speculative. As previously noted, because platelets are suspended in plasma, platelet transfusion also has the added risks and benefits associated with plasma transfusion.

MASSIVE EXSANGUINATION AND TRANSFUSION

Patients requiring massive transfusion are a unique cohort in whom aggressive transfusion is needed for hemodynamic support and reversal of coagulopathy (Table 81-7). The most commonly used definition of massive transfusion is transfusion of 10 units of PRBCs within 24 hours. This definition, though, does not direct attention to the coagulopathy that also exists in these patients and fuels the process underlying the hemorrhage.[59] Noncontrolled and retrospective studies suggest that aggressive transfusion using plasma/RBC ratios that approach 1:1 within a predefined massive transfusion protocol may result in earlier arrest of hemorrhage

Table 81-7 **Transfusion Guidelines for Patients Who Are Acutely Bleeding**

Clinical Situation	Recommended Response
Rapid acute hemorrhage without immediate control, estimated blood loss >30%-40%, *or* presence of symptoms of severe blood loss	Transfuse PRBCs; initiate massive transfusion protocol with 1:1 RBC/FFP transfusion*
Estimated blood loss <25%-30% without uncontrolled hemorrhage	Crystalloid resuscitation; proceed to blood transfusion if hemorrhage is not quickly arrested
Presence of comorbid factors	Consider transfusion with lesser degrees of blood loss

*May require uncrossmatched or type-specific blood.
FFP, fresh frozen plasma; *PRBC,* packed red blood cell; *RBC,* red blood cell.

Table 81-8 **Causes of Abnormal Bleeding in Surgery and Trauma**

Release of tissue thromboplastin
Massive transfusion
Autotransfusion
Disseminated intravascular coagulation
Platelet dysfunction
Hypothermia

and mortality benefit.[60-62] The PROMMTT (Prospective, Observational, Multicenter, Major Trauma Transfusion) trial prospectively evaluated 1245 trauma patients who received at least 1 unit of RBCs within 6 hours of admission. Increased ratios of plasma/RBCs and platelets/RBCs were independently associated with a decrease in 6-hour mortality. Patients with ratios less than 1:2 were 3 to 4 times more likely to die than patients with ratios of 1:1 or higher.[63] More recently, the PROPPR (Pragmatic, Randomized Optimal Platelet and Plasma Ratios) trial found no difference in mortality but a decrease in hemorrhage and transfusion need in trauma patients who received a 1:1 versus 1:2 transfusion strategy.[64] Until similar studies are performed in the nontrauma population, it may be prudent to treat exsanguinating, critically ill patients with aggressive transfusion of plasma and platelets in addition to RBCs while also preventing hypothermia, acidosis, and other causes of ongoing coagulopathy.[65] Common causes of abnormal bleeding in critically ill patients are noted in Table 81-8.

RECOMBINANT FACTOR VIIA

Mechanism of Action and Clinical Use

Recombinant factor VIIa is approved for use in hemophiliacs with antibodies to factor VIII or IX. Many case reports and small series, though, found that it also may have a role in arresting hemorrhage from other causes. Recombinant factor VIIa works by binding to exposed tissue factor in an area of endothelial injury, thereby activating platelets and forming a platelet plug. Factor VIIa then stimulates the coagulation cascade by activating thrombin on the platelet plug. Fibrinolysis is inhibited through factor VIIa–mediated activation of thrombin-activatable fibrinolysis inhibitor.

Factor VIIa has been shown to decrease or arrest hemorrhage after injury. Two parallel, randomized, blinded placebo-controlled studies found that the drug was associated with a 50% relative reduction in severity of hemorrhage in bluntly injured patients, but it did not have a transfusion-sparing effect in victims of penetrating trauma.[66] The doses used in these studies, though, were much higher than the commonly accepted dose of 90 µg/kg—a difference that has substantial cost implications for use of this expensive drug. The only large, randomized, blinded, placebo-controlled study on the use of factor VIIa in injured patients (CONTROL trial) was stopped early for futility when the control arm was noted to have a substantially lower mortality than anticipated (11% in lieu of 30%), thereby making the study too underpowered to detect a mortality difference.[67] As with previous studies, though, this study also found a decrease in the amount of blood products needed in the treatment arm, with the biggest blood-salvaging benefit noted in patients sustaining blunt trauma.

Off-label use of factor VIIa has also been studied in other conditions.[68] Despite initial reports that factor VIIa may decrease the severity of spontaneous intracranial hemorrhage,[69] a large randomized controlled trial did not find any difference in mortality or neurologic outcome with administration of this drug.[70] In a randomized study, recombinant factor VIIa was shown to decrease the incidence of rebleeding in patients with esophageal varices, but patients required a total dose of 800 µg/kg over 30 hours.[71] This finding again calls the cost efficacy of this agent into question. Many case reports and small series suggest that factor VIIa is also effective in arresting postpartum hemorrhage, but prospective studies are needed to validate these findings.[72-75] Finally, a series of case reports and retrospective reviews suggests that factor VIIa can be used to rapidly reverse the anticoagulant effects of warfarin. Once again, though, prospective studies have not been performed to validate these findings or to determine how the reversal affects the ultimate clinical outcome.

Uncontrolled case series and retrospective reports suggest that factor VIIa is most effective when administered early in exsanguinating patients (before 8 units of PRBCs have been transfused).[76] Furthermore, the efficacy of this agent is markedly diminished if the pH is less than 7.1, the platelet count is less than 50,000 cells/mL, the prothrombin time is greater than 17.6 seconds, or the lactate is greater than 13 mg/dL.[77]

Adverse Events Associated with Recombinant Factor VIIa

Factor VIIa has been associated with thromboembolic complications, particularly when used in an off-label fashion. This problem is especially pertinent in patients older than 55 years because this cohort is likely to have ulcerated plaque (with exposed tissue factor) due to atherosclerosis. Reports from the U.S. Food and Drug Administration suggest that the incidence of thromboembolic disease is 0.02%

in hemophiliacs, but the incidence of myocardial infarction, stroke, or pulmonary embolism may be as high as 8% when the agent is used in other populations.[78] Moreover, there is an almost equal incidence of arterial and venous thrombi after administration of the drug. The CONTROL trial, however, did not find any difference in complications between trauma patients who did and did not receive factor VIIa.[67]

TRANEXAMIC ACID

Mechanism of Action and Clinical Use

Tranexamic acid (TXA) is a synthetic lysine derivative that inhibits fibrinolysis by binding to and inhibiting plasminogen. A review of 53 studies incorporating 3836 persons undergoing elective operation found that administration of this agent resulted in a 39% decrease in transfusion need. More recently, the CRASH-2 (Clinical Randomization of an Antifibrinolytic in Significant Hemorrhage 2) trial, a multinational, randomized, blinded, placebo-controlled study that included 270 hospitals and enrolled over 20,000 injured patients, found that administration of TXA within 8 hours of injury resulted in a statistically significant 1.5% decrease in the risk of death from any cause.[79] Further analysis found that the biggest reduction was in hemorrhage-related death. However, subsequent subgroup analysis found that this benefit was confined to patients who received the drug within 3 hours of injury.[80] Persons who received the medication between 3 and 8 hours after injury actually had a higher mortality than the placebo group. The study has been criticized for enrolling both patients who were actually hemorrhaging and those perceived to be at risk of hemorrhage based on the judgment of the bedside clinician. Furthermore, although the study found a significant decrease in the probability of hemorrhage-related death, there was no difference in the amount of blood transfused in surviving patients.

The MATTERs (Military Application of Tranexamic Acid in Trauma Emergency Resuscitation) and MATTERs II trials are retrospective studies of the same patient cohort and evaluated the benefits of TXA in soldiers wounded in battle.[81,82] As with the CRASH-2 trial, these studies found a significant decrease in hemorrhage-related mortality, but the study cohort consisted solely of patients requiring a massive transfusion. Maximal benefit from administration of TXA was found in patients who received both a 1:1:1 ratio of PRBC/FFP as well as cryoprecipitate. The risk of venous thromboembolic disease was 2% to 3%. The number needed to treat to prevent one hemorrhage-related death in the MATTERs study was 1:7.

There are currently no good prospective studies on which to base guidelines for use of TXA in the civilian setting. A promising area of research is use of vesicoelastography as a means to measure the degree of thrombolysis in hemorrhaging patients and to direct use of antifibrinolytic agents, such as TXA.

CONCLUSION

There remains a paucity of high-level evidence to guide transfusion practice in the ICU. The robust studies performed to date argue for a restrictive policy of PRBC

transfusion in critically ill patients who are not hemorrhaging and are not manifesting signs of end-organ ischemia. Likewise, patients who have other asymptomatic derangements in coagulation should not undergo transfusion unless an invasive procedure with propensity for hemorrhage is planned, and use of PCC may be superior to use of FFP in this setting. Patients who require ongoing transfusion support should be treated aggressively with transfusion of PRBCs, plasma, and platelets. Future studies evaluating pharmacologic adjuncts and laboratory-guided transfusion therapy, particularly viscoelastogram-guided therapy, in hemorrhaging patients are needed.

AUTHORS' RECOMMENDATIONS

RBC transfusion
- It is used to augment the oxygen-carrying capacity of blood.
- Evidence-based transfusion trigger in critically ill, resuscitated patients is an Hb level of 7 g/dL.
- The transfusion trigger in patients with end-organ dysfunction or shock remains uncertain. Common practice uses an Hb level of 9 to 10 g/dL as a trigger for transfusion if the patient fails crystalloid resuscitation.
- Complications of transfusion can be grouped into transfusion reaction (clerical), volume overload (TACO), and immune dysfunction (TRALI and TRIM).

Plasma transfusion
- It is used to reverse diffuse coagulopathy.
- It is dosed as 10 to 15 mL/kg.
- It has the highest association with TRALI.
- Physicians should consider treating patients who have vitamin K–dependent coagulopathy with PCC.

Cryoprecipitate transfusion
- It contains factor VIII, von Willebrand factor, factor XIII, and fibronectin.
- It is used to treat DIC or to reverse thrombolytic-induced hemorrhage (i.e., hypofibrinogenemia).

Platelet transfusion
- It may be used to reverse clopidrogel (and possibly aspirin)–induced thrombocytopathy.
- A platelet count of 50,000 to 100,000 cells/dL are needed for operation, depending on the nature of the procedure planned.
- Other than TEG, there is not a readily available test to clinically evaluate platelet function.

Massive transfusion
- Retrospective studies suggest that a ratio approaching 1:1:1 of RBCs/FFP/platelets may decrease net transfusion needs.
- Recombinant factor VIIa may decrease net transfusion needs, but it has not been shown to affect survival.
  - It is associated with a high rate of thromboembolic arterial and venous complications in patients older than 55 years.
- TXA may be associated with a survival benefit in hemorrhaging patients.

REFERENCES

1. French CJ, Bellomo R, Finfer SR, Lipman J, Chapman M, Boyce NW. Appropriateness of red blood cell transfusion in Australasian intensive care practice. *Med J Aust.* 2002;177:548–551.
2. Walsh TS, Garrioch M, Maciver C, et al. Red cell requirements for intensive care units adhering to evidence-based transfusion guidelines. *Transfusion.* 2004;44:1405–1411.
3. Corwin HL, Gettinger A, Pearl RG, et al. The CRIT Study: Anemia and blood transfusion in the critically ill–current clinical practice in the United States. *Crit Care Med.* 2004;32:39–52.

4. Hebert PC, Wells G, Blajchman MA, et al. A multicenter, randomized, controlled clinical trial of transfusion requirements in critical care. Transfusion Requirements in Critical Care Investigators, Canadian Critical Care Trials Group. *N Engl J Med.* 1999;340:409–417.

5. Vincent JL, Baron JF, Reinhart K, et al. Anemia and blood transfusion in critically ill patients. *JAMA.* 2002;288:1499–1507.

6. Hayes M, Timmins A, Yau E, Palazzo M, Hinds C, Watson D. Elevation of systemic oxygen delivery in the treatment of critically ill patients. *N Engl J Med.* 1994;330:1717–1722.

7. Carson JL, Duff A, Poses RM, et al. Effect of anaemia and cardiovascular disease on surgical mortality and morbidity. *Lancet.* 1996;348:1055–1060.

8. Carson JL, Noveck H, Berlin JA, Gould SA. Mortality and morbidity in patients with very low postoperative Hb levels who decline blood transfusion. *Transfusion.* 2002;42:812–818.

9. Hajjar LA, Vincent JL, Galas FR, et al. Transfusion requirements after cardiac surgery: the TRACS randomized controlled trial. *JAMA.* 2010;304:1559–1567.

10. Murphy GJ, Pike K, Rogers CA, et al. Liberal or restrictive transfusion after cardiac surgery. *N Engl J Med.* 2015;372:997–1008.

11. Carson JL, Terrin ML, Noveck H, et al. Liberal or restrictive transfusion in high-risk patients after hip surgery. *N Engl J Med.* 2011;365:2453–2462.

12. Frisch NB, Wessell NM, Charters MA, Yu S, Jeffries JJ, Silverton CD. Predictors and complications of blood transfusion in total hip and knee arthroplasty. *J Arthroplasty.* 2014;29:189–192.

13. Rivers E, Nguyen B, Havstad S, et al. Early goal-directed therapy in the treatment of severe sepsis and septic shock. *N Engl J Med.* 2001;345:1368–1377.

14. Holst LB, Haase N, Wetterslev J, et al. Lower versus higher hemoglobin threshold for transfusion in septic shock. *N Engl J Med.* 2014;371:1381–1391.

15. Dietrich KA, Conrad SA, Hebert CA, Levy GL, Romero MD. Cardiovascular and metabolic response to red blood cell transfusion in critically ill volume-resuscitated nonsurgical patients. *Crit Care Med.* 1990;18:940–944.

16. Fernandes Jr CJ, Akamine N, De Marco FV, De Souza JA, Lagudis S, Knobel E. Red blood cell transfusion does not increase oxygen consumption in critically ill septic patients. *Crit Care.* 2001;5:362–367.

17. Lorente JA, Landin L, De Pablo R, Renes E, Rodriguez-Diaz R, Liste D. Effects of blood transfusion on oxygen transport variables in severe sepsis. *Crit Care Med.* 1993;21:1312–1318.

18. Deleted in review.

19. Chang H, Hall GA, Geerts WH, Greenwood C, McLeod RS, Sher GD. Allogeneic red blood cell transfusion is an independent risk factor for the development of postoperative bacterial infection. *Vox Sang.* 2000;78:13–18.

20. Claridge JA, Sawyer RG, Schulman AM, McLemore EC, Young JS. Blood transfusions correlate with infections in trauma patients in a dose-dependent manner. *Am Surg.* 2002;68:566–572.

21. Hill GE, Frawley WH, Griffith KE, Forestner JE, Minei JP. Allogeneic blood transfusion increases the risk of postoperative bacterial infection: a meta-analysis. *J Trauma.* 2003;54:908–914.

22. Malone D, Dunne J, Tracy K, Putnam AT, Scalea T, Napolitano L. Blood transfusion, independent of shock severity, is associated with worse outcome in trauma. *J Trauma.* 2003;54:898–907.

23. Shorr AF, Duh MS, Kelly KM, Kollef MH. Red blood cell transfusion and ventilator-associated pneumonia: a potential link? *Crit Care Med.* 2004;32:666–674.

24. Taylor RW, Manganaro L, O'Brien J, Trottier SJ, Parkar N, Veremakis C. Impact of allogenic packed red blood cell transfusion on nosocomial infection rates in the critically ill patient. *Crit Care Med.* 2002;30:2249–2254.

25. Vamvakas EC. Perioperative blood transfusion and cancer recurrence: meta-analysis for explanation. *Transfusion.* 1995;35:760–768.

26. Taylor RW, O'Brien J, Trottier SJ, et al. Red blood cell transfusions and nosocomial infections in critically ill patients. *Crit Care Med.* 2006;34:2302–2308. quiz 9.

27. Napolitano LM, Kurek S, Luchette FA, et al. Clinical practice guideline: red blood cell transfusion in adult trauma and critical care. *J Trauma.* 2009;37:3124–3157.

28. Rao SV, Jollis JG, Harrington RA, et al. Relationship of blood transfusion and clinical outcomes in patients with acute coronary syndromes. *JAMA.* 2004;292:1555–1562.

29. Alexander KP, Chen AY, Wang TY, et al. Transfusion practice and outcomes in non-ST-segment elevation acute coronary syndromes. *Am Heart J.* 2008;155:1047–1053.

30. Aronson D, Dann EJ, Bonstein L, et al. Impact of red blood cell transfusion on clinical outcomes in patients with acute myocardial infarction. *Am J Cardiol.* 2008;102:115–119.

31. Singla I, Zahid M, Good CB, Macioce A, Sonel AF. Impact of blood transfusions in patients presenting with anemia and suspected acute coronary syndrome. *Am J Cardiol.* 2007;99:1119–1121.

32. Salisbury AC, Reid KJ, Marso SP, et al. Blood transfusion during acute myocardial infarction: association with mortality and variability across hospitals. *J Am Coll Cardiol.* 2014;64:811–819.

33. Dutton RP, Shih D, Edelman BB, Hess J, Scalea TM. Safety of uncrossmatched type-O red cells for resuscitation from hemorrhagic shock. *J Trauma.* 2005;59:1445–1449.

34. Vamvakas EC. Possible mechanisms of allogeneic blood transfusion-associated postoperative infection. *Transfus Med Rev.* 2002;16:144–160.

35. Stainsby D, Cohen H, Jones H, et al. *Serious Hazards of Transfusion (SHOT) Annual Report*; 2003. Accessed 15.03.15 at http://www.shotuk.org/shot-reports/reports-and-summaries-2003/.

36. Carson J, Altman D, Duff A, et al. Risk of bacterial infection associated with allogeneic blood transfusion among patients undergoing hip fracture repair. *Transfusion.* 1999;39:694–700.

37. Dutton RP, Lefering R, Lynn M. Database predictors of transfusion and mortality. *J Trauma.* 2006;60:S70–S77.

38. Reed W, Lee TH, Norris PJ, Utter GH, Busch MP. Transfusion-associated microchimerism: a new complication of blood transfusions in severely injured patients. *Semin Hematol.* 2007;44:24–31.

39. Utter GH, Nathens AB, Lee TH, et al. Leukoreduction of blood transfusions does not diminish transfusion-associated microchimerism in trauma patients. *Transfusion.* 2006;46:1863–1869.

40. Utter GH, Owings JT, Lee TH, et al. Blood transfusion is associated with donor leukocyte microchimerism in trauma patients. *J Trauma.* 2004;57:702–707; discussion 7–8.

41. American College of Pathologists. Practice parameter for the use of fresh-frozen plasma, cryoprecipitate, and platelets. *JAMA.* 1994;271:777–781.

42. Pugent Sound Blood Center. *Blood Component Therapy*; 2012. Accessed 15.03.15 at http://www.psbc.org/therapy/ffp.htm.

43. Deleted in review.

44. Goldstein JN, Thomas SH, Frontiero V, et al. Timing of fresh frozen plasma administration and rapid correction of coagulopathy in warfarin-related intracerebral hemorrhage. *Stroke.* 2006;37:151–155.

45. Holbrook A, Schulman S, Witt DM, et al. Evidence-based management of anticoagulant therapy: Antithrombotic Therapy and Prevention of Thrombosis, 9th ed: American College of Chest Physicians Evidence-Based Clinical Practice Guidelines. *Chest.* 2012;141:e152S–e184S.

46. Sarode R, Milling Jr TJ, Refaai MA, et al. Efficacy and safety of a 4-factor prothrombin complex concentrate in patients on vitamin K antagonists presenting with major bleeding: a randomized, plasma-controlled, phase IIIb study. *Circulation.* 2013;128:1234–1243.

47. Dara SI, Rana R, Afessa B, Moore SB, Gajic O. Fresh frozen plasma transfusion in critically ill medical patients with coagulopathy. *Crit Care Med.* 2005;33:2667–2671.

48. Contreras M, Ala FA, Greaves M, et al. Guidelines for the use of fresh frozen plasma. British Committee for Standards in Haematology, Working Party of the Blood Transfusion Task Force. *Transfus Med.* 1992;2:57–63.

49. O'Shaughnessy DF, Atterbury C, Bolton Maggs P, et al. Guidelines for the use of fresh-frozen plasma, cryoprecipitate and cryosupernatant. *Br J Haematol.* 2004;126:11–28.

50. Lauzier F, Cook D, Griffith L, Upton J, C M. Fresh frozen plasma transfusion in critically ill patients. *Crit Care Med.* 2007;35:1655–1659.

51. Palfi M, Berg S, Ernerudh J, Berlin G. A randomized controlled trial of transfusion-related acute lung injury: Is plasma from multiparous blood donors dangerous? *Transfusion.* 2001;41:317–322.

52. Sarani B, Dunkman WJ, Dean L, Sonnad S, Rohrbach JI, Gracias VH. Transfusion of fresh frozen plasma in critically ill surgical patients is associated with an increased risk of infection. *Crit Care Med.* 2008;36:1114–1118.

53. NIH Consensus Conference. Platelet transfusion therapy. *JAMA.* 1987;257:1777–1780.

54. British Committee for Standards in Haematology and Blood Transfusion Task Force. Guidelines for the use of platelet transfusions. *Br J Haematol*. 2003;122:10–23.

55. Wohlauer MV, Moore EE, Thomas S, et al. Early platelet dysfunction: an unrecognized role in the acute coagulopathy of trauma. *J Am Coll Surg*. 2012;214:739–746.

56. Da Luz L, Nascimento B, Shankarakutty A, Rizoli S, Adhikari N. Effect of thromboelastography (TEG(R)) and rotational thromboelastometry (ROTEM(R)) on diagnosis of coagulopathy, transfusion guidance and mortality in trauma: descriptive systematic review. *Crit Care*. 2014;18:518.

57. Sakr M, Wilson L. Best evidence topic report. Aspirin and the risk of intracranial complications following head injury. *Emerg Med J*. 2005;22:891–892.

58. Vilahur G, Choi BG, Zafar MU, et al. Normalization of platelet reactivity in clopidogrel-treated subjects. *J Thromb Haemost*. 2007;5:82–90.

59. Holcomb JB, Jenkins D, Rhee P, et al. Damage control resuscitation: directly addressing the early coagulopathy of trauma. *J Trauma*. 2007;62:307–310.

60. Cotton BA, Reddy N, Hatch QM, et al. Damage control resuscitation is associated with a reduction in resuscitation volumes and improvement in survival in 390 damage control laparotomy patients. *Ann Surg*. 2011;254:598–605.

61. Young PP, Cotton BA, Goodnough LT. Massive transfusion protocols for patients with substantial hemorrhage. *Transfus Med Rev*. 2011;25:293–303.

62. Borgman MA, Spinella PC, Perkins JG, et al. The ratio of blood products transfused affects mortality in patients receiving massive transfusions at a combat support hospital. *J Trauma*. 2007;63:805–813.

63. Holcomb JB, del Junco DJ, Fox EE, et al. The prospective, observational, multicenter, major trauma transfusion (PROMMTT) study: comparative effectiveness of a time-varying treatment with competing risks. *JAMA Surg*. 2013;148:127–136.

64. Holcomb JB, Tilley BC, Baraniuk S, et al. Transfusion of plasma, platelets, and red blood cells in a 1:1:1 vs a 1:1:2 ratio and mortality in patients with severe trauma: the PROPPR randomized clinical trial. *JAMA*. 2015;313:471–482.

65. McDaniel LM, Neal MD, Sperry JL, et al. Use of a massive transfusion protocol in nontrauma patients: activate away. *J Am Coll Surg*. 2013;216:1103–1109.

66. Boffard KD, Riou B, Warren B, et al. Recombinant factor VIIa as adjunctive therapy for bleeding control in severely injured trauma patients: two parallel randomized, placebo-controlled, double-blind clinical trials. *J Trauma*. 2005;59:8–15; discussion -8.

67. Hauser CJ, Boffard K, Dutton R, et al. Results of the CONTROL trial: efficacy and safety of recombinant activated Factor VII in the management of refractory traumatic hemorrhage. *J Trauma*. 2010;69:489–500.

68. Scarpelini S, Rizoli S. Recombinant factor VIIa and the surgical patient. *CurR Opin Crit Care*. 2006;12:351–356.

69. Mayer SA, Brun NC, Broderick J, et al. Recombinant activated factor VII for acute intracerebral hemorrhage: US phase IIA trial. *Neurocrit Care*. 2006;4:206–214.

70. Mayer S, Brun N, Begtrup K. Randomized, Placebo controlled, double blind phase 3 study to assess rFVIIa efficacy in acute cerebral hemorrhage: The FAST Trial. *Cerebrovasc Disease*. 2007;23:1–147.

71. Bosch J, Thabut D, Bendtsen F, et al. Recombinant factor VIIa for upper gastrointestinal bleeding in patients with cirrhosis: a randomized, double-blind trial. *Gastroenterology*. 2004;127:1123–1130.

72. Alfirevic Z, Elbourne D, Pavord S, et al. Use of recombinant activated factor VII in primary postpartum hemorrhage: the Northern European registry 2000-2004. *Obstet Gynecol*. 2007;110:1270–1278.

73. Franchini M, Manzato F, Salvagno GL, Lippi G. Potential role of recombinant activated factor VII for the treatment of severe bleeding associated with disseminated intravascular coagulation: a systematic review. *Blood Coagul Fibrinolysis*. 2007;18:589–593.

74. Heilmann L, Wild C, Hojnacki B, Pollow K. Successful treatment of life-threatening bleeding after cesarean section with recombinant activated factor VII. *Clin Appl Thromb Hemost*. 2006;12:227–229.

75. Jirapinyo M, Manonai J, Herabutya Y, Chuncharunee S. Effectiveness of recombinant activated factor VII (rFVII a) for controlling intractable postpartum bleeding: report of two cases and literature review. *J Med Assoc Thai*. 2007;90:977–981.

76. Perkins JG, Schreiber MA, Wade CE, Holcomb JB. Early versus late recombinant factor VIIa in combat trauma patients requiring massive transfusion. *J Trauma*. 2007;62:1095–1099; discussion 9–101.

77. Stein DM, Dutton RP, O'Connor J, Alexander M, Scalea TM. Determinants of futility of administration of recombinant factor VIIa in trauma. *J Trauma*. 2005;59:609–615.

78. O'Connell KA, Wood JJ, Wise RP, Lozier JN, Braun MM. Thromboembolic adverse events after use of recombinant human coagulation factor VIIa. *JAMA*. 2006;295:293–298.

79. Shakur H, Roberts I, Bautista R, et al. Effects of tranexamic acid on death, vascular occlusive events, and blood transfusion in trauma patients with significant haemorrhage (CRASH-2): a randomised, placebo-controlled trial. *Lancet*. 2010;376:23–32.

80. Roberts I, Shakur H, Afolabi A, et al. The importance of early treatment with tranexamic acid in bleeding trauma patients: an exploratory analysis of the CRASH-2 randomised controlled trial. *Lancet*. 2011;377:1096–1101, 101 e1–2.

81. Morrison JJ, Dubose JJ, Rasmussen TE, Midwinter MJ. Military Application of Tranexamic Acid in Trauma Emergency Resuscitation (MATTERs) Study. *Arch Surg*. 2012;147:113–119.

82. Morrison JJ, Ross JD, Dubose JJ, Jansen JO, Midwinter MJ, Rasmussen TE. Association of cryoprecipitate and tranexamic acid with improved survival following wartime injury: findings from the MATTERs II Study. *JAMA Surg*. 2013;148:218–225.

82 Which Anticoagulants Should Be Used in the Critically Ill Patient? How Do I Choose?

Prakash A. Patel, Emily K. Gordon, John G. Augoustides

The critically ill patient in the intensive care unit (ICU) is at risk for arterial and venous thromboembolic events, including pulmonary embolism (PE), deep venous thrombosis (DVT), and acute coronary syndrome (ACS). The clinical features of these thromboembolic syndromes may defy prompt diagnosis, emphasizing the importance of maintaining a high level of clinical suspicion for these events. It is equally clear that appropriate use of anticoagulant prophylaxis and therapy is essential in ICU practice.

Arterial and venous thromboses are managed with anticoagulants. In addition, antiplatelet therapy is also a mainstay in arterial or intracardiac conditions such as ACS, atrial fibrillation, coronary artery disease, peripheral vascular disease, or the presence of vascular stents. Use of antiplatelet therapy is especially important when the risk of using full anticoagulation is prohibitive. Although antiplatelet therapy is important, this review focuses on anticoagulants capable of preventing blood clot formation by mechanisms outside of decreasing platelet aggregation. We examine many of the well-established anticoagulant agents (Table 82-1), including indications, safety profiles, monitoring, and reversibility, but greater emphasis is given to the newer oral anticoagulant agents that are gradually being introduced to the critical care setting.

WARFARIN

Warfarin is a frequently used classic vitamin K antagonist (VKA) for the prevention of thromboembolic events.[1] However, it is limited by its narrow therapeutic index; unpredictable pharmacokinetics and pharmacodynamics; multiple drug interactions; a need for frequent monitoring of levels; food interactions; adverse bleeding effects; and, unfortunately, the induction of hypercoagulable states.[2] In addition to these limitations, physicians rely heavily on patient compliance in regard to dosage and frequent monitoring.[2]

Warfarin is primarily metabolized by the CYP2C9 hepatic microsomal enzyme system. This system is inducible by many other medications and carries genetic variability that can alter activity (Table 82-1).[3] Warfarin is

strongly protein bound, and it is the non–protein-bound fraction that is biologically active. The drug is water soluble and is highly absorbed after oral administration, mostly in the proximal small bowel.[4-6] The biological half-life is 36 to 42 hours.[4-6]

Warfarin interferes with the biosynthesis of the vitamin-K-dependent coagulation factors II, VII, IX, and X[5,6] as well as the natural anticoagulant proteins C and S.[5-7] Because of these contradictory effects, warfarin and other VKAs produce procoagulant and prothrombotic effects.[5-7] The desired anticoagulant effects are delayed by approximately 36 to 72 hours depending on the clearance of normal clotting factors, particularly prothrombin, from the circulation.[6-8]

Monitoring of warfarin levels is done by measurement of the international normalized rate (INR), defined as the ratio of the patient's prothrombin time (PT) to a normal sample (control). A therapeutic INR is defined according to the indication for anticoagulation: For venous thromboembolism (VTE) prophylaxis, a therapeutic INR is typically in the range of 2.0 to 3.0.[5,6] In the setting of mechanical heart valves, higher therapeutic goals for the INR are recommended.[5,6]

UNFRACTIONATED HEPARIN

Unfractionated heparin (UFH) was discovered in 1916, and its first human trial was conducted in 1935.[9] UFH potentiates the action of antithrombin III, inactivating thrombin and activated coagulation factors IX, X, XI, XII and plasmin, thereby preventing the conversion of fibrinogen to fibrin.[9] Heparin is primarily metabolized by the liver, but it may be partially metabolized in the reticuloendothelial system. The elimination half-life of heparin when discontinued from a steady state is approximately 1 to 2 hours. Because anticoagulation with UFH can be challenging in the individual patient, it is common to use dosing protocols that guide dosing to reach a goal therapeutic activated partial thromboplastin time (aPTT) and thereafter to guide maintenance of the aPTT in the goal range.[10] Importantly, the efficacy of this approach has not been truly tested.

Table 82-1 Drugs Associated with Warfarin Interactions

ALTERED PLATELET FUNCTION

Aspirin

Clopidogrel

GASTROINTESTINAL INJURY

Nonsteroidal anti-inflammatory drugs

ALTERED VITAMIN K SYNTHESIS

Antibiotics

Trimethoprim sulfamethoxazole

Ciprofloxacin

Amoxicillin

Clarithromycin

ALTERED WARFARIN METABOLISM

Amiodarone

Gemfibrozil

Rifampin

Simvastatin

UFH has been the traditional parenteral agent for anticoagulation. It is ubiquitous in the ICU for prevention of DVT and PE in diverse acute patient populations.[11] UFH is also the preferred anticoagulant in severe renal failure (creatinine clearance <30 mL/min). The short half-life of UFH offers the advantage of quick reversal of anticoagulant effects when needed. UFH can be rapidly reversed with protamine sulfate (1 mg/100 U heparin). However, protamine can trigger anaphylaxis, particularly in patients with insulin-dependent diabetes and fish allergies.[9,11] Specific ICU conditions that require the use of UFH have not been identified.

A rare but serious complication of heparin exposure is heparin-induced thrombocytopenia (HIT), a syndrome in which antibodies to the complex of heparin and platelet factor IV trigger platelet activation that causes major arterial and/or venous thrombosis.[12] Treatment of this life-threatening complication is to terminate heparin exposure and to anticoagulate with a nonheparin alternative such as a direct thrombin inhibitor (DTI).[12]

LOW-MOLECULAR-WEIGHT HEPARINS

Heparin is a naturally occurring polysaccharide consisting of molecular chains of varying lengths or molecular weights.[13,14] The low-molecular-weight heparins (LMWHs) are fractionated from heparin to yield only short polysaccharide chains.[13,14] The main LMWHs in clinical practice are enoxaparin, dalteparin, and tinzaparin.[13] Tinzaparin is currently not available in the United States. The advantages of LMWH relative to UFH are greater bioavailability, longer duration of anticoagulant action, fixed dosing, a lack of need for laboratory monitoring, and a lower risk of HIT.[14,15] Multiple meta-analyses indicate that subcutaneous LMWH is more effective than UFH for the treatment of VTE, exhibiting higher rates of thrombus regression and lower rates of recurrent thrombosis, major bleeding, and mortality.[16-19] Despite these presumed clinical advantages of LWMH, randomized trials of LMWH versus UFH for thromboprophylaxis in the ICU have yielded inconsistent results.[20-23] A recently completed large, multicenter, randomized trial in 3754 ICU patients compared dalteparin with twice-daily UFH for thromboprophylaxis. There was no difference (hazard ratio 0.92; 95% confidence interval [CI], 0.68 to 1.23; $P = .57$) between groups in the primary outcome variable—the incidence of proximal leg DVT.[24] However, dalteparin significantly lowered the incidence of PE (hazard ratio 0.51; 95% CI, 0.30 to 0.88; $P = .01$) and HIT (hazard ratio, 0.27; 95% CI, 0.08 to 0.98; $P = .046$).[24,25] Importantly, UFH administered three times per day has been shown to be superior to twice-daily dosing, a fact not accounted for in the above trial.

LMWH can lower the risk of HIT. A recent meta-analysis identified a lower incidence of HIT in postoperative patients undergoing thromboprophylaxis with LMWH when compared with UFH (risk ratio 0.25; 95% CI, 0.07 to 0.82; $P = .02$).[26] In the analysis for HIT complicated by VTE, LMWH was associated with an 80% risk reduction for this complication compared with UFH (risk ratio 0.20; 95% CI, 0.04 to 0.90; $P = .04$).[26] Although these analyses are suggestive, further high-quality trials are essential.[26] There are disadvantages to the use of LMWH in the ICU. These include variations in efficacy in obese patients and underweight elderly patients. Furthermore, the lack of a routine test to measure the effects of LMWH can be problematic in patients in whom bleeding is particularly dangerous. In addition, although dalteparin (5000 IU/day) did not bioaccumulate in critically ill patients with severe renal dysfunction (creatinine clearance <30 mL/min),[27] other LMWHs that are known to be renally cleared have not been examined. The investigators demonstrated that dalteparin at a daily dose of 5000 IU did not bioaccumulate and that there was no excessive bleeding risk.[27] Overall, further large randomized trials are required to evaluate for clinical superiority over UFH in the critically ill before LWMH will be more widely adopted for thromboprophylaxis in the ICU.

INTRAVENOUS DIRECT THROMBIN INHIBITORS

In contrast to the heparins, DTIs provide anticoagulation regardless of antithrombin III levels[12,28,29] and have the ability to inhibit fibrin-bound thrombin, allowing more complete anticoagulant activity. DTIs also are more predictable because they do not bind to other plasma proteins.[28,29] Currently available intravenous DTIs include lepirudin, desirudin, bivalirudin, and argatroban. The last two are used most commonly because they have a broader range of approved indications.[12,28,29]

Bivalirudin is a hirudin analogue that directly binds to thrombin, leading to an anticoagulant effect within 5 minutes.[12] This binding is reversible because of cleavage by thrombin, which leads to a short half-life (25 minutes) in patients with normal or mildly reduced renal function. Metabolism of the drug is primarily hepatic and proteolytic, but 20% of bivalirudin's clearance is via the kidney,[28] slightly prolonging the half-life in patients with moderate renal dysfunction (creatinine clearance of 30 to 59 mL/min).[30] Monitoring of the anticoagulant effect can be performed with the activated clotting time (ACT). Although no rapid reversal agent exists, the drug is cleared by hemodialysis.[30] The role of this agent in cardiac catheterization and cardiac surgery is emerging, but its value in the ICU remains undefined.

In the ICU setting, argatroban is an alternative parenteral DTI to bivalirudin. This drug also reversibly binds to an active site on thrombin, causing direct inhibition. The primary use of this DTI in the ICU setting is for anticoagulation in critically ill patients with HIT.[31,32] Because of its rapid onset and short half-life, argatroban is typically given as an infusion.[33,34] It is primarily metabolized by the liver; thus, dosing must be adjusted in patients with hepatic failure, but this is not necessary in renal dysfunction.[33,34] Monitoring can be performed with either an ACT or aPTT. The goal aPTT is often 1.5 to 3 times that of the baseline value.[34] Because argatroban affects thrombin-dependent coagulation tests, PT and INR may be altered, an important consideration when transitioning to warfarin.[33] Formal studies of argatroban in critically ill patients have not been reported.

PARENTERAL INDIRECT SYNTHETIC FACTOR XA INHIBITORS

Fondaparinux is an indirect factor Xa inhibitor that is a synthetic analog of a natural pentasaccharide contained in heparin and LMWH that interrupts the coagulation cascade upstream of thrombin.[35] The lack of thrombin inhibition prevents rebound thrombin generation.

Fondaparinux has a half-life of 17 to 21 hours and is administered as a daily subcutaneous injection. Peak plasma concentrations are achieved within 2 hours of injection.[35] A recent trial demonstrated that the bioavailability of fondaparinux after subcutaneous injection was not significantly affected by vasopressor therapy in critically ill patients.[36] Clearance is significantly decreased in the setting of renal failure. The effects of fondaparinux can be followed with serial measurement of factor Xa activity, but routine monitoring is not recommended.[35,36] The PT, INR, and aPTT typically are not affected. There is no specific reversal agent for fondaparinux, although recombinant factor VIIa may reverse its effects.[37,38]

In a randomized controlled trial (N = 849 acute medical patients >60 years, 35 centers from 8 countries), fondaparinux as compared with placebo significantly reduced the risk of VTE by 46.7% from 10.5% to 5.6% (*P* < .05) with no increase in bleeding risk.[39] A meta-analysis (cumulative N > 13,000 medical and surgical patients, 8 randomized trials) confirmed a one-fifth reduction in mortality from VTE with fondaparinux as compared with the control groups of placebo or LMWH.[40] Beyond thromboprophylaxis for VTE, a series of randomized controlled trials have established a role for fondaparinux in the management of ACSs managed with and without PCI.[41-43] Fondaparinux may also have a role in the treatment of HIT in selected patients.[44]

ORAL DIRECT THROMBIN INHIBITORS

Dabigatran etexilate is an oral DTI. The oral form is a prodrug that is activated by nonspecific esterases.[45,46] As discussed previously, DTIs inhibit free and fibrin-bound direct thrombin inhibition, an advantage over heparin, which is less effective at inhibiting the latter. Dabigatran has a rapid onset, reaching peak plasma concentrations within 1.5 hours,[45] and a half-life of 12 to 14 hours.[45,46] Adjustment for renal dysfunction is required because 80% of the drug undergoes renal elimination.[45,46] There is no known hepatotoxicity.[47,48]

The clinical use of dabigatran is expanding, and applications can occur in the ICU setting. Current indications include prophylaxis and treatment of VTE as well as stroke and thromboembolic prophylaxis in nonvalvular atrial fibrillation.

A large randomized trial compared twice-daily dabigatran with warfarin in atrial fibrillation patients (N > 18,000) who were at increased risk for stroke.[51,52] In patients receiving a high dose (150 mg given twice daily), the incidence of stroke during the median 2-year follow-up was lower than warfarin, without an increased risk of major bleeding.[52] Given this promising data on this new oral anticoagulant option, recent guidelines now endorse dabigatran as an alternative to warfarin in selected patients with atrial fibrillation (Class I recommendation; level of evidence B).[53]

Monitoring is problematic: the thrombin time is oversensitive to dabigatran's effect.[45] The ecarin clotting time, another option, is not a routinely available test, and the absolute aPTT value does not correlate to actual concentrations of dabigatran.[54,55] Reversal may require activated charcoal or hemodialysis.[45,55] Fresh frozen plasma is not effective in reversing dabigatran-related bleeding, but clinical hemostasis can be achieved with activated prothrombin complex concentrates or recombinant factor VIIa.[50,56] Because use in the critical care environment is limited and because it is an oral agent (subject to unpredictable absorption in the critically ill) that lacks a method for monitoring anticoagulant activity, use of dabigatran in the ICU requires further investigation.

ORAL DIRECT FACTOR XA INHIBITORS

The oral direct factor Xa inhibitors are also a new class of anticoagulants that includes rivaroxaban and apixaban.[57] Both agents inhibit factor Xa, independent of antithrombin, which gives it a direct advantage over intravenous agents such as UFH, LMWH, and fondaparinux.[46] They also do not cause rebound thrombin generation. Both available direct factor Xa drugs possess high bioavailability and half-lives in the range of 11 to 12 hours.[57] Rivaroxaban is primarily eliminated via the kidneys, which comprise only approximately 25% of apixaban's multiple elimination pathways.[57] Current indications for rivaroxaban include the prevention and treatment of VTE. Use of rivaroxaban (15 mg twice daily followed by 20 mg once daily) for the treatment of symptomatic VTE or PE has been described and is associated with a lower rate of major bleeding than warfarin.[58] An advantage in the rivaroxaban-treated patients was the significantly lower rate of major bleeding during treatment (P = .002).[58] Apixaban has been used for the prevention and treatment of VTE and has recently been approved for use in the United States.[59-61] Both oral direct factor Xa inhibitors have been used for the prevention of stroke or systemic embolism in nonvalvular atrial fibrillation.[62,63] Similar to dabigatran, studies investigating further clinical use of the oral direct factor Xa inhibitors are ongoing. A potential role in the prevention of ACSs may exist, but the agents are not approved at this time for this indication.[57,64] Further trials are also required to establish whether these agents are safe and effective in the management of anticoagulation for mechanical heart valves.[57] Other ICU use requires additional investigation. The lack of a routine test for anticoagulation is potentially problematic. The PT or aPTT may be elevated in the presence of these drugs, but these tests are unreliable.[54] A more promising test, the chromogenic anti-factor Xa assay, is not widely available.[54,65,66] For urgent reversal or for immediate treatment of active bleeding, hemodialysis is not an option because these agents are highly protein bound.[46,57] There is currently no specific antidote for the anticoagulant effect of rivaroxaban or apixaban.[57] Further trials are required to explore the safety and efficacy of these agents.

How Do I Choose in the ICU: Which Anticoagulant for Which Patient?

Choosing the optimal anticoagulant for the ICU patient depends on multiple factors. Consideration of whether the need is for prophylaxis or treatment of VTE is of paramount importance. It may also be important to consider the patient's post-ICU anticoagulation goals. Short-term anticoagulation may be addressed with an intravenous or subcutaneous medication. However, if the patient is to be treated for thromboembolism or requires extended prophylaxis, a longer-acting oral agent may be preferable. A delayed peak effect may make provision of a temporary bridging agent necessary. Other factors related to the specific drug should be considered. These include half-life and primary metabolic and elimination pathways. Patient factors such as hepatic and renal function must be considered, and dose adjustment in the critically ill may be necessary. Concerns regarding the risk for HIT may eliminate the use of heparins.

The ability to monitor the degree of anticoagulation is an essential consideration in choosing an anticoagulant. The lack of routine monitoring, often advertised as a significant benefit of the newer anticoagulants, may be problematic in the critically ill patient. Likewise, the ability to reverse the anticoagulant effect should play a role in choosing a specific drug.

Evidence-based clinical practice guidelines offer recommendations on the various available drugs.[67,68] However, most of these recommendations do not reflect the demands of critical illness. As the indications for the newer oral anticoagulant agents continue to expand, drugs such as dabigatran, rivaroxaban, apixaban, and similar agents may play an increased role in the critical care setting. The ongoing studies comparing these newer drugs to the already well-established drugs demonstrate that anticoagulation is of crucial importance in all patients at risk for thromboembolism.

AUTHORS' RECOMMENDATIONS

- Anticoagulation in critically ill patients is necessary given the multiple factors that increase their risk for the development of thromboembolism.
- The choice of a particular anticoagulant in the ICU patient should be determined by the indication for therapy, patient factors, and drug factors, including reversibility.
- Intensivists should be aware of the spectrum of available anticoagulant agents while recognizing that the newer oral anticoagulant agents are just entering ICU practice and require further investigation.

REFERENCES

1. Flato UAP, Buhatem T, Merluzzi T, et al. New anticoagulants in critical care settings. *Rev Bras Ter Intensiva*. 2011;23:68–77.
2. Augoustides JG. Advances in anticoagulation: focus on dabigatran, an oral direct thrombin inhibitor. *J Cardiothorac Vasc Anesth*. 2011;25:1208–1212.
3. Johnson JA, Cavallari LH. Warfarin pharmacogenetics. *Trends Cardiovasc Med*. 2015;25:33–41.
4. Lee WT, Klein TE. Pharmacogenetics of warfarin: challenges and opportunities. *J Hum Gent*. 2013;59:334–338.
5. Ansell J, Hirsh J, Hylek E, et al. Pharmacology and management of the vitamin K antagonists: American College of Chest Physicians Evidence-Based Clinical Practice guidelines. 8th ed. *Chest*. 2008;133:160S–198S.
6. Freedman MD. Oral anticoagulants: pharmacodynamics, clinical indications and adverse effects. *J Clin Pharmacol*. 1992;32:196–209.
7. Thomasberry LA, LoSicco KI, English III JC. The skin and hypercoagulable states. *J Am Acad Dermatol*. 2013;69:450–462.
8. Warkentin TE. Anticoagulant failure in coagulopathic patients: PTT confounding and other pitfalls. *Expert Opin Drug Saf*. 2014;13:25–43.
9. Hirsh J, Bauer KA, Donati MB, et al. Parenteral anticoagulants: American College of Chest Physicians evidence-based clinical practice guidelines. 8th ed. *Chest*. 2008;133:141S–159S.
10. Hylek EN, Regan S, Henault LE, et al. Challenges to the effective use of unfractionated heparin in the hospitalized management of acute thrombosis. *Arch Intern Med*. 2003;163:621–627.
11. Alhazzari W, Lim W, Jaeschike RZ, et al. Heparin thromboprophylaxis in medical-surgical critically ill patients: a systematic review and meta-analysis of randomized trials. *Crit Care Med*. 2013;41:2088–2098.
12. Augoustides JG. Update in hematology: heparin-induced thrombocytopenia and bivalirudin. *J Cardiothorac Vasc Anesth*. 2011;25:371–375.
13. Casu B, Naggi A, Torri G. Re-visiting the structure of heparin. *Cardbohydr Res*. 2015;403:60–68.
14. Weitz JI. Low-molecular-weight heparins. *N Engl J Med*. 1997;337:688–698.
15. Linkins LA, Dans AL, Moores LK, et al. Treatment and prevention of heparin-induced thrombocytopenia: antithrombotic therapy and prevention of thrombosis, 9th ed: American College of Chest Physicians evidence-based clinical practice guidelines. *Chest*. 2012;141:e495S–e530S.
16. Erkens PM, Prins MH. Fixed dose subcutaneous low molecular weight heparins versus adjusted dose unfractionated heparin for venous thromboembolism. *Cochrane Database Syst Rev*. 2010 (9): CD001100.
17. Castellucci LA, Cameron C, Le Gal G, et al. Clinical and safety outcomes associated with treatment of acute venous thromboembolism: a systematic review and meta-analysis. *JAMA*. 2014;312:1122–1135.
18. Segal JB, Streiff MB, Hofmann LV, et al. Management of venous thromboembolism: a systematic review for a practice guideline. *Ann Intern Med*. 2007;146:211–222.
19. Gould MK, Dembitzer AD, Doyle RL, et al. Low-molecular-weight heparins compared with unfractionated heparin for treatment of acute deep venous thrombosis: a meta-analysis of randomized, controlled trials. *Ann Intern Med*. 1999;130:800–809.

20. Cade JR. High risk of the critically ill for venous thromboembolism. *Crit Care Med.* 1982;10:448–450.

21. Fraisse F, Holzapfel L, Couland JM, et al. Nadroparin in the prevention of deep vein thrombosis in acute decompensated COPD. *Am J Respir Crit Care Med.* 2000;161:1109–1114.

22. De A, Roy P, Garg VK, et al. Low-molecular weight heparin and unfractionated heparin in prophylaxis against deep vein thrombosis in critically ill patients undergoing major surgery. *Blood Coag Fibrinolysis.* 2010;21:57–61.

23. Shorr AF, Williams MD. Venous thromboembolism in critically ill patients: observations from a randomized trial in sepsis. *Thromb Haemost.* 2009;101:139–144.

24. Cook D, Meade M, Guyatt G, et al. Dalteparin versus unfractionated heparin in critically ill patients. *N Engl J Med.* 2011;364:1305–1314.

25. Warkentin TE, Sheppard JA, Heels-Ansdell D, et al. Heparin-induced thrombocytopenia in medical surgical critical illness. *Chest.* 2013;144:848–858.

26. Junqueira D, Perini E, Penholati R, et al. Unfractionated heparin versus low molecular weight heparin for avoiding heparin-induced thrombocytopenia in postoperative patients. *Cochrane Database Syst Rev.* 2012; 9: CD007557.

27. Cook D, Douketis J, Meade M, et al. Venous thromboembolism and bleeding in critically ill patients with severe renal insufficiency receiving dalteparin thromboprophylaxis: prevalence, incidence and risk factors. *Crit Care.* 2008;12:R32.

28. Lee CJ, Ansell JE. Direct thrombin inhibitors. *Br J Clin Pharmacol.* 2011;72:581–592.

29. Untereiner O, Seince PF, Chterev V, et al. Management of the direct oral anticoagulants in the perioperative setting. *J Cardiothorac Vasc Anesth.* 2015;29:741–748.

30. Reed MD, Bell D. Clinical pharmacology of bivalirudin. *Pharmacotherapy.* 2002;22:105S–111S.

31. Alatri A, Armstrong AE, Greinacher A, et al. Results of a consensus meeting on the use of argatroban in patients with heparin-induced thrombocytopenia requiring antithrombotic therapy – A European Perspective. *Thromb Res.* 2012;129:426–433.

32. Smythe MA, Koerber JM, Forsyth LL, et al. Argatroban dosage requirements and outcomes in intensive care versus non-intensive care patients. *Pharmacotherapy.* 2009:1073–1081.

33. Retter A, Barrett NA. The management of abnormal haemostasis in the ICU. *Anaesthesia.* 2015;70:121–e41.

34. Nutescu EA, Shapiro NL, Chevalier A. New anticoagulant agents: direct thrombin inhibitors. *Cardiol Clin.* 2008;26:169–187.

35. Sakr Y. Heparin-induced thrombocytopenia in the ICU: an overview. *Crit Care.* 2011;15:211.

36. Cumbo –Nacheli G, Samavati L, Guzman JA. Bioavailbility of fondaparinux to critically ill patients. *J Crit Care.* 2011;26:342–346.

37. Lu G, DeGuzman FR, Hollenbach SJ, et al. A specific antidote for reversal of anticoagulation by direct and indirect inhibitors of coagulation factor Xa. *Nat Med.* 2013;19:446–451.

38. Bijsterveld NR, Moons AH, Boekholdt SM, et al. Ability of recombinant factor VIIa to reverse the anticoagulant effect of the pentasaccharide fondaparinux in healthy volunteers. *Circulation.* 2002;106:2550–2554.

39. Cohen AT, Davidson BL, Gallus AS, et al. Efficacy and safety of fondaparinux for the prevention of venous thromboembolism in older acute medical patients: randomised placebo controlled trial. *BMJ.* 2006;332:325–329.

40. Eikelboom JW, Quinlan DJ, O'Donnell M. Major bleeding, mortality, and efficacy of fondaparinux in venous thromboembolism prevention trials. *Circulation.* 2009;120:2006–2011.

41. Karthikeyan G, Mehta SR, Eikelboom JW. Fondaparinux in the treatment of acute coronary syndromes: evidence from OASIS 5 and 6. *Exper Rev Cardiovasc Ther.* 2009;7:241–249.

42. Steg PG, Jolly SS, Mehta SR, et al. Low-dose vs standard-dose unfractionated heparin for percutaneous coronary intervention in acute coronary syndromes treated with fondaparinux: the FUTURE? OASIS-8 randomized trial. *JAMA.* 2010;304:1339–1349.

43. Van Rees Vellinga TE, Peters RJ, Yusuf S, et al. Efficacy and safety of fondaparinux in patients with St-segment elevation myocardial infarction across the age spectrum: results from the Organization for the Assessment of Strategies for Ischemic Syndromes (OASIS 6) trial. *Am Heart J.* 2010;160:1049–1055.

44. Warkentin TE, Pai M, Sheppard JI, et al. Fondaparinux treatment of acute heparin-induced thrombocytopenia confirmed by the serotonin-release assay: a 30-month, 16-patient case series. *J Thromb Haemost.* 2011;9:2389–2396.

45. Augoustides JG. Advances in anticoagulation: focus on dabigatran, an oral direct thrombin inhibitor. *J Cardiothorac Vasc Anesth.* 2011;25:1208–1212.

46. Levy JH, Faraoni D, Spring JL, et al. Managing new oral anticoagulants in the perioperative and intensive care unit setting. *Anesthesiology.* 2013;118:1466–1474.

47. Lee WM, Larrey D, Olsson R, et al. Hepatic findings in long-term clinical trials of ximelagatran. *Drug Saf.* 2005;28:351–370.

48. Sergent O, Ekroos K, Lefeuvre-Orfila L, et al. Ximelagatran increases membrane fluidity and changes membrane lipid composition in primary human hepatocytes. *Toxilcol In Vitro.* 2009;23:1305–1310.

49. Flato UAP, Buhatem T, Merluzzi T, et al. New anticoagulants in critical care settings. *Rev Bras Ter Intensiva.* 2011;23:68–77.

50. Hankey GJ, Eikelboom JW. Dabigatran etexilate: a new oral thrombin inhibitor. *Circulation.* 2011;123:1436–1450.

51. Ezekowitz MD, Connoly S, Parekh A, et al. Rationale and design of RE-LY: randomized evaluation of long-term anticoagulation therapy, warfarin, compared with dabigatran. *Am Heart J.* 2009;157:805–810.

52. Connoly S, Ezekowitz MD, Yusuf S, et al. Dabigatran versus warfarin in patients with atrial fibrillation. *N Engl J Med.* 2009;361:1139–1151.

53. Wann LS, Curtis AB, Ellenbogen KA, et al. ACCF/AHA/HRS focused update on the management of patients with atrial fibrillation (update on dabigatran): a report of the American College of Cardiology Foundation/American Heart Association task force on practice guidelines. *J Am Coll Cardiol.* 2011;57:1330–1337.

54. Miyares MA, Davis K. Newer oral anticoagulants: a review of laboratory monitoring options and reversal agents in the hemorrhagic patient. *Am J Health Syst Pharm.* 2012;69:1473–1484.

55. Vanden Daelen S, Peetermans M, Vanassche T, et al. Monitoring and reversal strategies for new oral anticoagulants. *Expert Rev Cardiovasc Ther.* 2015;13:95–103.

56. Babilonia K, Trujillo T. The role of prothrombin complex concentrates in reversal of target specific anticoagulants. *Thromb J.* 2014;12:8.

57. Augoustides JG. Breakthroughs in anticoagulation: advent of the oral direct factor Xa inhibitors. *J Cardiothorac Vasc Anesth.* 2012;26:740–745.

58. Prins MH, Lensing AWA, Bauersachs R, et al. Oral rivaroxaban versus standard therapy for the treatment of symptomatic venous thromboembolism: a pooled analysis of the EINSTEIN-DVT and PE randomized studies. *Thromb J.* 2013;11:21.

59. Lassen MR, Raskob GE, Gallus A, et al. Apixaban versus enoxaparin for thromboprophylaxis after knee replacement (ADVANCE-2): a randomised double-blind trial. *Lancet.* 2010;375:807–815.

60. Lassen MR, Gallus A, Raskob GE, et al. Apixaban versus enoxaparin for thromboprophylaxis after hip replacement. *N Engl J Med.* 2010;363:2487–2498.

61. Agnelli G, Buller HR, Cohen A, et al. Oral apixaban for the treatment of acute venous thromboembolism. *N Engl J Med.* 2013;369:799–808.

62. Patel MR, Mahaffey KW, Garg J, et al. Rivaroxaban versus warfarin in nonvalvular atrial fibrillation. *N Engl J Med.* 2011;365:883–891.

63. Granger CB, Alexander JH, McMurray JJV, et al. Apixaban versus warfarin in patients with atrial fibrillation. *N Engl J Med.* 2011;365:981–992.

64. Messori A, Fadda V, Gatto R, et al. New oral anticoagulants in acute coronary syndrome: is there any advantage over existing treatments? *Int Cardiovasc Res J.* 2014;8:124–126.

65. Samama MM. Which test to measure the anticoagulant effect of rivaroxaban: the anti-factor Xa assay. *J Thromb Haemost.* 2013;11:579–580.

66. Hillarp A, Gustafsson KM, Faxalv L, et al. Effects of the oral, direct factor Xa inhibitor apixaban on routine coagulation assays and anti-FXa assays. *J Throm Haemost.* 2014;12:1545–1553.

67. Holbrook A, Schulman S, Witt DM, et al. Evidence-based management of anticoagulant therapy: antithrombotic therapy and prevention of thrombosis, 9th ed: American College of Chest Physicians evidence-based clinical practice guidelines. *Chest.* 2012;141:e152S–e184S.

68. Ageno W, Gallus AS, Wittkowsky A, et al. Oral anticoagulant therapy: antithrombotic therapy and prevention of thrombosis, 9th ed: American College of Chest Physicians evidence-based clinical practice guidelines. *Chest.* 2012;141:e44S–e88S.

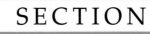

CRITICAL CARE RESOURCE USE AND MANAGEMENT

83 How Can Critical Care Resource Utilization in the United States Be Optimized?

Jason Wagner, Scott Halpern

Critical care resources should be allocated in ways that promote high-quality care, defined by the Institute of Medicine as care that is safe, effective, patient-centered, timely, efficient, and equitable.[1] However, utilization patterns in intensive care units (ICUs) often vary from ICU to ICU as well as within ICUs among individual providers. The source of this variation, while not fully understood, is likely undue—reflecting nonevidence-based practice patterns.[2-4] Given that ICU beds comprise a large proportion of the total number of hospital beds in the United States and that their utilization consumes a disproportionate amount of the gross domestic product compared with other developed nations,[5] numerous stakeholders have an increasingly vested interest in improving critical care delivery by aligning reimbursements with quality metrics. It is therefore of paramount importance both to accelerate the adoption of evidence-based critical care processes that are in line with patient values and to minimize both low-value and wasteful practices. With more attention to resource utilization, critical care outcomes will be improved, and there will be better matching of demand for, and supply of, ICU beds[6] in ways that adequately help prepare them for any strains on ICU capacity.[7,8]

ARE INTENSIVE CARE UNIT RESOURCES UNDERUSED?

Appropriate critical care resource utilization should be informed by evidence-based medicine, patient values, and social priorities. However, there is currently a large amount of variation in critical care utilization despite the existence of high-quality evidence.[9-11] One obvious way to remove much of this undue variation would be to quickly adopt evidence-based resources and promulgate these practices across the critical care spectrum. However, some suggest that it takes roughly 17 years for evidence to be fully implemented into clinical practice, suggesting that a significant proportion of critically ill patients are at risk for not receiving the standard of care due to a slow and capricious approach to implementation.[12] For the recommendation of specific areas within critical care where increased resource utilization is warranted, it is important to first discuss examples where high-value resources have been slowly adopted and then examine whether structural or organizational changes can lead to improvements in implementation.

Recent decades have seen substantial advancements in the care of many critically ill patients, such as those with septic shock and acute respiratory distress syndrome (ARDS)—two highly prevalent conditions that commonly result in both short-term and long-term mortality among patients admitted to ICUs.[13,14] Despite these improvements, there has been an obvious lag in the implementation of evidence. Almost 15 years after the seminal work demonstrating an impressive mortality benefit of low-stretch mechanical ventilation in ARDS patients,[15] studies suggest that providers still underuse lung protective strategies.[16,17] In a study of patients with lung injury, Needham et al. found that only 41% of patients meeting criteria to receive lung protective mechanical ventilation actually received this potentially lifesaving measure. In addition, there was a dose-response effect of adherence such that patients with high adherence had a much lower risk of mortality over a 2-year period compared with those patients with lower rates of adherence. If lung protective mechanical ventilation still suffers from delays in implementation, it is highly likely that other, more recent evidence-based strategies are also underutilized. These would include strategies relevant to almost all patients with respiratory failure, such as the daily interruption of sedation combined with a spontaneous breathing trial[18] and early ambulation,[19] as well as time-sensitive strategies reserved for patients with severe ARDS, such as early paralysis and prone positioning.[20,21]

It is worth noting that the evidence suggests that hospitals caring for higher numbers of patients undergoing mechanical ventilation have superior outcomes compared with lower volume hospitals—likely because of better adherence to evidence-based practices.[10] This volume–outcome relationship also appears to exist for severe sepsis, which has become a growing public health concern.[11,13,22] Many think that the volume-outcome relationship in severe sepsis exists because high-volume hospitals are better at adhering to evidence-based sepsis care,[23] such as the administration of early and appropriate broad-spectrum antibiotics and fluid resuscitation,[24,25] adherence to lung protective mechanical ventilation,[15] and restricted transfusion practices.[26]

Broadly, high-value resources exist beyond the scope of both ARDS and severe sepsis and extend to almost all patients admitted to ICUs with acute and reversible processes. One resource that may improve outcomes for critically ill patients is a multidisciplinary team led by an intensivist.[27] Much like the evidence for a volume–outcome relationship, the presence of an intensivist-led multidisciplinary team may increase adherence to evidence-based practices and improve patient outcomes, but some experts predict that there will be a growing shortage of board-certified critical care providers.[28] If this proves to be true, then efforts to benchmark ICUs based on the presence of an intensivist may be an ineffective undertaking.[29] With evidence lacking for the 24-hour presence of an intensivist,[30] more work needs to be done to determine how to deploy our projected staffing resources in ways that optimize patient outcomes. This includes an improved understanding of which patients derive the greatest benefit from being cared for by intensivists as well as how to think more broadly about critical care organization and structure. Given that it is unlikely that every critically ill patient will go to hospitals that employ intensivists, one possible solution to improve the overall quality of critical care would be the incorporation of checklists[31] and/or leverage defaults embedded in electronic medical records to help providers adhere to evidence-based processes. Examples include prophylaxis for deep venous thromboembolism and gastrointestinal bleeding, implementation of early enteral feeding, prevention of ventilator-associated pneumonias, early physical therapy, and the timely removal of intravascular and urinary catheters.[32] In addition, it is also possible that expanding the use of telemedicine to provide remote access to intensivists may help to bridge the intensivist-patient gap and add quality to our critical care system.[33]

Finally, in addition to increasing the utilization of evidence-based resources, it is equally if not more important that critical care practitioners effectively elicit patient preferences to ensure that the deployment of these resources is in line with patients' goals and values. Because of severity of illness, many patients in the ICU setting will die despite being exposed to evidence-based processes. Therefore it is important to emphasize that high-quality critical care should include a timely elicitation of patient values to help promote a patient-centered approach that minimizes unwarranted and overly aggressive care at the end of life.[34] Early meetings with patients or their surrogates to elicit goals and values, strategies that promote incorporating families/surrogates on ICU rounds, and the inclusion of palliative care experts in a multidisciplinary approach to patients faced with a high risk of morbidity and mortality all represent promising interventions in need of rapid study and, if successful, implementation.

ARE INTENSIVE CARE UNIT RESOURCES OVERUSED?

At any hour of the day approximately one third of U.S. ICU beds are vacant and available with roughly one in three beds

in use for patients receiving mechanical ventilation.[6] This surplus of U.S. critical care beds outnumbers the total number of ICU beds in many other modern countries. The concept of supply-induced demand,[35] or "if you build it, they will come," suggests that this excess in ICU beds results in the routine admission of patients that are either too well or too sick to benefit from critical care—signifying that many ICU admissions are likely examples of either low-value or no-value (wasteful) care. One suggestion to help optimize critical care resource utilization is to better determine who truly benefits from an admission to the ICU.

There are some data to suggest that the severity of illness of patients admitted to ICUs is inversely correlated with the number of ICU beds available at the time of admission.[9] This hypothesis begs the question: Do we admit patients who are too well to benefit from critical care when ICU beds are plentiful? This possibility of overutilization is supported by two recent observational studies of low-risk patients.[36,37] Gershengorn et al. published a retrospective study of 15,994 severity-adjusted patients with diabetic ketoacidosis and found that patients were more likely to be admitted to ICUs in hospitals that had higher overall rates of ICU utilization. Importantly, this greater use of ICU level care was not associated with improved outcomes such as reductions in hospital length of stay or in-hospital mortality. In a similar study, Admon et al. examined the relationship between ICU utilization in 61,249 patients with pulmonary embolism and a variety of outcomes and demonstrated that hospitals varied considerably in ICU admission rates for acute pulmonary embolus. They also found that patients admitted to ICUs in "high utilizing" hospitals were less likely to receive critical care procedures, suggesting that their indications for ICU admission were weaker—a notion supported by the additional finding that there was no relationship between ICU admission rate and risk-adjusted hospital mortality.

These are also data to suggest that there may be a subset of patients who are "too sick" to benefit from critical care.[38] Stelfox et al. performed a prospective study of clinically deteriorating floor-level patients for whom a medical emergency team was activated. They specifically looked at whether the number of ICU beds available at the time of the clinical deterioration was associated with a patient's time to ICU admission as well as subsequent changes in their goals of care and in-hospital mortality. They found that fewer available ICU beds were directly associated with patients being more likely to have their goals of care changed to comfort-based approach, but there was no association between the number of available ICU beds and the subsequent in-hospital mortality. These findings suggest that relative scarcity may expedite transitions of care toward palliation in a group of patients that is likely to die with or without ICU-level care.[39] Therefore, when examining the possibility that excess ICU beds may result in overutilization, it is worth considering whether *restricting the future expansion of our critical care bed supply* may paradoxically result in higher quality critical care.

In addition to considering how existing ICU beds are appropriated, it is also worth reflecting on whether there are common critical care practices that are either low value or wasteful. A common theme is emerging within the field of critical care: that *less is often more.*[40] Recently, there has been a palpable increase in the interest of multiple stake-holders to target inefficiencies in our health-care system. One example of this concerted effort is the American Board of Internal Medicine's Choosing Wisely Campaign. This campaign collectively embodies a professional societal spirit that leads on identifying areas of low-value or wasteful care by asking health-care providers to determine a list of five specialty-specific services that should not be routinely provided. Given the resource intensive nature of critical care, embracing these efforts may lead to improved quality.[41] Within critical care, the expert consensus suggests that health-care providers should reduce the reflexive use of diagnostic testing such as routine blood draws and chest imaging, the liberal use of blood products and total parenteral nutrition, deeply sedating mechanically ventilated patients without a specific indication, and continuing life support in high-risk patients without offering patients the alternative of a comfort-based approach.

Finally, critical care providers must continually reevaluate their practices and de-adopt practices that are no longer rooted in evidence. Within critical care, it is not uncommon for diagnostics and therapies to initially demonstrate a positive outcome only later to be shown to lack efficacy or be harmful. Examples would include the routine use of Swan-Ganz catheters,[42] the routine placement of central venous catheters in an algorithmic approach to sepsis,[43] and overly tight glucose control.[44] Although the notion of de-adoption is in the same vein as minimizing low-value and wasteful care, it merits acknowledgment given the evolving nature of critical care clinical trials. Our patients deserve a critical care system that praises the stewardship of resources as opposed to a system that promotes haphazard utilization patterns and wasteful practices. Thankfully, more high-quality research is being done to help us better understand how best to deploy our resources and has only served to strengthen the notion that a conservationist approach to critical care resource utilization is often the correct approach.[24-26,45]

What Is Needed and What Should Be Eliminated?

We discussed that focusing on correcting the underutilization or the slow adoption of evidence-based practices while simultaneously eliciting patient values would vastly improve the quality of critical care provided. To do this, we recommend focusing on four major areas. First, given the large degree of "negative" critical care trials, there needs to be a concerted effort among critical care researchers to improve the quality of critical care trial design to ensure that future trials are relevant, have patient-centered outcomes, possess high-quality statistical methodology that maximizes the likelihood of achieving enrollment and statistical power, and segue to comparative effectiveness research.[46]

Second, the lion's share of health-care research dollars currently targets "bench-to-bedside" or "Translational 1" research centered on technologic and pharmaceutical innovation while only a paucity of health-care dollars are set aside to improve health-care delivery, integration, and quality. Therefore more emphasis must be placed on "beside-to-policy" or "Translational 2" research that focuses on both disseminating knowledge across the critical care spectrum and advancing implementation science to ensure that knowledge dissemination is integrated into routine practice frameworks.[12]

Third, the transition from fee-for-service to value-based purchasing reimbursement mechanisms has helped to stress the importance of patient safety and quality improvement by ensuring that best practices are sought. Given that cost-awareness and appropriate resource stewardship is an important component of quality, formal training structures must be put in place at the graduate medical education level that serve to train future providers how to conduct quality improvements and incorporate cost-awareness into their practice.[47,48] Much of how physicians ultimately practice stems from their early training environment so it is possible that focusing on quality improvement by distinguishing high-value from low-value care may translate into long-lasting improvements in critical care resource utilization.

Fourth, it is worth conceptually exploring the notion of a "net ICU benefit" by improving our understanding of who benefits most (or not at all) from receiving critical care. ICU admissions are costly and should be reserved for severely ill patients with reversible disease processes. Efforts to help further elucidate who best benefits from critical care may require advancements in predictive models that generate probabilities of in-hospital mortality based on the presenting diagnosis and various comorbidities. In turn, the promotion of standardized ICU admission guidelines may then help to implement these findings. For those who may not be sick enough to benefit, hospital organization and staffing efforts to redistribute these patients to lower acuity settings would undoubtedly improve critical care utilization without compromising patient care. For those patients that are too sick to benefit from critical care, rather than act primarily as obstructionists or ICU gatekeepers, we believe a more long-lasting benefit may be achieved by fostering improvements in the end-of-life decision sciences, educating high-risk patients and their surrogates on the risks and benefits of ongoing critical care, and promoting the timely and early elicitation of patient values.

In an effort to avoid overutilization of resources, critical care providers should be circumspect in adopting the newest technology or drug unless it is rooted in high-quality evidence. Although every new technology, device, and drug is marketed as truly innovative, what enters into practice may often be pseudoinnovative. Pseudoinnovative critical care services increase costs without clearly improving patient outcomes. These technologically advanced but low-value services then compete with evidence-based practices and threaten the delivery of high-quality critical care. One suggestion for optimizing resource utilization would be for hospitals to establish ICU resource utilization review committees. These committees would continually appraise critical care evidence, leverage electronic medical records and incorporate defaults to make it more difficult for providers to adopt pseudo-innovation, streamline the adoption of best practices, and prompt providers to de-adopt services later proven to lack evidence. In addition to aligning reimbursement mechanisms with quality and performance metrics[49] and increasing the transparency of provider practice patterns,[50] focusing on optimizing resource utilization as we have outlined previously will help maximize the provision of high-quality critical care.

AUTHORS' RECOMMENDATIONS

- Appropriate critical care resource utilization ought to be informed by evidence-based medicine, patient values, and social priorities. This may take many years.
- The application of EB practice may be advanced by a highly trained multidisciplinary critical care team led by an intensivist.
- It is important that patients' goals and values are elicited when making decisions regarding expensive intensive therapies.
- In the United States, a large number of ICU beds are vacant at any time. The severity of illness of patients admitted to ICUs is inversely correlated with the number of ICU beds available at the time of admission. This may result in overutilization.
- Many critical care interventions appear to be low value or wasteful ("less may be more").
- Critical care providers must continually re-evaluate their practices and de-adopt practices that are no longer rooted in evidence.
- In an effort to avoid overutilization of resources, critical care providers should be circumspect in adopting the newest technology and/or drug unless it is rooted in high-quality evidence.

REFERENCES

1. Insitute of Medicine. *Crossing the Quality Chasm. A New Health System for the 21st Century.* Washington, DC: National Academy Press; 2001.
2. Admon AJ, Cooke CR. Will Choosing Wisely(R) improve quality and lower costs of care for patients with critical illness? *Ann Am Thorac Soc.* 2014;11(5):823–827.
3. Seymour CW, Iwashyna TJ, Ehlenbach WJ, Wunsch H, Cooke CR. Hospital-level variation in the use of intensive care. *Health Serv Res.* 2012;47(5):2060–2080.
4. Garland A, Shaman Z, Baron J, Connors Jr AF. Physician-attributable differences in intensive care unit costs: a single-center study. *Am J Respir Crit Care Med.* 2006;174(11):1206–1210.
5. Wunsch H, Angus DC, Harrison DA, et al. Variation in critical care services across North America and Western Europe. *Crit Care Med.* 2008;36(10):2787–2793, e2781–2789.
6. Wunsch H, Wagner J, Herlim M, Chong DH, Kramer AA, Halpern SD. ICU occupancy and mechanical ventilator use in the United States. *Crit Care Med.* 2013;41(12):2712–2719.
7. Gabler NB, Ratcliffe SJ, Wagner J, et al. Mortality among patients admitted to strained intensive care units. *Am J Respir Crit Care Med.* 2013;188(7):800–806.
8. Wagner J, Gabler NB, Ratcliffe SJ, Brown SE, Strom BL, Halpern SD. Outcomes among patients discharged from busy intensive care units. *Ann Intern Med.* 2013;159(7):447–455.
9. Chen LM, Render M, Sales A, Kennedy EH, Wiitala W, Hofer TP. Intensive care unit admitting patterns in the Veterans Affairs health care system. *Arch Intern Med.* 2012;172(16):1220–1226.
10. Kahn JM, Goss CH, Heagerty PJ, Kramer AA, O'Brien CR, Rubenfeld GD. Hospital volume and the outcomes of mechanical ventilation. *N Engl J Med.* 2006;355(1):41–50.
11. Gaieski DF, Edwards JM, Kallan MJ, Mikkelsen ME, Goyal M, Carr BG. The Relationship between Hospital Volume and Mortality in Severe Sepsis. *Am J Respir Crit Care Med.* 2014;190(6):665–674.
12. Green LW, Ottoson JM, Garcia C, Hiatt RA. Diffusion theory and knowledge dissemination, utilization, and integration in public health. *Ann Rev Public Health.* 2009;30:151–174.
13. Liu V, Escobar GJ, Greene JD, et al. Hospital deaths in patients with sepsis from 2 independent cohorts. *JAMA.* 2014;312(1):90–92.
14. Herridge MS, Tansey CM, Matte A, et al. Functional disability 5 years after acute respiratory distress syndrome. *N Engl J Med.* 2011;364(14):1293–1304.
15. Ventilation with lower tidal volumes as compared with traditional tidal volumes for acute lung injury and the acute respiratory distress syndrome. The Acute Respiratory Distress Syndrome Network. *N Engl J Med.* 2000;342(18):1301–1308.
16. Umoh NJ, Fan E, Mendez-Tellez PA, et al. Patient and intensive care unit organizational factors associated with low tidal volume ventilation in acute lung injury. *Crit Care Med.* 2008;36(5):1463–1468.
17. Needham DM, Colantuoni E, Mendez-Tellez PA, et al. Lung protective mechanical ventilation and two year survival in patients with acute lung injury: prospective cohort study. *BMJ.* 2012;344:e2124.
18. Girard TD, Kress JP, Fuchs BD, et al. Efficacy and safety of a paired sedation and ventilator weaning protocol for mechanically ventilated patients in intensive care (Awakening and Breathing Controlled trial): a randomised controlled trial. *Lancet.* 2008;371(9607):126–134.
19. Schweickert WD, Pohlman MC, Pohlman AS, et al. Early physical and occupational therapy in mechanically ventilated, critically ill patients: a randomised controlled trial. *Lancet.* 2009;373(9678):1874–1882.
20. Papazian L, Forel JM, Gacouin A, et al. Neuromuscular blockers in early acute respiratory distress syndrome. *N Engl J Med.* 2010;363(12):1107–1116.
21. Guerin C, Reignier J, Richard JC, et al. Prone positioning in severe acute respiratory distress syndrome. *N Engl J Med.* 2013;368(23):2159–2168.
22. Walkey AJ, Wiener RS. Hospital case volume and outcomes among patients hospitalized with severe sepsis. *Am J Respir Crit Care Med.* 2014;189(5):548–555.
23. van Zanten AR, Brinkman S, Arbous MS, et al. Guideline bundles adherence and mortality in severe sepsis and septic shock. *Crit Care Med.* 2014;42(8):1890–1898.
24. Pro CI, Yealy DM, Kellum JA, et al. A randomized trial of protocol-based care for early septic shock. *N Engl J Med.* 2014;370(18):1683–1693.
25. ARISE Investigators, A.C.T. Group, Peake SL, et al. Goal-directed resuscitation for patients with early septic shock. *N Engl J Med.* 2014;371(16):1496–1506.
26. Holst LB, Haase N, Wetterslev J, et al. Lower versus higher hemoglobin threshold for transfusion in septic shock. *N Engl J Med.* 2014;371(15):1381–1391.
27. Kim MM, Barnato AE, Angus DC, Fleisher LA, Kahn JM. The effect of multidisciplinary care teams on intensive care unit mortality. *Arch Intern Med.* 2010;170(4):369–376.
28. Angus DC, Kelley MA, Schmitz RJ, et al. Caring for the critically ill patient. Current and projected workforce requirements for care of the critically ill and patients with pulmonary disease: can we meet the requirements of an aging population? *JAMA.* 2000;284(21):2762–2770.
29. Lawrence AC. Implementations of the Leapfrog Group's ICU physician staffing standard may adversely affect the excellence of graduate medical education. *Crit Care Med.* 2013;41(5):e55.
30. Kerlin MP, Small DS, Cooney E, et al. A randomized trial of nighttime physician staffing in an intensive care unit. *N Engl J Med.* 2013;368(23):2201–2209.
31. Rosen MA, Pronovost PJ. Advancing the use of checklists for evaluating performance in health care. *Acad Med.* 2014;89(7):963–965.
32. Hart J, Halpern SD. Default options in the ICU: widely used but insufficiently understood. *Curr Opin Crit Care.* 2014;20(6):627–662.
33. Lilly CM, McLaughlin JM, Zhao H, et al. A multicenter study of ICU telemedicine reengineering of adult critical care. *Chest.* 2014;145(3):500–507.
34. Curtis JR, Engelberg RA, Bensink ME, Ramsey SD. End-of-life care in the intensive care unit: can we simultaneously increase quality and reduce costs? *Am J Respir Crit Care Med.* 2012;186(7):587–592.
35. Gooch RA, Kahn JM. ICU bed supply, utilization, and health care spending: an example of demand elasticity. *JAMA.* 2014;311(6):567–568.
36. Gershengorn HB, Iwashyna TJ, Cooke CR, Scales DC, Kahn JM, Wunsch H. Variation in use of intensive care for adults with diabetic ketoacidosis. *Crit Care Med.* 2012;40(7):2009–2015.
37. Admon AJ, Seymour CW, Gershengorn HB, Wunsch H, Cooke CR. Hospital-level variation in intensive care unit admission and critical care procedures for patients hospitalized for pulmonary embolism. *Chest.* 2014;146(6):1452–1461.
38. Stelfox HT, Hemmelgarn BR, Bagshaw SM, et al. Intensive care unit bed availability and outcomes for hospitalized patients with sudden clinical deterioration. *Arch Intern Med.* 2012;172(6):467–474.
39. Wagner J, Halpern SD. Deferred admission to the intensive care unit: rationing critical care or expediting care transitions? *Arch Intern Med.* 2012;172(6):474–476.

40. Kox M, Pickkers P. "Less is more" in critically ill patients: not too intensive. *JAMA Intern Med*. 2013;173(14):1369–1372.

41. Halpern SD, Becker D, Curtis JR, et al. An official american thoracic society/american association of critical-care nurses/american college of chest physicians/society of critical care medicine policy statement: the choosing wisely(R) top 5 list in critical care medicine. *Am J Respir Crit Care Med*. 2014;190(7):818–826.

42. Wiener RS, Welch HG. Trends in the use of the pulmonary artery catheter in the United States, 1993-2004. *JAMA*. 2007;298(4):423–429.

43. Rivers E, Nguyen B, Havstad S, et al. Early goal-directed therapy in the treatment of severe sepsis and septic shock. *N Engl J Med*. 2001;345(19):1368–1377.

44. Wiener RS, Wiener DC, Larson RJ. Benefits and risks of tight glucose control in critically ill adults: a meta-analysis. *JAMA*. 2008;300(8):933–944.

45. Harvey SE, Parrott F, Harrison DA, et al. Trial of the route of early nutritional support in critically ill adults. *N Engl J Med*. 2014;371(18):1673–1684.

46. Harhay MO, Wagner J, Ratcliffe SJ, et al. Outcomes and statistical power in adult critical care randomized trials. *Am J Respir Crit Care Med*. 2014;189(12):1469–1478.

47. Sofka CM. Developments and innovations in resident and fellowship education: review article. *HSS J*. 2014;10(3):225–229.

48. Anstey MH, Weinberger SE, Roberts DH. Teaching and practicing cost-awareness in the intensive care unit: a TARGET to aim for. *J Crit Care*. 2014;29(1):107–111.

49. Berwick DM. Donald Berwick, M.D.: connecting finance and quality. *Healthc Financ Manage*. 2008;62(10):52–55.

50. Lindenauer PK, Remus D, Roman S, et al. Public reporting and pay for performance in hospital quality improvement. *N Engl J Med*. 2007;356(5):486–496.

84 Does ICU Admission Improve Outcome?

Andrea Carsetti, Hollmann D. Aya, Maurizio Cecconi, Andrew Rhodes

Critically ill patients require different types of organ support. These include invasive therapies such as orotracheal intubation, mechanical ventilation, inotropic/vasoactive support, invasive monitoring, or continuous renal replacement therapy. This care can usually be implemented only in an intensive care unit (ICU) that has the skills, technology, and human resources to be able to perform them in a safe and effective manner.

WHICH OUTCOMES ARE WE CONSIDERING?

When looking at critical care outcomes, there are two aspects to consider: first, we need to select and measure a suitable outcome, and second, we need to compare the intervention with an appropriate alternative.

In recent years we have witnessed many advances, such as the implementation of protective lung strategies[1] and the initiation of early goal-directed therapy (GDT) in septic[2,3] and surgical patients,[4-8] and now these are our current standards of care. These are processes where the alternative would be providing care without the same protocols/strategy. In other cases such as life-threatening respiratory failure, airway obstruction or profound hypoxia, or renal failure requiring hemofiltration, there is no alternative.

Traditionally, the principal outcome studied in the ICU is mortality (either at the ICU or hospital discharge). However, there are a number of different endpoints that might also be considered.[9,10] These alternatives include longer term mortality and morbidity, neurocognitive dysfunction, impaired mental health, poor functional status, decreased quality of life, decreased return to work and usual activities, burden and stress on families, and economic costs to the patient, the family, and society. Many of these items reflect the entire hospital course, the intensive care management of which is only a small part. Quality of life and functional outcome, such as long-term survival, depend on the effectiveness of the entire health-care system, including convalescent care and rehabilitation in the community.[11] The difficulties in measuring longer term outcomes lead us to believe that short-term benefits may persist later, but this is not always true.

Critical illness carries a substantial mortality. Despite medical advances, patients continue to die. This does not mean that our treatments are ineffective. Indeed, outcomes such as mortality must be benchmarked against national and international standards. For example, the mortality of patients with septic shock may have been reduced significantly in recent years. A 2014 meta-analysis showed that observed mortality decreased from 46.9% during years 1991-1995 to 29% during years 2006-2009 (3.0% annual change).[12]

Outcomes from critical care can be viewed from at least three perspectives: that of patients, that of health-care professionals, and that of health managers.[11]

OUTCOME FOR SPECIFIC TREATMENTS

Mortality is logically an important outcome for patients, but sometimes it may not be the best choice to appropriately assess an intervention. Cardiovascular optimization, for example, requires continuous hemodynamic monitoring, and many studies have demonstrated its efficacy. Some authors have questioned the benefit of pulmonary arterial catheters,[13-16] and several clinicians prefer to use less invasive monitoring systems (e.g., pulse contour analysis) to follow the trend in a number of variables and to assess the response to therapy. It is not the monitoring system, though, that affects outcome, but rather the therapeutic protocol used and the correct interpretation of the data are paramount.

In 2001, Rivers et al.[2] showed that early GDT reduced mortality in patients with severe sepsis or septic shock compared with patients treated with standard therapy (30.5% vs. 46.5%). This study was very original at that point and focused on an aspect of emergency medicine/critical care therapy that greatly affects outcome: the timing of intervention. Previously, sepsis investigators had up to 48 to 72 hours to enroll patients.[17] Rivers and colleagues reached hemodynamic goals in the first 6 hours of patient assessment in the emergency department (ED). Consequently, international guidelines on sepsis management maintain this advice.[18] In 2014, Peake et al.[19] showed that the mortality of septic patients treated without a specific protocol was lower than that observed by Rivers, but this study was conducted in the "post-Rivers age," when clinicians realized that timely treatment is very important. Recently, different resuscitation strategies have been compared, and

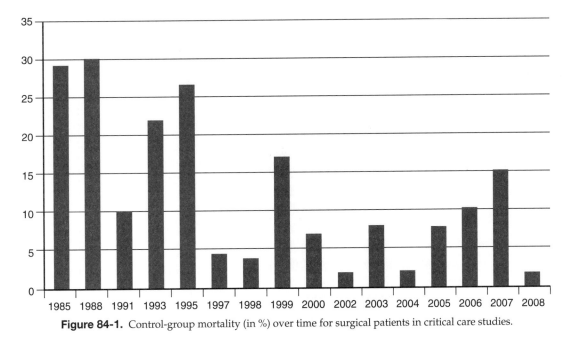

Figure 84-1. Control-group mortality (in %) over time for surgical patients in critical care studies.

Rivers' protocol was not found to be superior to usual care.[20] This difference should be viewed in a context that accounts for the overall improvement in the quality of standard ICU care in the interim. A recent meta-analysis demonstrated that reaching resuscitation goals within the first 6 hours[3] and compliance with a resuscitation bundle were associated with a lower overall mortality (29.3% vs. 38.6%, $P < .01$).[21]

In other cases, mortality can be a very illustrative outcome. In a study of patients with community-acquired pneumonia in the ED, delayed transfer to the ICU was associated with a substantial increase in hospital mortality (odds ratio [OR], 2.07; 95% confidence interval [CI], 1.12 to 3.85).[22] A similar study by Chalfin et al.[23] found that delaying transfer from the ED to the ICU for more than 6 hours increased the risk of hospital death and lengthened hospital stay.

Early GDT may also improve outcome in surgical patients. Three recent meta-analysis revealed that early GDT significantly reduced perioperative complications. A mortality benefit was found, though, only in the highest risk groups, findings that must be tempered by recognition of a mortality reduction in controls, suggesting improvements in the underlying standard care (Fig. 84-1).[5,6,8] The implementation of GDT is clinically effective and cost effective[24]. Manecke et al.[25] estimated a cost savings of $569 to $970 per patient when this strategy was implemented.

In recent years the survival of cardiac surgical patients has benefited from improvements in postoperative care. Stamou et al.[26] showed that implementation of a quality improvement program decreased mortality after cardiac surgery (2.6% vs. 5.0%, $P < .01$). Radbel et al.[27] conducted a 15-year retrospective analysis on mortality in patients with acute respiratory distress syndrome (ARDS). This study identified 174,180 patients from the National Inpatient Sample database between 1996 and 2011 and demonstrated an absolute mortality reduction of 14.6% (from 46.8% to 32.2%) and a relative reduction of 31%. Interestingly,

there was an 8.9% absolute reduction from 2000 to 2005. The authors suggested that the improvements in critical care medicine, such as the introduction of low tidal volume ventilation, contributed to this decline.

IMPACT OF BED AVAILABILITY ON OUTCOME: MANAGERS' OUTLOOK

There is a high variability in the provision of ICU beds among different countries even when corrected for population size. In a 2012 study of bed availability in Europe, Germany (29.2/100,000) had the highest, whereas Portugal had the lowest (4.2/100,000) number of ICU beds (Fig. 84-2).[28] The overall number of critical care beds for Europe was 11.5/100,000. This is in contrast to the number for the United States (28/100,000).[29] Although definitional differences make interpretation of these data problematic, there appears to be a relationship between the availability of beds and the outcome. Wunsch et al. demonstrated that patients admitted to U.S. ICUs had lower APACHE (Acute Physiology and Chronic Health Evaluation) II scores and lower rates of mechanical ventilation than patients admitted to ICUs in the United Kingdom.[30] At any given time, approximately two thirds of ICU beds in the United States are occupied, and approximately one third of the total are for patients requiring mechanical ventilation. These results suggest that the United States has a significant excess of ICU beds.[31]

The number of ICU beds per capita is highly correlated with hospital beds across all countries, excluding the United States.[32] It is logical that the patient population in resource-poor areas is sicker, and therefore poorer outcome is to be expected. Quality of care, however, may not differ. Wunsch et al.[33] compared the organizational characteristics of intensive care in England and the United States and found important differences, especially in end-of-life care. This study also demonstrated that the percentage of patients admitted

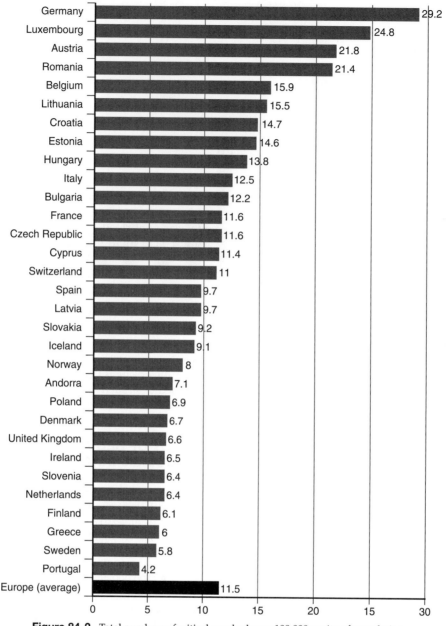

Figure 84-2. Total numbers of critical care beds per 100,000 capita of population.

to ICUs in England is substantially lower (2.2% vs. 19.3%) than in the United States. Furthermore, patients in critical care units account for 10.1% of hospital deaths in the United Kingdom but for 47.1% in the United States. This discrepancy reflects minimal use of ICU resources by elderly patients (1.3% in the United Kingdom vs. 11% in the United States). The two countries, though, have similar rates of intensive care use among children and young adults. The practice of discharging ill and ventilator-dependent patients to skilled nursing care facilities or chronic respiratory units outside of hospitals likely reduces the percentage of deaths that occur in U.S. ICUs. The differences between the largely public health-care system in the United Kingdom and the essentially private system in the United States may also explain the differences found by Wunsch et al.

It is difficult to estimate what constitutes optimal provision of ICU beds in a given population. Recently Wunsch[34] described a "Starling curve" for intensive care, speculating that exceeding a certain limit of beds per capita results in poorer outcome and an increase in health-care spending. Therefore, in countries with lower availability of beds, the triage of patients for ICU admission plays a fundamental role.

IMPACT OF ADMISSION/DISCHARGE CRITERIA ON OUTCOME: HEALTH-CARE PROFESSIONALS' OUTLOOK

Critically ill patients use resources disproportionately. Expense relates to the high costs of staffing ICUs, where

Table 84-1 **Early and Late Effect of ICU Admission on 30-Day Mortality**			
Effect of Department on Mortality	**Category**	**Hazard Ratio**	***P* value**
During early period (0-3 days)	ICU	0.262	.000
	SCU	0.308	.000
	Regular department	1.000	Reference
During late period (4-30 days)	ICU	1.083	.84
	SCU	0.405	.005
	Regular department	1.000	Reference

ICU, intensive care unit; *SCU*, special care unit.

a higher nurse/patient ratio is essential. Thus, ICU admission criteria that identify patients who are truly likely to benefit are a matter of considerable importance.[35] Some national societies have produced guidelines for admission criteria to the ICU.[36,37] These guidelines suggest that the categories of patients who do not take benefit from the ICU are those "too well to benefit" and those "too sick to benefit."

The benefit from ICU admission can best be determined by comparing similar patients admitted or not admitted to the ICU. A number of studies demonstrate that there are times when patients are not admitted to the ICU because beds are not available. Sinuff et al.[38] systematically reviewed 10 studies and found that patients denied admission to an ICU were at considerably higher risk of dying (OR, 3.04; 95% CI, 1.49 to 6.17). A report by Simchen et al.[39] demonstrated poor outcomes in patients meeting ICU admission criteria but managed elsewhere because of bed shortages. In this study, only 27% of eligible patients were admitted to the ICU within 24 hours, when survival benefit was greatest. These findings were confirmed by the same authors years later (Table 84-1).[40]

These studies highlight the potential for long-term ICU survival. Iatrogenic complications, a risk of ICU-acquired infections, and the difficulties inherent in prolonged immobilization may all add to the risks of intensive care, particularly in patients at low risk of death. O'Callaghan et al.[41] presented a contrary picture, though. During a period of 5 years, patients whose ICU admission was delayed by more than 3 hours did not have an increased length of ICU stay, ICU mortality, or hospital mortality rate. Iapichino et al.[42] evaluated triage decisions and outcomes of patients referred for admission to ICU who were either accepted or were refused and treated on the ward. No bed availability was the cause of refusal of ICU admission in 47.1% of cases. ICU admission was associated with lower mortality at 28 (OR, 0.73; *P* < .001) and 90 days (OR, 0.79; *P* < .005).

Postoperative monitoring in a high dependency unit (HDU) may lower the risk of complications. Mathew et al.[43] reported a 6% complication rate among patients admitted to an HDU after maxillofacial surgery. Over the years, the number of patients undergoing major vascular surgery and managed in an HDU postoperatively has increased.[44] Alternatively, postanesthesia care units (PACUs) have been used to manage selected patients after uncomplicated major surgery. Schweizer et al.[45] showed that PACU use was associated with lower ICU admission rates after elective major noncardiac surgery. No negative impact on the quality of care was associated with this different setting of care.

The timing of discharge from the ICU can affect outcome. Schweizer at al. demonstrated a 21.4% mortality rate in patients discharged with a Therapeutic Intervention Scoring System (TISS) of 20, whereas those whose TISS was less than 10 had a rate of only 3.7%.[46] This finding was confirmed by the work of Beck et al.; patients with a TISS more than 30 discharged to hospital wards had a higher risk (1.31; 95% CI, 1.02 to 1.83) of in-hospital death than patients discharged to HDUs.[47] Daly et al.[48] developed a discharge triage model to reduce mortality after discharge, using objective data in a logistic regression equation to identify patients at risk from inappropriate early discharge. Mortality was 14% in at-risk patients but only 1.5% among those not at risk. These investigators also found that post-ICU mortality could be reduced by nearly 39% by an extra 2 days in the ICU. Conversely, late discharge from ICU presents a problematic economic burden. Late discharge also reduces bed availability for other patients.

CONCLUSION

Intensive care can improve patient-related outcomes when applied early in selected and appropriate patients (life-threatening conditions). All the interventions used in the ICU have complications, though, and the risk/benefit balance must be carefully assessed.

AUTHORS' RECOMMENDATIONS

- Traditionally, the principal outcome studied in ICU is mortality (either at ICU or hospital discharge). However, qualitative research in critical care now looks at a variety of measures that affect quality of life, functional outcome, and economic costs.
- Outcomes from critical care can be viewed from at least three perspectives: that of patients, that of health-care professionals, and that of health managers.
- Critical care mortality has decreased over the past two decades, principally because of increased awareness of sepsis and iatrogenic complications. This has been mirrored by improved outcomes in surgical patients (cardiac, vascular, upper gastrointestinal) who use critical care (including intermediate care units).
- There are significantly more ICU beds per capita in the United States compared with other Western countries, with associated higher utilization. This translates to significantly more hospital deaths in the ICU in the United States compared with, for example, the United Kingdom.
- Certain subgroups of patients do not benefit from critical care because they are either too sick or too well to benefit.

- Early versus delayed admission to ICU appears to improve outcomes; early discharge appears to negatively affect outcomes. Delayed ICU discharge has significant economic costs and reduces bed availability to others.
- Intensive care can improve patient-related outcomes when applied early in selected and appropriate patients (e.g., those with life-threatening conditions). However, all the interventions used in the ICU have complications, and the risks/benefit balance needs to be carefully assessed.

REFERENCES

1. Ventilation with lower tidal volumes as compared with traditional tidal volumes for acute lung injury and the acute respiratory distress syndrome. The Acute Respiratory Distress Syndrome Network. *N Engl J Med.* 2000;342(18):1301–1308.
2. Rivers E, Nguyen B, Havstad S, et al. TMEG-DTCG. Early goal-directed therapy in the treatment of severe sepsis and septic shock. *N Engl J Med.* 2001;345(19):1368–1377.
3. Gu WJ, Wang F, Bakker J, Tang L, Liu JC. The effect of goal-directed therapy on mortality in patients with sepsis-earlier is better: a meta-analysis of randomized controlled trials. *Crit Care.* 2014;18(5):570.
4. Donati A, Loggi S, Preiser JC, et al. Goal-directed intraoperative therapy reduces morbidity and length of hospital stay in high-risk surgical patients. *Chest.* 2007;132(6):1817–1824.
5. Hamilton M, Cecconi M, Rhodes A. A systematic review and meta-analysis on the use of preemptive hemodynamic intervention to improve postoperative outcomes in moderate and high-risk surgical patients. *Anesth Analg.* 2011;112(6):1392–1402.
6. Cecconi M, Corredor C, Arulkumaran N, et al. Clinical review: Goal-directed therapy-what is the evidence in surgical patients? The effect on different risk groups. *Crit Care.* 2013;17(2):209.
7. Salzwedel C, Puig J, Carstens A, et al. Perioperative goal-directed hemodynamic therapy based on radial arterial pulse pressure variation and continuous cardiac index trending reduces postoperative complications after major abdominal surgery: a multicenter, prospective, randomized study. *Crit Care.* 2013;17(5):R191.
8. Benes J, Giglio M, Brienza N, Michard F. The effects of goal directed fluid therapy based on dynamic parameters on post-surgical outcome: a meta-analysis of randomized controlled trials. *Crit Care.* 2014;18(5):584.
9. Angus DC, Carlet J. Surviving intensive care: a report from the 2002 Brussels Roundtable. *Intensive Care Med.* 2003;29(3):368–377.
10. Modrykamien AM. The ICU follow-up clinic: a new paradigm for intensivists. *Respir Care.* 2012;57(5):764–772.
11. Ridley S. Critical care outcomes. *Anaesthesia.* 2001;56:1–3.
12. Stevenson EK, Rubenstein AR, Radin GT, Wiener RS, Walkey AJ. Two decades of mortality trends among patients with severe sepsis: a comparative meta-analysis. *Crit Care Med.* 2014;42(3):625–631.
13. Hadian M, Pinsky MR. Evidence-based review of the use of the pulmonary artery catheter: impact data and complications. *Crit Care.* 2006;10(suppl 3):S8.
14. National Heart, Lung, and Blood Institute Acute Respiratory Distress Syndrome (ARDS) Clinical Trials Network, Wheeler AP, Bernard GR, Thompson BT, et al. Pulmonary-artery versus central venous catheter to guide treatment of acute lung injury. *N Engl J Med.* 2006;354(21):2213–2224.
15. Sandham JD, Hull RD, Brant RF, et al. A randomized, controlled trial of the use of pulmonary-artery catheters in high-risk surgical patients. *N Engl J Med.* 2003;348(1):5–14.
16. Rhodes A, Cusack RJ, Newman PJ, Grounds RM, Bennett ED. A randomised, controlled trial of the pulmonary artery catheter in critically ill patients. *Intensive Care Med.* 2002;28(3):256–264.
17. Gattinoni L, Brazzi L, Pelosi P, Latini R, Tognoni G, Pesenti A. A trial of goal-oriented hemodynamic therapy in critically ill patients. SvO2 Collaborative Group. *N Engl J Med.* 1995;333(16):1025–1032.
18. Dellinger RP, Levy MM, Rhodes A, et al. Surviving sepsis campaign: international guidelines for management of severe sepsis and septic shock: 2012. *Crit Care Med.* 2013;41(2):580–637.
19. ARISE Investigators; ANZICS Clinical Trials Group, Peake SL, Delaney A, Bailey M, et al. Goal-directed resuscitation for patients with early septic shock. *N Engl J Med.* 2014;371(16):1496–1506.
20. Yealy DM, Kellum J, Huang DT, et al. A randomized trial of protocol-based care for early septic shock. *N Engl J Med.* 2014;370(18):1683–1693.
21. Levy MM, Rhodes A, Phillips GS, et al. Surviving Sepsis Campaign: association between performance metrics and outcomes in a 7.5-year study. *Crit Care Med.* 2015;43(1):3–12.
22. Renaud B, Santin A, Coma E, et al. Association between timing of intensive care unit admission and outcomes for emergency department patients with community-acquired pneumonia. *Crit Care Med.* 2009;37(11):2867–2874.
23. Chalfin DB, Trzeciak S, Likourezos A, Baumann BM, Dellinger RP. Impact of delayed transfer of critically ill patients from the emergency department to the intensive care unit. *Crit Care Med.* 2007;35(6):1477–1483.
24. Ebm C, Cecconi M, Sutton L, Rhodes A. A cost-effectiveness analysis of postoperative goal-directed therapy for high-risk surgical patients. *Crit Care Med.* 2014;42(5):1194–1203.
25. Manecke GR, Asemota A, Michard F. Tackling the economic burden of postsurgical complications: would perioperative goal-directed fluid therapy help? *Crit Care.* 2014;18(5):566.
26. Stamou SC, Camp SL, Stiegel RM, et al. Quality improvement program decreases mortality after cardiac surgery. *J Thorac Cardiovasc Surg.* 2008;136(2):494–499.
27. Radbel J, Mehta K, Shah N, Soni R, Singh J. The Sharp Decline in ARDS Mortality: Analysis of 856,293 National Inpatient Sample Admissions. *Chest.* 2014;146:210A. 4_MeetingAbstracts.
28. Rhodes A, Ferdinande P, Flaatten H, Guidet B, Metnitz PG, Moreno RP. The variability of critical care bed numbers in Europe. *Intensive Care Med.* 2012;38(10):1647–1653.
29. Carr BG, Addyson DKKJ. Variation in critical care beds per capita in the United States: implications for pandemic and disaster planning. *JAMA.* 2013;303(14):1371–1372.
30. Wunsch H, Angus DC, Harrison D, Linde-Zwirble WT, Rowan KM. Comparison of medical admissions to intensive care units in the United States and United Kingdom. *Am J Respir Crit Care Med.* 2011;183(12):1666–1673.
31. Wunsch H, Wagner J, Herlim M, Chong DH, Kramer A, Halpern SD. ICU occupancy and mechanical ventilator use in the United States. *Crit Care Med.* 2013;41(12):2712–2719.
32. Wunsch H, Angus DC, Harrison D, et al. Variation in critical care services across North America and Western Europe. *Crit Care Med.* 2008;36(10):2787–2793.
33. Wunsch H, Linde-Zwirble WT, Harrison D, Barnato AE, Rowan KM, Angus DC. Use of intensive care services during terminal hospitalizations in England and the United States. *Am J Respir Crit Care Med.* 2009;180(9):875–880.
34. Wunsch H. Is there a Starling curve for intensive care? *Chest.* 2012;141(6):1393–1399.
35. Capuzzo M, Moreno RP, Alvisi R. Admission and discharge of critically ill patients. *Curr Opin Crit Care.* 2010;16(5):499–504.
36. Guidelines for intensive care unit admission, discharge, and triage. Task Force of the American College of Critical Care Medicine, Society of Critical Care Medicine. *Crit Care Med.* 1999;27:633–638.
37. SIAARTI guidelines for admission to and discharge from Intensive Care Units and for the limitation of treatment in intensive care. *Minerva Anestesiol.* 2003;69(3):101–118.
38. Sinuff T, Kahnamoui K, Cook DJ, Luce JM, Levy MM. Rationing critical care beds: a systematic review. *Crit Care Med.* 2004;32(7):1588–1597.
39. Simchen E, Sprung CL, Galai N, et al. Survival of critically ill patients hospitalized in and out of intensive care units under paucity of intensive care unit beds. *Crit Care Med.* 2004;32(8):1654–1661.
40. Simchen E, Sprung CL, Galai N, et al. Survival of critically ill patients hospitalized in and out of intensive care. *Crit Care Med.* 2007;35(2):449–457.
41. O'Callaghan DJP, Jayia P, Vaughan-Huxley E, et al. An observational study to determine the effect of delayed admission to the intensive care unit on patient outcome. *Crit Care.* 2012;16(5):R173.

42. Iapichino G, Corbella D, Minelli C, et al. Reasons for refusal of admission to intensive care and impact on mortality. *Intensive Care Med.* 2010;36(10):1772–1779.

43. Mathew SA, Senthilnathan P, Narayanan V. Management of post-operative maxillofacial oncology patients without the routine use of an intensive care unit. *J Maxillofac Oral Surg.* 2010;9(4):329–333.

44. Teli M, Morris-Stiff G, Rees JR, Woodsford PV, Lewis MH. Vascular surgery, ICU and HDU: a 14-year observational study. *Ann R Coll Surg Engl.* 2008;90(4):291–296.

45. Schweizer A, Khatchatourian G, Ho L, Romand J, Licker M. Opening of a new postanesthesia care unit : impact on critical care utilization and complications following major vascular and thoracic surgery. *J Clin Anesth.* 2002;8180(02):486–493.

46. Smith L, Orts CM, O'Neil I, Batchelor AM, Gascoigne ADBS. TISS and mortality after discharge from intensive care. *Intensive Care Med.* 1999;25(10):1061–1065.

47. Beck DH, McQuillan P, Smith GB. Waiting for the break of dawn? The effects of discharge time, discharge TISS scores and discharge facility on hospital mortality after intensive care. *Intensive Care Med.* 2002;28(9):1287–1293.

48. Daly K, Beale R, Chang RWS. Reduction in mortality after inappropriate early discharge. *BMJ.* May 2001;322:1–5.

85 How Should Care Within an Intensive Care Unit or an Institution Be Organized?

Ho Geol Ryu, Todd Dorman

In this chapter, we review the evidence for the association between intensive care unit (ICU) organization and optimal care delivery. In addition, we review the evidence for ICU organization within a hospital and across a health system. We recognize up front that only a few issues regarding organization of care have strong evidence based on high-quality publications. We remind the reader, though, that evidence-based medicine also allows for the consideration of lower levels of evidence, such as experience and observational data. Various models of critical care delivery (ICU level and institution level) have been tested regarding the structure and process of ICU care, including the personnel responsible for providing care and their associated workload. This chapter addresses all organization-related practices at the ICU through the health system level and will attempt to be clear where the evidence is the strongest and where the evidence is more observational.

HIGH-INTENSITY PHYSICIAN STAFFING

In a 2002 systematic review, Pronovost and colleagues demonstrated that high-intensity physician staffing was associated with reduced ICU and hospital length of stay and lower ICU mortality (relative risk [RR], 0.61; 95% confidence interval [CI], 0.50 to 0.75) and hospital mortality (RR, 0.71; 95% CI, 0.62 to 0.82).[1] Since then, many studies have confirmed these findings or uncovered additional benefits of high-intensity physician staffing in the ICUs of different types in various settings.[2,3] As a result, the high-intensity approach is considered to be the staffing model of choice in most ICU settings. It is now being applied worldwide and in atypical settings. Institution of high-intensity physician staffing in an Army hospital ICU deployed in Afghanistan was associated with decreases in mortality, the duration of mechanical ventilation, and the incidence of ventilator-associated pneumonia.[4] Likewise, high-intensity physician staffing in a mixed ICU serving a regional nonteaching medical center was associated with a decrease in hospital length of stay, better compliance with evidence-based practices, and a significant increase in survival from sepsis.[5] However, Levy et al. performed a retrospective analysis of 101,832 ICU patients entered into the Surviving Sepsis Campaign database and compared outcomes in ICUs where critical care physicians provided more than 95% of the care with those in ICUs where intensivists managed less than 5% of patients.[6] Even when data were adjusted for severity of illness and patients were matched with propensity scores, intensivist-led care was associated with a higher standardized mortality ratio (RR, 1.09; 95% CI, 1.05 to 1.13 vs. RR, 0.91; 5% CI, 0.88 to 0.94) and resulted in more interventions. These results stand in stark contrast to numerous investigations and reports that showed an association between high-intensity physician staffing and outcome in ICUs of all types. Although the authors acknowledge the study's significant limitations (unclear definition of "critical care physician," significant gaps in the dataset, unmeasured confounders), the large number of patients and the magnitude of the dataset cannot be ignored. Since the publication of the report by Levy and colleagues, a retrospective cohort study of medical ICU patients (n = 107,324) that compared high-intensity physician staffing and multidisciplinary care teams with low-intensity physician staffing without multidisciplinary care teams reported that the former was associated with lower 30-day mortality (odds ratio [OR], 0.78; 95% CI, 0.68 to 0.89).[7] In addition, a recent meta-analysis that included the study described previously[6] indicated that high-intensity physician staffing was associated with lower ICU (RR, 0.81; 95% CI, 0.68 to 0.96) and hospital mortality (RR, 0.83; 95% CI, 0.70 to 0.99).[8] These results also suggested that surgical and combined medicosurgical ICUs received most of the benefits of high-intensity physician staffing.

Despite the overwhelming body of literature (>30 studies) touting the superiority of high-intensity physician staffing, the processes that link this approach to improved outcomes remain obscure. It seems reasonable to postulate that consistent and reliable delivery of care using evidence-based standardized protocols by experienced and trained personnel contributed. Indeed, daily rounds by a multidisciplinary team were associated with a reduction in adjusted mortality,[7,9] and high-intensity physician staffing was associated with increased compliance with evidence-based practices.[5] It has been suggested that other aspects of care delivery, such as interprofessional communication, are positively altered by high-intensity staffing, but supporting data are lacking.

NIGHTTIME INTENSIVIST STAFFING

In an effort to further improve patient care in the ICU, some institutions have attempted to move beyond the Leapfrog standards[10] and toward 24/7 intensivist coverage or nighttime intensivist coverage. A survey of ICU program directors at academic medical centers in the United States indicated that one third (37%) of the respondents' ICUs were covered 24/7 by board-certified or board-eligible in-house intensivists. More than half of the respondents thought that 24/7 coverage is associated with better patient care and improved education for training fellows, although they did raise concerns about reductions in autonomy and the opportunity to make independent decisions.[11]

The assumption underlying the move to 24/7 staffing is that the intensity of physician staffing ("dose") will improve patient outcomes ("response"). It is essential that this dose–response relationship remains sufficiently positive so that the benefit is worth the additional cost. A randomized trial in an academic ICU running under a high-intensity physician staffing model compared the addition of nighttime in-hospital intensivists with a model in which the nighttime intensivist (often the same one who covered in house during the day) provided coverage via telephone.[12] The study did not demonstrate a difference in any of the selected outcome variables—ICU or hospital length of stay, mortality (OR, 1.08, $P = .78$), or readmission within 48 hours. A retrospective cohort study showed that adding a nighttime intensivist to an ICU using a low-intensity physician staffing model during the day resulted in a reduction in mortality (OR, 0.62, $P = .04$).[13] Thus the current evidence is not sufficient to justify 24/7 intensivist coverage in ICUs with daytime high-intensity physician staffing. One could argue that the retrospective arm of the previous study indicates that nighttime coverage may be of benefit in ICUs operating under a low-intensity daytime model. In addition, there are other reported benefits associated with 24/7 intensivist coverage (e.g., earlier decision making regarding end-of-life care,[14] improvement in the quality of end-of-life care[14,15]) that have not been subjected to evidence-based investigation.

COPING WITH SHORTAGE OF INTENSIVISTS

The demand for intensivists has been increasing and is projected to continue to do so. There is an ongoing shortage of intensivists, though, that has been foreseen for some time.[16,17] The projected shortages have engendered strategies to provide enhanced coverage without a need for additional personnel. Models under evaluation include telemedicine for remote or underserved ICUs and deployment of alternative providers—nonintensivist physicians (hospitalists) or nonphysicians (nurse practitioners, physician assistants).

INTENSIVE CARE UNIT TELEMEDICINE

The initial report by Rosenfeld and colleagues that showed a significant reduction in mortality, length of stay, and costs[18] demonstrated that ICU telemedicine is a potential solution to ICU workforce shortages. Several publications have addressed the issue. A systematic review and meta-analysis using a preobservational and postobservational study design showed that telemedicine was associated with lower ICU (RR, 0.79; 95% CI, 0.65 to 0.96) and hospital mortality (RR, 0.83; 95% CI, 0.73 to 0.94) as well as a significant decrease in ICU and hospital length of stay when compared with standard care.[19] However, a more recent study that evaluated ICU telemedicine using a pre- and postcomparison and a concurrent control ICU in a network of Veterans Affairs hospitals failed to show any improvement in ICU, hospital, or 30-day mortality or in ICU or hospital length of stay.[20] A similar nonrandomized, unblended, preassessment and postassessment of ICUs involving 118,990 patients in 56 U.S. ICUs showed that ICU telemedicine was associated with lower adjusted ICU and hospital mortality, as well as a reduction in ICU and hospital length of stay that was particularly pronounced in patients with very long ICU courses.[21] ICU telemedicine was also associated with higher adherence to clinical practice guidelines.[22]

As is often the case in medicine, the clinical benefit to patients managed with ICU telemedicine is not a product of the technology alone. In an observational, before-and-after comparison of ICU telemedicine use in six ICUs within a single health-care system, ICU telemedicine was not associated with any discernible benefit.[23] Proposed explanations, including minimal delegation to the telemedicine team, a lack of access to clinical notes, and computerized physician order entry, suggest that the degree of integration of the telemedicine team into the ICU is an important determinant of efficacy. The presence of an ICU culture dedicated to outcome improvement and the impact leadership models have also been touted, but they have not been sufficiently investigated.

Although ICU telemedicine may provide clinical benefits, it is an expensive undertaking that mandates careful financial consideration.[24] Capital expenditures and maintenance costs for ICU telemedicine are not trivial, and to date the care in the United States is not subject to direct reimbursement. Thus, use of ICU telemedicine will expand only if enhanced ICU use can offset the cost[25] or if changes in health-care delivery and reimbursement (i.e., bundled payments) translate into an enhanced margin.

COPING WITH SHORTAGE OF INTENSIVISTS WITH NONINTENSIVISTS: HOSPITALISTS AS INTENSIVE CARE UNIT WORKFORCE

Hospitalists have a primary focus on the general medical care of hospitalized patients. They have increasingly been asked to care for patients with a lower severity of illness in the ICU and in step-down units. A single small, prospective, observational study found no significant differences in ICU or hospital mortality or length of stay between medical ICU patients cared for by a hospitalist team and those cared for by an intensivist-led team.[26]

CAREGIVER WORKLOAD OF CAREGIVERS IN THE INTENSIVE CARE UNIT

Although the concept seems intuitively obvious, only limited and controversial data support the suggestion that patient outcome is negatively affected by an increase in the workload or census in the ICU. In a retrospective study examining the records of more than 200,000 ICU patients, Dara and Afessa were unable to identify an association between the ICU census and patient mortality.[32] Likewise, a retrospective cohort study in a medical ICU of a tertiary hospital compared patient outcomes when the intensivist-to-patient ratio was 1:7.5 with those observed when the ratio was 1:15. Hospital and ICU mortality was similar, whereas a ratio of 1:15 was associated with a relatively increased ICU length of stay.[33] Appropriately, the report prepared by the Society of Critical Care Medicine's Task Force on ICU staffing declined to recommend a limit on the number of ICU patients that an individual intensivist should care for, suggesting instead that common sense be used.[34]

Studies on the contribution of critical care nurses to patient outcome provide a more consistent picture. A study conducted in the United Kingdom reported that a heavy nursing workload was associated with a twofold increase in adjusted mortality.[35] In addition, in a cross-sectional analysis of more than 55,000 patients in more than 300 hospitals in the United States, Kelly et al. found an association between outcomes in elderly mechanically ventilated patients and both more nurturing critical care nurse environments and the presence of nurses with a higher level of education.[36]

Adverse drug events are common in the ICU, likely reflecting the severity of illness and the large number of drugs used per patient.[37] Participation of pharmacists on ICU rounds was associated with a decreased rate of adverse drug events.[38] It has been proposed that respiratory therapists contributed to improved outcomes by standardizing care and contributing to the consistent application of evidence-based principles and by reducing the workload of other team members.[39] Physical therapists may contribute to improved clinical outcome through redistribution of workload, especially when rehabilitation is started early.[40] Palliative care providers may also affect hospital and ICU length of stay while maintaining family satisfaction.[41]

ORGANIZATION OF INTENSIVE CARE UNIT CARE: INSTITUTIONAL AND HEALTH SYSTEM LEVELS

The impact of ICU organizational structures on care at either the institutional or health system level has been subject to significant evidence-based investigation. Consequently, this aspect of care remains fertile ground for study.

The most common institutional model is a distributed system of independent ICUs, in which each ICU is managed by a different group or department. Indeed, different groups or departments manage different beds within a single ICU. It is likely that standardization and protocols are very difficult if not impossible to achieve under these circumstances. An arrangement of this sort, though, might enhance specialty practice and thus achieve high-level outcomes, especially at the interprofessional level. Concerns about institutional objectives and improved service delivery have led to the creation of critical care committees with representation across the different ICUs. This approach might also facilitate bed-sharing arrangements between

ICUs to maximize specialty care while still addressing institutional objectives regarding efficient bed use.

There are several critical care centers in the United States. These typically attempt to bind units across the institution in a formal construct and are clearly aimed at maximizing interprofessional care and outcomes while leveraging efficiency. In some organizations, this approach has resulted in formation of a department of critical care medicine. The impact of these approaches on providers, teams, and patients in such models remains unknown. There are even fewer data addressing organizational characteristics across a health system. At present, system-wide integration reflects the organization within the component hospitals. There are several health systems that have successfully integrated ICUs within an institution and are attempting to extend this model across the health system via a center or a department. Some systems are using telemedicine to more broadly leverage knowledge and experience.

AUTHORS' RECOMMENDATIONS

- High-intensity physician staffing has consistently been shown to significantly improve mortality and ICU and hospital length of stay over a wide range of conditions; however, these studies to date have failed to demonstrate the value of expanding the high-intensity staffing to 24/7 coverage.
- Hospitalists and nonphysician providers seem to be comparable to each other as alternatives to intensivists and house staff in ICUs caring for lower acuity patients.
- Telemedicine seems to be an attractive alternative model for care delivery. However, cost considerations may limit its utility.
- Integration of ICU services across a health system has been insufficiently studied, but it may be the next step for further improving delivery of critical care.

REFERENCES

1. Pronovost PJ, Angus DC, Dorman T, et al. Physician staffing patterns and clinical outcomes in critically ill patients: a systematic review. *JAMA*. 2002;288(17):2151–2162.
2. O'Malley RG, Olenchock B, Bohula-May E, et al. Organization and staffing practices in US cardiac intensive care units: a survey on behalf of the American Heart Association Writing Group on the Evolution of Critical Care Cardiology. *Eur Heart J Acute Cardiovasc Care*. 2013;2(1):3–8.
3. Suarez JI, Zaidat OO, Suri MF, et al. Length of stay and mortality in neurocritically ill patients: impact of a specialized neurocritical care team. *Crit Care Med*. 2004;32(11):2311–2317.
4. Lettieri CJ, Shah AA, Greenburg DL. An intensivist-directed intensive care unit improves clinical outcomes in a combat zone. *Crit Care Med*. 2009;37(4):1256–1260.
5. Iyegha UP, Asghar JI, Habermann EB, et al. Intensivists improve outcomes and compliance with process measures in critically ill patients. *J Am Coll Surg*. 2013;216(3):363–372.
6. Levy MM, Rapoport J, Lemeshow S, et al. Association between critical care physician management and patient mortality in the intensive care unit. *Ann Intern Med*. 2008;148(11):801–809.
7. Kim MM, Barnato AE, Angus DC, et al. The effect of multidisciplinary care teams on intensive care unit mortality. *Arch Intern Med*. 2010;170(4):369–376.
8. Wilcox ME, Chong CA, Niven DJ, et al. Do intensivist staffing patterns influence hospital mortality following ICU admission? A systematic review and meta-analyses. *Crit Care Med*. 2013;41(10):2253–2274.

9. Checkley W, Martin GS, Brown SM, et al. Structure, process, and annual ICU mortality across 69 centers: United States Critical Illness and Injury Trials Group Critical Illness Outcomes Study. *Crit Care Med*. 2014;42(2):344–356.

10. Pronovost PJ, Needham DM, Waters H, et al. Intensive care unit physician staffing: financial modeling of the Leapfrog standard. *Crit Care Med*. 2006;34(suppl 3):S18–S24.

11. Diaz-Guzman E, Colbert CY, Mannino DM, et al. 24/7 in-house intensivist coverage and fellowship education: a cross-sectional survey of academic medical centers in the United States. *Chest*. 2012;141(4):959–966.

12. Kerlin MP, Small DS, Cooney E, et al. A randomized trial of nighttime physician staffing in an intensive care unit. *N Engl J Med*. 2013;368(23):2201–2209.

13. Wallace DJ, Angus DC, Barnato AE, et al. Nighttime intensivist staffing and mortality among critically ill patients. *N Engl J Med*. 2012;366(22):2093–2101.

14. Reineck LA, Wallace DJ, Barnato AE, et al. Nighttime intensivist staffing and the timing of death among ICU decedents: a retrospective cohort study. *Crit Care*. 2013;17(5):R216.

15. Wilson ME, Samirat R, Yilmaz M, et al. Physician staffing models impact the timing of decisions to limit life support in the ICU. *Chest*. 2013;143(3):656–663.

16. Halpern NA, Pastores SM, Oropello JM, et al. Critical care medicine in the United States: addressing the intensivist shortage and image of the specialty. *Crit Care Med*. 2013;41(12):2754–2761.

17. Angus DC, Kelley MA, Schmitz RJ, et al. Caring for the critically ill patient. Current and projected workforce requirements for care of the critically ill and patients with pulmonary disease: can we meet the requirements of an aging population? *JAMA*. 2000;284(21):2762–2770.

18. Rosenfeld BA, Dorman T, Breslow MJ, et al. Intensive care unit telemedicine: alternate paradigm for providing continuous intensivist care. *Crit Care Med*. 2000;28(12):3925–3931.

19. Wilcox ME, Adhikari NK. The effect of telemedicine in critically ill patients: systematic review and meta-analysis. *Crit Care*. 2012;16(4):R127.

20. Nassar BS, Vaughan-Sarrazin MS, Jiang L, et al. Impact of an intensive care unit telemedicine program on patient outcomes in an integrated health care system. *JAMA Intern Med*. 2014;174(7):1160–1167.

21. Lilly CM, McLaughlin JM, Zhao H, et al. A multicenter study of ICU telemedicine reengineering of adult critical care. *Chest*. 2014;145(3):500–507.

22. Lilly CM, Cody S, Zhao H, et al. Hospital mortality, length of stay, and preventable complications among critically ill patients before and after tele-ICU reengineering of critical care processes. *JAMA*. 2011;305(21):2175–2183.

23. Thomas EJ, Lucke JF, Wueste L, et al. Association of telemedicine for remote monitoring of intensive care patients with mortality, complications, and length of stay. *JAMA*. 2009;302(24):2671–2678.

24. Kruklitis RJ, Tracy JA, McCambridge MM. Clinical and financial considerations for implementing an ICU telemedicine program. *Chest*. 2014;145(6):1392–1396.

25. Breslow MJ, Rosenfeld BA, Doerfler M, et al. Effect of a multiple-site intensive care unit telemedicine program on clinical and economic outcomes: an alternative paradigm for intensivist staffing. *Crit Care Med*. 2004;32(1):31–38.

26. Wise KR, Akopov VA, Williams Jr BR, et al. Hospitalists and intensivists in the medical ICU: a prospective observational study comparing mortality and length of stay between two staffing models. *J Hosp Med*. 2012;7(3):183–189.

27. Deleted in review.

28. Deleted in review.

29. Deleted in review.

30. Deleted in review.

31. Deleted in review.

32. Iwashyna TJ, Kramer AA, Kahn JM. Intensive care unit occupancy and patient outcomes. *Crit Care Med*. 2009;37(5):1545–1557.

33. Dara SI, Afessa B. Intensivist-to-bed ratio: association with outcomes in the medical ICU. *Chest*. 2005;128(2):567–572.

34. Ward NS, Afessa B, Kleinpell R, et al. Intensivist/patient ratios in closed ICUs: a statement from the Society of Critical Care Medicine Taskforce on ICU Staffing. *Crit Care Med*. 2013;41(2):638–645.

35. Tarnow-Mordi WO, Hau C, Warden A, et al. Hospital mortality in relation to staff workload: a 4-year study in an adult intensive-care unit. *Lancet*. 2000;356(9225):185–189.

36. Kelly DM, Kutney-Lee A, McHugh MD, et al. Impact of critical care nursing on 30-day mortality of mechanically ventilated older adults. *Crit Care Med*. 2014;42(5):1089–1095.

37. Cullen DJ, Sweitzer BJ, Bates DW, et al. Preventable adverse drug events in hospitalized patients: a comparative study of intensive care and general care units. *Crit Care Med*. 1997;25(8):1289–1297.

38. Leape LL, Cullen DJ, Clapp MD, et al. Pharmacist participation on physician rounds and adverse drug events in the intensive care unit. *JAMA*. 1999;282(3):267–270.

39. Durbin Jr CG. Therapist-driven protocols in adult intensive care unit patients. *Respir Care Clin N Am*. 1996;2(1):105–116.

40. Schweickert WD, Pohlman MC, Pohlman AS, et al. Early physical and occupational therapy in mechanically ventilated, critically ill patients: a randomised controlled trial. *Lancet*. 2009;373(9678):1874–1882.

41. Aslakson R, Cheng J, Vollenweider D, et al. Evidence-based palliative care in the intensive care unit: a systematic review of interventions. *J Palliat Med*. 2014;17(2):219–235.

86 What Is the Role of Advanced Practice Nurses and Physician Assistants in the ICU?

Ruth Kleinpell, W. Robert Grabenkort

At present, the U.S. population uses 23.2 million intensive care unit (ICU) days at an estimated cost of $81.7 billion each year.[1] This equates to 13.4% of hospital costs and 4.1% of the national health expenditure.[1] It has been suggested that $3.3 million in annual cost savings could be realized for each 12- to 18-bed ICU if care were delivered by intensivist-led teams. Currently, though, less than 40% of all ICU patients are treated with this model.[1] The Association of American Medical Colleges expects a shortage of more than120,000 physicians by the end of this decade.[2] A deficit of this magnitude is likely to threaten access to care, including ICU care.

One strategy for meeting ICU workforce needs is the addition of advanced practice professionals to ICU teams.[3,4] Advanced practice providers, including nurse practitioners (NPs) and physician assistants (PAs), are an increasingly important component of the nation's health-care workforce. More than 250,000 (>180,000 NPs and >85,000 PAs) practice in the U.S. health-care system.[5,6] Consistent with the Institute of Medicine's report,[7] NPs and PAs play a vital role in delivering patient care, promoting multiprofessional collaboration, and advancing team approaches to care. These clinicians provide primary, acute, and specialty care services to patients in countless acute and nonacute care settings.

NURSE PRACTITIONER AND PHYSICIAN ASSISTANT ROLES

NPs are registered nurses who are prepared at either the master's or doctoral level, have an independent license, and are required to pass a national certification examination in most states to practice. NPs practice autonomously in most states with a scope of practice that is dependent on education, licensure, accreditation, and certification. To be in compliance with the National Council of State Boards of Nursing's recommendations for the Advanced Practice Registered Nurse Consensus Model for practice in the ICU setting, NPs should be certified in either acute care or adult gerontology acute care.[8] Similarly, PAs are health-care professionals who are certified by a national examination

process. Most PAs are prepared at the graduate level, but some have bachelor's degrees.[6] PAs are licensed health-care professionals who practice under the supervision of a responsible physician who must be available for consultation by phone or in person.[6]

NPs and PAs often have similar roles in the ICU, but in some settings differences exist. PAs focus on direct medical management or surgical assistance, whereas NP care encompasses direct patient care in addition to continuity of care components such as discharge planning; nursing, patient, and family education; and quality improvement/research, among other subroles (Table 86-1).[9-11]

USE OF NURSE PRACTITIONERS AND PHYSICIAN ASSISTANTS IN THE ICU

Data from national surveys on the use of NPs and PAs indicates that utilization in hospital settings has increased because of the higher acuity of hospitalized patients, restrictions placed on medical resident work hours, the need for continuity of care, and workforce shortages.[12] In university-based hospital settings where the new Accreditation Council for Graduate Medical Education duty-hour regulations for physicians in training have been implemented, the integration of NPs and PAs into multidisciplinary provider models represents a solution to the gap in coverage.[12] A study of 25 academic medical centers indicated that an additional role for NP and PA care has resulted from the need for improved access, improved continuity of care, patient throughput, and medical resident training restrictions, among others (Fig. 86-1).[12] Role components of NPs and PAs in the ICU are detailed in Table 86-2.[14]

Several studies have linked improved quality and reduced costs to the participation of NPs and PAs in care (Table 86-3). Because ICU care is often team based, assessing the impact of NPs and PAs in the ICU can be difficult. Several studies, though, have demonstrated that NP- and PA-provided care resulted in improved outcomes (Table 86-4).[15-27]

On the basis of reports of established and developing models of care with NPs and PAs and research demonstrating

Table 86-1 **NP and PA Role Comparisons**

Category	PA	NP
Definition	Health-care professionals licensed to practice medical care with physician supervision.	Registered nurses with advanced education and training who have independent license.
Philosophy/model	Medical/physician model, disease centered, with emphasis on the biological/pathologic aspects of health, assessment, diagnosis, treatment. Practice model is a team approach relationship with physicians.	Medical/nursing model, biopsychosocial centered, with emphasis on disease adaptation, health promotion, wellness, and prevention. Practice model is a collaborative relationship with physicians.
Education	Affiliated with *medical schools*. Previous health-care experience required; most require entry-level bachelor's degree. The program curriculum is advanced science based. Approximately 2000 clinical hours. All PAs are trained as generalists (a primary care model), and some receive postgraduate specialty training. Education is procedure and skill oriented with emphasis on diagnosis, treatment, surgical skills, and patient education. Currently, more than 50% of programs award master's degrees and all are currently transitioning to the master's level.	Affiliated with *nursing schools*. BSN is prerequisite and education is at master's or doctoral level; curriculum is biopsychosocial based, based on behavioral, natural, and humanistic sciences. Approximately 750 to 1000 clinical hours. NPs choose a specialty training track in adult, acute care, pediatric, women's health, or gerontology.
Certification/licensure	Separate accreditation and certification bodies require successful completion of an accredited program and NCCPA national certification exam.	National certification is required in majority of states.
Recertification	Recertification requires 100 hr of CME every 2 years and exam every 10 years. All PAs are licensed by their State Medical Board and the Medical Practice Act provisions.	Recertification requires, on average, 75 CEUs every 5-6 years. NPs are licensed by their State Board of Nursing.
Scope of practice	The supervising physician has relatively broad discretion in delegating medical tasks within his/her scope of practice to the PA in accordance with state regulations. PAs in Maryland may prescribe Schedule II-V controlled substances if the physician delegates this. On-site supervision is not required.	NP scope of practice is based on licensure, accreditation, certification, and education. NPs have independent practice in majority of states; some states have physician collaboration requirements. NPs may prescribe controlled substances. On-site supervision is not required.
Third-party coverage and reimbursement	PAs are eligible for certification as Medicaid and Medicare providers. Commercial payer reimbursement is currently variable.	NPs are eligible for certification as Medicaid and Medicare providers and generally receive favorable reimbursement from commercial payers.

Adapted from: Maryland Academy of Physician Assistants. http://www.mdapa.org/maryland/differences.asp.
BSN, bachelor of science in nursing; *CEU*, continuing education unit; *CME*, continuing medical education; *NCCPA*, National Commission on Certification of Physician Assistants; *NP*, nurse practitioner; *PA*, physician assistant.

their effectiveness, the use of NPs and PAs in the ICU is now a recognized solution to workforce challenges in managing critically ill patients.[28] Integrating NPs and PAs in the ICU can help to facilitate the delivery of high-quality medical care and can provide continuity of care. NPs and PAs can become important elements of multiprovider ICU teams.[29]

CONCLUSIONS

NPs and PAs are increasingly being integrated into ICUs. Care provided by teams that include NPs and PAs has been demonstrated to be comparable to that provided in other staffing models.[30,31] Increasing patient acuity levels, burgeoning requirements for ICU care, and a need to have ICU-trained clinicians provide for critically ill patients presents an important opportunity to integrate NPs and PAs as ICU care providers. Continued dissemination of successful ICU staffing models integrating NPs and PAs as well as additional research on ICU staffing models that include NPs and PAs is needed to identify best strategies for promoting optimal care for critically ill patients.

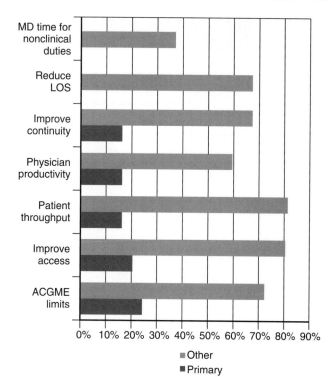

Figure 86-1. Reasons for hiring nurse practitioners and physician assistants as reported by 25 academic medical centers. *ACGME,* Accreditation Council for Graduate Medical Education; *LOS,* length of stay; *MD,* medical doctor. (*Adapted from Moote M, Krsek C, Kleinpell R et al. Physician assistant and nurse practitioner utilization in academic medical centers. Am J Med Qual. 2011;5:1–9.*[11])

Table 86-2 **Roles of NPs and PAs in the ICU**
Patient care management
Rounding
Obtaining history and performing physical examinations
Diagnosing and treating illnesses
Ordering and interpreting tests
Initiating orders, often under protocols
Prescribing and performing diagnostic, pharmacologic, and therapeutic interventions consistent with education, practice, and state regulations
Performing procedures (as credentialed and privileged, such as arterial line insertion, suturing, and chest tube insertion)
Assessing and implementing nutrition
Collaborating and consulting with the interdisciplinary team, patient, and family
Assisting in the operating room
Education of staff, patients, and families
Practice guideline implementation
Lead, monitor, and reinforce practice guidelines for ICU patients (e.g., central line insertion procedures, infection prevention measures, stress ulcer prophylaxis)
Research
Data collection
Enrollment of subjects
Research study management
Quality assurance
Lead quality-assurance initiatives such as ventilator-associated pneumonia bundle, sepsis bundle, rapid response team
Communication
Promote and enhance communication with ICU staff, family members, and the multidisciplinary team
Discharge planning
Transfer and referral consultations
Patient and family education regarding anticipated plan of care

Adapted from Kleinpell RM, Ely EW, Grabenkort R. Nurse practitioners and physician assistants in the ICU: an evidence-based review. *Crit Care Med.* 2008;26:2888–2897.

ICU, intensive care unit, *NP,* nurse practitioner, *PA,* physician assistant.

Table 86-3 Selected Studies on NP and PA Care in the ICU

Study	Method/Focus	Main Results
Burns et al, 2002; Burns et al, 2003	Before and after comparison of ventilator days, LOS, and per-patient cost after adding an NP as compared to before NP role comparing 125 patients in 5 ICUs after to 575 before.	Decreased ventilator days by 1 day, ICU LOS by 3 days, hospital LOS by 2 days, and mortality rate from 38% to 31%. Over $3,000,000 in cost savings.
Cowan et al, 2006	Quasiexperimental design comparing NP-led group to control group of usual care. LOS and hospital profit determined from cost savings.	Average LOS of NP group = 5 days, usual care = 6 days. Hospital profit NP group = $1591 per patient, usual care = $639 per patient.
Ettner et al, 2006	Comparison of 1207 patients randomized to either an NP/MD group or an MD-only group.	NP/MD group had net cost savings of $978 per patient over MD-only group.
Gershengorn HB et al, 2011	Retrospective review of 590 daytime admissions to 2 MICUs with use of NPs and PA coverage.	No significant difference in hospital mortality, ICU LOS, or hospital LOS. Discharge to a skilled care facility was similar for NP/PA care compared with medical resident care.
Gershengorn HB et al, 2012	Literature review of the use of NP and PA providers in the ICU.	NPs and PAs have been used in ICUs as a replacement for physicians in training or to provide onsite semiclosed staffing to care for critically ill patients. Data suggest that use of NPs and PAs is safe and equally efficacious for patient care.
Kapu et al, 2014	Evaluation of impact of adding NP to the rapid response team.	In 2011, the new teams responded to 898 calls, averaging 31.8 min per call. The most frequent diagnoses were respiratory distress (18%), postoperative pain (13%), hypotension (12%), and tachyarrhythmia (10%). The teams facilitated 360 transfers to intensive care and provided 3056 diagnostic and therapeutic interventions. Communication with the primary team was documented on 97% of the calls. After implementation, charge nurses were surveyed, with 96% expressing high satisfaction associated with enhanced service and quality.
Kapu et al, 2014	Retrospective, secondary analysis of return on investment after adding NPs to 5 teams.	Gross collections compared with expenses for 4 NP-led teams for 2-year time periods were 62%, 36%, 47%, and 32%. Average risk-adjusted LOS for the 5 time periods after adding NPs decreased and charges decreased.
Kawar and DiGiovine, 2011	Comparison of clinical outcomes between patients admitted to a resident-run MICU and a PA-run MICU with retrospective analysis of prospectively collected data for 5346 patients admitted to an MICU from January 2004 through January 2007; 3971 patients were admitted to a resident-run MICU (resident group) and 1375 to a PA-run MICU (PA group).	There was no difference in hospital mortality or in ICU mortality between the two groups either in uncontrolled or controlled analyses. Survival analyses showed no difference in 28-day survival between the 2 groups.
McMillen et al, 2012	Surgical ICU care for 13,020 patients by PA team in 12-bed stepdown unit.	Annual surgical mortality decreased and surgical volume increased.
Meyer et al, 2005	Retrospective comparison of 1-year outcomes of NP care for postoperative CV surgery patients.	After NPs added, LOS decreased by 1.91 days and total cost decreased by $5039 per patient.
Russell et al, 2002	Prospective analysis of LOS, rates of UTIs, and skin breakdown before and after addition of NPs to the practice. The baseline included randomized sample of 122 patients admitted to a neurologic ICU over 12 months as compared with 402 patients admitted in first 6 months of the following year after NPs added.	LOS after NP = 8 days vs. baseline = 11 days. UTI NP = 2% vs. baseline 6%; skin breakdown NP = 0% vs. baseline = 2%. Patient days showed 2306 fewer days than baseline group with total cost savings of $2,467,328.
Sirleaf et al, 2014	Comparison of procedures by NPs, PAs, and MDs for 1404 patients.	MDs performed 1020 procedures, with 21 complications (complication rate, 2%). NP/PAs completed 555 procedures; with 11 complications (complication rate, 2%). There was no difference in the mean ICU and hospital LOS. Mortality rates were also comparable between the 2 groups (MD 11% vs. NP/PA 9.7%).
Sise et al, 2011	Prospective analysis of adding NPs to level 1 trauma center. Analysis of demographics, injury severity scores, LOS, complications, total direct costs of care, and outcomes.	After addition of NPs, a decrease in complications by 28.4%, LOS by 36.2, and costs of care by 30.4%.

CV, cerebrovascular; *ICU,* intensive care unit; *LOS,* length of stay; *MD,* medical doctor; *MICU,* medical intensive care unit; *NP,* nurse practitioner; *PA,* physician assistant; *UTI,* urinary tract infection.

Table 86-4 NP- and PA-Performed Tasks That Enhance the Quality of Care[15-27]

Reduced length of stay
Reduced rates of urinary tract infections
Reduced rates of skin breakdown
Reduced time to bladder catheter removal
Reduced time to mobilization
Reduced duration of mechanical ventilation
Increased compliance with clinical practice guidelines
Reduced rates of reintubation
Increased time in coordination of care activities and cost-effective care

NP, nurse practitioner; *PA*, physician assistant.

AUTHORS' RECOMMENDATIONS

- ICU models of care that incorporate NPs and PAs should be disseminated through publications and presentations to promote replication and extension.
- Additional research that demonstrates the effect of NP and PA care for ICU patients is needed.
- Funding should be allocated for research that explores optimal ICU workforce and staffing models that include NPs and PAs.

REFERENCES

1. Gupta R, Zad O, Jimenez E. Analysis of the variations between Accreditation Council for Graduate Medical Education requirements for critical care training programs and their effects on the current critical care workforce. *J Crit Care*. 2013;28:1042–1047.
2. Association of American Medical Colleges. *AAMC Physician Workforce Policy Recommendations*. AAMC; 2012.
3. Pastores SM, O'Connor MF, Kleinpell RM, et al. The ACGME resident duty-hour new standards: history, changes, and impact on staffing of intensive care units. *Crit Care Med*. 2012;39:2540–2549.
4. Ward N, Afessa B, Kleinpell R, et al. Intensivist/patient ratios in closed ICUs: A statement from the society of critical care medicine taskforce on ICU staffing. *Crit Care Med*. 2013;41:638–645.
5. American Association of Nurse Practitioners (AANP). Nurse Practitioner Fact Sheet http://www.aanp.org/all-about-nps/np-fact-sheet. Accessed 20.09.14.
6. American Academy of Physician Assistants (AAPA). What is a Physician Assistant? http://www.aanp.org/all-about-nps/np-fact-sheet.
7. Institute of Medicine. *The Future of Nursing: Leading Change, Advancing Health*. Washington, DC: National Academies Press; 2011:638–645.
8. National Council of State Boards of Nursing. *Advanced Practice Registered Nurse (APRN) Consensus Model*. Chicago: NCSBN; 2008.
9. Kleinpell R. Acute care nurse practitioner practice: results of a 5 year longitudinal study. *Am J Crit Care*. 2005;14:211–219.
10. Kleinpell R, Buchman T, Boyle WA, eds. *Integrating Nurse Practitioners and Physician Assistants in the ICU: Strategies for Optimizing Contributions to Care*. Society of Critical Care Medicine; 2012.
11. Moote M, Krsek C, Kleinpell R, et al. Physician assistant and nurse practitioner utilization in academic medical centers. *Am J Med Qual*. 2011;5:1–9.
12. Nurse practitioners and physician assistants: Do you know the difference? *Medsurg Nurs*. 2007;16:404–407.
13. Deleted in review.
14. Kleinpell RM, Ely EW, Grabenkort R. Nurse practitioners and physician assistants in the ICU: an evidence based review. *Crit Care Med*. 2008;26:2888–2897.
15. Gershengorn HB, Johnson MP, Factor P. The use of nonphysician providers in adult intensive care unit. *Am J Respir Crit Care Med*. 2012;185:600–605.
16. Russell D, VorderBruegge M, Burns SM. Effect of an outcomes-managed approach to care of neuroscience patients by acute care nurse practitioners. *Am J Crit Care*. 2002;11:353–362.
17. Gracias VH, Sicoutris CP, Satwicki SP, et al. Critical care nurse practitioners improve compliance with clinical practice guidelines in semi-closed surgical intensive care unit. *J Nurs Care Qual*. 2008;23:338–344.
18. Hoffman LA, Miller TH, Zullo TG, Donahoe MP. Comparison of 2 models for managing tracheotomized patients in a subacute medical intensive care unit. *Respir Care*. 2006;51:1230–1236.
19. Dubayo BA, Samson MK, Carlson RW. The role of physician assistants in critical care units. *Chest*. 1991;99:89–91.
20. Kapu AN, Kleinpell R, Pilon B. Quality and financial impact of adding nurse practitioners to inpatient care teams. *J Nurs Adm*. 2014;44:87–96.
21. Paton A, Stein D, D'Agostino R, Pastores S, Halpern NA. Critical care medicine advanced practice provider model at a comprehensive cancer center: successes and challenges. *Am J Crit Care*. 2013;22:439–443.
22. Kawar E, DiGiovine B. MICU care delivered by PAs versus residents: do PAs measure up. *J Am Acad Physician Assistants*. 2011;24:36–41.
23. Gershengorn HN, Wunsch H, Wahab R, et al. Impact of nonphysician staffing on outcomes in a medical ICU. *Chest*. 2011;139:1347–1353.
24. Sirleaf M, Jefferson B, Christmas AB, et al. Comparisons of procedural complications between resident physicians and advanced clinical providers. *J Trauma Acute Care Surg*. 2014;77:143–147.
25. Barocas DA, Kulahalli CS, Ehrenfeld JM, et al. Benchmarking the use of a rapid response team by surgical services at a tertiary care hospital. *J Am Coll Surg*. 2014;218:66–72.
26. Kapu AN, Wheeler AP, Lee B. Addition of acute care nurse practitioners to medical and surgical rapid response: a pilot program. *Crit Care Nurse*. 2014;34:51–59.
27. Kapu AN, Kleinpell R, Pilon B. Quality and financial impact of adding nurse practitioners to inpatient care teams. *J Nurs Adm*. 2014;44:87–96.
28. Perlmutter L, Nataraja S. *Developing the Sustainable Critical Care Team*. Washington, DC: The Advisory Board Company Physician Executive Council; 2012.
29. McCarthy C, O'Rourke NC, Madison JM. Integrating advanced practice providers into medical care teams. *Chest*. 2013;143:847–850.
30. Garland A, Gershengorn HB. Staffing in ICUs. *Chest*. 2013;143.
31. Hing E, Uddin S. Physician Assistant and Advance Practice Nurse Care in Hospital Outpatient Departments: United States, 2008-2009. U.S. Department of Health and Human Services Centers for Disease Control and Prevention National Center for Health Statistics (NCHS) Data Brief No. 77.

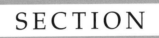

SECTION XX

CRITICAL CARE
ETHICS

87 What Factors Influence a Family to Support a Decision Withdrawing Life Support?

Randall J. Curtis, Margaret Isaac

Most patients who die in the intensive care unit (ICU) do so after having life-sustaining interventions withheld or withdrawn.[1] Evidence suggests that more than 70% of elderly patients in the United States require a surrogate decision maker at the end of life,[2] and involving surrogates in medical decision making at the end of life can be exceedingly challenging. For families of patients with life-threatening illnesses in the ICU, many factors can affect decisions to either continue or withdraw life-sustaining interventions. Clinical status and prognosis can affect how both surrogate decision makers and physicians approach such end-of-life decisions. Patient and family factors, including race, ethnicity, culture, language, religion, and spirituality, and socioeconomic status can also shape how these decisions are approached. Fortunately, advance care planning can help both surrogate decision makers and clinicians better understand the wishes of patients who lack decisional capacity. Physician factors, including their own race, religion, and geographic location, can shape attitudes toward end-of-life care decisions and specifically toward opinions about withholding or withdrawing life-sustaining interventions. Communication strategies used by clinicians and institutional and system factors can also have an effect on surrogates' experiences with decision making.

PATIENT FACTORS

Medical/Health Status and Prognosis

Only a small minority of patient surrogates cite physicians' explicit statements of prognosis as their sole source of information on possible outcomes—reporting reliance on their own perceptions of patient factors (e.g., the patient's character and will to live, the patient's history of illness and resilience, and the patient's physical appearance)[3] and surrogate factors such as their own personal outlook, faith, and intuition.[4] In addition, most surrogate decision makers express doubt in physicians' ability to prognosticate accurately,[5,6] which may be understandable given that doctors are often poor at prognostication for individual patients and have been shown to overestimate prognosis in terminally ill patients by a factor of 5.3.[7] Advanced patient age, functional limitations, and comorbidities appear to have

an important effect on the intensity of care at the end of life—influencing both patients and clinicians' approaches[8] to these types of care decisions.

Patient Characteristics, Values, and Preferences

Race, Ethnicity, and Culture

Broad differences in preferences for end-of-life care have been noted across racial and ethnic groups, although there is great heterogeneity within groups. As such, clinicians are advised to address treatment preferences specifically with patients and surrogates rather than relying on broad generalizations about group preferences and values. In general, African Americans tend to prefer more aggressive use of life support at the end of life[9] when compared with other racial and ethnic groups.[8] Nonwhite patients use more life-sustaining interventions at the end of life than white patients.[8,10] Asians and Latinos[9,11] are more likely to favor a family-centered decision-making process, and nonwhite racial and ethnic groups are less likely to have knowledge of and support with advance care planning.[9] One study comparing white and African American caregivers of patients with advanced lung cancer suggested that African American caregivers had more optimistic expectations for treatment outcomes, which may be part of what shapes these observed differences in expressed preferences by patients and their surrogates.[12] Another study of families of critically ill patients compared family perceptions among patients of similar severity of illness and found that African Americans tended to perceive the illness as less enduring and serious, reported more confidence in treatment efficacy, and reported lower illness comprehension compared with whites.[13] A review found that some of the differences between African American patients and non-Hispanic white patients were related to historic mistrust of the health-care system, differences in knowledge and access to services, and differences in spiritual beliefs between these two groups.[14] In addition, clinicians appear to be influenced by patient race, with physicians being more likely to recommend withdrawal of life support with nonwhite patients, although nonwhite patients are more likely to die with full life support in place.[15]

In a study of U.S. caregivers, those who were less "Americanized" or acculturated to the United States (as determined by language preference and questions related to cultural identity) expressed different preferences for end-of-life care, including a more positive preference for feeding tubes/artificial nutrition, a feeling that they received too much information from physicians, and a desire to receive additional services, including complementary therapies and mental health and nutritional counseling.[16]

Language Fluency

Families with limited English proficiency receive less information and fewer explicit statements of support in family conferences,[17] although it is not clear how this affects their decisions about issues such as withdrawal of life support. Use of professional interpreters rather than ad hoc interpreters (e.g., family members) can foster accurate communication and minimize errors in translation, particularly when discussing emotionally charged topics such as end-of-life care.[18] Interpreted family conferences also contain fewer elements of shared decision making and a greater ratio of physician/family speech,[19] which has been associated with decreased family satisfaction.[20]

Religious and Spiritual Beliefs

Patients who identify as religious or spiritual or who identify as using spiritual coping strategies are more likely to choose life-prolonging treatments at the end of life[21-23] and are more likely to oppose do-not-attempt-resuscitation (DNAR) orders.[24] Specifically, individuals who believe strongly that the length of one's life is controlled by a higher power are less likely to engage in advance care planning,[25] and those who express deference to God's will tend to choose more life-prolonging treatments (e.g., continuation of life support).[26] There is great variability in the approaches to medical decision making dictated by theology and by religious authorities, and increasingly, religious authorities have been called on to weigh in on matters related to use of medical technology, medical ethics, and end-of-life care. Furthermore, there is considerable heterogeneity in the application and interpretation of religious tenets within individual religious traditions, and many of the approaches common to specific religious groups are more appropriately attributed to cultural beliefs, not being grounded in specific religious doctrine or teachings.[27] In addition, when patients' or families' spiritual care needs go unmet, patients rate their care more poorly.[28,29] Indeed, evidence suggests that unmet spiritual care needs are associated with increased medical costs at the end of life.[30]

Socioeconomic Status and Education

Socioeconomic status and education may also impact end-of-life care, although very few studies have examined these specific factors in this context. A systematic review found that uninsured patients were more likely to have life support withdrawn in the ICU.[31] In one study, uninsured ICU patients, when compared with those with insurance being cared for at the same hospital, received fewer procedures, including hemodialysis and placement of central venous catheters, and had increased mortality despite being younger in age, having fewer comorbidities, and having a lower probability of death at the time of admission to the ICU.[32] Low literacy has been identified as a risk factor for not having an advance directive in place,[33] which can limit surrogates' abilities to understand patients' values and wishes. In addition, low or marginal health literacy has been shown to be associated with a preference for more aggressive care at the end of life.[34]

Role of Advance Directives and Advance Care Planning

Advance care planning generally and advance directives specifically can be helpful for surrogates in clarifying the wishes of their loved one. Indeed, the absence of an advance directive has been identified by ICU directors as a barrier to optimal end-of-life care.[35] Historically, the prevalence of advance directives has been low, ranging from 5% to approximately one third of patients.[36-39] Several more recent studies demonstrate much higher rates of advance directive use,[2,40,41] a change that has been attributed in part to the aging of the U.S. population, as well as increased familiarity with and growing public discourse around the importance of advance care planning.[40] Some evidence suggests that patients who have engaged in advance care planning or who have advance directives are more likely to receive care that mirrors their stated preferences[2,42] and less likely to receive technologically aggressive interventions.[2] In addition, the presence of a living will has been shown to improve families' assessments of the quality of death and dying for their loved one in the ICU.[43] Importantly, there is a growing understanding that advance directives are most helpful in the context of a broader process of advance care planning that helps patients and their families prepare to be able to make the best "in the moment" decisions about life-sustaining treatments.[44]

SURROGATE DECISION MAKER/FAMILY FACTORS

Surrogate Preferences for Control, Role, and Decision Making

Historically, physicians have used a parentalist approach to medical decision making. Calls for increased patient and family autonomy have led to implementation of alternate models of decision control. Decision control can be viewed as a spectrum, with patient and family autonomy/informed consent at one end and clinician parentalism at the other. In between these extremes is shared decision making, a model in which clinicians share medical information; patients and/or surrogate decision makers share information about values, goals, and preferences; and both parties discuss and come to an agreement about an optimal plan of care. Although shared decision making has been endorsed by critical care societies as the preferred default approach,[45-47] clinicians should recognize that patient/surrogate preferences related to decision control can vary widely and are influenced by factors that include gender, personality, education, socioeconomic status, and culture.[9,48,49] To optimize communication, clinicians must assess preferences related to decision control for each patient and family and modify their approach to reflect these preferences. Although it is not clear how these different approaches might affect choices specifically around the withdrawal of life-sustaining interventions, it is important to consider what approach might be preferred and be most effective with surrogate decision makers before beginning family conferences focused on these decisions.

In addition, surrogates use varying approaches to their role as a proxy decision maker. Many medical ethicists and clinicians suggest that surrogates apply the principle of substituted judgment,[50,51] in other words, asking surrogates to use their knowledge of the patient's values, goals, and preferences to articulate what the patient would choose were the patient able to participate in medical decision making. Evidence, though, suggests that many surrogate decision makers have difficulty in determining what the wishes of their loved one might be, with about a third of surrogates incorrectly predicting the treatment preferences of patients.[52,53] This may be in part because some patients' wishes change and evolve,[54-56] although most patients show stability in medical preferences over time.[57,58] In addition, in cases in which surrogates inaccurately predict the wishes of their loved one, their preferences on behalf of their loved one more closely approximate their own personal wishes about end-of-life care,[59,60] highlighting the challenges of applying a substituted judgment standard. Surrogates use different factors in medical decision making, including factors other than the patient's perceived wishes; these factors include their own personal values, religious beliefs and preferences, family consensus, and shared experiences with the patient.[4,61,62]

Family relationships seem to have an impact on the accuracy of proxies to predict the wishes of their loved one. Spouse proxies have been found to be more accurate than adult children of patients.[63] Patients with highly supportive and well-functioning families are more likely to engage in advance care planning,[64,65] and lower levels of family conflict have also been associated with higher proxy–patient accuracy in medical decision making.[63]

Patient Preferences for Surrogate Latitude in Decision Making

In addition to the difficulty in implementing substituted judgment as a surrogate decision maker, patients vary in the latitude they choose to give to their surrogate decision makers. Most patients, in the event of decisional incapacity, would want decisions made on their behalf using both substituted judgment and best interest standards and involving both surrogates and physicians.[66] Many patients show a great deal of trust in the decisions of surrogates as well—with more than three quarters of patients in one study preferring that physicians follow the preferences of their surrogate even when those preferences were at odds with previously stated wishes.[67] The fact, though, that some patients prefer that advance directives be followed even if surrogates disagree highlights the importance of discussing surrogate latitude as part of advance care planning.

CLINICIAN FACTORS

Physician Bias and Influence

Many clinician factors can influence decisions around the withholding and withdrawing of life support. For example, clinicians' overall religiosity and specific religious affiliation can influence the likelihood that life-sustaining interventions are either withheld or withdrawn, with religious physicians more likely to favor more aggressive interventions and less likely to favor withdrawal of life-sustaining interventions.[68] In one European study, withdrawal of life support was more common among physicians who identified as Catholic, Protestant, or nonreligious, whereas a decision to withhold rather than withdraw life support was more common among Jewish, Greek Orthodox, and Muslim physicians.[69]

Most physicians select DNAR status for themselves when presented with a hypothetical end-of-life scenario[70,71] and express a personal preference to receive less aggressive care in general.[8] It remains unclear why physician and layperson preferences are so different and whether these personal preferences have an impact on treatment approaches toward patients. It seems reasonable, though, that clinical experiences and witnessed suffering might affect physicians' personal preferences. This hypothesis suggests a possible opportunity for physicians to better communicate with patients and their families about their own clinical experiences and to offer to make recommendations to families who likely have considerably less experience with both critical care and end-of-life care.

Physician factors such as white race, residence in North American or northern Europe, more clinical experience, and experience in ICU care predict provision of less technologically aggressive end-of-life care,[8] although there are conflicting data about the effect that physician age might have on comfort with DNAR orders and, in general, on treatment decisions in patients with advanced illness.[72-74] Medical residents have been found to be marginally more likely than attending physicians to promote aggressive end-of-life care,[75] with the least experienced residents the most likely to prescribe technologically aggressive care at the end of life.[72]

Communication Strategies and Skill

Communication strategies and skill can have a major influence on surrogates' medical decision making. There is significant variability in physicians' roles in navigating complex medical decision making, and few physicians explicitly negotiate their roles with individual families.[76] Patient families are also highly variable in their preferences regarding physicians' recommendations about care decisions at the end of life.[77] One study found that most physicians think that making recommendations about end-of-life care is appropriate, although there is significant heterogeneity in whether physicians actually make these recommendations to families.[78]

Prognostic information can also be easily misunderstood, and some data suggest that surrogates' interpretation of a report of a poor prognosis may be overly optimistic.[3] Furthermore, in one study nearly a third of surrogates stated that they would choose to continue life-sustaining interventions even in the face of poor prognosis (<1% chance of survival), and 18% opined that they would choose to continue these measures given a physician's assessment that there was "no chance of survival."[6] Estimating prognosis accurately for individual patients is incredibly challenging, and, as a rule, physicians tend to be overly optimistic.[7,79] More experienced physicians and physicians with shorter physician–patient relationships also tend to be more accurate,[7] and prognostication is more accurate as patients approach the end of life.[80] Although accurate prognostication is difficult, using numerical estimates rather than vague language, framing prognosis from both a positive and a negative perspective, and using consistent denominators when estimating risk can all promote better understanding by patients and their surrogates.[81]

Provision of Emotional Support

Explicit statements of empathy by clinicians for family members have been shown to increase family satisfaction with communication,[82] and although effective communication strategies can promote trust on the part of family members,[83] it is not clear how these statements might affect decisions around life-sustaining interventions. Many family conferences do not contain any explicit empathic statements or statements of support for family members.[82,84] Specific communication tools, such as the NURSE (Name, Understand, Respect, Support, Explore) mnemonic for acknowledging and validating emotion[85] and the facilitated values history,[86] may help in both supporting family members and enhancing the ability of surrogates to understand their role in decision making and to contribute to decision making that reflects the authentic values and wishes of their family member.

Role of Palliative Care Providers

Not surprisingly, ICU patients for whom palliative care providers are consulted tend to be sicker, with longer lengths of stay in the ICU and higher mortality;[87] that is, the sickest patients with the poorest prognosis seem to be identified as those who would benefit most from palliative care services. A randomized controlled trial evaluating the impact of an inpatient palliative care consultation service found no differences in survival or symptom management, although patients seen by the consult service had fewer ICU admissions on hospital readmission and sustained lower costs over a 6-month time horizon. In addition, patients themselves were more satisfied with their care experience and with provider communication specifically.[88]

INSTITUTIONAL/SYSTEM FACTORS

There is some evidence that institutional and system factors may play a role in end-of-life care, including the decision to withdraw life support. Access to information and physicians has been associated with fewer family–physician conflicts related to prognosis,[89] which might have an impact on a family's support of a decision to withdraw

life-sustaining interventions. Family members of patients with private ICU rooms have been found to experience lower rates of anxiety and depression.[90] In addition, the lack of regular family conferences with physicians and even the absence of a dedicated room for family conferences have been associated with anxiety symptoms in caregivers,[91] though it is unclear how these factors might shape surrogates' approach to a decision to withdraw life-sustaining interventions.

AUTHORS' RECOMMENDATIONS

- Many factors influence decisions by patients and their families to withdraw life-sustaining interventions.
- Although surrogate decision makers are influenced by physicians' estimates of prognosis, they are also often guided by other factors. Personal factors such as race, ethnicity, and culture may shape assumptions and preferences at the end of life for both patients and their caregivers or surrogate decision makers.
- Religiosity and specific spiritual beliefs can affect not only end-of life decisions, but also preferences around advance care planning and decision control.
- Advance care planning has the potential to assist both surrogate decision makers and physicians caring for ICU patients who lack decisional capacity.
- Patients who complete advance directives are more likely to want less aggressive medical care at the end of life, and those who engage in advance care planning are more likely to have care that reflects their stated preferences.
- Clinician factors can also shape decisions around withdrawal of life-sustaining interventions, with differences associated with geographic regions of practice, religious background, and race/ethnicity.
- Specific communication approaches that support patients and family members, involvement of palliative care specialists, and other institutional and systemic factors can also improve family decision making around end-of-life care, as well as family/surrogate satisfaction, and psychological burden.

REFERENCES

1. Sprung CL, et al. End-of-life practices in European intensive care units: the Ethicus Study. *JAMA.* 2003;290(6):790–797.
2. Silveira MJ, Kim SY, Langa KM. Advance directives and outcomes of surrogate decision making before death. *N Engl J Med.* 2010;362(13):1211–1218.
3. Zier LS, et al. Surrogate decision makers' interpretation of prognostic information: a mixed-methods study. *Ann Intern Med.* 2012;156(5):360–366.
4. Boyd EA, et al. "It's not just what the doctor tells me:" factors that influence surrogate decision-makers' perceptions of prognosis. *Crit Care Med.* 2010;38(5):1270–1275.
5. Zier LS, et al. Doubt and belief in physicians' ability to prognosticate during critical illness: the perspective of surrogate decision makers. *Crit Care Med.* 2008;36(8):2341–2347.
6. Zier LS, et al. Surrogate decision makers' responses to physicians' predictions of medical futility. *Chest.* 2009;136(1):110–117.
7. Christakis NA, Lamont EB. Extent and determinants of error in doctors' prognoses in terminally ill patients: prospective cohort study. *BMJ.* 2000;320(7233):469–472.
8. Frost DW, et al. Patient and healthcare professional factors influencing end-of-life decision-making during critical illness: a systematic review. *Crit Care Med.* 2011;39(5):1174–1189.
9. Kwak J, Haley WE. Current research findings on end-of-life decision making among racially or ethnically diverse groups. *Gerontologist.* 2005;45(5):634–641.

10. Hanchate A, et al. Racial and ethnic differences in end-of-life costs: why do minorities cost more than whites? *Arch Intern Med.* 2009;169(5):493–501.

11. Yennurajalingam S, et al. A multicenter survey of Hispanic caregiver preferences for patient decision control in the United States and Latin America. *Palliat Med.* 2013;27(7):692–698.

12. Zhang AY, Zyzanski SJ, Siminoff LA. Ethnic differences in the caregiver's attitudes and preferences about the treatment and care of advanced lung cancer patients. *Psychooncology.* 2012;21(11): 1250–1253.

13. Ford D, et al. Factors associated with illness perception among critically ill patients and surrogates. *Chest.* 2010;138(1):59–67.

14. Wicher CP, Meeker MA. What influences African American end-of-life preferences? *J Health Care Poor Underserved.* 2012;23(1):28–58.

15. Muni S, et al. The influence of race/ethnicity and socioeconomic status on end-of-life care in the ICU. *Chest.* 2011;139(5):1025–1033.

16. DeSanto-Madeya S, et al. Associations between United States acculturation and the end-of-life experience of caregivers of patients with advanced cancer. *J Palliat Med.* 2009;12(12):1143–1149.

17. Thornton JD, et al. Families with limited English proficiency receive less information and support in interpreted intensive care unit family conferences. *Crit Care Med.* 2009;37(1):89–95.

18. Flores G, et al. Errors of medical interpretation and their potential clinical consequences: a comparison of professional versus ad hoc versus no interpreters. *Ann Emerg Med.* 2012;60(5):545–553.

19. Van Cleave AC, et al. Quality of communication in interpreted versus noninterpreted PICU family meetings. *Crit Care Med.* 2014;42(6):1507–1517.

20. McDonagh JR, et al. Family satisfaction with family conferences about end-of-life care in the intensive care unit: increased proportion of family speech is associated with increased satisfaction. *Crit Care Med.* 2004;32(7):1484–1488.

21. Phelps AC, et al. Religious coping and use of intensive life-prolonging care near death in patients with advanced cancer. *JAMA.* 2009;301(11):1140–1147.

22. Balboni TA, et al. Religiousness and spiritual support among advanced cancer patients and associations with end-of-life treatment preferences and quality of life. *J Clin Oncol.* 2007;25(5):555–560.

23. True G, et al. Treatment preferences and advance care planning at end of life: the role of ethnicity and spiritual coping in cancer patients. *Ann Behav Med.* 2005;30(2):174–179.

24. Jaul E, Zabari Y, Brodsky J. Spiritual background and its association with the medical decision of, DNR at terminal life stages. *Arch Gerontol Geriatr.* 2014;58(1):25–29.

25. Garrido MM, et al. Pathways from religion to advance care planning: beliefs about control over length of life and end-of-life values. *Gerontologist.* 2013;53(5):801–816.

26. Winter L, Dennis MP, Parker B. Preferences for life-prolonging medical treatments and deference to the will of god. *J Relig Health.* 2009;48(4):418–430.

27. Bülow HH, et al. The world's major religions' points of view on end-of-life decisions in the intensive care unit. *Intensive Care Med.* 2008;34(3):423–430.

28. Astrow AB, et al. Is failure to meet spiritual needs associated with cancer patients' perceptions of quality of care and their satisfaction with care? *J Clin Oncol.* 2007;25(36):5753–5757.

29. Wall RJ, et al. Spiritual care of families in the intensive care unit. *Crit Care Med.* 2007;35(4):1084–1090.

30. Balboni T, et al. Support of cancer patients' spiritual needs and associations with medical care costs at the end of life. *Cancer.* 2011;117(23):5383–5391.

31. Fowler RA, et al. An official American Thoracic Society systematic review: the association between health insurance status and access, care delivery, and outcomes for patients who are critically ill. *Am J Respir Crit Care Med.* 2010;181(9):1003–1011.

32. Lyon SM, et al. The effect of insurance status on mortality and procedural use in critically ill patients. *Am J Respir Crit Care Med.* 2011;184(7):809–815.

33. Waite KR, et al. Literacy and race as risk factors for low rates of advance directives in older adults. *J Am Geriatr Soc.* 2013;61(3): 403–406.

34. Volandes AE, et al. Health literacy not race predicts end-of-life care preferences. *J Palliat Med.* 2008;11(5):754–762.

35. Nelson JE, et al. End-of-life care for the critically ill: A national intensive care unit survey. *Crit Care Med.* 2006;34(10):2547–2553.

36. Kavic SM, et al. The role of advance directives and family in end-of-life decisions in critical care units. *Conn Med.* 2003;67(9): 531–534.

37. Johnson RF, Baranowski-Birkmeier T, O'Donnell JB. Advance directives in the medical intensive care unit of a community teaching hospital. *Chest.* 1995;107(3):752–756.

38. Goodman MD, Tarnoff M, Slotman GJ. Effect of advance directives on the management of elderly critically ill patients. *Crit Care Med.* 1998;26(4):701–704.

39. Tillyard AR. Ethics review: 'Living wills' and intensive care–an overview of the American experience. *Crit Care.* 2007;11(4):219.

40. Silveira MJ, Wiitala W, Piette J. Advance directive completion by elderly Americans: a decade of change. *J Am Geriatr Soc.* 2014;62(4):706–710.

41. Teno JM, et al. Association between advance directives and quality of end-of-life care: a national study. *J Am Geriatr Soc.* 2007;55(2):189–194.

42. Detering KM, et al. The impact of advance care planning on end of life care in elderly patients: randomised controlled trial. *BMJ.* 2010;340:c1345.

43. Glavan BJ, et al. Using the medical record to evaluate the quality of end-of-life care in the intensive care unit. *Crit Care Med.* 2008;36(4):1138–1146.

44. Sudore RL, Fried TR. Redefining the "planning" in advance care planning: preparing for end-of-life decision making. *Ann Intern Med.* 2010;153(4):256–261.

45. Joosten EA, et al. Systematic review of the effects of shared decision-making on patient satisfaction, treatment adherence and health status. *Psychother Psychosom.* 2008;77(4):219–226.

46. Davidson JE, et al. Clinical practice guidelines for support of the family in the patient-centered intensive care unit: American College of Critical Care Medicine Task Force 2004-2005. *Crit Care Med.* 2007;35(2):605–622.

47. Carlet J, et al. Challenges in end-of-life care in the ICU. Statement of the 5th International Consensus Conference in Critical Care: Brussels, Belgium, April 2003. *Intensive Care Med.* 2004;30(5):770–784.

48. Moselli NM, Debernardi F, Piovano F. Forgoing life sustaining treatments: differences and similarities between North America and Europe. *Acta Anaesthesiol Scand.* 2006;50(10):1177–1186.

49. Johnson SK, et al. An empirical study of surrogates' preferred level of control over value-laden life support decisions in intensive care units. *Am J Respir Crit Care Med.* 2011;183(7):915–921.

50. Curtis JR, White DB. Practical guidance for evidence-based ICU family conferences. *Chest.* 2008;134(4):835–843.

51. Luce JM. End-of-life decision making in the intensive care unit. *Am J Respir Crit Care Med.* 2010;182(1):6–11.

52. Shalowitz DI, Garrett-Mayer E, Wendler D. The accuracy of surrogate decision makers: a systematic review. *Arch Intern Med.* 2006;166(5):493–497.

53. Foo AS, Lee TW, Soh CR. Discrepancies in end-of-life decisions between elderly patients and their named surrogates. *Ann Acad Med Singapore.* 2012;41(4):141–153.

54. Wittink MN, et al. Stability of preferences for end-of-life treatment after 3years of follow-up: the Johns Hopkins Precursors Study. *Arch Intern Med.* 2008;168(19):2125–2130.

55. Weissman JS, et al. The stability of preferences for life-sustaining care among persons with AIDS in the Boston Health Study. *Med Decis Making.* 1999;19(1):16–26.

56. Danis M, et al. Stability of choices about life-sustaining treatments. *Ann Intern Med.* 1994;120(7):567–573.

57. Pruchno RA, et al. Stability and change in patient preferences and spouse substituted judgments regarding dialysis continuation. *J Gerontol B Psychol Sci Soc Sci.* 2008;63(2):S81–S91.

58. Martin VC, Roberto KA. Assessing the stability of values and health care preferences of older adults: A long-term comparison. *J Gerontol Nurs.* 2006;32(11):23–31. quiz 32–3.

59. Moorman SM, Hauser RM, Carr D. Do older adults know their spouses' end-of-life treatment preferences? *Res Aging.* 2009;31(4):463–491.

60. Marks MA, Arkes HR. Patient and surrogate disagreement in end-of-life decisions: can surrogates accurately predict patients' preferences? *Med Decis Making.* 2008;28(4):524–531.

61. Vig EK, et al. Beyond substituted judgment: how surrogates navigate end-of-life decision-making. *J Am Geriatr Soc.* 2006;54(11):1688–1693.

62. Fritsch J, et al. Making decisions for hospitalized older adults: ethical factors considered by family surrogates. *J Clin Ethics.* 2013;24(2):125–134.

63. Parks SM, et al. Family factors in end-of-life decision-making: family conflict and proxy relationship. *J Palliat Med.* 2011;14(2):179–184.

64. Boerner K, Carr D, Moorman S. Family relationships and advance care planning: do supportive and critical relations encourage or hinder planning? *J Gerontol B Psychol Sci Soc Sci.* 2013;68(2):246–256.

65. Carr D, Moorman SM, Boerner K. End-of-life planning in a family context: does relationship quality affect whether (and with whom) older adults plan? *J Gerontol B Psychol Sci Soc Sci.* 2013;68(4):586–592.

66. Sulmasy DP, et al. How would terminally ill patients have others make decisions for them in the event of decisional incapacity? A longitudinal study. *J Am Geriatr Soc.* 2007;55(12):1981–1988.

67. Covinsky KE, et al. Communication and decision-making in seriously ill patients: findings of the SUPPORT project. The Study to Understand Prognoses and Preferences for Outcomes and Risks of Treatments. *J Am Geriatr Soc.* 2000;48(suppl 5):S187–S193.

68. Bülow HH, et al. Are religion and religiosity important to end-of-life decisions and patient autonomy in the ICU? The Ethicatt study. *Intensive Care Med.* 2012;38(7):1126–1133.

69. Sprung CL, et al. The importance of religious affiliation and culture on end-of-life decisions in European intensive care units. *Intensive Care Med.* 2007;33(10):1732–1739.

70. Periyakoil VS, et al. Do unto others: doctors' personal end-of-life resuscitation preferences and their attitudes toward advance directives. *PLoS One.* 2014;9(5):e98246.

71. Gallo JJ, et al. Life-sustaining treatments: what do physicians want and do they express their wishes to others? *J Am Geriatr Soc.* 2003;51(7):961–969.

72. Kelly WF, et al. Do specialists differ on do-not-resuscitate decisions? *Chest.* 2002;121(3):957–963.

73. Christakis NA, Asch DA. Physician characteristics associated with decisions to withdraw life support. *Am J Public Health.* 1995;85(3):367–372.

74. Alemayehu E, et al. Variability in physicians' decisions on caring for chronically ill elderly patients: an international study. *CMAJ.* 1991;144(9):1133–1138.

75. Walter SD, et al. Confidence in life-support decisions in the intensive care unit: a survey of healthcare workers. Canadian Critical Care Trials Group. *Crit Care Med.* 1998;26(1):44–49.

76. White DB, et al. Expanding the paradigm of the physician's role in surrogate decision-making: an empirically derived framework. *Crit Care Med.* 2010;38(3):743–750.

77. White DB, et al. Are physicians' recommendations to limit life support beneficial or burdensome? Bringing empirical data to the debate. *Am J Respir Crit Care Med.* 2009;180(4):320–325.

78. Brush DR, et al. Recommendations to limit life support: a national survey of critical care physicians. *Am J Respir Crit Care Med.* 2012;186(7):633–639.

79. Glare P, et al. A systematic review of physicians' survival predictions in terminally ill cancer patients. *BMJ.* 2003;327(7408):195–198.

80. Brandt HE, et al. Predicted survival vs. actual survival in terminally ill noncancer patients in Dutch nursing homes. *J Pain Symptom Manage.* 2006;32(6):560–566.

81. Paling J. Strategies to help patients understand risks. *BMJ.* 2003;327(7417):745–748.

82. Selph RB, et al. Empathy and life support decisions in intensive care units. *J Gen Intern Med.* 2008;23(9):1311–1317.

83. Torke AM, et al. Communicating with clinicians: the experiences of surrogate decision-makers for hospitalized older adults. *J Am Geriatr Soc.* 2012;60(8):1401–1407.

84. Curtis JR, et al. Missed opportunities during family conferences about end-of-life care in the intensive care unit. *Am J Respir Crit Care Med.* 2005;171(8):844–849.

85. Pollak KI, et al. Oncologist communication about emotion during visits with patients with advanced cancer. *J Clin Oncol.* 2007;25(36):5748–5752.

86. Scheunemann LP, Arnold RM, White DB. The facilitated values history: helping surrogates make authentic decisions for incapacitated patients with advanced illness. *Am J Respir Crit Care Med.* 2012;186(6):480–486.

87. Hsu-Kim C, et al. Integrating Palliative Care into Critical Care: A Quality Improvement Study. *J Intensive Care Med.* 2015;30(6):358–364.

88. Gade G, et al. Impact of an inpatient palliative care team: a randomized control trial. *J Palliat Med.* 2008;11(2):180–190.

89. Fumis RR, Nishimoto IN, Deheinzelin D. Families' interactions with physicians in the intensive care unit: the impact on family's satisfaction. *J Crit Care.* 2008;23(3):281–286.

90. Pochard F, et al. Symptoms of anxiety and depression in family members of intensive care unit patients before discharge or death. A prospective multicenter study. *J Crit Care.* 2005;20(1):90–96.

91. Pochard F, et al. Symptoms of anxiety and depression in family members of intensive care unit patients: ethical hypothesis regarding decision-making capacity. *Crit Care Med.* 2001;29(10):1893–1897.

Index

A

Abdominal compartment syndrome (ACS), 94, 551–555
  adjunctive measurements of, 551–552
  cardiovascular system and, 552
  central nervous system and, 553
  development of, risk factors for, 552t
  diagnosis of, 551–552
  management of, 553–554
  mechanism of action of, 551
  nonrenal viscera and, 553
  ocular system and, 553
  pathophysiology of, 551
  renal system and, 552–553
  respiratory system and, 552
  systemic impact of, 552–553
Abnormal bleeding, causes of, 599t
ACCEPT trial. *see* Algorithms for Critical Care Enteral and Parenteral Therapy (ACCEPT) trial
ACCM. *see* American College of Critical Care Medicine (ACCM)
ACEP. *see* American College of Emergency Physicians (ACEP)
Acetaminophen (APAP), 579f
  ALF and, 497, 499
  for fever, 119–121
  poisonings from, 578–579
N-acetyl-β-$_D$-glucosaminidase (NAG), 386
N-acetylcysteine (NAC), 233
  for acetaminophen toxicity, 499
  for AKI, 393
  for APAP poisoning, 577
  for ARDS, 242
  for mushroom poisoning, 499
  for non-acetaminophen-induced ALF, 504–505
N-acetyl-p-benzoquinoneimine (NAPQI), 578
Acid base disturbances, 410, 411t
Acid-base chemistry, analytical tools used in, 413
Acid-base disorders, 407–418
  acute metabolic acidosis, 411–412
  acute metabolic alkalosis, 412–413
  acute respiratory acidosis, 410–411
  acute respiratory alkalosis, 410–411
  analytical tools used in, 413
  anion gap approach, 413–414, 413f
  classification of, 411t
  in critical illness, 412–413
  descriptive carbon dioxide-bicarbonate approach, 413, 413t
  disturbances in, 410, 411t
  scientific background of, 409–410
  semiquantitative approach, 414–415
  Stewart-Fencl approach, 415–416
  strong ions, 410
  tools and outcome prediction, 416
  weak acids, 410
Acid-base status, AKI and, 394–395
ACS. *see* Abdominal compartment syndrome (ACS)

Activated charcoal (AC), single-dose, 581
Activated partial thromboplastin time (aPTT), 171
Activated protein C (APC), 9, 231, 243
Acute Dialysis Quality Initiative (ADQI), 383
Acute fatty liver of pregnancy, 499
Acute heart failure (AHF)
  description of, 343
  management of, 341–346
    improving cardiac function in, 345–346
    reducing extracellular volume in, 344–345
    vasodilators in, 343, 344t
  mechanism of actions and hemodynamic effects in, 344t
Acute hypoxemic respiratory failure, 31
Acute ischemic stroke (AIS)
  blood pressure control in, 463
  cardiac care in, 463
  complications of, 466–467
  critical care management of, 462–463
  in emergency setting, 461–462
  fluid management in, 463
  glucose control in, 463–464
  hemoglobin management in, 464
  hemorrhagic transformation of, 466–467
  in intensive care unit, 461–469
  seizure after, 467
  temperature in, 464
  thrombolytic therapy for, 466–467
Acute kidney injury (AKI), 262–263, 381–387
  AKIN classification of, 383–384, 384t
  with ALF, 503
  biomarkers of, 385–386
    cell-cycle arrest, 386
    clinical uses of, 386
    specific, 385–386
  clinical, 383–384, 385f
    limitations of, 384
  evaluation, 388–391
    history, 388
    imaging studies, 391
    laboratory studies, 388–391
    physical examination, 388
  KDIGO classification of, 384, 384t
  management of, 394–395
  MAP and, 279
  metabolic acidosis with, 399
  precipitating factors for, 388, 389t
  prevention of, 391–394
    interventions for, 392–394, 393t
  prognosis of, 395
  with pulmonary edema, 399
  RIFLE classification of, 383, 384t
  subclinical, 384–385, 385f
  ultrafiltration for, 402–403
Acute Kidney Injury Network (AKIN), 383–384, 384t, 388, 389t
Acute liver failure (ALF), 497–509
  from APAP, 578
  causes of, 498t
  clinical presentation of, 497

Acute liver failure *(Continued)*
  coagulopathy and, 502
  epidemiology of, 497
  gastrointestinal bleeding and, 503–504
  hemodynamic support for, 503
  hypothermia for, 504
  infection with, 502–503
  initial assessment and management of, 497
  living donor liver transplantation for, 505
  management guidelines for, 505t
  mechanical ventilation for, 503
  metabolic concerns in, 504
  NAC for, 504–505
  nutrition and, 504
  prognosis for, 498–499, 498t
  studies on, 506t
  therapy for, 499
  transplantation and, 504
Acute lung injury/acute respiratory distress syndrome (ALI/ARDS), 184, 190–194
  NIV for, 39
  ventilator management in, 5
Acute Physiology and Chronic Health Evaluation (APACHE), 178
  SDD and, 313t–317t
Acute Physiology and Chronic Health Evaluation IV (APACHE IV) model, 9
Acute respiratory distress syndrome (ARDS), 12, 61, 75–80, 181–189, 326, 611
  airway pressure release ventilation in, 201
  anti-inflammatory therapies in, 239–246
  Berlin definition of, 184–186, 184t
    acuity of onset, 184
    ancillary variables, 185–186
    chest radiographic findings, 185
    limitations in, 186t
    origin of edema, 185
    oxygenation, 184–185
    performance of, 186–187
    redressals in, 186t
  characteristics of, 62
  CPP and, 442
  definition of, 183–184, 326
    achieving consensus on, 183–184
    as clinical entity, 183
  description of, 239
  direct vs, indirect injury, 241–242
  elevation of head of bed, 214
  etiology of, 13
  events in, 326
  extracorporeal life support for, 66–74
    clinical trial for, 69–72
    economic feasibility, 69
    history of patient survival in, 68–69
    insufficient critical care evidence in, 66–67
    meta-analysis for, 71f
    protocols for clinical trials, 67–68
    randomized controlled trials of, 67t
  H1N1 epidemic associated with, 68
  HFOV in, 200
  high frequency ventilation for, 199–200

Acute respiratory distress syndrome
(*Continued*)
    hospital-acquired exposures, 77–78
    hypothesis for, 75–77
    inhaled nitric oxide for, 224–226, 225f
    inhaled vasodilators in, 224–228
    interventions in, 326t
    key research landmarks in, 195, 196t
    lateral position in, 213–214
    low *vs.* high tidal volume in, mechanical
        ventilation with, 197t
    "low-stretch" approach for, 196
    lung recruitment maneuvers and, 197–199
    management of, 68–69, 195
    mechanical ventilation for, 195–203
    neuromuscular blockade in, 201
    nonventilatory strategies for, 229–238,
        234t
    open lung approach for, 196–197
    outcomes of severe, 63
    pathogenesis of, 75
    pathologic changes in, 192–193, 193f
    pathophysiologic changes in, 190–191
    pathophysiologic consequences in, 192
    patient positioning in, 212–218
    permissive hypercapnia and, 204–211,
        206t
    pharmacologic ineffectiveness with,
        234–235
    physiologic rationale, 224
    predisposing conditions, 75, 76f
    in pregnancy, 574–575
    pressure *vs.* volume-controlled ventilation
        in, 199
    prone positioning in, 200–201, 214–217
    prostaglandins for, 226
    pulmonary hypertension in, 219
    pulmonary vasodilator therapies for,
        220–222
    reconciling the rationale with clinical
        research findings, 226
    risk modifiers, 75–77, 76f
    risk prediction models, 77
    sepsis and, 262–263
    steroids for, 239–241
        in early stage, 239–240, 240t
        in late stage, 240–241
    subphenotypes, 187
    ventilator-induced lung injury and, 195
Acute respiratory failure, treatment of, 33
Acute traumatic central cord syndrome
    (ATCCS), 587, 587f
Acute-phase proteins, 495
Acute-phase response, 495–496
ACV. *see* Assist-control mechanical
    ventilation (ACV)
Adenosine diphosphate (ADP), 335
Adenosine triphosphate (ATP), 130, 335
Administrative data, for critical care
    outcomes, 11
Adrenal insufficiency, ALF and, 503
β$_1$-Adrenergic receptors, 285
Advance care planning, role of, 634
Advance directives, role of, 634
Adverse events, 21
Adynamic ileus, GBS and, 482
Aerodigestive tract colonization, of bacteria,
    prevention of, 311
AFC. *see* Alveolar fluid clearance (AFC)
AFFIRM trial. *see* Atrial Fibrillation
    Follow-up Investigation of Rhythm
    Management (AFFIRM) trial
Afterload, 172
Agitation, after TBI, 445
Airspace mechanics, 212–213

Airway, stroke and, 462–463
Airway management, morbid obesity and,
    144–151
Airway occlusion pressure, 47
Airway opening pressure (PAo), 45
Airway pressure release ventilation (APRV),
    in ARDS, 201
AIS. *see* Acute ischemic stroke
AKI. *see* Acute kidney injury (AKI)
AKIN. *see* Acute Kidney Injury Network
    (AKIN)
ALBIOS. *see* Albumin Italian Outcome
    Sepsis (ALBIOS) study
Albumin, 410
    administration of, 564
Albumin Italian Outcome Sepsis (ALBIOS)
    study, 126, 392
Albuminocytologic dissociation, 475
Alcohol, 526
    elevated lactate and, 421
    sepsis and, 75
ALF. *see* Acute liver failure (ALF)
ALF Early Dynamic (ALFED) model,
    498–499
ALFED model. *see* ALF Early Dynamic
    (ALFED) model
Alfentanil, for morbid obesity, 148
Algorithm, definition of, 160
Algorithms for Critical Care Enteral and
    Parenteral Therapy (ACCEPT) trial, 489
ALI/ARDS. *see* Acute lung injury/acute
    respiratory distress syndrome
Allergic interstitial nephritis (AIN), 389–390
Almitrine, 231
Alveolar dead space, 43
Alveolar edema, 229–230
Alveolar fluid clearance (AFC)
    for ARDS, 205
    maximizing, 230–232
Alveolar overdistension, 61
Alveolar-capillary barrier dysfunction, in
    ARDS, 191
Alveolar-capillary membrane, 191
Amanita phalloides, 499
American Association for Thoracic Surgery,
    postoperative atrial fibrillation
    prevention guidelines, 363
American College of Critical Care Medicine
    (ACCM), 118
American College of Emergency Physicians
    (ACEP), F-TTE and, 88
American Society of Echocardiography
    (ASE), F-TTE and, 88
American Spinal Injury Association (ASIA),
    583, 584t
American Thoracic Society (ATS), 267, 269
American-European Consensus Conference
    (AECC)
    acute lung injury definition and, 183–184
    ARDS definition and, 183
        limitations in, 186t
        redressals in, 186t
Amino acid hypothesis, 536
Aminoglycosides, 109–110
Amiodarone, 363
Ammonia, 500
Amphotericin, 311
Anabolic hormones, 515–522
    androgens, 517–518, 518f
    growth hormone, 519–520
    insulin, 518–519
    thyroid hormones, 520
Anabolic processes, 424
Anabolism, definition of, 517
Anaerobic bacteria, 267

Analgesia
    for critical illness, 327
    epidural, for atrial fibrillation, 364
Analgesics
    for HE, 501
    for morbid obesity, 148
    for TBI, 445
Androgens, 517–518
    biosynthesis of, 518f
Anemia, 456, 464
    oxygen delivery in, mechanisms to
        increase, 596t
    postoperative outcomes of, in Jehovah's
        witnesses, 596t
Anesthetics, for TBI, 445
Aneurysmal subarachnoid hemorrhage,
    management of, 450–460
Angiotensin-converting enzyme inhibitors,
    233–234
Anhedonia, 331–332
Anion gap approach, 413–414, 413f
ANP. *see* Atrial natriuretic peptide (ANP)
Antacids, 114
Antiadhesion molecule therapy, 233
Antibiotics, 391
    for COPD, 177
    for critically ill patient, 103–111
    pharmacodynamic considerations of,
        105–106, 106t
    pharmacokinetic considerations of,
        105–106, 106t
    resistance, 106–107, 107t, 272
        minimizing, effective approaches in,
            109t
    for sepsis, 262–277
        in pregnancy, 573
    specific classes of, 107–110
Antibiotic susceptibility testing, 106–107,
    109t
Anticoagulants, 603–608
    for ARDS, 231
    for atrial fibrillation, 367–368
    intravenous direct thrombin inhibitors,
        604–605
    low-molecular-weight heparins, 604
    for morbid obesity, 149
    oral direct factor Xa inhibitors, 605–606
    oral direct thrombin inhibitors, 605
    parenteral indirect synthetic factor Xa
        inhibitors, 605
    unfractionated heparin, 603–604
    used in ICU, 606
    warfarin, 603, 604t
Antiepileptic drug (AED), 452
Anti-factor Xa, 149
Antifibrinolytic agents, 450–451, 451t
Anti-infective strategies, in iatrogenic
    disorder, 327
Anti-inflammatory therapies, 259
    for ARDS, 232–234, 239–246
Antioxidants, for ARDS, 233, 242
Antithrombin III, 231
Antithrombotics, 464–465
Anxiety, 17
AOD. *see* Atlanto-occipital dislocation
    (AOD)
APACHE. *see* Acute Physiology and Chronic
    Health Evaluation (APACHE)
APACHE IV. *see* Acute Physiology and
    Chronic Health Evaluation IV
    (APACHE IV) model
APAP. *see* Acetaminophen (APAP)
Apixaban, for VTE, 605–606
Apoptosis, 257–258, 257f
Arachidonic acid, 232

ARDS. *see* Acute respiratory distress syndrome (ARDS)
ARDS Clinical Trial Network, 240
Argatroban, for critically ill patient, 605
ARISE trial. *see* Australasian Resuscitation in Sepsis Evaluation (ARISE) trial
ARMA. *see* Autoregressive moving average model (ARMA)
Arrhythmias
  with SAH, 456
  supraventricular, 361, 363–364
ART trial, in ARDS, 199
Arterial blood gas (ABG) analysis, 409
Arterial lactate, 419
Arterial pressure monitoring, invasive or noninvasive, 83
ASA. *see* Salicylates
ASE. *see* American Society of Echocardiography (ASE)
ASIA. *see* American Spinal Injury Association (ASIA)
Assist-control mechanical ventilation (ACV), 56
Asthma
  acute severe, permissive hypercapnia and, 205
  NIV for, 39
Asynchrony, 48, 48f
ATC. *see* Automatic tube compensation (ATC)
Atelectasis, 62
  role of, 62
Atelectrauma, 61, 200
Atlanto-occipital dislocation (AOD), 584, 584f
Atracurium, for morbid obesity, 146, 148
Atrial fibrillation, 361–369
  hemodynamic stability with, 365–366
  pathogenesis of, 361, 362t
  rate control *vs.* rhythm control, 362t
  risk factors for, 361, 362t
Atrial Fibrillation Follow-up Investigation of Rhythm Management (AFFIRM) trial, 365
Atrial natriuretic peptide (ANP), 394
Atrial pacing, 364
Atrial septostomy, 376
ATS. *see* American Thoracic Society (ATS)
Atypical respiratory infections, 75
Australasian Resuscitation in Sepsis Evaluation (ARISE) trial, 84, 264–265
Autoimmune hepatitis, 499
Automated weaning, 56
Automatic tube compensation (ATC), 55–56
Autonomic dysfunction, 330–334
  critical illness in, 330–331
    cardiovascular dysfunction, 332–333
    immune dysfunction, 333
    modern critical care strategies for, 331–332
    onset of, 331, 332f
  definition of, 330, 331t
  spinal cord injury and, 589
Auto-PEEP. *see* Auto-positive end-expiratory pressure (auto-PEEP)
Auto-positive end-expiratory pressure (auto-PEEP), 94, 178
Autoregressive moving average model (ARMA), 62, 205
Autoregulation, 278
"Auto-regulation zone", 278
Awakening and Breathing Controlled Trials, 539
Azotemia, 400

B
BAL. *see* Bronchoalveolar lavage (BAL)
BALTI. *see* Beta-Agonist Lung Injury Trial (BALTI)
Barbiturates, for morbid obesity, 146
Baroreflex control, loss of, 331
Barotrauma, 61, 200
Base deficit gap, 415t
BEAT examination. *see* Bedside Echocardiographic Assessment in Trauma/Critical Care (BEAT) examination
Bed availability, impact on outcome, 617–618, 618f
Bed rest, 327
Bedside Echocardiographic Assessment in Trauma/Critical Care (BEAT) examination, 89
Benchmark Evidence from South American Trials: Treatment of Intracranial Pressure (BEST TRIP), 434, 437
Benzodiazepine
  for delirium, 539
  for morbid obesity, 148
  for status epilepticus (SE), 471–472
BEST TRIP. *see* Benchmark Evidence from South American Trials: Treatment of Intracranial Pressure (BEST TRIP)
Beta agonists, inhaled, 77–78
Beta blockers
  for atrial fibrillation, 362–363
  HHS from, 526
  for hypertension, 356
  withdrawal from, 358
Beta-2 adrenoreceptor agonists, for ARDS, 243
Beta-Agonist Lung Injury Trial (BALTI), 243
Beta-hydroxybutyrate, 523
Bickerstaff brainstem encephalitis, 475
Biotrauma, 61
Bivalirudin, for critically ill patient, 604–605
Blood clot integrity, 115
Blood cultures, 263, 573
Blood flow, distribution of, 213
Blood glucose, in intensive care unit, 128–132
  presentation of available data based on systematic review, 129–130
Blood glucose control
  by intensive insulin therapy, RCTs in, 129, 129t
    interpretation of data in, 130–131
  outcomes of, 302
Blood pressure
  control of, 463
  systemic, 441
Blood transfusion. *see* Transfusion
BNP. *see* B-type natriuretic peptide (BNP)
Body temperature, 118
  AIS and, 464
Brain Trauma Foundation (BTF), 433
British Thoracic Society (BTS), 267
Bronchoalveolar lavage (BAL), 239
Bronchodilators, for chronic obstructive pulmonary disease, 176–177
Bronchoscopy, flexible, NIV and, 38
BTF. *see* Brain Trauma Foundation (BTF)
BTS. *see* British Thoracic Society (BTS)
B-type natriuretic peptide (BNP), 53
Buffering, permissive hypercapnia and, 208
Bundles
  definition of, 297
  need of, in severe sepsis, 297–299
  in septic shock, 297–299
  in severe sepsis, 297–299
  Surviving Sepsis Campaign, 298t
    application of, 297–298, 298f

BUN-to-creatinine ratio, 390–391
Burns, 556–562
  cardiac performance in, 556
  elevated lactate and, 421
  estimation of, size, 557f
  fluid resuscitation for, 556–558, 557f, 557t–558t
  fluid therapy for, 126
  glucose control in, 560
  hormonal and endocrine response, modulation of, 560
  infection/sepsis in, 558, 558t
  inhalation injury in, 558
  initial assessment and emergency treatment of, 556
  metabolic response and nutritional support, 559–560, 559t
  wound excision with, 559

C
CABG. *see* Coronary artery bypass graft (CABG)
Calcium channel blockers, 363, 454
  for AKI, 393
CAM-ICU. *see* Confusion Assessment Method for Intensive Care Unit (CAM-ICU)
cAMP. *see* Cyclic adenosine monophosphate (cAMP)
Campylobacter jejuni, 475
Candida albicans, 272
CAP. *see* Community-acquired pneumonia (CAP)
Capillary lactate, 419–420
Capnograms, different characteristic of, 44f
Capnometry (ETCO$_2$), 43, 155
Carbapenems, 107
Carbon dioxide (CO$_2$)
  acid-base disorders and, 410
  intracellular action of, 205
  invasive and noninvasive, monitoring of, 43–45
  management of, 206t
  measurement of, partial rebreathing technique of, 44
  transcutaneous, monitoring of, 44–45
Carbon dioxide-bicarbonate (Boston) approach, 413, 413t
Carbon monoxide, cytochrome oxidase and, 337
Cardiac arrest (CA), hypothermia in, 133, 135–136, 138t–139t
Cardiac dysfunction, SAH and, 456
Cardiac failure, autonomic dysfunction and, 330–331
Cardiac function curve, 99, 100f
Cardiac function index (CFI), 85
Cardiac index, 347
Cardiac output (CO), 552
  measurement of, 84
Cardiac preload, static indices of, 99
Cardiac support, ultrafiltration for, 403
Cardiac tamponade, 95, 348–349
Cardiogenic pulmonary edema, acute, NIV for, 37–38
Cardiogenic shock (CS), 95, 347–352, 348f, 547
  causes of, 348t
  definition of, 347
  diagnosis of, 347
  elevated lactate and, 421
  epidemiology and etiology of, 347–349, 348t
  evidence-based approach, 349–351
  mechanical therapy for, 349–350

Cardiogenic shock *(Continued)*
  pharmacologic therapy for, 349
  revascularization therapy for, 350–351
  treatment of, 95, 96f
Cardiomyopathy, SAH and, 456
Cardiopulmonary arrest, F-TTE during, 88
Cardiovascular hypertensive emergencies,
  356–357, 356t
Cardiovascular system
  ACS and, 552
  dysfunction of, autonomic dysfunction
    and, 332–333
  hypercapnia and, 204
  IAH and, 552
  metabolism and, 425
Cardioversion, 367–368
Caregivers, workload in intensive care unit,
  623–624
Carotid endarterectomy (CEA), 357
CARS. *see* Compensatory anti-inflammatory
  response syndrome (CARS)
CAST. *see* Chinese Acute Stroke Trial (CAST)
Catabolic processes, 424
Catabolism, 424
  definition of, 517
Catecholamine, 134, 331, 333, 356t, 357–358
  overload, 288–289
Catheter-based embolectomy, 172
Catheter-related bloodstream infection
  (CRBSI), 305–310
  diagnosis of, 307
  incidence of, 307
  organisms identified in, 307
  pathogenesis of, 307
  prevention of, 308–309
  reducing, central line "bundle", 308t
  risk factors for, 308
CBF. *see* Cerebral blood flow (CBF)
CBFV. *see* Cerebral blood flow velocity
  (CBFV)
CDAD. *see* Clostridium difficile-associated
  diarrhea (CDAD)
CDH. *see* Congenital diaphragmatic hernia
  (CDH)
CEA. *see* Carotid endarterectomy (CEA)
Cecal ligation and puncture (CLP),
  335–336
cEEG. *see* Continuous
  electroencephalography (cEEG)
Cell-mediated immunity, metabolism and,
  426
Central nervous system (CNS)
  ACS and, 553
  hypercapnia and, 205
  IAP and, 553
Central venous pressure (CVP), 6, 83–84,
  229, 553
  CS and, 348–349, 349f
  hypothermia and, 134
Cephalosporins, third-generation, 311
Cerebellar infarction, 466
Cerebral autoregulation, 442, 536
Cerebral blood flow (CBF), 442
Cerebral blood flow velocity (CBFV), 453
Cerebral edema, 498, 524
  HE and, 499–500
Cerebral hyperperfusion syndrome, 357
Cerebral perfusion pressure (CPP), 442
  ACS and, 552
  maintenance of, 501
Cerebrospinal fluid (CSF), 443, 452
CESAR trial. *see* Conventional Ventilation
  for Severe Adult Respiratory Failure
  (CESAR) trial
CFI. *see* Cardiac function index (CFI)

CGAO-REA (Computerized Glucose
  Control in Critically Ill Patients) study,
  129
cGMP. *see* Cyclic guanosine monophosphate
  (cGMP)
CHD. *see* Congenital heart disease (CHD)
Checklist for Lung Injury Prevention (CLIP),
  77
CHF. *see* Congestive heart failure (CHF)
Chinese Acute Stroke Trial (CAST), 464
Chlorhexidine, for catheter-related
  bloodstream infection, 308
Cholesterol, 517
Cholestyramine, 528t
Cholinergic deficiency hypothesis, 536
Chronic critical illness (CCI), 284
  definition of, 328
Chronic obstructive pulmonary disease
  (COPD)
  exacerbations of, 37
    assisted ventilation for, 177–178
    end-of-life decisions in, 179
    in intensive care unit, 175–180
    management of, 176–177
    outcomes, 178–179
    oxygen therapy for, 177
    prognosis of, 178–179
    prognostic indicators in, 176
  extubating patients with, 38
  permissive hypercapnia and, 207
  prevalence of, 175
  respiratory failure in, 175–176
  precipitants of, 175–176
CI-AKI. *see* Contrast-induced acute kidney
  injury (CI-AKI)
Circulation
  monitoring-defined assessment of, 99–102
  tools to optimize, 99–102
Clevidipine, 354t, 357
Clinical microbiology laboratory, role in
  sepsis, 263–264
Clinical observational data, for critical care
  outcomes, 11
Clinical Randomization of an
  Antifibrinolytic in Significant
  Hemorrhage 2 (CRASH-2) trial, 600
Clinical trials, in extracorporeal life support
  (ECLS) for acute respiratory distress
  syndrome, 69–72
  protocols for, 67–68
CLIP. *see* Checklist for Lung Injury
  Prevention (CLIP)
Clonidine, 358
Clostridium difficile infection, 116, 511
Clostridium difficile-associated diarrhea
  (CDAD), 270
Clotting factor replacement, in hemorrhagic
  trauma, 565t–566t
CLP. *see* Cecal ligation and puncture (CLP)
CNS. *see* Central nervous system (CNS)
Cocaine, 526
Cockcroft-Gault (CG) equation, 395
Cognitive impairment, 16–17
Colchicine, for atrial fibrillation, 364
COlchicine for Prevention of
  Postcardiotomy Syndrome (COPPS-1)
  trial, 364
Colistin, 110, 311
Colloid osmotic pressure (COP), 191
Colloids, 124
Community-acquired pneumonia (CAP),
  265, 267–268
Compartment syndrome, 553. *see also*
  Abdominal compartment
  syndrome (ACS)

Compensated shock, 563
Compensatory anti-inflammatory response
  syndrome (CARS), 256–257
Complement receptor 1, 232
Compliance, decreased, in ARDS, 192
Compliance, Respiratory rate, arterial
  Oxygenation, and maximal inspiratory
  Pressure (CROP) index, 54
Computed tomography angiography (CTA),
  453
Computed tomography (CT)
  for acute ischemic infarct of cerebellar
    hemisphere, 466f
  for ARDS, 185, 195, 196f
  for cervical spine trauma, 583
  for HE, 500
  of lung, in ARDS, 326, 326f
  of middle cerebral artery, 465f
  for pulmonary embolism, 171
  for respiratory function, 49
Computer technology
  to advise physicians, 160–161
  in implementation of sepsis management
    guidelines, 161f–163f, 162–164
  role of, in medicine, 161
Computerized algorithms
  development and implementation of, 163f
  in managing critically ill patient, 160–166
  as models of medical reasoning, 161–162
  protocols and, 162–164, 163f
Computerized Patient Record System
  (CPRS), 161
Computerized protocols, 160
  to guide shock resuscitation of trauma
    patients, 162
Concentration-dependent killing kinetics, of
  antibiotic, 105
Confusion Assessment Method for Intensive
  Care Unit (CAM-ICU), 537, 537f
Congenital diaphragmatic hernia (CDH),
  207
Congenital heart disease (CHD), 207
Congestive heart failure (CHF), 499
Continuous electroencephalography (cEEG),
  453–454
Continuous positive airway pressure
  (CPAP), 56, 199
Continuous renal replacement therapy
  (CRRT), 395, 503
  anticoagulation types of, 404
  IHD *vs.*, 403
Continuous veno-venous-hemodiafiltration
  (CVVHDF), 402–403
Contrast-induced acute kidney injury
  (CI-AKI), 392
Conventional Ventilation for Severe Adult
  Respiratory Failure (CESAR) trial, 67t,
  69–70
Cooling methods, 133–134
COP. *see* Colloid osmotic pressure (COP)
COPD. *see* Chronic obstructive pulmonary
  disease (COPD)
COPPS-1 trial. *see* COlchicine for Prevention
  of Postcardiotomy Syndrome
  (COPPS-1) trial
Coronary artery bypass graft (CABG), 347,
  362
Corticosteroids, 447
  for ALF, 499
  for atrial fibrillation, 364
  for COPD, 176
Cortisol, 529
  gluconeogenesis and, 128
CPAP. *see* Continuous positive airway
  pressure (CPAP)

CPP. *see* Cerebral perfusion pressure (CPP)
CPRS. *see* Computerized Patient Record System (CPRS)
Craniotomy, 356
CRASH-2 trial. *see* Clinical Randomization of an Antifibrinolytic in Significant Hemorrhage 2 (CRASH-2) trial
CRBSI. *see* Catheter-related bloodstream infection (CRBSI)
CRISTAL trial, 124–125, 125t
Critical care medicine, 11
Critical care outcomes, 11–15
  in critically ill populations, 11, 12t
  mortality and, 12–13
  sources of data for, 11
    administrative data, 11
    clinical observational data, 11
Critical Care Outreach Teams, 23
Critical care resources, 609–615
  elimination in, 613
  need in, 613
Critical illness
  chronic, definition of, 328
  critical care *vs.*, 1–7, 4f
  inflammation and, 4
    biologic perspectives, 4
    therapeutic perspectives, 4–6
  persistent, as iatrogenic disorder, 323–329
  specific, trends for, 12–13
  survivors of, problems of, 16–17
    compensation, 19
    consequences of, 17–18
    enhancement, 19
    prevention of, 18
    protection, 18
    remediation, 18
    treatment, 18
CROP index. *see* Compliance, Respiratory rate, arterial Oxygenation, and maximal inspiratory Pressure (CROP) index
CRRT. *see* Continuous renal replacement therapy (CRRT)
Cryoprecipitate, transfusion of, 598, 598t
Crystalloids, 124, 573
  for fluid resuscitation, 563–564
CS. *see* Cardiogenic shock (CS)
CSF. *see* Cerebrospinal fluid (CSF)
CT. *see* Computed tomography (CT)
CTA. *see* Computed tomography angiography (CTA)
Culture
  as aid to empirical antibiotic therapy, 263
  end-of-life care and, 633–634
CURB-65 score, 176
CVP. *see* Central venous pressure (CVP)
CVVHDF. *see* Continuous veno-venous-hemodiafiltration (CVVHDF)
Cyclic adenosine monophosphate (cAMP), 221
Cyclic guanosine monophosphate (cGMP), 220
CYP3A4, 146–148
Cystatin C, 385, 391
Cytochrome, 146–148
Cytochrome oxidase (complex IV), 335–336
  metabolic downregulation and, 336–337
  suspended animation and, 337
Cytokines, gluconeogenesis and, 128

D
"Da Nang lung", 563
Dabigatran etexilate, for VTE, 605
DAD. *see* Diffuse alveolar damage (DAD)
Damage control resuscitation, 564–567

Daptomycin, 109
Data sources, for critical care outcomes, 11
  administrative data, 11
  clinical observational data, 11
DCI. *see* Delayed cerebral ischemia (DCI)
Dead space, in ARDS, 192
DECAF score, 176
Decision making
  communication strategies and skill in, 635–636
  patient preferences for surrogate latitude in, 635
  surrogate preference for, 634–635
Decompensation, hemodynamic
  in critically ill patients, 92–98
  targets of treatment of, 92
Decompressive craniectomy, 444
Decongestive agents, characteristics of, 345t
Deep vein thrombosis (DVT), 169
  GBS and, 482
  prophylaxis for, morbid obesity and, 146, 147t–148t
De-escalation, 273
Delayed cerebral ischemia (DCI), 453–454
Delayed ischemic neurologic deficits (DINDs), 453, 455t
Delirium, 533–542
  amino acid hypothesis in, 536
  awakening and breathing controlled trial for, 539
  benzodiazepine for, 539
  cholinergic deficiency hypothesis in, 536
  definition of, 535
  exercise and early mobility, 539, 540f
  impaired oxidative metabolism in, 536–537
  management of, 539
  monoamine axis hypothesis in, 536
  neuroinflammatory response hypothesis in, 536
  pathogenesis of, 535–536
  pharmacologic intervention, 539–541
  primary prevention, 538–539
  recognition of, 537–538
  risk factors of, 535, 536t
  spontaneous breathing trials for, 539
Delirium protocol, 540f
Delta up (dUp), 92–93
Deoxyhemoglobin slope (DeO₂), 292
Depression, 17
Dexamethasone in Cardiac Surgery (DECS), 364
Dexmedetomidine, 445
Diabetes mellitus, ARDS and, 75
Diabetic ketoacidosis (DKA), 523–525
  clinical presentation, 523
  complications of, 524–525
  diagnostic criteria for, 524t
  fluid and electrolyte replacement for, 523–524
  HHS and, 525–526
  insulin therapy for, 524
  pathophysiology of, 523
  precipitating factors of, 524
  therapy for, 523–524
Diagnostic and Statistical Manual of Mental Disorders (DSM-V), delirium definition, 535
Dialysis, renal acidosis and, 412
Diaspirin cross-linked Hb, 564
Diazepam, for SE, 471–472
Diffuse alveolar damage (DAD), 192
Digital subtraction angiography (DSA), 453
Digoxin, 363, 578
Diltiazem, 527, 528t

DINDs. *see* Delayed ischemic neurologic deficits (DINDs)
Direct lung injury, 241–242
Direct thrombin inhibitors (DTIs)
  intravenous, 604–605
  oral, 605
Distributive shock, 503
Diuretics
  loop
    for AHF, 344, 345t
    for AKI, 392, 394
  thiazide, 526
DKA. *see* Diabetic ketoacidosis (DKA)
DNAR. *see* Do-not-attempt-resuscitation (DNAR)
Dobutamine, 286–287
  for AHF, 345
Docosahexaenoic acid, 232
Do-not-attempt-resuscitation (DNAR), 634
Dopamine, 285–286
  for AHF, 345
  for AKI, 392
Dopamine-resistant septic shock (DRSS), 286
Dorsal perfusion, predominance of, 214
Dosing weight correction factor (DWCF), 146
Douglas bag method, 43
Doxycycline, 105–106
DRSS. *see* Dopamine-resistant septic shock (DRSS)
Drug(s)
  elevated lactate and, 421
  withdrawal, 358
DSA. *see* Digital subtraction angiography (DSA)
DTIs. *see* Direct thrombin inhibitors (DTIs)
Durotomy, 444
DVT. *see* Deep vein thrombosis (DVT)
Dynamic pressure-time curve, 45

E
Early Acute Lung Injury Score, 77
Early goal-directed therapy (EGDT), 8, 84, 251, 264, 280, 420
  outcomes of, 302
Early *versus* Delayed Enteral nutrition (EDEN) study, 488–489
Early warning scores, 22–23
  adverse events, 21
  help identify patients at risk, 21–23
  for outcome improvement, 21–28
EARLYDRAIN trial, 452
ECCO₂R. *see* Extracorporeal carbon dioxide removal (ECCO₂R)
Echocardiography, 172, 348, 371
  for cardiogenic shock, 95
  in hemodynamic monitoring, 83
  in management of critically ill, 88–91
ECLS. *see* Extracorporeal life support (ECLS)
ECMO. *see* Extracorporeal membrane oxygenation (ECMO)
EDEN. *see* Early *versus* Delayed Enteral nutrition (EDEN) study
EEG. *see* Electroencephalogram (EEG)
EELV. *see* End-expiratory lung volume (EELV)
Effector cell inhibition, for ARDS, 233
Efficacy of Volume Substitution and Insulin Therapy in Severe Sepsis (VISEP) trial, 129, 519
EGDT. *see* Early goal-directed therapy (EGDT)
EGF. *see* Epidermal growth factor (EGF)
EGOS. *see* Erasmus GBS Outcome Score (EGOS)

EGRIS. *see* Erasmus GBS Respiratory Insufficiency Score (EGRIS)
Eicosanoids, 232
Eicosapentaenoic acid, 232
Electrical impedance tomography, 49
Electroencephalogram (EEG), for status epilepticus, 470
Electrolyte disorders, in hypothermia, 134
Electrolytes
    AKI and, 394–395
    for DKA, 523–524
    for HHS, 525
    metabolism and, 425
Electron transport system (ETS), 335
Electronic medical record (EMR), 160
Emotional support, provision of, 636
Empirical antibiotic therapy
    assays to guide, 264
    of community-acquired IAIs, 271
    Gram stain and culture as an aid to, 263
    for ICU infections, 108t, 110t
    rapid microbiological diagnostics to, role of, 263–264
    selection, 266–272
    for sepsis, 262–277
Empirical antifungal therapy, 271–272
EMR. *see* Electronic medical record (EMR)
Enalapril, 354t
End-expiratory lung volume (EELV), 48
End-expiratory occlusion test, 100, 100f–101f
Endocrine system
    emergencies with, 523–532
    metabolism and, 426
Endothelial repair, ARDS and, 230–231
Endothelin receptor antagonists, 376
Endothelin-1, 231
Endotracheal intubation, 33–34
    potential indications for, 34t
Endovascular Treatment for Small Core and Proximal Occlusion Ischemic Stroke (ESCAPE) trial, 462
Endpoints resuscitation, in trauma, 563, 565t–566t, 567
Enteral nutrition, 115–116
    early, 489–490
    vs. delayed, 488–489
    hypocaloric nutrition and, 487
    randomized controlled trials of, 489–490
EOLIA trial, 71
Epidermal growth factor (EGF), 512
Epidural analgesia, for atrial fibrillation, 364
Epilepsia partialis continua, 470
Epinephrine, 287
Epithelial cells, 511f, 512
Epithelial repair , ARDS and, 230–231
Epoprostenol, 376
Epsilon-aminocaproic acid, 450–451
Erasmus GBS Outcome Score (EGOS), 477, 479t, 480f
Erasmus GBS Respiratory Insufficiency Score (EGRIS), 475, 479t
ESCAPE trial. *see* Endovascular Treatment for Small Core and Proximal Occlusion Ischemic Stroke (ESCAPE) trial
Escherichia coli, 266–267, 336
Esmolol, 354t, 528t
Esophageal pressure, 47
Ethnicity, end-of-life care and, 633–634
Evidence-based medicine, 8–10
    accountability in, 9
    do less, not more, 9
    it is not just the intensivist, 9
    single randomized controlled trials, 8–9
    small things make a big difference, 9
EVLW. *see* Extravascular lung water (EVLW)

Excretory impairment, incidence of, 495
Expiratory reserve volume, 145
External cooling, for fever, 119
Extracellular volume, reduction of, in AHF, 344–345
Extracorporeal blood purification, 402
Extracorporeal carbon dioxide removal (ECCO$_2$R), 67t, 69, 208
Extracorporeal life support (ECLS)
    for acute respiratory distress syndrome, 66–74
        clinical trial for, 69–72
        economic feasibility, 69
        history of patient survival in, 68–69
        insufficient critical care evidence, 66–67
        meta-analysis of, 71f
        protocols for clinical trials, 67–68
        randomized controlled trial (RCT), 66, 67t
    criteria for, 69
    principles and objectives of, 69
Extracorporeal membrane oxygenation (ECMO), 67t, 68, 207, 349–350, 575
    HFOV and, 200
Extravascular lung water (EVLW), 229
    measurement of, 48
Extubation, 56

F

Facilitation therapy, 57–58
Family ICU syndrome, 18
FATE examination. *see* Focused Assessed Transthoracic Echocardiography (FATE) examination
Fenoldopam, 354t
    for AKI, 392, 394
Fentanyl, for morbid obesity, 148
Fever, 118–123
    with ALF, 502
    control of
        neurologic critically ill patients, 120t
        nonneurologic critically ill patients, 120t
        RCTs for, 118–122, 122t
    in critically ill patients
        large-scale observational studies assessing, 121–122, 121t
        ongoing RCT assessing, 121–122, 122t
    definition of, 118–119
    with SAH, 456
    TBI and, 445
FFAs. *see* Free fatty acids (FFAs)
FFP. *see* Fresh frozen plasma (FFP)
Filtration gradient, 553
Flexible bronchoscopy, NIV and, 38
Flow-volume loop, characteristics of, 48, 49f
Fluctuating blood pressure, GBS and, 481
Fluid
    administration of, algorithm of, 101f
    for critical illness, 327
    management of, in trauma, 563–570
    metabolism and, 425
Fluid challenge, 100, 100f
Fluid resuscitation
    for burns, 556–558, 557f
        adult, 557t
        pediatric, 558t
    crystalloids for, 563–564
    for DKA, 523–524
    formulas for estimating of, 557t
    for HHS, 525
    in sepsis, 4–5
    for trauma, 563
        uncontrolled, 565t–566t

Fluid therapy
    for burn injury, 126
    for critically ill patients, 124–127
    for general ICU patients, 124–125, 125t
    for hemorrhagic shock, 126
    for sepsis, 125–126
    for trauma, 126
Focused Assessed Transthoracic Echocardiography (FATE) examination, 88
Focused bedside transthoracic echocardiography (F-TTE), 88
    during cardiopulmonary arrest, 88
    case scenarios in, 89–90
    case stem in, 89–90, 90f
    future in, 89
    history of, 88
    in postcardiac surgery patient, 89
    training in, 89
    in trauma and surgical ICU, 89
Fondaparinux, for HIT, 605
Fosphenytoin, for SE, 472–473
Fraction of inspired oxygen (F$_i$O$_2$), 32, 68–69
Fractional excretion of sodium (FeNa), 390
Fractional excretion of urea (FeUN), 390
Frank hypotension, 463
"Frank-Starling" approach, 293–294
FRC. *see* Functional residual capacity (FRC)
Free fatty acids (FFAs), ARDS and, 242
Fresh frozen plasma (FFP), 597
F-TTE. *see* Focused bedside transthoracic echocardiography (F-TTE)
Functional residual capacity (FRC), 48, 145, 212
Fungi, 264

G

Gadolinium-based contrast agents, 395
Galactomannan (GM), 264
Gas exchange, monitoring of, 45
Gastric acid production, and effect of acid reduction therapy, 114f
Gastric acid secretion, 114
Gastric emptying (GE), 581
Gastric intraluminal acidity, 113
Gastric mucosal blood flow (GMBF), 287
Gastrointestinal system
    bleeding in
        acute, from gastric erosions, 327
        ALF and, 503–504
    metabolism and, 425–426
    myxedema coma and, 529
GBS. *see* Guillain-Barré syndrome (GBS)
GCSE. *see* Generalized convulsive status epilepticus (GCSE)
G-CSF. *see* Granulocyte colony-stimulating factor (G-CSF)
GDT. *see* Goal-directed therapy (GDT)
GE. *see* Gastric emptying (GE)
GEDVI. *see* Global end-diastolic volume index (GEDVI)
Generalized convulsive status epilepticus (GCSE), 452–453
GFP. *see* Glomerular filtration pressure (GFP)
GH releasing hormone (GHRH), 519
GH releasing peptide-2 (GHRP-2), 519–520
Ghrelin, 519
GHRH. *see* GH releasing hormone (GHRH)
GHRP-2. *see* GH releasing peptide-2 (GHRP-2)
GIK. *see* Glucose-insulin-potassium (GIK)
Glasgow Outcome Scale (GOS), in intracranial pressure, 431
GLD. *see* Good lung down (GLD)

Global end-diastolic volume index (GEDVI), 85

Global Initiative for Chronic Obstructive Lung Disease (GOLD), 177

Glomerular filtration pressure (GFP), 553

Glomerular filtration rate (GFR), 383

β-Glucan, 264

Glucocorticoids
   for ARDS, 232
   HHS from, 526

Gluconeogenesis, 128

GluControl trial, 129, 519

Glucose
   blood, 128–132
   control, in burns, 560

Glucose-insulin-potassium (GIK), 130

Glutamine, 500

Glycosylated proteins, 512

GMBF. see Gastric mucosal blood flow (GMBF)

GM-CSF. see Granulocyte-macrophage colony-stimulating factor (GM-CSF)

GnRH. see Gonadotropin-releasing hormone (GnRH)

Goal-directed therapy (GDT), 616, 617f

Gonadotropin-releasing hormone (GnRH), 517

Good lung down (GLD), 213

GOS. see Glasgow outcome scale (GOS)

G-protein-coupled receptor (GPCR) recycling, disruption of, 330

GRADE system, for traumatic brain injury, 442t

Gram stain, 263

Granulocyte colony-stimulating factor (G-CSF), 301–302

Granulocyte-macrophage colony-stimulating factor (GM-CSF), 233, 259

Growth factors
   KGF, 230
   TGF-α, 230
   VEGF, 230

Growth hormone (GH), 519–520

Guanethidine, 528t

Guanosine 5′-triphosphate, 220

Guillain-Barré syndrome (GBS), 475–484
   clinical features of, 477t
   diagnosis of, 475, 477t–478t
   immunopathogenesis of, 476f
   management of, 478–482
      immunotherapy, 481–482
      monitoring, 478–480
      temporary pacing, indication for, 481
      ventilatory, 480–481
   mortality in, 477
   pathogenesis of, 475
   poor long-term outcome of, 477
   predictors of, 475–477
      mechanical ventilation, 475–476
   supportive treatment of, 482

Gut, 510–514
   alterations in intestinal integrity, 512
   critical illness in, 512
      role of intestinal lymph in, 512
   definitions of, 510
   epithelial layer, 512
   intestinal integrity, 512
   microbiome for therapeutic benefit in, 510–511

H

H1N1 epidemic, in acute respiratory distress syndrome, 68

H$_2$ blockers, for morbid obesity, 146

H$_2$-receptor antagonists, 114

Haloperidol, 148
   for delirium, 539

HARP-2 trial, for ARDS, 242

HBOCs. see Hemoglobin-based oxygen carriers (HBOCs)

HDU. see High dependency unit (HDU)

HE. see Hepatic encephalopathy (HE)

Head of bed, elevation of, 214

Head-up positioning, in respiratory failure, 213

Health-care associated infections (HAIs), prevention of, 308

Health-care-associated pneumonia, ATS and IDSA treatment guidelines for, 269

Heart failure, right, pulmonary hypertension and, 219–220

Heart monitoring, 6

Hemodialysis, for ALF, 505

Hemodynamic decompensation
   in critically ill patients, 92–98
   targets of treatment of, 92

Hemodynamic monitoring, invasive, 81–87

Hemodynamic support, for critical illness, 327

Hemofiltration
   for AHF, 344–345, 345t
   for ALF, 505

Hemoglobin-based oxygen carriers (HBOCs), 564

Hemorrhagic shock
   fluid therapy for, 126
   hypertonic saline for, 565t–566t
   pathophysiology of, 563–564
   transfusion for, 564, 565t–566t
   uncontrolled, 567–568

Hemostatic resuscitation, 564–567

Heparin-induced thrombocytopenia (HIT), 604

Hepatectomy, 505

Hepatic encephalopathy (HE), 499–502
   grades of, 500t
   treatment of, 500–502

Hepatic gluconeogenesis, 425

Hepatobiliary transport systems, 495

Hepatocellular excretory dysfunction, 494–495

HFOV. see High frequency oscillation ventilation (HFOV)

HHS. see Hyperosmolar hyperglycemic state (HHS)

Hibernation, 258, 335
   cardiac function during, 336
   sepsis and, 336–337

Hibernation-like state, in sepsis, 336–337

HIE. see Hypoxic-ischemic encephalopathy (HIE)

High dependency unit (HDU), postoperative monitoring in, 619

High frequency oscillation ventilation (HFOV), for ARDS, 200

High output respiratory syndrome, 326

High vasopressor load, effect of, 279

HIT. see Heparin-induced thrombocytopenia (HIT)

HMG CoA. see 3-Hydroxy-3-methylglutaryl-coenzyme A (HMG CoA)

Hydralazine, 354t

Hydration status, in AKI, 384

Hydrocephalus, 452

Hydrocortisone, 528t
   for septic shock, 8–9

Hydrogen sulfide (H$_2$S), 337

3-Hydroxy-3-methylglutaryl-coenzyme A (HMG CoA), 233

Hypercapnea, in chronic obstructive pulmonary disease, 175

Hypercapnia, 62–63
   physiology and molecular biology of, 204–205, 206f

Hypercapnic acidosis, 204
   ARDS and, 75

Hypercarbia, 32–33
   symptoms and signs of, 31, 32t

Hypercarbic ventilatory failure, 31
   causes of, 32t

Hyperchloremic acidosis, clinical relevance of, 412

Hyperglycemia, 128, 463–464
   pathophysiology and mechanism of action of, 128
   stress, 128

Hyperkalemia, with RRT, 399

Hyperlactatemia, 419

Hypernatremia, 134

Hyperosmolar hyperglycemic state (HHS), 525–526
   clinical presentation of, 525
   complications with, 526
   diagnostic criteria for, 525–526
   fluid and electrolyte replacement for, 525
   pathophysiology of, 525
   precipitating factors for, 526
   therapy for, 525–526

Hyperosmolar therapy, for TBI, 444

Hyperphosphatemia, AKI and, 395

Hyperpyrexia, 528

Hypertension, 353–360
   with acute coronary syndrome, 356–357
   after carotid revascularization, 357
   after craniotomy, 356
   with aortic dissection, 357
   with left heart failure, 356–357
   in perioperative period, 357
   SE and, 471

Hypertensive crisis
   classification of, 353
   drugs for, 354t

Hypertensive emergency, 353, 354t
   cardiovascular, 356–357, 356t
   catecholamine and, 354t, 356t, 357–358
   clinical features of, 353–358
   neurologic, 353–356, 355t
   renal, 357

Hyperthermia, SE and, 471

Hyperthyroidism, 526

Hypertonic saline, for ALF, 501–502

Hyperventilation, 502
   in TBI, 443–444

Hypoalbuminemia, ARDS and, 75

Hypocalcemia, 134
   AKI and, 395

Hypocaloric nutrition, 487–488
   for morbid obesity, 149–150

Hypoglycemia, 464
   myxedema coma and, 529
   neuroglycopenia and, 130
   SE and, 471

Hypokalemia, 134

Hypomagnesemia, 134, 454

Hyponatremia, 529
   with SAH, 454

Hypoperfusion, 112

Hypophosphatemia, 134

Hypotension, 441
   AKI and, 392
   myxedema coma and, 529
   orthostatic, after spinal cord injury, 589
   pulmonary embolism and, 170
   right ventricle dysfunction and, 172

Hypotension (*Continued*)
  SE and, 471
  sepsis-induced, 572
  vasopressors and, 284–285
Hypothermia, 133–143, 445
  after spinal cord injury, 588
  for ALF, 504
  for ARDS, 234
  in cardiac arrest, 135–136, 138t–139t
  cooling methods and, 133–134
  for hypoxic-ischemic encephalopathy, 137–139
  for ischemic stroke, 136, 138t–139t
  mechanism of action of, 134–135
  for myocardial infarction, 137
  myxedema coma and, 529
  for percutaneous coronary intervention, 137
  for spinal cord injury, 136–137
  temperature monitoring with, 133
  therapeutic, 138t–139t
    complications associated with, 134
  for traumatic brain injury, 137, 138t–139t
Hypothyroidism, 529
Hypoventilation, 529
Hypovolemia, 92–94
Hypovolemic shock, 92, 546
  treatment of, 93–94
Hypoxemia, 32, 192, 441
  ARDS and, 183
  myxedema coma and, 529
Hypoxemic respiratory failure, 31
  causes of, 32t
Hypoxia, symptoms and signs of, 31, 32t
Hypoxic-ischemic encephalopathy (HIE), hypothermia for, 137–139, 138t–139t
Hysteresis, 45

I

IABPs. *see* Intraaortic balloon pumps (IABPs)
IAH. *see* Intra-abdominal hypertension (IAH)
IAIs. *see* Intra-abdominal infections (IAIs)
IAP. *see* Intra-abdominal pressure (IAP)
Iatrogenic disorder, 323–329
  critical illness in, 327–328
  organ dysfunction as, 325–327
Iatrogenic injury, in ARDS, 191
Ibuprofen, 119, 232
ICOPER. *see* International Cooperative Pulmonary Embolism Registry (ICOPER)
ICP. *see* Intracranial pressure (ICP)
ICU. *see* Intensive care unit (ICU)
IDSA. *see* Infectious Diseases Society of America (IDSA)
IGF-1. *see* Insulin-like growth factor-1 (IGF-1)
IGFBP-7. *see* Insulin-like growth factor binding protein-7 (IGFBP-7)
IHD. *see* Intermittent hemodiafiltration (IHD)
IIT. *see* Intensive insulin therapy (IIT)
IL-7. *see* Interleukin-7 (IL-7)
IL-10. *see* Interleukin-10 (IL-10)
IL-15. *see* Interleukin 15 (IL-15)
IL-18. *see* Interleukin-18 (IL-18)
Iloprost, 172
Imaging, for evaluation and monitoring of respiratory function, 49
Immune effector cells, apoptosis of, 257f
Immune suppression, 256–261

Immune system
  dysfunction of, 257–259
    autonomic dysfunction and, 333
    mechanisms of, 257–259, 257t
    in septic patient, 258–259
  in sepsis, 256–257
Immunocompromised patients, NIV for, 38
Immunonutrition, for ARDS, 232–233
Impaired excretory function, 494
Impaired oxidative metabolism, 536–537
Incident dark-field (IDF), 292–293
Incremental cost-effectiveness ratio, 299
Indirect lung injury, 241–242
In-dwelling catheter, infection of, 307
Ineffective triggering, asynchrony and, 48, 48f
Infection. see also *specific types of infection*
  with ALF, 502–503
  in burns, 558, 558t
  catheter-related bloodstream, 305–310
  HHS from, 526
  in-dwelling catheter, 307
Infectious Diseases Society of America (IDSA), 118, 267, 269
Inferior vena cava (IVC), 171
  bedside ultrasound of, 93
Inflammation, and critical illness, 4
  biologic perspectives, 4
  therapeutic perspectives, 4–6
Inflammatory injury, in ARDS, 190
Inflammatory response, to surgery, modulation of, 364
Inhalation injury, in burns, 558
Inhaled nitric oxide
  for ARDS, 224–226, 225f
  prostaglandin *vs.*, 226
  for pulmonary hypertension, 220
Injury severity score (ISS), 433
Innate immune cells, 256
Inotropes, 331
  for AHF, 345
INR. *see* International normalized rate (INR)
Insulin, 134, 518–519
  for AKI, 393
  for DKA, 524
  for HHS, 525–526
  meta-analyses on, 130t
  resistance, 128
  studies on, 130t
Insulin-like growth factor binding protein-7 (IGFBP-7), urinary, 386
Insulin-like growth factor-1 (IGF-1), 518–519
Integrative weaning index (IWI), 54
Intensive care delirium screening checklist, 538t
Intensive care unit (ICU), 3
  early and late effect of, on 30-day mortality, 619t
  mortality and, 616
  number of bed in, 617–618, 618f
  organization of care in, 622–625
    caregivers workload in, 623–624
    high-intensity physician staffing, 622
    hospitalists as workforce in, 623
    institutional and health system levels of, 624
    nighttime intensivist staffing, 623
    telemedicine, 623
  outcome, 616–621
  overused, 612–613
  role of practice nurse and physician assistants in, 626–630, 627t–628t
    comparison between, 627t
    selected studies on, 629t
    use of, 626–627, 628f, 630t

Intensive care unit (*Continued*)
  trends for diagnoses with variable admission to, 13
  trends for patients admitted to, 12
  underused, 611–612
Intensive insulin therapy (IIT), 5–6
  tight glucose control by, RCTs in, 129, 129t
    interpretation of data in, 130–131
Intensivists
  coping with shortage of, 623
  nonintensivists, 623
  nighttime staffing, 623
Intentional underfeeding, controlled trials of, 488
Interferon β-1a, 232
Interhospital transport, 155
  adverse effects of, 155
  adverse events during, 155
  equipment and monitoring for, 156
  mode of, 156
  mortality from, 155
  personnel selection for, 156
  planning for, 155–156
Interleukin-7 (IL-7), 260
Interleukin-10 (IL-10), 258–259
Interleukin-15 (IL-15), 512
Interleukin-18 (IL-18), 385–386, 391
Intermittent hemodiafiltration (IHD), 399
  CRRT *vs.*, 403
Intermountain Healthcare Intensive Medicine Clinical Program, 297
International Cooperative Pulmonary Embolism Registry (ICOPER), 169
International normalized rate (INR), 603
International Standards for Neurological Classification of Spinal Cord Injury (ISNICSCI), 583
International Subarachnoid Aneurysm Trial (ISAT), 451–452
Internist-I, in medical informatics, 161
Interstitial lung disease, NIV for, 40
Intestinal epithelium, 512
Intestinal microbiome, 511f
Intra-abdominal hypertension (IAH), 551
  cardiovascular system and, 552
    grading classification of, 552t
    management of, 553–554
    respiratory system and, 552
Intra-abdominal infections (IAIs), 270–271
  health-care-associated *vs.* community-acquired, 270–271
Intra-abdominal pressure (IAP)
  CNS and, 553
  renal system and, 553
Intraaortic balloon pumping (IABP), 346
Intraaortic balloon pumps (IABPs), 347
Intracellular zonula occludens, 512
Intracranial hemorrhage, 356
Intracranial hypertension, survivors of, 436
Intracranial pressure (ICP)
  ACS and, 552
  in brain-injured patients, 429–440
  CPP and, 433, 500
  elevated, treatment for, 500–502
  HE and, 500–502
  interpretation of, approaches to, 436
  magnitude of, 436
  monitoring of, 433, 501
    advantages of, 437
    center-based studies for, 433
    indications for, 432t
    management protocols in, 433
    and outcome of, 433
    patient-based studies for, 433–434
  prognosis and, 431–432

Intracranial pressure (*Continued*)
  regulation of, permissive hypercapnia and, 207
  responsive to routine treatment, 434–435
  on "second-tier" therapies, 435
  severe traumatic brain injury with, 436–437
  shortcomings of, 438t
  successful management of, 434
  threshold of, 435–436
Intrahospital transport, 154
  adverse effects of, 154
  adverse events during, 154–155
  management of, 155
  risk-to-benefit ratio of, 155
  transport ventilation during, 155
Intratidal pressure-volume loop, 45
Intravascular volume overload, 399
Intravenous direct thrombin inhibitors, 604–605
Intravenous fluids
  hyperchloremic and dilutional acidosis associated with, 411
  therapy, 325
Intravenous immunoglobulin (IVIG), for GBS, 481
Intubation
  actual need for, 31–34
    signs of, 31
    symptoms of, 31
  endotracheal, 33–34
    potential indications for, 34t
  for GBS, 480–481
  impending needs for, 31, 33–34
  indications for, in critically ill patient, 29–35
  preoxygenation before, 38
Iodine, 527
Iopanoic acid, 528t
Ipratropium, for chronic obstructive pulmonary disease, 177
ISAT. *see* International Subarachnoid Aneurysm Trial (ISAT)
Ischemic stroke, hypothermia for, 136, 138t–139t
ISNICSCI. *see* International Standards for Neurological Classification of Spinal Cord Injury (ISNICSCI)
Isotonic saline, 124
ISS. *see* Injury severity score (ISS)
IVC. *see* Inferior vena cava (IVC)
IVIG. *see* Intravenous immunoglobulin (IVIG)
IWI. *see* Integrative weaning index (IWI)

J
Jabour pressure time product, 54
Jefferson fracture, 585, 585f
Jugular bulb catheter, 446

K
Kayser-Fleischer rings, 499
KDIGO. *see* The Kidney Disease: Improving Global Outcome (KDIGO)
Keratinocyte growth factor (KGF), 230
Ketoconazole, 232
  for ARDS, 242
Kidney Disease: Improving Global Outcomes (KDIGO) classification, 384, 384t
Kidney injury molecule-1 (KIM-1), 385
KIM-1. *see* Kidney injury molecule-1 (KIM-1)
Kinetic therapy, 213
King's College criteria, 498–499

L
L1 burst fracture, 586f
Labetalol, 354t
β-Lactam/β-lactamase inhibitors (BL/BLIs), 270
β-Lactams, 107
Lactate
  clearance, 420–421
  elevated, 419
    clinical approach to, 421
  goal-directed therapy, 420–421
  measurement of, 419
    in emergency department, 420
    in intensive care unit, 420
    limitations, 421
    prehospital, 419–420
  production of, 419
D-Lactate, 419
L-Lactate isomer, 419
Lactic acidosis, 419–423
Large-scale observational studies, for fever, 121–122, 121t
LARMA trial. *see* Lisofylline and Respiratory Management of Acute Lung Injury (LARMA) trial
Lateral positioning, in respiratory failure, 213–214
Left ventricle (LV), pulmonary embolism and, 169
Left ventricular end-diastolic pressure (LVEDP), 347–348
Legionella pneumophila, 268
Leukopenia, 134
Levetiracetam, for SE, 472–473
Levosimendan, 221–222, 288, 349
  for AHF, 346
LH. *see* Luteinizing hormone (LH)
Liberation
  definition of, 52
  from mechanical ventilation, 52–60
Life support, factors withdrawing, 631–638
  clinician, 635–636
  institutional/system, 636
  patient factors, 633–634
    advance directives and advance care planning, 634
    characteristics of, 633–634
    education, 634
    language fluency, 634
    medical/health status, 633
    preferences of, 633–634
    prognosis of, 633
    religious and spiritual beliefs, 634
    socioeconomic status, 634
    values of, 633–634
  surrogate decision maker/family, 634–635
Linezolid, 108
  for MRSA, 269
γ-Linolenic acid, 232
Lipid metabolism, 425
Lipopolysaccharide (LPS), 119f
Lipopolysaccharide (LPS)-induced ARDS model, 230–231
LIPS. *see* Lung Injury Prediction Score (LIPS)
Lisofylline, 233
Lisofylline and Respiratory Management of Acute Lung Injury (LARMA) trial, for ARDS, 242–243
Lisofylline, for ARDS, 242
Listeria monocytogenes, 106
Lithium carbonate, 528t
Liver. *see also* Acute liver failure (ALF)
  acute fatty liver of pregnancy, 499
  acute-phase response and, 495–496
  alterations in, 494–496

critical illness of, 494–496
  dysfunction of, 494–495
    impact of critical care pharmacology in, 495
    manifestation in, 494–495
    mechanisms in, 494–495
  ischemic damage to, 494
  OLT, 497, 504
  support systems, 505
  transplantation of, 504
  ultrafiltration for, 404
Liver-type fatty acid binding protein, 385
Living donor liver transplantation, for ALF, 505
LMWHs. *see* Low-molecular-weight heparins (LMWHs)
Loop diuretics
  for AHF, 344, 345t
  for AKI, 392, 394
Lorazepam
  for morbid obesity, 148
  for SE, 471–472
Low left ventricular ejection fraction (LVEF), 53
"Low resistance potential" antibiotics, 105
"Low stretch" approach, for ARDS, 196, 197t
Lower driving pressures (delta P), ARDS and, 199
Low-molecular-weight heparinoids, for DVT, 482
Low-molecular-weight heparins (LMWHs), 604
  for atrial fibrillation, 366
  for morbid obesity, 149
  for pulmonary embolism, 171
LPS. *see* Lipopolysaccharide (LPS)
Lugol solution, 528t
Lung, in acute respiratory distress syndrome, 326
  computed tomography of, 326, 326f
Lung damage, minimizing, 62–64
Lung Injury Prediction Score (LIPS), 77, 77t
Lung injury score, 183
Lung recruitment maneuvers, 197–199
Lung strain, 61
Lung support, ultrafiltration for, 404
Lung ultrasound, 49
Lung volume measurement, 48
Lung-protective ventilation, for ARDS, 68, 77
Luteinizing hormone (LH), 517
LVEDP. *see* Left ventricular end-diastolic pressure (LVEDP)
LVEF. *see* Low left ventricular ejection fraction (LVEF)

M
Macrolides, for ARDS, 242–243
Magnesium, 134, 454
  for atrial fibrillation, 363–364
Magnetic resonance imaging (MRI), 453, 583–584
Malignant infarction, 465–466
Mannitol
  for ALF, 501
  for lowering ICP, 444
MAOIs. *see* Monoamine oxidase inhibitors (MAOIs)
MAP. *see* Mean arterial pressure (MAP)
MARS. *see* Molecular adsorbent recirculating system (MARS)
Massachusetts General Hospital Utility Multi Programming System (MUMPS), 161

Massive transfusion, 598–599
MATTERs II trial. *see* Military Application of Tranexamic Acid in Trauma Emergency Resuscitation (MATTERs) II trial
Maximal inspiratory pressure, 47, 53
MDAC. *see* Multiple-dose activated charcoal
MDCT. *see* Multidetector computed tomography (MDCT)
MDRD. *see* Modification of Diet in Renal Disease (MDRD) Study group
Mean arterial pressure (MAP), 92, 278, 442, 501, 572
    acute kidney injury and, 279
    autoregulation and, 278
    in controlled randomized trials, 280–281
    vasopressors and, 284–285
Mechanical therapy, for cardiogenic shock, 349–350
Mechanical ventilation, 34
    for ALF, 503
    for ARDS, 195–203
    for GBS, 479f, 480–481
    low *vs.* high tidal volume, 197t
    pregnancy and, 574–575
    SIMV, 56–57
    stroke volume variations induced by, 99–100
    weaning from, 52–60
        assessment for, 52–56
        with difficult-to-wean patient, 56–58
        spontaneous breathing trial for, 54–56
        success predictors for, 53–54, 53t
        tracheostomy and, 58
Mechanical ventilatory support, for RV failure, 373
Medical Emergency Team (MET), 23
Medical informatics, decision support and, 160–161
Medical Literature Analysis and Retrieval System (MEDLARS), 160
Medical Literature Analysis and Retrieval System Online (Medline), 160
Medical Research Council (MRC), 475
Medication dose adjustments, AKI with, 395
MEDLARS. *see* Medical Literature Analysis and Retrieval System (MEDLARS)
mEGOS. *see* Modified Erasmus GBS Outcome Score (mEGOS)
MERIT trial, 24
Messenger RNA (mRNA), 335–336
MET. *see* Medical Emergency Team (MET)
Metabolic acidosis
    acute, 411–412
        due to unmeasured anions, 411–412
    AKI and, 395, 399
Metabolic alkalosis, acute, 412–413
Metabolic concerns, ALF and, 504
Metabolic downregulation, 336–337
    mitochondria and, 335–337
Metabolism, 424–428
    burns and, 559–560, 559t
    data
        available, 426
        interpretation of, 426–427
    drug, hypothermia and, 134
    mechanism of, 424–426
    pathophysiology of, 424–426
Methicillin-resistant *Staphylococcus aureus* (MRSA)
    ALF and, 502–503
    CAP and, 267
Methimazole, 527, 528t
Methylprednisolone, 447
    for morbid obesity, 146

Methylxanthines, for chronic obstructive pulmonary disease, 177
MFS. *see* Miller Fisher syndrome (MFS)
mHLA-DR, 259
Microcirculation, 291
    alterations in, quantification of, 293
    assessment of
        direct methods, 292–293
        indirect methods, 292
    clinical examination in, 292
    monitoring, in sepsis, 291–296
        current methods, 291–292
        outcome of, 291–296
        resuscitation in, 293–294
        during sepsis, 278–279
Microcirculatory failure, manifestation of, 284
Microvascular flow index (MFI), 293
Microvascular perfusion, evaluation of, 292–293
Midazolam
    for morbid obesity, 148
    for SE, 471–472
Middle cerebral artery, computed tomography scan of, 465f
Military Application of Tranexamic Acid in Trauma Emergency Resuscitation (MATTERs) II trial, 600
Miller Fisher syndrome (MFS), 475
    clinical features of, 477t
    diagnosis of, 477t
        criteria for, 478t
Milrinone, 172
    for AHF, 345–346
Mineralocorticoid receptor antagonists (MRAs), for AHF, 344
Minute ventilation, 53
Mitochondria
    biogenesis of, 337–338
    dysfunction of, 284
    sepsis and, 335–337
Mitochondrial DNA (mtDNA), 335
Mitophagy, 338
MLCK. *see* Myosin light chain kinase (MLCK)
Modification of Diet in Renal Disease (MDRD) Study group, 146–148
Modified Denver Screening Criteria, 588, 588t
Modified Erasmus GBS Outcome Score (mEGOS), 477, 479t, 480f
MODS. *see* Multiple organ dysfunction syndrome (MODS)
Molecular adsorbent recirculating system (MARS), 404, 505
Monoamine axis hypothesis, 536
Monoamine oxidase inhibitors (MAOIs), 358
Monocyte deactivation, 333
Monotherapy, combination therapy and, 267
Morbid obesity, 144–153
    airway management and, 144–151
    anticoagulants for, 149
    deep venous thrombosis prophylaxis and, 146, 147t–148t
    diagnostic imaging for, 150, 150t
    drug dosing for, 149t
    neuromuscular blockade for, 148
    nutrition for, 149–150
    outcomes for, 150–151
    respiratory system and, 145–146
    and sepsis, 151
    trauma and, 151
Mortality, 11
    improvement of, 13–14
    trends in, 12–13

MRAs. *see* Mineralocorticoid receptor antagonists (MRAs)
MRC. *see* Medical Research Council (MRC)
MRI. *see* Magnetic resonance imaging (MRI)
mRNA. *see* Messenger RNA (mRNA)
MRSA. *see* Methicillin-resistant *Staphylococcus aureus* (MRSA)
mtDNA. *see* Mitochondrial DNA (mtDNA)
Multidetector computed tomography (MDCT), for pulmonary embolism, 171
Multiple organ dysfunction syndrome (MODS), 247–255, 325–326
    autonomic dysfunction and, 330
    RRT for, 402
Multiple-dose activated charcoal (MDAC), 581
MUMPS. *see* Massachusetts General Hospital Utility Multi Programming System (MUMPS)
Mycin, in medical informatics, 161
Myocardial depression, sepsis and, 336
Myocardial hibernation, 336
Myocardial infarction, hypothermia for, 137
Myosin light chain kinase (MLCK), 512
Myxedema coma, 529–530
    clinical presentation of, 529
    hormonal replacement therapy for, 529–530
    monitoring therapy for, 530
    pathophysiology of, 529
    precipitating factors for, 530
    therapy for, 529–530

N
NAC. *see* N-acetylcysteine (NAC)
NADH. *see* Nicotinamide adenine dinucleotide (NADH)
NAG. *see* N-acetyl-β-D-glucosaminidase (NAG)
NAPQI. *see* N-acetyl-p-benzoquinoneimine (NAPQI)
NASCIS. *see* National Acute Spinal Cord Injury Study (NASCIS)
National Acute Spinal Cord Injury Study (NASCIS), 587
National Early Warning Score (NEWS), 22, 23t
National Heart, Lung, and Blood Institute (NHLBI), 185
Natriuresis, 344
Natriuretics, for AKI, 392, 394
Near-infrared spectroscopy (NIRS), 292, 568
Neomycin, 500
Neonatal respiratory distress syndrome, 207
NephroCheck, 391
Nephrotoxic agents, 391, 392t
Nervous system, metabolism and, 425
Nesiritide, for AHF, 343, 344t
Neurocritical care society consensus guidelines, on antifibrinolytic therapy, 450–451
Neurogenic shock, 547
Neurogenic stunned myocardium, 456
Neuroinflammatory response hypothesis, 536
Neurologic hypertensive emergencies, 353–356, 355t
    vasodilator management in, 355t
Neuromuscular blockade
    ARDS and, 201, 232
    for autonomic dysfunction, 331
    for morbid obesity, 148
Neuromuscular blocking agents, for SE, 471–472

Neuromuscular disease, NIV for, 39
Neuropathic pain, in GBS, 482
Neutrophil, role of, in ARDS, 190
Neutrophil elastase inhibitors, for ALI, 243
Neutrophil gelatinase-associated lipocalin (NGAL), 385
NEWS. *see* National Early Warning Score
NF-κB. *see* Nuclear factor-κB (NF-κB)
NHLBI. *see* National Heart, Lung, and Blood Institute (NHLBI)
Nicardipine, 354t, 454
NICE SUGAR (Normoglycemia in Intensive Care Evaluation Survival Using Glucose Algorithm Regulation) trial, 5–6, 129
Nicotinamide adenine dinucleotide (NADH), 335
NIPPV. *see* Noninvasive positive pressure ventilation (NIPPV)
NIRS. *see* Near-infrared spectroscopy (NIRS)
Nitric oxide (NO)
    for ARDS, 231
    inhaled
        for ARDS, 224–226
        for pulmonary hypertension, 220
        for right ventricle dysfunction, 172
        for RV failure, 373–376, 375t
Nitroglycerin, 354t
    for AHF, 343, 344t
NIV. *see* Noninvasive ventilation (NIV)
NO. *see* Nitric oxide; Nitric oxide (NO)
Nonabsorbable enteral antibiotics, 311
Nonadrenergic inotropic agents, 345–346
Nonconvulsive status epilepticus, 452–453, 470
Noninvasive positive pressure ventilation (NIPPV), 176
Noninvasive ventilation (NIV), 57, 176
    applications of, 36–38
    contraindications to, 36, 37t
    facilitation therapy with, 57–58
    as first-line therapy, 37–38
    indications for, 37t
    palliative care, 39
    postextubation respiratory failure and, 40
    prophylactic therapy with, 57
    rescue therapy with, 57
    risk factors for failure of, 37t
    role of, in intensive care unit, 36–42
    selecting patients for, 36
Nonrenal viscera, ACS and, 553
Non-ST-elevation myocardial infarction (NSTEMI), 347
Nonsteroidal anti-inflammatory drugs (NSAIDs), 391
Norepinephrine, 134, 285, 573
    for AHF, 345
    for septic shock, 279
NPs. *see* Nurse practitioners (NPs)
NSAIDs. *see* Nonsteroidal anti-inflammatory drugs (NSAIDs)
NSTEMI. *see* Non-ST-elevation myocardial infarction (NSTEMI)
N-terminal pro-BNP, 53
Nuclear factor-κB (NF-κB), 205
Nurse practitioners (NPs), 626
    comparisons between PAs and, 627t
    reasons for hiring, 628f
    role of, 626, 628t
    selected studies on, in ICU, 629t
    use of, in ICU, 626–627, 628f, 630t
NUTRIC score. *see* NUTrition Risk in the Critically ill Score (NUTRIC score)

Nutrition
    ALF and, 504
    for burns, 559–560, 559t
    hypocaloric, 487–488
    metabolism and, 425
    for morbid obesity, 149–150
    for TBI, 447
NUTrition Risk in the Critically ill Score (NUTRIC score), 490

O
Obesity, ARDS and, 75
Obesity hypoventilation syndrome, NIV for, 38–39
Obstructive shock, 94–95
Occlusion pressure, 53
Ocular system, ACS and, 553
Odontoid fracture, 585, 585f
OI. *see* Oxygenation index (OI)
Oliguria, 388–389, 400
Omeprazole, for peptic ulcer, 115
"Open loop" control system, 162
Open lung approach, for ARDS, 196–197, 198t
Opiates
    for HE, 501
    for morbid obesity, 148
Oral direct factor Xa inhibitors, 605–606
Oral direct thrombin inhibitors, 605
Organ dysfunction
    as adaptive prosurvival response, 335–340
    sepsis and, 250–254, 335–340
Orthogonal polarization spectral (OPS), 292–293
Orthostatic hypotension, after spinal cord injury, 589
Orthotopic liver transplantation (OLT), 497, 504
OSCAR study, in ARDS, 200
OSCILLATE trial, in ARDS, 200
Outcomes
    critical care, 11–15
        in critically ill populations, 11, 12t
        mortality and, 12–13
        sources of data for, 11
    determination of, 5
    impact of admission/discharge criteria on, 618–619, 619t
    impact of bed availability on, 617–618, 618f
    measures, in Rapid Response Systems (RRSs), 23–24, 25t–26t
    sources of data for
        administrative data, 11
        clinical observational data, 11
    for specific treatment, 616–617
Oxidative phosphorylation, 335
    inhibition of, 338
Oxygenation, 441
    ARDS and, 184–185
    prone positioning in ARDS and, 214
    standardized assessment of, 187
    stroke and, 462–463
    tissue, evaluation of, 292
Oxygenation index (OI), 187

P
PAC. *see* Pulmonary artery catheter (PAC)
Packed red blood cells (PRBCs), transfusion of, 595–597
Paco$_2$ (partial pressure of carbon dioxide in arterial blood), 443–444
    permissive hypercapnia and, 208

PAE. *see* Prolonged postantibiotic effect (PAE)
Pain, after TBI, 445
Palliative care, noninvasive ventilation and, 39
Palliative care providers, role of, 636
PAMPs. *see* Pathogen-associated molecular patterns (PAMPs)
Pao$_2$ (partial pressure of oxygen in arterial blood), 32
PAOP. *see* Pulmonary artery occlusion pressure (PAOP)
Parenteral indirect synthetic factor Xa inhibitors, 605
Partial rebreathing technique, of carbon dioxide measurement, 44
Partial thromboplastin time (PTT), 134
PAs. *see* Physician assistants (PAs)
Passive leg raising test, 100f–101f, 101–102
Pathogen-associated molecular patterns (PAMPs), 118
Patient positioning
    in ARDS, 212–218
    in respiratory failure, 213–214
"Patient-at-Risk Team", 23
PAWP. *see* Pulmonary artery wedge pressure (PAWP)
PCI. *see* Percutaneous coronary intervention (PCI)
PCIRV. *see* Pressure-controlled inverse ratio ventilation (PCIRV)
PCV. *see* Pressure-controlled ventilation (PCV)
PD-1, 259
PDT. *see* Percutaneous dilational tracheostomy (PDT)
PE. *see* Pulmonary embolism (PE)
PEEP. *see* Positive end-expiratory pressure (PEEP)
PEITHO (Pulmonary Embolism Thrombolysis) trial, 172
Penicillin G, for mushroom poisoning, 499
Pentoxifylline, 233
Percentage E$_2$ (distension index), 45, 46f
Percutaneous coronary intervention (PCI), hypothermia for, 137
Percutaneous dilational tracheostomy (PDT), 145
Percutaneous transluminal coronary angioplasty (PTCA), 373
Perfused vessel density (PVD), 293
Perfusion, microvascular, evaluation of, 292–293
Perfusion lung scans (V/Q scans), 171
Pericardial effusion, 95
Perioperative Ischemia Evaluation (POISE), 362–363
Peripheral autonomic sensing, of inflammation, 332f
Permeability pulmonary edema, in ARDS, 191
Permissive hypercapnia, 195, 204–211
    in adult critical care, 205–207
    at bedside, 208–209
    controversies and areas of uncertainty, 207–208
    description of, 204
    in pediatric critical care, 207
Permissive Hypercapnia, Alveolar Recruitment and Limited Airway Pressure (PHARLAP) trial, 199
Persistent critical illness, 3–4, 254
Persistent pulmonary hypertension, of newborn, 207
PET. *see* Positron-emission tomography (PET)
PGE$_2$. *see* Prostaglandin E$_2$
PGI$_2$. *see* Prostaglandin I$_2$

PHARLAP trial. *see* Permissive Hypercapnia, Alveolar Recruitment and Limited Airway Pressure (PHARLAP) trial
Pharmacodynamic, of antibiotic, 105–106, 106t
Pharmacokinetic, of antibiotic, 105–106, 106t
  in ICU, 107t
Pharmacologic therapy, for cardiogenic shock, 349
Pharmacy, 548
Phenobarbital, for SE, 471–472
Phentolamine, 354t
Phenylephrine, 287
Phenytoin, 526
  for SE, 471–473
Pheochromocytoma, 357
Phosphodiesterase, 376
Phosphodiesterase inhibitors, 172, 221, 288
Phosphoinositide 3-kinase, 518
Physical therapy, 548
Physician assistants (PAs), 626
  comparisons between NPs and, 627t
  reasons for hiring, 628f
  role of, 626, 628t
  selected studies on, in ICU, 629t
  use of, in ICU, 626–627, 628f, 630t
Physician bias, withdrawing life support and, 635
Physiologic dead space, 43
PICS. *see* Post-intensive care syndrome; Post-intensive care syndrome (PICS)
Plasma, transfusion of, 597
  indications for, 598t
Plasma exchange, for GBS, 481–482
Plateau pressure (P_{plat}), 196
Platelet, transfusion of, 598
Pneumonia. *see also* Community-acquired pneumonia (CAP); Ventilator-associated pneumonia (VAP)
  NIV for, 39
Pneumothorax, tension, 94–95
POISE. *see* Perioperative Ischemia Evaluation (POISE)
Poisonings, 577–582
  dangerous, 578–580
  decontamination for, 581
  diagnosis of, 577–578
  elimination for, 581
  laboratory, 577–578
  management of, 580–581
  from salicylates, 577
Polyacrylonitrile filters, 402
Polycythemia, 464
PolyHeme, 564
Positive end-expiratory pressure (PEEP), 62
  alveolar recruitment and, 199
  for ARDS, 183, 195
  static compliance and, 53
Positron-emission tomography (PET), 456
Postcardiac surgery patient, F-TTE in, 89
Postextubation respiratory failure, NIV for, 40
Post-intensive care syndrome (PICS), 16
Postoperative respiratory failure, NIV for, 38
Posttraumatic seizure (PTS), 443
Posttraumatic stress disorder (PTSD), 17
PPVs. *see* Proportion of perfused vessels (PPVs)
PRBCs. *see* Packed red blood cells (PRBCs)
Pregnancy, 571–576
  acute respiratory distress syndrome in, 574–575
  mechanical ventilation with, 574–575
  sepsis in, 571

Prehospital transport, 156
  interventions in, 157
  mode of, 156
  personnel for, 156–157
  prehospital time and, 157
  receiving care facility for, 157
  retrieval systems for, 156–157
Preoptic area (POA), 118
Preoxygenation, before intubation, 38
Prerenal azotemia, 386
Pressure reactivity index (PRx), of ICP, 436
Pressure support ventilation (PSV), 55, 57
Pressure-controlled inverse ratio ventilation (PCIRV), 67t, 70
Pressure-controlled ventilation (PCV), for ARDS, 199
Pressure-volume curve, 45
Pressure-volume metrics, 551
Procalcitonin, 264
  for SIRS and sepsis, 259
ProCESS study, 264–265, 280
Procysteine, 233, 242
Proinflammatory mediator inhibition, 232
Prolonged postantibiotic effect (PAE), 105
Prone positioning
  in ARDS, 63, 200–201, 214–217, 216t
  physiology and physiopathology of, 214–217
Prone ventilation, in ARDS, 215
Prophylaxis
  for pulmonary embolism, 172–173
  specific ulcer, 114–115, 114f
  for stress ulceration, 114–116
    infectious complications, 115–116
Propofol
  for ALF, 501
  for morbid obesity, 148
  for TBI, 445
Proportion of perfused vessels (PPVs), 293
Propranolol, 426, 528t
Propylthiouracil, 527, 528t
PROSEVA trial, in ARDS, 200
Prostacyclin, 172, 231, 376
Prostaglandin E_1 (PGE_1), 220–221, 231, 242
Prostaglandin E_2 (PGE_2), 224
Prostaglandin I_2 (PGI_2), 224, 231
Prostaglandins
  for ARDS, 226
  inhaled nitric oxide *vs.*, 226
  for pulmonary hypertension, 220–221
Prostanoids, 376
Protein, in urine, 389
Proteomic technologies, 263–264
Prothrombin complex concentrate (PCC), 597
Prothrombin time (PT), 603
Protocol, definition of, 160
Proximal tubular pressure (PTP), 553
PRx. *see* Pressure reactivity index (PRx)
Pseudomonas, 267
Pseudomonas aeruginosa, 107, 233
PSV. *see* Pressure support ventilation (PSV)
PT. *see* Prothrombin time (PT)
PTCA. *see* Percutaneous transluminal coronary angioplasty (PTCA)
PTS. *see* Posttraumatic seizure (PTS)
PTSD. *see* Posttraumatic stress disorder (PTSD)
PTT. *see* Partial thromboplastin time (PTT)
Pulmonary artery catheter (PAC), 84–85
  for CS, 348
  hemodynamic optimization with, 85
Pulmonary artery occlusion pressure (PAOP), 229, 347
  measurement of, 84

Pulmonary artery wedge pressure (PAWP), 183–184
  measurement of, 84
Pulmonary edema, 524
  acute cardiogenic, NIV for, 37–38
  AKI with, 399
  permeability, in ARDS, 191
  refractory to diuretic therapy, 399
Pulmonary embolectomy, 172
Pulmonary embolism (PE), 167–174
  asymptomatic, silent group with incidental finding and, 170
  clinical presentation of, 169–170
  diagnosis of, 169–171
  diagnostic tools for, 171
  epidemiology of, 169
  hemodynamically stable and symptomatic group and, 170
  hemodynamically unstable group and, 170
  history of, 169
  pathophysiology of, 169
  prophylaxis for, 172–173
  respiratory failure caused by, 176
  treatment for, 171–172
Pulmonary glutathione, 233
Pulmonary hypertension
  in ARDS, 192, 219
  chronic, vasodilator for, 374t–375t
  death and, 219–220
  inhaled nitric oxide for, 220
  persistent, of newborn, 207
  phosphodiesterase inhibitors for, 221
  prostaglandins for, 220–221
  right heart failure and, 219–220
Pulmonary system, metabolism and, 425
Pulmonary vascular resistance, permissive hypercapnia and, 208
Pulmonary vasodilator therapies, for ARDS, 220–222
Pulse pressure variation, 92–93
Pulse wave analysis, 85
Purple glove syndrome, 472–473
PVD. *see* Perfused vessel density (PVD)
Pyelonephritis, 389–390

Q
Quinolones, 107–108
Quorum sensing, 510

R
Race, end-of-life care and, 633–634
RACE trial. *see* Rate Control *versus* Electrical Cardioversion (RACE) trial
RAI. *see* Renal angina index (RAI)
Randomized controlled trials (RCTs), 267
  of early enhanced enteral nutrition, 489–490
  of ECLS for acute respiratory distress syndrome, 66, 67t
  for fever control, 118–122, 120t, 122t
  of intentional underfeeding, 488
  for intracranial pressure monitoring, 434
  in prone positioning in ARDS, 216t
  single, 8–9
  in tight glucose control by intensive insulin therapy, 129, 129t
    interpretation of data in, 130–131
  of trophic feeds, 488–489
  of underfeeding full feeding, meta-analysis of, 490, 491f
Rapid Response Systems (RRSs), 23
  clinical trials of, 24
  composition of, 22f

Rapid Response Systems (*Continued*)
  effect on clinical outcomes, 25t–26t
  ethical issues of, 24–26
  general principles of, 23
  for improvement outcomes, 21–28
  outcome measures in, 23–24
  physiologic functions of, 21
  potential benefit of, 26
Rapid shallow breathing index (RSBI), 47, 53–54
RAS. *see* Renin-angiotensin system (RAS)
RASS. *see* Richmond Agitation-Sedation Scale (RASS)
Rate control, in atrial fibrillation, 365, 365t
Rate Control *versus* Electrical Cardioversion (RACE) trial, 367
RCTs. *see* Randomized controlled trials (RCTs)
Rebleeding, with SAH, 450–452
Receiver operator characteristic (ROC) curves, 279
Recombinant factor VIIa
  adverse events associated with, 599–600
  for ALF, 502
  transfusion and, 599–600
Recreational drug use, 357–358
Recruitment maneuvers (RM), 197–199
Refractory status epilepticus, definition of, 470
Regional wall motion abnormalities (RWMAs), 456
Remifentanil, for morbid obesity, 148
Remote ischemic preconditioning (RIPC), 394
Renal acidosis, dialysis and, 412
Renal angina index (RAI), 388, 388t
Renal hypertensive emergencies, 357
Renal Optimization, Strategies Evaluation in Acute Heart Failure (ROSE) trial, 343
Renal parenchymal disease, 391
Renal perfusion pressure, 553
Renal replacement therapy (RRT), 229, 399–406
  azotemia and, 400
  drug intoxication with, 400
  hyperkalemia with, 399
  indications for, in AKI, 399–400, 400t
  for MODS, 402
  oliguria and, 400
  prior to complications, 400–402
  role of, in intensive care unit, 399–406
  for sepsis, 402
  severe electrolyte derangements with, 400
  for SIRS, 402
  timing of, 401t–402t
  uremic state with, 399–400
Renal system
  ACS and, 552–553
  IAP and, 552–553
  metabolism and, 426
Renal tubular acidosis, 411
Renin-angiotensin system (RAS), 233
Reoxygenation slope (ReO$_2$), 292
Reserpine, 528t
Resistance potential, of antibiotic, 106–107, 107t
Resistive index (RI), 391
Respiratory acidosis
  acute, 410–411
  myxedema coma and, 529
Respiratory alkalosis, acute, 410–411
Respiratory failure
  in COPD, 175–176
    chronic hypercapnic, 176
    clinical precipitants of, 175–176

Respiratory failure (*Continued*)
  diagnosis of, 32–33
  hypoxemic, 31
    causes of, 32t
  indications for endotracheal intubation in absence of, 34t
  lateral position, 213–214
  patient positioning in, 213–214
  postextubation, NIV and, 57
  respiratory effects of frequent posture changes in, 213
  treatment of, 33
Respiratory function, in intensive care unit, evaluation and monitoring of, 43–51
  applications and limitations, 47
  imaging in, 49
Respiratory mechanics, 45–46
Respiratory system
  ACS and, 552
  compliance, 45
  hypercapnia and, 204
  IAH and, 552
  morbid obesity and, 145–146
  physiology of, effects of position on, 212–213
  resistance, 45
Respiratory variation
  in inferior vena cava, 100
  of stroke volume, 100
  of vena caval diameter, 100
Resuscitation
  in microcirculation, 293–294
  sepsis, impact of targeting microcirculation in, 294–295
Resuscitation Outcomes Consortium (ROC), 564
Revascularization therapy, for cardiogenic shock, 350–351
Rhythm control, in atrial fibrillation, 366
RI. *see* Resistive index (RI)
Richmond Agitation-Sedation Scale (RASS), 537, 537f
Rifaximin, 500
RIFLE classification, of AKI, 383, 384t
Right ventricle (RV)
  acute dysfunction of, management for, 172
  failure of, 370–380
    causes of, 371–372, 372f
    conclusion for, 377
    diagnosis of, 370–371, 371f
    management of, 372
    mechanical support, atrial septostomy, and transplantation, 376
    mechanical ventilatory support for, 373
    miscellaneous therapy for, 376–377
    pathophysiology of, 370, 371f
    physiology of, 370
    prognosis for, 377
    pulmonary hypertension and, 219–220
    vasodilator therapy for, 373–376, 374t–375t
  myocardial infarction, 372–373
  pulmonary embolism and, 169
Right ventricular assist devices (RVADs), 95, 376
Right-sided shock, management of, 95
RIPC. *see* Remote ischemic preconditioning (RIPC)
Risk prediction models, for acute respiratory distress syndrome (ARDS), 77
Risk Stratification Scoring Systems, 366, 366t
Rivaroxaban, for VTE, 605–606
ROC. *see* Resuscitation Outcomes Consortium (ROC)

ROSE trial. *see* Renal Optimization, Strategies Evaluation in Acute Heart Failure (ROSE) trial
RRSs. *see* Rapid response systems (RRSs)
RRT. *see* Renal replacement therapy (RRT)
RSBI. *see* Rapid shallow breathing index (RSBI)
Rule of nines, for burns, 557f
Rules of thumb, for Boston approach to acid-base balance, 413t
RVADs. *see* Right ventricular assist devices (RVADs)
RWMAs. *see* Regional wall motion abnormalities (RWMAs)

S

SAH. *see* Subarachnoid hemorrhage (SAH)
Salicylates (ASA), 579–580, 580f
  poisonings from, 577
S$_a$O$_2$ (oxygen saturation in arterial blood), 45
SAPS II. *see* Simplified Acute Physiology Score (SAPS) II
Saturated solution of potassium iodide (SSKI), 528t
SBT. *see* Spontaneous breathing trial (SBT)
SCI. *see* Spinal cord injury (SCI)
S$_{cv}$O$_2$ (central venous oxygen saturation), 83–84, 92
SDD. *see* Selective decontamination of the digestive tract (SDD)
Sedation, for critical illness, 327
Sedatives
  for delirium, 539
  for HE, 500–501
  for morbid obesity, 148
  for TBI, 445
Seizure, 467
  with ALF, 502
  classification of, 470
  prophylaxis for, 443
  with SAH, 452–453
Selective decontamination of the digestive tract (SDD), 311–322, 511
  details of, 311
  evidence on efficacy of, 311–312
  examples of, 312t
  opposition in, 319–320
  reviews and meta-analyses of, 317t–319t
  SOD *vs.*, 311–319
  treatment of, 313t–317t
  trials for, 313t–317t
Selective oral decontamination (SOD), 311
  examples of, 312t
  SDD *vs.*, 311–319
Semiquantitative approach, 414–415, 414t–415t
Sepsis, 247–255, 269–270, 291, 301
  acute organ dysfunction in, 262–263
  in alcoholics, 75
  altered microcirculation in, 291, 293
  antibiotic for, 262–277
    resistance, 272
  in burns, 558, 558t
  clinical criteria in identification of, 252
  CLP and, 335
  definitions of, 250–254
    availability of patient data, 251
    healthcare practitioners, 251
    lay public, 251
    nature of the problem in, 251
  diagnostic issues, 262–264
    assays to guide empirical antibiotic therapy, 264
    clinical features, 262–263

Sepsis (*Continued*)
empirical therapy, Gram stain and culture, 263
rapid microbiological diagnostics, role of, 263–264
drug selection for, 265–266
early treatment, 264–265
empirical antimicrobial selection for, 266–272
extracorporeal blood purification and, 402
fluid resuscitation in, 4–5
fluid therapy for, 125–126
gut and, 511f
hemodynamic derangement in, 284
hibernation-like state in, 336–337
immune dysfunction in, 258–259, 259t
immune system in, 256–257
immunosuppression in, 257t
management guidelines for, computer technology for, 161f–163f, 162–164
microbiology of, 266–267
microcirculation monitoring in, 291–296
current methods, 291–292
mitochondria and, 335–337
morbid obesity and, 151
multidisciplinary response teams in, 302–303
myocardial depression and, 336
organ dysfunction and, 250–254, 335–340
outcome determination in, 5
outcome improvement in, 301, 302t
outcome success in, 302–303
pathobiology of, 250–251
in pregnancy, 571
diagnosis of, 571–572, 572t
induced hypotension, 572
nonobstetric, 571
resuscitation for, 572
SSC Guidelines for, 572–574
resuscitation, impact of targeting microcirculation in, 294–295
RRT for, 402
severe, 249–251
bundles in, 297–299
epidemiologic features of, 13
source of, 266–267
SSC Guidelines, 297, 298f
variability in terminology, 250
vasopressors for, 284–290
Sepsis in Obstetrics Score, 572, 572t
Sepsis Occurrence in Acutely Ill Patient (SOAP) study, 286
Sepsis-induced immunosuppression
diagnostic markers of, 259t
potential therapies aimed at, 259–260
SEPSISPAM study, 281
Septic shock, 12, 94, 250, 278, 546–547
bundles in, 297–299
clinical criteria in identification of, 253–254
definitions of, 251–254
dopamine for, 286
hydrocortisone treatment for, 8–9
MAP and, 278–283
autoregulation and, 278
high vasopressor load, effects of, 279
interventional studies of, 279–280, 281t
microcirculation and, 278–279
observational studies of, 279
physiologic rationale, 278–279
SEPSISPAM study and, 281
norepinephrine for, 285
resuscitation
clinical care process for, 161f–163f
goal of, 278

Sequential compression devices, for DVT, 482
Serotonin, in delirium, 536
Serum creatinine, 390–391
SHINE trial. *see* Stroke Hyperglycemia Insulin Network Effort (SHINE) trial
Shock, 112. *see also* Cardiogenic shock (CS); Septic shock
after arrest, elevated lactate and, 421
distributive, 503
hypovolemic, 546
neurogenic, 547
pulmonary embolism and, 170
special considerations of, 546–547
"Shock lab", 302–303
Shunt, ARDS and, 192
SIADH. *see* Syndrome of inappropriate secretion of antidiuretic hormone (SIADH)
Sidestream dark-field (SDF), 292–293
Sildenafil, 221
Silibinin, for mushroom poisoning, 499
Simplified Acute Physiology Score (SAPS) II, 39, 279
SIMV. *see* Synchronized intermittent mechanical ventilation (SIMV)
Simvastatin, 454
SIRS. *see* Systemic inflammatory response syndrome (SIRS)
SIRS trial. *see* Steroids In caRdiac Surgery (SIRS) trial
Sivelestat, for ALI, 243
SLED. *see* Slow, low-efficiency dialysis (SLED)
Slow, low-efficiency dialysis (SLED), 402–403
SMART. *see* Study for Monitoring Antimicrobial Resistance Trends (SMART)
SOAP study. *see* Sepsis Occurrence in Acutely Ill Patient (SOAP) study
SOD. *see* Selective oral decontamination (SOD)
Sodium bicarbonate, for poisoning, 580
Sodium nitroprusside, 354t
for AHF, 343, 344t
Sodium valproate, for SE, 472–473
Sodium-potassium adenosine triphosphatase (Na⁺,K⁺-ATPase), 230
Soluble guanylate cyclase, 220
Sotalol, 363
Spinal cord injury (SCI)
acute, management of, 583–592
airway and pulmonary, 589
assessment of
clinical, 583, 584t
radiographic, 583–584
atlanto-occipital dislocation, 584, 584f
autonomic dysfunction and, 589
corticosteroid therapy for, 587
Hangman's fracture, 585, 585f
hemodynamic support in, 589
hypothermia for, 136–137, 588
injury patterns of, 584–586
Jefferson fracture, 585
odontoid fracture, 585, 585f
orthostatic hypotension after, 589
pathophysiology of, 583
penetrating, 588–589, 588f
subaxial cervical, 586f
surgical decision making in, 586–587
Spontaneous breathing trial (SBT)
for delirium, 539
failure of, 54t
for mechanical ventilation weaning, 54–56
success of, 55t
SRMD. *see* Stress-related mucosal damage (SRMD)

SSC. *see* Surviving Sepsis Campaign (SSC)
SSKI. *see* Saturated solution of potassium iodide (SSKI)
Staff Time and Resource Intensity Verification (STRIVE) study, 243
Staphylococcus aureus infection
incidence of, 266–267
SDD and, 311
Staphylococcus pneumoniae, SDD and, 311
Static compliance, 45
PEEP and, 53
Static pressure-volume curve analysis, 45
Statins
for ARDS, 233, 242
for atrial fibrillation, 364
for CI-AKI, 392
for SAH, 454
Status epilepticus (SE), 470–474
causes of, 471
classification of, 470
definition of, 470
epidemiology of, 470
first-tier (emergency) therapies, 471–472
management of, 471, 471f
natural history and prognosis, 473–474
pathophysiology of, 471
second-tier (control) therapies for, 472–473
systemic complications of, 471
third-tier therapies (for refractory SE), 473
treatment algorithm for, 472f
Steroids
for ALI/ARDS, 239–241
in early stage, 239–240, 240t
in late stage, 240–241
dosage of, 241
timing with, 241
physiologic response to, 241
for TBI, 447
treatment duration with, 241
trial appraisal with, 241–242, 244t
Steroids In caRdiac Surgery (SIRS) trial, 364
Stewart-Fencl approach, 415–416, 415f
Stress hyperglycemia, 128
Stress index, 45–46, 46f
physiologic background, 46–47
Stress metabolism, 426–427
Stress response
curve, 425f
perioperative/postinjury, 3
Stress ulceration
development of, 113f
infectious complications in, 115–116
prevention of, 113
prophylaxis for, 113–115
in iatrogenic disorder, 327
infectious complications, 115–116
risk factors for, 114t
Stress-related mucosal damage (SRMD), 112
definitions of, 112
epidemiology of, 113
management of, 113
pathophysiology of, 112–113, 113f
risk factors of, 113, 114t
STRIVE study. *see* Staff Time and Resource Intensity Verification (STRIVE) study
Stroke. *see also* Acute ischemic stroke
ischemic, hypothermia for, 136, 138t–139t
oxygenation and, 462–463
ventilation and, 462–463
Stroke Hyperglycemia Insulin Network Effort (SHINE) trial, 463–464
Stroke volume, 85, 284
respiratory variation of, 100
variations of, induced by mechanical ventilation, 99–100

Strong ions, 410
Study for Monitoring Antimicrobial
    Resistance Trends (SMART), 270–271
Subarachnoid hemorrhage (SAH),
    aneurysmal
  complications with, 450–456
  emergency setting, 450
  endovascular measures of, 451–452
  management of, 450–460
  surgical measures of, 451–452
  timing of, 452
Subaxial cervical spine injury, 586f
Subaxial Cervical Spine Injury
    Classification, 587
Subjective "worried" criterion, 22
Suboccipital decompressive craniectomy
    (SDC), 466
Suboptimal antibiotic therapy, consequences
    of, 110t
Sucralfate, 114
SUPPORT trial. see Surfactant, Positive
    Pressure, and Oxygenation
    Randomized Trial (SUPPORT)
Supraventricular arrhythmias, 361, 363–364
Surfactant, 192
Surfactant, Positive Pressure, and
    Oxygenation Randomized Trial
    (SUPPORT), 178
Surfactant deficiency, ARDS and, 229
Surgery, abnormal bleeding in, 599t
Surgical decompressive therapy, 444–445
Surrogate preference, for decision making,
    634–635
Surviving Sepsis Campaign (SSC)
    Guidelines, 5, 297, 298t
  cost saving from implementation of, 299f
  for sepsis in pregnancy, 572–574
Suspended animation, 337
SvO₂ (venous oxygen saturation),
    45, 92, 284
SVR. see Systemic vascular resistance (SVR)
Synchronized intermittent mechanical
    ventilation (SIMV), 56–57
Syndrome of inappropriate secretion of
    antidiuretic hormone (SIADH), 454
  GBS and, 482
Synthetic androgen oxandrolone, 518
Systematic error, 66
Systemic inflammatory response syndrome
    (SIRS), 249, 256–257, 262
  RRT for, 402
Systemic vascular resistance (SVR), 134, 347
Systolic pressure variation, 92–93

T
T regulatory cells, 258
Tachycardia, 331
TACO. see Transfusion-associated
    circulatory overload (TACO)
TBI. see Traumatic brain injury (TBI)
TCD. see Transcranial Doppler ultrasound
    (TCD)
TEE. see Transesophageal echocardiography
    (TEE)
TEG. see Thromboelastography (TEG)
Telemedicine, 623
Tension pneumothorax, 94–95
Testosterone, 517
TFPI. see Tissue factor pathway inhibitor
    (TFPI)
TGF-α. see Transforming growth factor-α;
    (TGF-α)
The Kidney Disease: Improving Global
    Outcome (KDIGO), 392

Therapeutic Intervention Scoring System
    (TISS), 619
Thiazide diuretics, 526
Thionamides, 527
Thoracic spine, fracture dislocation injury
    of, 586f
Thoracolumbar Injury Classification and
    Severity Scale (TLICS), 587
Threshold, intracranial pressure, 435–436
Thromboelastography (TEG), 134, 598
Thromboembolism-deterrent hose, for DVT,
    482
Thrombolytics, 172, 466–467
Thrombomodulin, 231
Thyroid hormones, 520
  antagonize adrenergic effects of, 527
Thyroid storm
  diagnostic scoring system for, 527t
  pharmacologic management for, 528t
Thyroid-releasing hormone (TRH), 520
Thyroid-stimulating hormone (TSH), 520
  myxedema coma and, 529
Thyrotoxic crisis, 526–529
  clinical presentation of, 526
  definitive treatment for, 528–529
  diagnostic scoring system for, 527t
  pathophysiology of, 526
  precipitating factors of, 528
  supportive care for, 527–528
  treatment of, 526–529, 528f, 528t
Thyrotropin-releasing hormone, 526
Tidal volume (V_T), 62, 196
Tigecycline, 109
Time-dependent killing kinetics, of
    antibiotic, 105
TIMP-2. see Tissue inhibitor of
    metalloproteinase-2 (TIMP-2)
TISS. see Therapeutic Intervention Scoring
    System (TISS)
Tissue factor pathway inhibitor (TFPI), 231
Tissue hypoperfusion, markers of, 102t
Tissue inhibitor of metalloproteinase-2
    (TIMP-2), urinary, 386
Tissue oxygenation
  evaluation of, 292
  hypercapnia and, 204–205
Tissue plasminogen activator, 172
TLICS. see Thoracolumbar Injury
    Classification and Severity Scale
    (TLICS)
TLR-4. see Toll-like receptor 4 (TLR-4)
TNF-α. see Tumor necrosis factor α; (TNF-α)
Tobramycin, 311
Toll-like receptor 4 (TLR-4), fever and, 118
Tonic-clonic movements, 470
Torpor, 335
Toxidromes, 577, 578t
T-piece, 54–55, 57
Tracheostomy
  for GBS, 481
  mechanical ventilation weaning and, 58
TRALI. see Transfusion-related acute lung
    injury (TRALI)
Tranexamic acid, 450–451, 567, 600
Transcranial Doppler ultrasound (TCD), 453
Transcutaneous carbon dioxide monitoring,
    44–45
Transesophageal echocardiography (TEE),
    366
Transforming growth factor-α (TGF-α), 230
Transfusion, 327, 593–602
  benefits and risks of, 595–598
  of cryoprecipitate, 598
  guidelines in acute bleeding, 599t
  for HS, 568

Transfusion (Continued)
  massive, 598–599
  of plasma, 597
  of platelet, 598
  of PRBCs, 595–597
  of recombinant factor VIIa, 599–600
  thresholds for, 596t
  tranexamic acid and, 600
  for trauma, 564
Transfusion Requirements in Critical Care
    (TRICC) trial, 327
Transfusion-associated circulatory overload
    (TACO), 597
Transfusion-related acute lung injury
    (TRALI), 597
Transfusion-related immunomodulation
    (TRIM), 597
Translational Research Investigating
    Biomarker Endpoints (TRIBE) study,
    386
Transplantation, ALF and, 504
Transportation, 154–159
  interhospital, 155
  intrahospital, 154
  prehospital, 156
Transpulmonary pressure, 47
Transpulmonary thermodilution, 85
  hemodynamic optimization with, 85
Trauma, 543–550
  abnormal bleeding in, 599t
  biomarkers of, 546
  elevated lactate and, 421
  endpoints resuscitation in, 563, 565t–566t,
    567
  fluid resuscitation for, 563
  fluid therapy for, 126
  F-TTE in, 89
  ICU
    extended team in, 548
    infrastructure of, 545
    protocols of, 547–548
  invasive hemodynamic monitoring in,
    546
  morbid obesity and, 151
  noninvasive hemodynamic monitoring
    in, 546
  open cavity, 547
  resuscitation, 545–547
  special considerations of, 547
  tertiary examination for, 548
  traction/immobility, 547
  transfusions for, 564
Traumatic brain injury (TBI), 441–449
  brain oxygen monitoring in, 446–447
  cerebral perfusion thresholds and, 442
  hyperosmolar therapy for, 444
  hyperventilation for, 443–444
  hypothermia for, 134, 137, 138t–139t
  ICP and, 433
  intracranial pressure thresholds and,
    443
  normothermia for, 445–446
  nutrition for, 447
  oxygenation and, 441
  prophylactic hypothermia, 445–446
  seizure prophylaxis and, 443
  severe, considerations for, 436–437
  steroids for, 447
  surgical decompressive therapy for,
    444–445
  systemic blood pressure and, 441
Treprostinil, 376
TRH. see Thyroid-releasing hormone
    (TRH)
Trial sequential analysis (TSA), 71

TRIBE study. *see* Translational Research Investigating Biomarker Endpoints (TRIBE) study
TRICC trial. *see* Transfusion Requirements in Critical Care (TRICC) trial
Trigger systems, 22
TRIM. *see* Transfusion-related immunomodulation (TRIM)
Tromethamine, 208
Trophic feeds, randomized controlled trials of, 488–489
TSH. *see* Thyroid-stimulating hormone (TSH)
T-tube, 54–55
Tumor necrosis factor α (TNF-α), in immune system, 256

U
UFH. *see* Unfractionated heparin (UFH)
UIP. *see* Upper inflection point (UIP)
Ultra-early tranexamic acid after subarachnoid hemorrhage (ULTRA), 450–451
Ultrafiltration, 403–404
Ultrasound
    bedside, of inferior vena cava (IVC), 93
    contrast-enhanced, for AKI, 391
    lung, 49
UMLS. *see* Unified Medical Language Program (UMLS)
Uncontrolled hemorrhagic shock, 567
Underfeeding, 485–493
    meta-analysis of randomized controlled trials of, 490, 491f
    search strategy of, 490–492
    vs. full feeding, 490, 491f
Unfractionated heparin (UFH), 603–604
    for atrial fibrillation, 366
    for pulmonary embolism, 171
Unified Medical Language Program (UMLS), 160
United Network for Organ Sharing (UNOS), 499
United States, critical care resource utilization in, 609–615
UNOS. *see* United Network for Organ Sharing (UNOS)
Upper inflection point (UIP), 45
Uremic state, 399–400
Urinalysis, for AKI, 389, 390t
Urine alkalinization, 580
Urine creatinine, measurement of, 389
Urine microscopy, 389–390
Urine sodium concentration, 390
Urine urea nitrogen, measurement of, 389

V
VAD. *see* Ventricular assist device (VAD)
Valsalva retinopathy, 553
Vancomycin, 105, 108
    for MRSA, 269
VAP. *see* Ventilator-associated pneumonia (VAP)

Vascular endothelial growth factor (VEGF), 230
Vascular occlusion test (VOT), 292
Vasoactive agents, 327
    for AKI, 392, 394
Vasoconstrictors, 231
Vasodilators, 231
    for AHF, 343, 344t
    inhaled, in ARDS, 224–228
    pulmonary, for ARDS, 220–222
    for right ventricular failure, 373–376, 374t–375t
Vasogenic amine, 172
Vasoplegia, 284
Vasopressin, 287–288
    for ALF, 503
    antagonists, for AHF, 344, 345t
Vasopressin and Septic Shock Trial (VASST), 94, 280
Vasopressors
    catecholamine, 288–289
    dobutamine, 286–287
    dopamine, 285–286
    epinephrine, 287
    hypotension and, 284–285
    MAP and, 284–285
    norepinephrine, 285
    phenylephrine, 287
    for sepsis, 284–290
    therapy, 284–288
    vasopressin, 287–288
Vasospasm, 453, 455t
VASST. *see* Vasopressin and Septic Shock Trial (VASST)
Vecuronium, 331
    for morbid obesity, 148
VEGF. *see* Vascular endothelial growth factor (VEGF)
Venoarterial (VA) cannulation, 69
Venous lactate, 419
Venous thromboembolism (VTE), 169, 547
    prophylaxis for, 547, 589–590
    risk factors for, 170t
Veno-venous (VV) cannulation, 69
Ventilation
    lung-protective, for ARDS, 68, 77
    stroke and, 462–463
Ventilation perfusion ratio, distribution of, 213
Ventilation-perfusion mismatch, ARDS and, 192
Ventilator-associated pneumonia (VAP), 9, 115, 268–269
Ventilator-induced lung injury (VILI), 61, 195, 215, 326
Ventilators, 61–65
    liberation, in GBS, 481
    lung damage and, 61–62
    transport, 155
Ventilatory dead space, measurement of, 43
Ventilatory management, for GBS, 480–481
Ventricular assist device (VAD), 349–350
Ventricular fibrillation (VF), with hypothermia, 134

Vertebral artery injury
    diagnosis of, 588
    management of, 588
Veterans Health Information Systems and Technology Architecture (VistA), 161
Videomicroscopy, 292–293
VILI. *see* Ventilator-induced lung injury (VILI)
Viral hepatitis, 499
VISEP trial. *see* Efficacy of Volume Substitution and Insulin Therapy in Severe Sepsis (VISEP) trial
VistA. *see* Veterans Health Information Systems and Technology Architecture (VistA)
Vitamin C, for ARDS, 233
Vitamin E, for ARDS, 233
Vitamin K, for ALF, 502
Vitamin K antagonist (VKA), 603
VKA. *see* Vitamin K antagonist (VKA)
Volume expanders, for AKI, 392
Volume loading, 172
Volume responsiveness, 92–94
    algorithm for, 93, 93f
    dynamic parameters to predict, 99–102
    static indices of cardiac preload to predict, 99, 100f
Volume-controlled ventilation (VCV), for ARDS, 199
Volutrauma, 61, 195, 200
V/Q. *see* Perfusion lung scans (V/Q scans)
V_T. *see* Tidal volume (V_T)
VTE. *see* Venous thromboembolism (VTE)

W
Warfarin, 597
    for critically ill patient, 603
Waveform monitoring, 48
WBI. *see* Whole bowel irrigation
Weak acids, 410
Weaning
    definition of, 52
    in GBS, 481
    from mechanical ventilation, 52–60
        assessment for, 52–56
        with difficult-to-wean patient, 56–58
        factors reducing success in, 57t
        predictors for success in, 53–54, 53t
        spontaneous breathing trial for, 54–56
        success in, 55t
    tracheostomy and, 58
    parameters during, 47
White blood cells, 128
WHO. *see* World Health Organization (WHO)
Whole bowel irrigation (WBI), 581
"Will Rogers phenomenon", 13
Wilson disease, 499
WOB. *see* Work of breathing
Work of breathing (WOB), 47
World Health Organization (WHO), COPD and, 175